Handbook of Experimental Pharmacology

Continuation of Handbuch der experimentellen Pharmakologie

Vol. 72

Antitumor Drug Resistance

Contributors

N. K. Ahmed · B. Barlogie · W. T. Beck · A. Begleiter
A. K. Belousova · J. R. Bertino · J. M. Boyle · J. Brennand
C. T. Caskey · T. A. Connors · B. Drewinko · M. Fox · H. Fuji
G. J. Goldenberg · J. F. Henderson · B. T. Hill · J. A. Houghton
P. J. Houghton · M. M. Ip · J. G. McVie · M. Moore · P. S. Schein
D. Scott · K. D. Tew · D. M. Tidd · M. J. Tisdale · J. R. Uren
J. V. Watson · A. D. Welch · J. M. Whitehouse

Editors

B. W. Fox and M. Fox

Springer-Verlag
Berlin Heidelberg New York Tokyo 1984

Professor BRIAN W. FOX, Ph. D.
Dr. MARGARET FOX

Paterson Laboratories, Christie Hospital and Holt Radium Institute, Wilmslow Road, Withington, Manchester M20 9BX, Great Britain

With 99 Figures

ISBN-13:978-3-642-69492-9 e-ISBN-13:978-3-642-69490-5
DOI: 10.1007/978-3-642-69490-5

Library of Congress Cataloging in Publication Data. Main entry under title: Antitumor drug resistance. (Handbook of experimental pharmacology; v. 72) Includes bibliographical references and index. 1. Antineoplastic agents. 2. Drug resistance. 3. Tumors – Chemotherapy. I. Ahmed, N.K. II. Fox, Brian W. III. Fox, Margaret. IV. Series. [DNLM: 1. Drug resistance. 2. Antineoplastic agents – Pharmacodynamics. 3. Neoplasms – Drug therapy. W1 HA51L v. 72/QZ 267 A633] QP905.H3 vol. 72 615'.1s [616.99'4061] 83-27139 [RC271.C5]

Softcover reprint of the hardcover 1st edition 1984

2122/3130-543210

List of Contributors

N. K. Ahmed, Division of Biochemical and Clinical Pharmacology, St. Jude Children's Research Hospital, 332 North Lauderdale, P.O. Box 318, Memphis, TN 38101/USA

B. Barlogie, Medical Oncology, The University of Texas System Cancer Center, M. D. Anderson Hospital and Tumor Institute, 6723 Bertner, Houston, TX 77030/USA

W. T. Beck, Division of Biochemical and Clinical Pharmacology, St. Jude Children's Research Hospital, 332 North Lauderdale, P.O. Box 318, Memphis, TN 38101/USA

A. Begleiter, The Manitoba Institute of Cell Biology and the Department of Medicine, University of Manitoba, 100 Olivia Street, Winnipeg, Manitoba R3E OV9, Canada

A. K. Belousova, Laboratory of Biochemical Pharmacology, All-Union Cancer Research Center, Moscow 115478, USSR

J. R. Bertino, Departments of Internal Medicine and Pharmacology, Yale University School of Medicine, 333 Cedar Street, P.O. Box 3333, New Haven, CT 06510/USA

J. M. Boyle, Paterson Laboratories, Christie Hospital and Holt Radium Institute, Wilmslow Road, Withington, Manchester M20 9BX, Great Britain

J. Brennand, Paterson Laboratories, Christie Hospital and Holt Radium Institute, Wilmslow Road, Withington, Manchester M20 9BX, Great Britain

C. T. Caskey, Howard Hughes Medical Institute Laboratories, Departments of Medicine, Cell Biology and Chemistry, Baylor College of Medicine, Houston, TX 77030/USA

T. A. Connors, MRC Toxicology Unit, Medical Research Council Laboratories, Woodmansterne Road, Carshalton, Surrey SM5 4EF, Great Britain

B. Drewinko, Section of Hematology, Department of Laboratory Medicine, Box 73, The University of Texas System Cancer Center, M. D. Anderson Hospital and Tumor Institute, 6723 Bertner, Houston, TX 77030/USA

M. Fox, Paterson Laboratories, Christie Hospital and Holt Radium Institute, Wilmslow Road, Withington, Manchester M20 9BX, Great Britain

H. Fuji, Molecular Immunology, Roswell Park Memorial Institute, New York State Department of Health, 666 Elm Street, Buffalo, NY 14263/USA

G. J. Goldenberg, The Manitoba Institute of Cell Biology and the Department of Medicine, University of Manitoba, 100 Olivia Street, Winnipeg, Manitoba R3E OV9, Canada

J. F. Henderson, Cancer Research Unit, The University of Alberta, Edmonton, Alberta T6G 2H7, Canada

B. T. Hill, Laboratory of Cellular Chemotherapy, Imperial Cancer Research Fund Laboratories, P.O. Box 123, Lincoln's Inn Fields, London WC2 3PX, Great Britain

J. A. Houghton, Division of Biochemical and Clinical Pharmacology, St. Jude Children's Research Hospital, 332 North Lauderdale, P.O. Box 318, Memphis, TN 38101/USA

P. J. Houghton, Division of Biochemical and Clinical Pharmacology, St. Jude Children's Research Hospital, 332 North Lauderdale, P.O. Box 318, Memphis, TN 38101/USA

M. M. Ip, Department of Experimental Therapeutics, Grace Cancer Drug Center, Roswell Park Memorial Institute, New York State Department of Health, 666 Elm Street, Buffalo, NY 14263/USA

J. G. McVie, Clinical Research Unit, Netherlands Cancer Institute, Plesmanlaan 121, 1066 CX Amsterdam, The Netherlands

M. Moore, Immunology Division, Paterson Laboratories, Christie Hospital and Holt Radium Institute, Wilmslow Road, Withington, Manchester M20 9BX, Great Britain

P. S. Schein, Division of Medical Oncology, Department of Pharmacology, Georgetown University Hospital, 3800 Reservoir Road, N.W., Washington, DC 20007/USA

D. Scott, Paterson Laboratories, Christie Hospital and Holt Radium Institute, Wilmslow Road, Withington, Manchester M20 9BX, Great Britain

K. D. Tew, Division of Medical Oncology, Department of Medicine, Georgetown University Hospital, 3800 Reservoir Road, N.W., Washington, DC 20007/USA

D. M. Tidd, School of Biological Sciences, University of East Anglia, Norwich, Norfolk NR4 7TJ, Great Britain

M. J. Tisdale, CRC Experimental Chemotherapy Group, Department of Pharmacy, University of Aston in Birmingham, Gosta Green, Birmingham B4 7ET, Great Britain

J. R. Uren, Genex Corporation, 16020 Industrial Drive, Gaithersburg, MD 20877/USA

J. V. Watson, MRC Clinical Oncology and Radiotherapeutics Unit, Medical Research Council Centre, The Medical School, University of Cambridge, Hills Road, Cambridge CB2 2QH, Great Britain

A. D. Welch, National Cancer Institute (National Institutes of Health), Drug Evaluation Branch, Division of Cancer Treatment, Blair Building, Room 428, 900 Rockville Pike, Bethesda, MD 20205/USA

J. M. Whitehouse, Department of Medical Oncology, CRC and Wessex Regional Medical Oncology Unit, Centre Block CF99, Southampton General Hospital, Southampton SO9 4XY, Great Britain

Preface

The study of tumour resistance to anticancer drugs has been the subject of many publications since the initial discovery of the phenomenon by J. H. Burchenal and colleagues in 1950. Many papers have been published since then reporting development of resistance to most of the well-known anticancer agents in many different animal tumour systems, both in vivo and in vitro. Many different mechanisms of resistance have been described, and it is clear that the tumour cell has a wide diversity of options in overcoming the cell-killing activity of these agents.

Definition of the magnitude of the phenomenon in the clinic is, however, much more problematical, and it is with this in mind that the initial chapter, seeks to outline the problem as the clinicians see it. It appears that the phenomenon of true resistance to a drug, as the biochemist would recognise it, is an important cause of the failure which clinicians experience in treating the disease. The extent of the contribution of this phenomenon to the failure of treatment cannot easily be evaluated at the present time, but it is hoped that the development and application of new and more sophisticated techniques for the analysis of cellular subpopulations may help to give a more exact estimate and to shed some light on the causes of failure of many of the present therapeutic techniques.

The purpose of this book is to bring together in a single volume the results of many years' work by key people in this field. The different studies of the mechanisms of resistance are considered; in a separate section, the ways in which tumours adapt to different drug groups, taken primarily from the experimental field, but also – where recognised – from the clinical field, are described. The armoury of experimental techniques is rapidly expanding; along with improved methods of measuring drug transport and DNA repair, monoclonal and polyclonal antibodies are being employed in different ways. One of the main aims has been to identify specific changes which take place in the biochemistry of the tumour cell, especially at the cell surface, when it exhibits resistance to an anticancer drug. We are already learning about the changing levels of specific proteins, e.g. enzymes and cell-surface glycoproteins; with the newer concepts in immunology and the application of powerful techniques such as flow cytometry, a better understanding of the depth and extent of the problem of resistance is being achieved. The greatest emphasis in this book has been placed on the individual mechanisms determined to be those by which tumours have become resistant to specific drugs, and on the experimental observations and arguments that have led to the present understanding of these mechanisms.

A detailed study of the origin of resistance is basic to further progress in the treatment of cancer. It could not only modify the course of treatment, but may also, as our knowledge of "intrinsic resistance" increases, modify the type of initial treatment used, based as it is on a rapid analysis of the spectrum of sensitivity of the tumour. Although, to some extent, clonogenic assays, xenografts and renal capsule implant systems are being used for the initial analysis, the need for speed is paramount in making the early decision required for effective therapy. It is clear that some indicator of drug sensitivity at the time of the pathological investigation would be ideal, and in order to arrive at this level of diagnostic efficiency, flow cytometry will be a necessary intermediate stage in the study of properties of tumour subpopulations. Identifying a spectrum of sensitive and resistant cells in a tumour will provide a more rational basis for the choice of a drug or drug combination. More detailed pharmacokinetic data in humans are also needed if we are to take advantage of the sensitivity pattern obtained by subpopulation studies at the pathological level.

A knowledge of the genetics of the tumour, as well as that of the host, is important to understanding the sensitivity spectrum of a new tumour, and a knowledge of these factors could ultimately provide a basis for optimising the therapeutic index of the drug. The flow cytometry analytical technique will, again, be a useful tool for the effective manipulation of these factors.

During the preparation of this book it has become clear that the word "resistance" requires further description. It seems to us that "resistance" is a word that can justifiably be related only to the property of a single cell. It could be defined as the ability of a single tumour cell to survive a local concentration of a damaging drug that would otherwise have been expected to kill it. This could be an innate property of the cell (intrinsic resistance) or could have been acquired by a rapid adaptive response (adaptive resistance). If a cell were to survive a low concentration of a damaging agent and divide, probably in the face of the loss of many similar cells within the population of which it is a part, it could form the basis of a new population of resistant cells through a series of divisions. These may be further selected for reduced sensitivity (selected resistance) or actively become adapted by expressing alternative biochemical pathways, enhanced protective group synthesis, etc. (acquired resistance). In all such cases the type of resistance would merely describe the property of a single cell within the system being studied.

The tumour mass, which includes the population of tumour cells within its matrix, exhibits an overall sensitivity – usually measured according to changes in volume, number or weight – part of which may be a reflection of the tumour cell population it contains. The overall response of the tumour-cell population depends on the average sensitivity of the cells within it. The acquisition of resistance by a whole tumour could thus be the result of a shift in the proportion of intrinsically sensitive and resistant cells, influencing the overall average sensitivity of the population. The term "resistant tumour" is so widely used, however, that to speak of the "population resistance" of a tumour or tumour-cell population in this context would seem to be more accurate. It must be recognised that this is an average property of the tissue, and may not involve anything other than a change in the proportion of existing cells.

This collection of chapters, we believe, achieves the interim aim of bringing together the many parameters that are presently considered to constitute the nature of resistance in tumour populations; we hope that they will provide a basis for further discussions to substantially improve the efficacy of drug treatment of cancer in humans.

We would like to thank the many authors who adhered very closely to the timetable for submission of their chapters; we regret the omission of two of the originally planned chapters from the latter half of the book at such a late date that alternatives could not be found. However, much of the material that was to be presented in these is well covered in other contributions.

In particular we thank the Chief Editor, Professor A. D. Welch, for his continued vigilance, Mr. Ric Swindell for the indexing and Ms. Gillian A. Simpson for the typing of the necessary correspondence. Finally, the courtesy and efficiency of Mrs. Doris Walker of Springer-Verlag is much appreciated.

Manchester

BRIAN W. FOX
MARGARET FOX

Contents

Section I: Concepts of Drug Resistance

CHAPTER 1

Clinical Setting. J. M. WHITEHOUSE

CHAPTER 2

Experimental Setting. J. F. HENDERSON

CHAPTER 5

The Molecular Basis of Genetically Acquired Resistance to Purine Analogues in Cultured Mammalian Cells. J. BRENNAND and C. T. CASKEY

Section III: Cellular Aspects

CHAPTER 6

Cell Cycle Perturbation Effects. B. DREWINKO and B. BARLOGIE. With 14 Figures

CHAPTER 7

Tumour Resistance and the Phenomenon of Inflammatory-Cell Infiltration
M. MOORE. With 2 Figures

CHAPTER 8

Flow Cytometric Methods for Studying Enzyme Activity in Populations of Individual Cells. J.V. WATSON. With 12 Figures

CHAPTER 9

Chromosome Studies. D. SCOTT. With 17 Figures

CHAPTER 10

Alterations of Drug Transport. G. J. GOLDENBERG and A. BEGLEITER

CHAPTER 11

Cell Hybridisation. J. M. BOYLE. With 5 Figures

Section IV: Modification of Tumor Biochemistry

CHAPTER 12

Drug Resistance and DNA Repair. M. FOX. With 4 Figures

CHAPTER 13

Cyclic AMP and Prostaglandins. M. J. TISDALE. With 5 Figures

CHAPTER 14

Properties of Mitochondria. A. K. BELOUSOVA. With 4 Figures

CHAPTER 15

Mechanism of "Resistance" Towards Specific Drug Groups. T. A. CONNORS. With 10 Figures

CHAPTER 16

Nitrosoureas. K. D. TEW and P. S. SCHEIN

Section V: Antimetabolites

CHAPTER 17

Antipurines. D. M. TIDD. With 6 Figures

CHAPTER 18

Ribofuranose-containing Analogues of Uridine and Cytidine
A. D. WELCH and N. K. AHMED. With 1 Figure

CHAPTER 19

5-Halogenated Pyrimidines and Their Nucleosides
J. A. HOUGHTON and P. J. HOUGTHON. With 2 Figures

Section VI: Antifolates

Section I:
Concepts of Drug Resistance

CHAPTER 1

Clinical Setting

J. M. WHITEHOUSE

A. Introduction

The development of different classes of drugs with anticancer activity has radically altered the patterns of cancer management over the past few decades and continues to do so. As could have been anticipated, no universally successful agent acting solely and specifically on the neoplastic cells has emerged or is likely to. Nonetheless, an improved understanding of the biology of human cancer and the recognition of its disseminated nature in all but a few situations emphasises the growing dependence on systemic therapies. Given the right conditions no tumour cell is totally resistant to the effects of available anticancer drugs. In reality, any consequence of drug therapy depends on its contrasting influence on normal and neoplastic tissues.

Fundamental to the problem is therefore the drug's degree of selectivity for the tumour cell and its subsequent influence upon it (ZUBROD 1978). It is the qualitative failure of this selectivity which varies from drug to drug when used against different tumours which equates with resistance.

This apparently straightforward observation masks very real problems of interpretation, which will be explored in this chapter.

A whole medical discipline – medical oncology – has grown from the consequences of drug resistance. Were it not for drug resistance, the problem of the management of a spectrum of varied and occasionally serious effects on normal tissues would not arise, and, indeed, local therapies such as radiotherapy and surgery would have dwindling relevance. Despite the introduction of some 25–30 agents into common usage in clinical practice over the past 40 years (Table 1) and the existence of many others undergoing preliminary assessment or in experimental use, very few indeed are without significant effects on bone marrow, gastrointestinal epithelium or gonadal tissue. The spectrum of toxicity varies considerably with the drug and the dosage, some affecting more tissues than others, but virtually no tissue is immune. Short-term reversible toxicity to normal tissues may be of little consequence where the antitumour effect is substantial and durable. Such a clear benefit is not often apparent and in many situations the margins of therapeutic benefit may be narrow when weighed against the consequences of toxicity to normal tissues. Few drugs have a specific antagonist which may be used to hasten recovery, and indeed such an antagonist might compromise the antitumour effect. While prolonged but reversible toxicity is an undoubted management problem, improved survival of patients treated with intensive or long-term chemotherapy has highlighted late and potentially serious complications

Table 1. Introduction of drugs with anticancer activity

	1940–1949	1950–1959	1960–1969	1970–1979
Alkylating agents	Mustine	Busulphan Chlorambucil	Cyclophosphamide Melphalan	
Anti-metabolites	Methotrexate	6-Mercaptopurine 5-Fluorouracil	Cytosine arabinoside 6-Thioguanine	5-Azacytidine Pyrazofurin
Antibiotics		Actinomycin D	Mithramycin Daunorubicin Bleomycin Adriamycin	
Plant alkaloids		Vinblastine Vincristine		Vindesine VP-16–213 VM-26
Miscellaneous			1,3-bis(2-Chloroethyl)-3-cyclohexyl-1-nitrosourea (BCNU) 5-(3,3-Dimethyl-1-triazeno)-imidazole-4-carboxamide (DTIC) Procarbazine Hydroxyurea Asparaginase Streptozotocin	*cis*-Platinum

which are likely to influence future treatment planning. Since these side effects can be identified only in patients who survive for long periods, they are found by definition among patients whose tumours show significant and durable sensitivity to the drugs used.

Resistance of tumour cells to the effects of individual drugs delivered orally or parenterally can be seen to be inextricably related to the effects on normal tissue. If drug delivery could be improved so that the exposure of tumour tissues was significantly greater than that of normal tissues, resistance could more clearly be regardedd comparatively between tumours, rather than as a contrasting phenomenon between normal and abnormal cells in the same host. Unfortunately, such selective administration remains problematic, and tumour resistance must continue to be viewed within the framework of the effects of therapy on host tissues.

B. Resistance – A Clinical Phenomenon?

Tumour regression rarely occurs spontaneously, although there are a number of well-quoted established instances in the literature (EVERSON and COLE 1956; EVERSON 1964; SUMNER and FORAKER 1960). Local treatment with radiotherapy may result in a reduction of measurable tumour size, or even complete disappearance. Similarly, intralesional therapy using a sensitising agent, i.e. dinitrochlorobenzene (DNCB) or Bacille Calmette Guerin (BCG) may result in a diminution of tumour size (HOLMES et al. 1975). Stimulation of immunological mechanisms has also been reported to reduce the incidence of relapse (McKNEALLY et al. 1976). The administration of anticancer drugs may produce similar regressions and disease control but on a more widespread and reproducible scale. Not unreasonably, such a phenomenon is attributed collectively to sensitivity of the entire tumour-cell population to the agents used. Where the response is complete, such a conclusion is certainly justified. Anything less than total disappearance of the tumour implies a degree of "resistance". However, this term is used more frequently in a clinical situation to describe either minimal change or continuing tumour enlargement despite therapy. These interpretations do not take account of the multifactorial characteristics influencing response nor of the variables associated with therapy.

In only one tumour – choriocarcinoma – is single-agent chemotherapy capable of producing cure (GOLDSTEIN et al. 1976). Maximal tumour regression sufficient to produce complete eradication of disease requires the use of different drugs not only in combination, but in adequate dosage. Even under these circumstances many tumours remain resistant and the natural history of the disease and also survival are unaffected.

The enormous impact of cancer chemotherapy on the management of malignant disease cannot be measured by cure alone. Much of the benefits have come from improved survival and effective palliation. In reviewing the rationale for single-agent versus combination chemotherapy, DEVITA et al. (1975) categorised tumours (Table 2) into:

Table 2. Categorisation of cancers according to drug response. (After DE VITA et al. 1975)

Group 1. Cancers in which drugs have been responsible for some patients achieving a normal life span	Group 2. Cancers in which responders to chemotherapy have had demonstrated improvement in survival
Acute leukaemia in children	Ovarian carcinoma
Hodgkin's disease	Breast carcinoma
Histiocytic lymphoma	Adult acute leukaemias
Skin cancer	Multiple myeloma
Testicular carcinoma	Endometrial carcinoma
Embryonal rhabdomyosarcoma	Prostatic cancer
Ewing's sarcoma	Lymphocytic lymphomas
Wilms' tumour	Neuroblastoma
Burkitt's lymphoma	Adrenal cortical carcinoma
Retinoblastoma	Malignant insulinoma
Choriocarcinoma	
Group 3. Cancers responsive to drugs for which clinically useful improvement in survival of responders has not been clearly demonstrated	Group 4. Cancers only marginally responsive or unresponsive to chemotherapeutic agents
Head and neck cancers	Hypernephroma
Gastrointestinal cancer	Bladder carcinoma
Central nervous system cancer	Cancer of the oesophagus
Endocrine gland tumours	Epidermoid carcinoma of the lung
Malignant melanoma	Pancreatic carcinoma
Oat-cell carcinoma of the lung	Hepatocellular carcinoma
Malignant carcinoid tumours	Thyroid carcinoma
Osteogenic sarcomas	
Soft tissue sarcomas	

1. Those where drugs had been responsible for some patients achieving normal life span
2. Those where responders had demonstrated improved survival
3. Those where a clinically useful improvement in survival had not been seen among responders
4. Those marginally responsive or unresponsive to chemotherapeutic agents

Though only 5 years have elapsed, substantial improvements in survival are now seen in some patients in group 3, namely head and neck cancers and oat-cell carcinoma of the lung. Bladder carcinoma, rated as unresponsive, is now being reported to show significant response to some combinations (S. D. WILLIAMS et al. 1978).

Thus it is possible to identify by tissue of origin tumours which remain essentially resistant to the drug therapies we have in common use today, but even among those cancers widely regarded to be sensitive, resistance is found and the converse is true of those regarded to be generally resistant. Resistance should therefore be considered not only within the spectrum of tumours arising from particular tissues, but also as a phenomenon associated with an individual tumour and host. To assess resistance the consequence of therapy upon the overall behaviour of the tumour must be meticulously assessed. Any attempt to do so is dependent on a careful documentation of disease extent at the outset so that all known sites of disease may be scrutinised for evidence of change.

C. Disease Assessment

High relapse rates at distant sites, despite total excision or radical radiotherapy of tumours which appear well localised at presentation, are a feature of many common malignancies. This implies early dissemination of the disease. Since many tumour cells are motile with an invasive capacity (MAREEL 1979), exhibit lack of contact inhibition in vitro (ABERCROMBIE 1975) and have a capacity for replication, it is not entirely surprising that in a 1-cm diameter tumour containing 1×10^9 cells some should disseminate either by local infiltration or by lymphatic or haematogenous routes and lodge to form micrometastases. The high relapse rate among women with carcinoma of the breast, even when the primary is apparently entirely localised within the excised tissue, emphasises the systemic nature of the disease and the limitations of local therapy. It also underlines the very profound problems of assessment, for if undetectable but distant mestastases are established in a significant proportion of patients, these must presumably be influenced by systemic therapy, but the effect upon them cannot easily be monitored.

Modern investigative techniques have greatly increased the ability to detect metastases, but there remain "occult" micrometastases beyond the detectable range of sensitivity of these methods. These ultimately declare themselves, but achieve significance in the definition of "relapse-free survival" (the time from complete disappearance of all detectable disease to its reappearance), which is in itself a measure of disease control.

Patterns of spread and relapse are, however, similar in certain conditions, so facilitating both assessment and management planning. In Hodgkin's disease, for example, disease appears to spread to contiguous lymph node groups, and in cancer of the ovary the tumour may remain within the abdominal cavity for the major part of the coursc of tumour growth. In other tumours, particular tissues or organs are recognised as favoured targets for metastases. Examples are the lungs in patients with sarcomas, cancers of the breast, thyroid and kidney. Assessment of therapeutic effect must therefore take account of alterations in patterns of metastases.

Any attempt to measure tumour response must be prefaced by a meticulous definition of disease extent. Investigations selected will depend largely on a knowledge of the natural history and behavioural characteristics of the tumour. Solid tumours therefore pose different assessment problems from the leukaemias. Table 3 compares the investigations used to define disease extent in Hodgkin's disease, the acute leukaemias, carcinoma of the breast, carcinoma of the ovary and small-cell carcinoma of the lung. Definition of tumour extent prior to therapy

Table 3. Comparison of staging investigations

	Acute leukaemia	Hodgkin's disease	Breast cancer	Ovarian cancer	Small-cell lung cancer
Clinical documention of:					
Lymphadenopathy	0	++	++	++	++
Splenomegaly	0	++	0	0	0
Hepatomegaly	0	++	++	++	++
Local tumour characteristics (i.e. skin tethering, lateral extension, local infiltration)	0	+ (Skin, extranodal)	++	++	+
Blood					
Indices	++	+	+	0	+
Bone marrow	++	++	++	0	++
Chemistry	0	+ (Hepatic disease)	+ (Hyper-calcaemia)	0	+ Hepatic disease
Miscellaneous					
Lymphangiogram	–	+	–	0	–
Ultrasound (abdomen and liver)	–	–	+	+	+
CT scan	–	+	+	+	+
Bone scan	–	0	++	–	++
Surgical staging	–	++	++	++	0

++, essential for staging; +, helpful in staging; 0, not essential for staging but may be useful; –, not required

Table 4. Change in stage following laparotomy in Hodgkin's disease. (SUTCLIFFE et al. 1976)

Clinical stage	No. of patients	Pathological stage		
		Same	Increased	Decreased
IA	23	16	7	0
IB	1	0	1	0
IIA	22	14	8	0
IIB	4	3	1	0
IIIA	18	11	3	4
Total	68	44 (64%)	20 (30%)	4 (6%)

has been finalised by the introduction of staging systems (HARMER 1978; CARBONE et al. 1971). To be of relevance, a staging system should have prognostic significance and be of consequence in therapy planning, or both. In some diseases the staging outlines appear to have limited relevance but may play a useful role in providing a standardised format or comparison of disease characteristics. The Ann Arbor modification of the Rye staging system for Hodgkin's disease is perhaps the one most completely fulfilling these criteria at the present time. This is largely due to the unusually predictable mode of spread and the fact that intra-abdominal extension through the lymphoid system is defined microscopically following a detailed staging laparotomy in those patients who do not appear to have widespread disease (i.e. IIIB or IV) by clinical assessment. The significance of this investigation is demonstrated in Table 4, which summarises the change in stage as a result of laparotomy in 68 patients with clinical stage I-IIIA Hodgkin's disease (SUTCLIFFE et al. 1976).

In the leukaemias the extent of bone marrow infiltration can be quantified crudely following bone marrow examination, but the peripheral blood count and extent of lymphadenopathy, splenomegaly or skin infiltration may reflect the differing consequences of the process.

Although a bone scan may detect metastases in patients with breast cancer, and thus result in documentation of more extensive disease, some surgeons do not perform this investigation, since the management they intend to apply is unaltered by a positive result. Where a systemic therapy is to be applied, however, monitoring canot be carried out without adequate documentation. Prior to therapy, all investigation results should be reviewed for accuracy, completeness and consistency, and if possible the disease stage should be documented formally. Not all staging systems take account of the precise location of metastases, nor their volume – these should also be recorded and each subsequently scrutinised for evidence of change. Problems may arise in defining the limits of a diffusely infiltrating tumour, such as a fibrosarcoma, a mobile intra-abdominal tumour or a radiological lesion with surrounding lung collapse, fibrosis or infection. Eventual response assessment in such circumstances, particularly when this is incomplete, may be crude, and the conclusions therefore cannot be evaluated.

D. Drug Selection

The need to compare the relative merits of available therapies applies throughout medicine. However, in the field of cancer the ready availability of new therapies lends some urgency to comparative studies. It is both the development of anticancer drugs and the greater understanding of the biological behaviour of different cancers which have led to marked changes in patterns of cancer management. The widespread dissemination of many cancers at the time of presentation, the ultimate relapse despite effective local control by radiotherapy or surgery and the activity of drugs comparable to that of radiotherapy in many tumours have collectively encouraged critical evaluation of chemotherapy as an alternative or complementary treatment. Clinical trials have an established place in cancer medicine, but the characteristics which may make a study both valid and acceptable are subject to extremes of definition (PETO et al. 1976, 1977; FREIREICH and GEHAN 1979).

The past 40 years have seen an initially slow and unmethodical but, more recently, an intensive and critical evaluation of drugs active in cancer therapy. Despite this, only some 30 are in current or everyday use, although many others are under experimental evaluation.

The process of evaluating a new drug is extremely complex and beyond the scope of this chapter. Once nominated for use in man it proceeds through a well-defined system of three phases:

1. Phase I clinical trial: The purpose of a phase I clinical trial is to determine maximum tolerated dose (MTD) at the schedule and route chosen, and to determine if human toxicity is predictable, reversible and treatable. The evaluation of antitumour activity is not required, but is carefully documented once noted. The starting dose in man is taken as one-tenth of the LD_{10} in mice. Patients entered must have cancer which is no longer responsive to available treatment. These patients must not have major hepatic, renal or bone marrow dysfunction and must have a survival expectancy of at least 2 months.
2. Phase II clinical trial: At this level the aim is to identify therapeutic activity in different tumour types and to define an optimum drug schedule.
3. Phase III clinical trials: Here the purpose is to confirm activity seen in phase II studies in much larger numbers of patients, to compare activity with other potential therapies and to define the major application of a drug in relation to tumour type.

The phase I, II and III concept of evaluating new drugs has produced much useful information concerning toxicity and antitumour activity, although the latter is inevitably modified by the inability to study activity against untreated tumours. Much currently accepted management has been derived from informal observation of gross response in different tumour types. These reports are historical, the dosages were non-standard and the mode of administration variable. Nonetheless, these studies cannot be repeated and the associations between individual agents and the therapy of specific tumours have now become widely accepted. These associations, again largely empirically derived, are well exemplified by the alkylating agents – the use of mustine is now almost exclusively confined to the treatment of Hodgkin's disease, melphalan to multiple myeloma (although it is now widely used in adjuvant chemotherapy of carcinoma of the breast), chlorambucil to the lymphomas and carcinoma of the ovary, and busulphan to chronic myeloid leukaemia. Only cyclophosphamide is widely used throughout a broad spectrum of malignancies. Similar associations exist for drugs of other classes. Since the choice of drug for use in combination is influenced by single-agent activity, such rigid associations may well have compromised the selection and identifiction of alternative useful agents. Toxicity to normal tissues increases when drugs with the same mode of action are combined. This summation of activity against normal tissues can to some extent be minimised by combining agents of differing classes, so maintaining a tolerable degree of toxicity while potentiating the antitumour effect. The dependence on clinical evaluation has meant, however, that the ability to select drugs on a rational basis is constrained by the interpretative difficulties of such an evaluation. Three- and four-drug combinations are used where two drugs may produce the same response with only minor dose escalation of one drug alone. Drug synergism is difficult to detect in clinical systems where patient differences, tumour differences and the changes induced by a previous treatment compound the problems of assessment. Equally, apparent resistance of a tumour to combination chemotherapy could result, not from resistance to both drugs, but from antagonism of one drug negating the activity of the other. In experimental systems, synergism and antagonism can be clearly demonstrated. C. J. WILLIAMS et al. (1979), using a TLX5 lymphoma model, showed that 5-azacytidine and pyrazofurin had a synergistic antitumour effect, while the use of a number of antimetabolites in combination with pyrazofurin antagonised the antitumour effect. Unfortunately the increased cell kill achieved when 5-azacytidine and pyrazofurin were used in combination was associated with an equivalent increase in toxicity.

Another factor which influences drug selection arises when a major metabolic or excreting organ can be shown to have a significant reduction in function. Drugs such as Adriamycin, which are excreted via the liver, should be given at a modified dose, or an alternative agent given, when there is obstructive jaundice or a markedly raised alkaline phosphatase or 5′-nucleotidase. Where there is demonstrable renal functional impairment, *cis*-diammine dichloroplatinum and cyclophosphamide should be used with caution, or be replaced by other active agents. Factors such as drug cost or the problems of toxicity monitoring may also influence drug selection but are not considered here.

The clonogenic stem-cell assay of SALMON and HAMBURGER (SALMON et al. 1978) is the most promising of the in vitro predictive tests for resistance available despite its technical problems. It has proved reproducible and to have a predictive correlation accurate to 90% between in vitro testing and in vivo effect where resistance to individual drugs is examined. If satisfactorily developed, this approach offers great potential for selecting out drugs to which a tumour is resistant and thus avoiding unnecessary toxicity.

E. Measurement of Response

There is only one tumour in which a tumour product can be directly correlated with the number of tumour cells with a precision which is relevant to therapy; this is the choriocarcinoma. Beta human chorionic gonadotrophin (HCG) levels not only assist in diagnosis of this tumour, but provide a means to a definitive therapeutic end point (LANGE and FRALEY 1977). Attempts have been made to use beta-HCG and alpha-fetal protein to monitor the therapy of testicular teratomas and other germ-cells tumours, but the heterogeneous nature of these neoplasms has limited the value of this approach. DURIE and SALMON (1975) have used the rate of production of idiotypic immunoglobulin in an attempt to calculate tumour mass and subsequently cellular number, but this has proved of limited therapeutic relevance.

In other tumours the response to anticancer therapy can only be measured in terms of changes in tumour volume, changes in the degree of infiltration, and less specifically in terms of improvement in anticipated survival. Assuming adequate drug access and optimal dosage, failure to achieve complete eradication implies drug resistance. The maximum response achieved over several treatments is regarded as a measure of the effectiveness or otherwise of the primary treatment. This maximum response can then be used to compare identical treatments in patients with similar malignancies, and also as a key temporal point in management when a subsequent treatment decision is indicated.

Since the objective of therapy is total eradication of disease, and in consequence cure, any re-evaluation must be comprehensive and include a repeat of all original investigations which showed abnormality. "Complete remission" implies that all investigations are normal. However, in practice some minimal abnormality may be accepted. For example, in almost all patients with acute myelogenous leukaemia (AML) the disease eventually recurs (LISTER et al. 1981). If bone marrow transplant patients are excluded, complete eradication of AML using chemotherapy is extremely rare, and, furthermore, interpretation of the bone marrow with minimal residual disease is complicated by the presence of "blast" cells, which are precursor cells of the "normal" marrow. Although defined some years ago criteria including infiltration of the bone marrow with up to 5% blast cells have formed the basis of an internationally accepted standard for "complete remission" (HEWLETT et al. 1964). Complete remission status demands a value judgment by the observer which may not be justified by subsequent events. Indeed it may prove exceptionally difficult to be entirely objective in defining complete remission, as for example in responding patients with carcinoma of the lung where minimal change at the site of the primary tumour on chest X-ray may be felt to be due to residual fibrosis. Transbronchial biopsy at this site may be negative, but it is a common experience that relapse occurs frequently at the site of primary disease (C. J. WILLIAMS et al. 1977).

Despite these and many other qualifying situations, complete remission has real significance in terms of survival. This is well established in the acute leukaemias (WEINSTEIN et al. 1980), bad prognosis lymphomas (LISTER et al. 1978 b), particular histiocytic lymphomas (R. I. FISHER et al. 1977), small-cell lung cancer (OLDHAM and GRECO 1980), cancer of the ovary (YOUNG et al. 1978), the teratomas (EINHORN and DONOHUE 1979), carcinoma of the breast (CANELLOS et al. 1976) and certain childhood tumours, including rhabdomyosarcoma and Wilms tumour (D'ANGIO et al. 1980).

Delay in achieving complete remission greater than might be anticipated for a particular treatment may be interpreted to indicate a degree of resistance. However, poor drug access, insufficient dosage and delayed tumour resolution (even after the death of the malignant cells) may all contribute to this picture. Their separate influence is difficult both to identify and quantify.

Continued tumour growth, despite therapy, is readily identifiable if rapid, but less so in a slowly growing tumour. Indeed it may require several cycles of therapy to identify an apparent total resistance to treatment. The latter may be difficult to distinguish from a situation where the influence on the tumour is modest – perhaps a slowing in the rate of growth rather than a marginal regression. For the purposes of documentation, definite disease progression is labelled "progressive disease" and the distinction made from "stable" or "minimal change", in which only marginal differences in tumour volume can be detected. Gradations of response between that of minimal change and that of complete remission are much harder to define consistently. Table 5 lists commonly used terminology defining clinical responses and their definitions.

A large tumour volume may be greatly diminished by therapy, but a small residue remains, while in another situation the apparent tumour volume may be small at the outset and become only slightly smaller with therapy. Both leave minimal residual disease, but the response in the former is a substantial one and in the latter only minor. Resistance to therapy in the latter is clinically significant, but both eventually (in that minimal residual disease persists in the face of therapy with active agents) manifest comparable degrees of resistance despite very different responses.

The nodular lymphomas are frequently widespread at presentation and respond to therapy with single agents, but complete eradication of disease is almost unknown (QAZI et al. 1976). Indeed the survival of those patients who achieve a

Table 5. Definitions of responses to therapy

1. *Complete Response* (CR): Complete disappearance of all clinically detectable disease and return to normal of all laboratory tests and X-rays for at least 4 weeks
2. *Good Partial Response* (GPR): Greater than, or equal to, 90% decrease in tumour size in at least 90% of involved sites, without increase in size of any area of known disease or appearance of new lesions
3. *Poor Partial Response* (PPR): Greater than, or equal to, 50% decrease in tumour size (measured as product of two diameters) of bidimensional measurable disease, or 30% decrease of unidimensional measurable disease, in at least 50% of involved sites without increase in size of any area of known disease or appearance of new lesions
4. *Minimal Change* (MC): No significant change in measurable or evaluable disease for at least 6 weeks and no new lesions
5. *Disease Progression* (PD): Significant increase in the size of lesions present at the start of therapy, or appearance of new metastatic lesions known not to be present at the start of therapy

minimal residual disease state parallels that of those patients achieving complete remission (LISTER et al. 1978 a). From this it can be assumed that undetectable disease persists and remains resistant to therapy. Why it is that the disease can be sublimated effectively, but not eradicated, has yet to be satisfactorily explained, and it is indeed one of the reasons for exploring resistance in depth in this book.

F. Can Resistance be Quantified Clinically?

The response criteria outlined in the previous section give only the simplest appreciation of the antitumour effect of the agents used. Failure to produce any measurable degree of tumour regression, despite adequate exposure to a drug at MTD, is an indication for aborting therapy with that agent and substituting another. Failure to respond, despite substitution of alternative therapies, may justifiably be interpreted as total resistance. This is a common feature of gastrointestinal tract malignancy, renal carcinoma and brain tumours, but is also seen sporadically in tumours where response is anticipated, such as the lymphomas, teratomas and breast carcinoma. It is appropriate to make a distinction between resistance to all drug classes, and that of resistance to one drug but sensitivity to another. The problem arises in attempting to define anything less than apparent absolute resistance or absolute sensitivity. Measuring the volume change of a solid tumour or the diminishing degree of infiltration of the bone marrow in acute leukaemia is an indicator of drug activity, but takes little account of the residual tumour-cell population in which resistance to further therapy may be most apparent. Ultimately, it is the capacity to maintain continued disease regression which is the justification for continuing therapy, but once a plateau state is achieved resistance is implied and therapy should be changed. Here also quantification of resistance is unsatisfactory, for the rate of tumour regression varies with each disease process and with the therapy used. For example, in the good prognosis lymphomas complete and good partial remission may be achieved more quickly using combination chemotherapy than when chlorambucil is used alone (LISTER et al. 1978 a). That is to say, the ultimate residual disease volume is similar using either therapeutic approach. Since substituting the alternative regime does not affect the outcome, the assumption is made that the resistant population remaining is also similar. Thus in clinical terms it is the change in rate of tumour regression or failure to achieve regression which equates with resistance. The combined total dosage of drugs required to produce an effect may allow comparison between similar patients and tumours, indicating a dose relationship between response and therapy. However, in the situation where residual disease persists despite originally effective therapy, resistance is manifested as a dose-unrelated problem within the limits of toxicity.

Clinical quantification of resistance in isolation can only be recorded as dose or drug-related and interpreted in the simplest terms.

G. Factors Influencing Changes in Tumour Volume

I. Heterogeneous Target Populations of Tumour Cells

Cell kinetic studies show very clearly that any tumour contains cells distributed throughout the cell cycle. There is therefore an inbuilt heterogeneity of the tumour-cell population, which may be made more or less relevant to the outcome of therapy by the class of drugs selected for treatment. This whole area is the subject of Chap. 5. Histopathological studies have also shown that many tumours are infiltrated by macrophages and lymphocytes. These may represent a significant proportion of the total tumour-cell population. In experimental animal tumours the macrophage content may be responsible for a significant part of the tumour volume. Tumour volume will thus be influenced by the size of this non-neoplastic-cell population.

While changes in tumour volume due to variations in the proportion of infiltrating non-neoplastic cells may result in misinterpretation of the effectiveness of therapy, so too may confusion arise from the response of a mixed population of neoplastic cells. Few tumours contain tissue of such obviously different origin as the malignant teratomas. Chemotherapy may result in a radical change in the histological picture, with elimination of one or more elements, but leaving a residual tissue or cellular population which is unaffected by therapy. Proliferation of this tissue may lead to demise of the host. Such a change usually declares itself clinically with enlarging tumour masses, perhaps a rise in alpha-fetal protein, beta-HCG, or both, and the appearance of new metastases. In some patients bulky tumour may remain following therapy, the marker proteins may be within normal limits, but until proven otherwise tumour is presumed to persist. In 17 patients who came to laparotomy in these circumstances, six had complete excision of residual active tumour, five necrotic tissue and fibrosis only and six benign teratoma (EINHORN and DONOHUE 1979). In some patients with Hodgkin's disease the lymphangiogram returns to normal very slowly and repeat biopsy shows fibrosis but no evidence of tumour. A persisting localised mass which remains despite initial tumour regression and which appears static in size when treatment is discontinued may not necessarily represent tumour. Were treatment of the tumour to be continued in these circumstances it would certainly be labelled as resistant. Rebiopsy may therefore be justified to assist in defining approximate therapy.

II. Changes in Histology

This is a feature which is manifest particularly in the lymphomas – and should be considered in patients with poorly differentiated nodular lymphoma where lymphadenopathy develops through previously effective therapy. Rebiopsy is essential (CULLEN et al. 1979). Occasionally, where a large number of lymph nodes are sampled as in a laparotomy, the majority will be found to contain poorly differentiated nodular lymphoma, but in a diffuse lymphoma – the converse may be found, suggesting a more advanced disease transformation. Diffuse lymphoma involving part of a lymph node is well recognised. This statement has been justified by observation of the more aggressive nature of the disease having this characteristic. In such patients the disease may appear resistant to chlorambucil, but respond when combination chemotherapy is given. With the exception of the diffuse histiocytic lymphomas few patients are cured, suggesting that a resistant population of cells persists despite eradication of the majority.

With the exception of the well-differentiated lymphomas and chronic lymphocytic leukaemia, a marked degree of differentiation tends to be associated with poor response to chemotherapy. In some tumours poor differentiation is associated with chemotherapy responsiveness. It follows that changes in differentiation either spontaneously or as a consequence of therapy may influence the apparent responsiveness and hence the resistance to anticancer therapy.

III. Second Malignancy

The late consequences of chemotherapy in long survivors are now the subject of intense scrutiny. Second malignancy is a feature of some tumours and is well recognised to be associated with a number of cancers, including retinoblastoma, chronic lymphocytic leukaemia and myeloma. Second primary tumours are found in 10% of women with carcinoma of the breast. Acute leukaemia and non-Hodgkin lymphoma are found at increased incidence after a latent period of 4–10 years in patients with Hodgkin's disease who received combined modality therapy with chemotherapy plus radiotherapy (BORUM 1980; KRIKORIAN et al. 1979). Patients with ovarian cancer receiving continuous alkylating agent therapy for several years also are at a greatly increased risk of developing acute myelogenous leukaemia (EINHORN 1978).

Treatment-induced second malignancy is therefore uncommon during the early treatment phase, but concomitant second malignancy or, in woman with breast carcinoma, a second primary must be considered where the pattern of response exhibits a striking regional difference. Biopsy may clarify the situation.

IV. Miscellaneous Factors Contributing to Tumour Volume

The hazards of using tumour volume as an indicator of resistance to therapy have been outlined above. These are compounded by the fact that some masses fluctuate in size in the absence of therapy. This may occur particularly in regional lymph nodes draining a variety of primaries early in the spread of the disease. Generalised lymphadenopathy in patients with poorly differentiated nodular lymphomas may fluctuate considerably over a period of years in the absence of treatment. Necrosis and inflammation or haemorrhage may result in a rapid increase in tumour size and, if occurring during therapy, may lead to misinterpretation and the conclusion of tumour resistance. Fibrosis of a tumour mass may eventually make clinical assessment impossible, so that biopsy is required to define remission or to confirm the presence of a resistant population of cells. To assume resistance in the latter situation ignores the possibility that drug access to cells trapped within a fibrous matrix may be impaired. Concomitant therapy should not be ignored when assessing overall response to therapy. Steroids, in particular dexamethasone, may produce a marked reduction in tumour size when given alone. Hormonal preparations may also influence tumour growth quite independently as a specific anticancer therapy.

Some drugs may also potentiate the activity of antitumour agents and, while this may influence interpretation of response, this is of minor consequence compared with the potentially increased toxicity. Some of the interactions with commonly used drugs are listed in Table 6.

Table 6. Some of the more commonly recognised drug interactions

Actinomycin D	–	Radiotherapy
Adriamycin	–	6-Mercaptopurine
Asparaginase	–	Vincristine
5-Azacytidine	–	Pyrazofurin
Cyclophosphamide	–	Allopurinol
Hydroxyurea	–	CNS depressants
6-Mercaptopurine	–	Adriamycin, allopurinol
Methotrexate	–	Aspirin
cis-Platinum	–	Gentamycin
Procarbazine	–	Monoamine oxidase inhibitors
Pyrazofurin	–	5-Azacytidine
Vincristine	–	Asparaginase aspirin
VP-16-213	–	Chloroquine

H. Influence of Clinically Determined Drug Resistance on Management

I. Resistance and Toxicity

As the dosage administered of a compound is increased, so the effect on normal tissues may be expected to become more pronounced. Some of the most important dose-limiting side effects are summarised in Table 7. The tolerance by the patient of the toxicity determines both the dosage and duration of therapy and these must both be influenced by a realistic appraisal of potential benefits. Toxicity is a consequence both of tumour resistance and the lack of drug specificity for neoplastic cells – thus dosage must be escalated to the point where tumour-cell kill can be achieved without irreversible damage to the normal tissues. In practice the drug is administered to the point where toxicity to the normal tissue reaches a maximal tolerable point. Failure to influence tumour growth at this point equates with resistance, and alternative drugs are tried. Cumulative toxicity may, however, result in a drug having to be discontinued after several administrations, despite showing a therapeutic effect, and an unproven agent substituted for it. Quality of life is appropriately regarded as a major moderator of therapeutic initiative. In tumours with a long natural history, prolonged therapy with agents producing life-threatening side effects or considerable morbidity is unacceptable. Late side effects, such as second malignancy, pulmonary fibrosis, cardiac toxicity or renal toxicity, should also be pre-empted by dose modification. Rapid disease progression requires to be treated intensively, and short-term but severe side effects can be anticipated and a high level of supportive care given. Where response can be expected, but does not materialise, dose escalation to overcome resistance can be attempted.

In the face of marked resistance despite a rapid tumour growth, as for example in terminal malignant melanoma, it is unjustifiable to persist with intensive therapy which is more damaging to the host than to the tumour.

Table 7. Dose-limiting side effects

	Bone marrow suppression	Nausea/vomiting	Chemical irritant	Haemorrhagic cystitis	Infertility	Bone pain	Cardiotoxicity	Renal toxicity	Ototoxicity	Pulmonary fibrosis	Pulmonary infiltrates	Skin pigmentation	Stomatitis	Abdominal pain	Neuropathy	Inappropriate antidiuretic hormone syndrome	Alopecia	Diabetes mellitus	Hypoproteinaemia	Mental upset
Alkylating agents																				
Busulphan	+									+		+								
Chlorambucil	+																			
Cyclophosphamide	+	+		+			+										+			
Melphalan	+																			
Mustine	+	+	+														+			
Antimetabolites																				
Methotrexate	+									+	+		+							
6-Mercaptopurine	+																			
5-Fluorouracil	+																			
Cytosine arabinoside	+														+					
6-Thioguanine	+																			
Antibiotics																				
Actinomycin D	+	+	+				+													
Daunorubicin	+	+	+														+			
Adriamycin	+	+	+				+						+				+			
Bleomycin										+		+								
Plant alkaloid																				
Vinblastine	+		+											+	+		+			
Vincristine	+		+			+								+	+	+	+			
VP-16-213																				
Miscellaneous																				
BCNU	+	+	+														+			
DTIC	+	+	+														+			
Procarbazine	+																			+
Hydroxyurea	+																			+
cis-Platinum	+	+						+	+						+					
Asparaginase																		+	+	

The Karnofsky status can be used to monitor the patient's condition throughout therapy. As treatments become more selective and the prediction of resistance to drugs more accurate, it should be possible to reduce toxicity to a minimum and to maintain quality of life at an acceptable level throughout the early intensive phase of therapy. In some conditions it is now recognised to be one of the most important prognostic factors (YATES et al. 1980; GRECO and OLDHAM 1979).

II. Resistance and Survival

In the sense that disease recurrence represents failure of the primary treatment, it must be regarded as equating with resistance. This is not always obviously so, for in conditions such as acute lymphoblastic leukaemia, the lymphomas and some testicular tumours, it is possible to re-treat effectively with the original drug combination. In the majority of situations, however, when disease recurs the tumour appears much less sensitive not only to the original therapy, but often to all others. This cross-resistance, whatever the cause, is largely unaffected by dose escalation, and inevitably progressive tumour growth eventually compromises the host, resulting in death.

It is the eventual emergence of apparent total resistance despite initial sensitivity which has led some clinicians to the belief that the primary treatment should be intensive. The concept of further reducing the tumour-cell population by additional therapy after the achievement of complete remission gained favour in the acute leukaemias, but has not so far influenced disease-free survival in solid tumours. Indeed "consolidation" therapy has been poorly evaluated in the acute leukaemias, although some reports do suggest that in AML duration of complete remission might be influenced by consolidation therapy (CLARKSON 1972).

Few bulky tumours regress completely following chemotherapy, whereas minimal disease may resolve to produce complete remission. Tumour bulk and the potential advantages of effecting a reduction in tumour volume have been clearly demonstrated by GRIFFITHS et al. (1979) for carcinoma of the ovary. In patients who had their tumours reduced to metastases of less than 1.5 cm in diameter, the survival equalled that of patients with a residual tumour size below this limit. In another study, while Adriamycin had no effect on survival in patients with bulky disease, in those in whom there was minimal residual disease a significant improvement in survival could be documented (EDMONNSON et al. 1979). Several factors, namely the presumed existence of micrometastases, the advantages of treating the well patient with low-volume disease and the experimental data from SKIPPER (SKIPPER et al. 1964), implying the death of a fixed proportion of cells with each treatment, have long encouraged the concept of treating to prevent disease recurrence. In acute lymphoblastic leukaemia of childhood, low-dose "maintenance" therapy once complete remission is obtained is an established part of management. The drugs used in maintaining the remission differ from those used in remission induction and when relapse does occur in patients while on maintenance therapy, the prognosis declines, but second and subsequent remissions are frequently and readily obtained (ANONYMOUS 1981). However, this is in contrast to AML, where only 10% of those maintained with chemotherapy achieve a second remission. In Hodgkin's disease, the value of maintenance or "adjuvant" chemotherapy is not proven. In some studies disease-free survival was improved, but not overall survival.

Adjuvant chemotherapy has achieved greatest notoriety in the management of carcinoma of the breast. At least two controlled clinical trials have now shown some benefit in those patients receiving chemotherapy (Fisher et al. 1977; Bonadonna et al. 1978) (either with melphalan or with cyclophosphamide plus methotrexate and 5-fluorouracil) after radical mastectomy. The 5-year disease-free survival is 15% greater in the treated group in the Italian study and shows a 30% difference at 4 years in the National Surgical Adjuvant Breast Program (NSABP) study. Despite the initial enthusiasm, it now appears that certain subgroups of patients are responsible for the major influence on both disease-free and overall survival. These are the premenopausal and those with three or less positive lymph nodes. However, when total dosage of therapy administered was considered, the limitation of benefit to premenopausal patients was abolished.

Inevitably, some patients in these studies would not relapse and so receive excessive treatment, but since the majority eventually develop metastatic disease if untreated, it is essential that the role of adjuvant chemotherapy be properly evaluated.

If adjuvant chemotherapy only suppresses growth of micrometastases, then relapse will eventually follow. The possibility remaining is that continued exposure at low dosage may facilitate the emergence of a resistant clone of cells. This fear is to some extent borne out in practice, for those relapsing while on adjuvant chemotherapy may have disease which is less readily controlled by alternative drug treatment.

In osteogenic sarcoma, high-dose methotrexate used as an adjuvant to surgery and radiotherapy appeared to offer a significant survival advantage. Although doses of methotrexate used in conjunction with leucovorin rescue reached high levels, the overall improvement in survival seen in some centres which use radiotherapy and surgery alone was comparable and has thrown the value of adjuvant therapy of this kind into question (Anonymous 1977). For all the encouraging information on adjuvant therapy in these and other tumours, the most useful guides to prognosis remain the tissue of origin of the tumour and the degree of apparent clinical resistance following initial therapy. The return to clinical normality carries a survival advantage as yet unexplained in terms of drug resistance alone.

References

Abercrombie M (1975) In: Cellular membranes and tumor cell behavior. Williams and Wilkins, pp 21–37

Anonymous (1977) Combined therapy and childhood sarcomas. Br Med J 5097:1241–1242

Anonymous (1981) Second remissions in childhood acute lymphoblastic leukaemia. Br Med J 282:760–761

Bonadonna G, Valagussa P, Rossi A et al. (1978) Are surgical adjuvant trials altering the course of breast cancer? Semin Oncol 5:450–464

Borum (K (1980) Increasing frequency of acute myeloid leukemia complicating Hodgkin's disease. Cancer 46:1247–1252

Canellos GP, DeVita VT, Gold GL, Chabner BA, Schein PS, Young RC (1976) Combination chemotherapy for advanced breast cancer: response and effect on survival. Ann Intern Med 84:389–392

Carbone PP, Kaplan HS, Musshof K. Smithers DW, Tubiana M (1971) Report of the committee on Hodgkin's disease. Cancer Res 31:1860–1861

Clarkson BD (1972) Acute myelocytic leukemia in adults. Cancer 30:1572–1582

Cullen MH, Lister TA, Brearley RC, Shand WS, Stansfeld AG (1979) Histological transformation of non-Hodgkins lymphoma – a prospective study. Cancer 44:645–651

D'Angio GJ, Beckwith JB, Breslow NE, Bishop HC, Evans AE, Farewell V, Fernbach D, Goodwin WE, Jones B, Leape LL, Palmer NF, Tefft M, Wolff JA (1980) Wilm's tumor: an update. Cancer 45:1791–1798

DeVita VT, Young RC, Canellos GP (1975) Combination versus single agent chemotherapy: a review of the basis for selection of drug treatment of cancer. Cancer 35:98–110

Durie BGM, Salmon SE (1975) A clinical staging system for multiple myeloma: correlation of measured myeloma cell mass with presenting clinical features, response to treatment, and survival. Cancer 36:842–854

Edmonson JH, Fleming TR, Decker DG, Malkasian GD, Jorgensen EO, Jefferies JA,, Webb MJ, Kvols LK (1979) Different chemotherapeutic sensitivities and host factors affecting prognosis in advanced ovarian carcinoma versus minimal residual disease. Cancer Treat Rep 63:241

Einhorn LH, Donohue JP (1979) Combination chemotherapy in disseminated testicular cancer: the Indiana University experience. Semin Oncol 6:87–93

Einhorn N (1978) Acute leukemia after chemotherapy (melphalan). Cancer 41:444–447

Everson TC (1964) Spontaneous regression of cancer. Ann NY Acad Sci 114:721–735

Everson TC, Cole WH (1956) Spontaneous regression of cancer: preliminary report. Ann Surg 144:366–380

Fisher B, Glass A, Redmond C et al. (1977) L-phenylalanine mustard (L-PAM) in the management of primary breast cancer: an update of earlier findings and a comparison with those utilizing L-PAM plus 5-fluorouracil (5-FU). Cancer 39:2883–903

Fisher RI, DeVita VT, Johnson BL, Simon R, Young RC (1977) Prognostic factors for advanced diffuse histiocytic lymphoma following treatment with combination chemotherapy. Am J med 63:177

Freireich EJ, Gehan EA (1979) The limitations of the randomised trial. Methods Cancer Res 17:277–310

Goldstein DP, Goldstein PR, Bottomley P, Osathanondh R, Marean AR (1976) Methotrexate with alnovorum factor rescue for non-metastatic gastrational trophoblastic neoplasms. Obstet Gynecol 48:321–323

Greco FA, Oldham RK (1979) Current concepts in cancer: small-cell lung cancer. N Engl J med 301:355–358

Griffiths CT, Parker LM, Fuller AF (1979) Role of cytoreductive surgical treatment in the management of advanced ovarian cancer. Cancer Treat Rep 63:235

Harmer MH (ed) (1978) TNM classification of malignant tumours. UICC, Geneva

Hewlett JS, Battle JD, Bishop RC (1964) Phase II study of A-8103 (NSC-25154) in acute leukemia in adults. Cancer Chemother Rep 42:25–28

Holmes EC, Eilber FR, Morton DL (1975) Immunotherapy of malignancy in humans. JAMA 232:1052–1055

Krikorian JG, Burke JS, Rosenberg SA, Kaplan HS (1979) Occurrence of non-Hodgkin's lymphoma after therapy for Hodgkin's disease. N Engl J Med 300:452–458

Lange PH, Fraley EE (1977) Serum alpha-fetoprotein and human chorionic gonadotropin in the treatment of patients with testicular tumors. Urol Clin north Am 4:394–405

Lister TA, Cullen MH, Beard MEJ, Brearley RL, Whitehouse JMA, Wrigley PFM, Stansfeld AG, Sutclive SBJ, Malpas JS, Crowther D (1978 a) Comparison of combined and single-agent chemotherapy in non-Hodgkin's lymphoma of favourable histological type. Br Med J 1:533–537

Lister TA, Cullen MH, Brearley RB, Beard MEJ, Stansfeld AG, Whitehouse JMA, Wrigley PFM, Ford JM, Malpas JS, Crowther D (1978b) Combination chemotherapy for advanced non-Hodgkin's lymphoma of unfavourable histology. Cancer Chemother Pharmacol 1:107–112
Lister TA, Johnson SAN, Bell R, Henry E, Malpas JS (1981) Progress in acute myelogenous leukaemia. In: Neth R, Gallo RC, Graf T, Mannweiler K, Winkler K (eds) Modern trends in human leukaemia 4. Springer, Berlin Heidelberg New York
Mareel MMK (1979) Mini-review: is invasiveness in vitro characteristic of malignant cells? Cell Biol Int Rep 3:627–640
McKneally MF, Maver C, Kansel MW (1976) Regional immunotherapy of lung cancer with intrapleural BCG. Lancet 1:377–379
Oldham RK, Greco FA (1980) Small-cell lung cancer: a curable disease. Cancer Chemother Pharmacol 4:173–177
Peto R, Pike MC, Armitage P, Breslow NE, Cox DR, Howard SV, Mantel N, McPherson K, Peto J, Smith PG (1976) Design and analysis of randomized clinical trials requiring prolonged observation of each patient. I. Analysis and examples. Br J Cancer 34:585–612
Peto R, Pike MC, Armitage P, Breslow NE, Cox DR, Howard SV, Mantel N, McPherson K, Peto J, Smith PG (1977) Design and analysis of randomized clinical trials requiring prolonged observation of each patient. II. Analysis and examples. Br J Cancer 35:1–39
Qazi R, Aisenberg AC, Long JC (1976) The natural history of nodular lymphoma. Cancer 37:1923–1927
Salmon SE, Hamburger AW, Soehnlein B, Durie BCM, Alberts DS, Moon TE (1978) Quantitation of differential sensitivity of human-tumor stem cells to anticancer drugs. N Engl J Med 298:1321–1327
Skipper HE, Schabel FM, Wilcox WS (1964) Experimental evaluation of potential anticancer agents XIII. On the criteria and kinetics associated with "curability" of experimental leukemia. Cancer Chemother Rep 35:1
Sumner WC, Foraker AG (1960) Spontaneous regression of human melanoma. Cancer 13:79–81
Sutcliffe SBJ, Wrigley PFM, Smyth JF, Webb JAW, Tucker AK, Beard MEJ, Irving M, Stansfeld AG, Malpas JS, Crowther D, Whitehous JMA (1976) Intensive investigation in management of Hodgkin's disease. Br Med J 2:1343–1347
Weinstein HJ, Meyer RJ, Rosenthal DS, Camitta BM, Coral FS, Nathan DG, Frei E (1980) Treatment of acute myelogenous leukemia in children and adults. N Engl M Med 303:473–478
Williams CJ, Alexander M, Glatsein EJ, Daniels JR (1977) role of radiation therapy in combination with chemotherapy in extensive oat cell carcinoma of the lung. A randomised study. Cancer Treat Rep 16:1427
Williams CJ, Swan A, Al-Atia G, Whitehouse JMA (1979) Synergistic antitumor activity and toxicity of pyrazofurin (PZ) and 5-azacytidine (AzaCyd). In: Weinhouse S (ed) Proceedings 15th AACR, vol 20, No. 226, p 56. Waverly, Baltimore
Williams SD, Rohn RJK, Donohue JP, Einhorn LH (1978) Chemotherapy of bladder cancer with *cis*-diammine-dichloroplatinum (DDP), adriamycin (ADR) and 5-fluorouracil (5-FU). Proceedings 14th ASCO, vol 19, C-37, p 316. Waverly, Baltimore
Yates JW, Chalmer B, McKegney FP (1980) Evaluation of patients with advanced cancer using the Karnofsky performance status. Cancer 45:2220–2224
Young RC, Chabney BA, Hubbard SP, Fisher RI, Bender RA, Anderson T, Simon RM, Canellos GP, DeVita VT (1978) Advanced ovarian adenocarcinoma: a prospective clinical trial of melphalan (L-PAM) versus combination chomtherapy. N Engl J Med 299:1261–1266
Zubrod CG (1978) Selective toxicity of anticancer drugs: presidential address. Cancer Res 38:4377–4384

CHAPTER 2

Experimental Setting

J. F. HENDERSON

A. Introduction

Three basic questions provide the focus for experimental studies of antitumor drug resistance. First, how does a population change from a state of drug sensitivity to one of insensitivity? This is the question of the *origins* of resistance. Second, why do resistant cells no longer respond to drug treatment? This is the question of the *mechanisms* or bases of resistance. Third, how can resistance be overcome or circumvented therapeutically?

These are the questions to be considered here, not in great detail, drug by drug – this will be the task of other chapters – but rather by laying out the concepts at issue and by sketching the larger picture of drug resistance. The several phenomena and experimental conditions that are loosely termed resistance or insensitivity will be dissected and defined in detail elsewhere; here, however, we may be content with rather broad and experiential definitions. Two points should be noted, however. First, resistance is a relative term, with high, intermediate, and low degrees, as defined by the investigator in terms of individual experimental systems. Second, resistance is not the property of an individual tumor cell or tumor-cell population. At the very least it is the property of some tumor-drug system, and in vivo it is characteristic of particular tumor-drug-host combinations.

Because this chapter concerns concepts, and because details of studies of individual drugs are to be covered in subsequent chapters, no references will be made here to the original experimental literature.

B. Origins of Resistance

Antitumor drug resistance may arise through changes in the tumor, through changes in the host, or through changes in one or another parameter relating to the drug treatment. Certainly, emphasis both conceptually and experimentally has heretofore been placed on changes in the tumor; yet the other potential origins of resistance require serious consideration as well.

I. Changes in the Tumor

Resistance usually is thought of in terms of genetic, and mostly permanent, changes in individual tumor cells and in the tumor-cell population as a whole. In addition, however, a variety of nongenetic origins of resistance either have been documented experimentally or at least remain theoretically possible. Both genetic and nongenetic origins of resistance will be considered here.

1. Nongenetic Origins

Among potential nongenetic origins of antitumor drug resistance are the location in which the tumor grows, its size and growth characteristics, and adaptive (i.e. nongenetic and impermanent) biochemical changes.

a) Location of Tumor Cells

The localization of tumor cells in the animal body clearly affects their responsiveness to drug treatment and can effectively be an origin of drug insensitivity. It is well known, for example, that the brain (and a few other sites) affords a "pharmacological sanctuary" for tumor cells, inasmuch as many water-soluble drugs cannot penetrate the so-called blood-brain barrier. In other cases the amount of drug that reaches tumor cells will be affected by the blood supply to the anatomical region, by the extravascular distance through which the drug must diffuse, by drug metabolism by extracellular enzymes and normal cells that surround the tumor, etc. In addition the location in which tumor cells grow may affect various characteristics of tumor growth; this point will be discussed below.

Except for the case of tumors growing in the brain, the role of tumor-cell localization in drug insensitivity has been relatively little investigated.

b) Effect of Tumor Size

It is well known in both experimental and clinical cancer chemotherapy that it usually is easier to treat a small tumor (or a small number of tumor cells) than a large one. Effectively, therefore, insensitivity is related to tumor size or mass, and four possible nongenetic bases for this may be noted. First, a particular drug treatment regimen will kill only so many logs of tumor cells and with a larger tumor a number of viable cells may remain unscathed. If the drug treatment cannot be repeated soon enough, due to problems of host toxicity, then the tumor cannot be totally eradicated. Second, in large tumors not only drug concentration is important, but also the total amount of drug administered, inasmuch as a large tumor mass "soaks up" drug. Again, if host toxicity limits the amount of drug that can safely be given, it may not be possible to achieve sufficiently toxic drug concentrations. Third, the death of some or many tumor cells may lead to release of metabolites that can effectively protect other cells from the toxic effects of the drug; the larger the tumor the more important this "cross-feeding" is likely to be. Fourth, tumor size also has consequences for the growth characteristics of at least portions of the total cell population, as will be considered below. Genetic factors related to tumor size will be considered below.

c) Growth Characteristics

Biological features that are or may be important determinants of drug effectiveness include the "form" of growth, whether as single-cell suspensions or as solid tumors; the fraction of the total population that is growing (growth fraction); the cell cycle time of the growing portion of the population; the duration of different phases of the cell cycle; and the gradients of oxygen, glucose, and nutrients within solid tumors. Viable but nongrowing tumor cells may remain insensitive to treatment with many anticancer drugs, and hypoxic cells may be insensitive to drugs that would affect even nongrowing oxygenated cells. Growing cells may be sensitive or insensitive depending upon the phase of the cell cycle they are in at the time of drug treatment. Though cell kinetic considerations are no longer thought to be the main factor determining drug effectiveness, their importance should not be minimized.

d) Adaptive Biochemical Changes

Though little attention has been paid to this point, the possibility is great that at least some tumor cells may respond to drug treatment by adaptive, nonpermanent metabolic changes of a sort that may effectively lead to drug resistance. One example of an adaptive biochemical change is the increased activity of several enzymes of pyrimidine biosynthesis de novo (and increased rate of the initial portion of this pathway) in cells treated with inhibitors of its terminal reactions (e.g. azauridine). These changes apparently are due to derepression of enzyme synthesis as a result of lowered concentrations of pyrimidine nucleotides such as uridine triphosphate and cytidine triphosphate.

In addition, exposure of cells to low doses of some purine analogs may lead to a relatively low level of resistance in a high proportion of the cells. This resistance apparently is not due to loss of key enzymes, but rather to less drastic metabolic alterations of unknown character. In the absence of continued exposure to drug, resistance is lost within a few weeks. Clearly, this type of resistance deserves further investigation.

2. Genetic Origins

a) Mutation and Selection

The first hypothesis regarding the origin of drug resistance in tumor cells, based on previous studies of microbial systems, was that resistant mutant cells, already present in very small numbers prior to initiation of drug treatment, were being selected for by the pressure of the drug treatment. There is indeed evidence in favor of this view, though it is technically difficult to demonstrate it in tumor-bearing animals in vivo.

With the realization that many anticancer drugs are themselves mutagenic, the original viewpoint was broadened to include selection of resistant mutant cells produced during drug treatment by the drug used itself. Thus the drug treatment not only provided the selection pressure, but also increased the mutation rate.

Again, the genetic origin of drug resistance was originally thought of in terms of point, frameshift, and deletion mutations in the nuclear genetic material. In recent years, however, this picture has been expanded in two respects. First, drug resistance due to gene amplification has been discovered. In this case mutant cells are selected that have duplicated portions of their genetic materials so that increased amounts of gene products are made from the multiple gene copies. These mutants are rare and require carefully applied selection pressures in order for them to come to dominate the total picture. Resistance to methotrexate due to elevated levels of dihydrofolate reductase, and resistance to *N*-phosphonacetyl-L-aspartate (PALA) due to increased amounts of aspartate transcarbamylase, have been shown to be due to gene amplification.

In addition, mutations in mitochondrial DNA have been shown to confer resistance to certain agents (e.g. chloramphenicol, rutamycin, antimycin A) that act on mitochondria. To date, no case of resistance in tumors to an anticancer drug has been found to fall into this category.

In all types of resistance of genetic origin, the emergence of a drug-resistant population will depend on a number of factors: the frequency of mutation to resistance in the untreated population together, with the additional frequency of drug-induced mutation (if any), whether the mutation is dominant or recessive, the ploidy of the cells, and perhaps the location of the responsible gene in the chromosome. In addition, the selection pressure that is imposed upon the population is important, as is the actual degree of resistance associated with the predominant mutation to resistance in any particular experimental system. Frequencies of mutation to drug resistance that commonly are observed (10^{-7}–10^{-5}) are such that large tumor masses in vivo may be expected to contain such subpopulations at the time of initiation of treatment. The relative importance of this factor in the observed insensitivity of large tumors, compared with the effects of the nongenetic factors considered above, is not clear.

High degrees of resistance may arise readily after short periods of treatment, or gradually as a result of treatment over prolonged periods. Stepwise increases in resistance may indicate the involvement of multiple genes or alleles in the development of the highly resistant phenotype. Finally populations may remain resistant even without maintenance of the original selection pressure, or may be unstable and revert to sensitivity if drug treatment is not continued.

b) Tumor Heterogeneity

Spontaneous tumors in animals and humans are genetically very heterogeneous, and within a single tumor-cell population such characters as morphology, karyotype, doubling time, antigenicity, ability to metastasize, and drug sensitivity may vary widely. This property of tumors means that drug treatment does not have to play the same role in selecting rare drug-resistant cells as in studies using cultured cell lines in vitro; instead, the resistant cells may already constitute an appreciable fraction of the tumor-cell population, and hence resistance may arise quickly and relatively easily. Studies of this phenomenon are still at an early stage.

II. Changes in the Host

The potential role of the host in the phenomenon of resistance has not been studied in any detail, and the plethora of studies using cell culture systems in recent years has tended to take attention away from this member of the tumor-drug-host triad.

In the most general way, changes in the host which potentially may lead to insensitivity may be said to include (a) altered absorption, distribution, or excretion of the drug so that less reaches the tumor, (b) increased synthesis, decreased inactivation, or altered distribution of enzymes that inactivate the drug, and (c) increased sensitivity of normal tissues to drug effects so that lower doses have to be given.

In many experimental situations, in which host animals are of the same genetic stock and healthy at the beginning of the experiment, and in which drug treatment is given for only a short period of time, it is unlikely that changes in the host would lead to insensitivity. If drug treatment is prolonged, however, or in the usual circumstances of clinical chemotherapy, the possible role of the host deserves more serious consideration.

Host effects may be considered to be adaptive in nature, of the sort already discussed above in terms of nongenetic changes in the tumor. In addition, consideration must also be given to individual variation in any of the factors important for drug actions; this is based at least in part on genetic variation among host animals.

III. Changes in Pharmacological Parameters

Though it is quite elementary to state this, for the sake of completeness it must be added that insensitivity may result simply from drug doses, treatment schedules, or routes of administration that are inappropriate or inadequate.

IV. Experimental Systems

The relevance of different kinds of origins of drug resistance in experimental systems, to the origins of resistance in the clinic, is not known. Similarly, the relevance of different types of origins to chemotherapeutic circumvention by different approaches is not yet clear. In general, however, it seems likely that the relatively high selection pressures exerted in many experimental studies of drug resistance are higher than those exerted in human cancer patients undergoing chemotherapy; however, there is no certainty on this point. The relative role of adaptive biochemical changes and one-step and multistep mutation-selection mechanisms in the evolution of clinical resistance remains to be established; in view of a more recent appreciation of initial heterogeneity in spontaneous tumors, perhaps all of these laboratory models are grossly oversimplified. The most important lacuna in this field remains the development of experimental models that do realistically reflect the origins of the kind or kinds of resistance encountered clinically.

C. Mechanisms of Resistance

Whether resistance or insensitivity arises out of changes in the tumor, in the host, or in pharmacological parameters, certain basic biochemical and pharmacological principles usually are involved in the actual mechanism of resistance. Most studies of this topic have been focused on the resistant tumor cell, and this discussion will continue this emphasis.

Before considering biochemical mechanisms in more detail, however, it seems appropriate to note that at least potentially a genetic change in the tumor population could also provide an immunological mechanism of resistance. Thus in the chemotherapy of some tumors growing in noninbred animals, an immunological component has been shown to have a role in the overall therapeutic effect. If such a tumor were to become more compatible with the host through mutation and selection, then an overall decrease in drug effectiveness would be noted. Apparently there are no actual examples of this type of mechanism.

In biochemical terms, resistance may be the result of differences between sensitive and insensitive cells of any of the factors required for drug action. Thus there may be differences in the concentration of the active form of the drug at the intracellular site of action, differences in the interaction of the drug with its biochemical target, or differences in the importance of the target for cell growth or viability.

I. Differences in Drug Concentration

As already mentioned, insensitivity of nongenetic origins may in some cases be due to the presence at the site of tumor growth of ineffectively low drug concentrations. These cases include those of pharmacological sanctuary and other localization effects, altered drug metabolism by the host, and inappropriate pharmacological parameters.

1. Drug Uptake

One factor that may lead to resistance in tumor-cell populations whose resistance is of genetic origin is decreased drug uptake. Many examples of this mechanism of resistance are known, and two types of changes have been observed. First, some drugs, especially some antimetabolites and some alkylating agents, enter cells by specific carrier-mediated transport mechanisms, either of the concentrative or facilitated diffusion type. In these cases resistance may be caused by changes in the specificity of the transport mechanism, leading effectively to an increased apparent Michaelis constant for uptake. Alternatively, the maximum velocity of uptake may be decreased.

A second subtype pertains to drugs which enter cells by nonspecific mechanisms, usually free diffusion. In these cases resistance has been shown to be due to changes in the cell surface or plasma membrane that reduce either the original binding of drug to the cell surface or its subsequent diffusion into the cell. Such changes usually lead to resistance to a variety of structurally unrelated drugs, most of which tend to have relatively large and complex structures.

Drug uptake by carrier-mediated mechanisms may be inhibited by the naturally occurring permeants (e.g. nucleosides, amino acids). Thus elevated concentrations of these permeants in the host or simply within the tumor may be another mechanism of insensitivity.

2. Nucleotide Formation

Nucleoside monophosphates are the active forms, or intermediates in the synthesis of the active forms, of most growth inhibitory purine and pyrimidine analogs and derivatives, and numerous examples of resistance due to decreased rates of drug nucleotide formation have been reported.

Thus adenine analogs may be converted to nucleoside monophosphates by adenine phosphoribosyltransferase, hypoxanthine and guanine analogs by hypoxanthine-guanine phosphoribosyltransferase, adenosine analogs by adenosine kinase, and deoxyadenosine and deoxyguanosine analogs by kinases whose specificity and number vary among tissues and have not yet been clearly defined.

Among pyrimidines, uracil analogs may be converted to nucleoside monophosphates by uracil phosphoribosyltransferase and by the sequential action of uridine phosphorylase and uridine kinase, uridine and cytidine analogs by uridine-cytidine kinase, deoxycytidine analogs by deoxycytidine kinase, and deoxyuridine and thymidine analogs by one or two kinases, depending on the cell studied.

In most cases of resistance due to decreased drug nucleotide formation, the activating enzymes listed above are simply absent or present in reduced amounts. Sometimes the enzyme is still present, however, but with altered substrate specificity, so that its apparent Michaelis constant for the substrate analog is very much increased. At a fixed drug concentration, therefore, less drug nucleotide is formed.

A quite different mechanism by which drug nucleotide formation could be depressed is inhibition of activating enzymes by elevated concentrations of normal nucleotide metabolites. Thus high concentrations of uridine triphosphate or cytidine triphosphate could inhibit drug nucleotide formation via uridine-cytidine kinase, and high concentrations of deoxycytidine triphosphate could inhibit drug nucleotide formation via one or another pyrimidine deoxyribonucleoside kinase. The latter situation has, for example, been associated with resistance to arabinosylcytosine and to thymidine in certain systems.

Finally, many drug nucleoside monophosphates are metabolized by other reactions of nucleotide metabolism, including phosphorylation, interconversion, ribonucleotide reduction and incorporation into RNA, DNA, or both. Resistance could potentially be due to changes in any of these reactions, if they are involved in growth inhibition; however, this area is more technically difficult to study, and in general resistance has not yet been associated with such mechanisms.

3. Drug Catabolism

A third determinant of pharmacologically efficacious drug concentrations in cells is the rate at which drugs are catabolized, and several examples of resistance and insensitivity due to increased rates of drug inactivation are known. Most of these cases involve resistance to purine and pyrimidine analogs, and they may be divided into two subclasses. Thus the drugs may be catabolized prior to conversion to nucleotides (thus, usually, in the form actually administered), or it may be the activated nucleotide derivative whose rate of catabolism is accelerated.

Important catabolic enzymes for purine bases and nucleoside analogs and derivatives include adenosine deaminase, guanine deaminase, purine nucleoside phosphorylase, and xanthine oxidase. Many cases of insensitivity to adenosine analogs have been associated with high levels of adenosine deaminase activity, though genetically altered tumor-cell populations with elevated amounts of this enzyme have not been described. Guanine deaminase activity has also been shown to be a determinant of the activity of several guanine analogs; again, mutants with elevated activities of this enzyme have not been found. The possible roles of purine nucleoside phosphorylase and xanthine oxidase in insensitivity have not received much study.

The principle enzyme of pyrimidine nucleoside catabolism, at least so far as resistance is concerned, is cytidine deaminase, and high activities of it have been associated with resistance to arabinosylcytosine. The enzymes of pyrimidine ring catabolism are also important in the metabolism of fluorouracil in some tissues. The possible role of pyrimidine nucleoside phosphorylases in insensitivity has not been much studied.

Increased dephosphorylation of nucleotides of thioguanine and methylmercaptopurine ribonucleoside has been associated with resistance to these agents in a few tumors, and recent studies have shown that the rate of dephosphorylation is an important determinant of sensitivity to deoxyadenosine. Study of such systems is complicated because a number of enzymes exist which are able to dephosphorylate nucleoside mono-, di-, and triphosphates; not all of these have been well characterized, and their occurrence varies among tumors and normal tissues. Alkaline phosphatase has been implicated in some cases of resistance, intracellular 5′-nucleotidase(s) in others, and ecto-5′-nucleotidase(s) in others; the situation remains confused, however.

Much less is known about inactivation of other classes of antineoplastic agents in resistant cells. In a few cases, an increased content of sulfhydryl compounds has been associated with resistance to alkylating agents, though the evidence is not strong. In some cells, inactivation of methotrexate may be a determinant of sensitivity, though again there really is not much evidence on this point.

II. Differences in Drug-Target Interaction

After a significant concentration of the active form of a drug has been attained within a cell, the drug must then interact in some way with its biochemical "target," which usually is an enzyme or other protein or one or another species of ribo- or deoxyribonucleic acid. In a few cases, resistance has been attributed to alterations in their interaction. It may also be noted that drugs may interact with more than one cell constituent, but only those interactions that lead to growth inhibition are relevant to cancer chemotherapy.

1. Drug-Enzyme Binding

The affinity of target enzyme (or other target species) clearly is an important determinant of sensitivity, and in a few cases resistant tumor-cell populations have been shown to contain species of enzymes that bind drug less tightly than do the respective enzymes in sensitive cells. Thus altered forms of dihydrofolate reductase, thymidylate synthetase, and glutamine amidophosphoribosyltransferase have been shown to have decreased affinities for methotrexate, fluorodeoxyuridylate, and methylmercaptopurine ribonucleotide, respectively.

2. Drug-Cell Interaction

In some cases, particularly those in which the precise target of the drug is not known, comparisons have been made of drug binding to cell constituents or to cellular fractions of sensitive and resistant cells. The interpretation of these observations is necessarily less certain than when drug-enzyme interactions can be studied. In some cases, these results also cannot clearly be distinguished from decreased retention of bound drug, as discussed below.

3. Metabolite Concentrations

Interaction of drug and target may be affected not only in changes in the target but also by differences in the concentration of normal metabolites that might, in effect, protect the target from the drug. There are several cases, for example, in which resistance to arabinosylcytosine has been attributed to increased concentrations of deoxycytidine triphosphate. This metabolite may compete with the active form of the drug for binding to DNA polymerase.

III. Differences in Importance of Biochemical Target

The next determinant of drug sensitivity that needs to be considered is the significance of the interaction of drug and target for cell growth and viability. This is an important mechanism of resistance and insensitivity of nongenetic origin, especially in cases dependent on the growth characteristics of tumors. Thus binding to targets related to growth or to particular phases of the cell cycle may not be detrimental in tumors with low growth fractions or to cells in other phases of the cell cycle, respectively. To give another example, drugs that affect oxidative energy metabolism or that inhibit glycolysis, respectively, may or may not impair viability depending on the oxygen tension and glucose concentration in the tumor or in individual tumor cells.

1. Recovery from Drug Effects

The rate of repair of damage or of recovery from the initial effects of the drug is one factor that may modify the chemotherapeutic significance of drug-target interactions. For example, several cases of resistance to alkylating agents have been attributed to increased rates of DNA repair. Increased rates of synthesis of certain enzymes of purine and pyrimidine have also been associated with resistance to specific drugs which inhibit these enzymes. Finally, several studies of drug binding to cellular constituents or subcellular fractions (in cases in which the precise target of drug action was not known) have also revealed differences between sensitive and resistant cells in the length of time drug was bound.

2. Alternative Pathways

Some tumors appear to have become resistant because of accelerated rates of pathways which are, or may be, alternatives to those affected by the drugs in question. Thus certain tumors resistant to purine or pyrimidine base analogs have accelerated rates of purine or pyrimidine nucleotide biosynthesis de novo; however, the true relationship of these changes to the resistance observed remains uncertain. Observations that the activity of asparagine synthetase is elevated in some tumors that are resistant to asparaginase are more convincing, however.

In addition to these cases of increased enzyme activity, usually in resistance that is of genetic origin, various cases of resistance of nongenetic origin may be due to the increased availability of the substrates of alternative pathways. Thus the effectiveness of chemotherapy using inhibitors of the pathways of purine or pyrimidine nucleotide biosynthesis de novo is limited by the extent of nucleotide formation via the alternative, so-called salvage pathways. The substrates of the latter are purine and pyrimidine bases and nucleosides, which may be derived both from intracellular and extracellular sources. (Little is known in quantitative terms about the supply of these substrates.) The concentrations of some of these substrates in plasma varies widely among animal species and among human subjects. They are also produced as a result of cell death, and hence in a solid tumor dead cells can feed and thereby protect nearby living cells.

3. Concentration of Target

Drug effectiveness may also be affected by the concentration of the biochemical target, inasmuch as a given amount of drug-target complex may be a large percentage of a small absolute amount or a small percentage of a large amount of target. The best known examples are those cases of resistance to methotrexate that are associated with elevated cellular concentrations of dihydrofolate reductase. Finally, some enzymes vary in concentration according to state of growth or phase of the cell cycle. Hence if these are targets of drug action, one would expect such variations to be associated with sensitivity and insensitivity.

IV. Experimental Systems

Several general remarks may be made regarding the experimental study of mechanisms of resistance, especially as related to cases of genetic origin. First, it should be clear from the preceding discussion that resistance to individual drugs may arise due to several different mechanisms; hence each experimental system and situation has to be examined individually. In addition, the frequency with which particular mechanisms of resistance may arise with respect to any particular tumor-drug or tumor-drug-host system is not known. The mechanisms of resistance of most resistant or insensitive tumors simply are not known, and the apparent relatively high frequency of certain mechanisms (e.g. decreased nucleotide formation from purine and pyrimidine analogs) may reflect the ease with which this mechanism can be identified experimentally rather than its true frequency. A third point to be noted is that the frequency with which individual mechanisms of resistance occur in experimental studies, whether in culture or in vivo, cannot be taken as indicating the likely mechanisms of clinical resistance to anticancer drugs. At the present time, the relationship between experimental resistant systems and the resistance that is observed in human cancer patients is an open question.

Fourth, the possibility that resistance may be due to the combined effects of multiple biochemical changes of genetic or nongenetic origins (or both) should be considered; there may not be a single mechanism of resistance in some tumors. A fifth and very important point is that resistant tumor-cell populations of genetic origin may be expected to vary biochemically in features other than those responsible for resistance and selection. Other random changes may also be present, and these may account for otherwise unexplained patterns of cross-resistance, collateral sensitivity, and intermediary metabolism. These secondary alterations can introduce considerable confusion and uncertainty into experimental studies.

The study of mechanisms of resistance and insensitivity may be approached from two related but distinct directions, that of the metabolism of the drug and that of the mechanism of action of the drug. More progress usually is made in the former case, as more is known about drug metabolism than about mechanisms of action, and the methods for studying drug metabolism often are less difficult.

Studies of drug metabolism should account for all drug metabolites, and the ability to do so will depend first upon the limits of detection of the methods used; to what extent can quantitatively minor metabolites be detected? It is clear that such minor metabolites (e.g. purine or pyrimidine analogs incorporated into nucleic acid) may be very important with respect to growth inhibition. In addition, the sophistication of the extraction and separation procedures are important.

Drug uptake studies and measurements of drug nucleotide formation from purine and pyrimidine analogs form a very common aspect of investigations of resistance mechanisms, and several common experimental problems deserve some comment. First, drug "uptake" should not be confused with drug "transport." The latter term refers to the actual passage of drug from one side of the cell membrane to another, and for technical reasons it sometimes is quite difficult to determine accurately. In contrast, uptake may be influenced not only by the true rate of transport, but also by intracellular drug metabolism, by binding to intracellular constituents, and by binding to the outside of the cell, if this occurs. Thus the interpretation of the results of uptake measurements in sensitive and resistant cells must be more qualified than is the case if only rates of transport are determined.

Comparisons of drug nucleotide formation in sensitive and resistant cells may be made in several different ways, which have different degrees of validity. One approach is to assay the activity of the enzyme in question according to conventional techniques. This may establish that the enzyme activity is substantially lowered, but the data obtained are limited (a) because the assay conditions are not exactly those under which the enzyme operates inside the cell and (b) because the enzyme usually is in excess within the cell, and the degree of decrease in assayable activity may not be the same as the degree of decrease of functional activity within the cell. It certainly should not be assumed that drug resistance in itself means that the enzyme concerned is completely lacking.

A second approach is to measure the extent to which the metabolism of the naturally occurring purine or pyrimidine substrate differs in sensitive and resistant cells. This has the advantage that the data are from experiments using intact cells. However, it cannot simply be assumed that the decrease in rate of metabolism of the antimetabolite in the mutant cells is exactly the same as that of the natural substrate. In most cases some residual enzyme activity is present, and this activity may have a different substrate specificity than the enzyme in the parental cells; even if this is not the case, the Michaelis constants of natural substrate and antimetabolite are likely to be different.

In the final analysis it is best always to measure the rate of metabolism of the drug itself in the sensitive and resistant cell lines, at concentrations that are growth inhibitory.

As mentioned above, it is more difficult to study mechanisms of resistance that involve the mechanism of action of the drug rather than its metabolism. First, the mechanisms of action of many antitumor drugs are not known with certainty. In addition, whether or not the mechanism of action is known, it is always necessary to distinguish between this mechanism and other biochemical effects that may not be directly related to growth inhibition, and not to confuse these two types of effects in comparing sensitive and resistant cells. Finally, studies of resistance mechanisms related to the mechanism of action of the drug will always depend both upon the detail in which the particular area of cellular metabolism is understood and upon the sophistication of the methods with which the resistance mechanism is studied.

D. Chemotherapy of Resistant Tumors

Though it has been relatively simple to isolate lines of tumor cells that are resistant to one or another antitumor drug, and though there has been considerable progress in the elucidation of the mechanisms of resistance and insensitivity, there has been much less success in the very basic and practical problem of the therapy – especially chemotherapy – of resistant tumors.

The chemotherapy of resistant tumors may either take into account knowledge of the origins and mechanisms involved in particular cases, or may proceed in ignorance of this information; only the former case will be considered here. Similarly, a major distinction may be made between resistance or insensitivity of genetic and nongenetic origin. In the latter case, insensitivity associated with pharmacological sanctuary is being approached through the use of more lipid-soluble drugs that can penetrate the blood-brain barrier. Insensitivity due to large tumor mass is being approached through drug treatment regimens that maximize log cell kill, while insensitivity associated with growth characteristics is being approached through drugs that kill nongrowing cells, through drugs that affect hypoxic cells, through drugs that synchronize cells with respect to the cell cycle, etc. These situations will not be considered further.

I. Cross-Resistance

Tumors that are resistant or insensitive to one drug often are found to be resistant to others as well. Frequently cross-resistance extends only to structurally related drugs, but this in fact depends on the actual mechanism of resistance in a particular case. Thus as already mentioned, resistance to a wide variety of structurally complex (though dissimilar) drugs is associated with altered plasma membrane-cell surface composition and decreased drug uptake. In the case of most other mechanisms, however, the range of drugs affected by the phenomenon of cross-resistance is much narrower.

In addition to cross-resistance that can be understood in terms of the basis of origins and mechanisms of resistance, there are also examples of cross-resistance that occur unexpectedly. This situation apparently arises from the existence of secondary and nonspecific biochemical changes that have arisen in the tumor-cell population but which have not been directly involved in the selection of the original resistant population. For example, a tumor that was resistant to 5-azacytidine because of decreased uridine kinase activity also had lowered deoxycytidine kinase activity and hence was also resistant to substrates of this enzyme.

Another tumor was selected for low hypoxanthine-guanine phosphoribosyltransferase activity, but also had increased nucleotidase activity and altered glutamine amidophosphoribosyltransferase. Other examples of unexpected cross-resistance could be given.

II. Collateral Sensitivity

This term refers to an increased sensitivity to one drug that is or may be a direct consequence of the biochemical changes that led to resistance to another drug. In the early days of the study of resistance, there was considerable optimism that mechanisms of resistance could be used against the tumor through this phenomenon of collateral sensitivity. This has not been very successful, however, and it has not been possible to make reliable predictions regarding collateral sensitivity. Certainly resistant tumors have often been found to have an increased sensitivity to one or several other drugs; however, the biochemical bases of such observations have seldom been elucidated or related to the original mechanism of resistance.

One successful approach to the question of collateral sensitivity may be mentioned. In this case advantage was taken of the observation that many tumors that are resistant to cytidine and deoxycytidine analogs have elevated activities of cytidine deaminase. The relatively inactive compound bromodeoxycytidine was therefore prepared with the idea that its deamination by this enzyme would lead to the formation of the much more potent antimetabolite, bromodeoxyuridine.

III. Circumvention of Resistance

The first approach that should be taken to the therapeutic circumvention of resistance or insensitivity is simply to increase the dose of the original drug. The efficacy of this approach will of course be limited by host toxicity and by the degree of resistance manifested, but it could be of value in situations of low degrees of resistance; this probably is the case in many, if not most, cases of clinical resistance. This approach might also be effective if insensitivity were due to altered drug metabolism by the host, leading to lowered drug concentrations in the tumor.

Two other approaches are related to specific mechanisms of resistance. Thus when resistance or insensitivity is associated with high rates of deamination of purine or pyrimidine analogs, inhibitors of adenosine deaminase (such as deoxycoformycin), guanine deaminase (e.g. aminoimidazole carboxamide), or cytidine deaminase (e.g. tetrahydrouridine) have been used in combination with the appropriate cytotoxic antimetabolites. A second example concerns resistance or insensitivity due to alternative pathways, especially alternative pathways of purine or pyrimidine nucleotide synthesis. Thus there have been numerous efforts to inhibit various "salvage" pathways of nucleotide formation, though unfortunately these have so far not been very successful.

Few other attempts to circumvent resistance or insensitivity based on knowledge of the mechanisms responsible appear to have been made and these have not been very effective. The only resort in most cases, therefore, is simply to initiate therapy using drugs whose metabolism, mechanism of action, or both are different from those originally used. At the present time, therefore, the chemotherapy of resistant tumors remains an empirical matter.

Acknowledgment. The preparation of this review was supported by the National Cancer Institute of Canada.

Section II:
Modification of Host-Tumor Interaction

CHAPTER 3

Drug Disposition and Pharmacology

J. G. McVie

A. Introduction

The relevance of drug disposition to resistance studies is not at first sight obvious.

In most drug resistance studies, particularly those carried out in vitro as described elsewhere in this book, the broad assumptions are made that the free active drug or drugs can be delivered to the target site, be it tumour-cell membrane, nuclear DNA or nucleotides, that duration of exposure can then be regulated and that the drug or drugs can eventually be cleared from the target site by metabolism or excretion. The application of such in vitro studies to the human situation is impossible without consideration of bioavailability. It is unlikely that pharmacology studies in patients will add to the understanding of natural resistance to cytostatic drugs.

Rather, knowledge of drug disposition is essential when applying in vitro studies to the in vivo reality. It is now possible to test the sensitivity of a patient's tumour to a variety of drugs in an assortment of culture systems. When the in vitro experiment is paralleled by a therapeutic trial, the results may agree, or may show striking disparity. Drug-sensitive tumours are common in Petri dishes, not so in patients. The gulf between the systems is partly bridged by the understanding of drug handling by an individual patient, which can explain such discrepancies, or through lack of absorption of drug, too rapid clearance or dose-limiting toxicity.

For instance, it has been reported that several drugs are inactive in perfusion experiments in limbs, where the drug infused was known to require activation by liver enzymes. Resistance of cells due to inadequate drug delivery through to the classical sanctuary sites of testis, ovary and brain is not to be confused with concepts of naturally resistant clones of cells which will remain resistant, regardless of their exposure to drug. One of the few persuasive advantages of the tumour-colony-forming assay, as applied to hundreds of patients' tumours by von Hoff et al. (1981), is the splendid correlation with resistance. In other words, negative results in vitro go with negative results in patients.

If this assay could be improved so that meaningful pharmacological variables were brought to bear on the method – bearing in mind the limitation that the target-cloning cells are only a few percent of the original tumour mass – variables such as drug dose, drug exposure, the degree of metabolism and the possibility of rescue could be more satisfactorily correlated with resistance and with the overcoming of such resistance in vitro.

The equivalent studies in vivo have only recently been begun due to lack of sensitive drug assays, and so in the past the clinican has had little control over those variables in any given patient (Ehrlichman et al. 1980). Considering the application of drug characteristics to the study of acquired resistance, one of the reasons which makes drug characteristics important is the experimental evidence (Schabel 1976) that tumour cells can acquire resistance extremely quickly, particularly if they are exposed to non-toxic doses of a cytostatic drug.

Drug disposition studies therefore become relevant assuming that better schedule design would alleviate this problem. Ideal design would ensure the delivery of an appropriate toxic dose of drug or its active metabolites to the tumour cell as fast as possible, thus minimizing the chance of sublethal damage to the tumour cell and emergence of resistant clones. The problem of all resistance studies in tumours in man is the narrow therapeutic ratio of the group of cytostatic drugs, due to the obscurity of definition of the real target for drug action. Discussion of the role of pharmacodynamics is on the whole theoretical until more precise characterization of target receptors can be carried out; thus discussion of selectivity of antitumour effect is highly relative and indeed almost meaningless.

With the exception of the overquoted example of asparaginase, which was designed to exploit a relative inability of certain tumour cells to survive asparagine depletion, and perhaps the application of oestrogen or antioestrogen therapy to oestrogen-receptor-positive tumour cells, this area of research is depressingly bleak.

To ask the drug disposition expert for new solutions, with this paucity of knowledge of targets, is unrealistic. Indeed in a recent review (Mihich 1980) it was clearly pointed out that the application of knowledge of pharmacological parameters as sole determinants of selectivity was not reasonable.

It is possible, however, to narrow the odds against the tumour by a variety of manipulations of drug delivery and, with the use of first- and second-order targeting and better regulation of metabolism and excretion, at least safer cytostatic chemotherapy can be given without compromising antitumour effect or risking the emergence of resistance. The advantage and indeed perhaps one of the most important applications of the knowledge of drug handling by patients has proved to be the lessening of drug toxicity, which secondarily has improved the therapeutic ratio.

Dedrick et al. (1975) considered aspects of methotrexate kinetics such as blood flow, membrane transport, protein and cell binding, enzyme binding and enzyme synthesis, using data which are in plentiful supply for methotrexate. Also available from the literature on methotrexate is the cytotoxic concentration required, the optimal exposure time of a variety of cell lines to methotrexate and also at least three ways of inactivating or detoxifying methotrexate after it has had its effect (viz. folinic acid, thymidine, carboxypeptidase). Dedrick went on to build what he called a theoretical model framework for prediction of resistance to the drug. Such a model may in future be available to predict the optimal characteristics of a drug, which will ensure maximal antitumour effect with minimum antihost effect. The scheme is yet to be proven and its reproduction with respect to other antitumour drugs is not yet possible due to the lack of knowledge of those drug parameters. Hopefully, with the accelerated application of high-pressure liquid chromatography with or without mass spectrometry to determine the real concentrations of active drugs and active and inactive metabolites in plasma, in tissues and target tumour cells, this data bank will soon be built up.

It must be re-emphasized that schedules of administration, dosage, timing and duration for the large majority of cytostatic drugs given singly or in combination have been empirically based on clinical experiences with barely an occasional nod to the existence of a plethora of cell kinctic data and the rapid emergence of new pharmacological data.

With this background of the limited clinical application of pharmacological principles to the study of resistance, be it natural or acquired, this chapter will review the existing evidence concerning changes in the mode of absorption, delivery, distribution or clearance of a drug that may be advantageous. It is possible that by alterations of dosage, scheduling, awareness of drug interactions and their exploitation the possibility of acquired resistance could be minimized.

B. Drug Absorption

A drug may be delivered by a variety of routes: into the gut per os or per rectum, directly into the blood via a vein or artery, into a body cavity such as the pleura, pericardium or the peritoneum or directly into the target site, such as a skin tumour nodule, a bladder papilloma or a small bronchial tumour.

Drugs must pass through a minimum of one cell membrane before entry into the body and this can occur by active transport, filtration or diffusion, facilitated or along a concentration gradient.

Since cell membrane function is at least partially dependent on a lipid layer, lipid solubility of a given drug as well as any concentration gradient which exists become major determinants in drug access.

That there are wide interindividual differences in these characteristics is immediately obvious from any absorption study reported in the literature. Even with the seemingly simple oral administration of one tablet of melfalan, hexamethylmelamine, methotrexate or cyclophosphamide, up to 100-fold differences in absorption have been reported (TATTERSALL et al. 1978; D'INCALCI et al. 1978; STUART et al. 1979a; JUMA et al. 1979).

These variations reflect not only variations of cell membrane transport of the particular cytostatic agent from the gut, but also other problems related to gastric and jejuno-ileal motility, which can in turn be affected not only by presence of tumour or metastases but also by concomitant therapy with narcotics (NIMMO et al. 1975) or by previous surgery to the gastrointestinal tract.

Administration of methotrexate by mouth has been studied in a Latin square dose study over the ranges 25, 50, 75, and 100 mg given in a bicarbonate-based syrup to minimize alterations of gastric emptying. In only one of four patients was there a linear increase in absorption over the four doses.

In one patient the area under the time concentration curve (AUC) after 25 mg was only 10% less than the dose after 100 mg (MCVIE et al. 1981).

A cohort of six patients was studied after a single dose of 100 mg and, 2 weeks later, the same dose, divided into four 25-mg portions each separated by 4 h. The resulting area (AUC) for the divided-dose schedule was two to three times greater than after the individual dose (Steele et al. 1979a). This was thought to be due to the probability that methotrexate absorption occurs by the same mechanism as folic acid absorption, which is either flooded by the high-dose methotrexate or else is impeded by the direct cytostatic actions of the drug.

Bioavailability studies comparing oral absorption to that obtained after intravenous injection are on the whole consistent. They show a superiority for the intravenous route of administration.

The best bioavailability ratio for methotrexate was 50% (Stuart et al. 1979 a). An exception, however, was seen with cyclophosphamide; alkylating activity was 3.5 times higher after an oral dose, compared with an identical dose given intravenously. The half-lives of plasma alkylating activity were identical after both oral and intravenous administration.

Labelled 1,3-bis(2-chloroethyl)3-cyclohexyl-1-nitrosourea (BCNU) was cleared with a half-life of 34 h after oral administration compared with 67 h after intravenous injection. Both the BCNU and cyclophosphamide results may be due to a combination of hepatic metabolism and plasma protein binding; the contribution of enterohepatic circulation was not measured in either study (Juma et al. 1979; Oliverio 1976).

Plasma levels of 5-fluorouracil are usually lower after oral administration than after intravenous administration. In one recent study (Finch et al. 1979), the kinetics of the drug given intravenously were shown to be dose dependent. Doubling of the intravenous dose from 0.5 to 1 g produced a doubling in initial plasma drug concentration and an increase of 1.5 in the plasma half-life.

It has been suggested by Craft et al. (1977) that one possible reason for the development of resistance of childhood acute lymphocytic leukaemia to maintenance therapy might be the intrinsic malabsorption of oral maintenance therapy, particularly methotrexate, or else the development of secondary malabsorption due to the direct enterotoxic effect of cytostatics (Pinkerton et al. 1981). A pilot survey of peak plasma levels of methotrexate was conducted after a maintenance dose of oral methotrexate and there was a broad split into two groups, showing relatively good absorption in one group and relatively poor absorption in the other group (Craft 1981). A relationship appeared to exist between poor absorbers and poorer survival figures. The study group was too small to draw any statistically valid conclusions. One publication has suggested that methotrexate given in a twice-weekly schedule can alter absorption of xylose. It has subsequently been pointed out that xylose absorption is not a good marker for methotrexate absorption. Indeed there is now evidence supporting very rapid recovery of gastrointestinal epithelium from high-dose oral methotrexate. McVie et al. (1981) treated 12 patients with 250 mg methotrexate (50 mg every 2 h for 10 h), repeated 2-weekly for 16 weeks. Measurement of 72-h absorption curves of methotrexate were carried out on the first, third, fifth and seventh courses of oral methotrexate and the areas under the subsequent time concentration curves for each individual patient were not altered throughout the course of therapy. If malabsorption had been induced by high-dose oral methotrexate, it had clearly recovered within a 2-week period.

Also of note from this study is that six of the twelve patients – all with head and neck cancer – responded to this relatively simple medication, and this response rate compares favourably with evidence in the literature on intravenous methotrexate at doses ranging from 50 mg to 10 g. A common feature of these publications is the exceptionally fast appearances of "resistance" to methotrexate based on the median duration of remission in patients treated with methotrexate as a single agent, which, regardless of dose or schedule, is of the order of 3–5 months. It would appear therefore in this situation that optimization of dose or schedule does not prevent emergence of "resistance". After the first remission is complete, induction of a second is often extremely difficult, leading to a clinical implication of "acquired cross-resistance."

The majority of cytostatic drugs are given parenterally, usually intravenously. Methotrexate, cytarabine and bleomycin can be given intramuscularly or subcutaneously, and the kinetics certainly of methotrexate and bleomycin are similar, irrespective of intramuscular or intravenous administration (STUART et al. 1979 b). The use of the arterial approach for tumour targeting, in order to deliver the highest possible dose to a tumour site, has been explored empirically by many groups.

There is little doubt that intra-arterial methotrexate in treatment of head and neck tumours is as effective as intravenous treatment, but it is not more effective. After hepatic artery administration the pharmacokinetics of methotrexate are identical to patterns seen after intravenous administration (IGNOFFO et al. 1981), which in theory would negate further use of this less accessible route. The authors, however, correctly point out that although the pharmacokinetics may not be seen to differ, this does not rule out the pharmacodynamic advantage for the delivery of a high dose of methotrexate to the target organ.

Better methods of measuring the retention of active methotrexate, for instance with sequential gamma camera-scans of the labelled drug, will be needed to defend this idea and ideally a clinical trial comparing intra-arterial and intravenous methotrexate should be carried out.

GARNICK et al. (1979) have compared the hepatic extraction of doxorubicin given either into the hepatic artery or into a peripheral vein.

They showed a marked difference in the degree of systemic exposure to doxorubicin in the sense that plasma levels were consistently 25% lower after hepatic arterial doxorubicin, compared with the identical dose given through a peripheral vein.

This study had the advantage of measuring hepatic venous anthracycline levels during the experiment, including seven patients with primary metastatic liver cancer, and the hepatic venous levels of the drug were consistently higher after it had been given through the artery than through the arm vein.

They calculated therefore a clear increase in the therapeutic index of doxorubicin, implying that an identical dose of the drug could be given into the hepatic artery with 25% sparing of distant target organ toxicity. It is of note that they are one of the first groups to point out a direct correlation between plasma levels of doxorubicin reached and the subsequent development of bone marrow suppression.

LEE et al. (1980), however, carried out a similar experiment and showed no obvious differences in five patients who received doxorubicin, either through the hepatic artery or through the systemic circulation. When the concentrations of metabolites of doxorubicin, however, were measured, these were definitely higher after intra-arterial administration than after intravenous administration. This group also measured doxorubicin in samples of tissue and showed, after an intravenous bolus, high levels of doxorubicin in liver and tumour, compared with lymph node, muscle and bone marrow. The amount of doxorubicin in fat and skin tissue was relatively low.

In a review of the theoretical advantages of drug delivery by intra-arterial infusion, Chen and Gross (1980) concluded that out of a group of agents consisting of doxorubicin, bleomycin, 5-fluorouracil (5-FU), melfalan and methotrexate, only 5-FU gave an increase in response rate in the treatment of liver tumours when the drug was given intra-arterially, compared with intravenously. Their conclusion was that this route of administration should not be routinely used until further substantiated by controlled studies, preferably linked with pharmacokinetic and pharmacodynamic investigation.

That 5-FU intra-arterially may indeed overcome resistance was indicated by Buroker et al. (1976), who noted remissions in patients previously unresponsive to intravenous 5-FU.

The rather unusual use of arterial infusion to overcome established resistance to cytarabine is reported by Canellos et al. (1979). They reported the use of splenic artery infusion of cytarabine in five patients who had massive splenomegaly, associated with blast crisis of chronic granulocytic leukaemia. These patients were resistant to conventional intravenous cytostatic chemotherapy, including vincristine, prednisolone in all patients and cytarabine in three of the five. Cytarabine was administered in conventional doses ranging from 40 to 200 mg in 24 h daily, during 5–11 days. All five patients experienced reduction in spleen size, which was accompanied by benefit in terms of symptom relief in four of the five and by improvement of hypersplenism (thrombocytopenia) in one of the five patients. Transient leukopenia was the only side effect noted and that occurred in one patient out of the five. The lack of systemic side effects accompanied by the treatment may have been due to rapid deamination of cytarabine in the peripheral blood.

The clinical effect was, although dramatic, short lasting and no patient was submitted to splenectomy while the spleen remained small.

This study does demonstrate the possibility of realizing an antitumour effect in the face of clinical resistance by giving the usual dose of a drug directly to a target organ.

Ideally the delivery of high doses of a drug to an organ which does not metabolise the drug should then be accompanied by drainage of the effluent. This amounts in fact to perfusion, a technique which has long been described for the treatment of melanoma and sarcoma in peripheral limbs.

Today, there is no convincing clinical evidence from controlled trials or pharmacokinetic evidence from the uncontrolled trials that perfusion is indeed a better form of therapy than infusion.

One of the principal problems of limb perfusion remains the non-selective nature of the toxicity of the high doses applied, and indeed in one series two patients out of fifteen had their limbs amputated because of drug-induced toxicity to normal tissue, particularly muscle and skin (T. Wieberdink 1981, personal communication). In a rat model of limb perfusion with doxorubicin (C. BENCKHUISEN 1981, personal communication) rats developed sarcomas around 30 weeks after the perfusion experiment in a frequency from 30% to 80% according to dose and schedule.

It appears therefore that high-dose perfusion therapy may have a chronic toxicity in the form of carcinogenesis, as well as the local non-selective toxicity. Control of drug and tissue concentrations of perfused drugs by pharmacological monitoring should improve the therapeutic ratio of drugs given in this manner, and then the technique should be compared in randomized trials with conventional intravenous therapy.

Intracavitary administration of cytostatics has been performed in an attempt to provide high local concentrations of drugs and therefore maximum change of cell kill without emergence of resistance. In the management of superficial transitional cell carcinoma of the bladder, for instance, intracavitary thiotepa, methotrexate, actinomycin-D, 5-fluorouracil, podophyllotoxin, doxorubicin, cyclophosphamide and even BCG vaccine have at some time been tried.

Almost all of these drugs produce transient partial or complete remissions in either transitional-cell carcinoma or the premalignant phase of this tumour. There is little evidence that this technique is more effective than intravenous or oral therapy and there have been very few attempts made to measure the systemic exposure due to absorption from the bladder of these cytostatic agents (BANKS et al. 1977; NEEDLES et al. 1981).

Whereas all experimental chemotherapists are familiar with intraperitoneal administration in small rodents, not a great deal of comparative work has been done either in small rodents or in man to demonstrate pharmacodynamic or kinetic advantages over intravenous administration.

In small rodents it is of course considerably simpler to inject a drug intraperitoneally and it is a common fault to extrapolate such drug results to the human given the same substance intravenously.

OZOLS et al. (1979) have, however, shown that doxorubicin given intraperitoneally to mice with a transplantable ovarian cancer gives better results than the same dose given intravenously.

This may be explained partly by the direct examination of tumour cells in the ascitic fluid in the mice. Doxorubicin fluorescence was easily detected in tumour cells minutes after an intraperitoneal dose, but was never detected in tumour cells after an equivalent intravenous dose. The ascites fluid levels of doxorubicin and its metabolites reached a peak level 30 times higher after intraperitoneal administration than after intravenous administration, and over a 48-h period the exposure of the tumour cells to the drug and/or its metabolites was consistently one log higher after the local route of administration. The measurement of doxorubicin in the tumour cells, apart from by direct fluorescent examination, confirmed that the ascites fluid levels were reflected in the intracellular concentrations of the drug. In the same study, peak drug levels were examined in other distant organs such as liver, kidney and heart, and the peaks were three times higher after intravenous injection than after intraperitoneal injection in heart and kidney, and eight times higher after intravenous injection in liver.

After 24 h these differences had disappeared, so that concentrations of the drug and its metabolites remained the same, regardless of the route of administration. The equivalent but preliminary human studies with doxorubicin are reported by Roboz et al. (1981) and Ozols et al. (1980).

Experience with intraperitoneal administration and pharmacokinetic studies in patients treated with methotrexate and 5-FU have recently been presented (Jones et al. 1981; Speyer et al. 1979, 1981). Five patients were treated with intraperitoneal methotrexate to achieve steady-state levels of 7.5–50 μ*M* through a peritoneal dialysis apparatus. The methotrexate concentration was concurrently measured in peritoneum and plasma and was consistently 20–36 mol higher in peritoneal fluid than in plasma.

The plasma level of methotrexate was never over 3 μ*M*. In 29 treatment cycles myelosuppression was only noted in six and was moderate in all. No therapeutic benefit was achieved, nor in the subsequent study with 5-FU. Four patients were given 5-FU by the peritoneal route to maintain peak portal vein concentrations of 60 μ*M*. Drug exposures expressed as concentration against time during the first exposure to 5-FU were four times higher in the portal vein than in the peripheral vein, hepatic artery or hepatic vein. The calculated amount of fluorouracil extracted by the liver after absorption from peritoneum through the portal vein was around 67%. Although these studies demonstrated the feasibility of intraperitoneal chemotherapy using established dialysis techniques and although pharmacological advantages have been demonstrated in both studies, more information is required about the uptake of these antimetabolites into tumour both in peritoneum and in liver, the degree of subsequent metabolism in those tumour cells and the assurance that giving the drug at those concentrations and in this delivery system constitutes a reality for overcoming natural resistance or preventing acquired resistance. A caveat on the use of intracavitary drugs comes from a study by Trotter et al. (1981). They demonstrated that bleomycin was an effective treatment for recurrent ascites or pleural effusion in that over 70% of patients so treated had satisfactory symptomatic and measurable disappearance of fluid. Five patients, however, out of 47 so treated died shortly after administration of bleomycin and those patients portrayed an exceptionally high absorption into the peripheral circulation. For the majority of this group of patients absorption of bleomycin into the systemic circulation in this study agreed with the data of Alberts et al. (1978) in that around 40% of the dose given was absorbed. This calculation was initially carried out with the intention of predicting the contribution of intracavitary bleomycin to the total cumulative exposure of the lungs (as target organ for toxicity of bleomycin). The area under the time concentration curve for the patients who died in the Trotter study was more than twice as high as in the larger group who showed no toxicity after bleomycin. There was an intermediate group who suffered side effects of bleomycin in the form of severe shivering, sometimes rigors and high temperature, and their areas under the time concentration curves were halfway between the fatal group and the non-toxic group. The clinical features which separated the group of patients who died were on the whole advanced age and poor Karnofsky status. On the other hand this finding emphasizes the interindividual variability of drug handling by patients and the explanation, in this instance, of toxicity.

There was no obvious correlation between the pharmacokinetics of bleomycin in patients who were resistant to the therapy and those who responded.

C. Distribution

The pharmacologist uses distribution studies to answer two questions: how much drug reaches the tumour and how much drug reaches the host organs?

The relative balance between the answers to these two questions can also be a reflecton of the therapeutic ratio described above, and can have an important bearing on the dosage schedule chosen.

Ideally a drug should have affinity for the target only, but, as previously discussed, for cytostatic drugs this is not the case, and indeed there are some tumours (in sanctuary sites) which, because of physiological or anatomical barriers, remain completely out of contact with a circulating drug. A common problem of tumour access is the large fungating solid tumour with an anoxic, partly necrotic relatively avascular centre. It is difficult to visualize adequate drug concentrations in such masses; nevertheless it is clinical experience that large masses of teratoma, for instance in the lung, will respond completely to combination chemotherapy such as cisplatin, vinblastine and bleomycin, whereas in the same patient smaller masses of para-aortic lymph nodes or liver metastases will remain partly or completely resistant to therapy. Not only is the site of tumour obviously important, but a further complication is the existence of fibrotic tissue either due to previous surgery or extensive X-irradiation.

Pelvic tumours, particularly carcinoma of the cervix, have been notoriously resistant to chemotherapy and this may be because most patients with these tumours are primarily treated by surgery or radiotherapy. The fact that it may not necessarily be due to primary resistance of cervical cancer to cytostatics has been shown in a recent study of combination chemotherapy including cisplatin, vincristine, mitomycin and bleomycin in which a high complete remission rate was achieved, but all complete remissions were in patients who had metastatic disease rather than local residual tumor. Indeed in several patients who had local residual tumour and clearly measurable metastases such as in lung, soft tissue or liver, a complete remission was observed in metastases with no effect whatsoever on the size or viability of the pelvic tumour (VERMORKEN et al. 1981). A possible explanation for both these examples is the different intrinsic sensitivity of metastases in certain organs compared with their sister cells in other organs or in a primary tumour. That cells can be cloned from a primary tumour to metastasize to a particular given organ on command has been shown in an animal model (FIDLER and KRIPKE 1977). The extent of application of this model, however, to the human situation or to a wide variety of alternative animal tumours is awaited.

Of interest moreover is the study by DONELLI et al. (1976), where doxorubicin was shown to concentrate in hearts of mice previously injected with Lewis lung cancer to a greater degree than in hearts of control animals; this was thought to be due to an alteration of pulmonary circulation secondary to the lung metastases associated with the tumour.

On the other hand it was also noted in B16 melanoma in mice but not with a C3H mammary cancer or a rat Walker carcinosarcoma. The same group, Do-

Nelli et al. (1977), showed in the Lewis lung tumour that a peak level of doxorubicin was five times higher in lung metastases than in subcutaneously transplanted primary tumours.

A similar phenomenon was noted for daunorubicin and to a lesser extent for hydroxyurea and methylnitrosourea. Alkylating metabolites of cyclophosphamide were also noted to be higher in metastases than in primary tumour in this model, but methotrexate was present in equal concentrations in both.

Rats bearing the Brown Norway acute myeloid leukaemia were reported (Sonneveld and van Bekkum 1981) to have lower doxorubicin concentrations than normal only in organs infiltrated by leukaemia cells, thus indicating either model or tumour-type dependence if compared with the above work.

Chadwick and Rogers (1972) carried out a similar sort of experiment with radio-labelled 5-FU administered to mice bearing solid L1210 lymphocytic leukaemia. They measured fluorodeoxyuridine monophosphate (one of the active metabolites) of 5-FU and showed that it was considerably more concentrated in tumour compared with other tissues.

Chadwick and Chang (1976) used the same tumour model and measured 5-fluorodeoxyuridine (FUDR) and the parent 5-FU and showed once again that a higher concentration of both drug and metabolite were to be found in the tumour compared with normal tissues such as the small intestine. Cytarabine, another antimetabolite which requires phosphorylation for its antitumour activity, has been studied in L1210 leukaemia in mice.

Although no differences between tumour cells and normal cells were seen with respect to araC, araC MP or araC DP, the levels of araC TP were consistently tenfold higher than in liver cells or in small intestine cells [araC MP, DP and TP are the mono-, di- and triphosphate respectively of cytarabine (Chou et al. 1971)].

Examples abound of the increased and selective uptake of cytostatic drugs into sensitive cell lines compared with resistant cell lines. For instance, L-phenyl alanine mustard (L-PAM), doxorubicin and daunorubicin are all measurable in higher concentrations in sensitive cell lines than in resistant cell lines (Hill and Montgomery 1980). Whether these or the above in vivo data reflect pharmacological differences or pharmacodynamic differences or merely differences in cell kinetics or even biochemistry between the different types of cells is not completely clear. It is known for instance that different tumour cells have widely varying resting nucleotide pool sizes (Leyva et al. 1982).

With extensive pharmacological information in animals and limited plasma and occasional tissue levels of drugs in man, pharmacokinetic predictive models can be constructed which indeed may have more than a hypothetical chance of assisting in drug planning. Chan et al. (1978) developed a ten-compartment pharmacokinetic model, derived from rabbit tissue distribution data for doxorubicin. They then predicted reasonably accurately from plasma doxorubicin concentrations in 23 patients the appropriate tissue uptake confirmed at biopsy in nine of them. They also correctly predicted the change in profile of doxorubicin decay caused by pre-existing abnormalities in liver function leading to impaired metabolism and excretion of the drug. A similar model for methotrexate was mentioned in the introduction (Dedrick et al. 1975). A practical application of this latter has been the work of Cano, who used a computerized model to predict from a single

50-mg intravenous dose of methotrexate in a given patient the maximum dose of the drug in that patient with or without folinic acid rescue.

In over 30 patients studied, toxicity was averted by the application of the predicted dose schedule (MONJANEL et al. 1979). This seems an interesting direction for further pursuit in the future.

The problem of sanctuary sites of tumour cells is strictly speaking not relevant to a discussion of resistance, although it is conceivable that leukaemia cells, for instance nestling in the testis, ovary or central nervous system of the patient, become resistant to a drug due to exposure to small suboptimal concentrations of that drug and, at a later date, metastasize into the systemic circulation and lead to drug-resistant relapse.

An attempt to overcome the obstacle provided by one of these sanctuary sites, the brain, has been the use of higher and higher doses of drugs such as methotrexate.

In theory, if the dose of methotrexate is high enough in the peripheral blood, cytotoxic concentrations will be achieved in the cerebrospinal fluid.

Whether those concentrations can also be achieved in the parenchyma of the brain is quite another matter, however, and indeed there are now disappointing clinical results, for instance in the adjuvant use of high doses of methotrexate in place of prophylactic brain radiation in the treatment of patients with small-cell lung cancer who are in complete systemic remission (SCHEIN 1981, personal communication).

Rescue of bone marrow and mucous membrane toxicity by subsequent delivery of folinic acid or carboxypeptidase (the latter does not cross the blood-brain barrier) seems an attractive way of delivering methotrexate selectively to the brain. Another approach, however, has been through attempts to disrupt the blood-brain barrier osmotically, just before administration of methotrexate.

OHNO et al. (1979) showed in the rat that intracarotid arterial infusion of a 1.6 *M* solution of the sugar arabinose led to an increase of methotrexate permeation to the brain by a factor of 7. A study in dogs by NEUWELT et al. (1979) employed hypertonic mannitol instead of arabinose. This drug was delivered through the carotid artery 5–15 min before intra-arterial injection of methotrexate. Methotrexate brain levels were increased from 90–216 ng/g tissue before mannitol to a range of 350–2200 ng/g tissue, 3–6 h after mannitol. Assuming that the therapeutic tissue concentration of methotrexate is in the region of 300 ng/g tissue, this method would appear to be relevant, as a therapeutic tissue concentration of methotrexate is in the region of 300 ng/g tissue; this method would appear to be relevant as a therapeutic study. It is of interest that this group showed no correlation whatever between cerebrospinal fluid levels of methotrexate and brain levels. The same group (NEUWELT et al. 1981) then reported their clinical experience in six patients treated a total of 33 times with methotrexate after blood-brain barrier disruption in the same manner. All these patients had metastatic or primary brain tumours and were followed by computerized tomography (CT) scans, enhanced by contrast. Plasma methotrexate levels did not correlate with the degree of barrier disruption nor did the concentration of methotrexate in the CSF.

Barrier disruption seemed to be achieved in all patients as indicated by a persistence of contrast agent, seen on CT scan, both in and around the brain tumour.

Complications of the procedure of disruption by mannitol were seen in two patients who experienced brief epileptiform fits, but no systemic toxicity was reported. This remains an experimental model and might be further expanded to include other drugs. It is indeed the minority of drugs which reach the brain without such blood-brain barrier interference. They include the *Vinca* alkaloids, the nitrosoureas, procarbazine and the lipophilic analogues of methotrexate and fluorouracil, 2,4-diamino-5-(3′,4′-dichlorophenyl)-6-methylpyrimidine (DDMP) and ftorofur respectively.

In addition to lipophilicity disadvantages, most cytotoxic drugs are only limitedly available to the CNS due to their degree of ionization, protein binding or their molecular weight (MELLETT 1977). In contrast to the plethora of information concerning access of drugs to the central nervous system, very little is known of their access to the other sanctuary sites such as ovary and testis, and to previously radiated tumours. In a small study on two patients suffering from malignant peritoneal mesothelioma and one patient suffering from mesothelioma affecting both peritoneum and pleura, doxorubicin in a dose of 25 mg/m^2 was given intravenously and followed by analysis of plasma and intracavitary concentrations of the drug and its metabolites (ROBOZ et al. 1981). Of considerable interest was the complete absence of detectable doxorubicin in the pleural space in one patient and in the peritoneum in two out of the three patients. The detection limit for the assay was reported as 0.018 μM.

Mesothelioma is a notoriously resistant tumour and the only responses reported in the literature have been to doxorubicin.

D. Metabolism

The plasma decay of a drug is described by pharmacokineticists in series of half-lives ($t_{1/2}$). The $t_{1/2}$ is an index of the elimination process, but as it depends on the volume of distribution of the drug as well as elimination due to clearance, it is more useful when discussing the disappearance of a drug from the blood to discuss clearance specifically rather than $t_{1/2}$ indexes.

The clearance of a drug can be achieved by metabolism and/or excretion. Most metabolism of cytostatic drugs is carried out in the liver, although there is evidence that tumours can metabolize drugs and recently a study of 5-FU pharmacology indicated extrahepatic metabolism of the drug probably in muscle (SPEYER et al. 1981). The "intrinsic clearance" describes activity of enzymes in the liver which metabolize cytostatic drugs either to more active compounds as in the case notably with cyclophosphamide, etoposide, mitomycin, carminomycin and procarbazine or to inactive alcohols or conjugates (review: MENARD et al. 1980). The total "hepatic clearance" of the drug depends not only on the intrinsic clearance by liver microsomal and other enzymes, but also on the concentration of free drug in the liver which in turn is dependent on the blood flow rate and the degree of drug binding to protein and cells in the blood.

Where a drug is totally removed from the blood by hepatic clearance, then the "systemic clearance" equals the hepatic clearance. Usually there is also extrahepatic metabolism or excretion through other routes than the bile, for instance tears, saliva, exhaled air or urine (STEELE et al. 1979 b; LANKELMA et al. 1981).

The action of a drug is often related to the amount of free drug available, and its excretion is dependent on the degree of binding to proteins of, for example, methotrexate and cisplatin and to cells (*Vinca* alkaloids bind avidly to platelets).

Further calculations from the pharmacokinetic profiles of a drug therefore must take free drug concentrations as most relevant. In cancer patients there are a host of variables which may alter drug handling such as the presence of the tumour itself.

SOTANIEMI et al. (1977) showed quite clearly in a patient with primary liver tumours or metastatic deposits in the liver that metabolism of a compound antipyrine (a model for cytochrome P-450 liver enzymes) was seriously disrupted and delayed when compared with patients with no liver cancer.

Similarly extensions of the plasma half-lives of antipyrine or phenylbutazone have been noted with increasing age and it need not be reiterated that cancer is a disease predominantly of elderly people (ANONYMOUS 1975). Alterations in the same model compound antipyrine have been seen in normal volunteers fed on varying diets (ALVAREZ et al. 1976). The mean plasma half-life for antipyrine was 9.2 h when these volunteers ate a low carbohydrate: high protein diet, compared with 17.5 h in the same people fed on a high carbohydrate: low protein diet.

A further in vitro study of 18 assorted drugs was carried out using serum from kwashiorkor patients, who had extremely low albumin levels (BUCHANAN 1977); no alterations in protein binding were noted. One of the few experiments in vivo carried out with a cytostatic drug was reported by KAPELANSKI et al. (1981). This group showed in male Sprague-Dawley rats, maintained on protein free diets and then given an injection of doxorubicin, significantly lower serum concentrations measured at several times up to 48 h, when compared with a group of identical animals treated with a normal diet.

These lower serum concentrations were reflected in lower liver, lung and heart concentrations, but higher kidney concentrations than in the normal group. The latter corresponded with an increase in urinary excretion of doxorubicin in the protein-free diet animals. The relevance of these animal findings to the commonly cachectic cancer patient has yet to be explored adequately, but remains a possible explanation for the non-optimal handling of cytotoxic drugs in such patients.

Interestingly, depletion of any of the amino acids, glutamic acid, aspartic acid, arginine, citrulline or ornithine, has a profound reversing effect on the cytotoxic effect of vinblastine in cell culture (JOHNSON et al. 1960).

Studies of hepatic extraction of cytostatic drugs are also few. The 5-FU intraperitoneal study has been alluded to above (SPEYER et al. 1981), and in this study the calculated hepatic extraction of 5-FU after intraperitoneal administration was 67% with a range from 23%–89%. ENSMINGER and FREI (1978) reported a dose-dependent extraction of thymidine, viz. $<99\%$ at a dose of 8 g/m^2 per day and $>54\%$ at 32 g/m^2 per day. A comparative figure for the extraction of doxorubicin by the liver is provided by the study of GARNICK et al. (1979), using a calculation of the hepatic arterial doxorubicin level minus the hepatic venous level, divided by the hepatic level, and their ratio was between 0.45 and 0.5 according to the dose of doxorubicin chosen. It has commonly been advised that patients with abnormal liver function tests should receive a 50% dosage of doxorubicin (BENJAMIN et al. 1974). What precisely, however, is implied by "abnormal liver function" is not stated in this or in a variety of other commentaries on the subject. What is clear is that even with a lower dose of doxorubicin the therapeutic effect may be retained in the presence of abnormal liver function tests (Brenner et al. 1980), such as in patients with elevated bromsulphthalein excretion times. Predictability of how an individual patient will metabolize doxorubicin or for that matter any other drug, cytotoxic or not, appears to be impossible without actually administering the drug to the individual patient.

Nebert (1981) has recently reviewed the existing evidence which suggests that drug-metabolizing capacity is a genetically determined phenomenon. Thus a patient may be a fast metabolizer of drug A and a slow metabolizer of drug B, regardless of the fact that both drugs, A and B, may be 4-hydroxylated or o-dealkylated or n-deoxidated. It would appear therefore that the cancer physician is in a dilemma. On one hand he wishes to give the highest possible dose immediately, so as to limit the likelihood of secondary resistance, but, on the other hand, in the face of abnormal liver function he is not able to predict, without giving a safe small dose of the drug, what sort of toxicity pattern he is likely to provoke. Clinical experience has shown that full doses of anthracyclines can be tolerated in the face of abnormal liver function tests, especially when these abnormalities are due to presence of tumour in the liver and that response of this tumour is accompanied by normalization of the liver function.

The same problem is theoretically present, but in reverse, when considering another group of drugs, typified by cyclophosphamide; it is an inactive compound until metabolized to a series of metabolites, of which the most important, with respect to antitumour effect, are probably 4-hydroxy-cyclophosphamide, aldophosphamide and phosphoramide mustard.

The interesting discovery that urothelial toxicity accompanying cyclophosphamide administration is due to another metabolite, namely acrolein, which has no antitumour effect, has led to the specific antagonism of the toxic metabolite by administration of mesnum, while the cytotoxic metabolites remain intact and effective.

It is not difficult to visualize an imbalance of metabolism by a given genetically determined microsomal system in a patient, which would appear to the clinician as primary resistance of the drug in the face of toxicity.

There are several drugs which have been shown to accelerate cyclophosphamide metabolism; notably Sladek (1972) showed that phenobarbitone increased metabolism to both toxic and inactive metabolites of the drug. There is no evidence that coadministration of hepatic enzyme inducers increases the therapeutic index of cyclophosphamide, or for that matter any of the other drugs mentioned earlier which require hepatic metabolism for their antitumour activity (Bagley et al. 1973).

Cyclophosphamide is itself capable of inducing several liver enzyme systems and of interest in this regard is a recent study in children (Sladek et al. 1980), which showed that daily administration of cyclophosphamide in a dose of 50 mg/kg per day by mouth led to significant sequential reduction in the plasma half-life of cyclophosphamide and the urinary excretion of cyclophosphamide. This suggests that the drug has induced its own metabolism. Whether that metabolism is accelerated towards phosphoramide mustard, acrolein or both has not yet been determined in patients receiving daily cyclophosphamide, though it is likely to be to both, as the last steps in the metabolism of cyclophosphamide are probably chemical and not enzyme mediated. A further example of the importance of hepatic metabolism for activation of a cytostatic drug is carminomycin, an anthracycline analogue. This drug is metabolized to carminomycinol within minutes, and in a study of nine patients the plasma levels of the metabolite were higher than those of the parent drug within 10–30 min of an intravenous administration of the drug (LANKELMA et al. 1982).

Carminomycinol was detectable up to 7 days in the plasma of patients, whereas carminomycin was rarely seen in plasma after 24 h. This may be significant in that carminomycinol would appear in several in vitro systems to be more cytotoxic than its parent. Of further interest in this study was the finding of two distinct patterns of hepatic clearance of carminomycin. Three patients cleared the drug very quickly and the other six patients cleared it slowly. The relative degree of metabolism was equal in all patients. The areas under the time concentration curves for carminomycin and carminomycinol in the fast-clearing group were 30% of those found in this slower group. When these patients were closely studied for toxicity, according to the World Health Organization toxicity gradings, there was also a threefold difference in total toxicity – the fast clearance group had very little toxicity compared with the slower clearance group, who suffered considerable myelosuppression and gastrointestinal toxicity. All these patients had received an identical dose of the drug and were matched for tumour type, extent of tumour and pre-existing liver function. It appears therefore that pharmacokinctic parameters can give insight into pharmacogenetic differences in a group of patients. Until now these differences have not been shown to correlate with primary or secondary resistance to an antitumour drug but have been shown to correlate with production of toxicity.

E. Renal Excretion

In order to extrapolate from the in vitro drug sensitivity test to a patient, it would be ideal to add a drug to a patient's tumour in culture at a given dose for a given time and then to remove it. This removal or excretion process in vivo can be extremely complicated and is not always predictable.

The kidney is a major excretory organ which secretes or filters drugs in different proportions dependent on each individual drug. Interference with renal clearance of a drug will lead to its accumulation and probable increase of cytotoxic or toxic effects or both. There are countless examples of increased toxicity due to drugs such as methotrexate or cisplatin given to patients who had inadequate renal function.

Although creatinine clearance gives a reasonably good prediction for the safety or otherwise of bleomycin and cisplatin administration at conventional doses, the same cannot be said for methotrexate. Several authors including STOLLER et al. (1976) and STUART et al. (1979a) have shown that the serum creatinine or the creatinine clearance gives no indication of the renal excretion of methotrexate. Monitoring of the plasma methotrexate level is important, particularly when high doses of this drug have been given, in order to predict patients who excrete the drug slowly and who must be given higher and more prolonged rescue schedules. The elimination of methotrexate after an injection of a bolus of the drug is dose dependent (Lawrence et al. 1980). Renal clearance of the drug was markedly lower after a dose of 100 mg (18 ± 6 ml/min) than after 25 mg (53 ± 19 ml/min) in the same patient.

It is possible that the proximal tubular transport system for methotrexate can be saturated by higher doses of the drug; thus the drug inhibits its own elimination.

Cisplatin is a nephrotoxic drug, which essentially causes a progressive fall of creatinine clearance and leads to a slowing of subsequent clearance of cisplatin. Excretion in the urine is schedule dependent (Gullo et al. 1980), less drug being excreted in the urine when cisplatin is administered over a 20-h infusion than in a 1-h infusion. A variety of techniques have been used to alleviate or ameliorate cisplatin nephrotoxicity as this inhibits the use of the drug in higher, more effective doses.

Hydration is mandatory when the drug is given in doses higher than 20 mg/m^2, and different schedules have employed mannitol or frusemide diuresis in addition to hydration. Neither frusemide nor mannitol seems to alter the toxicity of the drug or the pharmacokinetics (Ostrow et al. 1981). It is possible to give cisplatin to an anuric patient if haemofiltration is used at the same time, and indeed a patient has been reported who went on to have a partial tumour response after two treatment courses in this manner (Gouyette et al. 1981). Renal excretion in the kidney, however, is largely irrelevant to the concept of drug resistance except in the contribution it makes to the toxicity side of the therapeutic ratio; thus in a patient with non-optimal clearance of a drug added toxicity due to persistence of the drug may cancel out any cytostatic effect which has been achieved.

F. Dose

Much of the foregoing discussion has revolved round the thesis that an increase in effective dose of the active anticancer compound at the target in the cancer cell will either minimize some forms of primary resistance or will stop the evolution of secondary resistance.

The dose of the drug which reaches the target cell is of course dependent on the dose given to the patient, and the dose-limiting factor in cancer chemotherapy is usually toxicity.

A recent review of dose and dose response in cancer chemotherapy (Frei and Canellos 1980) summarizes the literature by pointing out that the dose response curve is extremely steep and mostly linear for highly sensitive tumours such as leukaemia in children, non-Hodgkin lymphoma, Hodgkin's disease, testicular teratoma, breast cancer and small-cell lung cancer.

The same cannot be said for tumours which remain primarily resistant to conventional chemotherapy, and sadly these tumours, such as cancer of the colon, non-small-cell cancer of the lung and melanoma, constitute the majority in clinical practice.

Dose-response evaluation has been attempted clinically for individual drugs such as doxorubicin (O'Bryan et al. 1977), but this is difficult to extract from the literature because of the varieties of dosage schedules employed.

The importance of schedule in the attainment of effect both positive and negative has been mentioned in the foregoing text and will be further expanded in the next section. Maintenance of complete remission according to FREI and CANELLOS may not now be required in several tumour types, viz. acute lymphocytic and myeloid leukaemias, teratoma, choriocarcinoma or Burkitt's lymphoma; nor do they consider further prolonged schedules in adjuvant breast cancer necessary.

There is a relative lack of evidence from the clinical literature that increase in the dose of drug overcomes refractory tumour. High-dose cytarabine, though, produced four remissions in eleven patients who had previously been refractory to conventional doses of cytarabine (RUDNICK et al. 1979) and this small paper is supported by another showing six complete remissions in acute leukaemia achieved with megadose cytarabine (3 g/m^2 twice daily for 6 days) out of eleven patients considered resistant to conventional doses of the drug (100 mg/m^2 per day for 5–10 days) (WILLEMZE et al. 1981).

The main problem about increasing the dose of a drug such as cytarabine is that the pattern of toxicity is generally altered. The predominant toxicity of cytarabine in very high doses is gastrointestinal and unexpected respiratory failure. Aplasia of the bone marrow is of course achieved but recovery is not a great deal delayed when compared with conventional therapy. Similar problems have been shown by several authors reporting high-dose single-agent chemotherapy with autologous bone marrow rescue.

TAKVORIAN et al. (1980) used high-dose BCNU to treat gliomas of the brain resistant to conventional therapy and, whereas bone marrow toxicity was rescued by the infusion of bone marrow, fatal toxicity due to liver failure and/or respiratory failure became the new dose-limiting criteria. A possible explanation for this is the alteration in pharmacokinetics accompanied by increases in dose of a variety of cytostatic drugs (review: POWIS et al. 1981).

DISTEFANO et al. (1980) also rescued patients from myelotoxicity by autologous marrow reinfusion after high doses of mitomycin, and renal and pulmonary complications were again reported. Of interest, however, were six objective responses in breast cancer patients resistant to conventional doses of mitomycin. Reference has been made earlier in this chapter to the non-linearity of oral absorption of a drug on a dose basis and the non-linearity of its elimination by the kidney, which is clearly saturable by higher doses (MCVIE et al. 1981; LAWRENCE et al. 1980).

The incidence of primary resistance to methotrexate is very high, and increasing the dose after resistance has developed, for instance in head and neck cancer, has rarely been shown to lead to a second response. As is amplified elsewhere in this book, with particular respect to methotrexate, there are many other known mechanisms of methotrexate resistance which would explain the lack of effect by a simple adjustment of dose.

The drug is therefore useful in combination chemotherapy because much of the toxicity is preventable by rescue techniques and because dose reduction of the other component drugs in the combination is not required. This is a continuous practical problem when trying to optimize the dose of drugs in a combination scheme.

On one hand there is evidence for a dose-response effect of certain drugs; on the other hand there is also evidence that these drugs are better used in combination than singly and sequentially, and combinations at the maximal dose of each component drug are rarely possible.

The synergistic and antagonistic interactions which are involved in such combinations have to a large extent been ignored in clinical practice, most clinicians believing that cancer can be likened to tuberculosis and that on this ground resistance is minimized by giving more than one or, preferably, more than two compounds at one particular time. Also not fully appreciated or fully evaluated in the use of combinations of drugs is the actual total dose delivered over a course of therapy, expressed as a percentage of the ideal dose.

Rossi et al. (1981) have retrospectively studied their ability in this respect, to deliver cyclophosphamide, methotrexate and 5-fluorouracil (CMF) in an adjuvant programme for breast cancer, and have found striking improvement in the disease-free and total survival in patients who were able to take the optimal dose of the combination CMF.

Patients in whom the dosage of the combination was less than 65% of the calculated total showed the same survival rates as the patients in the other arm of the randomized study who received no drugs at all. Although this is a retrospective analysis it supports the evidence obtained from the treatment of advanced disease which would indicate that higher doses of combinations are better than lower doses.

G. Schedule Dependence

Discussion of the dose of a drug is incomplete without reference to the timing of its administration. A drug can be given in a bolus or by infusion and can be given on a repeated schedule hourly, weekly or monthly. Response of murine tumours to cytostatic drugs both singly and in combination is schedule dependent (Schabel 1976; Schabel et al. 1978, 1979). The number of clinical trials which have proved an advantage for one schedule over another is extremely limited. Schedules in the clinic have been chosen to fit the clinic work rotas, for patient convenience or according to trial and error. An obvious and now classic experiment of Selawry et al. (1965) showed that methotrexate given twice a week was more effective and safer than when the drug was given daily. Credit for this result can be given to the cell kineticist or the pharmacokineticist or both, according to one's bias.

The leading proponent of the first school was probably Skipper, who very elegantly pointed out that for the treatment of experimental leukaemia models high-dose intermittent therapy was optimal (Skipper 1971). It is only recently, however, that in some areas, such as treatment of ovarian cancer with alkylating agents, such theory has been proved in practice; thus daily single-dose alkylating agent such as cyclophosphamide or melphelan, while leading to good partial and occasional complete remissions in ovarian cancer, accompanied by minimal toxicity is probably inferior to combination chemotherapy employing drugs in high dose intermittently (Young et al. 1978). Regimes combining cyclophosphamide, cisplatin, hexamethylmelamine and doxorubicin have now repeatedly been shown to produce high complete remission rates, although accompanied by toxicity, which for the complete responders led to meaningful prolongation of survival (VOGL et al. 1981).

Alterations in clinical schedule or in the mode of administration of a drug may lead to differences in toxicity but rarely lead to improved response. An exception to the rule is etoposide (VP 16213), which in a daily or alternate-day schedule gives better therapeutic results in animal tumours (M. D'INCALCI 1981, personal communication) and also in the treatment of small-cell lung cancer in man (CAVALLI et al. 1978).

A comparison of continuous infusion of 5-FU with bolus injection for treatment of colon cancer demonstrated well the superiority of the infusion because of the absence of myelotoxicity, accompanied by maintenance of the same sort of numbers of responses as were obtained in the bolus group (SEIFERT et al. 1975).

ANSFIELD et al. (1977) on the other hand using the same drug in the same tumour compared four different schedules and observed an improvement in response rate and duration of response following the introduction of an intravenous loading course of the drug. Overall survival was not, however, lengthened, nor was there any sign of difference between the four treatment schedules applied to breast cancer patients.

Other drugs sometimes given by infusion rather than intravenous bolus are bleomycin, 5′-azacytidine and cytarabine, on the grounds that the therapeutic index of all three can be improved by the infusion, at least when the experiment is carried out in the mouse system. In man azacytidine is probably best given by infusion to lessen gastrointestinal toxicity, not evident in the mouse (VOGLER et al. 1976). SIKIC et al. (1978) showed an improvement of tumour inhibition in mice, all bearing Lewis lung carcinoma, when bleomycin was infused subcutaneously, continuously, compared with animals given the identical total dose divided in either a twice daily or in a twice weekly schedule. This group measured pulmonary toxicity due to bleomycin by measurement of the hydroxyproline levels in the lung and reported a high incidence of increased lung hydroxyproline concentration in the intermittent group. The net result was an increase in therapeutic index due to a higher tumour effect and a lower pulmonary toxicity.

The equivalent clinical experiment has yet to be carried out, although some authors report that the administration of bleomycin by infusion leads to less pulmonary interstitial fibrosis than expected after intravenous bolus (KRAKOFF et al. 1977; PENG et al. 1980) while others claim that response rates may also be improved by the manoeuvre (BLUM et al. 1973; CARTER and TORTI 1980; CORTES et al. 1980).

In the absence of controlled trials it can, however, be said that bleomycin used singly or alone in continuous infusion still produces remissions and the incidence of pulmonary fibrosis may be lessened.

A similar controversy surrounds doxorubicin. Whereas there is no claim that resistance can be overcome or antitumour effect improved by giving doxorubicin in a divided dose schedule or by infusion, several authors believe that the drug can be more effectively given in these ways because of a lesser incidence of cumulative cardiotoxicity.

Weiss and Manthel (1977) first reported that doxorubicin in combination schedules given weekly could be possibly less cardiotoxic than the conventional three-weekly schedule and Benjamin et al. (1981) claim the same protection from cardiotoxicity when the drug is given by prolonged infusion. The theory behind these experiments is that the high uptake of doxorubicin by cardiac tissue may be lessened if the high bolus dose of the drug leading to peak plasma concentration was cut down. Till now there is no evidence of lack of efficacy of the drug when given in lower doses more frequently or by infusion, but a detrimental effect might by predicted as decreased cell membrane transport of doxorubicin may be a source of resistance to the drug. A high bolus dose may be optimal in preventing resistance or overcoming resistance in the cancer cell. Once more controlled trials are called for.

Lastly on the topic of infusion, it has been shown that cytarabine by infusion certainly retains as good an antitumour effect as when it is given in an intravenous bolus (Bottino et al. 1979), although there would appear to be no superiority in terms of prevention of toxicity by giving the drug in this fashion. If infusions prove better than bolus injection several implantable infusion systems are now under trial which should add to their efficiency and patient acceptability.

Another approach to controlled delivery of cytarabine has been the use of liposomes made of a variety of phospholipids as carrier vesicles.

Liposomes have two possible advantages over the use of a drug by direct injection. Firstly the liposomes act as a reservoir in vivo and bring about slow release of the entrapped drug at a fairly constant rate. Secondly, liposomes of a particular size and charge may be pinocytosed more readily by tumour cells than by normal cells (review Gregoriadis 1976). In practice, however, there is considerable dispute over the second claim and the problems of regulating the manufacture and sterilization of stable liposomes containing a regulated amount of drug are only now being solved.

Liposomes tend to distribute mostly in the reticuloendothelial system, and a tumour localization study, for instance using technetium radio-labelled liposomes, has shown disappointing tumour uptake (Richardson et al. 1979).

Nevertheless, in animal models an advantage of entrapment of cytarabine within liposomes has been shown by Mayhew et al. (1978) and the same has been shown for actinomycin D by Papahajopoulos et al. (1976) and Rahman et al. (1975), and for 1-β-D arabinofuranosylcytosine 5′-triphosphate by Mayhew et al. 1976; combined with local hyperthermia, selective delivery of methotrexate has been claimed when encapsulated inside liposomes (Weinstein et al. 1979; Magin et al. 1979).

A distinctly different use of liposome-encapsulated doxorubicin has been reported by Rahman et al. (1979), who showed that whereas liposomes did not enhance the uptake of doxorubicin by tumour cells, positively charged liposomes selectively decreased the uptake of the drug in cardiac muscle, compared with the same dose of drug given either alone or in negatively charged liposomes in a mouse model.

Other larger vesicles such as microspheres from 40 to 100 μM in diameter, usually made of starch or ethyl cellulose, have been used as carriers for 5-FU (Ar-

FORS et al. 1979), mitomycin (KATO et al. 1980) and carmustine (ENSMINGER et al. 1980).

KATO et al. (1981) reported responses in a variety of pelvic tumours to mitomycin wrapped up in ethyl cellulose microcapsules and then delivered through a percutaneous arterial catheter.

Several of these patients had previously been shown to be resistant to conventional chemotherapy and responded to the combination of mitomycin and chemoembolization, which is temporarily produced by the use of large microspheres of the order 250 μM. Smaller microspheres (40 μM) containing carmustine were injected through the hepatic artery in three patients (ENSMINGER et al. 1980). Systemic carmustine levels were 70%–90% lower (as expressed by the area under the time concentration curve) when the carmustine was so given than when the same dose was given to the same patients by an intravenous bolus. Two of the three patients responded to this selective regional chemotherapy, although it is not clear if these patients had previously been resistant to intravenous carmustine.

In conclusion, just as there is as yet little conclusive evidence that tumour resistance can be overcome by direct intra-arterial delivery of chemotherapy by bolus or infusion, there is also need for controlled studies of the same drugs given by the same route with or without the use of carriers such as microspheres or liposomes.

There are theoretical advantages both for regional administration of chemotherapy, provided the tumour is known only to flourish in that region, and for the controlled exposure to high doses of cytostatic drug, which can then be removed by normal excretion, metabolism or dialysis. The question of binding to carriers need not be restricted to the use of small spheres. ZAHARKO et al. (1979) have reviewed the theoretical advantages of a host of low-molecular-weight carriers, macromolecules such as albumin, fibrinogen and globulin, dextrans and antibodies. The last is of renewed interest since the revival of the concept of tumour-specific antibodies made possible by the new technology associated with the production of monoclonal antibodies directed against tumour antigens.

This would appear to offer the ultimate in tumour targeting as monoclonal antibodies need not be cytotoxic intrinsically; all they need to do is carry the cytostatic compound linked directly or via a liposome or microsphere selectively to the tumour leading to high concentrations of the drug at the desired site of action. The teething problems surrounding the use of monoclonal antibodies in humans include the disappearance of tumour antigens, the multiplicity of different antigens on single tumour cells, the formation of antigen-antibody complexes in plasma and the subsequent hepatorenal and reticuloendothelial blockade, subsequent to complex formation. In theory, however, the use of monoclonal antibodies remains an attractive idea for increasing localization of drugs and, as a consequence, the minimization of resistance.

H. Drug Interactions

An essay on the application of pharmacokinetics to any topic must focus at some time on the problems of interaction between the drugs under study.

As has been the case in the history of pharmacokinetic studies there are considerably more examples of theoretical drug interactions or else interactions which are only reproducible in vitro than there are practical problems which come to the attention of the clinician. An obvious interaction, which all oncologists know and many use to advantage, is the exacerbation of the effect of 6-mercaptopurine by the coadministration of allopurinol. It is probable that due to the effect of allopurinol on xanthine oxidase, which blocks the degradation of 6-mercaptopurine, an increase in therapeutic ratio of the drug of 1.5 can be gained by reducing the dose of 6-mercaptopurine and adding allopurinol, a relatively non-toxic substance. Other examples are more empirical. It is obviously not optimal practice to use together two drugs which have identical toxicity on the same target organ, for instance the use of cisplatin and methotrexate together, where both drugs are cleared predominantly by the kidney. A mention has been made above of the fact that phenobarbitone accelerates metabolism of cyclophosphamide and doxorubicin. This may be of more or less clinical consequence. Thymidine has been combined with 5-FU in order to produce a biochemical modulation. If thymidine is given just before 5-FU the half-life of the latter is increased 12-fold (Woodcock et al. 1978).

The use of amphotericin B, an antifungal agent, has remarkably been shown by Presant et al. (1977, 1980) to reverse resistance to doxorubicin-containing chemotherapy regimes. Thus seven patients, all of whom were resistant to a particular chemotherapy regime, were treated with an identical regime with the addition of amphotericin B in the hope that its interference with cholesterol binding in the plasma membrane of tumour cells might lead to increased uptake of one or other of the cytostatic drugs.

A complete remission in acute myelomonocytic leukaemia and partial remissions in a patient with cancer of the breast and a patient with myeloma were then observed.

Four patients out of the seven suffered in addition, however, increased myelosuppression while being treated with amphotericin in combination with the cytostatic drugs. There are therefore a handful of clinical examples of the relevance of drug interaction studies. Few of them show any benefit; the majority point to theoretical antagonistic interaction with respect to additive toxicity.

Mihich and Grindey (1977) have recently expounded the theoretical basis of intentional modulation of pyrimidine or purine metabolism prior to or at the same time as administration of an antimetabolite. Thus, *N*-phosphonacetyl-L-aspartate (PALA) or pyrazofurin treatment may lead to enhanced efficiency of uptake and phosphorylation of cytarabine or 5-FU. Also of interest is the possible differential rate of recovery between tumour and normal cells after blockade of nucleotide synthesis, which theoretically would also lead to more specificity of subsequent antimetabolite effect. Methotrexate might also be used to advantage by such an interaction, though most of that work remains to be proven.

Bender et al. (1978) list 18 possible drug interactions involving methotrexate. Considerable caution must be exercised in interpretation and application of these examples. Some are of potential interest to the study of resistance, e.g. Divema, a copolymer, will increase the therapeutic index of methotrexate when given together, or better still when bound to the drug (Przybylsky et al. 1978), and poly-

L-lysine conjugation will render methotrexate-resistant mouse lymphosarcoma sensitive (RYSSER et al. 1979).

On the other hand, probenecid, which improves the pharmacokinetic profile of methotrexate by increasing delivery to brain and blocking renal transport (ISRAELI et al. 1978), also blocks tumour-cell uptake of methotrexate (GANGJI et al. 1979). It is important therefore on a theoretical and practical basis to explore possible drug interactions fully, not only to seek synergy but also to ensure that a detrimental result is not achieved.

J. Conclusion

The study of drug disposition fills the gap which exists between the experimental work on drug resistance and clinical experience. It goes some way to explaining some sorts of resistance. It can be exploited to yield better therapy and certainly safer therapy and can provide data complementary to those of the cell kineticist and experimental biologist, all of which are necessary for new understanding of drug resistance.

References

Alberts D, Chen HS, Liu R, Chen J, Mayersohn M, Perrier D, Moon T, Cross J, Broughton A, Salmon S (1978) Systemic absorption of bleomycin (bleo) after intracavitary (ic) administration. Proc AACR 18:77

Alvares AP, Anderson KE, Conney AH, Kappas A (1976) Interactions between nutritional factors and drug biotransformations in man. Proc Natl Acad Sci USA 73:2501–2504

Anonymous (1975) Drug metabolism and increasing age. Br Med J 1:581

Ansfield F, Klotz J, Nealon Th, Ramirez G, Minton J, Hill G, Wilson W, Davis H Jr, Cornell G (1977) A phase III study comparing the clinical utility of four regimens of 5-fluorouracil. Cancer 39.34–40

Arfors K, Aronsen K, Rothman U, Regelson W (1979) The use of amylase biodegradable starch microspheres as a tumor infarcting and delivery system for chemotherapy: intermittent hepatic arterial occlusion and the delivery of regionalized chemotherapy to hepatic metastases. Proc ASCO 20:370

Bagley CM Jr, Bostick FW, DeVita VT Jr (1973) Clinical pharmacology of cyclophosphamide. Cancer Res 33:226–233

Banks MD, Pontes JE, Izbicki RM, Pierce JM Jr (1977) Topical instillation of doxorubicin hydrochloride in the treatment of recurring superficial transitional cell carcinoma of the bladder. J Urol 118:757–760

Bender RA, Zwelling LA, Doroshow JH, Locker GY, Hande KR, Murinson DS, Cohen M, Myers CE and Chabner BA (1978) Antineoplastic drugs: clinical pharmacology and therapeutics. Drugs 16:46–87

Benjamin RS, Wiernik PH, Bachur NR (1974) Adriamycin chemotherapy – efficacy, safety, and pharmacologic basis of an intermittent single high-dosage schedule. Cancer 33:19–27

Benjamin RS, Legha S, Mackay B, Ewer M, Wallace S, Valdevieso M, Rasmussen S, Blumenschein G, Freireich E (1981) Reduction of adriamycin cardiac toxicity using a prolonged continuous intravenous infusion. Proc AACR 22:179

Blum RH, Carter SK, Agre K (1973) A clinical review of bleomycin – a new antineoplastic agent. Cancer 31:903–914

Bottino J, McCredie KB, Ho DWH, Freireich EJ, Buckles R, Herbst S, Lawson M (1979) Continuous intravenous arabinosyl cytosine infusion system. Cancer 43:2197–2201

Brenner D, Chang P, Bachur N, Wiernik P (1980) Adriamycin dosing: relationship to pretreatment liver function, pharmacokinetics and response in leukemia patients. Proc AACR 20:177

Buchanan W (1977) Drug-protein binding and protein energy malnutrition. S Afr Med J 52:733
Buroker T, Samson M, Correa J (1976) Hepatic artery infusion of 5 FUDR after prior systemic 5-fluorouracil. Cancer Treat Rep 60:1277–1279
Canellos GP, Sutcliffe SB, De Vita VT, Lister TA (1979) Treatment of refractory splenomegaly in myeloproliferative disease by splenic artery infusion. Blood 53:1014–1017
Carter SK, Torti FM (1980) Combination Chemotherapy of nonseminomatous testicular cancer. Cancer Chemother Pharmacol 4:71–77
Cavalli F, Sonntag RW, Jungi F, Senn HJ, Brunner KW (1978) VP16-213 monotherapy for remission induction of small cell lung cancer. Cancer Treat Rep 62:473
Chadwick M, Chang C (1976) Comparative physiologic disposition of 5-fluoro 2'deoxyuridine and 5-fluorouracil in mice bearing solid L1210 lymphocytic leukemia. Cancer Treat Rep 60:845–855
Chadwick M, Rogers WI (1972) The physiological disposition of 5-fluorouracil in mice bearing solid L1210 lymphocytic leukemia. Cancer Res 37:4297–4303
Chan KK, Cohen JL, Cross JF, Himmelstein KJ, Bateman JR, Tsu-Lee Y, Marlis AS (1978) Prediction of adriamycin disposition in cancer patients using physiologic pharmacokinetic model. Cancer Treat Rep 62:1161–1171
Chen HG, Cross JF (1980) Intra-arterial infusion of anti cancer drugs: theoretic aspects of drug delivery and review of responses. Cancer Treat Rep 64:31–40
Chou TC, Hutchison DJ, Schmid FA, Philips FS (1975) Metabolism and selective effects of 1-beta-D-arabinofuranosylcytosine in L1210 and host tissues in vivo. Cancer Res 35:225–236
Cortes EP, Kalra J, James R, Marchiony A, Walczak M (1980) Chemotherapy for head and neck cancer in relapse after prior radiotherapy and evaluation of method of bleomycin administration on anti tumour effect. Proc ASCO 21:364
Craft AW, Rawkin A, Aherne W (1981) Methotrexate absorption in children with acute lymphoblastic leukaemia. Cancer Treat Rep 65[Suppl 1]:77–81
Craft AW, Kay HEM, Lawson DN, McElwain TJ (1977) Methotrexate-induced malabsorption in children with acute lymphoblastic leukemia. Br Med J 2:1511–1512
Dedrick RL, Zaharko DS, Bander RA, Bleyer WA, Lutz RJ (1975) Pharmacokinetic considerations on resistance to anti cancer drugs. Cancer Chemother Rep 59:795–804
D'Incalci M, Bolis G, Mangioni C, Garattini S (1978) Variable oral absorption of hexamethylmelamine in man. Cancer Treat Rep 62:2177–2180
Distefano A, Spitzer G, Schell F, Blumenschein GR (1980) Phase I study of high dose mitomycin (MM) with autologous bone marrow transfusion (ABMT) in resistant breast adenocarcinoma. Proc ASCO 21:408
Donelli MG, Martini A, Colombo T, Bossi A, Garattini S (1976) Heart levels of adriamycin in normal and tumor-bearing mice. Eur J Cancer 12:913–923
Donelli MG, Colombo T, Brogini M, Garattini S (1977) Differential distribution of antitumour agents in primary and secondary tumour. Cancer Treat Rep 61:1319–1324
Ehrlichman C, Donehower RC, Chabner BA (1980) The practical benefits of pharmacokinetics in the use of antineoplastic agents. Cancer Chemother Pharmacol 4:139–145
Ensminger WD, Frei E III (1978) High dose intravenous and hepatic artery infusions of thymidine. Clin Pharmacol Ther 24:610–615
Ensminger WD, Dakhil S, Cho KG (1980) Improved regional selectivity of hepatic arterial bichlorethylnitrosurea plus degradable starch microspheres. Clin Res 28:742
Fidler IJ, Kripke ML (1977) Metastasis results from pre-existing variant cells within malignant tumour. Science 197:893–895
Finch RE, Bending MR, Lant AF (1979) Plasma levels of 5-fluorouracil after oral and intravenous use in cancer patients. Br J Clin Pharmacol 7:613–617
Frei E III, Canellos GP (1980) Dose: critical factor in cancer chemotherapy. Am J Med 69:585–594
Gangji D, Ross WE, Poplack DG, Levine AS, Kohn KW, Glaubiger D (1979) Effect of probenecid on methotrexate cytotoxicity. Proc AACR 20:244
Garnick MC, Ensminger WD, Israel M (1979) A clinical pharmacological evaluation of hepatic arterial infusin of adriamycin. Cancer Res 39:4105–4110

Gouyette A, Lemoine R, Adhemar JP, Kleinknecht D, Man WK, Droz JP, Macquet JP (1981) Kinetics of cisplatin in an anuric patient undergoing hemofiltration. Cancer Treat Rep 65:665–668

Gregoriadis G (1976) The carrier potential of liposomes in biology and medicine. N Eng J Med: 704–770

Gullo JJ, Litterst CL, Maguire PJ, Sikic BI, Hoth DF, Woolley PV (1980) Pharmacokinetics and protein binding of cis-dichlorodiammine platinum administered as a one hour or as a twenty hour infusion. Cancer Chemother Pharmacol 5:21–26

Hill DL, Montgomery JA (1980) Selective uptake and retention of anticancer agents by sensitive cells. Cancer Chemother Pharmacol 4:221–225

Ignoffo RJ, Oie S, Friedman MA (1981) Pharmacokinetics of methotrexate administered via the hepatic artery. Cancer Chemother Pharmacol 5:217–220

Israeli ZH, Soliman AM, Cunningham RF, Plowden JF, Keller JW (1978) The interaction of methotrexate and probenecid in man and dog. Proc AACR 19:194

Johnson IS, Armstrong JC, Gorman M (1960) The *Vinca* alkaloids: a new class of oncolytic agents. Cancer Res 32:2761–2764

Jones RB, Collings JM, Myers CE, Brooks AR, Hubbard SM, Balow JE, Brennan MF, Dedrick RL, De Vita VT (1981) High-volume intraperitoneal chemotherapy with methotrexate in patients with cancer. Cancer Res 41:55–59

Juma FD, Rogers HJ, Trounce JR (1979) Pharmacokinetics of cyclophosphamide and alkylating activity in man after intravenous and oral administration. Br J Clin Pharmacol 8:209–217

Kapelanski DP, Daly JM, Copeland EM, Dudrick SJ (1981) Doxorubicin pharmacokinetics – the effects of protein deprivation. J Surg Res 30:331–337

Kato T, Nemoto R, Mori H, Kumagai I (1980) Sustained release properties of microencapsulated mitomycin C with ethylcellulose infused into the renal artery of the dog. Cancer 46:14–21

Kato T, Nemoto R, Mori H, Takahashi M, Harada M (1981) Arterial chemoembolization with mitomycin C microcapsules in the treatment of primary or secondary carcinoma of the kidney, liver, bone and intrapelvic organs. Cancer 48:674–680

Krakoff IH, Vitkovic E, Currie V, Yeh S, Lamonte C (1977) Clinical pharmacological and therapeutic studies of bleomycin given by continuous infusion. Cancer 40:2027–2037

Lankelma J, Penders PGM, Leyva A, Kleeberg UR, Kenny JB, McVie JG, Pinedo HM (1981) Concentrations of *n*-(phosphonacetyl)-L-aspartate (PALA) in plasma and tears of man. Europ J Cancer Clin Oncol 17:1199–1204

Lankelma J, Penders PGM, McVie JG, Leyva A, ten Bokkel huinink WW, de Planque MM, Pinedo HM (1982) Plasma concentrations of carminomycin and carminomycinol in man, measured by HPLC. Eur J Cancer Clin Oncol

Lawrence JR, Steele WH, Stuart JFB, McNeill CA, McVie JG, Whiting B (1980) Dose dependent methotrexate elimination following bolus intravenous injection. Eur J Clin Pharmacol 17:371–374

Lee YTN, Chan KK, Harris PA, Cohen JL (1980) Distribution of adriamycin in cancer patients. Tissue uptakes, plasma concentration after IV and hepatic IA administration. Cancer 45:2231–2239

Leyva A, Appel H, Pinedo HM (to be published) Deoxynucleotide pool sizes in relation to thymidine sensitivity. Cancer Res

Magin RL, Weinstein JN, Yatvin MB, Blumenthal R (1979) Selective localization of liposomal encapsulated methotrexate in locally treated murine tumors. Proc AACR 19:250

Mayhew E, Papahadjopoulos D, Rustum YM, Dave C (1976) Inhibition of tumor cell growth in vitro and in vivo by 1-β-D arabinofuranosylcytosine entrapped within phospholipid vesicles. Cancer Res 36:4406–4411

Mayhew E, Papahadjopoulos D, Rustum YM, Dave C (1978) Use of liposomes for the enhancement of the cytotoxic effects of cytosine arabinoside. Ann NY Acad Sci 308:371–386

McVie JG, Stuart JFB, Calman KC, Steele WS (to be published) Pharmacology of high dose oral methotrexate. Cancer Treat Rep

Mellett LB (1977) Physiochemical considerations and pharmacokinetic nervous system. Cancer Treat Rep 61:527–531

Menard DB, Gisselbrecht C, Marty M, Reyes F, Dhumeaux D (1980) Antineoplastic agents and the liver. Gastroenterology 78:142–164

Mihich E (1980) Biochemical pharmacological determinants of drug action in cancer therapeutics. Oncology 37:28–33

Mihich E, Grindey GB (1977) Multiple basis of combination chemotherapy. Cancer 40:534–543

Monjanel S, Rigault JP, Cano JR, Carcassonne Y, Favre R, Baratier F (1979) High dose methotrexate: preliminary evaluation of a pharmacokinetic approach. Cancer Chemother Pharmacol 3:189–196

Nebert DW (1981) Possible clinical importance of genetic difference in drug metabolism. Br Med J 283:531–542

Needles B, Blumenreich M, Yagoda A, Sogani P, Whitmore WF (1981) Intravesical cisplatin for superficial bladder cancer. Proc AACR and ASCO 22:158

Neuwelt EY, Hill S, Rapoport S, Sheehan R, Maywood M, Frenkel EP, Kirkpatrick J, Clark WK (1979) Delivery of therapeutic levels of methotrexate to the brain after reversible disruption of the blood brain barrier. Proc AACR 19:99

Neuwelt EA, Diehl JT, Vu LH, Hill SA, Michael AJ, Frenkel EP (1981) Monitoring of methotrexate delivery in patients with malignant brain tumors after osmotic blood-brain barrier disruption. Ann Intern Med 94:449–454

Nimmo WS, Wilson J, Prescott LF (1975) Narcotic analgesics and delayed gastric emptying during labour. Lancet 1:890–891

O'Bryan RM, Baker LH, Gottlieb JE, Rivkin SE, Balcerzak SP, Grumet GN, Salmon SE, Moon TE, Hoogstraten B (1977) Dose response evaluation of adriamycin in human neoplasia. Cancer 39:1940–1948

Ohno K, Fredericks WR, Rapoport SI (1979) Osmotic opening of the blood-brain barrier to methotrexate in the rat. Surg Neurol 12:323–328

Oliverio VT (1976) Pharmacology of the nitrosoureas: an overview. Cancer Treat Rep 60:703–707

Ostrow S, Egorin MJ, Hahn D, Markus S, Aisner J, Chang P, Leroy A, Bachur NR, Wiernik PH (1981) High-dose cisplatin therapy using mannitol versus furosemide diuresis: comparative pharmacokinetics and toxicity. Cancer Treat Rep 65:73–78

Ozols RF, Locker GY, Doroshow JH, Grotzinger KR, Myers CE, Young RC (1979) Pharmacokinetics of adriamycin and tissue penetration in murine ovarian cancer. Cancer Res 39:3209–3214

Ozols RF, Young RC, Speyer JL, Weltz M, Collings JM, Dedrick RL, Myers CE (1980) Intraperitoneal adriamycin in ovarian carcinoma. Proc ASCO 20:425

Peng YM, Alberts DS, Chen HSA, Mason N, Moon TE (1980) Antitumour activity and plasma kinetics of bleomycin by continuous and intermittent administration. Br J Cancer 41:644–647

Pinkerton TR, Glasgow JFT, Bridges JM, Welshman SG (1981) Enterotoxic effect of methotrexate. Br Med J 1:1276–1277

Powis G, Ames MM, Kovach JS (1981) Dose-dependent pharmacokinetics and cancer chemotherapy. Cancer Chemother Pharmacol 6:1–9

Presant CA, Garrett S (1980) Drug resistance: reversal by amphotericin B (AmB). Proc AACR 20:138

Presant CA, Klahr C, Santala R (1977) Amphotericin B induction of sensitivity to adriamycin, 1,3-bis(2-chloroethyl)-1-nitrosourea (BCNU) plus cyclophosphamide in human neoplasia. Ann Intern Med 86:47–51

Przybylski M, Zaharko DS, Chirigos MA, Adamson RH, Schultz RM, Ringsdorf H (1978) Divema-methotrexate – immune adjuvant role of polymeric carriers linked to antitumor agents. Cancer Treat Rep 62:1837–1843

Rahman Y, Kisicleski WE, Buess EM, Cerny EA (1975) Liposomes containing 3H-actinomycin D. Differential tissue distribution by varying the mode of drug incorporation. Eur J Cancer 11:883–889

Rahman A, Kessler A, MacDonald J, Waravdekar O, Schein P (1979) Liposomal delivery of adriamycin. Proc AACR 19:228

Richardson OJ, Ryman BE, Jewkes RF, Jeyasingh K, Tattersall MNA, Newlands ES, Kaye SB (1979) Tissue distribution and tumour localization of 99m-technetium-labelled liposomes in cancer patients. Br J Cancer 40:35–43

Roboz J, Jacobs AJ, Holland JF, Deppe G, Cohen CJ (1981) Intraperitoneal infusion of doxorubicin in the treatment of gynecologic carcinoma. Med Pediatr Oncol 9:245–250

Rossi A, Bonadonna G, Valagussa P, Veronesi U (1981) Multimodal treatment in operable breast cancer: five-year results of the CMF programme. Br Med J 282:1427–1431

Rudnick SA, Cadman EC, Capizzi RL, Skeel RT, Bertino JR, McIntosh S (1979) High dose cytosine arabinoside (HDARAC) in refractory acute leukemia. Cancer 44:1189–1193

Rysser HJP, Pritchard D, Sen WC (1979) Methotrexatepoly(L-lysine) conjugates injected i.v. overcome drug resistance of sub-cutaneous P1798 lymphosarcoma in BALB/C mice. Proc AACR 20:203

Schabel FM Jr (1976) Nitrosoureas: a review of experimental antitumor activity. Cancer Treat Rep 60:665–698

Schabel FM Jr, Tradder MW, Laster WR Jr, Wheeler GP, Witt MHC (1978) Patterns of resistance and therapeutic synergism among alkylating agents. Antibiot Chemother 23:200–216

Schabel FM Jr, Tradder WM, Laster WR Jr, Corbett TH, Griswold DP Jr (1979) *cis*-Dichlorodiammineplatinum (II): combination chemotherapy and cross-resistance studies with tumors of mice. Cancer Treat Rep 63:1459–1473

Seifert P, Baker LH, Reed ML, Vaitkevicius VK (1975) Comparison of continuously infused 5-fluorouracil with bolus injection in treatment of patients with colorectal adenocarcinoma. Cancer 36:123–128

Selawry OS, Hananian J, Wolman IJ, Abir E, Chevalier L, Gourdeau R et al. (1965) New treatment schedule with improved survival in childhood leukemia and intermittent parenteral vs. daily oral administration of methotrexate for maintenance of induced remission. JAMA 194:75–81

Sikic BJ, Collings JM, Mimnaugh EG, Gram TE (1978) Improved therapeutic index of bleomycin when administered by continuous infusion in mice. Cancer Treat Rep 62: 2011–2017

Skipper HE (1971) Clowes memorial lecture. Cancer Res 31:1173–1180

Sladek NE (1972) Therapeutic efficacy of cyclophosphamide as a function of its metabolism. Cancer Res 32:535–542

Sladek NE, Priest J, Doeden D, Mirocha CJ, Pathre S, Krivit W (1980) Plasma half-life and urinary excretion of cyclophosphamide in children. Cancer Treat Rep 64:1061–1066

Sonneveld P, van Bekkum DW (1981) Different distribution of adriamycin in normal and leukaemic rats. Br J Cancer 43:464–470

Sotaniemi EA, Olavipelkonen R, Mokka RE, Auttunen R, Viljakainen E (1977) Impairment of drug metabolism in patients with liver cancer. Eur J Clin Invest 7:269–274

Speyer JL, Collings JM, Dedrick RL, Brennan MF, Londer H, De Vita VT Jr, Myers CE (1979) Phase I and pharmacological studies of intraperitoneal (I.P.) 5-fluorouracil (5-FU). Proc ASCO 19:352

Speyer JL, Sugarbaker PH, Collings JM, Dedrick RL, Klecker RW jr, Myers CE (1981) Portal levels and hepatic clearance of 5-fluorouracil after intraperitoneal administration in humans. Cancer Res 41:1916–1922

Steele WH, Stuart JFB, Lawrence JR, McNeill CA, Sneader WE, Whiting B, Calman KC, McVie JG (1979a) Enhancement of methotrexate absorption by subdivision of dose. Cancer Chemother Pharmacol 3:235–237

Steele WH, Stuart JFB, Whiting B, Lawrence JR, Calman KC, McVie JG, Baird GM (1979b) Serum, tear and salivary concentrations of methotrexate in man. Br J Clin Pharmacol 7:207–211

Stoller RG, Drake JC, Jacobs SA (1976) Monitoring high dose methotrexate, value of serum creatinine. Proc ASCO 17:255

Stuart JFB, Calman KC, Watters J, Paxton J, Whiting BW, Lawrence J, Steele WH, McVie JG (1979a) Bioavailability of methotrexate: implications for clinical use. Cancer Chemother Pharmacol 3:239–241

Stuart JFB, Aherne W, Prasad L, James S, Trotter JM, McVie JG (1979b) Pharmacokinetics of bleomycin following intramuscular, intravenous or intracavitary administration. Br J Cancer 40:316

Takvorian T, Parker LM, Hochberg FH, Zervas NP, Frei E, Canellos GP (1980) Single high doses of BCNU with autologous bone marrow: a phase I study. Proc ASCO 4:341

Tattersall MHN, Jarman M, Newlands ES, Holyhead L, Milstead RAV, Weinberg A (1978) Pharmacokinetics of melphalan following oral or intravenous administration in patients with malignant disease. Eur J Cancer 14:507–509

Trotter J, Calman KC, Stuart JFB, Aherne W, McVie JG (to be published) Pharmacology and clinical effect of intracavitary bleomycin. Cancer Chemother Pharmacol

Vermorken JB, van Oosterom AT, ten Bokkel Huinink WW, Mangioni C, Hoff AM, Rotmensz N (1981) Phase II study of vincristine, bleomycin mitomycin and cisplatin in disseminated squamous cell carcinoma of the uterine cervix. Proc of 3rd NCI-EORTC Symposium, EORTC, Brussels

Vogl S, Kaplan B, Pagano M (1981) CHAD (cyclophosphamide, hexamethylmelamine, adriamycin and diamminedichloroplatinum) is superior to melphalan in the therapy of bulky advanced ovarian cancer – Eastern Cooperative Oncology Group randomised trial. Proc UICC conference, Lausanne

Vogler WR, Miller DS, Keller JW (1976) 5 azacytidine: a new drug for the treatment of myeloblastic leukaemia. Blood 48:331–337

von Hoff DD, Casper J, Bradley E, Sanbach J, Jones D, Makuch R (1981) Association between tumor colony-forming assay results and response of an individual patient's tumor to chemotherapy. Am J Med 70:1027–1032

Weinstein JN, Magin RL, Yatvin MB, Zaharko DS (1979) Liposomes and local hyperthermia: selective delivery of methotrexate to treated tumors. Science 204:188–191

Weiss AJ, Manthel RW (1977) Experience with the use of adriamycin in combination with other anticancer agents using a weekly schedule, with particular reference to lack of cardiac toxicity. Cancer 40:2046–2052

Willemze R, Zwaan FE, Keuning JJ, Colpin G (1982) Treatment of refractory acute leukaemia with high dose cytosine arabinoside. Br J Haematol 51:497

Woodcock TM, Martin DS, Kemeny N, Young CW (1978) Phase I evaluation of thymidine plus fluorouracil in patients with advanced cancer. Proc AACR 18:351

Young RC, Chabner BA, Hubbard SP, Fisher RI, Bender RA, Anderson T, Simon RM, Canello GP, De Vita VT (1978) Advanced ovarian adenocarcinoma. N Engl J Med 299:1261–1266

Zaharko DS, Przybylski M, Oliverio VT (1979) Binding of anticancer drugs to carrier molecules. Methods Cancer Res 14:347–380

CHAPTER 4

Immunological Changes

H. Fuji

A. Introduction

Since the initial demonstrations that experimental tumors bear antigens different from those of the normal adult host (Prehn and Main 1957; Klein et al. 1960), evidence has accumulated for the occurrence of tumor-associated antigens (TAAs) in tumors of both animal and human origins. The observation that increased immunogenicity is associated with a mouse L1210 lymphoma subline resistant to a drug (Mihich 1969) stimulated much interest as to the basis of the observed phenomenon and the characteristics of the immunological changes occurring in such tumor sublines. Studies have also been directed toward determining the nature of host immune responses to the TAA in the tumor sublines and toward exploring the manner in which the growth of these tumors is affected by these responses.

This chapter summarizes the available information on the immunological changes associated with various drug-resistant tumor sublines of animals and the procedures used to determine the immunogenicity and antigenicity of tumors. In addition, some attention has been given to possible mechanisms for the occurrence of the increased immunogenicity of the resistant sublines. The phenomenon is still not completely understood, however, and the discussions in the literature are largely speculative.

B. Tumor-Associated Antigens

Tumor cells express several different types of TAAs (see Ting and Herberman 1976). The precise nature of most TAAs is unknown.

In carcinogen-induced tumors, the tumor-associated transplantation antigens (TATAs) are demonstrated by means of the transplantation method (Prehn and Main 1957; Klein et al. 1960). The unique feature of the TATA in carcinogen-induced tumors is its distinct specificity to individual tumors. Thus, TATA of one tumor does not usually cross-react with that of others (Prehn and Main 1957).

The TAAs of tumors induced by murine leukemia viruses (MuLVs) include those related to the virions which bud continuously from transformed cells and those related to non-virion products controlled by the viral genome. The virally induced tumors are cross-reactive due to the presence of these antigens on the surface of their cells (Klein and Klein 1964; Old et al. 1965; Ting and Herberman 1976).

Antibodies to TATAs that are unique to each chemically induced tumor have been extremely difficult to demonstrate. The fact that some non-virus-induced tumors, e.g., chemically or radiation-induced tumors, may also express MuLV-related antigens of exogenous or endogenous origins (GRANT et al. 1974; SATO et al. 1973; BROWN et al. 1978) complicates the determination of the nature of the TAA in these tumors. However, DELEO et al. (1977) characterized the TAA of a MuLV-negative chemically induced BALB/c sarcoma, Meth A, using syngeneic antisera and showed that the antigens are unique to Meth A. It is still not clear whether the serologically detected antigens in their study are identical to the TATA defined by the transplantation method.

Many tumors have been shown to express so-called oncofetal antigens which are present not only in tumors but also in embryo tissue or even at low levels in adult tissue of different species (TING and HERBERMAN 1976). Fetal antigens with the same specificity were shown to be present in tumors of different origins. The oncofetal antigens do not usually produce in vivo resistance to tumor growth and, if they do, it is often weaker than that induced by other TATAs.

Some studies have suggested that the TATA of chemically induced murine tumors represents derepressed or modified H-2 alloantigens (INVERNIZZI and PARMIANI 1975; GARRIDO et al. 1976; MARTIN et al. 1976). Recent chemical studies provided evidence that the alien H-2^k molecules present on a BALB/c (H-2^d) tumor are very similar to the normal H-2^k molecules (ROGERS et al. 1979). However, the expression of alien antigens on tumor cells seems to be rather rare. In several cases, the detection of the alien antigens was traced to the presence of C-type viral proteins or to the existence of unidentified public H-2 specificities (KLEIN 1975; FLAHERTY and RINCHIK 1978; PRAT et al. 1978). The immunogenetic drift of histocompatibility antigens during tumor passages may also be a reason for the observed histocompatibility disparity.

The relationship between the expression of the TAA and normal cell-surface antigens has been investigated in several mouse tumors. An inverse relationship between TAA and H-2 antigens has been described in some tumors (HAYWOOD and MCKHANN 1971; TING and HERBERMAN 1971; BOYSE and OLD 1969). Whether this relationship is a general phenomenon or not is unclear.

As recent studies have demonstrated, relationships between the H-2 histocompatibility complex and immune responses are multiple. The recognition of virally induced TAAs by cytotoxic lymphocytes is restricted by the H-2 complex in mouse model systems, indicating that H-2 products and TAAs may interact on the cell surface to form the actual antigen seen by the particular effector cell (DOHERTY et al. 1976). The H-2 complex influences cell to cell interactions (MITCHISON 1971), antigen presentation (ROSENTHAL and SHEVACH 1973; BENACERRAF and GERMAIN 1978), and induction of suppressor T cells (TADA et al. 1975). It has been proposed that the major histocompatibility complex is responsible for diversification of T-cell specificities (JERNE 1971; VON BOEHMER et al. 1978). All these functions of the major histocompatibility complex have potential relevance to host antitumor responses.

C. Altered Transplantability of Drug-Resistant Tumor Sublines

I. Tumor Transplantation in Unimmunized Animals

A possible change in the immunological characteristics of a drug-resistant tumor subline was first demonstrated in a study (MIHICH 1969) comparing the growth of DBA/2 lymphoma L1210 and a L1210 subline resistant to methylglyoxal-bis-guanylhydrazone (CH_3–G) in unimmunized DBA/2 mice that were under treatment with arabinosylcytosine (araC). The L1210 subline resistant to CH_3–G (L1210/CH_3–G) was developed by serial intraperitoneal transplantations of the parent L1210 cells in DBA/2 mice treated with CH_3–G (MIHICH 1967a).

As illustrated in Fig. 1, treatment with low doses of araC (5 mg/kg per day for 6 days) led to 50-day cures in a much higher percentage of DBA/2 mice inoculated with the L1210/CH_3–G cells than in those inoculated with the parent L1210 cells. This enhanced chemotherapeutic effects of araC in the animals bearing the resistant subline, i.e., "collateral sensitivity", was abolished in animals that had been X-irradiated with a total dose of 300 R 1 day prior to the i.p. inoculation of tumor cells, indicating that the radiosensitive defense mechanism of the host, most likely the host immune response, was responsible for the therapeutic difference noted in nonirradiated mice (MIHICH 1969).

Subsequently, BONMASSAR et al. (1970) demonstrated a change in transplantability of L1210 cells during the development of resistance to 5-(3,3-dimethyl-1-triazeno)imidazole-4-carboxamide (DTIC). After several serial transplantations in (BALB/c × DBA/2) F1 mice (CDF1), treated with DTIC, the L1210 subline re-

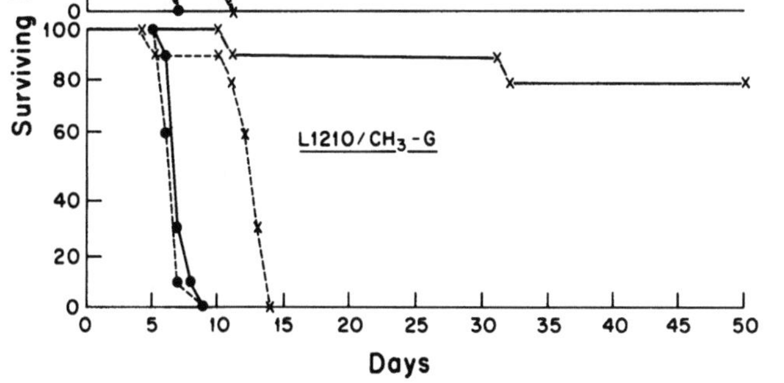

Fig. 1. Effects of araC against lymphoma L1210 and a variant resistant to L1210/CH_3–G. AraC was injected i.p. once a day for 6 days at the daily dose of 5 mg/kg, starting the day after the i.p. inoculation of 1×10^6 lymphoma cells. Total body radiation was administered the day before tumor implantation. (MIHICH 1969)

sistant to DTIC (L1210/DTIC) failed to grow in normal CDF1 mice even with an inoculum of 10^5 viable cells. In contrast, the L1210/DTIC did grow well in those CDF1 mice that had been immunosuppressed by the administration of cyclophosphamide or DTIC. It was also found that treatment with 1,3-bis(2-chloroethyl)-1-nitrosourea (BCNU) was more effective against the L1210/DTIC than against the L1210.

The results in these initial studies suggested that the drug-resistant L1210 sublines have acquired either a high immunogenicity or a high susceptibility to host immune effectors. It has since been established that both L1210/CH_3–G and L1210/DTIC have an increased immunogenicity in comparison to the parent L1210 as detailed in this and other sections (see Sects. C.II, D, E).

Table 1. Drug-resistant tumor sublines with altered transplantability

Drugs	Tumors	Host of tumor origin	References
CH_3-G	L1210	DBA/2	MIHICH (1969)
DTIC	L1210	DBA/2	BONMASSAR et al. (1970)
DDUG	L1210	DBA/2	MIHICH and KITANO (1971)
6-MP	L1210	DBA/2	NICOLIN et al. (1972)
Cytoxan	L1210	DBA/2	NICOLIN et al. (1972)
5-Fluorouracil	L1210	DBA/2	NICOLIN et al. (1972)
Methotrexate and derivatives	L1210	DBA/2	NICOLIN et al. (1972)
araC	L1210	DBA/2	NICOLIN et al. (1972)
Terephthanilide-2-chloro-4′,4″-di-2-imidazolin-2-yldihydrochloride	L1210	DBA/2	NICOLIN et al. (1972)
Isoquinaldehyde thiosemicarbazone	L1210	DBA/2	NICOLIN et al. (1972)
Imidazole-4(or 5)-carboxamide, 5(or 4)-(3-methyl-1-triazeno)	L1210	DBA/2	NICOLIN et al. (1972)
araC, cytoxan	L5178Y	DBA/2	SCHMID and HUTCHISON (1972)
6-MP	L1210	DBA/2	SCHMID and HUTCHISON (1972)
1-Phenyl-3,3-dimethyltriazene	L1210	DBA/2	SCHMID and HUTCHISON (1973)
1-Phenyl-3-monoethyltriazene	L1210	DBA/2	SCHMID and HUTCHISON (1973)
Nitrogen mustard	Yoshida sarcoma[a]	Donryu	TSUKAGOSHI and HASHIMOTO (1973)
Actinomycin D	EPO	C57BL/6	BELEHRADEK et al. (1974)
6-MP, methotrexate	L1210	DBA/2	CALMAN et al. (1974)
GZL	L1210	DBA/2	FUJI and MIHICH (1975)
DTIC	S-1033	C57BL/10	BONMASSAR ET AL. (1975)
DTIC	LSTRA	BALB/c	HOUCHENS et al. (1976)
DTIC	RBL5	C57BL/6	HOUCHENS et al. (1976)
DTIC	EL4	C57BL/6	NICOLIN et al. (1977)
DTIC	GL	C3H	NICOLIN et al. (1977)
DTIC	K36	AKR	BONMASSAR et al. (1979)

[a] A rat ascites sarcoma

The above findings were confirmed and extended later to tumor sublines resistant to a wide variety of chemotherapeutic agents, as listed in Table 1. The phenomenon was found in tumors of various host origin that included six different inbred strains carrying three different H-2 haplotypes, i.e., $H\text{-}2^b$, $H\text{-}2^d$, and $H\text{-}2^k$; in at least one case, it was demonstrated in a rat sarcoma (TSUKAGOSHI and HASHIMOTO 1973). With regard to the types of tumor inductions, those murine tumors that had been induced by chemicals (MIHICH 1969; BONMASSAR et al. 1970; SCHMID and HUTCHISON 1973; BELEHRADEK et al. 1974; NICOLIN et al. 1976a, 1977), by radiation (BONMASSAR et al. 1975), and by MuLVs (HOUCHENS et al. 1976; NICOLIN et al. 1977; SANTONI et al. 1978; BONMASSAR et al. 1979) were generally affected although some tumors such as EL4, GL, and K36 were shown to be less susceptible than other tumors to the DTIC treatment (NICOLIN et al. 1977; BONMASSAR et al. 1979). Among the various drugs listed in Table 1, DTIC appears to be the most effective drug in generating the immunogenicity change. However, in view of the fact that the immunological changes have been demonstrated for a considerable number of drugs and in a variety of tumor lines, it would seem reasonable to assume that such changes could occur generally during the development of resistance to chemotherapeutic agents.

Immunological changes develop with time following transplant generations during drug treatments (BONMASSAR et al. 1970; SCHMID and HUTCHISON 1973; TSUKAGOSHI and HASHIMOTO 1973; HOUCHENS et al. 1976). In most cases, the altered immunological characteristics of the drug-resistant sublines were very stable and were retained after many transplant generations in syngeneic or histocompatible F1 mice without administration of maintenance doses of drugs (BONMASSAR et al. 1970; MIHICH and KITANO 1971; SCHMID and HUTCHISON 1973; FUJI and MIHICH 1975; NICOLIN et al. 1976a, 1977), indicating that the changes are genetically determined. This, in turn, ruled out the possibility that the drug itself serves as a haptenic determinant by attaching to the cell surfaces and thereby enhancing the immunogenicity of the tumor cells (MITCHISON 1970; PRAGER and BAECHTEL 1973).

In some cases (SCHMID and HUTCHISON 1972, 1973; BELEHRADEK et al. 1974), a decrease in "oncogenic potential", i.e., the capacity for infiltrative cell growth, has been suggested in several tumor sublines resistant to different drugs since the inhibited growth of the resistant subline cells was observed even in immunosuppressed hosts of allogeneic as well as xenogeneic origins. However, when the cell growth rate was determined in vitro, no significant difference was found between the parent line and the resistant sublines (SILVESTRINI et al. 1977). Moreover, in immunosuppressed syngeneic animals, the growth of the resistant subline was comparable to that of the parental cells, as mentioned before. Therefore, it does not seem likely that reduced "oncogenic potential" is a major contributing factor in the reduced transplantability associated with these resistant subline cells.

II. Tumor Transplantation in Preimmunized Animals

Further evidence for an increased immunogenicity in drug-resistant sublines was obtained by the more direct approach of determining the ability of irradiated DTIC-resistant tumor subline cells to induce transplantation immunity in host animals (Nicolin et al. 1977). It was found that the immunization of (C57BL/6×DBA/2) F1 mice (BDF1) with a single i.p. injection of 4×10^7 irradiated cells of a DTIC-resistant subline of C57BL/6 lymphoma EL4 (EL4/DTIC) elicited a marked transplantation immunity in BDF1 mice against a challenge with EL4/DTIC cells, as evidenced by the survival of the host mice, but not against a challenge with the parent EL4 cells. Preimmunization with the same number of irradiated cells of the parent EL4 failed to elicit significant immunity against the challenge with either the EL4 or the EL4/DTIC, indicating a marked difference in immunogenicity between the parent EL4 and the EL4/DTIC. Similar results were obtained in the experiments conducted with DTIC-resistant sublines of DBA/2 lymphoma L5178Y and L1210 (Nicolin et al. 1976a, b).

A similar approach was employed in this laboratory (Fuji et al. 1979) in order to differentiate the immunogenicity of the parent L1210 and three L1210 sublines each resistant to different antileukemic agents, namely, L1210 sublines resistant to CH_3–G, 4,4′-diacetyldiphenylurea-bis-guanylhydrazone (DDUG) (Mihich 1967b), and guanazole (GZL) (Dave et al. 1978). It was found that a single i.p. injection of 3×10^7 irradiated cells of each resistant subline into syngeneic DBA/2 mice elicited transplantation immunity not only toward the immunizing but also toward the other two L1210 sublines, indicating the expression of common TATA(s) by these sublines. Under these conditions the parent L1210 cells were negative, either as immunizing cells or challenging cells. The demonstration of common TATA(s) on three L1210 sublines, each resistant to different drugs, indicates that immunological alterations of drug-resistant tumor sublines are not directly related to the development of resistance to a specific drug.

The increased immunogenicity of drug-resistant subline cells and the apparent lack of activity in the parent cells, as demonstrated by the transplantation method, may indicate a qualitative change in antigenic characteristics such as the acquisition of new transplantation antigens by the resistant sublines (Bonmassar et al. 1970; Nicolin et al. 1976a, 1977). Alternatively, the amount of antigen(s) present on the parent cells could have been below the level of detectability by the assay method employed. Although one injection of irradiated L1210 cells failed to induce significant transplantation immunity against the parent L1210, L1210/CH_3–G, L1210/DDUG, or L1210/GZL, multiple injections of irradiated parent cells induced a strong immunity that rejected the challenging L1210 as well as L1210 subline cells, indicating that the parental cells shared the TATA with the resistant sublines (Fuji et al. 1979). The relationship of the common TATA(s) detected by the primary immunization among the sublines and those detected by the hyperimmunization in the above experiments is not known.

In the case of Moloney leukemia virus-induced BALB/c lymphoma LSTRA, it was found that DTIC-resistant sublines of LSTRA (LSTRA/DTIC) retained a TATA(s) present on the parental cells. Experiments were designed to determine whether the host CDF1 mice rendered "tolerant" to the TATA of the parental LSTRA [by an injection of 5×10^7 irradiated LSTRA followed 24 h later by cyclophosphamide (250 mg/kg)] would still reject the LSTRA/DTIC by virtue of the possible presence of new antigens on the latter cells (Houchens et al. 1976). The CDF1 mice rendered "tolerant" to the parent LSTRA were capable of rejecting a challenge of viable LSTRA/DTIC cells (but not the LSTRA cells), as evidenced by the survival of the host mice, whereas those mice rendered "tolerant" to the LSTRA/DTIC showed a markedly reduced resistance to a challenge of either LSTRA/DTIC or LSTRA cells. It was concluded that LSTRA/DTIC express new antigen(s) that are not detectable on the parent cells as well as common antigen(s) which are shared by the parent LSTRA. It should be emphasized, however, that the "tolerant" state of the experimental animals induced in this study should be corroborated by additional assays with higher sensitivity.

III. Adoptive Transfer of Transplantation Immunity

The adoptive-cell transfer method was employed to compare the immune activity of spleen cells derived from mice that had been immunized against either the parent L1210 or L1210/DTIC (NICOLIN et al. 1974a). CDF1 mice that had been immunosuppressed and injected with spleen cells immune to L1210/DTIC showed transplantation resistance against an L1210/DTIC challenge but not against an L1210 challenge: the transfer of spleen cells immune to the parent cells or to unrelated syngeneic or allogenic tumors was not effective. It was shown that the demonstrated resistance was dependent on the number of immunizing tumor cells, the number of immune spleen cells inoculated, and the timing of immune spleen-cell transfer relative to the time of the tumor challenge.

It was shown that the immunity elicited in CDF1 mice by a single injection of 10^7 L5178Y/DTIC cells can be long lasting since an adoptive transfer of spleen cells obtained 6 months after the immunization could still protect the recipient mice against a challenge with L5178Y/DTIC (NICOLIN et al. 1976a). The capacity to transfer transplantation immunity was abolished by exposing the immune spleen cells in vitro to X-irradiation (500 R) indicating that cell proliferation is involved.

The results of the adoptive-cell transfer experiments provide evidence that large numbers of specific lymphocytes are indeed produced in the host spleens by immunization with L1210/DTIC cells. The adoptive-cell transfer experiments added, however, no new information concerning the question of the antigenic change in drug-resistant sublines discussed in the previous section.

D. Immunological Changes in Drug-Resistant Tumor Sublines Defined by Antibodies

I. Changes in Tumor Antigenicity Defined by Antisera

Serological analysis of cell-surface properties of tumor cells has been conducted on several drug-resistant tumor sublines. In the initial study comparing the L1210 and the L1210/CH_3–G (KITANO et al. 1972) the capacity of tumor cells to bind antibodies was investigated by means of the paired label radioantibody technique (TANIGAKI et al. 1967) using immunoglobulins of DBA/2Ha-DD hyperimmune antiserum that had been raised against either the L1210 or the L1210/CH_3–G as a source of antibodies. It was found that the L1210/CH_3–G cells have higher antibody-binding capacity than the parent L1210 cells as shown by differences in the specific uptake of radioiodine-labeled immunoglobulins of anti-L1210/CH_3–G serum. In addition, anti-L1210/CH_3–G serum was shown to have more specific antibody than anti-L1210, which suggested a higher immunogenicity of L1210/CH_3–G as compared with L1210. With regard to antigenic specificities, the repeated absorptions of anti-L1210/CH_3–G immunoglobulins with the parent L1210 caused a partial removal of the antibodies reacting with the L1210/CH_3–G; the residual antibody activity was not removed by further absorptions with L1210 cells as completely as by comparable absorptions with the L1210/CH_3–G, suggesting that the resistant cells have different as well as common antigenic specificities in comparison with the parent L1210 cells.

The possible presence of new antigens on resistant subline cells has also been suggested by the serological studies on an L1210 subline resistant to araC (NICOLIN et al. 1972) and the C57BL/6 sarcoma EPO subline resistant to actinomycin D (BELEHRADEK et al. 1974) that were carried out by the cytotoxicity test and the membrane immunofluorescence technique, respectively. However, in the case of L1210/CH_3–G, the possibility exists that the failure by L1210 cells to absorb out completely anti-L1210/CH_3–G antibodies could have been due to a relatively insufficient number of absorbing cells or of sequential absorptions.

In subsequent studies (FUJI and MIHICH 1975; FUJI et al. 1979), three drug-resistant sublines, L1210/CH_3–G, L1210/DDUG, and L1210/GZL, were analyzed by the cytotoxicity tests with syngeneic DBA/2J antisera and complement in attempts to resolve the following questions:

1. Do L1210 sublines resistant to various antileukemic agents carry different TAAs or a common TAA(s)?
2. If they carry a common TAA(s), to what extent would this antigen contribute to their increased immunogenicity?
3. Is the common TAA(s) also shared with the parental L1210 cells?

It was found that cells of all three resistant sublines, but not of the parent L1210, are highly susceptible to specific lysis by the primary DBA/2J antisera directed against different resistant sublines (raised by a single injection of 10^8 irradiated cells of each subline), indicating the presence of common TAA(s) on all three sublines.

The fact that in the quantitative absorption tests with graded numbers of tumor cells the complete and specific removal of the anti-L1210/GZL antibody activity was achieved by a large number of the parent L1210 cells and that approximately ten times more L1210 cells than L1210/GZL cells were required to absorb out the antibody activity indicated that the common TAA(s) is expressed also on the parent L1210 cells though in a lesser degree. Consistent with the above observations was the demonstration that, although no cytotoxic antibody activity was detectable in the serum of DBA/2 mice after primary stimulation with L1210 cells, strong antibody activity was shown after hyperimmunization with L1210 cells. Furthermore, hyperimmune DBA/2 anti-L1210 antibody was more cytotoxic against all three sublines than against the parent L1210; similar cytotoxic patterns were exhibited by hyperimmune DBA/2 anti-L1210/GZL antibody (Fig. 2). Quantitative absorption of antiparent and antisubline antisera with tumor cells revealed that, although either the subline cells or the parental cells removed the antibody activity of both antisera completely, subline cells were more

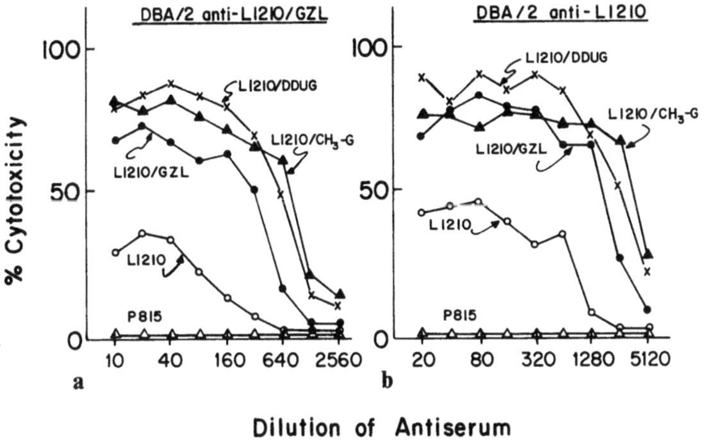

Fig. 2a, b. Cytotoxic activity of hyperimmune **a** DBA/2 anti-L1210/GZL and **b** DBA/2 anti-L1210 sera as measured by a ^{51}Cr-release assay with complement. Note that cells of the parental L1210 line are less effective as target cells than are cells of the sublines L1210/GZL, L1210/DDUG, and L1210/CH_3–G. DBA/2 mastocytoma P815 cells served as controls. (FUJI et al. 1979)

efficient. Normal spleen cells, fetal livers, or another DBA/2 tumor, i.e., P815 (mastocytoma), did not remove the activity. Taken together, these results indicate that all three resistant sublines have an increased expression of common TAA(s) and an increased susceptibility to lysis by the antisera as compared with the parent L1210. The differential expression of the common TAA on the parent L1210 and the resistant sublines appears to be selective because no marked difference was observed between these two cell types in their expression of H-2D and H-2K antigens as evidenced by the lack of difference in their susceptibility to anti-H-2D or K cytotoxic activity or in their capacities to absorb the activity from the anti-H-2 antisera.

To investigate the possibility that the TAA expressed strongly on L1210 subline cells may be related to antigens associated with either endogenous or exogenous MuLV, the reactivity of the DBA/2 anti-L1210 serum to several murine lymphomas known to express distinct MuLV-associated antigens was tested. These lymphomas included Rauscher virus-induced RBL5 (McCOY et al. 1967), Gross-virus-induced E♂G2 (OLD et al. 1965), and Gross-cell surface antigen-positive EL4(G^+) (HERBERMAN et al. 1974) as well as radiation-induced lymphoma RL♂1 which expressed endogenous MuLV antigen X.1 (SATO et al. 1973). Both cytotoxicity tests and quantitative absorption tests were negative with these lymphoma cells. Thus, no evidence was obtained for a possible relationship of the TAA with the known MuLV-associated antigens. This does not exclude the possibility of its having an unknown viral origin (FUJI et al. 1979).

In comparing the immunological properties of L1210/DTIC and L5178Y/DTIC (NICOLIN et al. 1976b), serological cross-reactivity between these two lines was demonstrated by the cytotoxicity test with the hyperimmune CDF1 antisera directed against each resistant line or with similar hyperimmune rabbit antiserum after proper absorption. The cross-reactivity between these two resistant lines was also demonstrated by a cell-mediated cytotoxicity assay in vitro with immune spleen cells or by tumor transplantation in vivo in CDF1 mice immunized against each resistant subline. It is not known whether similar cross-reactivity exists among other tumor sublines resistant to DTIC, however.

II. Changes in Tumor Antigenicity Defined by Monoclonal Antibody

The recent development of the hybridoma technique (Köhler and Milstein 1975) provides a method by which cell-surface antigenic properties can be analyzed by monoclonal antibody with defined specificity. This approach has been employed to investigate further the antigenic relationships between the parent L1210 and the L1210 sublines, L1210/CH_3–G, L1210/DDUG, and L1210/GZL (Fuji 1980, 1981; Rapp and Fuji 1983). Three hybridomas that produce monoclonal antibody recognizing the TAA on these tumor lines were developed by fusing spleen cells from DBA/2 mice immunized against either the parent L1210 or the L1210/GZL to cells of a nonimmunoglobin secreting variant of a BALB/c myeloma derived line (P3-NS-1/1-Ag4-1), using polyethylene glycol as the fusing agent.

After the cell fusion, three stable clones of antibody-producing hybridomas were selected for analysis of antigenic characteristics of the tumor cells; one hybridoma clone, designated as 3A6, was derived from spleen cells immunized against the L1210, and two other hybridomas, designated as 2B2 and 1C3, were derived from spleen cells immunized against the L1210/GZL. These hybridoma clones that had been established in vitro produced a large amount of monoclonal antibody in ascites fluids when they were propagated intraperitoneally in CDF1 mice. The supernatants of hybridoma-bearing ascites as well as the supernatants of hybridoma cultures were used as a source of monoclonal antibody.

The most direct and definitive information on differential antigenic expression of these tumor cells was obtained in the experiments conducted by the use of the anti-L1210 monoclonal antibody (3A6) and membrane immunofluorescence as determined by the fluorescence-activated cell sorter (Fuji 1981; Rapp and Fuji 1983). The immunofluorescence profiles of tumor cells treated with monoclonal anti-L1210 antibody (3A6) plus fluorescein isothiocyanate (FITC)-labeled $F(ab')_2$ of rabbit antimouse immunoglobulins and analyzed by the fluorescence-activated cell sorter are shown in Fig. 3. Cells of L1210/GZL and L1210/CH_3–G were strongly fluorescent after indirect staining with the 3A6 antibody whereas similar treatment caused only a weak immunofluorescence on the parent L1210 cells. The fluorescence intensity of individual cells showed a broad distribution, indicating heterogeneity in the expression of the TAA (85% of the L1210/GZL cells, 55% of L1210/CH_3–G cells, and only 10% of the parent cells showed specific fluorescence). Control staining of the tumor cells that was performed with nonspecific mouse myeloma protein (MOPC-195), replacing the 3A6 antibody, gave little fluorescence (data not shown in Fig. 3). Cells of another L1210 subline, L1210/DDUG, were also strongly immunofluorescent (70% of the tumor cells were specifically stained) after similar staining. These data establish that the monoclonal antibody-defined TAA is expressed in a greater amount

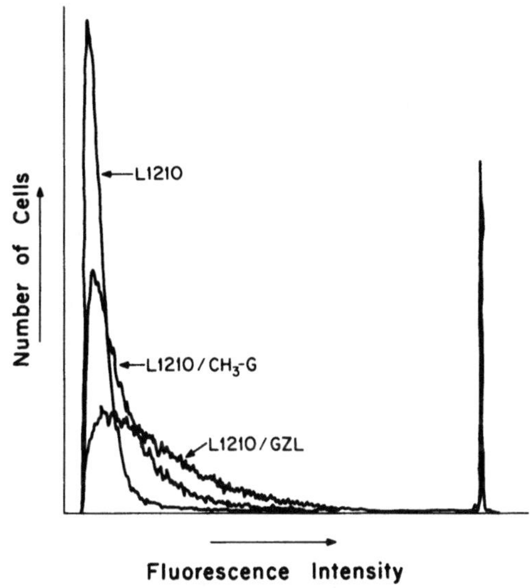

Fig. 3. Membrane immunofluorescence analysis of the expression of the TAA recognized by monoclonal DBA/2 anti-L1210 antibody, 3A6. Cells of L1210, L1210/CH_3–G, and L1210/GZL were treated with the monoclonal antibody and were stained with the FITC-labeled $F(ab')_2$ of rabbit antimouse immunoglobulin. The immunofluorescence analysis was carried out by means of the fluorescence-activated cell sorter

on the surfaces of L1210/CH_3–G, L1210/DDUG, and L1210/GZL cells than on the parent L1210 cells and that the cells of each tumor line are heterogeneous with respect to the expression of the TAA on cell surfaces.

Cytotoxicity tests conducted with 3A6, 2B2 as well as 1C3 monoclonal antibodies against the above tumor cells and quantitative absorptions of the monoclonal antibodies with the tumor cells gave results that are consistent with the above conclusions.

These monoclonal antibodies showed no detectable reactivity either with normal mouse tissues (liver, kidney, spleen, and thymus) or with most control mouse tumors of syngeneic and allogeneic origins including those induced by Rauscher- and Gross-mouse leukemia viruses. However, two DBA/2 tumors, i.e., L5178Y and P388-D1, showed a weak cross-reaction with all three monoclonal antibodies. In addition, these monoclonal antibodies reacted significantly with several spontaneous mammary tumors from C3H/St mice as well as with murine mammary tumor virus preparations (Rapp and Fuji 1983). These results and those of a recent study by Strzadala et al. (1981), who used a conventional antiserum directed to the mammary-leukemia antigen (Stück et al. 1964), indicate that the TAA may be related to an antigen which is associated with the murine mammary tumor virus. However, the exact nature of the antigen is still unknown. The availability of the hybridomas producing the antibody recognizing the TAA will facilitate the isolation and chemical characterization of the antigen as well as the finer analysis of tumor antigenicity.

E. Cellular Immune Responses Against Drug-Resistant Tumor Sublines

I. Antibody-Forming Cell Responses

Antibody-forming cell responses against the TAA on the drug-resistant L1210 sublines were demonstrated in the spleens of immunized DBA/2 mice by means of the modified Jerne plaque assay using the resistant subline cells as targets (Fuji and Mihich 1975). After a single i.p. injection of 10^8 irradiated cells of L1210/GZL, L1210/CH_3–G, or L1210/DDUG, the presence of as many as 5,000 plaque-forming cells (PFC) were demonstrated in the entire spleen of DBA/2 mice at the peak of the PFC response 5 days after the injection of the immunogen. Immunization of DBA/2 mice with the parental L1210 cells resulted in no more than 100 PFC in the total spleen under such conditions.

An entirely in vitro primary PFC response against the TAA was induced in cultures in which spleen cells derived from normal DBA/2 mice were incubated together with irradiated cells of the drug-resistant L1210 sublines (Fuji et al. 1977). Because of its flexibility, the in vitro system permitted conducting various quantitative analyses of the cellular immune responses. Dose-response experiments showed that cells of all three sublines had a similar capacity to evoke the PFC responses and were more efficient than the parental cells in this capacity. The difference between the parental and subline cells was primarily quantitative. Thus, high doses of the parental cells did, indeed, elicit responses comparable to those elicited by the subline cells. The responses are specific to the L1210 and its sublines inasmuch as DBA/2 P815 mastocytoma did not elicit a response detectable on the L1210 sublines.

The PFC response in the spleen-cell cultures was elicited not only by the stimulation with irradiated tumor cells but also by the stimulation with certain immunogenic components that are present in the supernatants of 24-h cultures of L1210/GZL cells and are presumably shed from the tumor-cell surfaces (Fuji 1981). The immunogenic components are apparently not the soluble TAA because the immunogenic activity can be removed from the culture supernatants by ultracentrifugation at 100,000 g for 1 h (Fuji, unpublished). The in vivo immunogenicity of this component is not known. The relationships between the immunogenicity and the membrane dynamics of these tumor sublines is a subject to be explored in the future.

II. Cell-Mediated Cytotoxic Responses

An in vitro analysis of the cell-mediated immunity against drug-resistant tumor sublines has been performed in several studies using DTIC-resistant tumor sublines: L5178Y/DTIC (Nicolin et al. 1974b), L1210/DTIC, and EL4/DTIC (Testorelli et al. 1978), and LSTRA/DTIC (Santoni et al. 1978). Using L5178Y/DTIC, it was shown that strong secondary cell-mediated cytotoxicity directed against the DTIC-resistant subline was elicited in cultures of CDF1 spleen cells that had been preimmunized against the L5178Y/DTIC in vivo and stimulated in vitro against the same tumor cells. The specificity of the cytotoxic activity of these cultured spleen cells was indicated by the demonstration that no significant cytotoxicity was detectable with the parent L5178Y and control tumors as the target, and no significant inhibition of the cytotoxic activity resulted in the inhibition assay with unlabeled cells of the parental line and other control tumors. Essentially similar results were obtained with L1210/DTIC, EL4/DTIC, and LSTRA/DTIC. The susceptibility of L1210/DTIC and L5178Y/DTIC to the cytotoxic effects of allogeneic and xenogeneic lymphocytes immunized against DBA/2 histocompatibility antigens were not different from the susceptibility of corresponding parental line to the same cytotoxic effects, indicating that there is no significant difference between the parent and the sublines with respect to their susceptibility to cell-mediated cytotoxicity (NICOLIN et al. 1976c). These data seem to support the conclusion derived from the in vivo experiments that new antigens are present on the DTIC-resistant tumor sublines.

Although primary cell-mediated cytotoxic response in vitro was either undetectable or marginal in the mixed cultures of normal CDF1 spleen cells and inactivated cells of drug-resistant sublines, the subline cells elicited a marked specific lymphocyte proliferative response in such cultures 96 h after the stimulation with the subline cells; no lymphocyte stimulation was observed with the parental cells (TESTORELLI et al. 1978).

Some drug-resistant sublines were shown to have cross-reactivity demonstrable by cell-mediated cytotoxicity. L1210/DTIC and L5178Y/DTIC were cross-reactive when tested by cell-mediated cytotoxicity with CDF1 spleen cells immunized against either tumor line, and the cross-reactivity between these two lines was also demonstrated by the serological test as mentioned earlier (NICOLIN et al. 1976b). In a study of the secondary cell-mediated cytotoxic response in vitro, cross-reactivity was demonstrated among L1210/DDUG, L1210/CH_3–G, and L1210/GZL by syngeneic T-lymphocytes immunized against L1210/GZL, indicating the expression of a T-cell-defined common TAA on these cells, whereas the presence of the antigen on the parent L1210 has yet to be established (FUJI and PRESSMAN 1977; Fuji, unpublished).

It is not known whether the T-cell-defined common TAA, the common TATA defined by the transplantation method, and the monoclonal antibody-defined TAA are the same antigens. In a recent study (FUJI 1981), data were obtained suggesting an apparent dissociation between the antibody-defined TAA and the T-cell-defined TAA; a cultured cell line derived from L1210/GZL exhibited a markedly reduced expression of the antibody-defined TAA but it showed a susceptibility to the T-cell-mediated cytotoxicity comparable to that of the in vivo L1210/GZL. To resolve whether or not the TAA or its antigenic determinants recognized by the antibody are different from those recognized by the cytotoxic T cell, further analysis should be carried out at the level of the antigen molecules.

F. Other Immunobiological Characteristics and Possible Mechanisms of Immunological Changes

Strong influence of the host genetic composition on the natural host resistance toward the drug-resistant tumor subline has been demonstrated (FUJI and MURAKAMI 1983). Upon testing the transplantability of the L1210 and the L1210/GZL in different histocompatible F1 hybrids of DBA/2 mice crossed with other strains of mice, it was found that certain F1 hybrids were strongly resistant toward tumor growth whereas other F1 hybrids were as susceptible as syngeneic mice. The resistant hybrids always showed a higher resistance toward the L1210/GZL than the parental L1210. The immunogenetic analysis with F1 hybrids between DBA/2 and congenic H-2 recombinant strains showed that genes linked to the H-2K-IA regions and certain non-H-2 loci confer a strong influence on the observed natural resistance against L1210/GZL. The resistance was abolished by injections of silica, an antimacrophage agent, or rabbit antimouse thymocyte serum. These results suggest that the resistance is immunological and that the genetically controlled host resistance may be directed to surface changes related to the increased expression of the TAA.

Although much information concerning the immunological characteristics of drug-resistant sublines has accumulated to date, the mechanisms underlying the emergence of high immunogenic drug-resistant sublines are still not clear. The important unique feature of the immunological change associated with drug-resistant sublines is their stability even in the absence of drug administration, which indicates that the change is genetically determined (BONMASSAR et al. 1970; MIHICH and KITANO 1971; SCHMID and HUTCHISON 1973; FUJI and MIHICH 1975; NICOLIN et al. 1976a, 1977).

Increased immunogenicity was demonstrated in three L1210 sublines, each resistant to different drugs, CH_3–G, DDUG, and GZL (MIHICH and KITANO 1971; KITANO et al. 1972; FUJI and MIHICH 1975). The sites of the antiproliferative actions of the drugs are different from each other (MIHICH 1967a, b, 1975; BROCKMAN et al. 1970). Thus, it was considered unlikely that the immunological change is specifically related to the development of resistance to each drug. Consistent with this notion is the fact that, in the case of DTIC, even a tumor subline (L1210Ha) naturally resistant to the drug can be rendered immunogenic by treatment with the drug (BONMASSAR et al. 1973), indicating that the immunogenicity change is independent of the development of drug resistance. Such results have not yet been demonstrated in the case of drugs other than DTIC, however.

As mentioned earlier, the possibility that a reduction in the oncogenic potential is a major factor contributing to the reduced tumor transplantability associated with resistant subline cells (SCHMID and HUTCHISON 1972, 1973) is unlikely in view of the fact that the complete reversal of the inhibited growth of the resistant subline cells was often demonstrated in immunosuppressed syngeneic animals. In addition, the analysis of cell growth kinetics did not show any significant difference between the parental line and the resistant sublines (SILVESTRINI et al. 1977).

The possibility that an increase in the susceptibility to immune lysis is a main factor responsible for the impaired growth of the resistant tumor cells (TSUKAGOSHI and HASHIMOTO 1973) can be excluded. In fact, the parent cells and the resistant subline cells are equally susceptible to the cytotoxic effects of antiserum (or immune lymphocytes) derived from allogeneic or xenogeneic animals that had been immunized against normal cell-surface antigens present on the tumor cells (FUJI and MIHICH 1975; FUJI et al. 1979; NICOLIN et al. 1976c; SANTONI et al. 1978; BONMASSAR et al. 1975). The above results indicate also that no major change occurs in the expression of histocompatibility antigens in drug-resistant sublines.

Studies on the sialic acid content on the surface of cells from the L1210 and the resistant L1210 sublines (L1210/CH_3–G, L1210/DDUG, and L1210/GZL) showed no correlation between surface sialic acid content and susceptibility to lysis (BERNACKI et al. 1974).

Since both CH_3–G and DDUG have been shown to be immunosuppressive (MIHICH et al. 1970; MIHICH 1963, 1964, 1967 b), the possibility was considered that the L1210-resistant cell populations with increased immunogenicity may develop consequent to immunosuppression by drug treatments selecting for drug resistance (MIHICH and KITANO 1971). The results using anti-TAA antibodies that demonstrated the presence of a greater amount of the common TAA in all three L1210 sublines (L1210/CH_3–G, L1210/DDUG, and L1210/GZL) and the pre-existence of the TAA in the parent L1210 are consistent with this hypothesis (FUJI and MIHICH 1975; FUJI et al. 1977, 1979; FUJI 1980; RAPP and FUJI 1983) (Figs. 2, 3). The positive immunoselective pressure favoring the growth of a pre-existent, high-TAA-density cell subpopulation may conceivably be provided by the host's weak immunity (PREHN 1972) that is a result of drug-induced immunosuppression during selection for drug resistance.

Data apparently contradictory to the above hypothesis have been obtained in the following study. Using naturally immunodeficient athymic (nude) mice as hosts for L1210 and LSTRA lymphomas, it was found that no increase in the immunogenicity of these lymphomas occurred during the maintenance in such hosts. Highly immunogenic tumor lines were obtained, however, after nude mice were treated with DTIC (CAMPANILE et al. 1975). Therefore, the presence or absence of host immune capability was considered not essential for the development of high immunogenicity as a result of the DTIC treatment. However, the fact that nude mice do have a high level of natural killer cell (HERBERMAN et al. 1975; KIESSLING et al. 1975) and B-cell activities (PREHN and OUTZEN 1977) makes the argument not very definitive.

The alternative possibility could be an altered expression of tumor-associated and/or virus-related antigens on the resistant subline cells resulting from direct drug action. This hypothesis cannot be entirely ruled out if such altered expression is genetically determined and stable in the absence of drug.

A hypothesis that new antigens may be produced by resistant subline cells as a result of somatic mutations through direct drug actions has been postulated (BONMASSAR et al. 1970). The data favoring this hypothesis may be found in a recent study that showed an antagonistic effect of quinacrine on DTIC-mediated immunogenic changes of tumor cells, presumably through its antimutagenic activity (GIAMPIETRI et al. 1980). A possibility should be considered, however, that the antagonistic activity of quinacrine shown in this experiment might be related to mechanisms other than the antimutagenic activity of the compound. The data showing increased expression of common TAA on the L1210 sublines resistant to CH_3–G, DDUG, and GZL and the pre-existence of the TAA in the parent L1210 (Figs. 2, 3) are inconsistent with the hypothesis.

Immunological changes have been shown in tumor sublines that had been developed by exposure of tumor cells to drugs in vitro (TSUKAGOSHI and HASHIMOTO 1973; BELEHRADEK et al. 1974; CONTESSA et al. 1979). In the report by BELEHRADEK et al. (1974), a marked change in the morphology was noted in the drug-resistant subline. In such cases, it might be possible that the mechanisms involved in generating the immunological changes may not necessarily be the same as those involved in vivo.

It should be noted here that an apparent decrease in immunogenicity was observed in the case of Sarcoma 180/MP, a subline of Sarcoma 180 resistant to 6-mercaptopurine (6-MP) (FERRER and MIHICH 1967), and Sarcoma 180/B_6, a subline capable of growing in vitamin-B_6-deficient mice, namely under conditions in which S-180 is rejected through the mechanism of host defense (MIHICH and NICHOL 1960). An apparent loss of antigenicity was demonstrated in the case of two L1210 sublines resistant to either MTX or 6-MP: the BDF1 mice hyperimmunized against the parent L1210 cells showed a substantial degree of immunity against the challenge with the parent L1210 cells whereas only a weak immunity was demonstrated against the challenge with either MTX-resistant or 6-MP-resistant L1210 subline cells (CALMAN et al. 1974).

Taken together, these examples indicate the possibility that changes in immunogenicity may occur in either direction during drug treatment selecting for resistance and that multiple mechanisms may be involved in such changes.

Recent findings that suggested differential recognition of the TAA(s) or TAA determinants of the L1210-resistant subline cells by the host's T- and B-lymphocytes point out the need for a comprehensive analysis with regard to contributions of various subpopulations of host immune cells in host-tumor interactions (FUJI 1981). As noted before, the host's ability to reject the L1210/GZL is influenced strongly by the host's histocompatibility genes (FUJI and MURAKAMI 1983). Therefore, the possibility that the host's genetic composition may affect the occurrence of immunological changes in drug-resistant tumor sublines should also be considered.

Tumor-cell lines with well-defined antigenicity and distinct immunogenicity provide an experimental tumor model suitable for investigating host antitumor immune responses and their regulatory mechanisms. Studies conducted in this laboratory indicate that the spleen cells from animals bearing the parent L1210 cells may have stronger suppressor-cell activity than those bearing the L1210/GZL cells (FUJI and PRESSMAN 1977). Thus, there was an inverse relationship between a tumor's immunogenicity and its ability to induce suppressor cell activity.

G. Conclusions

An increase in immunogenicity has been found in many animal tumor sublines resistant to a variety of chemotherapeutic agents.

The immunological change(s) develops with time during treatment with drugs selecting for resistance. Once established, the change is stable during many transplant generations without maintenance drug treatment, indicating that the change is genetically determined. Some drugs are more effective than others in generating the increased immunogenicity and some tumors appear to be more susceptible to such change.

The increased immunogenicity of the resistant sublines has been defined by the tumor transplantation method, by the analysis with humoral antibodies including monoclonal antibody, and by the cell-mediated cytotoxicity response in vitro.

The change may be attributable to an increased expression, on tumor sublines resistant to different drugs, of common tumor-associated antigens that are preexistent in the parent tumor, as in the cases of the L1210 sublines resistant to CH_3–G, DDUG, and GZL. In other cases, such as tumor sublines resistant to DTIC, it may be due to a possible acquisition by the sublines of new antigens not detectable in the parent line. Yet in another case, the immunological change may be reflected in an apparent loss of tumor antigenicity in the resistant sublines.

There is no detectable change in the expression of normal cell-surface antigens associated with drug-resistant sublines.

The mechanisms underlying the emergence of the highly immunogenic resistant subline cells are not yet understood. Several possibilities have been postulated: (a) altered immunoselection during immunosuppression by drug treatment selecting for resistance, (b) altered expression of tumor-associated antigens by direct drug actions, and (c) an expression of new antigens through somatic mutations by direct drug actions; these are mostly speculative at this time.

Differences in membrane turnover, membrane shedding, and interactions among membrane antigenic components are considered potentially important for tumor immunogenicity changes.

The host's genetic composition affecting natural host resistance and lymphocyte subpopulations exerting selective regulatory functions should also be taken into consideration in order to elucidate comprehensively the basis for the differential tumor immunogenicity. Recent technical developments such as the hybridoma technology, the fluorescence-activated cell sorter, as well as sensitive analytical procedures should facilitate further studies in this area and enhance the usefulness of the drug-resistant sublines as an experimental model for the study of the immunobiology of tumors, as well as for possible chemotherapeutic or immunotherapeutic implications.

References

Belehradek J Jr, Biedler JL, Thornier M, Barski G (1974) Actinomycin D-resistant in vitro mouse cell line derived from a methylcholanthrene-induced sarcoma: decrease of malignancy and antigenic characteristics. Int J Cancer 14:779–788

Benacerraf B, Germain RN (1978) The immune response genes of the major histocompatibility complex. Immunol Rev 38:70–119

Bernacki RJ, Fuji H, Mihich E (1974) A comparison of plasma membrane sialic acid content, ectosialyltransferase activity, and immunogenicity of leukemia L1210 cells and three drug resistant sublines. Proc Am Assoc Cancer Res 15:132

Bonmassar E, Bonmassar A, Vadlamudi S, Goldin A (1970) Immunological alteration of leukemic cells in vivo after treatment with an antitumor drug. Proc Natl Acad Sci USA 66:1089–1095

Bonmassar E, Bonmassar A, Vadlamudi S, Goldin A (1973) Antigenic changes of L1210 leukemia in mice treated with 5-(3,3-dimethyl-1-triazeno)-imidazole-4-carboxamide. Cancer Res 32:1446–1450

Bonmassar E, Testorelli C, Franco P, Goldin A, Cudkowicz G (1975) Changes of the immunogenic properties of a radiation-induced mouse lymphoma following treatment with antitumor drugs. Cancer Res 5:1957–1962

Bonmassar A, Franti L, Floretti MC, Romani L, Giampietri A, Goldin A (1979) Changes of the immunogenic properties of K36 lymphoma treated in vivo with 5(3,3-dimethyl-1-triazeno) imidazole-4-carboxamide (DTIC). Eur J Cancer 15:933–939

Boyse EA, Old LJ (1969) Some aspects of normal and abnormal cell surface genetics. Annu Rev Genet 3:269–290

Brockman RW, Shaddix S, Laster WR Jr, Schabel FM Jr (1970) Inhibition of ribonucleotide reductase, DNA synthesis, and L1210 leukemia by guanazole. Cancer Res 30:2358–2368

Brown JP, Klitzman JM, Hellström I, Nowinski RC, Hellström KE (1978) Antibody response of mice to chemically induced tumors. Proc Natl Acad Sci USA 75:955–958

Calman NS, Eng B, Slater LM, Wallerstein H (1974) Antigenic changes associated with resistance to methotrexate and 6-mercaptopurine in L1210 ascites lymphoma. JNCI 52:997–998

Campanile F, Houchens DP, Gaston M, Goldin A, Bonmassar E (1975) Increased immunogenicity of two lymphoma lines after drug treatment of athymic (nude) mice. JNCI 55:207–209

Contessa AR, Giampietri A, Bonmassar A, Goldin A (1979) Increased immunogenicity of L1210 leukemia following short-term exposure to 5-(3,3-dimethyl-1-triazeno) imidazole-4-carboxamide (DTIC) in vivo or in vitro. Cancer Immunol Immunother 7:71–76

Dave C, Paul MA, Rustum YM (1978) Studies on the selective toxicity of guanazole in mice. Eur J Cancer 14:33–40

DeLeo AB, Shiku H, Takahashi T, John M, Old LJ (1977) Cell surface antigens of chemically induced sarcomas of the mouse. I. Murine leukemia virus-related antigens and alloantigens on cultured fibroblasts and sarcoma cells: description of a unique antigen on Balb/c Meth A sarcoma. J Exp Med 146:720–734

Doherty PC, Blanden RV, Zinkernagel RM (1976) Specificity of virus-immune effector T cells for H-2K or H-2D compatible interactions: implications for H-antigen diversity. Transplant Rev 29:89–124

Ferrer JF, Mihich E (1967) Relationship between tumor incompatibility and therapeutic response. Proc Soc Exp Biol Med 126:402–405

Flaherty L, Rinchik E (1978) No evidence for foreign H-2 specificities on the EL4 mouse lymphoma. Nature 273:52–53

Fuji H (1980) Monoclonal antibody recognizing tumor-associated antigen of DBA/2 mouse lymphoma L1210 and its sublines. Transplant Proc 12:388–390

Fuji H (1981) Differential recognition of tumor cell variants by B- and T-Lymphocytes. In: Steinberg C, Lefkovits I (eds) The immune system, vol 2. Karger, Basel, pp 431–437

Fuji H, Mihich E (1975) Selection for high immunogenicity in drug-resistant subline of murine lymphomas demonstrated by plaque assay. Cancer Res 35:946–952

Fuji H, Murakami M (1983) Differential tumor immunogenicity of DBA/2 mouse lymphoma L1210 and its sublines. III. Control of host resistance to drug-resistant L1210 sublines by H-2-linked and non-H-2-linked genes. JNCI 70:119–125

Fuji H, Pressman D (1977) Differential tumor immunogenicity of L1210 and its sublines. An inverse relationship between immunogenicity and an ability to elicit splenic "suppressor" activity. Fed Proc 36:1204

Fuji H, Mihich E, Pressman D (1977) Differential tumor immunogenicity of L1210 and its sublines. I. Effect of an increased antigen density on tumor cell surfaces on primary B cell responses *in vitro*. J Immunol 119:983–986

Fuji H, Mihich E, Pressman D (1979) Differential tumor immunogenicity of DBA/2 mouse lymphoma L1210 and its sublines. II. Increased expression of tumor-associated antigens on subline cells recognized by serologic and transplantation methods. JNCI 62:1503–1510

Garrido F, Festenstein H, Schirrmacher V (1976) Further evidence for derepression of H-2 and Ia-like specificities of foreign haplotypes in mouse tumor cell lines. Nature 261:704–706

Giampietri A, Fioretti MC, Goldin A, Bonmassar E (1980) Drug-mediated antigenic changes in murine leukemia cells: antagonistic effects of quinacrine, an antimutagenic compound. JNCI 64:297–301

Grant JP, Bigner DD, Fischinger PJ, Bolognesi DP (1974) Expression of murine virus structural antigens on the surface of chemically induced murine sarcomas. Proc Natl Acad Sci USA 71:5037–5041
Haywood GR, McKhann CF (1971) Antigenic specificities on murine sarcoma cells. Reciprocal relationship between normal transplantation antigens (H-2) and tumor-specific immunogenicity. J Exp Med 133:1171–1187
Herberman RB, Aoki T, Nunn M, Lavrin DH, Soares N, Gazdar A, Holden H, Chang KSS (1974) Specificity of ^{51}Cr-release cytotoxicity of lymphocytes immune to murine sarcoma virus. JNCI 53:1103–1111
Herberman RB, Nunn ME, Lavrin DH (1975) Natural cytotoxic reactivity of mouse lymphoid cells against syngeneic and allogeneic tumors. I. Distribution of reactivity and specificity. Int J Cancer 16:216–229
Houchens DP, Bonmassar E, Gaston MR, Kende M, Goldin A (1976) Drug-mediated immunogenic changes of virus-induced leukemia in vivo. Cancer Res 36:1347–1352
Invernizzi G, Parmiani G (1975) Tumor-associated transplantation antigens of chemically induced sarcomata cross reacting with allogeneic histocompatibility antigens. Nature 254:713–714
Jerne NK (1971) The somatic generation of immune recognition. Eur J Immunol 1:1–9
Kiessling R, Klein E, Pross H, Wigzell H (1975) Natural killer cells in the mouse. II. Cytotoxic cells with specificity for mouse Moloney leukemia cells. Characteristics of the killer cells. Eur J Immunol 5:117–121
Kitano M, Mihich E, Pressman D (1972) Antigenic differences between leukemia L1210 and a subline resistant to methylglyoxal-bis(guanylhydrazone). Cancer Res 32:181–186
Klein PA (1975) Anomalous reactions of mouse alloantisera with cultured tumor cells. I. Demonstration of widespread occurrence using reference typing sera. J Immunol 115:1254–1260
Klein E, Klein G (1964) Antigenic properties of lymphomas induced by the Moloney agent. JNCI 32:547–568
Klein G, Sjögren HO, Klein E, Hellstrom KE (1960) Demonstration of resistance against methylcholanthrene-induced sarcomas in the primary autochthonus host. Cancer Res 20:1561–1572
Köhler G, Milstein C (1975) Continuous cultures of fused cells secreting antibody of predefined specificity. Nature 256:495–497
Martin WJ, Gipson TG, Martin SE, Rice JM (1976) Derepressed alloantigen on transplantally induced lung tumor coded for H-2 linked gene. Science 194:532–533
McCoy JL, Fefer A, Glynn JP (1967) Comparative studies on the induction of transplantation resistance in BALB/c and C57BL/6 mice in three murine leukemia systems. Cancer Res 27:1743–1748
Mihich E (1963) Current studies with methylglyoxal-bis(guanylhydrazone). Cancer Res 23:1375–1389
Mihich E (1964) Impairment of host defenses by methylglyoxal-bis(guanylhydrazone) (CH_3–G). Fed Proc 23:388
Mihich E (1967a) Recent studies with new antileukemic bisguanylhydrazone. In: Goldin A, Kaziwara K, Kinosita R, Yamamura Y (eds) Cancer chemotherapy, Gann monograph, vol 2. Maruzen, Tokyo, pp 167–175
Mihich E (1967b) Antileukemic action of new aromatic bisguanylhydrazone derivatives. Cancer 20:880–884
Mihich E (1969) Modification of tumor regression by immunologic means. Cancer Res 29:2345–2350
Mihich E (1973) Tumor immunogenicity in therapeutics. In: Mihich E (ed) Drug resistance and selectivity. Biochemical and cellular basis. Academic, New York, pp 391–412
Mihich E (1975) Bis-guanylhydrazones. In: Sartorrelli AC, Jones DG (eds) Antineoplastic and immunosuppressive agents II. Springer, Berlin Heidelberg New York, pp 766–788
Mihich E, Kitano M (1971) Differences in the immunogenicity of leukemia L1210 sublines in DBA/2 mice. Cancer Res 31:1999–2003
Mihich E, Nichol CA (1960) Development of a sub-line of mouse Sarcoma-180 capable of growing in pyridoxine-deficient animals. Nature 188:379–382

Mihich E, Bross I, Mihich RM, Nichol CA (1970) A model system for detecting drug impairment of antitumor host defenses. Cancer Res 30:1376–1383

Mitchison NA (1970) Immunologic approach to cancer. Transplant Proc 2:92

Mitchison NA (1971) The carrier effect in the secondary response to hapten-protein conjugates. II. Cellular cooperation. Eur J Immunol 1:18–27

Nicolin A, Vadlamudi S, Goldin A (1972) Antigenicity of L1210 leukemic sublines induced by drugs. Cancer Res 32:653–657

Nicolin A, Canti G, Goldin A (1974a) Adoptive immunotherapy in BALB/c×DBA/2CrF1 mice bearing an immunogenic subline of L1210 leukemia. Cancer Res 34:3044–3048

Nicolin A, Bini A, Coronetti E (1974b) Cellular immune response to a drug-treated L5178Y lymphoma subline. Nature 251:654–655

Nicolin A, Spreafico F, Bonmassar E, Goldin A (1976a) Antigenic changes of L5178Y lymphoma after treatment with 5-(3,3-dimethyl-1-triazeno) imidazole-4 carboxamide in vivo. JNCI 56:89–93

Nicolin A, Bini A, Padova FD, Goldin A (1976b) Immunologic cross-reactivity of antigen(s) induced by drug treatment in two leukemic sublines. J Immunol 116:1347–1349

Nicolin A, Franco P, Testorelli C, Goldin A (1976c) Immunosensitivity and histocompatibility antigens in drug-altered leukemic cells. Cancer Res 36:222–227

Nicolin A, Cavalli M, Missiroli A, Goldin A (1977) Immunogenicity induced in vivo by DIC in relatively non-immunogenic leukemias. Eur J Cancer 13:235–239

Old LJ, Boyse EA, Stockert E (1965) The G (Gross) leukemia antigen. Cancer Res 25:813–819

Prager MD, Baechtel FS (1973) Methods for modification of cancer cells to enhance tumor antigenicity. In: Busch H (ed) Methods in Cancer research, vol 9. Academic, New York, pp 339–400

Prat M, Rogers MJ, Appella E (1978) Alloantisera reacting with tumor cells of inappropriate haplotype. I. Characterization of target antigen. JNCI 61:527–534

Prehn RT, Main JM (1957) Immunity to methylcholanthrene-induced sarcomas. JNCI 18:769–775

Prehn RT (1972) The immune reaction as stimulator of tumor growth. Science 176:170–171

Prehn LM, Outzen HC (1977) Primary tumor immunity in nude mice. Int J Cancer 19:688–691

Rapp L, Fuji H (1983) Differential antigenic expression of the DBA/2 lymphoma L1210 and its sublines: cross-reactivity with C3H mammary tumors as defined by syngeneic monoclonal antibodies. Cancer Res 43:2592–2599

Rogers MJ, Appella E, Pierotti MA, Invernizzi G, Parmiani G (1979) Biochemical characterization of alien H-2 antigens expressed on a methylcholanthrene-induced tumor. Proc Natl Acad Sci USA 76:1415–1419

Rosenthal AS, Shevach EM (1973) Function of macrophages in antigen recognition by guinea pig T lymphocytes. I. Requirement for histocompatible macrophages and lymphocytes. J Exp Med 138:1194–1212

Santoni A, Kinney Y, Goldin A (1978) Secondary cytotoxic response in vitro against Moloney lymphoma cells antigenically altered by drug treatment in vivo. JNCI 60:109–112

Sato H, Boyse EA, Aoki T, Iritani C, Old LJ (1973) Leukemia-associated transplantation antigens related to murine leukemia virus. The X.1 system: immune response controlled by a locus linked to H-2. J Exp Med 138:593–606

Schmid FA, Hutchison DJ (1972) Collateral sensitivity of resistant lines of mouse leukemias L1210 and L5178Y. Cancer Res 32:808–812

Schmid FA, Hutchison DJ (1973) Decrease in oncogenic potential of L1210 leukemia by triazenes. Cancer Res 33:2161–2165

Silvestrini R, Testorelli C, Goldin A, Nicolin A (1977) Cell kinetics and immunogenicity of lymphoma cells treated with 5-(3,3-dimethyl-1-triazeno) imidazole-4-carboxamide (DIC) in vivo. Int J Cancer 19:664–669

Strzadala L, Opolski A, Radzikowski C, Mihich E (1981) Differential expression of murine leukemia antigen on L1210 parental and drug-resistant sublines. Cancer Res 41:4934–4937

Stück B, Boyse EA, Old LJ, Carswell EA (1964) ML: a new antigen found in leukaemias and mammary tumours of the mouse. Nature 203:1033–1034
Tada T, Taniguchi M, Takemori T (1975) Properties of primed suppressor T cells and their products. Transplant Rev 26:106–129
Tanigaki N, Yagi Y, Pressman D (1967) Application of the paired label radioantibody technique to tissue section and cell smears. J Immunol 98:274–280
Testorelli C, Franco P, Goldin A, Nicolin A (1978) In vitro lymphocyte stimulation and the generation of cytotoxic lymphocytes with drug-induced antigenic lymphomas. Cancer Res 38:830–834
Ting CC, Herberman RB (1971) Inverse relationship of polyoma tumour specific surface antigen to H-2 histocompatibility antigens. Nature New Biol 232:118–120
Ting CC, Herberman RB (1976) Humoral host defense mechanisms against tumors. Int Rev Exp Path 15:93–152
Tsukagoshi S, Hashimoto Y (1973) Increased immunosensitivity in nitrogen mustard-resistant Yoshida sarcoma. Cancer Res 33:1038–1042
von Boehmer H, Haas W, Jerne NK (1978) Major histocompatibility complex-linked immune-responsiveness is acquired by lymphocytes of low-responder mice differentiating in thymus of high-responder mice. Proc Natl Acad Sci USA 75:2439–2442

CHAPTER 5

The Molecular Basis of Genetically Acquired Resistance to Purine Analogues in Cultured Mammalian Cells

J. Brennand and C. T. Caskey

A. Introduction

The gene coding for the enzyme hypoxanthine-guanine phosphoribosyltransferase (HPRT; inosine monophosphate: pyrophosphate phosphoribosyltransferase, EC 2.4.2.8) has been the focus of considerable attention in somatic-cell mutation studies for a number of reasons. Seegmiller et al. (1967) demonstrated that the absence of, or deficiency in, HPRT within mammalian cells was the primary biochemical lesion in cells of patients suffering from Lesch-Nyhan syndrome (Lesch and Nyhan 1964). This disease is an inborn error of purine metabolism and is characterized by patients who are mentally retarded and prone to self-mutilation, spasticity and severe neurological dysfunction. These authors also proved that this disease is heritable in an X-linked recessive manner. Further studies have conclusively assigned this gene to the X chromosome of human (Pai et al. 1980), hamster (Westerveldt et al. 1972) and mouse (Franke and Taggart 1980). The gene for HPRT is therefore hemizygous in male cells and functionally hemizygous in female cells, rendering the locus particularly amenable to the study of recessive mutation. Furthermore, in mammalian cells growing in culture HPRT is a non-essential enzyme (Sect. C); thus, there are few limitations on the types of mutation which can occur in this gene and permit the cell to survive. Well-defined selection systems have been developed which can select for growth of cells containing the enzyme while eliminating cells that do not, and vice versa (Sect. C). Thus, over the past 15 years there has been a considerable amount of analysis of the HPRT gene as a model system for investigating the mechanisms of mutation and drug resistance in mammalian cells. This chapter describes the HPRT selection system in detail and reviews the evidence that changes in the sequence and organisation of DNA within the HPRT gene lead to drug resistance.

B. The HPRT Enzyme

HPRT is one of the enzymes responsible for the "salvage" of preformed purine and pyrimidine bases, present within the cell as a result of normal nucleic acid turnover. It catalyses the transfer of phosphoribose from 5′-phosphoribosyl-1-pyrophosphate (PRPP) to the 9-position of hypoxanthine or guanine, yielding inosine monophosphate or guanosine monophosphate, respectively, and pyrophosphate. Native HPRT is a eumerism of identical subunits of molecular weight ~25,000 (Olsen and Milman 1974; Holden and Kelley 1978; Hughes et al. 1975). Although the subunits are of identical molecular weight, there are several reports of multiple peaks of activity following isoelectric focusing in polyacrylamide gels (ARNOLD and KELLEY 1971; OLSEN and MILMAN 1974; CASKEY and KRUH 1979), which probably reflect differences is subunit charge. The reasons for such differences are unclear, although deamination occurring during the purification procedure is possible while post-translational modification is unlikely (CASKEY and KRUH 1979). The number of subunits associated in the native enzyme is not conclusively established. Molecular weight determinations of 78,000–85,000 for hamster HPRT (OLSEN and MILMAN 1974), 68,000 for human HPRT (ARNOLD and KELLY 1971) and 80,000 for mouse HPRT (HUGHES et al. 1975) suggest that the enzyme exists in trimeric form. However, the report by HOLDEN and KELLEY (1978) suggests that human HPRT may exist in the native state as a tetramer.

The kinetics of the reaction for human and hamster HPRT follow linear Michaelis-Menten kinetics (KONG and PARKS 1974; OLSEN and MILMAN 1974), and GIACOMELLO and SALERMO (1974) demonstrated a sequential mechanism for the human enzyme. They observed that the PRPP forms a complex with magnesium ions and binds to the enzyme prior to the binding of the purine Mg^{++} complex. Reaction products subsequently dissociate at random.

The HPRT gene was first localized to the X chromosome in man by pedigree analysis of families with Lesch-Nyhan syndrome (SEEGMILLER et al. 1967). Somatic-cell hybridisation studies have assigned the gene more precisely to the distal end of the long arm (Xq27–Xq28) of the human X chromosome (RICCIUTTI and RUDDLE 1973; PAI et al. 1980), the distal end of Xp in the hamster (WESTERVELD et al. 1972; FARRELL and WORTON 1977; FENWICK 1980) and the Xcen-XD region of the mouse X chromosome (CHAPMAN and SHOWS 1976; FRANKE and TAGGART 1980).

C. Biochemical Basis of Drug Resistance

Mammalian cells can synthesize purine nucleotides for nucleic acid synthesis by two different pathways. Firstly, the purine ring can be synthesised de novo from ribose-5′-phosphate, glutamine, glycine, aspartate, and carbon dioxide in a series of eleven enzymic reactions. Alternatively, cells can "salvage" preformed purines, such as adenine, guanine, and hypoxanthine, by single-step enzymic phosphorylation reactions. HPRT is responsible for the "salvage" of hypoxanthine and guanine, while (APRT) adenine phosphoribosyl transferase (EC 2.4.2.7) catalyzes the phosphorylation of adenine to AMP. Only one functional pathway is required for the normal growth of mammalian cells in vitro. Purine analogue drugs such as 6-thioguanine (6TG) and 8-azaguanine (8AZ) are phosphorylated by HPRT to their corresponding monophosphates 6TGMP and 8AZMP (WAY and PARKES 1958) by mammalian cells with functional HPRT. Exposure of cells to these drugs leads to incorporation of the purine analogue nucleotides into nucleic acid with toxic consequences. It appears that the toxic effect of 6TG is mediated primarily by its incorporation into DNA while the toxicity of 8AZ is attributable to its incorporation into RNA (LEPAGE and JONES 1961; NELSON et al. 1975). It follows, therefore, that variants with a functional de novo purine biosynthesis pathway but defective or deficient in HPRT will survive in the presence of appropriate concentrations of drug where wild-type cells would not. This property has facilitated the study of forward mutation from the $HPRT^+$ phenotype to the $HPRT^-$ phenotype, where cells without functional HPRT are selected out of a population of wild-type cells by growth in the appropriate concentration of drug.

The de novo pathways of purine and pyrimidine biosynthesis require a supply of tetrahydrofolic acid as cofactor. This is supplied by the reduction of folic and dihydrofolic acids by the enzyme dihydrofolate reductase. The folate analogue methotrexate (amethopterin) inhibits this enzyme and prevents replenishment of the tetrahydrofolate pool, thus inhibiting de novo nucleotide synthesis (McBurney and Whitmore 1975). Wild-type cells will survive in the presence of methotrexate, providing an exogenous supply of purine and pyrimidine precursors is made available as substrates for the "salvage" systems. The addition of methotrexate and purine and pyrimidine bases to the culture media is termed HAT (hypoxanthine, amethopterin, thymidine) selection and HPRT-deficient cells will not survive under these conditions as they will have no means of synthesising nucleotides for nucleic acid synthesis. Thus, wild-type cells can be selected from a population of HPRT-deficient variants by growth in HAT media, forming the basis of the reverse mutation assay.

When mammalian cells are exposed in vitro to increasing concentrations of purine anologues their ability to grow and form colonies decreases linearly with dose until a plateau region of zero slope is attained which reflects the frequency of resistant cells present in the population as a result of spontaneous mutation at the HPRT locus. The region of transition between the two phases of this curve has been termed the Ds (Thompson and Baker 1974) and is of the order of 0.2–0.5 µg/ml for 6TG and 2–5 µg/ml for 8AZ. This difference is a reflection of the lower K_m of HPRT for 6TG than for 8AZ (van Diggelen et al. 1979). It is essential that selection for resistant variants be carried out in media containing concentrations of drug well into the "plateau" region, as lower concentrations can result in the survival of variants containing HPRT activity (Carson et al. 1974; van Zeeland et al. 1974; Fox and Radacic 1978, 1982).

D. Drug Resistance as a Consequence of Mutation Within the HPRT Gene

I. Phenotypic Variation Resulting from Non-mutational Events

The evidence that purine analogue resistance in cultured mammalian cells occurs as a direct consequence of alteration in the DNA of the HPRT structural gene has recently been reviewed by Siminovich (1976) and Caskey and Kruh (1979) and will be discussed in detail below. Other mechanisms have been postulated to explain enhanced resistance based on non-mutational shifts in gene expression.

The concept that variation in somatic cells might be mainly of non-mutational, or epigenetic, nature was argued by Harris (1971). He had demonstrated that the frequency of spontaneous resistance to 8AZ in Chinese hamster V79 cells was independent of ploidy. This was unexpected on the basis of the known recessive character of the HPRT locus. However, this author did not determine the number of active X chromosomes present in the tetraploid and octaploid lines used and an investigation by CHASIN and URLAB (1975) provided an explanation for these unexpected findings. They studied alkylating-agent-induced mutation to 6TG resistance in a tetraploid Chinese hamster ovary cell line which was homozygous for HPRT but heterozygous for the closely linked glucose-6-phosphate dehydrogenase (G6PD) gene. They found that HPRT-deficient clones with active G6PD occurred at approximately the same frequency as those deficient in both enzyme activities. A result compatible with the explanation that chromosomal segregation and loss occurred before mutation in the single remaining gene. FOX and RADACIC (1978, 1982) isolated variants of Chinese hamster cells from marginally toxic concentrations of purine analogue. Such cells were resistant to challenge with a higher dose of drug. If the exposure was continued for up to 3 weeks, the cells acquired resistance to even higher doses and also became sensitive to HAT medium with a concomitant loss of HPRT activity. When these variants were maintained for up to 8 weeks in the absence of selective pressure, the mutant phenotype disappeared and the cells acquired a wild-type phenotype and normal HPRT activity. A similar response has been reported in cultured human fibroblasts by VAN ZEELAND et al. (1974) and in Chinese hamster cells resistant to bromodeoxyuridine by HARRIS and COLLIER (1981).

These authors have postulated that shifts in gene expression might have been induced by treatment of the cells with these drugs and that no alteration within the HPRT gene has taken place. Other possible explanations have been forwarded. Increased levels of one or more purine catabolic enzymes, e.g., alkaline phosphatase (WOLPERT et al. 1971; LEE et al. 1980), 5′-nucleotidase (WILLIAMS et al. 1978) or guanase (BERMAN et al. 1980), might increase the rate of catabolism of purine analogues, thus lowering the effective concentration and conferring a resistant phenotype. Such increases could be brought about by a shift in gene expression, gene dosage effects or from amplification of the genes coding for these enzymes, in an analogous manner to the situation which can occur with methotrexate resistance (ALT et al. 1978; KAUFMAN et al. 1979).

MORROW (1977) has proposed that chromosomal rearrangements might lead to gene inactivation and hence a drug-resistant phenotype although the structural gene for the enzyme of interest may be intact within the genome. Hybridisation of HPRT-deficient rat hepatoma cells with normal human fibroblasts produced 7 out of 15 hybrid clones which expressed rat HPRT (CROCE et al. 1973). In six of these the enzyme was expressed in the absence of the human X chromosome, and human HPRT and G6PD were undetectable. These data suggested that human material contributed a factor towards the reactivation or depression of the rat HPRT gene and that the structural gene for HPRT was intact within the rat genome.

There are few conclusive data concerning the extent to which such mechanisms play a role in the resistance of mammalian cells to purine analogues, while there is a considerable body of evidence which shows conclusively that classical mutational mechanisms can be directly involved in the development of drug resistance.

II. Evidence that Drug Resistance Results from Mutation Within the HPRT Gene

Since the early observations of CHU and MALLING (1968) and CHU et al. (1969) that the frequency of purine-analogue-resistant variants among mammalian cells is markedly increased by treatment with known mutagens, many studies have attempted to demonstrate that such treatment results in an altered gene product as a result of structural gene mutation. One of the earlier pieces of work was conducted in another system by ADETUGBO et al. (1977). They undertook to characterize the peptides released upon tryptic and peptic digestion of the H chain of immunoglobulin G (IgG), secreted by four mouse myeloma cell lines. The four lines were spontaneous mutants secreting IgG which differed with respect to the positions of focusing upon polyacrylamide gel electrophoresis. Further characterisation was facilitated by analysis of the products of in vitro translation of the IgG mRNA. They were able to classify these four mutations as (a) a nonsense mutation due to a premature chain termination codon, (b) an internal deletion, (c) a frameshift mutation and (d) a point mutation.

Similar approaches have been directed towards the classification of induced mutants at the HPRT locus and have made possible the identification of mutants with altered subunit molecular weight and peptide composition (CHASIN and URLAB 1976; CAPECCHI et al. 1977; MILMAN et al. 1977; CASKEY and KRUH 1979; KRUH et al. 1981; WILSON et al. 1981). The latter report is perhaps the most elegant study of this type. These workers isolated HPRT protein from erythrocytes from five unrelated patients who have a partial deficiency of HPRT activity. They demonstrated alterations in specific activity, immunological reactivity towards antibodies raised against HPRT, molecular weight and altered isoelectric point of the variant proteins. They concluded that they had identified four different mutant forms of HPRT enzyme resulting from four different mutations in the HPRT structural gene. The report of CAPECCHI et al. (1977) is also particularly interesting because they were able to demonstrate an alteration in the carboxy terminal peptide of HPRT from mutagen-induced purine-analogue-resistant mouse L cells. This suggested that the structural gene for HPRT might contain a premature chain termination mutation. Enzyme activity could be restored in the mutant cells by the microinjection of ochre suppressor tRNA, indicating that this line might contain an ochre nonsense codon (UAA) within the HPRT mRNA.

An alternative approach to the study of altered gene product has been facilitated by the preparation of highly specific antibodies against HPRT protein from a number of species including hamster, mouse, and human (BEAUDET et al. 1973; WAHL et al. 1974; GHANGAS and MILMAN 1975; FENWICK et al. 1977a, b; CASKEY and KRUH 1979). The HPRT activity in a cell-free extract can be determined by measuring the quantitative displacement of wild-type HPRT from the immune complex into the supernatant upon addition of the extract. The presence of cross-reacting material (CRM) in the extract is evidence for the presence of HPRT protein with intact antigenic determinants. BEAUDET et al. (1973) identified three HPRT-deficient Chinese hamster cell lines induced by monofunctional alkylating agents which possessed cross-reacting material (CRM^+) to HPRT protein. They interpret this as being good evidence for the presence of a structural gene mutation. A refinement of this technique, where in vivo radiolabelled HPRT is precipitated by antibody and subsequently characterized by denaturing sodium dodecyl sulphate (SDS) polyacrylamide gel electrophoresis, enabled FENWICK et al. (1977 a) to identify two CRM^+ purine-analogue-resistant Chinese hamster V79 cell lines as possessing HPRT of reduced molecular weight. One of the clones has a reduction of approximately 1,000 daltons (eight to ten amino acids) in its protein, which was active. The second clone possessed inactive HPRT with a reduction in its molecular weight of some 500 daltons (four to five amino acids). From these data, and analysis of the tryptic peptides of these mutant proteins (KRUH et al. 1981), these authors concluded that the former clone probably contains a small deletion or missense mutation, while the latter clone is probably a missense mutant.

Despite the application of such sensitive biochemical and immunological techniques to the study of the gene product, this is not direct evidence that resistance to purine analogues has resulted from molecular alterations within the HPRT gene. Such evidence is now available.

III. Molecular Analysis of the HPRT Gene

Conclusive evidence that gene mutation has occurred can only come from direct analysis of the gene itself and the primary gene product, messenger RNA. With the advent of recombinant DNA technology such studies are now possible for any gene of interest. The cloning of many genes of clinical relevance has now been accomplished and a wide variety of mutational events have been fully characterized. A review of these data is beyond the scope of this chapter; instead we will concentrate on molecular variation within the HPRT gene.

The isolation of sequences of the HPRT gene has proved to be a difficult undertaking. The two principal methods of isolating the gene, (a) gene transfer and (b) cDNA cloning, have not been straightforward due to (a) the large size of the gene (see below) and (b) the scarcity of the protein within most cells (OLSEN and MILMAN 1974). This leads to low HPRT mRNA levels (cDNA sequences are copies of the mRNA molecules) and presents immense difficulty in identifying the complementary DNA sequence. Our laboratory made use of a mouse neuroblastoma cell line which had previously been shown to contain elevated levels of a variant HPRT protein (MELTON 1981). We suspected that this cell line would also contain elevated levels of HPRT mRNA; this was demonstrated (MELTON et al. 1981). Using standard recombinant DNA techniques we successfully identified HPRT cDNA sequences of this mouse HPRT gene (BRENNAND et al. 1982). The same report demonstrated that these sequences also recognized HPRT sequences from other species including human and Chinese hamster. The cell line that we used produced elevated levels of a thermolabile protein by virtue of amplification of its HPRT genomic sequences. We speculated that under appropriate selective pressure the amplification of genomic sequences of a gene producing a temperature-sensitive protein might be a common event. Amplification of the HPRT gene would not be expected to lead to purine analogue resistance in mammalian cells but it is one more example in a rapidly growing list (SCHIMKE 1982) where gene amplification is a major mechanism of drug resistance among mammalian cells. However, it is not inconceivable that amplification of other genes responsible for purine nucleoside catabolism might lead to increased purine analogue turnover and development of drug resistance. Indeed, it is interesting to note that acute lymphocytic leukemia cells of many patients who have developed resistance to 6-thioguanine therapy still contain detectable HPRT activity (SARTORELLI et al. 1974). These cells often contain elevated alkaline phosphatase levels which might possibly have resulted from this type of mechanism.

One classical type of mutation within a gene is its total or partial deletion. X-chromosomal alterations have been reported in HPRT-deficient cells following their exposure to ionizing radiation (COX and MASSON 1978; THACKER 1981). The lack of a nucleic acid probe prevented correlation of these changes with loss of HPRT genomic sequences. Using the procedure of SOUTHERN (1975), 2 of 19 spontaneously arising or ultraviolet-light-induced purine-analogue-resistant Chinese hamster cell lines have been shown to have lost all, or most, of their HPRT genomic sequences and no longer produce functional HPRT mRNA (FUSCOE et al. 1982). Thus, gene deletion is a major cause of purine analogue resistance in cultured mammalian cells. This does not appear to be the case in vivo, however. A preliminary study of the HPRT gene in 15 Lesch-Nyhan patients has failed to reveal any major rearrangements within the locus (NUSSBAUM et al. 1982). However, the methodology employed in these studies is not likely to reveal any small deletions or insertions within the gene, and the possibility that these mechanisms play a role in this disease cannot be excluded. These studies have revealed several interesting features about the HPRT gene. The gene is very large, probably on the order of 40 kilobases of DNA and contains multiple non-coding intervening sequences. Although there is considerable sequence homology between the coding regions of the mouse and Chinese hamster HPRT genes (KONECKI et al. 1982), Southern analysis of the HPRT genes of these species (and human) reveals considerable differences within the HPRT genomes. This is probably due to DNA sequence alterations within the intron sequences.

Despite the preliminary nature of these studies, the data accumulated so far in our laboratories conclusively demonstrate, for the first time, that resistance to purine analogues in cultured mammalian cells can result from classical mutational mechanisms, i.e., alterations in sequence and organization of DNA.

E. Perspectives

This chapter has reviewed the data that resistance to a particular drug can result by mutation. The power of recombinant DNA technology in determining these molecular alterations has only just begun to be applied, but already significant data have been accumulated. It should soon be possible to identify the precise molecular lesion which results in purine analogue resistance in any cell of choice. This might be applied to both cultured mammalian cells and to cells from patients known to be at risk of producing affected offspring. Furthermore, the extensive polymorphism that exists within the HPRT gene of man (NUSSBAUM et al. 1982) might prove useful in the study of closely linked disease-related genes, e.g. hemophilia A and Fragile X syndrome. The resistance of cultured mammalian cells to this drug and now the availability of cloned sequences of the HPRT gene should facilitate the development of a model system for the study of the introduction of cloned genes into enzyme-deficient cells. At present the integration and control of the expression of foreign sequences of DNA within the genome of receptor cells is poorly understood. If such a model system can be developed, many of the questions which preclude the use of gene replacement therapy for individuals defective in any particular gene might be overcome.

References

Adetugbo E, Milstein C, Secher DS (1977) Molecular analysis of spontaneous somatic mutants. Nature 265:299–304

Alt FW, Kellems RE, Bertino JR, Schimke RT (1978) Selective multiplication of dihydrofolate reductase genes in methotrexate-resistant variants of cultured murine cells. J Biol Chem 253:1357–1370

Arnold WJ, Kelly WN (1971) Human hypoxanthine guanine phosphoribosyltransferase. J Biol Chem 246:7398–7404

Beaudet AL, Roufa DJ, Caskey CT (1973) Mutation affecting the structure of hypoxanthine guanine phosphoribosyltransferase in cultured Chinese hamster cells. Proc Natl Acad Sci USA 70:320–324

Berman JJ, Tong C, Williams GM (1980) Differences between rat liver epithelial cells and fibroblast cells in sensitivity to 8-azaguanine. In Vitro 16:661–668

Brennand J, Chinault AC, Konecki DS, Melton DW, Caskey CT (1982) Cloned cDNA sequences of the hypoxanthine-guanine phosphoribosyltransferase gene from a mouse neuroblastoma cell line found to have amplifield genomic sequences. Proc Natl Acad Sci USA 79:1950–1954

Capecchi MR, Vonder-Haar RA, Capecchi NE, Sveda MM (1977) The isolation of suppressible nonsense mutants in mammalian cells. Cell 12:371–381

Carson MP, Vernick D, Morrow J (1974) Clones of Chinese hamster cells not permanently resistant to azaguanine. Mutat Res 24:47–54

Caskey CT, Kruh GD (1979) The HPRT locus. Cell 16:1–9

Chapman VM, Shows TB (1976) Somatic cell genetics. Evidence for X chromosome linkage of 3 enzymes in the mouse. Nature 259:665–667

Chasin LA, Urlab G (1975) Chromosome-wide event accompanies the expression of recessive mutation in tetraploid cells. Science 187:1091–1093

Chasin LA, Urlab G (1976) Mutant alleles for HPRT codominant expression, complementation and segregation in hybrids. Somatic Cell Genet 2:453–457

Chu EHY, Malling HV (1968) Mammalian cell genetics II. Chemical induction of specific locus mutation in Chinese hamster cells in vitro. Proc Natl Acad Sci USA 61:1306–1312

Chu EHY, Brimer P, Jacobson KB, Merriam EV (1969) Mammalian cell genetics I. Selection and characterisation of mutations auxotrophic for L-glutamine or resistant to 8-azaguanine in Chinese hamster cells in vitro. Genetics 62:359–377

Cox R, Masson WE (1978) Do radiation-induced thioguanine-resistant mutants of cultured mammalian cells arise by HGPRT gene mutation or X-chromosome rearrangement? Nature 276:629–630

Croce CM, Bakey B, Nyhan WL, Kuprowsky H (1973) Re-expression of the rat hypoxanthine phosphoribosyltransferase gene in rat-human hybrids. Proc Natl Acad Sci USA 70:2590–2594

Farrel SA, Worton RG (1977) Chromosome loss is responsible for segregation at the HPRT locus in Chinese hamster cell hybrids. Somatic Cell Genet 3:539–551

Fenwick RG (1980) Reversion of a mutation affecting the molecular weight of HGPRT: Intragenic suppression and localization of X linked genes. Somati Cell Genet 6:477–494

Fenwick RG, Sawyer TH, Kruh GD, Astrin KH, Caskey CT (1977a) Forward and reverse mutations affecting the kinetics and apparent molecular weigh of mammalian HPRT. Cell 12:383–391

Fenwick RG, Wasmuth JJ, Caskey CT (1977b) Mutations affecting the antigenic properties of hypoxanthine guanine phosphoribosyltransferase in cultured Chinese hamster cells. Somatic Cell Genet 3:207–216

Fox M, Radacic M (1978) Adaptional origin of some purine analogue resistant phenotypes in cultured mammalian cells. Mutat Res 49:275–296

Fox M, Radacic M (1982) Variations in chromosome numbers and their possible relationship to the development of 8-azaguanine resistance in Chinese hamster cells. Cell Biol Int Rep 6:39–48

Franke U, Taggart RT (1980) Comparative gene mapping: order of loci on the X-chromosome is different in mice and humans. Proc Natl Acad Sci USA 77:3595–3599

Fuscoe JC, Fenwick RG Jr, Ledbetter DH, Caskey CT (1983) Deletion and amplification of the HGPRT locus in Chinese hamster cells. Mol Cell Biol 3:1086–1096

Ghangas GS, Milman G (1975) Radioimmune determination of HGPRT cross-reacting material in erythrocytes of Lesch-Nyhan patients. Proc Natl Sci USA 72:4147–4150

Giacomello A, Salerno C (1974) Human hypoxanthine guanine phosphoribosyltransferase. J Biol Chem 253:6038–6044

Harris M (1971) Mutation rates in cells of different ploidy levels. J Cell Physiol 78:177–184

Harris M, Collier K (1981) Phenotypic evolution of cells resistant to bromodeoxyuridine. Proc Natl Acad Sci USA 77:4206–4210

Holden JA, Kelly WN (1978) Human hypoxanthine guanine phosphoribosyltransferase. J Biol Chem 250:120–126

Hughes SH, Wahl GM, Capecchi MR (1975) Purification and characterization of mouse hypoxanthine guanine phosphoribosyltransferase. J Biol Chem 250:120–126

Kaufman RJ, Brown PC, Schimke RT (1979) Amplified dihydrofolate reductase genes in unstably methotrexate-resistant cells are associated with double minute chromosomes. Proc Natl Acad Sci USA 76:5669–5673

Konecki DS, Brennand J, Fuscoe JC, Caskey CT, Chinault AC (1982) Sequence analysis of cDNA recombinants of the mouse and Chinese hamster hypoxanthine-guanine phosphoribosyltransferase genes. Nucleic Acids Res 10:6763–6775

Kong CM, Parks RE (1974) Human erythrocytic hypoxanthine guanine phosphoribosyltransferase: effect of pH on the enzymatic reaction. Mol Pharmacol 10:648–656

Kruh GD, Fenwick RG Jr, Caskey CT (1981) Structural analysis of mutant and revertant forms of Chinese hamster hypoxanthine guanine phosphoribosyltransferase. J Biol Chem 256:2878–2886

Lee SH, Shansky CW, Sartorelli AC (1980) Evidence for the external localization of alkaline phosphatase activity on the surface of sarcoma 180 cells resistant to 6 thioguanine. Biochem Pharmacol 29:1859–1861

LePage GA, Jones M (1961) Further studies on the mechanism of action of 6-thioguanine. Cancer Res 21:1590–1594

Lesch M, Nyhan WL (1964) A familial disorder of uric acid metabolism and nervous system disorder. Am J Med 36:561–570

McBurney MW, Whitmore GF (1975) Mechanism of growth inhibition by methotrexate. Cancer Res 35:586–590

Melton DW (1981) Cell fusion-induced mouse neuroblastoma HPRT revertants with variant enzyme and elevated HPRT protein levels. Somatic Cell Genet 7:331–344

Melton DW, Konecki DS, Ledbetter DH, Hejtmancik JF, Caskey CT (1981) In vitro translation of hypoxanthine guanine phosphoribosyltransferase mRNA; characterization of a mouse neuroblastoma cell line that has elevated levels of hypoxanthine guanine phosphoribosyltransferase protein. Proc Natl Acad Sci USA 78:6977–6980

Milman G, Krauss SW, Olsen AS (1977) Tryptic peptide analysis of normal and mutant forms of HGPRT from HeLa cells. Proc Natl Acad Sci USA 74:926–930

Morrow J (1977) Gene inactivation as a mechanism for the generation of variability in somatic cell cultivated in vitro. Mutat Res 44:391–400

Nelson JA, Carpenter JW, Rose LM, Adamson DJ (1975) Mechanisms of action of 6-thioguanine and 8-azaguanine in selecting resistant mutants from 2 V79 Chinese hamster cells in vitro. Mutat Res 35:279–288

Nussbaum RL, Caskey CT, Gilbert F, Nyhan W (1982) Southern analysis of the Lesch-Nyhan locus in man. In: deBruyn CHMM (ed) Proceedings of the international symposium on human purine and pyrimidine metabolism. Plenum, New York

Olsen AS, Milman G (1974) Chinese hamster hypoxanthine guanine phosphoribosyltransferase. J Biol Chem 249:4030–4037

Pai GS, Sprenkle JA, Do TT, Mareni CE, Migeon BR (1980) Localization of loci for hypoxanthine phosphoribosyltransferase and glucose-6-phosphate dehydrogenase and biochemical evidence of non-random X chromosome expression from studies of a human X-autosome translocation. Proc Natl Acad Sci USA 77:2810–2813

Ricciuti F, Ruddle FH (1973) Assignment of nucleoside phosphorylase to D-14 and localization of X linked loci in man by somatic cell genetics. Nature (New Biol) 241:180–182

Sartorelli AC, Lee MH, Rosman M, Agrawal KC (1974) In: Pharmacological basis of cancer chemotherapy. Williams and Wilkins, Baltimore, p 643

Schimke R (1982) Gene amplification. Cold Spring Harbor, New York

Seegmiller JE, Rosenbloom FN, Kelly WN (1967) Enzyme defect associated with a sex-linked human neurological disorder and excessive purine synthesis. Science 155:1682–1684

Siminovich L (1976) On the nature of hereditable variation in cultured somatic cells. Cell 7:1–11

Southern EM (1975) Detection of specific sequences among DNA fragments generated by gel electrophoresis. J Mol Biol 98:503–517

Thacker J (1981) The chromosomes of a V79 Chinese hamster line and a mutant subline HPRT activity. Cytogenet Cell Genet 29:16–25

Thompson LH, Baker RM (1974) Isolation of mutants of cultured mammalian cells. In: Prescott DH (ed) Methods in cell biology, vol 6. Academic, London, pp 209–281

Van Diggelen OP, Donahue TF, Shin SJ (1979) Basis for differential cellular sensitivity to 8-azaguanine and 6-thioguanine. J Cell Physiol 98:59–72

Van Zeeland AA, DeRuijter YCEM, Simons JWIM (1974) The role of 8-azaguanine in the selection from human diploid cells of mutants deficient in hypoxanthine guanine phosphoribosyltransferase (HGPRT). Mutat Res 24:55–68

Wahl GM, Hughes SH, Capecchi MR (1974) Immunological characterization of HPRT mutants of mouse L cells. Evidence for mutation at different loci in the HPRT gene. J Cell Physiol 85:307–320

Way JL, Parkes RE (1958) Enzymatic synthesis of 5′-phosphate nucleotides of purine analogues. J Biol Chem 231:467–480

Westerveldt A, Visser RPLS, Freeke MA, Bootsma D (1972) Evidence for linkage of 3-phosphoglycerate kinase, hypoxanthine guanine phosphoribosyltransferase and glucose 6-phosphate dehydrogenase loci in Chinese hamster cells studied by using a relationship between gene multiplicity and enzyme activity. Biochem Genet 7:33–40

Williams GM, Tong C, Berman JJ (1978) Characterisation of analogue resistance and purine metabolism of adult rat liver epithelial cell 8-azaguanine resistant mutants. Mutat Res 49:103–115

Wilson JM, Baugher BW, Landa L, Kelley WN (1981) Human hypoxanthine-guanine phosphoribosyltransferase. J Biol Chem 256:10306–10312

Wolpert MD, Damle SP, Brown JE, Sznycer E, Agrawal KC, Sartorelli AC (1971) The role of phosphohydrolates in the mechanism of resistance of neoplastic cells to 6-thiopurines. Cancer Res 31:1620–1626

Section III: Cellular Aspects

CHAPTER 6

Cell Cycle Perturbation Effects

B. DREWINKO and B. BARLOGIE

A. Introduction

I. General

The proliferative status of a cell population and its kinetics of proliferation recovery following treatment with antitumor agents are important determinants in the final outcome of the drug-cell interaction. Antitumor agents generate two types of unrelated effects in treated cells: cell kill and delayed transit through the mitotic cycle (DREWINKO and BARLOGIE 1976b; MADOC-JONES and MAURO 1975). Therefore, cell proliferation may be decreased because of actual cell kill or because of perturbation of the normal rate of progression through the cycle. This perturbation may be manifested in various forms including cycle stage traverse delay, a reversible or irreversible block in a particular stage of the cycle, or, more commonly, a combination of these factors. This temporary lag in the multiplication rate may increase the doubling time of the treated population and produce results indistinguishable from those obtained in populations whose cells are actually killed (ROPER and DREWINKO 1976). In addition, the reassortment and new distribution in different proliferative compartments or stages of the cell cycle experienced by the population will influence profoundly the effect of the same or another agent administered at subsequent intervals, thus resulting in either increased or decreased sensitivity to the agent (DETHLEFSEN 1975, 1979).

II. Proliferating and Quiescent Cells

Most malignant cell populations, both in vivo and in vitro, are composed of at least two classes of cells with distinct proliferative characteristics: overtly proliferating and nonproliferating, quiescent cells. The relative proportion of each class compartment fluctuates constantly with a trend to increasing numbers of cells in the quiescent compartment as the population expands. Thus, cell cultures and in vivo tumors initially proliferate very rapidly in a logarithmic fashion but eventually the multiplication rate slows down and the population becomes composed mostly of cells in the quiescent state. These quiescent cells are fully viable and capable of renewed proliferation under appropriate conditions, i.e., decreased cell number.

There is generalized agreement concerning the increased sensitivity of rapidly proliferating tumors to most anticancer regimens with respect to the inadequate response shown by tumors with low proliferating fractions (CLARKSON 1974; VAN PUTTEN 1974; TUBIANA et al. 1977; ZUBROD 1969). These clinical conclusions are supported by a vast array of experimental evidence obtained in a variety of systems ranging from bacterial and mammalian cell cultures to transplanted rodent tumors (BRUCE et al. 1966; DREWINKO et al. 1981 b; EPIFANOVA 1977; PITTILO et al. 1970; RAJEWSKY 1975; RAY et al. 1973; SCHABEL 1969; VALERIOTE and VAN PUTTEN 1975; VAN PUTTEN 1974; VAN PUTTEN et al. 1972).

The difference in cell killing efficacy is generally attributed to the ability of quiescent cells to repair or bypass drug-induced damage before it becomes a fixed, lethal event at mitosis (HAGEMANN et al. 1973; HAHN et al. 1973; PAPIRMEISTER and DAVIDSON 1965; ROBERTS et al. 1971) and can sometimes be overcome by massive doses of the antitumor agent (VALERIOTE 1973).

III. Age-Dependent Response

For the exponentially growing populations, the position in the cycle occupied by a cell at the time of drug administration is an important determinant for survival. Most antitumor drugs demonstrate significant differences in efficacy at each stage of the cell cycle (the so-called age-dependent response) (BHUYAN et al. 1972; DREWINKO and BARLOGIE 1976 b; MADOC-JONES and MAURO 1975) and these age-dependent differences may have a significant impact in the development of improved clinical chemotherapeutic regimens. The kinetics of cell killing may guide dose and time manipulations of clinical scheduling for different combinations of drugs given simultaneously or in sequence. Thus, it is theoretically possible to accumulate a large population of cells in a given stage of the cell cycle and utilize a second drug (or combination of drugs) the main killing effect of which occurs in that specific stage to sterilize the tumor more efficiently. On the other hand, agents with widely different activities in distinct stages of the cycle can be combined in a paired delivery to attack all of the cells composing the tumor population.

IV. Cell Synchronization

To analyze cell age-dependent cytotoxic and cell cycle traverse perturbation effects, so-called synchronized cells are exposed to the antitumor agents at regular intervals throughout their cell-cycle transit. Strictly, a synchronized population of cells is that in which all elements pass through a specific point of the cycle at the same time. Current available methods impose several technical limitations in the achievement of this purpose and no technique provides more than partial synchrony. Thus, although cells in one stage of the cycle may predominate, the population is actually spread at various points through that stage and even other stages of the cycle. Therefore, the operational term "synchronization" does not imply the phasing of all cellular processes, but refers to the simultaneous manifestation of some distinct marker, such as the synthesis of DNA or the presence of a mitotic apparatus. While the cell population may appear phased with respect to one biochemical process, other biochemical activities, which should normally occur in subsequent stages, may have already taken place during the interval required to obtain the "synchronous" population, a phenomenon manifested by a shorter cell cycle following the synchronization procedure (BARLOGIE et al. 1976a;

DREWINKO et al. 1973; DETHLEFSEN 1977; DETHLEFSEN and RILEY 1973a, b; ROTI ROTI and DETHLEFSEN 1975; TILL et al. 1963). In addition, synchronization is an ephemeral event since mammalian cells have random rates of transit through the cycle stages, and synchrony rapidly decays, preventing clear-cut interpretation of results obtained after the release of the synchrony induction. Hence, diversities in age-dependent response patterns obtained by different investigators on different cell types may only reflect an assortment of factors unrelated to actual cell cycle sensitivity (i.e., methods used to synchronize cells, degree of synchrony achieved, rate of synchrony decay, etc.).

V. Cell Cycle Perturbation

In addition to cell kill, most antitumor agents exert a profound influence on the traverse rate through one or more stages of the cell cycle. These cycle traverse perturbation effects are not necessarily associated with the killing activity of the drug as they may be elicited at concentrations much lower than those required for cytotoxicity and can be induced in stages of the cycle where cytotoxicity is minimal (DREWINKO and BARLOGIE 1976b; MADOC-JONES and MAURO 1970). The manifestations of the perturbation effect can range from short, reversible delays in the traverse through a particular stage of the cell cycle to complete irreversible blocks in transit. The magnitude and duration of these effects depend on drug concentration, length of treatment, and stage of the cycle occupied by the cells at the time of drug administration. In addition, many agents may exert additional perturbations at different points of the cell cycle as the concentration and/or the length of exposure is increased (BERGERAT et al. 1979; BARLOGIE and DREWINKO 1976, 1980; DREWINKO and BARLOGIE 1976a; DETHLEFSEN et al. 1979).

Evaluation of drug-induced cell cycle perturbation effects was difficult, tedious, and inconclusive until the advent of flow cytometry (FCM) technology about 20 years ago. This technology, coupled to development of ancillary methodology for cell preparation and staining, provided the means for rapid analysis of a large number of cells concerning their distribution throughout the entire cell cycle, either during normal growth or under the influence of antitumor drugs. For details of these methods the reader is referred to the excellent treatise on the subject edited by MELAMED et al. (1979). Suffice it to say that the method is based on the stoichiometric staining of cellular DNA with a fluorescent dye. The stained cells are then passed in a narrow flow sheath through a sensor that measures light pulses elicited by the activation of the fluorescent dye of each cell. The magnitude of the pulse is considered directly proportional to the DNA content of the examined cell, and thus a histogram revealing the distribution of the cell population in the various compartments of the cell cycle (based on DNA content) is generated. However, the analysis cannot yet distinguish quiescent (G_0) from G_1 cells, and cells in G_2-phase from those in mitosis as their DNA content is nearly identical. An important assumption of this method for the study of drug-treated cells is that stoichiometric affinity of DNA to the fluorescent ligand will be the same throughout the cell cycle before and after drug treatment, an assumption which may not always be true (ALABASTER et al. 1978). By following fluctuations in compartment distribution during and after terminating drug treatment, perturbations in cycle traverse and accumulations in particular stages can be demonstrated. However, in certain cases where perturbations may occur at various sites of the cycle, additional maneuvers consisting of continuous labeling with [^{3}H] thymidine (dThd) and/or treatment with antimitotic drugs (i.e., Colcemid) must be applied to the cells in order to detect subtle or multiple changes occurring simultaneously (BARLOGIE and DREWINKO 1980; BERGERAT et al. 1979; DOSIK et al. 1978, 1981). Under these conditions, changes of the rate of entry into the various stages can be analyzed from variations in the evacuation rate of the preceding compartment or from the increments in the proportion of labeled cells.

VI. In Vitro Systems

Cell cultures provide a rapid, efficient, and economic assay system for the screening of antitumor agents, allowing elucidation of the mode of action of a drug in a controlled, systematic fashion with a high degree of resolution. The main assumption for in vitro studies with chemotherapeutic agents is that the responses of cultured cells will reflect that of in vivo cells *once* the drug reaches the neoplastic elements, thus circumventing the pharmacokinetics determinants of tumor response (i.e., absorption, transportation, combination, transformation, and degradation). While a direct translation from in vitro to in vivo systems is not possible, many survival and cycle progression perturbation responses of proliferating mammalian cells are reasonably similar in the two situations (DETHLEFSEN 1979; KANEKO and LE PAGE 1978; MADOC-JONES and MAURO 1970; ROSENBLUM et al. 1975). One great advantage of utilizing in vitro systems is that they afford the possibility of studying the behavior of cells of human origin, thus providing a closer approximation to the response of the desired clinical target: the human cancer cell. By applying the appropriate methods, dose and time-dependent effects can be analyzed quantitatively, since the exact concentration of the drug bathing the cells and the duration of exposure are known, and these quantitative responses can be used to compare the efficacy of different agents on a given cell type or the activity of a specific drug on different cell classes.

A major limitation of experiments involving in vitro cells resides in the difficulty of extrapolating information obtained on cultured exponentially growing cells to the expected responses of tumor cells in vivo, where large fractions of the population may be in the quiescent state (G_0 cells) (DREWINKO et al. 1981 b; RAJEWSKY 1975; STEEL 1977; VAN PUTTEN 1974). As indicated above, quiescent cells are usually less sensitive than proliferating cells to the lethal activity of most antitumor drugs. However, recent investigations suggest the usefulness of utilizing stationary phase cultures as an adequate in vitro model for the biological behavior of in vivo neoplasms with low fractions of proliferating cells (low growth fractions) (BARRANCO and NOVAK 1974; BARRANCO et al. 1979; BHUYAN et al. 1977; HAHN and LITTLE 1972; MAURO et al. 1974a). Cultures in stationary phase can be obtained by a variety of methods, all of which lead the exponentially growing cells to a state where net increments in cell number can no longer be demonstrated. By comparing the survival response of cells treated in these two phases of in vitro growth, a more clinically relevant evaluation of cell-drug interactions can be obtained.

VII. Cell Death

Drug-induced cell killing is the result of an interplay between the type, extent, and duration of the damaging effect caused by a drug to critical biosynthetic pathways or subcellular structures and the capacity of living elements to bypass or repair such damage. Because of this interplay, a lethally damaged cell may divide several times before the entire progency perishes from the damage inherited from the single ancestor (EHMANN and WHEELER 1979; PEEL and COWEN 1972). Conversely, cells showing severe metabolic and kinetic alterations immediately following drug exposure may recover and subsequently proliferate as if they had never been exposed to an injurious agent. For these reasons, cellular death in proliferating populations is best evaluated by the permanent loss of the reproductive integrity of the individual cells (BHUYAN et al. 1976; DREWINKO et al. 1979 b; ROPER and DREWINKO 1976, 1979). In vitro, this permanent loss is reflected in the inability of cells to proliferate indefinitely, forming colonies (clonogenic capacity) under the appropriate experimental conditions (PUCK and MARCUS 1955). In vitro clone formation implies a minimum of five to six (but usually eight to ten) cell divisions which represent at least at 32- to 64- (and up to 1 000-)fold increment in the number of cells initially exposed to the drug. Under these circumstances, colony formation is independent of the initial biochemical or transit-delay effects caused by the agent on the treated cell (for example, a colony may be small but will still represent the progeny of a surviving cell) and the assessment will be more accurate but the lethal efficacy of the agent may appear decreased.

VIII. Cell Cycle Traverse Rate-Dependent Lethality

In addition to the position of the cell cycle at the time of drug administration, the rate of progression through that cycle stage may also be an important factor determining the extent of cell kill. The in vitro lethal efficacy to sarcoma 180 cells by the S-phase-specific agents, hydroxyurea and araC (cytosine arabinoside), was noted to be directly related to the rate of DNA synthesis (FORD and SHACKNEY 1977, SHACKNEY et al. 1978). Methylglyoxal bis-guanyl-hydrazone (methyl-GAG), an inhibitor of polyamine synthesis needed for cell efflux from G_1-phase, and various protein synthesis inhibitors protected against myelosuppression and intestinal toxicity induced by nitrogen mustard, araC, hydroxyurea, and methotrexate (BEN-ISHAY and FARBER 1975; CAPIZZI 1974; CAPIZZI et al. 1971; LIEBERMAN et al. 1970; PARDEE and JAMES 1975; RUPNIAK and PAUL 1980; VERBIN et al. 1973; WEISSBERG et al. 1978).

It was theorized that this protective effect may be the result of cell cycle arrest of normal tissues, while the tumor cells continued to proliferate, possibly at a slower rate, thus remaining sensitive to cytotoxic therapy (BRADLEY et al. 1977; DUBROW et al. 1979; PARDEE and JAMES 1975; ROZENGURT and PO 1976; RUPNIAK and PAUL 1980). A similar mechanism may underlie the reduction by interferon of araC inactivation of colony forming units (CFUc) (GREENBERG and MOSNY 1977). Thus, cell cycle perturbation effects caused by an agent may counterbalance the lethal activity of that agent or that of another drug administered simultaneously, as to impose a limiting effect on a potentially greater cytotoxic response (DETHLEFSEN et al. 1975; SKIPPER 1970).

B. Materials and Methods

Two established human cell lines and a Chinese hamster ovary (CHO) cell line were used in these studies. One of the human cultures was an IgA-producing lymphoid cell line (T_1 cells) derived from a patient with lymphocytic lymphoma (DREWINKO et al. 1978 a). The other human line was a carcinoembryonic antigen-producing line (LoVo cells) derived from the metastatic nodule of a patient with colon carcinoma (DREWINKO et al. 1978 b). For details on culture methods, growth kinetics properties, and xenogeneic transplantation of these cells, the reader is referred to previously published data (DREWINKO et al. 1976, 1978 a, b; STRAGAND et al. 1980). Cytotoxic drug effects were measured by the inhibition of colony formation assay (ROPER and DREWINKO 1976, 1979).

Survival curve patterns were classified into five types: simple exponential (type A), biphasic exponential (type B), threshold exponential (type C), exponential plateau (type D), and ineffectual (type E) (DREWINKO et al. 1979 b). Because in many instances the shape of the survival curve obtained for LoVo cells in stationary phase differed substantially from that determined for the exponentially growing counterpart, we arbitrarily calculated the differences in efficacy of these two classes of cells as the ratio of the survival levels determined at the mid-range point of concentrations used for each drug (DREWINKO et al. 1981 b). Age-dependent cell survival was investigated by incubating synchronized cells (DREWINKO and BARLOGIE 1976 B; DREWINKO et al. 1973, 1978 b) with increasing concentrations of drug at regular intervals throughout the cell cycle. Cell cycle pertubation effects were monitored by serial DNA histograms obtained by FCM as previously described (BARLOGIE and DREWINKO 1976, 1978, 1980; BARLOGIE et al. 1976 a, b). Histograms were evaluated by a modification (JOHNSTON et al. 1978) of the model of FRIED (1976). All drugs (listed in Table 1) were obtained from the Cancer Chemotherapy Branch, Division of Cancer Treatment, National Cancer Institute, United States.

Table 1. List of antitumor agents

Common Name	Chemical Name	Abbreviation	NSC #
Adriamycin	14-Hydroxydaunorubicin	ADR	123127
Alanosine	2-Amino-3-(hydroxynitroso-amino)proprionic acid	–	153353
AMSA	Methanesulfon-*M*-anisidide, 4′ (acridinyl-amino)	AMSA	24992
Mitoxantrone	1,4-Dihydro-5,8-bis{{2-{(2-hydroxyethyl)amino -ethyl} amino}9,10-anthracenedione dihydrochloride	DHAQ.Cl	301739
Anguidine	Diacetoxyscirpenol	–	141537
Bleomycin	–	BLEO	125066
Camptothecin	–	CS	100880
Carmustine	1,3-bis(2-Chloroethyl)-1-nitrosourea	BCNU	409962
cis-Acid	4-(3-(2-Chloroethyl)-3-nitroso-ureido)-*cis*-cyclohexanecarboxylic acid	*cis*-Acid	153174

Table 1. (continued)

Common Name	Chemical Name	Abbreviation	NSC #
Cisplatin	*cis*-Diamminedichloroplatinum	*cis*-DDP	119875
Cytosine arabinoside	1-β-D-Arabinofuranosyl-cytosine	araC	63878
Epipodophyllotoxin (etoposide)	4'Demethylepipodophyllotoxin 9-(4,6-0-ethylidiene-β-D-glucopyranoside	VP-16-213	141540
5-Fluorouracil	–	5-FU	19893
Hycanthone	–	–	142982
Hydroxyurea	–	HU	32065
Lomustine	1-(2-Chloro-ethyl)-3-cyclohexyl-1-nitrosourea	CCNU	79037
Maytansine	–	MAYT	153858
Melphalan	3-[*p*-[bis(2-Chloroethyl) amino]phenyl]-L-alanine	L-PAM	740
Methotrexate	Glutamic acid,*N*-[*P*-[(2,4-diamino-6-pteridinyl)methyl]–methylamino]benzoyl]	MTX	740
Methyl-GAG	Methylglyoxal bis-guanyl-hydrazone	Methyl-GAG	32946
Mitomycin C	–	Mito C	26980
PALA	*N*-(phosphonacetyl)-L-aspartate	PALA	224131
PCNU	1-(2-Chloroethyl)-3-(2,6-dioxo-3-piperidyl)-1-nitrosourea	PCNU	95466
Peptichemio	*m*-[Di(2-chloroethyl)amino]-L-pheylalanine, multipeptide complex	PC	247516
Prednisolone	Pregna-1,4-diene-3,20-dione, 11β,17,21-trihydroxy	–	9900
Prospidine	–	–	166100
Pyrazolo-imidazole	2,3-Dihydro-1-*H*-imidazo-(1,2-b)-pyrazole	IMPY	51143
Rubidazone	Daunorubicin benzoylhydrazone hydrochloride	RUB	164011
Semustine	1-(2-Chloroethyl)-3-trans-(4-methyl-cyclohexyl)-1-nitrosourea	MeCCNU	95441
Transplatin	*trans*-Diamminedichloroplatinum	*trans*-DDP	–
Vinblastine	–	VBL	49842
Vincristine	–	VCR	67574
Vindesine	Desacetyl vinblastine amide sulfate	VDS	245467
Yoshi 864	1-Propanol, 3,3'-iminodi-, dimethanesulfonate (ester), hydrochloride	–	102627

C. Results

I. Proliferating Versus Nonproliferating Cells

Survival after drug-treatment for 1 h was compared for LoVo cells in exponential growth (2-3 days after subculture) and in stationary phase (8 days after subculture) (DREWINKO et al. 1979a, 1981b). Four drugs [*N*-phosphonacetyl-L-aspartate (PALA), pyrazolo-imidazole (IMPY), araC, and anguidine] failed to kill either cell class even at concentrations of 1,000 µg/ml when administered for 1 h, but were lethal when delivered in continuous treatment for periods longer than the duration of S-phase.

Cisplatin (*cis*-DDP) was more effective (efficacy ratio = 2.3) on cells in stationary phase than on exponentially growing cells after 1 h of treatment. This effect resulted from the abrogation of the shoulder region of the type C survival curve, while the slope was maintained essentially intact. Vindesine (VDS) was also more effective on cells in stationary phase (efficacy ratio = 18.9), but in this case the type B pattern of the survival curve was similar for both cell classes.

Methyl-GAG, hycanthone, and vinblastine (VBL) had a similar low killing effect (less than 90%) on both exponentially growing and stationary phase cells. Radiomimetic agents [mitomycin C, 1,3-bis(2-chloroethyl)-1-nitrosourea (BCNU), 1-(2-chloroethyl)-3-(2,6-dioxo-3-piperidyl)-1-nitrosourea (PCNU) and *cis*-acid] displayed the same powerful effect (greater than 90% cell kill) and the same type C survival curve on both cell classes. Four anthracenedione derivatives (NSC #279836; 287513; 299195; and 301739) also had a similar activity on both exponentially growing and stationary phase cells.

Agents considered to be cell cycle stage-sensitive and to act primarily on cells positioned in S-phase [5-fluorouracil (5-FU), methotrexate (MTX), and hydroxyurea (HU)] were considerably less lethal on stationary phase cells than on exponentially growing cells (Table 2). In fact, MTX completely failed to kill cells in stationary phase of growth. Prospidine, an antitumor drug with an unknown mechanism of action, and alanosine, an aspartic acid analog, showed greater than 95% cell kill on exponentially growing cells, when used at high concentrations (5,000 and 300 µg/ml respectively). Both agents had a marked decrease in lethal efficacy (efficacy ratio = 11.3 and 26 respectively) when applied to cells in stationary phase. Mitotic inhibitors [vincristine (VCR), maytansine (MAYT), and

Table 2. Differential efficacy of antitumor drugs on proliferating and nonproliferating LoVo cells

Drugs	Stationary/Exponential[a]
5-FU	1.3
MTX	1.9
HU	1.3
VCR	2.5
MAYT	2.6
VP-16	3.2
ADR	2.5
RUB	3.3
AMSA	3.8
trans-DDP	3.0
BLEO	8.0

[a] Ratio of survivals at mid-range dose point

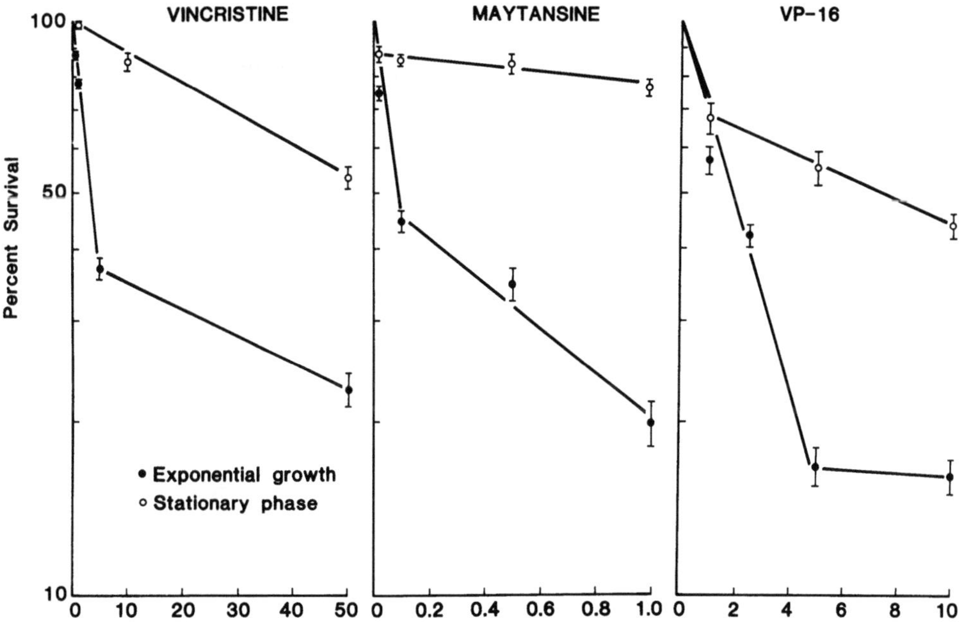

Fig. 1. Survival of proliferating and nonproliferating LoVo cells treated for 1 h with mitotic inhibitors. In this and subsequent charts, data points are mean values of at least two separate experiments, each with three replicates per concentration. *Bars* are standard errors

epipodophyllotoxin (VP-16)] all had similar type B survival curves and in all instances their efficacy on stationary phase cells was about 2.5- to 3-fold less than on exponentially growing cells (Fig. 1).

Similar differences in efficacy between exponential and stationary phase cells were observed for DNA-intercalating agents such as anthracycline derivatives [Adriamycin (ADR) and rubidazone (RUB)] and 9-acridinylamino-methansulfon-m-anisidide (AMSA). The ineffective transisomer of diamminedichloroplatinum was even less active when used on stationary cells, and the antibiotic bleomycin (BLEO) also showed markedly less activity (efficacy ratio = 8) on stationary phase cells than on exponentially growing ones.

II. Age-Dependent Survival Response

When synchronized cells were treated with antitumor drugs for 1 h at different stages of the cell cycle, a variety of age-dependent response patterns were observed. Both prednisolone and camptothecin had similar quantitative efficacies in G_2- and G_1-phases. However, while camptothecin displayed its greatest efficacy on cells in S-phase, such cells were completely refractory to prednisolone. HU and 5-FU, drugs considered to be S-phase specific, exerted their maximal lethal effect in early S. However, their efficacy decreased but did not totally disappear as the cells moved into G_2- and G_1-phase. MTX killed only about 20% of the cells in early S-phase, was even less effective in late S-phase, and totally ineffectual in G_2- and G_1-phase. Treatment with 500 µg/ml araC, IMPY, or PALA for 1 h

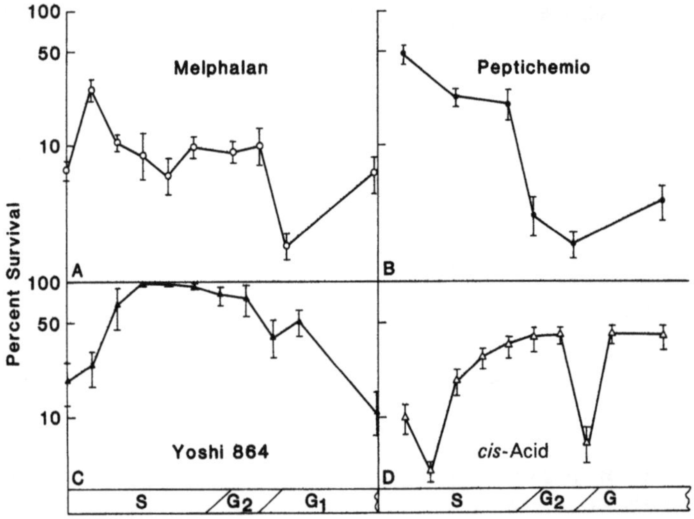

Fig. 2. Survival of synchronized T_1 cells treated for 1 h with alkylating agents: melphalan and peptichemio, 2.5 μg/ml; Yoshi 864 and *cis*-acid, 50 μg/ml

failed to decrease cell survival at every stage of the cell cycle. However, synchronized cells exposed for 14 h (length of S-phase) to these drugs, immediately after the synchronizing agent was removed, demonstrated a greater than 90% decrease in survival. Alanosine had the greatest lethal effect in S-phase but also killed cells in G_1 and G_2. VCR and VDS were equally effective in all stages of the cell cycle of synchronized LoVo cells.

There were considerable differences in the age-dependent response to alkylating agents (Fig. 2). While melphalan was most effective in early G_1-phase, peptichemio, its congener, had a greater efficacy in G_2-phase. Both agents were considerably less effective in S-phase. In contrast, Yoshi 864 and *cis*-acid, the latter an alkylating and carboamylating water-soluble nitrosourea derivative, had their greatest efficacy in early S-phase. Their efficacy persisted well into mid-S-phase, decreased during late S-phase, and increased again in late G_1-phase for Yoshi 864 and in G_2-phase for *cis*-acid.

Three nitrosourea derivatives killed T_1 cells in all stages of the cell cycle but each exerted preferential killing effects at different phases: BCNU in early S and G_2, methyl-1-(2-chloroethyl)3-cyclohexyl-1-nitrosourea (CCNU) in early S, and CCNU in early S and G_1. In the case of BCNU, age-dependent changes were reflected in modifications of both the extent of the shoulder region and the slope of the exponential part of the type C dose-dependent survival curve. Only the length of the shoulder region varied for cells treated with CCNU and only the slope changed for cells treated with methyl-CCNU. In contrast to the marked age-dependent cytotoxicities observed for nitrosourea derivatives on T_1 cells, LoVo cells exposed to BCNU, and *cis*-acid showed no significant increase in cell killing as a function of position in the cycle.

In many instances, the particular age-dependent pattern defined for a given drug did not change regardless of the concentration level employed in the analysis. For other agents, cell cycle stage sensitivity was either intensified or attenuated as the concentration of the agent was increased.

III. Cell Cycle Perturbation

1. Asynchronous Cell Populations

Seventeen agents (listed in Table 3) were investigated and each manifested individual changes in cell cycle perturbation that varied in a nonuniform manner as a function of treatment duration and concentration. The perturbation effects of each agent were too complex to be listed individually. Yet, there were sufficient similarities for many agents to permit grouping into general patterns.

Virtually every antitumor agent studied by us caused a delay in G_2 traverse leading to accumulation of cells in that stage. The onset, magnitude, and reversibility of this effect depended on both the length of treatment and the concentration of the drug. With increasing treatment periods and/or concentrations the delay became more pronounced, frequently yielding a complete block in traverse which for some agents was irreversible, leading to eventual cell death in that stage.

Table 3. Synopsis of major cytokinetic effects of antitumor drugs

Group classification	Drug	Traverse delay					
		G_1	S	Q_s	G_2	R	"Frozen" cycle
Intercalating	ADR	++	+	No	++++	No	No
	ADR-DNA	++	+	No	+++	No	No
	RUB	++	+	No	+++	No	No
	AMSA	–	–	No	+++	No	No
Alkylating	L-PAM	–	++	No	+++	No[a]	No
	Peptichemio	–	++	No	+++	No[a]	No
	Mito C	+	–	No	+++	Yes	Yes[b]
	Yoshi 864	–	–	[c]	+++	Yes	No
	cis-DDP	+	++	Yes	++++	No	Yes[b]
Antimitotics	VP-16	+	++	Yes[b]	+++	Yes[d]	Yes[b]
	VBL	–	+[b]	No	+++	Yes	No
	VCR	–	+	No	+++	Yes[d]	No
	VDS	–	+	No	+++	Yes[d]	No
Metabolic inhibitors	IMPY	++	+++	No	+[b]	Yes	No
	PALA	+++	++	[c]	+[b]	Yes	No
	Anguidine	+++	+++	Yes	+++	Yes	Yes
Undetermined	BLEO	–	+	Yes	+++	Yes	No

Q_s, marked discrepancy between LI and FCM-determined S-phase compartment; R, reversible G_2 block; +, slight delay; ++, moderate delay; +++, marked delay to partial block; ++++, complete block

[a] Yes at low concentrations
[b] At high concentrations
[c] Not studied
[d] Not at very high concentrations

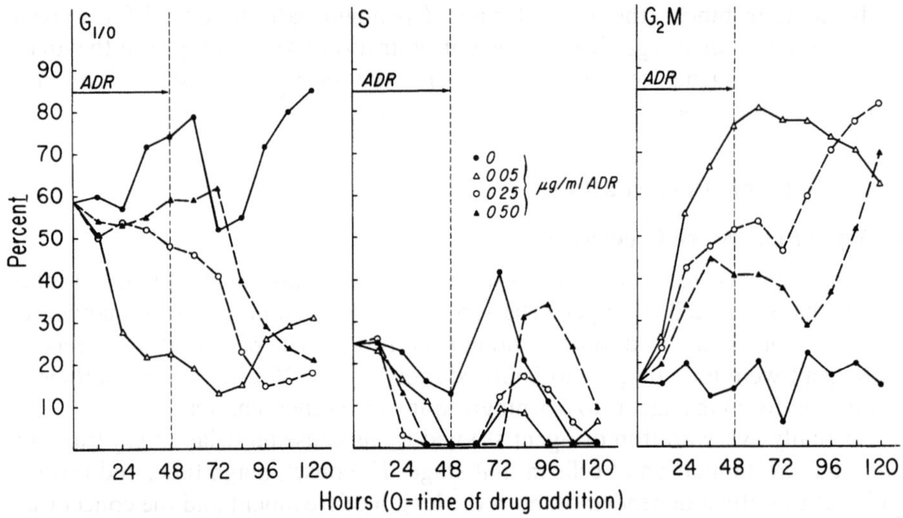

Fig. 3. Compartment distribution of asynchronous T_1 cells treated with ADR (0.05, 0.25, 0.5 μg/ml) for 48 h

Additionally, for some agents lengthier treatment periods and especially higher concentrations were also accompanied by additional delays or blocks in other stages of the cycle such as S-phase or at the G_1/S boundary.

Three anthracycline derivatives (ADR, ADR-DNA, and RUB) displayed a similar potent blocking action best exemplified by the effects induced by ADR (Fig. 3). Cells continuously incubated with 0.05 μg/ml demonstrated a steady decrease in the size of both $G_{1/0}$ and S compartments and an increase in the G_2+M compartment. The mitotic index (MI) was less than 0.1% for all drug-treated samples, indicating that the observed increase of the G_2+M fraction of the DNA histogram was due to accumulation of cells in G_2-phase. Removal of the drug at 48 h did not change this pattern, and the accumulation of cells in G_2 progressed, peaking at 60 h. Minimum values of $G_{1/0}$ and S-phase cells were reached at 72 and 48 h respectively. Treatment with 0.1 μg/ml induced similar compartment changes but at a slower rate, while depletion of the S-phase compartment proceeded slightly faster. Different patterns of compartment distribution were noted for cells incubated with both 0.25 and 0.50 μg/ml. No substantial change in the size of the $G_{1/0}$ compartment was observed until removal of the drug, but the percentage of S-phase cells decreased rapidly, reaching minimum values (<1%) at about 36 h, while the G_2 compartment increased to values of 40%–45%. Twenty-four hours after drug removal a steady decline of the $G_{1/0}$ fraction was observed, accompanied by a sudden rise in the S-phase compartment size from less than 1% to values of 20%–40%. These cells subsequently entered into G_2, demonstrated by a second increase of the G_2 compartment to 75%–82% 72 h after drug removal.

When treatment was interrupted after 1,3 and 12 h, the accumulation of cells in G_2+M occurred mostly at the expense of $G_{1/0}$ cells regardless of concentration

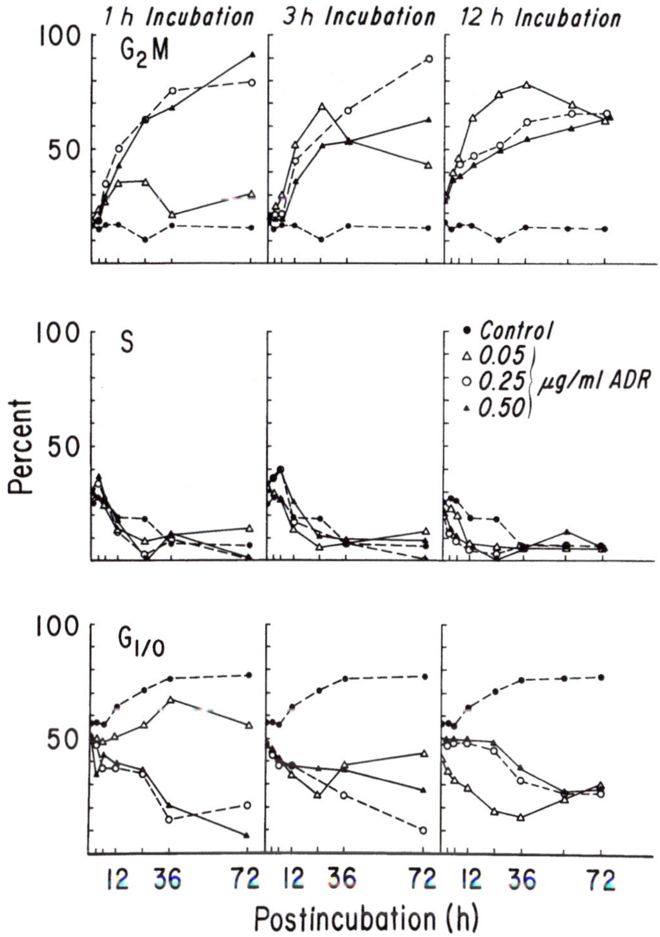

Fig. 4. Compartment distribution of asynchronous T_1 cells treated with ADR (0.05, 0.25, 0.5 µg/ml) for 1, 3, and 12 h

and exposure time (Fig. 4). Incubation with 0.05 µg/ml for 1 and 3 h caused a treatment increase of cells in G_2+M 24 h after drug release. Prolongation of treatment with 0.05 µg/ml to 12 h further increased the magnitude of G_2+M accumulation, which was maintained for the 72-h period of observation after drug removal. Higher concentrations (0.25 and 0.5 µg/ml) were required to induce a substantial accumulation of cells in G_2+M after 1 h of incubation. An inverse correlation of drug concentration with time interval required for maximal G_2 accumulation was noticed after 3 and 12 h of incubation. There was no significant difference between the labeling index and S-phase compartments determined by FCM for any concentration or incubation time period.

Although the perturbation effects of ADR-DNA and RUB were even more closely related to concentration and incubation time, the magnitude of their G_2 block was decreased.

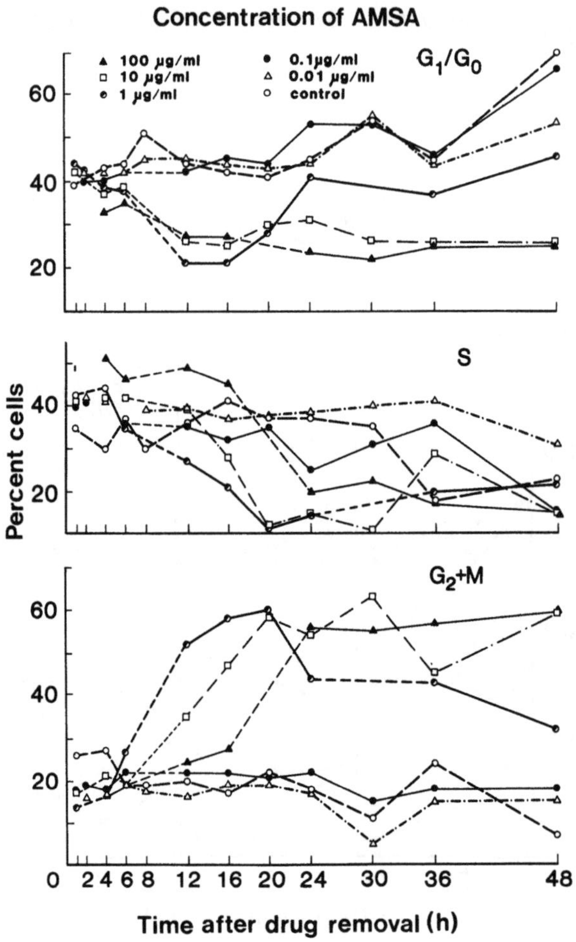

Fig. 5. Compartment distribution of asynchronous LoVo cells following treatment with various concentrations of AMSA for 1 h

Treatment for 1 h with another intercalating agent, AMSA, showed marked concentration-dependent fluctuations in subsequent cell cycle traverse rates (Fig. 5). Treatment with 0.01 and 0.1 µg/ml induced a steady decrease of the $G_{1/0}$ and S-phase compartments mirrored by an ever-increasing accumulation of cells in G_2, peaking 20 h after drug removal. At this time the magnitude of the G_2 compartment decreased while that of the $G_{1/0}$ compartment increased.

The effects of three alkylating agents [L-phenylalanine mustard (L-PAM), peptichemio, and Yoshi 864] were very similar and can be illustrated by the changes induced by melphalan. Treatment with 0.05 and 0.25 µg/ml of melphalan did not induce significant changes in DNA distribution, even when drug exposure was extended to 48 h. Incubation with ≧0.5 µg/ml resulted in an increase of the G_2+M compartment associated with a diminution of the $G_{1/0}$ population. The mitotic index at the time of peak G_2+M accumulation never exceeded control values.

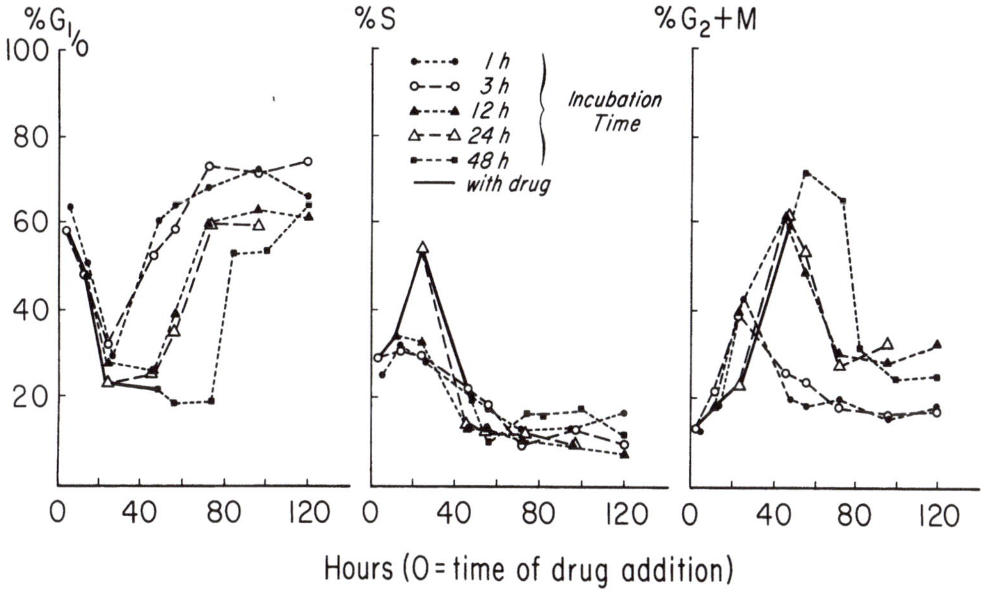

Fig. 6. Effect of melphalan (1.0 μg/ml) on the compartment distribution of exponentially growing T_1 cells. The *solid lines* indicate the presence of the drug; the *dotted lines* connect values obtained after drug removal

Treatment with 0.5 μg/ml induced completely reversible compartment shifts, independent of the length of drug exposure. Maximum $G_{1/0}$ evacuation and G_2 accumulation were observed 12 h after release from a 12-h treatment interval. The S-phase compartment showed a transient increase at the end of 24-h treatment and returned to pretreatment values in spite of continuous drug exposure.

Magnitude and duration of G_2 accumulation and $G_{1/0}$ evacuation of cells treated with 1 μg/ml clearly correlated to exposure time (Fig. 6). Treatment for 48 h induced transient compartment shifts with almost complete evacuation of $G_{1/0}$ with a transient rise of the fraction at 24 h followed by an increase of G_2. Earlier drug removal showed essentially the same decline of the $G_{1/0}$ compartment. However, termination of drug exposure after 1, 3, and 12 h led to a more rapid increase of the G_2 compartment without a significant preceding increase of the S-phase fraction. Twenty-four-hour drug exposure induced initial compartment shifts similar to that of a 48-h treatment. Incubation with 2.5 μg/ml of melphalan induced further enhanced and more persistent compartment transitions with little reversibility of these effects after 1- and 3-h treatments. The rate of efflux out of $G_{1/0}$ was equal for all exposure time studies. At the end of a 24-h drug exposure, an increase of cells in both S and G_2 was observed. Twenty-four hours after drug removal, the majority of cells had moved into G_2 with few cells left in $G_{1/0}$ and in S-phase. This DNA distribution profile was maintained during the ensuing 3 days while the untreated population was approaching the DNA distribution of cells in stationary phase. The course of S-phase compartment size fluctuations showed similar patterns after 24 and 48 h of incubation with 2.5 μg/ml of melphalan; in particular, there was a rapid decline from 24 to 48 h, independent of further drug exposure. While the rates of G_2 accumulation were essentially equal for all incubating times, the onset of G_2 increment for short-term treatment (1–12 h) by 12 h. The final compartment distribution in $G_{1/0}$-, S-, and G_2-phases was a function of exposure time. Thus, with extension of incubation time, G_2 compartment size increased from 60% after 1-h treatment to 90% after 48-h treatment; the $G_{1/0}$ fraction was inversely correlated to the period of drug exposure with 40% after 1-h treatment and 15% after 48-h treatment. The S-phase fraction comprised 10% after 1-h incubation and contained about 5% for longer periods of treatment. Treatment with 5.0 µg/ml produced compartment shifts with final values for $G_{1/0}$, S, and G_2 virtually identical for all exposure times, i.e., $G_{1/0}=2\%$–10%, $S=5\%$–10%, and $G_2=85\%$–90%. The pattern of compartment changes over time essentially followed that observed after treatment with 2.5 µg/ml. However, 28-h drug exposure maintained a prolonged S-phase accumulation with a rapid decline after drug removal. Likewise, the onset of G_2 accumulation was delayed for 24 more hours until drug release. Evacuation of $G_{1/0}$ was slightly slowed down after incubation for >12 h. There was no discrepancy between the LI and DNA histogram-derived S-phase compartment size for any concentration and exposure time studied.

Cell cycle traverse perturbations induced by a fourth alkylating agent, mito C, were even more complex. Figure 7 gives a synopsis of DNA compartment changes effected by the various treatment conditions. For the lowest concentration (0.1 µg/ml), 1-h treatment was virtually ineffective, while $\geqq 12$-h exposure produced a transient S-phase accumulation followed by an increase of ccells with a G_2 DNA content to a maximum of 50%. Increase in concentration to 0.5 µg/ml produced cell cycle effects comparable to those noted after treatment with 0.1 µg/ml, but after a shorter exposure time. After 24-h and 48-h treatment, there appeared to be a persistence of cells in S-phase (40%–50%), along with a larger retention of G_1 cells (20%–30%), both accounting for less pronounced increases of cells in G_2-phase in cases of prolonged drug exposure. Treatment with 50 µg/ml seemed to freeze the initial cycle distribution in cases of $\geqq 24$-h incubation. Treatment for 1 h produced cycle distribution changes very similar to those that occurred after 3-h treatment with the immediately lower concentration (1.0 µg/ml). Treatment for 3 and 12 h effectively delayed $G_{1/0}$ evacuation and maintained an S-phase accumulation of 40%–60%, thus progressively reducing the rate and magnitude of G_2 accumulation. Thus, from the point of view of equal efficacy of cycle perturbation effects, comparable interference with S- and G_2-phase traverse could be effected by different concentrations of mito C, provided that treatment duration was modified accordingly. Smaller exposure doses (above the *shaded area* of Fig. 7) are associated with largely reversible S- and G_2-phase delays, while higher exposure doses (below the *shaded area*) generate progressively irreversible accumulations of cells in S-phase and prevent G_1-S transition, thus ultimately leading to a "frozen" cell cycle distribution state.

Cell cycle distribution changes of such a complex nature, with different perturbation sites as a function of exposure dose, can be more readily appreciated in an experiment using continuous exposure to both mito C and Colcemid. Compared with Colcemid treatment alone, concurrent exposure to a concentration of 0.5 µg/ml of mito C was associated with an initial delay in $G_{1/0}$ evacuation, fol-

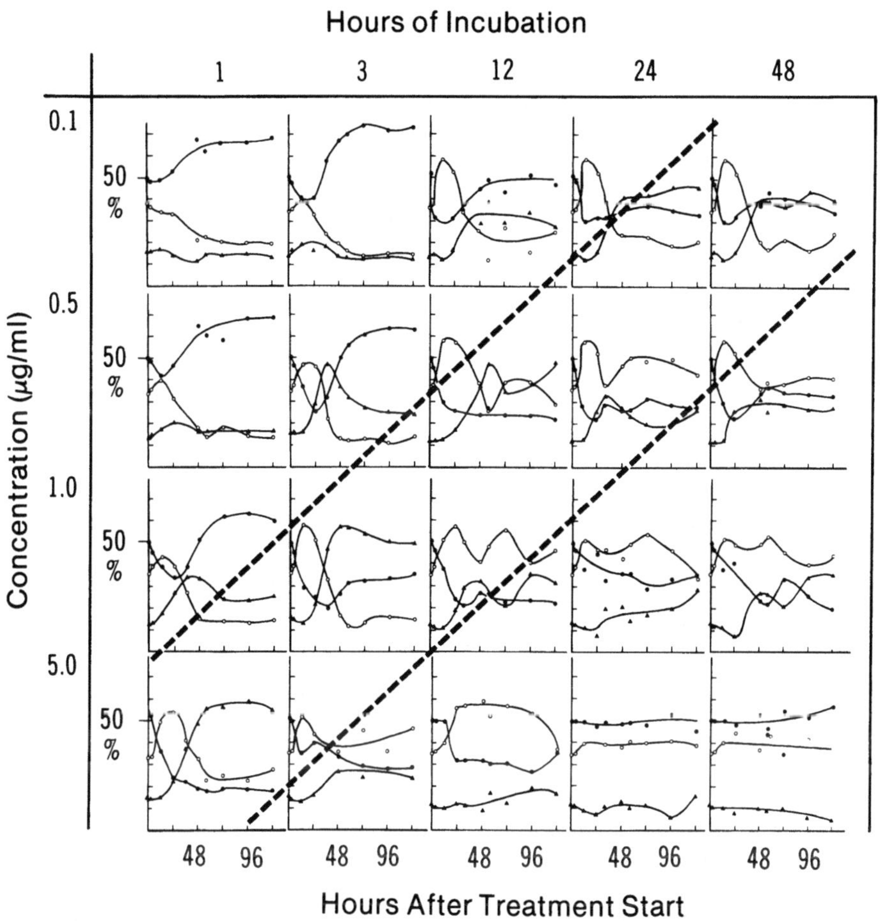

Fig. 7. Synopsis of cell cycle compartment distribution changes as a function of mito C concentration and exposure time. Curves were constructed from these original data points ●, G_1, ▲, G_2, ○, S. Smaller exposure doses (C × t) *above the upper line* are associated with largely reversible S- and G_2-phase delays. Treatment conditions *between the lines* reversibly delay S-phase traverse before institution of a partially irreversible G_2 block. Higher exposure doses (*below the lower line*) generate progressively irreversible accumulations of cells in S and prevent G_1-S transition, ultimately leading to a "frozen" cell cycle state in cases of ≧24-h treatment with 5.0 µg mito C/ml

lowed by a marked accumulation of cells in S-phase with subsequent transition into G_2-phase (Fig. 8). The MI in this experiment at the height of G_2+M accumulation was only 0.2%, suggesting an effective G_2 block. S-phase accumulation did not originate from a diffuse increase of cells throughout the entire S-phase but rather as a preferential accumulation in early S-phase. In the continuous presence of mito C this accumulation proceeded on through mid- and late S-phase into G_2-phase. Thus, under these treatment conditions, cycle progression was preferentially delayed in early S-phase, with subsequent prolonged traverse of synchronized cells into G_2-phase.

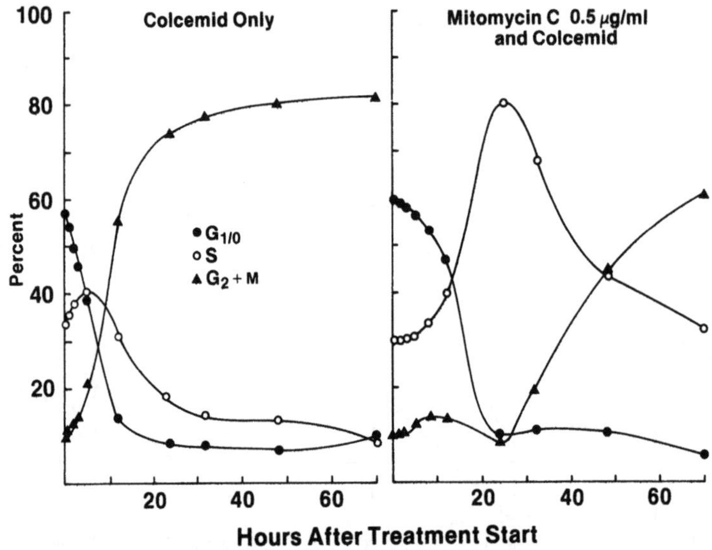

Fig. 8. Cell cycle distribution changes associated with continuous exposure of exponentially growing LoVo cells to Colcemid (0.05 µg/ml) alone (*right panel*) and in combination with mito C (0.5 µg/ml) (*left panel*)

So-called antimitotic agents (VP-16 and *Vinca* alkaloids) had a similar effect in blocking traverse through G_2-phase. During continuous incubation with 0.1 µg/ml of VP-16, a steady increase of cells in G_2 to 92% at 48 h ws observed with a concurrent decrease of both G_1- and S-phase fractions. Drug removal and incubation with fresh medium at earlier time points (1, 3, and 12 h) resulted in considerably smaller compartment changes when compared with the long-term incubation of 48 h. In all instances, the population distribution returned to control values about 48 h after drug release. No discrepancy was found between the size of the S-phase compartment determined by FCM and the labeling index (LI) for all exposure times. Continuous incubation with 0.5 µg/ml for 48 h induced a steady increase of cells in G_2, with a maximum accumulation similar to that achieved after treatment with 0.1 µg/ml. Both G_1- and S-phase compartments were almost completely evacuated at 48 h. The rate of G_2 accumulation and G_1 efflux during the 48-h exposure was equal to that observed for treatment with 0.1 µg/ml. The S-phase fraction showed a transient slight increase, peaking 12 h after drug addition. Earlier termination of drug treatment (after 1, 3, and 12 h) and subsequent culture in fresh medium showed progressively smaller degrees of G_2 accumulation and G_1 reduction. Thus, a 12-h treatment induced a G_2 maximum of 50% compared with 25% following a 3-h incubation. In addition, these short-term drug exposures resulted in a higher degree of reversibility of the G_2 accumulation resulting in a subsequent rapid increase of the G_1 fraction. There was no significant difference between the percentage values of the S-phase compartment determined by FCM and the LI.

The first kinetic perturbation effect observed during continuous incubation with 1.0 µg/ml for 48 h was a significant transient increase of cells in the S-phase compartment, reaching a maximum of 60% after 12 h. Concurrently, the G_1

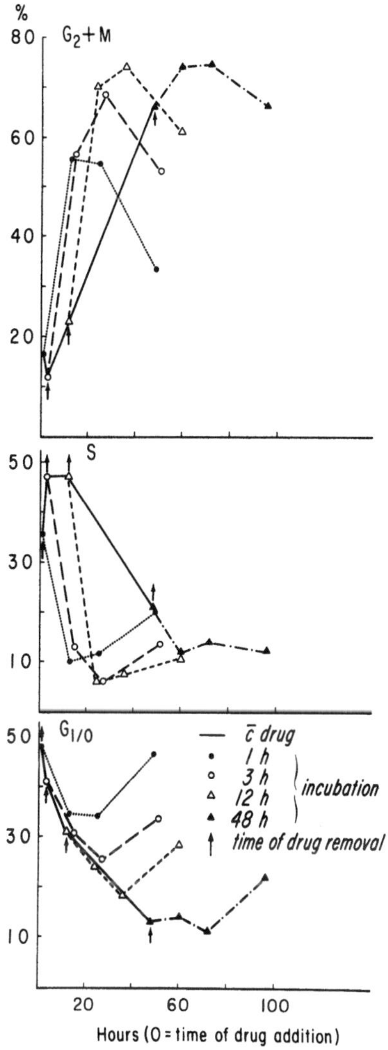

Fig. 9. Compartment distribution of asynchronous T_1 cells treated with 5 μg/ml of VP-16 for different time periods. *Arrows* indicate time of drug removal, washing, and reincubation with drug-free medium

compartment decreased, but no change of the G_2 fraction was noted. The final histogram distribution at the end of the 48-h treatment was not different from the distribution pattern obtained after treatment with 0.1 and 0.5 μg/ml. Drug release after either the 1-, 3-, or 12-h treatment resulted in an immediate evacuation of the S-phase compartment followed by a prompt increase of the G_2 fraction. Peaks of G_2 accumulation were distinctly correlated to the duration of treatment (1 h = 42%, 3 h = 57%, and 12 h = 65%). Similarly, the extent of reversibility of G_2 accumulation (with subsequent rise in G_1) was also related to the time of drug exposure. Further increase of drug concentration to 5 μg/ml (Fig. 9) showed profiles for G_1, S, and G_2 curves similar to those observed for treatment with 1.0 μg/ml.

Yet, in contrast, the slope and magnitude of G_2 accumulation during continuous 48-h treatment were reduced, and a G_2 maximum of 75% was achieved 12 h after drug release. Concomitantly, there were somewhat larger residual populations in both G_1- and S-phase (about 10% each). Drug removal after 1, 3, and 12 h did not accelerate the evacuation of the G_1 compartment when compared with prolonged treatment. G_2 peak values attained after these short-term drug exposures were again closely correlated to duration of treatment. The highest concentration was 10 μg/ml. Continuous drug exposure for 48 h induced only a slight and transient increase in the size of the S-phase compartment at the expense of the G_1 population. There was no increment of G_2 cells. Twenty-four hours after drug release a small decrease of the G_1 compartment and a similar increase of the G_2 fraction were observed. Drug release after 1- and 3-h treatments induced an immediate increase of the G_2 compartment (60%) which was only slightly smaller than that obtained with the lower concentrations of VP-16. At the end of the 12-h incubation, the increase of cells in S-phase was primarily due to accumulation in early S-phase. During the subsequent 12-h culture period in drug-free medium, a major shift from early into late S-phase (and further into G_2-phase) had occurred. Twelve hours later the G_2 maximum of 38% was reached. Thus, when compared with treatment with lower VP-16-213 concentrations, an opposite pattern of the effect of duration of treatment on maximal G_2 accumulation was observed. LI values were significantly smaller (two fold) than the corresponding S-phase fractions determined by FCM when treatment with 10 μg/ml was extended for longer than 3 h. Whereas the discrepancy between FCM-determined S fraction and LI values at the end of a 2-h incubation was resolved during the subsequent 12-h incubation in drug-free medium, the difference at the end of a 12- and 48-h treatment was maintained over the ensuing 48 h after drug removal. To test for further fluctuations in the compartment distribution subsequent to recovery from G_2 accumulation, long-term follow-up experiments over a total period of 200 h were carried out. After perturbation with 1 and 5 μg/ml for 3 h, second waves for S (at 48 h) and for G_2 (at 72 h) compartments were observed.

Three *Vinca* alkaloid derivatives (VBL, VCR, and VDS) showed a similar pattern of accumulation in the G_2+M compartment augmenting as the concentration and especially the incubation time increased. Yet, in all instances the MI was, at most, only one-third of the proportion of cells calculated by FCM (Table 4). In addition to this general pattern, each agent induced further unique changes. For low concentrations of VBL (0.05, 0,1, and 0.4 μg/ml) the accumulation in G_2 and in mitosis was accompanied by a similar decline in both G_1- and S-phase, suggesting a complete block in mitosis with no traverse delay in either G_1- or S-phase. When the concentration was increased to 50 μg/ml, evacuation of the G_1 compartment plateaued after 14 h and that of S after 24 h; in fact, there was a slight increase in cells with S-phase DNA content after 30 h. These additional delays in G_1- and S-phase transits were reflected by a decreased G_2 accumulation (in comparison to that achieved with lower drug concentrations) and especially the MI. For VCR, changes were more complex (Table 4). At a concentration of 0.05 μg/ml the G_2 accumulation proceeded for 14 h, at which time it declined to levels almost similar to that of control cells. The MI remained high while the G_1 compartment, which had steadily declined for 14 h, experienced in increment.

Table 4. DNA compartment distribution of asynchronous LoVo cells during continuous exposure to vincristine

Drug concentration (μg/ml)	Length of exposure (h)	G_1	S	G_2+M	MI	G_2
0.05	1	36.6[a]	41.0	22.4	2.5	19.9
	4	24.7	35.5	39.7	11.3	28.4
	6	18.3	33.5	48.2	19.9	28.3
	14	25.4	17.6	57.1	16.9	40.2
	24	34.0	27.0	39.0	16.6	22.4
	30	37.0	28.0	35.0	12.8	22.2
0.1	1	34.7	41.0	21.3	2.8	18.5
	4	22.7	35.8	41.5	10.4	31.1
	6	16.5	33.3	50.2	16.7	33.5
	14	19.0	19.0	62.0	19.7	48.3
	24	22.0	26.0	52.0	20.7	31.3
	30	20.0	36.0	44.0	23.0	21.0
0.4	1	33.9	41.1	24.7	3.3	21.4
	4	23.8	35.2	41.0	7.8	33.2
	6	15.4	32.8	51.6	15.1	36.5
	14	6.0	16.0	78.0	22.9	55.1
	24	10.0	16.0	74.0	50.8	23.2
	30	10.0	30.0	60.0	32.5	27.5
50	1	40.2	41.0	18.9	0.9	18.0
	4	33.0	38.2	28.7	2.4	26.3
	6	29.1	30.0	42.0	6.5	35.5
	14	16.2	21.6	61.2	4.1	57.1
	24	15.7	17.0	67.3	5.8	61.5
	30	15.3	15.7	68.9	5.4	63.5
	33	16.4	18.6	65.0	3.6	61.4

[a] Values are expressed in percent

Higher concentrations (0.1 and 0.4 μg/ml) caused a greater accumulation in G_2 and only a small decline after 14 h. The MI was even higher than that observed for 0.05 μg/ml, but only a small increment in the G_1 fraction was noted. After 24 h the S-phase compartment increased. Treatment with 50 μg/ml resulted in a complete block in G_2-phase with a very low MI and virtually no changes in the G_1- and S-phase compartments. Treatment with all concentrations of VDS yielded results very similar to those noted for VCR, although of different magnitude and with the exception that the G_2 delay induced by 50 μg/ml was not complete.

Continuous incubation with bleomycin (BLM) at concentrations of 5, 10, 25, 50, 100, and 500 μg/ml showed a concentration-dependent steady accumulation of cells in the G_2+M fraction, at the expense of both the $G_{1/0}$ and S-phase compartments, reaching 60% of the total population. After 24 h, there was no further change in the distribution of cells for any concentration. The MI of treated cells dropped drastically after 4 h, indicating that the compartment measured by FCM consisted virtually of G_2 cells. In these experiments, we noted a concentration-dependent dissociation between the percentage of cells in S-phase measured by FCM and that measured by the LI after 24-h incubation with BLM for concentrations greater than 25 μg/ml which was maintained over the ensuing period of the experiment. In other experiments, cells were incubated with 100 μg BLM/ml for 3, 6, 9, and 12 h. The drug was decanted and the cells were washed twice and reincubated with fresh medium. Compartment distribution was followed for the ensuing 60 h. The accumulation in G_2 was exposure time dependent, peaking at 12 h after drug removal, with a subsequent decline in the percentage of G_2 cells. This increment of the G_2 compartment occurred primarily at the expense of S-phase cells (reduced to three- to fourfold of control), while a minor contribution of G_1-phase cells (less than twofold) occurred only after incubations longer than 9 h. In these experiments, there was no dissociation of S-phase cells measured by FCM and LI.

The cytokinetic effects induced by *cis*-DDP were very complex and depended markedly on the concentration and length of exposure. Exposure to 1 μg/ml resulted in a transient accumulation of cells in S-phase, most pronounced after exposure for longer than 12 h, accompanied by a decline of the $G_{1/0}$ compartment and a constant G_2+M compartment. After 26 h, the size of the S-phase compartment declined, associated with a corresponding increase of the G_2+M compartment. During continuous exposure, the $G_{1/0}$ compartment decreased, and the S-phase accumulation occurred at a slower rate than that after earlier removal at 12 h. For this and other experiments listed below,, the G_2+M compartment increase resulted primarily from accumulation in G_2-phase, since the MI never exceeded control values. The constant size of the G_2+M compartment at the time of S-phase accumulation suggests an effective G_2 delay that becomes more pronounced once cells previously delayed in S-phase move into G_2-phase. While the rate of G_2 accumulation after longer than 12-h exposure was independent of treatment duration, there was a larger residual G_2+M compartment size after 24 and 48 h of treatment. This was mirrored by progressively slower and smaller recoveries of the $G_{1/0}$ compartment. Treatment with 5 μg/ml was associated with a strikingly different pattern of DNA compartment distribution over time, characterized by significantly less pronounced compartment fluctuations for incubation times longer than 12 h. In fact, for cells treated for 48 h, there was no further decline in $G_{1/0}$ and increase in S-phase beyond the values determined after 26 h,

Table 5. Cytokinetic effects induced by DDP

DDP concentration (μg/ml)	Exposure time (h) 1	3	12	24	48
0.1		○	○ △	○ △	○ △
0.5	○	○ △	○ △	○ ▲	○ ▲
1	○ △	○ △	○ ▲	○ ▲	○ ▲
5	○ △	○ ▲	● ▲ ■	● ▲ ■	● ▲ ■
10	○ ▲	● ▲ ■	● ▲ ■	● ▲ ■	● ▲ ■

○, S delay; ●, S block; △, G_2 delay; ▲, G_2 block; ■, G_1 or G_1-S block. Cell cycle phase "delay" is defined as a temporary increase in the proportion of cells in a particular cycle stage. "Block" denotes a permanent accumulation of cells in a given cycle stage without reversal during the observation period of the experiment (6–7 days) so that both $G_{1/0}$- and S-phase compartments plateaued around 40%. Rate and extent of G_2+M accumulation were inversely related to incubation time. Table 5 schematically summarizes the cytokinetic effects of *cis*-DDP as a function of exposure time and drug concentration. If sustained compartment shifts are considered evidence of a total block of cycle progression through a given stage, then both the S and G_2 delays are progressively converted into complete blocks as the concentration and exposure time increase. Apparently, treatment with concentrations equal or greater than 5 μg/ml are required to institute a block in G_1-phase or at the G_1-S boundary. For low concentrations (0.1–1 μg/ml), FCM-derived S-phase proportions, correlated with the magnitude of LI for all exposure times studied, and nearly identical values were obtained with both techniques. Exposure to higher concentrations produced a dissociation of S-phase and LI values after 24 h when the S-phase compartment size attained a plateau of 40%, and the LI progressively decreased to 2% at 150 h. The decrease in LI values was associated with a decrease in the mean grain count from 20 to 7.

To determine the effect of *cis*-DDP on the transition of cells from G_2-phase into mitosis, cultures were treated continuously with Colcemid (0.05 μg/ml) and increasing concentrations of *cis*-DDP. Cultures treated with Colcemid alone showed a linear accumulation of cells in mitosis at an approximate rate of 2.4% /h, attaining a plateau of about 76% after 48 h. MI determinations after this time were complicated by morphological alterations, so that later values may be underestimations. Simultaneous exposure to Colcemid and *cis*-DDP (1 μg/ml) initially showed a similar mitotic accumulation pattern. However, after 6 h, the mitotic rate was reduced to 1%/h, reaching a plateau of about 22% after 24 h. Further increase in DDP concentration to 5 μg/ml was associated with a decrease in the mitotic rate to 1.2%/h, and a plateau of 12% was reached after 12 h. Thus, increase in *cis*-DDP concentration lowered the entry rate of cells into mitosis and its final maximum value. For treatment with 10 and 15 μg/ml, the mitotic rate was similar to that of control cultures only during the first hour, and a plateau of 3%–9% was reached after 4 h.

FCM studies were also conducted for up to 120 h of continuous incubation with Colcemid (0.05 μg/ml) alone or in the presence of increasing concentrations of *cis*-DDP. Cultures exposed to Colcemid alone showed a rapid decrease of the $G_{1/0}$ compartment at a rate of approximately 3%/h, with a plateau of 16%–18% reached within 24 h of treatment. After 9 h, the S-phase compartment decreased from 30% to a plateau value of approximately 4%. The size of the G_2+M compartment increased at a rate of 3.5%/h, attaining a plateau of about 78% after 48 h. In the presence of *cis*-DDP (1 μg/ml), changes of $G_{1/0}$-phase compartment size were not significantly different from those obtained for cells treated with Colcemid alone. The S-phase compartment showed an initial increase from 30%–45% at 9 h, followed by a steep decrease to a plateau of approximately 15% at a rate similar to that for control cultures. The initial rate of increase in the G_2+M compartment was similar to that observed for cells treated with Colcemid alone, but with a lower plateau of 68% reached at 48 h. Continuous treatment with 5 μg/ml decreased the initial rate of $G_{1/0}$ evacuation and raised the minimum $G_{1/0}$ compartment size from 18%–25%. This concentration also produced a steep increase of the S-phase compartment to a maximum of 48% at 12 h, followed by a gradual decline to a plateau of around 32%. The rate of G_2+M accumulation was appreciably decreased after treatment with 5 μg/ml, and a considerably lower plateau value of some 40% was observed 72 h after starting treatment. Following a transient increase of control cells in the G_2 compartment to a maximum of 28% at 12 h, a plateau value of 6.4% was reached within one generation time of LoVo cells (about 30 h). For *cis*-DDP-treated cultures, there was a transient decline of the G_2 compartment (from 24%–16%) between 2 and 10 h of treatment, followed by a progressive increase to 57% after treatment with 1 μg/ml and to 28% after treatment with 5 μg/ml. Following continuous exposure to [^{3}H]dThd, there was a linear increase of LI values at an initial rate of 2.4%/h, which is *not* significantly different from that observed after continuous exposure of LoVo cells to *cis*-DDP (1 μg/ml) and is identical to the mitotic accumulation rate. Following treatment with 5 μg/ml, no appreciable difference in the initial LI rate was noted, while a plateau of 60% was achieved within 12 h. Further dose escalation to 10 μg/ml similarly did not change the initial LI rate per hour, but there was no further significant increase beyond 4 h.

Treatment with anguidine (1–50 μg/ml) yielded virtually no changes in DNA content compartment distribution for periods up to 72 h. However, simultaneous continuous exposure to [^{3}H]dThd or Colcemid revealed profound alterations caused by the agent on the efflux from G_1 into S and from G_2 into mitosis. Anguidine 1 μg/ml) reduced the rate of entry into S from 5%/h to about 1%/h over the first 10 h of exposure. Treatment with 50 μg/ml further reduced the initial rate to <0.75%/h. Additionally, there was a reduction of the initial labeling values, from 39% for control cultures to 27% and 18% for cells treated with 1 and 50 μg/ml of anguidine, respectively. The transit from G_2 into mitosis was severely delayed by a concentration of 1 μg/ml and completely suppressed by 50 mg/ml.

Continuous exposure (24 h) to 100 μg IMPY was associated with concentration-dependent delays in early S-phase or at the $G_{1/S}$ boundary. Treatment with 1,000 μg/ml induced a frozen cell cycle, as reflected by the virtual absence of DNA compartment distribution changes over time. Lack of G_2+M evacuation in the presence of an effective S-phase delay indicated a block in the premitotic phase as well. These effects were better appreciated when cultures were concurrently exposed to IMPY and Colcemid. Compared with controls, there was an immediate and effective concentration-dependent G_1/S delay. Lack of early S-phase evacuation reflects an S-phase delay, and the hindered concentration-dependent G_2 accumulation stemmed from delays in preceding cell cycle stages. Analysis by subcompartments in early, mid- and late S-phase showed that the S-phase delay was primarily due to interference with transition through early S-phase. Probably as a result of predominant delay in a rather small section of the entire cell cycle (i.e., G_1 and early S-phase), a tighter synchronized cohort of cells can be observed moving from early through mid- into late S- and G_2-phases (Fig. 10). These perturbation effects were further confirmed on exponentially growing CHO cells, as illustrated in Fig. 11. Because of less dispersion in cell cycle times, the concentration-dependent blocks in G_1, S, and G_2 can be more readily appreciated.

Exponentially growing LoVo cells exposed to various concentrations of PALA in the absence and presence of Colcemid showed a dose-dependent delay

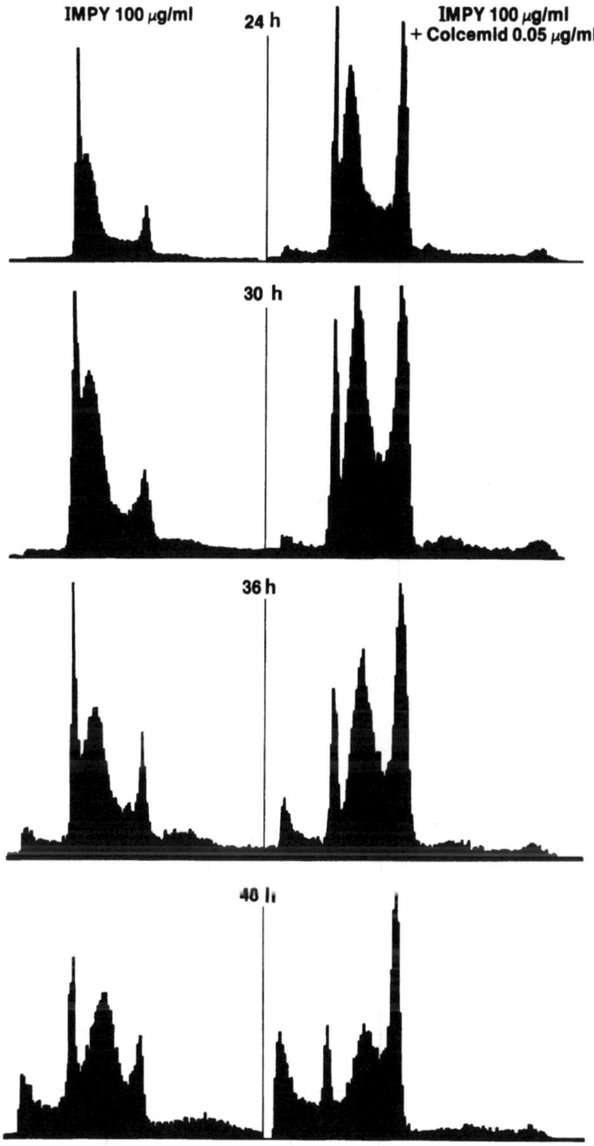

Fig. 10. DNA compartment distribution of asynchronous LoVo cells treated for 24 h with IMPY. Cells were then washed and reincubated with fresh medium alone or with medium containing Colcemid (0.05 µg/ml). FCM measurements were effected immediately after termination of treatment (*uppermost panel*, 24 h) and at 6 h (*2nd panel*, 30 h), 12 h (*3rd panel*, 36 h), and 24 h (*last panel*, 48 h) after terminating treatment

in G_1/S transition and in S-phase and to a minor extent in G_2 phase, not dissimilar from results obtained for IMPY (Fig. 12). Due to a more effective G_1/S delay after treatment with 2.5 mg/ml of PALA, S-phase accumulation occurred at a slower rate.

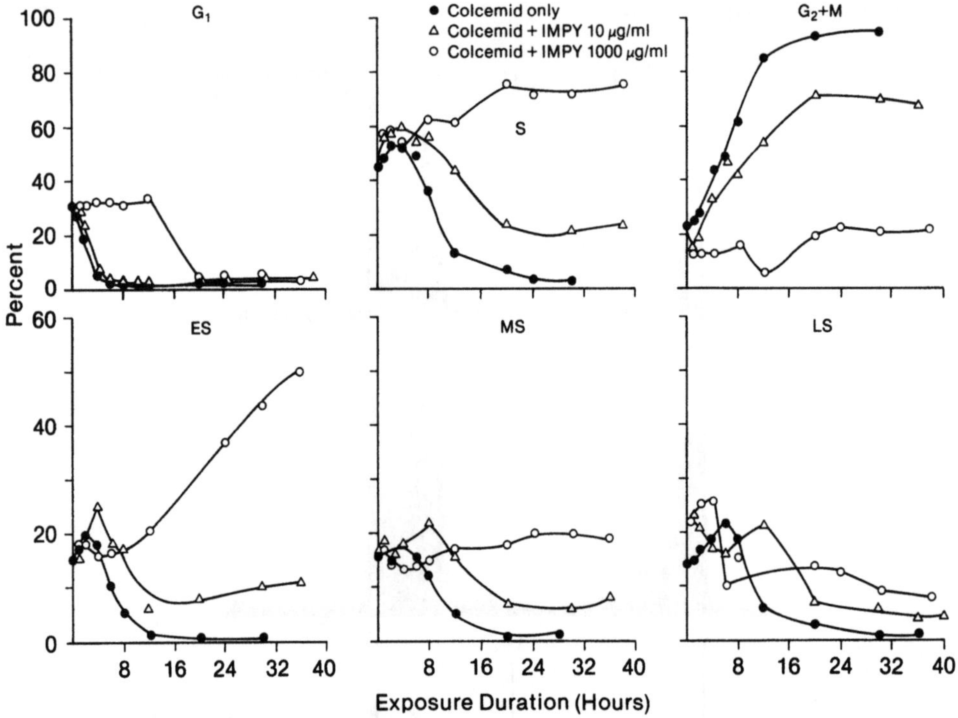

Fig. 11. DNA compartment distribution of CHO cells during treatment with IMPY and Colcemid (0.05 μg/ml)

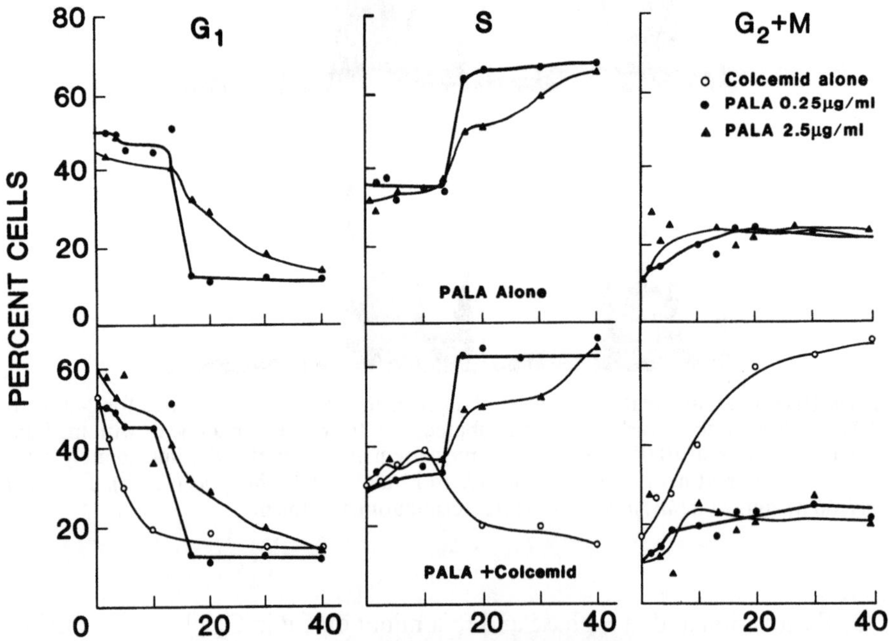

Fig. 12. DNA compartment distribution of LoVo cells treated continuously with PALA (*upper panel*) and with PALA and Colcemid, 0.05 μg/ml (*lower panel*)

2. Synchronized Cells

When synchronized cells were treated with anthracycline derivatives for 1 h at different stages of the cell cycle, striking age-dependent effects on G_2 accumulation were noted. ADR irreversibly accumulated more than 70% of the cell population in G_2-phase, independent of cycle stage of administration (Fig. 13). However, while drug exposure in S- and G_2-phase elicited an immediate accumulation, treatment in G_1-phase yielded a progressive G_2 increment over a period of 4 days. This effect suggests that some cells treated before the onset of DNA synthesis can escape the blocking effect of ADR during their life span. However, their progeny will be blocked in the subsequent G_2-phase, thus contributing to the total accumulation in that stage. When ADR was administered complexed to DNA, a phase-dependent sensitivity in G_2 arrest induction was observed (Fig. 13 b); treat-

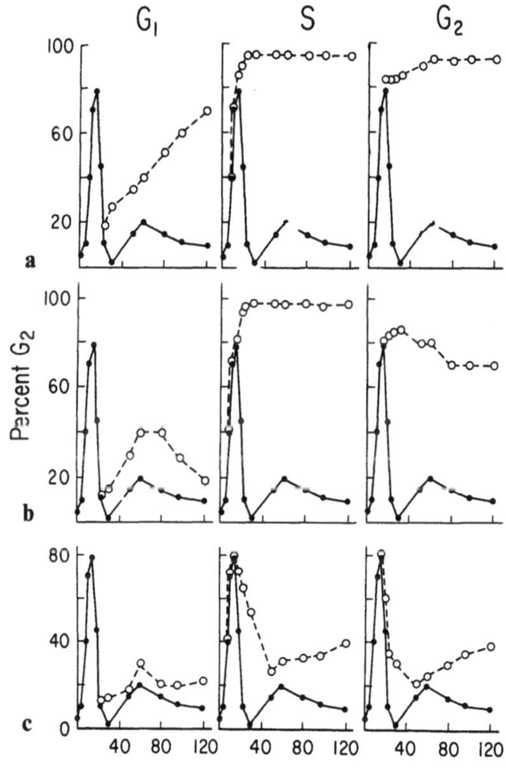

Fig. 13 a–c. Effect of anthracycline antibiotics on G_2 traverse of T_1 cells as a function of the stage of treatment (G_1-, mid-S-, and early G_2-phase). The *solid lines* (●——●) represent the proportion of control cells in G_2-phase, the *dashed lines* (○--○) connect values after 1 h of treatment in the three different phases. **a** ADR: 0.5 µg/ml, 1 h. Induction of high degree of irreversible G_2 accumulation of 70%–95%, independent of the cycle stage of drug exposure. The time of G_2 maximum is delayed for cells treated in G_1-phase. **b** ADR-DNA: 0.5 µg/ml, 1 h. Compared with ADR, initiation of treatment in G_1-phase causes only a transient G_2 accumulation of 40%. **c** RUB: 1.0 µg/ml, 1 h. S-phase cells are most effectively delayed during their traverse through G_2-phase, while exposure of cells in G_1-phase effects a minor increase of the G_2 compartment

ment of cells throughout S- and in early G_2-phase elicited a largely irreversible G_2 block of 80%–90%; in contrast, treatment in late G_2- and in G_1-phase caused a transient increment of cells in G_2 (20% and 40%, respectively). The degree and extent of the G_2 block following incubation with RUB was also an function of cell age; treatment of T_1 cells in early and mid-S-phase was most effective in interfering with the traverse through the subsequent G_2-phase (Fig. 13c).

For alkylating agents the time of manifestation of the delay in G_2 following treatment, whether during the life span of the treated cells or within that of their immediate progeny, varied with cell age at the time of drug exposure. Treatment with melphalan in G_1-phase effected a largely irreversible G_2 increment of 75% within the same life cycle. Drug incubation in S- and G_2-phase did not interfere with cycle traverse to mitosis and the subsequent progression through G_1- and S-phase of the progeny cells; yet, a significant block was noted in the consecutive G_2-phase. Thus, in all circumstances, DNA synthesis in drug-free medium preceded the induction of G_2 block by melphalan. Peptichemio mimicked very closely the kinetic effects of melphalan, where for a given drug concentration similar degrees of G_2 accumulations were observed. Yet, notable differences were noted on synchronized cells. Cells treated in both G_1- and early and mid-S-phase were effectively delayed upon their arrival in the immediate G_2-phase. Drug exposure of cells in late S- and G_2-phase transmitted this perturbation effect to the daughter cells. For Yoshi 864, similar, yet more transient cycle stage-dependent manifestations of G_2 delay were noted.

Induction of G_2 accumulation by VP-16 was also age dependent; for the lower concentration of 5 μg/ml sensitivity to the induction of a G_2 block decreased in the following order: early and mid-S-phase > later S-phase > early G_2- > late G_2- > G_1-phase. Dose escalation to 10 μg/ml partially abrogated the pronounced phase sensitivity: treatment in both early and late G_2-phase was equally effective as drug exposure in S-phase to produce maximal G_2 accumulation.

IV. Protection of Cell Kill by Inhibition of Cell Cycle Traverse

An effective cell cycle arrest was maintained for at least 12 h after a 4-h treatment with greater than 4 μg/ml of anguidine, conditions which were noncytotoxic to CHO cells (THEODORI et al. 1981). Treatment with araC alone required prolonged drug exposure intervals for effective cell killing. Pretreatment with 5 μg/ml of anguidine for 4 h reduced the lethal damage from 18-h treatment with araC by 30- to 100-fold over the entire concentration range of 5–50 μg/ml (Fig. 14). In the case of ADR, anguidine pretreatment also effected a significant reduction in cell kill. Preincubation with anguidine was crucial to elicit an antagonistic effect against cell inactivation by ADR, whereas concurrent or subsequent treatment with anguidine did not afford any protection. In the case of araC, which required prolonged continuous exposure for significant cytoreduction, postincubation with anguidine mimicked the survival pattern for araC treatment alone, while simultaneous exposure to araC and anguidine afforded protection of a similar extent as was observed after pretreatment with anguidine. Increasing time intervals between termination of anguidine exposure and treatment with ADR were associ-

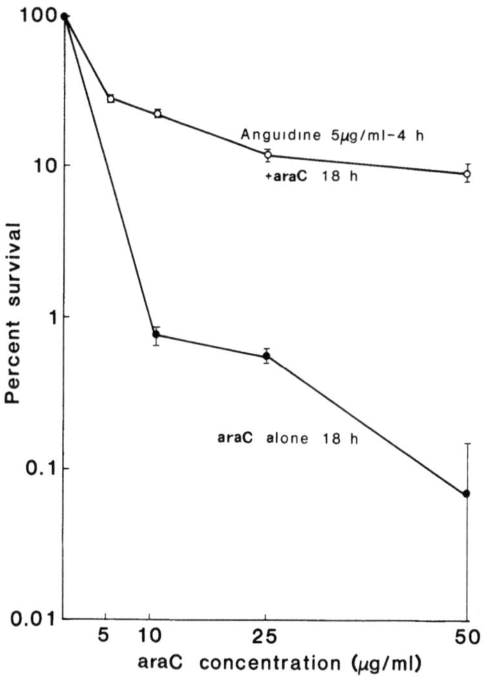

Fig. 14. Concentration-dependent survival of exponentially growing CHO cells following 18 h of araC treatment in the presence and absence of 4 h preincubation with 5 μg/ml anguidine. There is a 30- to 100-fold reduction in cell kill in case of preincubation with anguidine over the entire range of araC concentrations

ated with a decrease in cytoprotection by almost 1 log with 12 h, although still maintaining 1/4 log protection from cell kill by ADR alone. This decrease in cytoprotection was accompanied by a gradual increase in the labeling index following anguidine treatment from 0% at the end of a 4-h anguidine exposure to 13% and 51%, 6 h and 24 h after drug removal, respectively.

D. Discussion

There is considerable controversy concerning the ability of certain antitumor drugs to exert equal or greater cytotoxic effects on cultured nonproliferating cells than on proliferating ones (BARRANCO and NOVAK 1974; BARRANCO et al. 1973; BHUYAN et al. 1977; HAHN et al. 1974; MAURO et al. 1974b; SUTHERLAND 1974; THATCHER and WALKER 1979; TWENTYMAN 1976; TWENTYMAN and BLEEHAN 1973; VAN PUTTEN et al. 1972). Discrepancies in results among various investigators can be attributed in part to species-related biological differences. More important, perhaps, is the diversity in methodology used to obtain nonproliferating cultures (BARRANCO and NOVAK 1974; BARRANCO et al. 1979; EPIFANOVA et al. 1978; HAHN and LITTLE 1972; MAURO et al. 1974a; PARDEE 1974; TOBEY and LEY

1970; TWENTYMAN 1976), which can generate significant differences in physiological properties of the treated cells, in the metabolic disposition of the noxious agent (EPIFANOVA 1977; GLINOS and WERRLERN 1972; HAHN and LITTLE 1972; KOUNS 1975; MAURO et al. 1974a), and also lead to differences in sensitivity and clonogenicity as a function of the duration of the stationary growth (MAURO et al. 1974; TWENTYMAN and BLEEHEN 1975). Another equally important possibility resides in the fact that the stationary phase cultures used by different investigators differ significantly in their cell cycle compartment distribution (BARRANCO et al. 1973; BHUYAN et al. 1977; DREWINKO et al. 1979a, c; GELFANT 1977; MACIEIRA-COELHO 1967; MADOC-JONES and BRUCE 1967; ROSS and SINCLAIR 1972; THATCHER and WALKER 1969; TOBEY and LEY 1970); thus, it is possible that purported differences in drug sensitivity of stationary versus proliferating cells may actually reflect the sensitivity of cells accumulated in different stages of the cell cycle.

As shown by others for occasional agents, our cultured human cells also disclosed two drugs (*cis*-DDP and VDS) that were more effective on stationary phase cultures than on exponentially growing cells. In a manner similar to that observed by HAGEMAN et al. (1973) for BCNU on mouse plasmacytoma cells, the increased effectiveness of *cis*-DDP on the human tumor cells resulted from the abrogation of the shoulder region of the survival curve while the slope was retained intact. Such changes in the shape of the survival curve can also be observed in exponentially growing human cells if *cis*-DDP is administered at 41 °C (BARLOGIE et al. 1980), suggesting that the capacity to absorb drug-induced damage without expressing a lethal effect is thermosensitive and modulated by the proliferative status of the cells.

VDS was almost 20 times more effective on stationary phase cells than on exponentially growing ones. It is difficult to reconcile this observation with the lethal mode of action ascribed to *Vinca* alkaloids (i.e., inhibition of the mitotic spindle). Thus, it is possible that either VDS has an additional killing mechanism not shared by its congeners or that the activity of this particular agent persists long enough to inhibit division when the treated cells in stationary phase are allowed to proliferate exponentially for colony formation. In direct contrast to the findings of OLAH et al. (1978) for Chinese hamster cells, VCR was less sensitive on LoVo cells in stationary phase than on exponentially growing ones, and both our findings and those of OLAH et al. vary from the observations of HILL and WHELAN (1981) for Syrian hamster ovary cells where either VCR and VDS were totally ineffective against cells in stationary phase. Thus, it appears that species differences mediate important modifications of the interactions between antitumor drugs (at least *Vinca* alkaloids) and the target cells under various proliferative conditions.

In the manner described by others for alkylating agents (BLACKETT and ADAMS 1972; LAHIRI 1973; THATCHER and WALKER 1969), the efficacy of nitrosourea derivatives and mitomycin C was quite similar for both exponentially growing and stationary phase cells. This similar efficacy could originate from an intrinsic property of the interaction of alkylating agents and the target cells or result from the inability of stationary phase cells to repair potentially lethal damage before they are manipulated into exponential growth (HAHN et al. 1973).

Of great clinical importance, most antitumor drugs displayed decreased efficacy on cells in stationary phase of growth. The decreased efficacy was noted for cell cycle stage-sensitive agents, for mitotic inhibitors, and for DNA-intercalating agents. These findings reiterate the significance of quantifying cellular proliferation kinetics for determining resistance to tumor therapy and demonstrate that, in contrast to some cells of rodent origin, nonproliferating human tumor cells have decreased sensitivity to most antitumor agents. Although a rare drug may show increased activity on nonproliferating cells, in general only those agents that display alkylating properties can be expected, at most, to be as effective on nonproliferating as on proliferating cells.

As indicated before, position in the cycle at the time of exposure to a drug is an important determinant for survival of proliferating cells. Some drugs (i.e., MTX) may only kill cells positioned in the S-phase of the cycle, while virtually every drug exhibits preferential kill in a particular stage. Because most drugs exhibit preferential rather than specific cell kill in a given stage of the cycle, it is perhaps more appropriate to describe such agents as "cell cycle phase-sensitive" rather than with the commonly employed term "phase-specific." For instance, our studies with HU and 5-FU, agents considered to kill cells by inhibiting DNA synthesis, also displayed substantial killing in G_2- and G_1-phases, as also observed by BHUYAN et al. (1972) for DON cells. Conversely, T_1 cells synchronized in S-phase and exposed for 1 h to MTX showed a mere 20% decrease in survival, indicating that either all cells positioned in the cycle stage purportedly sensitive to an agent are not equally susceptible to its lethal action or that cell age alone is not sufficient to predict a lethal outcome. This fact is further emphasized by our results with araC, PALA, and IMPY. These agents completely failed to kill S-phase LoVo and T_1 cells when administered for only 1 h but readily decreased survival when treatment was extended for an interval equal to the length of S-phase. The reason for this finding can be ascribed, at least in part, to the lethal mode of action of the antitumor agent. Drugs that inhibit DNA synthesis kill cells by the mechanism of "unbalanced growth" (KIM et al. 1968; LAMBERT and STUDZINSKY 1976). To achieve lethality by this mechanism, inhibition of DNA synthesis must be maintained for a period longer than the generation time (BRACHETTI and WHITMORE 1969), lest the cells resume their growth, synchronized but still capable of unlimited proliferation. For drugs that bind irreversibly to their macromolecules, degrade slowly, and are exposed to cells which have a limited capacity to synthesize new macromolecules, continuous DNA inhibition may be achieved even after brief exposure to the drug. If one or more of these conditions are not satisfied, lethality can only be obtained if the cells are incubated continuously with the antitumor agent.

Some investigators (BHUYAN et al. 1972; MADOC-JONES and MAURO 1975) have analyzed the age-dependent response of different cell lines to a great number of antitumor agents with the intention of extracting generalizations useful in the classification of cell-drug interactions. For some agents, their observations on cell cycle stage sensitivity were similar. But for many drugs their conclusions disagreed not only with each other but also with the age-dependent patterns reported by other investigators employing the same drug (or their congener) on different cell lines. Our results serve to emphasize these discrepancies and the inadequacy of extrapolating results obtained on a given cell line to a generalized statement applicable to the response of al mammalian cells. For instance, both MADOC-JONES and MAURO (1975), and BHUYAN et al. (1972) considered that alkylating agents were characterized by a distinct preferential cell kill in G_1-phase or at the G_1/S transition. In our studies, this pattern was observed only for melphalan. Its congener, peptichemio, in addition to killing cells in G_1-phase, exhibited the greatest activity in G_2-phase. Other alkylating agents such as Yoshi 864 also killed cells in early S-phase, while *cis*-acid was most active in early S- and G_2-phase. *Vinca* alkaloids considered more efficacious in S-phase cells by other authors (OLAH et al. 1978; MACOC-JONES and MAURO 1969) showed almost equal activity in all stages of the cycle in our studies.

Minor structural modifications of a drug may generate profound changes in the age-dependent patterns. In the studies of MADOC-JONES and MAURO (1969) VCR and VBL, congeners whose molecular structure differs by only two H atoms showed distinct concentration-dependent activities and different age-dependent survival patterns, the latter characterized by particular modifications of the shape of the survival curve. These observations are similar to our present findings where three closely related nitrosourea congeners interacting with the same cell type (T_1 cells) each originated a unique age-dependent pattern of survival and a distinct modification of the capacity to absorb damage and/or sensitivity of the target molecule.

Several factors may be responsible for the disparity in results among different investigators. One such factor was indicated before and relates to the diversity of methods and degree of synchrony yield employed by different investigators. Another factor may relate to differences in species origin. Yet, even within a particular species, diversity in histological origin may originate distinct age-dependent response patterns. For instance, our human lymphoma (T_1) cells showed limited sensitivity (<20%) to MTX while the human colon carcinoma (LoVo) cells showed greater than 50% cell kill, a proportion greater than that of cells present in S-phase during the treatment interval. A similar age-dependent survival pattern was obtained for both BCNU and *cis*-acid when the target cells were colon carcinoma, a pattern that differed significantly from that obtained from lymphoma cells. However, the resonses of lymphoma cells to both agents were largely similar. These findings explain, in part, the distinct responses of different tissues elicited by a particular drug and could acquire significant value in treatment strategies requiring precise scheduling of antitumor agents.

It must also be considered that differences in age-dependent patterns among investigators may actually result from the dissimilar selection of concentration levels and unequal treatment intervals used to examine the sensitivity of the synchronized cells. Even if the treatment interval is maintained uniform, it may not be biologically equivalent. Different cell classes may have different generation and cell cycle stage transit times, and, therefore, during a given exposure interval, more cells of a faster cell type may pass through the sensitive stage of the cell cycle.

In addition to their cytotoxic effect, antitumor drugs induce profound alterations in the cycle traverse of the treated cells, usually manifested by a delay or block in one or more of the discrete stages of the cycle. These cytokinetic changes can be easily analyzed by serial FCM measurements of DNA content-dependent compartment distributions during and after treatment with the agent of interest. However, in many instances additional methods (i.e., continuous labeling with [^{3}H]dThd, mitotic block with Colcemid, LI, MI) are required to observe complex and multiple sites of cytokinetic perturbation in the cell cycle. For instance, the multiple-blocking effects of anguidine and those of the high concentrations of mitomycin C and *cis*-DDP could not have been elucidated on the basis of serial DNA histograms alone, as they failed to show significant fluctuations in DNA compartment distribution. Yet, by combining drug treatment with Colcemid block and LI determinations during continuous exposure to [^{3}H]dThd, we demonstrated delays at different stages of the cycle establishing what we called a "frozen" cycle. Similarly, by combining FCM with serial MI we demonstrated that, in contrast to previous beliefs, *Vinca* alkaloids, like epipodophilotoxine derivatives, exert their maximal cytokinetic delay in G_2-phase while the mitotic block is secondary and of a lesser magnitude than that occurring in the preceding compartment. At higher concentrations of *Vinca* alkaloid treatment, the delay in G_2 becomes an almost complete block and the MI actually drops to values closer of those of untreated cells.

Although for some agents, especially antimetabolites and protein inhibitors (i.e., MTX, HU, araC, thymidine, IMPY, etc.), the major cytokinetic effect is a delay at the boundary or in early S-phase (BARRANCO and HUMPHREY 1971; BORSA and WHITMORE 1969; DETHLEFSEN et al. 1977; DREWINKO et al. 1972; FORD and SHACKNEY 1977; GALAVAZI et al. 1966; GANAPATHI and KRISHAN 1978; SKIPPER 1970; TOBEY et al. 1966; WORTING and ROTI ROTI 1980), for most agents we investigated the major common end effect was a delay or complete block in G_2-phase; the onset, magnitude, and duration of this effect was directly related to the concentration and treatment interval with the drug. With increasing drug concentrations and/or treatment durations, additional delays at other stages of the cycle occurred, which could modify the degree of the G_2 accumulation. These cytokinetic effects appear unrelated to the mechanisms leading to cell death as marked perturbation of cycle traverse could be elicited at concentrations which yield minimal, if any, cytotoxicity and the age-dependent cytokinetic response pattern of most drugs differed from the cytotoxic age-dependent pattern. Although, when the cytokinetic effect led to a complete and irreversible block the eventual result was cell death, this phenomenon appears secondary to the principal mechanism of cell lethality as the stages of the cycle most susceptible to this effect differed from those where cytotoxicity was maximal.

In a manner similar to that described earlier for the cytotoxic effects of drugs, the cytokinetic effects of closely related analogs (i.e., anthracycline derivatives and *Vinca* alkaloids) or with similar putative modes of action (i.e., intercalating agents and alkylating drugs) displayed substantial differences in degree and duration of G_2 delays and induction of delays in other stages of the cycle. All of these facts reveal the multiplicity of biochemical events responsible for the orderly progression through the cycle and suggest that every agent interacts with one or more different molecular targets, each of which possesses a particular affinity for the drug "ligand" and has a significantly different role in facilitating cycle progression. In this context, it is interesting that different agents displayed distinct age-dependent efficacy in inducing accumulation in G_2-phase. Anthracycline derivatives exerted an immediate maximal blocking effect when applied in S- or G_2-phase, while treatment in G_1-phase resulted in a slower and lesser accumulation in the subsequent G_2-phase. For VP-16, sensitivity to the induction of a G_2 block decreased in the following order: early and mid-S-phase > later S-phase > early G_2- > late G_2- > G_1-phase. Dose escalation to 10 μg/ml partially abrogated the pronounced phase sensitivity, and treatment in both early and late G_2-phase was equally effective as drug exposure in S-phase to produce maximal G_2 accumulation. For BLEO, accumulation in G_2-phase could only be accomplished by continuous exposure (15 h) to the drug. When the cells were washed free of drug, treatment initiated in G_1-phase yielded a moderate accumulation in G_2-phase while treatment began in early or mid-S-phase produced a large long-lasting accumulation. Cells whose treatment was initiated in late S or in G_2 rapidly moved into mitosis and G_1. Alkylating agents administered for 1 h showed an unusual kinetic response pattern; the time of manifestation of the delay in G_2, whether evident during the life span of the treated cells or within that of their immediate progeny, varied with cell age at the time of drug exposure. Treatment in G_1-phase effected a largely irreversible G_2 increment within the same life cycle while incubation in S- and G_2-phase did not interfere with cycle traverse to mitosis and the subsequent progression through G_1- and S-phase of the progeny cells; yet, a significant block was noted in the consecutive G_2-phase. Thus, in all circumstances, DNA synthesis in drug-free medium preceded the induction of G_2.

These differential effects can be explained by postulating that orderly progression from G_2-phase into mitosis is modulated by one or more hypothetical "division-specific" enzymes (TOBEY et al. 1971). The synthesis of these "division-specific" enzymes (factor Y) starts in late S- or during G_2-phase, has a rapid turnover rate, and must attain a critical level at the end of G_2 to permit entry into mitosis. The synthesis of factor Y depends, in turn, on the production of a hypothetical factor X which may either be a series of precursor molecules of factor Y or one or more enzymes required for the synthesis of this factor. Synthesis of the relatively stable factor X proceeds throughout the cycle, albeit at a slow rate; factor X must also attain a critical level for initiating the production of factor Y and may be transmitted to the daughter cells at division. Thus, agents that inactivate or interfere with the synthesis of factor Y (i.e., anthracyclines and VP-16) will exert an immediate and sustained blocking effect when applied in G_2 while treatment in preceding stages will induce this effect only if the agent remains active at the time the cells initiate synthesis of factor Y. Agents that intefere with the synthesis of factor X (i.e., alkylating drugs) will not induce the G_2 block when applied in that stage since the level of factor X accumulated during G_1- and S-phase may permit the synthesis of sufficient factor Y to allow division. Because insufficient factor X is then shared by the daughter cells (and possibly because the drug remains active in the daughter cells) the level of factor X will not be sufficient to initiate synthesis of factor Y at the appropriate time and then the G_2 block is manifested in the progency of the treated cells. Treatment administered in G_1- or S-phase will not permit the cells to synthesize enough factor X to initiate production of factor Y upon reaching late S or G_2, and thus the block will be apparent during the same life cycle of the treated cells. In this manner, treatment with these antitumor drugs may provide a valuable probe for investigating the nature of the macromolecular mechanisms related to cell division.

From the preceding discussion, it is obvious that in addition to the proliferative status of the treated cells being a determinant for resistance to antitumor drugs, the simultaneously induced cytokinetic perturbation will affect the sensitivity of cells to the same or to other agents given subsequently. Not only can an agent such as anguidine protect against the cytotoxicity of another powerful antitumor drug by merely slowing down the rate of progression through the cell cycle, but the profound alterations in cycle traverse rates caused by most agents may determine whether administration of the same or other drugs will yield an antagonistic, additive, or synergistic effect simply on the basis of subsequent reassortment and kinetics of cells recovery. This fact has been exhaustively demonstrated in a series of elegant experiments conducted by VALERIOTE and his collaborators (EDELSTEIN et al. 1974, 1975; RAZEK et al. 1974, 1980; VALERIOTE and HSUI-SAN 1975) and by DETHLEFSEN and his collaborators (DETHLEFSEN et al. 1975). DETHLEFSEN's group has also endeavored to elucidate the time dependency of cell recovery of normal and malignant tissues in animal models in order to provide precise scheduling of the second drug administration and has shown the exactness in timing required for obtaining a therapeutic gain (DETHLEFSEN 1979; DETHLEFSEN et al. 1977; ROTI ROTI and DETHLEFSEN 1975).

If such critical precision is required for experimental tumors which posses relatively homogenous cytodynamic properties, it is evident that for human tumors with large variations in growth kinetics values, drug-induced small perturbations in cycle traverse or fluxes from the nonproliferating to the proliferating compartment may influence immensely the results of clinical treatments based on a growth kinetics rationale. Unfortunately, because substantial knowledge has already been accumulated on the cell cycle stage-dependent effects of a variety of antitumor agents, this information has been inappropriately utilized to develop so-called "kinetic" chemotherapeutic regimens which have thus far met with varying, mostly unsatisfactory, degrees of success in terms of improved clinical responses. The implementation of this information has obviously been too premature, not only because of the inadequacy of present knowledge, but also because of the vagaries of our current information regarding the cytodynamics of in vivo tumors. A clinical chemotherapeutic strategy based on a cell kinetics rationale requires accurate knowledge of the fraction of proliferating cells and of the durations of the phases of the cell cycle, features that may change continuously during the natural history of disease and, as indicated before, as a consequence of the perturbation induced by the therapeutic maneuvers. Such variations require alterations in the scheduling tactics of drugs in accordance with the fluctuating growth kinetics properties of the neoplastic and normal cells. Most "kinetic" protocols have thus far adhered to rigid schema of drug scheduling and were based on insufficient information on the growth kinetics properties of human tumors. Development of new and better techniques for studying these parameters and acquisition of a vast data bank on human tumor growth dynamics could alter this situation in the not too distant future. It is then when the full impact of the information on cytotoxic and cycle drug-induced perturbation effects may be finally attained.

Acknowledgments. This work was supported by the following grants: CA 14528 and CA 23272. We extend our sincere appreciation to Ms. Judy Johnson and Mrs. Lynette Weissman for excellent secretarial and editing skills.

References

Alabaster O, Tannenbaum E, Habersett MC, Magrath I, Herman C (1978) Drug-induced changes in DNA fluorescence intensity detected by flow microfluorometry and their implications for analysis of DNA content distributions. Cancer Res 38:1031–1035

Barlogie B, Drewinko B (1976) Cell cycle-related induction of cell progression delay. In: Drewinko B, Humphrey RM (eds) Growth kinetics and biochemical regulation of normal and malignant cells. Williams and Wilkins, Baltimore, p 315

Barlogie B, Drewinko B (1978) Cell cycle stage-dependent induction of G_2 phase arrest by different antitumor agents. Eur J Cancer 14:741–745

Barlogie B, Drewinko B (1980) Lethal and cytokinetic effects of mitomycin C on cultured human colon cancer cells. Cancer Res 40:1973–1980

Barlogie B, Drewinko B, Johnston DA, Buchner T, Hauss WH, Freireich EJ (1976a) Pulse cytophotometric analysis of synchronized cells in vitro. Cancer Res 36:1176–1181

Barlogie B, Drewinko B, Johnston DA, Freireich EJ (1976b) The effects of adriamycin on the cell cycle traverse of a human lymphoid cell line. Cancer Res 36:1975

Barlogie B, Corry P, Drewinko B (1980) In vitro thermochemotherapy of human colon cancer cells with cisplatinum and mitomycin C. Cancer Res 40:1165–1168

Barranco SC, Humphrey RM (1971) The effects of β-2'-deoxythioguanosine on survival and progression in mammalian cells. Cancer Res 31:583–586

Barranco SC, Novak JK (1974) Survival response of dividing and nondividing mammalian cells after treatment with hydroxyurea, arabinosylcytosine or adriamycin. Cancer Res 34:1616–1618

Barranco SC, Novak JK, Humphrey RM (1973) Response of mammalian cells following treatment with bleomycin and 1,3-bis(2-chloroethyl)-1-nitrosourea during plateau phase. Cancer Res 33:691–694

Barranco SC, Bolton WE, Novak JK (1979) A simple method for producing different growth fractions in vitro for use in anticancer drug studies. Cell Tissue Kinet 12:11–16

Ben-Ishay Z, Farber E (1975) Protective effects of an inhibitor of protein synthesis, cycloheximide on bone marrow damage induced by cytosine arabinoside or nitrogen mustard. Lab Invest 33:478–490

Bergerat J-P, Barlogie B, Gohde W, Johnston DA, Drewinko B (1979) In vitro cytokinetic response of human colon cancer cells to *cis*-dichlorodiammine-platinum (II). Cancer Res 39:4356–4363

Bhuyan BJ, Scheidt LG, Fraser TJ (1972) Cell cycle phase specificity of antitumor agents. Cancer Res 32:398–407

Bhuyan BK, Loughman BE, Fraser TJ, Day KJ (1976) Comparison of different methods of determining cell viability after exposure to cytotoxic compounds. Exp Cell Res 97:275–280

Bhuyan BK, Fraser TJ, Day KJ (1977) Cell proliferation kinetics and drug sensitivity of exponential and stationary populations of cultured L1210 cells. Cancer Res 37:1057–1063

Blackett NM, Adams K (1972) Cell proliferation and action of cytotoxic agents on haemopoietic tissue. Br J Haematol 23:751–758

Borsa J, Whitmore GF (1969) Cell killing studies on the mode of action of methotrexate on L-cells in vitro. Cancer Res 29:737–744

Brachetti S, Whitmore GF (1969) The action of hydroxyurea in mouse L-cells. Cell Tissue Kinet 2:193

Bradley MO, Kohn KW, Sharkey NA, Ewig RA (1977) Differential cytotoxicity between transformed and normal human cells with combinations of aminonucleosides and hydroxyurea. Cancer Res 37:2126–2131

Bruce WR, Meeker BE, Valeriote FA (1966) Comparison of the sensitivity of normal hematopoietic and transplanted lymphoma colony-forming cells to chemotherapeutic agents administered in vivo. J Natl Cancer Inst 37:233–245
Capizzi RL (1974) Biochemical interaction between asparaginase (A'ASE) and methotrexate (MTX) in leukemia cells. Proc Am Assoc Cancer Res 15:77
Capizzi RL, Summers WP, Bertino JR (1971) L-asparaginase-induced alteration of amethopterin (methotrexate) activity in mouse leukemia L5178Y. Ann NY Acad Sci 186:302 311
Clarkson BD (1974) The survival value of the dormant state in neoplastic and normal cell populations. In: Clarkson B, Baserga R (eds) Control of proliferation in animal cells. Cold Spring Harbor, New York, p 945
Dethlefsen LA (1979) Cellular recovery kinetic studies relevant to combined-modality research and therapy. Int J Radiat Oncol Biol Phys 5:1197–1203
Dethlefsen LA, Riley RM (1973a) Hydroxyurea effects in the C_3H mouse. I. Duodenal crypt cell kinetics. Cell Tissue Kinet 6:3–16
Dethlefsen LA, Riley RM (1973b) Hydroxyurea effects in the C_3H mouse. II. Mammary tumor cell kinetics. Cell Tissue Kinet 6:173–184
Dethlefsen LA, Sorensen SP, Riley RM (1975) Effects of double and multiple doses of hydroxyurea on mouse duodenum and mammary tumors. Cancer Res 35:694–699
Dethlefsen LA, Ohlsen JD, Roti Roti JL (1977) Cell synchronization in vivo: fact or fancy? In: Drewinko B, Humphrey RM (eds) Growth kinetics and biochemical regulation of normal and malignant cells. Williams and Wilkins, Baltimore, pp 491–507
Dethlefsen LA, Riley RM, Roti Roti (1979) Flow cytometric analysis of adriamycin-perturbated mouse mammary tumor. J Histochem Cytochem 27:463–469
Dosik GM, Barlogie B, Johnston DA, Murphy WK, Drewinko B (1978) Lethal and cytokinetic effects of anguidine on a human colon cancer cell line. Cancer Res 38:3304–3309
Dosik GM, Barlogie B, White A, Gohde W, Drewinko B (1981) A rapid automated stathmokinetic method for determination of in vitro cell cycle transit times. Cell Tissue Kinet 14:121–134
Drewinko B, Barlogie B (1976a) Survival and cycle progression delay of human lymphoma cells in vitro exposed to 4'demethylepipodophyllotoxin 9-(4,6-0-ethylidine-β-D-glucopyranoside) (NSC 141540; VP016). Cancer Treat Rep 60:1295
Drewinko B, Barlogie B (1976b) Age-dependent survival and cell-cycle progression of cultured cells exposed to chemotherapeutic agents. Cancer Treat Rep 60:1707
Drewinko B, Ho DHN, Barranco SC (1972) The effects of arabinosylcytosine on cultured human lymphoma cells. Cancer Res 32:2737–2742
Drewinko B, Lichtiger B, Trujillo JM (1973) Synchronization of cultured human lymphoid cells. Biomedicine 18:30–37
Drewinko B, Romsdahl MM, Yang L-Y, Ahearn MJ, Trujillo JM (1976) Establishment of a human carcinoembryonic antigen-producing colon adenocarcinoma cell line. Cancer Res 36:467–475
Drewinko B, Bobo B, Roper P, Malahy MA, Barlogie B, Jansson B (1978a) Analysis of the growth kinetics of a human lymphoma cell line. Cell Tissue Kinet 11:177–191
Drewinko B, Yang L-Y, Barlogie B, Romsdahl M, Meistrich M, Malahy MA; Giovanella B (1978b) Further biological characteristics of an established human carcino-embryonic antigen producing colon carcinoma cell line. J Natl Cancer Inst 61:75–83
Drewinko B, Barlogie B, Freireich EJ (1979a) Response of exponentially growing, stationary phase and synchronized cultured colon carcinoma cells to treatment with nitrosourea derivatives. Cancer Res 39:3630–3636
Drewinko B, Roper PR, Barlogie B (1979b) Patterns of cell survival following treatment with antitumor agents in vitro. Eur J Cancer 15:95–99
Drewinko B, Barlogie B, Mars W, Malahy MA, Jansson B (1979c) Proliferative characteristics of ARH-77 cells, an established human IgG-producing myeloma cell line. Cell Tissue Kinet 12:675
Drewinko B, Alexanian R, Boyer H, Barlogie B, Rubinow S (1981a) The growth fraction of human myeloma cells. Blood 57:333–338

Drewinko B, Patchen M, Yang L-Y, Barlogie B (1981 b) Differential killing efficacy of twenty antitumor drugs on proliferating and nonproliferating human tumor cells. Cancer Res 4:2328–2333

Dubrow R, Riddle VGH, Pardee AB (1979) Different responses to drugs and serum of cells transformed by various means. Cancer Res 39:2718–2726

Edelstein M, Vietti T, Valeriote F (1974) Schedule dependent synergism for the combination of 1-β-D-arabinofuranosyl cytosine and daunorubicin. Cancer Res 34:293–297

Edelstein M, Vietti T, Valeriote F (1975) The enhanced cytotoxicity of combinations of 1-β-D-arabinoguranosylcytosine and methotrexate. Cancer Res 35:1555–1558

Ehmann UK, Wheeler KT (1979) Cinemicrographic determination of cell progression and division abnormalities after treatment with 1,3 bis(2-chloroethyl)-1-nitrosourea (BCNU). Eur J Cancer 15:461–474

Epifanova OI (1977) Mechanisms underlying the differential sensitivity of proliferating and resting cells to external factors. Int Rev Cytol [Suppl] 5:303–335

Epifanova OI, Smolenskaya IN, Polunovsky VA (1978) Responses of proliferating and nonproliferating chinese hamster cells to cytotoxic agents. Br J Cancer 37:377–385

Ford SS, Shackney SE (1977) Lethal and sublethal effects of hydroxyurea in relation to drug concentration and duration of drug exposure in sarcoma 180 in vitro. Cancer Res 37:2628–2637

Fried J (1976) Method for the quantitative evaluation of data from flow microfluorometry. Computers Biomed Res 9:277–290

Galavazi G, Schenk H, Bootsma I (1966) Synchronization of mammalian cells in vitro by inhibition of the DNA synthesis. I. Optimal conditions. Exp Cell Res 41:428–433

Ganapathi R, Krishan A (1978) Cell cycle synchronization of L1210 and P388 ascites in vivo. Cell Tissue Kinet 11:681

Gelfant S (1977) A new concept of tissue and tumor cell proliferation. Cancer Res 37:3845–3862

Glinos AD, Werrlem RJ (1972) Density dependent regulation of growth on suspension cultures of L-929 cells. J Cell Physiol 79:79–90

Greenberg PL, Mosny SA (1977) Cytotoxic effects of interferon in vitro on granulocytic progenitor cells. Cancer Res 3:1794–1799

Hagemann RF, Schenken LL, Lesher S (1973) Tumor chemotherapy efficacy dependent on mode of growth. J Natl Cancer Inst 50:467–474

Hahn GM, Little LB (1972) Plateau-phase cultures of mammalian cells. An in vitro model for human cancer. Curr Top Radiat Res 8:39–83

Hahn GM, Ray GR, Gordon, DE, Kallman RF (1973) Response of solid tumor cells exposed to chemotherapeutic agents in vitro. Cell curvival after 2- and 24-hour exposure. J Natl Cancer Inst 50:529–533

Hill BT, Whelan RDH (1981) Comparative cell killing and kinetic effects of vincristine or vindesine in mammalian cell lines. J Natl Cancer Inst

Johnston DA, White RA, Barlogie B (1978) Automatic processing and interpretation of DNA distributions: comparison of several techniques. Comput Biomed Res 11:393–404

Kaneko T, LePage GA (1978) Growth characteristics and drug responses of a murine lung carcinoma in vitro and in vivo. Cancer Res 38:2084–2090

Kim LH, Perez AG, Djordjevic B (1968) Studies on unbalanced growth in synchronized HeLa cells. Cancer Res 28:2443–2447

Kouns A (1975) Differential effects of isoleucine deprivation on cell motility, membrane transport and DNA synthesis in N1L8 hamster cells. Exp Cell Res 94:15–22

Lahiri SK (1973) Response of mouse bone marrow colony-forming units in different stages of the cell cycle to in vitro incubation with mitomycin C. Cell Tissue Kinet 6:509–514

Lambert WC, Studzinsky G (1967) Recovery from prolonged unbalanced growth induced in HeLa cells by high concentration of thymidine. Cancer Res 27:2364–2370

Lieberman MW, Verbin RS, Landay MM, Liang H, Farber E, Lee TN, Starr R (1970) A probable role for protein synthesis in intestinal epithelial cell damage induced in vivo by cytosine arabinoside, nitrogen mustard or x-irradiation. Cancer Res 30:942–4951

Macieira-Coelho A (1967) Influence of cell density on growth inhibition of human fibroblasts in vitro. Proc Soc Exp Biol Med 125:548–552

Madoc-Jones, Bruce WR (1967) Sensitivity of L-cells in exponential and stationary phase to 5-fluorouracil. Nature 215:302–303

Madoc-Jones H, Mauro F (1969) Interphase action of vinblastine and vincristine: differences in their lethal action through the mitotic cycle of cultured mammalian cells. J Cell Physiol 72:185–196

Madoc-Jones H, Mauro F (1970) Age responses to x-rays, *Vinca* alkaloids and hydroxyurea of murine lymphoma cells synchronized in vivo. J Natl Cancer Inst 45:1131–1143

Madoc-Jones H, Mauro F (1975) Site of action of cytotoxic agents in the cell life cycle. In: Sartorelli A, Johns D (eds) Antineoplastic and immunosuppressive agents. Springer, Berlin Heidelberg New York, p 205 (Handbook of Experimental Pharmacology, vol 38)

Mauro F, Falpo B, Briganti G, Elli R, Zupi G (1974a) Effects of antineoplastic drugs on plateau-phase cultures of mammalian cells. I. Description of the plateau-phase system. J Natl Cancer Inst 52:705–713

Mauro F, Falpo B, Briganti G, Elli R, Zupi G (1974b) Effects of antineoplastic drugs on plateau-phase cultures of mammalian cells. II. Bleomycin and hydroxyurea. J Natl Cancer Inst 52:715–722

Melamed MR, Mullaney PF, Mendelsohn ML (1979) Flow cytometry and sorting. Wiley, New York

Olah E, Palyi I, Sugar J (1978) Effects of cytostatics on proliferating and stationary cultures of mammalian cells. Eur J Cancer 14:895–900

Papirmeister B, Davidson CL (1965) Unbalanced growth and latent killing of *Escherichia coli* following exposure to sulfur mustard. Biochim Biophys Acta 103:70–92

Pardee AB (1974) A restriction point for control of normal animal cell proliferation. Proc Natl Acad Sci USA 71:1286

Pardee AB, James LJ (1975) Selective killing of transformed baby hamster kidney (BHK) cells. Proc Natl Acad Sci USA 72:4994–4998

Peel S, Cowen DM (1972) The effect of cyclophosphamide on the growth and cellular kinetics of a transplantable rat fibrosarcoma. Br J Cancer 26:304–314

Pittillo RF, Schabel FM, Skipper HE (1970) The "sensitivity" of resting and dividing cells. Cancer Chemother Rep 54:137–142

Puck TT, Marcus PI (1955) A rapid method for viable cell titration and clone production with HeLa cells in tissue culture. Proc Natl Acad Sci USA 41:432–437

Rajewsky MF (1975) Proliferative parameters relevant to cancer therapy. In: Grundmann E, Gross R (eds) The ambivalence of cytostatic therapy. Springer, Berlin Heidelberg New York, pp 156–171 (Recent results in cancer research, vol 52)

Ray GR, Hahn GM, Bagshaw MA, Kurkjian S (1973) Cell survival and repair of plateau-phase cultures after chemotherapy – relevance to tumor therapy and to the in vitro screening of new agents. Cancer Chemother Rep 57:473–475

Razek A, Vietti T, Valeriote F (1974) Optimum time sequence for the administration of vincristine and cyclophosphamide in vivo. Cancer Res 34:1857–1861

Razek A, Valeriote F, Vietti T (1980) Effect of dose fractionation of daunorubicin on survival of leukemic cells. Cancer Res 40:2835–2838

Roberts JJ, Brent TP, Crathorn AR (1971) Evidence for the inactivation and repair of the mammalian DNA template after alkylation by mustard gas and half mustard gas. Eur J Cancer 7:515–524

Roper P, Drewinko B (1976) Comparison of in vitro methods to determine drug-induced cell lethality. Cancer Res 36:2182–2188

Roper PR, Drewinko B (1979) Cell survival following treatment with antitumor drugs. Cancer Res 39:1428–1430

Rosenblum ML, Wheeler KT, Wilson CB, Barker M, Kuebel KD (1975) In vitro evaluation of in vivo brain tumor chemotherapy with 1,3-bis(2-chloroethyl)-1-nitrosourea. Cancer Res 35:1387–1391

Ross DW, Sinclair WK (1972) Cell cycle compartment analysis of Chinese hamster cells in stationary phase cultures. Cell Tissue Kinet 5:1–14
Roti Roti JL, Dethlefsen LA (1975) Matrix simulation of duodenal crypt cell kinetics. II. Cell kinetics following hydroxyurea. Cell Tissue Kinet 8:335–353
Rozengurt E, Po CC (1976) Selective cytotoxicity for transformed 3T3 cells. Nature 261:701–702
Rupniak HT, Paul D (1980) Selective killing of transformed cells by exploitation of their defective cell cycle control by polyamines. Cancer Res 40:293–297
Schabel FM (1969) The use of tumor growth kinetics in planning "curative" chemotherapy of advanced solid tumors. Cancer Res 29:2384–2389
Shackney SE, Erickson BW, Lengel CE (1978) Schedule optimization of cytosine arabinoside (CA) and hydroxyurea (HU) in sarcoma 180 in vitro. Proc Am Assoc Cancer Res, Abstract 900
Skipper HE (1970) Leukocyte kinetics in leukemia and lymphoma. In: Clark RL (ed) Leukemia – Lymphoma. Year Book Medical Publishers, Chicago, p 27
Steel GG (1977) Growth kinetics of tumours. Clarendon, Oxford
Stragand JJ, Bergerat J-P, White RA, Hokanson J, Drewinko B (1980) Biological and cell kinetic characteristics of a human colonic adenocarcinoma (LoVo) growth in athymic mice. Cancer Res 40:2846–2852
Sutherland RM (1974) Selective chemotherapy of noncycling cells in an in vitro tumor model. Cancer Res 34:3501–3503
Teodori L, Barlogie B, Drewinko B, Swatzendruber D, Mauro F (1981) Reduction of ara-C and adriamycin cytotoxicity following cell cycle arrest by anguidine. Cancer Res 41:1263–1270
Thatcher CJ, Walker IG (1969) Sensitivity of confluent and cycling embryonic hamster cells to sulfur mustard, 1,3-bis(2-chloroethyl)-1-nitrosourea and actinomycin D. J Natl Cancer Inst 42:363–368
Till JE, Whitmore GF, Gulyas S (1963) Deoxyribonucleic acid synthesis in individual L-strain mouse cells. II. Effects of thymidine starvation. Biochim Biophys Acta 72:277–281
Tobey RA, Ley KD (1970) Regulation of initiation of DNA synthesis in Chinese hamster cells. I. Production of stable, reversible, G_1-arrested population in suspension culture. J Cell Biol 46:151–157
Tobey RA, Peterson DF, Anderson ED, Puck TT (1966) Life cycle analysis of mammalian cells. II. The inhibition of division in Chinese hamster cells by puromycin and actinomycin. Biophys J 6:567–572
Tobey RA, Petersen DF, Anderson ED (1971) Biochemistry of G_2 and mitosis. In: Baserga R (ed) The cell cycle and cancer, vol 1. Dekker, New York, p 309
Tubiana M, Guichard M, Malaise EP (1977) Determinants of cell kinetics in radiotherapy. In: Drewinko B, Humphrey RM (eds) Growth kinetics and biochemical regulation of normal and malignant cells. William and Wilkins, Baltimore, pp 827–842
Twentyman PR (1976) Comparative chemosensitivity of exponential-versus plateau-phase cells in both in vitro and in vivo model systems. Cancer Treat Rep 60:1719–1722
Twentyman PR, Bleehen NM (1973) The sensitivity of cells in exponential and stationary phases of growth to bleomycin and to 1,3-bis(2-chloroethyl)-1-nitrosourea. Br J Cancer 28:500–507
Twentyman PR, Bleehen NM (1975) Changes in sensitivity to radiation and to bleomycin occurring during the life history of monolayer cultures of a mouse tumour cell line. Br J Cancer 31:68–74
Valeriote F, Hsui-san L (1975) Synergistic interaction of anticancer agents; a cellular perspective. Cancer Chemother Rep 59:895–900
Valeriote F, van Putten L (1975) Proliferation-dependent cytotoxicity of anti-cancer agents: a review. Cancer Res 35:2619–2630
Valeriote FA, Vietti D, Tolen S (1973) Kinetics of the lethal effects of actinomycin D on normal and leukemic cells. Cancer Res 33:2658–2661
van Putten LM (1974) Are cell kinetic data relevant for the design of tumour chemotherapy schedules? Cell Tissue Kinet 7:493–504

van Putten LM, Lelieveld P, Kram Idsenga LKJ (1972) Cell-cycle specificity and therapeutic effectiveness of cytostatic agents. Cancer Chemother Rep 56:691–700
Verbin RS, Diluiso G, Farber E (1973) Protective effects of cycloheximide against 1-β-D-arabinosylcytosine-induced intestinal lesions. Cancer Res 33:2086–2093
Weissberg JB, Herion JC, Walker RI, Palmer JG (1978) Effect of cycloheximide on the bonemarrow toxicity of nitrogen mustard. Cancer Res 38:1523–1527
Wotring LL, Roti Roti JL (1980) Thioguanine-induced S and G_2 blocks and their significance to the mechanism of cytotoxicity. Cancer Res 40:1458–1462
Zubrod GC (1969) Trends in chemotherapy research. Can Cancer Conf 8:31–39

CHAPTER 7

Tumour Resistance and the Phenomenon of Inflammatory-Cell Infiltration

M. MOORE

A. Introduction

I. Heterogeneity of Tumour Cells

Tumours consist of a multiplicity of discrete cell populations which differ from each other in several physical, biological, and biochemical respects. Clonal analysis of proliferating tumour-cell populations has disclosed differences in morphology (DEXTER et al. 1978), karyotype (ITO and MOORE 1967; MITELMAN 1972; PÁLYI et al. 1977), growth rate and metastatic potential (FIDLER 1978; FIDLER and KRIPKE 1977), hormone receptors, enzyme characteristics, pigment production, metabolic activity and antigenicity (FIDLER 1978; SUGARBAKER and COHEN 1972; MIAN et al. 1974) in clones and subpopulations derived in vitro or in vivo from the original cell population.

The question whether the new biological characteristics of the derived clones pre-exist in the parent tumour population or result from an acquired genetic variability during proliferation has not been finally settled. It seems likely that most neoplasms arise from a single cell and that the subsequent heterogeneity is the consequence of mutation and selection, the latter process allowing for the emergence of subpopulations with an increased potential for survival (NOWELL 1976). On the other hand, carcinogen-induced tumours may be multifocal in origin and exhibit heterogeneity ab initio (PIMM and BALDWIN 1977).

The variety of biological and biochemical characteristics within a heterogeneous tumour-cell population is frequently accompanied by differences in drug sensitivity which also become apparent from experiments on isolated clones. Such differences have been found between cell clones isolated in vitro from established cell lines or between cell subpopulations derived from experimental tumours in vivo (HAKANSSON and TROPÉ 1974; PÁLYI et al. 1977; TROPÉ 1974). Similar differences have been documented for cell lines and in vivo-derived human neoplasms, as well as between primary cancers and their ascitic variants, different metastatic lymph nodes from the same patient tumour-bearing host and cells originating from various sites of the same tumour (UJHÁZY and SIRACKÝ 1980). The heterogeneity of tumour-cell populations represents a serious limitation on the rational design of chemotherapy based on the utilization of what might otherwise be adequate predictive pharmacological or biochemical assays.

In addition to the neoplastic cells, tumours comprise a vascular stroma derived from the host's tissues including, not infrequently, a heterogeneous lymphoreticular-cell [1] infiltrate the composition of which may vary widely between tumours of similar and dissimilar histological type, at different stages of tumour progression, and between primary and metastatic cancers (UNDERWOOD 1974).

II. Intratumour Lymphoreticular Cells: Biological Implications

The so-called "inflammatory" infiltrates of experimental and human tumours have been partially characterized by light microscopy of conventionally stained tissue sections, but recently disaggregation of tumours into single-cell suspensions has facilitated more definitive characterization of individual cell types and their associated functions. Both approaches are important for a comprehensive understanding of the way in which inflammatory cells relate to the biology of a neoplasm, though neither is free from limitations and potential artefacts which may be decisive for a critical evaluation of the phenomenon.

Recognition of lymphoreticular cells in human tumours goes back some 70 years when histopathologists first drew attention to "round-cell infiltration", which is a common, if somewhat inconsistent, feature of many epithelial neoplasms and some mesenchymal tumours as well. In the intervening years a favourable association between infiltration by lymphoreticular cells and prognosis has, in some quarters, tended to gain acceptance and has acquired immunological and defensive overtones (UNDERWOOD 1974). On the other hand there are many pathologists who have found no prognostic significance in the extent of leucocyte infiltration into tumours (TANAKA et al. 1970; CHAMPION et al. 1972; MORRISON et al. 1973). There is no direct evidence that the infiltrating cells are actively defensive in a conventional sense, except possibly in certain rare cases. Medullary carcinoma of the breast (O. S. MOORE and FOOTE 1949) and seminoma of the testis (SAUER and BURKE 1949) exemplify two such human tumour-host systems. There is a consensus that each has a more favourable prognosis than other types of neoplasm arising in the same organ. However, even in these situations it is difficult to determine whether the infiltrative cells exert any cytodestructive and/or cystostatic effects in situ.

Necrotic tissue can evoke a powerful inflammatory reaction and is undoubtedly responsible for polymorphonuclear leucocyte infiltration in some situations. However, there are numerous examples where the infiltrate (often devoid of polymorphs) has clearly been elicited independently of necrosis. One hypothesis, for which some experimental evidence is available, suggests that the intense leucocyte infiltration seen in some tumours may reflect concomitant immunity, i.e. the process whereby deposits of tumour cells in other organs or tissues are eliminated without significant destruction of the primary lesion (UNDERWOOD 1974). In other situations where an active cytodestructive role might be expected, evidence for infiltrating cells is lacking. The phenomenon was not observed to be a consistent feature in the cases of spontaneous tumour regression collected by EVERSON and COLE (1966) and in other situations (e.g. malignant melanoma) infiltration does not appear to be a necessary concomitant of tumour regression (BERG 1971). At a histopathological level, if infiltration indicates a host immune

1 Herein considered to include cells of the mononuclear phagocytic system, polymorphonuclear leucocytes, lymphocytes, and plasma cells

response, in the vast majority of cases, it would seem to represent a belated (or outmanoeuvred) effort to restrain a process which, apart from therapeutic intervention, has "escaped" beyond recall.

In theory this cellular "immunoresistance" could arise in several different ways (WOODRUFF 1980). At the level of the tumour, chromosomal changes, and alterations in cell surface antigen expression (by selective loss or modulation by antibody) represent two possible mechanisms by which attacking host cells may be deprived of their point d'appui. At the effector-cell level varying degrees of immune dysfunction might be envisaged to occur both systemically and in situ, in consequence of the early interaction between tumour and host. On this view, the presence of inflammatory cells in progressing neoplasms may be regarded as vestigial and experimental tumour-host systems in which identical neoplasms, depending on the conditions, spontaneously regress or progress of particular value for the elucidation of the biological role of inflammatory cells in situ.

Another school of thought, to which more recent experimental data (discussed later in Sects. C,IV, D.III) lend some support is that, in certain circumstances, lymphoreticular cells may actually favour and accelerate tumour growth. PREHN (1977) has argued that a weak cell-mediated immune response may actually be growth-stimulatory though it is not clear whether a persistent stromal relationship between lymphocytes and tumour cells is essential for growth stimulation to be sustained in an established lesion.

The prognostic and biological implications of inflammatory cells in tissue sections of experimental and human tumours, using conventional histological techniques, have been the subject of several reviews (e.g. UNDERWOOD 1974; TØNDER et al. 1980; IOACHIM 1976, 1980; IOACHIM et al. 1976). While these studies here failed to establish any systematic correlation between infiltration and biological behaviour of most neoplasms by these means, indications that host cells may be implicated in the regulation of tumour growth have provided the rationale for more detailed examination of the non neoplastic cells in a variety of experimental and human neoplasms. Host defences are believed to extend to a diversity of mechanisms, both immunological and non-immunological (APFFEL 1976). Immunological phenomena are thus only one facet of a complex, multifactorial situation.

III. Methodological Approaches

Notwithstanding the interpretative difficulties, histological examination is indispensable for information on the distribution of inflammatory cells within a neoplasm. Contact or close proximity between tumour cells and host cells is a likely prerequisite for the efficient expression of many tumour-inhibitory cell functions, especially cytotoxicity. Conventional microscopy may reveal whether host cells are relegated to the periphery of the tumour (LAUDER et al. 1977; RUSSELL and GILLESPIE 1977; SVENNEVIG et al. 1978), to bands of connective tissue separating lobules of neoplastic cells (ABRAHAM and BARBOLT 1978; SVENNEVIG and SVAAR 1979) or uniformly distributed and in intimate contact with tumour cells (LAUDER et al. 1977; RUSSELL and GILLESPIE 1977). Furthermore, the usefulness of this approach is enhanced if coupled with other techniques such as ultrastructural examination (CARR and UNDERWOOD 1974; UNDERWOOD and CARR 1972; KIKUCHI et al. 1976), immune haemadsorption (TØNDER et al. 1978; RUSSELL et al. 1980b), histochemistry (LAUDER et al. 1977; WOODS and PAPADIMITRIOU 1977; ABRAHAM and BARBOLT 1978; SVENNEVIG et al. 1979; SVENNEVIG 1980) or immunofluorescence (HUSBY et al. 1976; WOOD and GOLLAHON 1978) aimed at delineating specific cell types, provided the sampling is sufficiently representative of the lesion as a whole. Even so, the limitations of this approach are axiomatic. In man, particularly, tissue is rarely available for analysis at more than one instant in the pathogenesis of the lesion, and this is usually when the tumour is relatively advanced. The problem of subjectivity in making cell identifications based purely on morphological criteria and the attendant possibility that some inflammatory cells (e.g. macrophages) may actually be missed are further disadvantages of this approach. Above all, despite the inference from histology the functional attributes of in situ inflammatory cells cannot be ascertained. The morphological homogeneity of the lymphocyte, for instance, conceals an immense degree of functional diversity, and functional heterogeneity is also a feature of other inflammatory-cell types.

Recently, the availability of techniques for the recognition, fractionation and separation of subgroups of lymphoreticular cells within tumours from each other and from the neoplastic cells has disclosed a potential for understanding their biological role, which was inaccessible via conventional histopathology and associated refinements (RUSSELL et al. 1980a). Although it is recognized that tumour disaggregation raises new problems of a technical and interpretative nature, it is with the implications of these recent developments that we are here primarily concerned. In theory, disaggregation followed by separation of inflammatory cells from those of the tumour would appear to offer the prospect of more definitive qualitative and quantitative cellular characterization and delineation of functional roles than conventional histology. This assertion, however, is based on several assumptions: first, that tumour-cell suspensions are representative of the intact tissues from which they are derived; second, that the techniques for the differential characterization of the various cellular components are not adversely affected by the disaggregation procedures; third, that the isolated components of the inflammatory response retain their functional integrity; fourth and most important, that studies of cell-to-cell interactions in vitro bear some definitive relationship to those occurring in the microenvironment of the tumour from which they were isolated.

In recent years the validity of these assumptions has been critically examined for a wide variety of experimental tumours and for some human neoplasms as well (RUSSELL et al. 1980a). Mechanical and/or enzymatic dissolution of tumour is invariably traumatic, though frequently damage can be minimized. Even so, accurate quantification of cell yield has proved virtually impossible to attain: approaches based on comparison of DNA in the final cell suspension with that in the intact neoplasm, for instance, are complicated by an inability to distinguish DNA in viable cells from that in necrotic zones (RUSSELL et al. 1976a). An alternative approach, confined to use in laboratory animals, and based upon in vivo γ-isotopic labelling of cells within the tumour (BOERYD et al. 1965), is likewise not without difficulties. The diverse cells in neoplasms might be expected to take up the label in widely differing amounts and at different rates. Should selective loss of one or more cell types occur during dispersion, estimates of yield will be biased according to the amount of radioactivity associated with the host cell types.

While recovery is difficult to quantify, judicious combinations of enzymes and manoeuvres to minimize deleterious effects indicate that it is possible to obtain consistently single-cell suspensions of many experimental neoplasms which are grossly representative of the original in vivo population (RUSSELL et al. 1980a). Unfortunately, for many human cancers this may not be the case, not only because the requirements of histological diagnosis frequently render the greater part of the lesion unavailable, but also because replicate specimens cannot be obtained. Possible harmful effects of enzymes on inflammatory components, however, can usually be independently controlled by collateral studies of their effects on defined populations from normal lymphoid organs or peripheral blood, where high recovery of viable cells with retention of functional integrity is readily achieved.

Notwithstanding the advances which have been made in this field, now extending to a wide range of experimental and human neoplasms, identification of individual cell types and appraisal of their functional attributes in an isolated state should be made in the awareness that minor shifts in population distribution are probably unavoidable upon disaggregation and that these may be accompanied by subtle functional changes associated with, for example, the absence either of appropriate chemical mediators or of cooperative cells in the recovered populations.

B. Characterization of Intratumour Host-Cells

I. Total Host-Cell Component

Infiltrative inflammatory cells have been identified in freshly disaggregated tumour-cell suspensions by a variety of techniques, schematically represented in Fig. 1. For many of these actual physical separation of infiltrative cells from the neoplastic compartment is not a necessary requirement. A useful estimate of the total host-cell content of animal neoplasms can be obtained by serological analysis of parental tumours grown in F_1 hybrids. For instance, tumour cells originating in strain A of an animal and cultivated in vitro for a period (so as to effectively eliminate inflammatory cells contaminating the original explanted cells) may thereafter be injected into $(A \times B)$ F_1 hosts in which, as in strictly syngeneic hosts, any immune response is directed solely against tumour-associated antigens. The emergent tumour then comprises neoplastic cells of *A* genotype and non-neoplastic recipient host cells of $(A \times B)$ F_1 genotype. These latter can be readily distinguished from the progeny of the original inoculum and accurately quantified by immunofluorescent visualization with *A* anti-*B* alloantiserum (i.e. antiserum raised in strain *A* hosts by immunization with strain *B* antigens), or alternatively, by enumeration of cells killed in the presence of the antiserum and complement. This method has been applied to several rodent tumour systems where values obtained have corresponded remarkably well with cumulative estimates based upon other immunological criteria (KERBEL et al. 1975; K. MOORE and M. MOORE 1977).

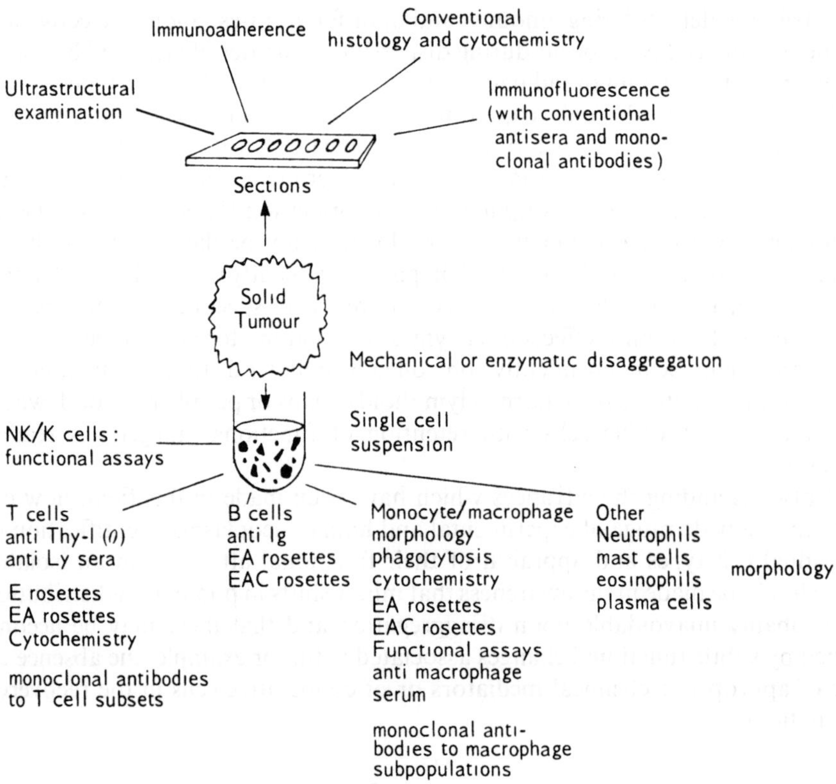

Fig. 1. Methodological approaches to the characterization and functional evaluation of leucocytes infiltrating solid tumours

II. Criteria for the Identification of Leucocyte Populations and Subpopulations

Exploitation of the receptor for the Fc portion of immunoglobulin G (FcγR) detected by formation of erythrocyte-antibody (EA) rosettes has been a particularly useful marker for infiltrating leucocytes by virtue of the variety of cells on which the FcR is found. The receptors are present on monocytes, macrophages and lymphocytes, as well as on polymorphonuclear leucocytes (Kerbel and Davies 1974). They are also present on a heterogeneous subpopulation of activated T cells (Rubin and Hertel-Wulff 1975). Not unexpectedly, FcR are present on some lymphoid neoplasms, but are apparently absent from solid tumour cells with which in this chapter we are mainly concerned (Kerbel et al. 1975). The virtual ubiquity of FcR on tumour-infiltrating leucocytes, particularly of some experimental tumours, has led some investigators to equate FcR^+ cells with the total leucocyte infiltrate. This assumption is likely to underestimate the total number of infiltrating cells since only a proportion of T cells, for example, are FcR^+. Since phagocytic cells and certain lymphoid cells all bear FcR, an estimate of the lymphoid contribution to the infiltrating cells can be made by subtraction of the percentage phagocytes from the total FcR^+ population. However, non-phagocytic FcR^+ cells should not be too rigidly equated with lymphoid cells since immature non-phagocytic monocytoid cells may also be FcR^+ (NATHAN et al. 1976).

Use of the receptor for the third component of complement (C3R), detected by formation of erythrocyte-antibody-complement (EAC) rosettes, has also facilitated the identification of infiltrating leucocytes. $C3R^+$ cells consist mainly of B-lymphocytes and monocytes and macrophages. There is evidence that in some situations tumour macrophages have their C3R blocked by a putative C3-containing complex which remains bound throughout the incubation period of the rosette test. Alternatively, by contrast with FcR, C3R may be lost through activation. These observations are based on the findings that the number of macrophages estimated in some tumours by functional and morphological criteria was not reflected by the estimates of C3R-bearing cells. Similar findings have been reported for macrophages and B cells recovered from acutely rejecting rat cardiac allografts (TILNEY et al. 1975), and emphasize that some properties of infiltrative cells whether of syngeneic tumour grafts or allografts may be influenced by their pathological environment and/or by the procedure used to retrieve them.

Cells of the mononuclear phagocytic system (MPS) are readily identified in Jenner-Giesma-stained cytocentrifuge preparations by morphology in short-term tissue culture (EVANS 1972), by their ability to phagocytose membrane-bound EA complexes after formation of rosettes and by uptake of polystyrene latex with which alternative parameter numerical correspondence is very close (K. MOORE and M. MOORE 1977). In addition macrophages may be demonstrated cytochemically by their non-specific esterase activity (YAM et al. 1971). Neutrophils phagocytosing latex are distinguished from macrophages by their characteristic nuclear structure, and other cell types (eosinophils, basophils, mast cells) are easily identified solely on morphological grounds.

Serological approaches to the identification of tumour inflammatory cells, additional to those already described, have utilized anti Thy-1 sera (originally anti θ sera) to quantify intratumoral thymus-derived lymphocytes in mice (e.g. PROSS and KERBEL 1976), heterologous antithymocyte sera (ATS) for similar evaluations in mice and other species (e.g. RUSSELL et al. 1976a, b; K. MOORE and M. MOORE 1977; WOOD and GOLLAHON 1978) and heterologous antimacrophage sera to delineate cells of the mononuclear phagocytic system (MPS) (ECCLES et al. 1976; GAUCI and ALEXANDER 1975). To date, almost all serological reagents used in this context have been generated by conventional means by xeno- or alloimmunization followed by appropriate absorption to remove unwanted specificities. In murine systems, the use of alloantisera directed against T-lymphocyte subsets has defined Ly alloantigens and cell surface marker profiles characteristic for T-helper and T-suppressor cells. These reagents and the monoclonal hybridoma reagents which are beginning to supersede them have yet to be applied to the delineation of intratumour murine lymphocytes. Labelled antiimmunoglobulin sera [or more usually the $F(ab')_2$ fragment of an anti Ig to prevent attachment to FcR] have been used to identify intratumour B cells which can usually be distinguished from tumour cells with cytophilic antibody on the basis of size or morphology.

Gross estimates of human T cells infiltrating solid neoplasms have been determined on the basis of their capacity to form spontaneous rosettes with sheep erythrocytes (HÄYRY and TÖTTERMAN 1978; SVENNEVIG et al. 1978); and α-naphthyl acetate esterase (ANAE) has been deployed as an additional cytochemical aid to distinguish T cells from B cells (SVENNEVIG 1980). Recently, T cells have been divided into several subpopulations on the basis of FcR for IgG, IgM, IgA, and IgE. T cells with IgG FcR (Tγ) are believed to represent a possible suppressor population, whereas T cells with IgM FcR (Tμ) have been shown to effect T-cell help. However, recent studies comparing a number of cell surface markers using monoclonal hybridoma reagents have emphasized the heterogeneity of Tγ cells, a subpopulation of which express I-region gene products, i.e. Ia antigens. In vitro studies in man have suggested that Ia^+ T cells may function as helpers.

Another population of cells often encountered in experimental and human tumours possesses neither B- nor T-cell markers. These cells – also known as "null" cells – are heterogeneous and in man a major subpopulation expresses FcR. Some cells of the "null" compartment (accounting for an estimated 2%–4% of normal human peripheral blood lymphocytes) are characterized operationally by their ability to lyse certain propagated tumour-cell lines – the so-called natural killer (NK) effect (HERBERMAN and HOLDEN 1978). The lineage of NK cells is presently undecided. In both mice and men there are grounds for identification with cells of myelomonocytic and lymphoid lineage, but current analyses with monoclonal antibodies may yet disclose a separate lineage with a precursor stem cell which is common to other peripheral blood cells. By presently available means these cells cannot be physically separated or distinguished by other criteria from "killer" or K cells, though they exert their cytotoxic functions via different mechanisms (Sect. D.I). K-cell function, which is synonymous with antibody-dependent cellular cytotoxicity (ADCC), involves the FcR for attachment to and lysis of the sensitized target, while NK function is, for the most part, antibody independent and the FcR is uninvolved (HERBERMAN et al. 1979).

Judicious combinations of the various procedures outlined above have confirmed the reports of pathologists made over half a century ago that many experimental and human neoplasms are frequently characterized by inflammatory infiltrates consisting variously of lymphocytes and plasma cells, monocytes, macrophages, and polymorphonuclear leucocytes. The relatively recent application of immunological techniques to the analysis of disaggregated tumours has introduced a quantitative dimension into the field and paved the way for functional analysis of the infiltrative cellular components. Even so it should be realized that the study of intratumour inflammatory cells is still in its infancy. Very few studies have appeared where the infiltrates have been characterized with the modern subclass-specific markers or monoclonal antibodies, the future application of which will be indispensable to the further elucidation of their biological significance.

C. Intratumour Leucocytes of Experimental and Human Neoplasms: Descriptive Studies

I. Preliminary Considerations

The main experimental tumours in which inflammatory cells have now been identified following disaggregation are summarized in Table 1. These comprise tumours induced by chemical carcinogens, radiation, and oncogenic viruses, as well as "spontaneous" neoplasms of unknown aetiology. For a given tumour, several variables will determine the qualitative and quantitative pattern of infiltrating cells, e.g. whether tested as primary tumour or transplant (and if the latter, the transplantation history); the immune status of the implanted host; the immunogenicity of the tumour; the nature of the implant (graft or cells), the degree of vascularization; and whether, as in most instances, tumour growth is destined to be inexorable or regressive. In the case of oncornavirus-induced tumours (e.g. Moloney sarcomas), the host strain may be critically important for the type of cellular infiltrate (BECKER 1980). However, under appropriately controlled conditions, the appearance of inflammatory cells within the same transplanted tumour and, more broadly, within the same tumour type (e.g. virus and chemically induced murine sarcomas) is a predictable phenomenon and therefore may be justifiably considered an intrinsic feature of the host reaction to the tumour in question.

II. Nature of Cells Infiltrating Experimental Neoplasms: Biological Correlates

Many chemically induced rodent sarcomas transplanted into syngeneic recipients are characterized by a macrophage infiltrate which occasionally numerically exceeds even the neoplastic population (EVANS 1972). The macrophage compartment tends to be greatest in primary tumours and declines progressively to a relatively stable level on serial transplantation (EVANS 1972; PROSS and KERBEL 1976). The macrophage content also varies as a function of time after transplantation of tumour cells (K. MOORE and M. MOORE 1977; M. MOORE and K. MOORE 1977). For some tumours, macrophages appear to form a greater proportion of the transplanted tumour mass when it is barely clinically detectable than when a tumour is well established. Events prior to the clinical detection (i.e. at the microscopic level) of a neoplasm have to date proved difficult to study, though there is evidence that here too, amidst the pleomorphic host cells, macrophages are also to be found (Woodruff, personal communication). Tumours which are immunogenic contain more macrophages than weakly- or non-immunogenic neoplasms (EVANS 1972) and the fact that some tumours in the latter categories spontaneously metastasize implies a relationship between tumour immunogenicity, macrophage infiltration and biological behaviour. The validity of this hypothesis has been tested by several investigators (ECCLES and ALEXANDER 1974, 1975; WOOD and GILLESPIE 1975). ECCLES and ALEXANDER (1974) observed that the capacity of rat fibrosarcomas to metastasize on transplantation in syngeneic hosts was inversely related to the immunogenicity and macrophage content of the tumour. In their model, control of metastatic spread was held to be regulated by the macrophage content

Table 1. Inflammatory cellular infiltrates of solid experimental neoplasms. I. Identification of host cells in primary and transplanted tumours; descriptive studies on disaggregated tumour-cell suspensions

Tumour/host system[a]	Host-cell population determined (%)[b]	Remarks	References
FS1, FS6, FS9 (C57Bl)	Macrophage; 20, 33, 45	All tumours immunogenic and non-metastatic except HSH and MC3	Evans (1972)
A, MCI, HSG, HSH, HSN, MC3 (hooded rat)	Macrophage; 53, 33, 9, 11, 46, 4		
Primary-1, -2, -3	Macrophage; 54, 45, 33		
FS9, Gardner[c] (CBA/H)	FcR^+; 54, 6	Many FcR^+ cells actively phagocytic, Tumour-cell cultures FcR^-	Kerbel et al. (1975)
CAD2[d], SAD2 (DBA/2)	FcR^+; 38, 61		
S-180 (BALB/c)	FcR^+; 42		
Primary MBQ-A, -B, -C, D, -E (CBA)	FcR^+ and θ^+; 68, 49, 55, 52, 39	Marker-bearing cells decreased to constant level on transplantation	Pross and Kerbel (1976)
MC3, HSH, ASPBI, MCI-M, HSN, HSBPA (hooded rat)	Macrophage; 8, 12, 22, 38, 40, 54	MØ content proportional to immunogenicity and inversely proportional to metastatic capacity in immunosuppressed hosts	Eccles and Alexander (1974), Eccles and Alexander (1975)
H-P[e], MCA-050, -060, MSV[f] (BALB/c)	FcR^+; >95, 50, 25, 95	Determined on primary cultures by absorption of sensitized ^{99m}Tc-labelled sheep red blood cells	Wood et al. (1975)
B16[e], (C57Bl)	FcR^+; 25		
Sarcoma I (A/J); MCA-43 (C3H)	FcR^+; 95, 95		
Walker 256 (Holtzman rat)	FcR^+; 50		
MSC[f] (BALB/c) Progressors:	N(4), Eo(1), T(7), MØ(9)	Neutrophils (N), eosinophils (Eo) T cells (T) and MØ proportions dependent on time postinoculation. Values given for day 14	Russell et al. (1976a, b)
Regressors:	N(4), Eo(3), T(27), MØ(9)		

Table 1 (Continued)

Tumour/host system[a]	Host-cell population determined (%)[b]	Remarks	References
Mc40A, Mc57, (W/not rat) AAF57[d], SPI[d], SP22[d] Primary MC2, MC3, MC5	FcR$^+$ and T cells; 42 45 $<$15, $<$15, $<$15 FcR$^+$; 41, 33, 44	Growth rate (s.c.) AAF57 > SP22 > > Mc40A Host-cell content reflects immunogenicity of tumours	K. Moore and M. Moore (1977); M. Moore and K. Moore (1977); M. Moore and K. Moore (1980)
MC (CBA)	FcR$^+$; 43	FcR$^+$ cells unchanged in T-cell-deprived mice	Szymaniec and James (1976)
MTV[d,f] (BALB/cf C3H and BALB/c) Primary: Transpl:	θ^+ (8–46): ALS$^+$ (34–46): FcR$^+$ ($\sim$15) θ^+ (14–47): ALS$^+$ (14–100): FcR$^+$ ($\sim$15)	Values are % (range) of lymphoid cells separated from tumour by isokinetic gradient centrifugation (fractions 4 to 6)	Blazar and Heppner (1978a, b)
B16[e] (C57Bl), Sa I (A/J), MCA-43 (C3H) Primary MCA-A, -B, -C, -D, -E, -F, -G (C3H)	Large FcR$^+$ (macrophage); 9, 34, 49 Large FcR$^+$ (macrophage); 27, 49, 36, 54, 27, 19, 47	Tumours depleted of macrophages display increased potential for metastasis	Wood and Gillespie (1975)
Primary MCA[(22)] (C3H/He)	$<$0.25 cm^3 T cells, 10%–83%; m∅, 0%–42% 0.25–1.0 cm^3 T cells, 10%–78%, M∅, 8%–38% $>$1.0 cm^3 T cells, 10%–24%, M∅, 38%–56%	M∅ content greater in larger tumours; T cells fewer, dispersed throughout tumour mass in small tumours, M∅ generally near tumour periphery	Wood and Gollahon (1978)

[a] Tumours cited are rodent sarcomas passaged in syngeneic hosts (strains in parentheses)
[b] As percentage of disaggregated tumour-cell suspensions, unless otherwise stated
[c] Lymphosarcoma
[d] Carcinoma
[e] Melanoma
[f] Virus (MSV or MTV)-induced tumours

of the tumour, which in turn was determined by specific T-cell responses evoked by tumour-associated antigens. This interpretation was supported by the fact that the frequency of metastases in tumour-bearing rats rendered T cell deficient by thymectomy and whole-body irradiation, but in which bone marrow function was normal, was greater than in their normal immunocompetent counterparts. These data also implied that, in the normal host, tumour cells with a propensity for metastasis frequently fail to do so on account of effective immune restraint. Consistent with the above findings WOOD and GILLESPIE (1975) found that the potential for metastasis in mice, of tumour-cell suspensions depleted of macrophages by adherence, was increased over that of suspensions in which macrophages were retained, and that this difference was reflected in the relative survival of the mice. PROSS and KERBEL (1976) also found in their series that the murine tumours with the least macrophages consistently appeared more rapidly and killed their hosts more quickly than those with the most macrophages.

Whether it is reasonable to assume that the many variables affecting the complex processes of tumour growth and metastasis allow for the formulation of simple bifactorial correlations has been questioned by several investigators, largely on the basis of the somewhat contradictory results in different tumour-host systems. Thus in some systems, depression of immunological reactivity decreases, or even prevents metastasis, or has no influence on the growth of a local or disseminated tumour (FIDLER 1974; UMIEL and TRAININ 1974; VAAGE 1978; HEWITT et al. 1976). The bases for these differences could lie in attempted comparison of tumours of disparate histological type, aetiology, strain or species. However, even under relatively uniform conditions, viz. evaluation of metastatic potential of three C_3H murine fibrosarcomas of different degrees of immunogenicity in normal, immunodepressed and immunoreconstituted mice the influence of the immune system varied for the different tumours (FIDLER et al. 1979). Experimentally, metastases do not appear to arise from random survival of cells released from the primary tumour but from the selective growth of specialized subpopulations of highly metastatic cells endowed with specific properties which befit them to complete each step of the metastatic process (POSTE and FIDLER 1980). The role of the macrophages in the complex multifactorial events has yet to be elucidated. In this context it is noteworthy that metastatic lesions usually contain far fewer macrophages than primary tumours.

A formal analysis of the relationship between tumour immunogenicity and host-cell content in transplanted neoplasms was undertaken by K. MOORE and M. MOORE (1977) and M. MOORE and K. MOORE (1977). Two immunogenic chemically induced rat sarcomas were found to contain significantly more host cells than a non-immunogenic chemically induced hepatoma and two spontaneous tumours. In the immunogenic tumours, and to a proportional extent in the non-immunogenic tumours as well, the host-cell compartment was found to comprise not only macrophages, but also non-phagocytic FcR^+ cells (?lymphoid ?monocytoid) and T cells, each in roughly equivalent proportions. Moreover, studies on infiltration of the tumours as a function of time after inoculation of pure tumour cells revealed that macrophages were as much a feature of early non-immunogenic tumours as of immunogenic tumours. These findings prompted the suggestion that the presence of macrophages at some stages of tumour development may be primarily determined by events of a non-immune nature. The propensity of these tumours to metastasize was not examined, but there was a broadly inverse relationship between the rate of subcutaneous growth and host-cell infiltration. For the non-immunogenic carcinomas, the absence of a significant antigenic stimulus was considered to be the more likely factor limiting the ingress of host leucocytes than that the rate of growth was so rapid as to completely outflank the immune response. In addition to macrophages, T cells have also been identified in primary murine chemically induced sarcomas (PROSS and KERBEL 1976; WOOD and GOLLAHON 1978) where their concentration appears to be largely a function of tumour size. Interestingly, in small chemically induced primary tumours ($<0.25\ cm^3$) T cells not infrequently account for the majority of the infiltrating population, whereas in larger neoplasms ($>1.0\ cm^3$) relatively more macrophages are to be found (WOOD and GOLLAHON 1978). T cells are also very much in evidence in chemically induced autochthonous rat sarcomas of high antigenicity undergoing regression (KIKUCHI et al. 1976). In primary mammary carcinomas and early generation transplants in BALB/c mice, the content of Thy 1^+ T cells although somewhat variable has a tendency to exceed that of FcR^+ cells of which the macrophage component is approximately half (BLAZAR and HEPPNER 1978a, b). The disparate nature of the cellular infiltrates among various tumour types underlines the need to take into account the basic individuality of each tumour-host system.

This point is further emphasized by consideration of the Moloney sarcoma virus (MSV) tumour system. Some morphological analyses of enzyme-dispersed MSV tumour material have revealed that only a minority of the cells ($<10\%$) could be identified as possible tumour cells (PLATA et al. 1975; BECKER and HASKILL 1981), the remaining cells consisting of inflammatory macrophages, polymorphs, and lymphocytes. These observations are consistent with several earlier histopathological studies of the lesion (STANTON et al. 1968; SIEGLER 1970; SIMONS and MCCULLY 1970) which emphasized the non-neoplastic nature of the cells, an interpretation consistent with the lack of success in the establishment of either transplantable tumour lines or the culture of the cells in vitro. On this view, it is argued that the MSV "tumour" is the manifestation of a response to a highly noxious virus infection rather than a tumour of dividing, transformed malignant cells.

An alternative view of the MSV sarcoma (RUSSELL and COCHRANE 1974) attributes the description of MSV tumours as atypical granulomas to experimental conditions in which dosage levels of MSV favoured the induction of regressing sarcomas, replete with the inflammatory response that is characteristic of the process. These investigators claimed that, depending upon the size of the inocula and the immune status of the recipients, tumours generated from a transplantable Moloney sarcoma line (MSC) (MASSICOT et al. 1971) could regress or progress with the development of secondary neoplasms. Inflammatory infiltrates of this tumour are composed exclusively of three broad cell types: neutrophils, T-lymphocytes, and macrophages; and the extent to which each was found varied with the time post inoculation of MSC. Neutrophils formed part of an early acute inflammatory response seen in both regressing and progressing sarcomas. The onset of regression was associated with the appearance of macrophages and T-lymphocytes, the latter always being present in greater porportion than in progressing sarcomas. Macrophage numbers were comparable in both progressors and regressors but histological examination indicated that there were differences in distribution: in the former they were confined to the periphery of the neoplasm, while in the latter they were distributed throughout. It is suggested that T-lymphocytes are instrumental in causing regression of Moloney sarcomas possibly through interactions with macrophages (RUSSELL et al. 1976 a, b).

A central issue between the two schools of thought about MSV sarcomas is whether the established tumour cell line (MSC) from which much of the inflammatory-cell data have been obtained has acquired characteristics, after extensive in vitro passage, different from those of the primary cells. In any event, studies of the inflammatory response to presumptive MSV sarcomas should be interpreted with the awareness that this lesion, although of intrinsic interest, is atypical of neoplasia in general. The growth of the majority of experimental neoplasms is relentless, and as such they are of seemingly greater relevance to the pervasive problem of human malignancy.

III. Nature of Cells Infiltrating Human Neoplasms: Clinicopathological Correlates

Several of the more common human malignancies have yielded evidence of infiltrating inflammatory cells following disaggregation (Table 2), and functional studies on preparations from which tumour cells have been largely removed are also now beginning to emerge. As was previously stressed, the study of human neoplasia suffers from the limitation that tumours can be analysed in this way only once and interpretation of the phenomena must rely to a large extent on what is observed in experimental systems with comparable patterns of infiltration.

In common with experimental tumours, macrophages, identified in cell suspensions by multiple criteria, are a common component of the non-neoplastic compartment. Numerically, the range of these cells is invariably wide (0%–30%), but where disease is localized (e.g. primary malignant melanoma or localized node-negative breast carcinoma) the macrophage content may approach 30% of the total cell suspension (GAUCI and ALEXANDER 1975). In benign disease and metastatic lesions, macrophages rarely account for >10% of the disaggregated tumour populations. This correlation is supported by cytochemical estimates of macrophages in infiltrating breast cancer, where significantly fewer cases with metastases were found among tumours with high numbers of macrophages and plasma cells (LAUDER et al. 1977). In this respect there is also a parallel with the relative macrophage content of some experimental tumours of metastasizing and non-metastasizing capability.

The range of human cancers found to be infiltrated by macrophages is apparent from the data of WOOD and GOLLAHON (1977), who identified FcR^+ cells in frozen sections from 39 tumours of various histopathological types, by adsorption of antibody-coated sheep erythrocytes. Their estimates by this technique, which varied from 5% to 100% of the tumour section covered, corresponded well with evaluation of FcR^+ after disaggregation of the corresponding tumours. The latter procedure enabled the vast majority of the FcR^+ cells to be identified morphologically, cytochemically and functionally as macrophages.

Systematic examination of human tumour-cell suspensions for leucocytes, in addition to macrophages, have to date been undertaken by a relatively small number of investigators (Table 2). Not unexpectedly, wide numerical variability is a conspicuous feature of these studies, which are drawn from a broad spectrum of untreated human cancers presenting at different stages in the pathogenesis of the disease.

SVENNEVIG and SVAAR (1979) found that lymphocytes and macrophages identified in mechanically prepared cell suspensions from 20 common solid human tumours comprised only a minority (< 10%) of the recovered populations. Studies of their distribution on cryostat sections indicated that both cell types were usually more numerous in the stroma surrounding the tumour tissue and in the stromal septa between the cords of malignant cells (peripheral infiltration) than in the central areas of the neoplasms. No signs of cell necrosis were seen near the lymphocyte zones or the stromal macrophages, though central necrotic areas contained aggregates of macrophages, lymphocytes and polymorphonuclear leucocytes.

Isolation of mononuclear cells from 20 such disaggregated tumours by a procedure similar to that used for the separation of mononuclear cells from peripheral blood permitted further characterization of the lymphocytic infiltrate in terms of T, B, and "null" cells (SVENNEVIG et al. 1979). Although there was much individual variation between tumours T cells, characterized by E rosette formation, constituted about 43% of these infiltrates, B cells, estimated by surface membrane immunoglobulin (SmIg) staining, constituted ~15% and null cells constituted ~41%, figures which closely concurred with earlier estimates on similar tumour types (SVENNEVIG et al. 1978). The proportion of T cells was consistently less among lymphocytes recovered from the tumours than in the peripheral blood of cancer patients (~58%) or normal donors (~80%). In some suspensions, typical clusters of lymphocytes and macrophages around tumour cells were observed.

HÄYRY and TÖTTERMAN (1978) selected ten tumours which displayed an unusually strong inflammatory reaction and enumerated different leucocyte populations and lymphocyte subpopulations after enzymatic digestion. Three distinct types of inflammatory infiltrates were documented which correlated to some extent with the type of neoplasm and tumour localization in the host. In three cases of thyroid papillary carcinoma and one of mammary carcinoma, the infiltrates comprised approximately equal proportions of monocytes and macrophages and lymphocytes, the last belonging almost exclusively to the null subset. By contrast, in three cases of testicular seminoma, the infiltrate was predominantly lymphocytic, though plasma cells and plasmablasts were also present in appreciable numbers. In these tumours, the lymphocytes were virtually all T cells. Finally, in two cases of papillary carcinoma of the ovary and one case of uterine carcinosarcoma, the infiltrate comprised approximately equal proportions of plasma cells, plus lymphocytes, macrophages and polymorphnuclear leucocytes. In the lymphocyte compartment of these neoplasms, T, B, and null cells were present to a similar

Table 2. Inflammatory cellular infiltrates of solid human neoplasms of various histological types. I. Identification of host cells in primary and metastatic tumours; descriptive studies on disaggregated tumour-cell suspensions

Histological type (No. studied)	Infiltrating cells identified[a, b]	Remarks	References
Breast carcinoma:			
Localized, node-negative	0%–30% Macrophages[a]	Macrophages identified by morphology in culture and staining with antimacrophage serum	GAUCI and ALEXANDER (1975)
node-positive	2%–9% Macrophages[a]		
Benign breast disease	0%–9% Macrophages[a]		
Malignant melanoma:			
Primary or local recurrence	9%–30% Macrophages[a]		
Metastases	0%–8% Macrophages[a]		
Primary breast carcinoma (13)		FcR^+ cells mainly macrophages	WOOD and GOLLAHON (1977)
Squamous-cell carcinoma			
Head and neck (5)	2%–5% FcR^+[a]		
Various others (21)	≦5% Lymphocytes[a]		
Carcinomas of colon (7), lung (3), breast (3), rectum (3), stomach (3), Wilms tumour (1)	0.2%–7% Macrophages[a] 0.2%–4% Lymphocytes[a] 1%–9% Polymorphs[a]	Macrophages and lymphocytes usually more numerous in stroma around tumour	SVENNEVIG and SVAAR (1979)
Carcinomas of stomach (2), colon (1), breast (4), lung (7)	0.5%–4% Mononuclear cells[a], mainly T cells and monocytes	Histology revealed variable distribution of mononuclear cells in tumours	SVENNEVIG et al. (1978)
Carcinomas of lung (11), colon-rectum (3), stomach (1), breast (1), kidney (1)	1%–28% Macrophages[a] 0.5%–5.0% Lymphocytes[a]	Lymphocyte component mainly T cells (E^+) and null cells	SVENNEVIG et al. (1979)
Thyroid papillary carcinoma (3) breast carcinoma (1)	Lymphocytes (~44%), macrophages (~63%), polymorphs (~6%)[b]	Lymphocytes mainly null cells	HÄYRY and TÖTTERMAN (1978)
Ovarian papillary carcinoma (2), uterine carcinosarcoma (1)	Plasma cells, plasmablasts (~10%); lymphocytes (~17%); macrophages (~42%); polymorphs (~30%)[b]	T ~ B ~ null	HÄYRY and TÖTTERMAN (1978)

Table 2 (Continued)

Histological type (No. studied)	Infiltrating cells identified[a, b]	Remarks	References
Seminoma (3)	Plasma cells, plasmablast (~25%); lymphocytes (~51%); macrophages (~27%)[b]	Lymphocytes mainly T cells (E^+, $ANAE^+$)	Häyry and Tötterman (1978)
Nasopharyngeal carcinoma (7)	87% T cells (76%–96%)[b], 8% B cells (2%–16%)	Cells of nasopharyngeal carcinoma carry EBV-DNA and express the nuclear antigen EBNA	Jondal and Klein (1975)
Lung carcinoma (16)	40%–91% T cells; 4%–35% FcR^{+b}	Conjugates of T-lymphocytes and tumour cells often seen. (Natural attachment)	Galili et al. (1979); Galili et al. (1980)
Lung metastases from:			
Kidney carcinoma (4)	65%–96% T cells: 3%–30% FcR^{+b}		
Sarcoma (3), melanoma (2)	60%–90% T cells; 2%–5% FcR^{+b}		
Seminoma (1)	75% T cells; 10% FcR^{+b}		
Various primary tumours (45) Mainly lung (14) and breast cancers (9)	Mainly T cells: Relatively high proportion of Tγ and Ia^+ T cells		Kaszubowski et al. (1980)

[a] Expressed as percentage of whole tumour-cell suspension [b] Expressed as percentage of semipurified leucocyte isolate

extent. The majority of the macrophages when present (fewest in seminoma) were FcR^+, as were the infiltrating monocytes.

These data demonstrate that the composition of the inflammatory infiltrate in different human cancers is highly variable, probably reflecting the type of tumour, its localization in the host, the stage of growth and the type of immune response. This latter point is taken up in a study by GALILI et al. (1980) on lymphocytes recovered from tumours and drainage nodes of nasopharyngeal carcinoma (NPC) the cells of which regularly carry EBV-DNA and express the nuclear antigen EBNA (E. KLEIN et al. 1974). The lymphocytes within the tumour are mostly T cells (JONDAL and KLEIN 1975). In view of the anti-EBV response of the patients (HENLE et al. 1973) and the presence of the virus DNA in the tumour cells, T-cell infiltration may represent the manifestation of a host immune response. T cells recovered from NPC and local nodes exhibit the following characteristics of immune activation: (a) stable E rosette formation; (b) natural attachment to various human cells; and (c) sensitivity in vitro to the lytic effect of glucocorticoids. Although the NPC T cells attach in vitro to various targets, they kill only the EBV-genome-carrying targets, suggesting the occurrence of a local cellular immune response in NPC, possibly directed to EBV-related antigens. The finding of activated T cells in carcinomas other than NPC (GALILI et al. 1979), notably of lung, provides further evidence for immunological recognition by the host.

Recently, T cells infiltrating a heterogeneous group of 45 primary untreated solid neoplasms have been subclassified on the basis of receptors for IgG and IgM, and expression of Ia antigen (see Sec. B.II) (KASZUBOWSKI et al. 1980). These authors found an increase in the percentage of peripheral blood $T\gamma$ cells and a decrease in $T\mu$ cells and Ia^+ cells in comparison with normal controls. In tumour tissue, the lymphoid infiltrates, which comprised mainly T cells, contained relatively high proportions of $T\gamma$ and Ia^+ cells. Low proportions of the latter population in blood were paralleled by a high percentage of such cells in tumour infiltrative lymphocytes (TIL). $T\gamma$ cells are believed to represent a possible suppressor population whereas $T\mu$ cells have been shown to mediate T-cell help. The significance of these infiltrates must await the development of reliable techniques for isolation and functional assessment of the various T-cell subsets from tumour tissues. Meanwhile the possibility that immunological effector or suppressor function may be concentrated within tumour tissues and reflected by numerical and functional changes in peripheral blood lymphocyte subsets remains an important question, the clarification of which could have profound implications for the balance of the host-tumour relationship. Since monoclonal antibodies are now available which react specifically with T-cell subsets expressing cytotoxic or suppressor functions, B cells and cells of monotype-macrophage lineage, their in situ characterization and localization in tissue sections is an immediate practical probability which will close the gap between classical histology and functional data generated by in vitro analysis.

In summary, despite the variation from tumour to tumour, cellular infiltration of experimental and human neoplasms is neither a random process, nor one which is due, more than minimally, to technical inconsistency, since the type and number of leucocytes entering the majority of animal tumours is a largely predictable phenomenon. The same argument may be sustained even for human tumours where the certain patterns of infiltration may be associated with particular types of neoplasm at certain stages of tumour growth. The identification of discrete patterns of infiltration has provided the rationale for systematic examination of functions putatively attributed to the infiltrating cells.

IV. Factors Which Determine Leucocyte Infiltration of Tumours

In both the experimental and human situations, leucocyte infiltration appears to be associated primarily, if not wholly, with the generation of an immune response to tumour-associated antigens. The presence of T cells is not inconsistent with this hypothesis, though in many tumours, as will be seen (Sects. D.III, E.II), detection of specifically cytotoxic T cells in situ has proved elusive. However, even in allografts the proportion of committed cells which ingress is small; the majority are probably unsensitized, appearing at random from the circulation by attraction into the grafts via chemical mediators emanating from the sensitized population.

The level at which the macrophage, the other major cell type, is maintained within tumours is likely to depend upon a multiplicity of factors favourable or unfavourable to continued recruitment from circulating monocyte precursors and upon the flux of macrophages within the tumour itself (EVANS 1977a, b, c; ECCLES 1978). From evidence already presented it is likely that immunity and macrophage ingress are closely linked, but the nature of the stimulae by which monocytes enter a tumour, and the extent to which such factors might be modified by antichemotactic, or anti-inflammatory factors and chemotactic inhibitors, remains obscure. The peripheral blood monocytes of tumour-bearing animals, levels of which are often raised, respond poorly to chemotactic and inflammatory stimulae in vivo (ECCLES et al. 1976; SNYDERMAN et al. 1976) and soluble tumour products (SNYDERMAN and PIKE 1976). Also immune complexes known to be present in the circulation of rats bearing tumours with a high macrophage content (THOMSON et al. 1973) may bind to monocytes via FcR to influence their extravasation and/or migration. In summary, it therefore seems likely, as EVANS (1977) has emphasized, that infiltration of tumours by leucocytes may be largely controlled by the interaction of protagonists and antagonists of chemotaxis, which in turn are under the control of the immune response. An antigenic tumour may thus be regarded as a putative chemotactic stimulus, but the relative importance of antigen, immune complexes, complement factors (SNYDERMAN and MERGENHAGEN 1976) or products of neoplastic cells (MELTZER et al. 1977) in this multifactorial process has yet to be evaluated. Paradoxically, recent reports that macrophages (whose role in a multiplicity of other phenomena is well recognized) once within the tumour may also stimulate proliferation or maturation of various normal and neoplastic cells by the release of soluble mediators, suggest that in some circumstances macrophages may be a requirement for tumour growth (EVANS 1979, 1980). Under the complex dynamic conditions of tumour development it is even possible to envisage the coexistence of opposing reactions in which different properties of similar cells serve mutually antagonistic ends.

Notwithstanding this inordinate degree of complexity, as a starting point it is a reasonable assumption that some of the answers may lie at the site of tumour growth, not necessarily to the exclusion of reactions occurring systemically, but in concert with them. The majority of investigators have subsumed a defensive role for the infiltrating cells in the design of their experiments; only a minority have entertained the possibility that they may be growth stimulatory, or at least that the latter effect might outweigh the former.

D. Effector Functions of Intratumour Leucocytes: Experimental Neoplasms

I. Systemic Effector Mechanisms

Of the many studies of tumour-directed immune responses almost all have concentrated on reactivity in peripheral blood, lymph node or spleen (reviewed by HERBERMAN 1974). From such studies it has become apparent that a wide variety of effector cells and types of immune functions may be involved (reviewed by LEVY and LECLERC 1977). Particular attention has been paid to T cells that may be directly cytotoxic against tumour cells or may proliferate upon stimulation with tumour antigens to produce a diversity of pharmacologically active substances, known generically as lymphokines, involved not only in the systemic regulation of the immune system, but also in the process of recruitment of other leucocytes to the tumour site. However, other effector mechanisms may also participate in host immune responses to tumours including B cells, which produce antibodies which affect tumour cells directly (reviewed by WITZ 1977) or interact with subpopulations of lymphoid cells ["killer" (K) cells] or macrophages and thereby mediate antibody-dependent cellular cytotoxicity (ADCC); monocytes and macrophages, which are spontaneously cytotoxic against tumour cells or can be activated to become so; and natural killer (NK) cells, a subpopulation of mononuclear cells whose functional ascription relates to the expression of cytotoxic activity against a wide range of tumour-derived targets. The interrelationship of the various mechanisms of natural and adaptive immunity operating at a systemic level is depicted in Fig. 2. Natural killer cells, whose action like that of cytotoxic T cells is independent of antibody, lack the specificity of the latter.

The experiments here to be reviewed have sought, for the most part, to delinate which of these effector mechanisms is represented within the tumour mass. Components of the immune system which are found in situ would be likely to play a more effective role in the regulation of tumour growth. Conversely, failure to find in tumours some immune reactivities which are present in central lymphoid tissues might provide important information on the usual inability of the immune response to limit tumour growth successfully. Such studies have revealed a considerable variety of effector-cell functions, with subpopulations of cells exerting antitumour activity, and with others actually suppressing immune responses such as lymphocyte proliferation and lymphokine production.

The major studies of cellular infiltration of experimental neoplasms which have incorporated a functional, as well as a descriptive, component are summarized in Table 3. In these experiments it was necessary to separate the putative effector cells from the remaining neoplastic and non-neoplastic elements. In practice such separations are rarely absolute, and morphologically "pure" popula-

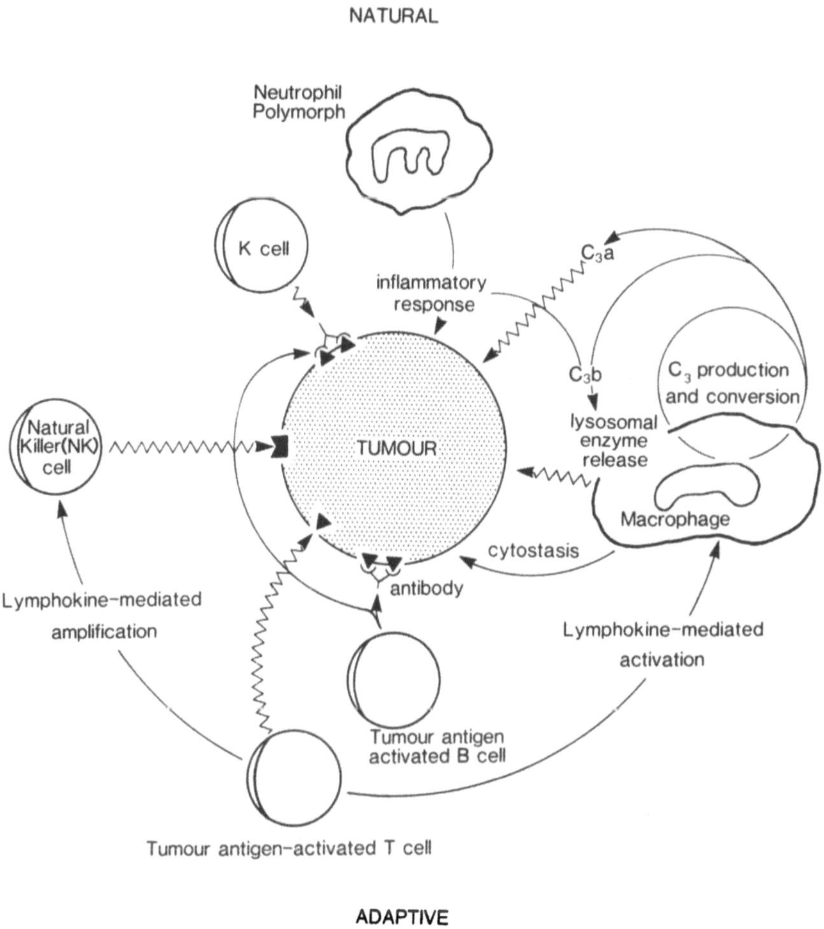

Fig. 2. Interaction between natural and adaptive immune mechanisms in the induction of antitumour effector function

tions of macrophages and lymphocytes are known to be heterogeneous in terms of maturation, differentiation and state of activation, etc. Many such studies have concentrated on the expression of "cytotoxicity" by infiltrative cells usually in comparison with those of central lymphoid tissues, in different in vitro assays and against different tumour targets. "Cytotoxicity" is an operational term and, depending on the assay, may connote different functions. Release of radioisotope from prelabelled target cells on encounter with effector cells during short-term coincubation, for example, provides a measure of tumour cytolysis. Enumeration by visual counting or postisotopic labelling of target cells surviving exposure to effector cells in longer-term assays on the other hand may measure both cytolysis and cytostasis (growth inhibition) or even growth stimulation. Macrophage "cytotoxicity" in some tumour systems is apparent against tumours only under these latter conditions.

Table 3. Inflammatory cellular infiltrates of solid experimental neoplasms. II. Separation of infiltrative cells and delineation of in vitro function

Tumour/host system	Effector cell[g]	Remarks	References
HSN (hooded rat) ASBPI (August)	Macrophage	Highly destructive	Evans (1973, 1976)
FS6 (C57B1) HSBPA (hooded rat)	Macrophage (short-lived)	Cytotoxicity induced or enhanced by endotoxin, lipid A, Poly I: Poly C, dsRNA. Weak labile cytotoxicity	Evans (1973, 1976)
SL2[c] (DBA/2) 448[b] (Wistar rat)	Macrophage Macrophage	Antigen-specific cytotoxicity	van Loveren and den Otter (1974)
MCA-1[a] (hooded rat) HSH[a]	Macrophage Macrophage precursors	Non-specific cytotoxicity	Haskill et al. (1975a, 1976)
T1699[d] (DBA/2)	Non-phagocytic FcR$^+$ (?lymphoid) (?monocytoid)	Antibody-dependent cellular cytotoxicity	Haskill et al. (1975b, 1976); Haskill and Fett (1976); Haskill and Parthenais (1978)
MCA2[a] (DBA/2)	T	Antigen-specific CTX	DeLustro and Haskill (1978)
Mc40A[a], Mc57[a] (W/not rat)	Natural killer, macrophage	Non-specific CTX	K. Moore and M. Moore (1979); M. Moore and K. Moore (1980)
MC7[a] (W/not rat)	?T	Active in Winn assays	Robins et al. (1979)
UV1316[a] (C3H) regressors: progressors:	T None detected	Antigen-specific CTX	Lill and Fortner (1978)
UV Tumours[a] (various)	Macrophage	Promotes generation of cytotoxic lymphocytes in vitro	Woodward and Daynes (1978)
MTV[d] (C3H)	Natural killer	Activity in lesions <20 mm diam greater than in lesions >30 mm	Gerson (1980); Herberman et al. (1980)

Table 3 (Continued)

Tumour/host system	Effector cell[g]	Remarks	References
MSV[e] (C57Bl/6) regressors	T Macrophage (cytotoxic) Macrophage (suppressor)	High antigen-specific CTX Non-specific CTX Suppress migration inhibition factor (MIF) production; inhibit lymphoproliferative response to mitogens	Herberman et al. (1980); Holden et al. (1976); Pucetti and Holden (1979); Varesio et al. (1979)
MSV[e] (C57Bl/6; regressors BALB/c) progressors nude progressors	Macrophage None: non-inducible with bacterial lipopolysaccharide	CTX regressors > progressors	Taniyama and Holden (1979)
MSC[e,f] (BALB/c) regressors progressors	T T (short-lived)	Antigen-specific cytotoxicity	Gillespie and Russell (1978)
MSC[e,f] (BALB/c) regressors progressors	Macrophage Macrophage; inducible with bacterial lipopolysaccharide	Non-specific cytotoxicity	Russell et al. (1976a, b)
MSV[e] (CBA, C57Bl A, etc.)	Natural killer	Activity dependent upon age and strain of mouse	Becker (1980); Becker and Klein (1976); Gerson (1980); Herberman et al. (1980)
MTV (BALB/cf C3H and BALB/c)	(For details, see Table 1, Ref. 1)	Lymphoid cells separated from tumour by isokinetic gradient centrifugation, markedly growth stimulatory in microcytotoxicity assay	Blazar et al. (1978a, b)

[a] Sarcomas
[b] Hepatoma
[c] Lymphoma
[d] Carcinoma
[e] Virus-induced (MSV or MTV) tumours
[f] Transplantable Moloney sarcoma line
[g] Purified by various fractionation procedures, after enzymatic disaggregation of tumours

For instance, STEWART and BEETHAM (1978) using time-lapse cinematography showed that macrophages separated from progressive EMT6 tumours could either be cytostatic (target cells neither divided nor lysed) or cytolytic. Prolonged contact between tumour and one or more macrophages was necessary for either effect to be seen. Targets in infrequent contact with macrophages, or in no contact at all, continued to divide. On the rare occasions when tumour cells divided after they had been in prolonged contact with macrophages, both daughter cells died synchronously within 1 h of division.

Many studies of experimental tumours utilize target cells passaged in tissue culture. These systems have a significant advantage over those of man, in that properties fundamental to their use as in vitro targets (i.e. neoplastic status, antigenic specificity) can be confirmed by in vivo experiments. In human tumour-host systems many similar studies with peripheral lymphoid effectors have been conducted in situations where the nature of the target cells, explanted from tumours and maintained in tissue culture, could not be confirmed. Recently, possible tissue culture artefacts have been avoided by the use of fresh tumour cells unadapted to tissue culture. Such populations, though more representative of the tumour from which they are derived, are nevertheless heterogeneous and contain variable, often undefined properties of non-neoplastic cells. Tumour-directed cytotoxic functions may thus be underestimated under these conditions.

In this context a factor of crucial importance, so little investigated, is the potential for interaction between the various cytotoxic effectors and the tumour stem-cell subset (SALMON 1980). Conceptual approaches to tumour stem cells are theoretical, since they depend on mathematical models to explain the stem-cell population dynamics from gross measurements of population parameters. These concepts have gained some validity from the recent development of techniques by which the capacity of a single cell to establish a clone can be estimated under artificial conditions (clonogenicity). Several such procedures have been described, including the ability of single-cell suspensions of tumour cells to form colonies in vitro and in recipient animals in vivo, or the capacity to repopulate the tumour in situ. However, there have been few studies on the interaction of clonogenic tumour cells with those of the immune system.

It should be emphasized that some assays of effector function (e.g. NK activity) not infrequently relate to rather specialized "NK-sensitive" targets, which have little relevance to the tumour from whence the lymphoid effector cells have been derived. In this situation, the assay serves as an operational indication of the presence of a certain subclass of effector cell, but has little or no relevance to biological behaviour, unless similar activity is also demonstrable against the relevant tumour.

II. Macrophage Function

Intratumour macrophages separated from progressive chemically induced neoplasms have been held to mediate specific (VAN LOVEREN and DEN OTTER 1974) and, more usually, non-specific cytotoxic effects in vitro (EVANS 1973; HASKILL et al. 1975a; M. MOORE and K. MOORE 1980), particularly if exposed to such agents as endotoxin, lipid A, poly I: poly C, or dsRNA, or after exposure to macrophage-activating factor (MAF), a lymphokine produced by sensitized T-lymphocytes (EVANS 1976; HIBBS 1976). This latter capacity and various other associated activities (such as increased bactericidal activity, enhanced FcR expression, increased enzyme secretion, etc.) constitute criteria by which macrophages are considered to be "activated". Activated macrophages do not kill tumour cells by phagocytosis, since cytochalasin B, a potent inhibitor of phagocytosis, has no effect on cytotoxicity. Inhibition of nucleic acid and protein synthesis are also incapable of suppressing macrophage-mediated cytotoxicity. HIBBS (1976) has formulated a hypothesis for the mechanism of macrophage cytotoxicity, which is compatible with these observations: target-cell damage is envisaged to result from the direct secretion of lyzosomal enzymes by the activated macrophage. The experimental evidence for this is broadly twofold and derives from morphological and biochemical observations. Phase contrast microscopy has revealed the transfer of a lyzosomal marker (dextran sulphate stained with toluidine blue) into target cells. Direct transfer of lyzosomal product was inferred from the total absence of cytotoxic factors in the milieu of the cultured cells. HIBBS is inclined toward the possibility that lysis occurs on account of direct membrane fusion between the effector macrophages and the target cell, but evidence for this is presently lacking. Not all macrophages recovered from tumours may be classified as "activated", however; their deficiency in this respect may be attributable to active inhibition by the tumour or its products, or to modulation under certain in vitro conditions (EVANS 1976). HASKILL et al. (1975a) found that, in addition to activated macrophages, the host cells of chemically induced rat sarcomas comprised macrophage precursors, able to proliferate in vitro, but apparently inhibited by the presence of tumour cells.

Macrophages recovered from regressing MSC tumours are capable of lysing a variety of tumour target cells, to varying degrees, suggestive of a difference in susceptibility among different tumours to macrophage-mediated killing (RUSSELL et al. 1977). Virus-induced, as distinct from cell-induced, Moloney sarcomas undergoing regression have yielded at least two populations of non-specifically cytotoxic macrophages (separated by velocity sedimentation at unit gravity), indicative of heterogeneity in this system, with regard to size (HOLDEN et al. 1976; PUCETTI and HOLDEN 1979).

Macrophages recovered from MSV progressors, on the other hand, kill tumour targets with greatly reduced efficiency (RUSSELL et al. 1977; TANIYAMA and HOLDEN 1979), observations which, together with the negative cytotoxic status of macrophages from other tumour types (EVANS 1976), raise several intriguing questions. For instance, is the phenomenon a failure of the activation process due to absence of appropriate stimulae, or have the macrophages been fully activated at one time but for some reason have lost their capability in vivo, much as activated tumour macrophages do upon explantation? (EVANS 1976; RUSSELL et al. 1977). Some insight into these questions was recently attempted through the use of lipopolysaccharide (LPS) as a probe of macrophage activation, with somewhat equivocal results (RUSSELL et al. 1977; TANIYAMA and HOLDEN 1979). Non-cytolytic macrophages from two different kinds of progressor mouse tumours responded to concentrations of LPS in the pg–ng/ml range by expressing high levels of non-specific cytolytic activity within a few hours. Comparable treatment had no detectable effect on thioglycollate-elicited peritoneal macrophages. Accordingly, it was proposed that non-cytolytic macrophages in some progressors are partially activated or "primed". The use of this terminology was intended to convey that these macrophages exist in a state of readiness with respect to cytotoxic function, which they fail to exert in the absence of a final stimulus(ae). Taniyama and Holden (1979) failed to confirm this hypothesis, however, since inactive macrophages from MSV tumours of nude or conventional mice did not develop detectable cytolytic activity on exposure to LPS.

The properties of macrophages are so diverse, that on presently available information the question of whether their intratumour role is primarily that of cytotoxic effector cells must remain open (Eccles 1978). Macrophages are involved at all stages of the immune response and have the capacity to respond to many different stimulae including the elaboration of a wide range of biologically active substances which influence or condition the tumour microenvironment (James 1977). Recent data on macrophages from tumour bearers suggest that a predominant activity of suppressor macrophages is inhibition not only of lymphoproliferative responses to tumour antigens, but of proliferation-independent immune responses as well (Klimpel and Henney 1978; Varesio et al. 1979). In addition macrophages appear to be involved in the in vivo regulation of NK activity (Oehler and Herberman 1978).

III. T-Cell Function

Cytotoxic T-lymphocytes (CTL) have been demonstrated at a systemic level, in populations variously derived from regional lymph nodes, spleen, blood, and the peritoneal cavity (Cerottini and Brunner 1974).

T-cell-mediated lysis is effected by cells with a membrane-associated receptor for the antigen(s) expressed on the tumour target cells. Under optimal conditions these cells cause rapid lysis in vitro (less than 1 h) and each effector is capable of killing more than one target. The overall reaction is energy dependent, most of this requirement apparently being involved in effector-target interaction. Cytolysis is inhibited by ethylenediaminetetra-acetic acid (EDTA), by the cytochalasins A and B and by drugs which increase intracellular cAMP levels. De novo protein and DNA synthesis are unnecessary for lysis, which is dependent on intimate association between effector and target cell rather than on the secretion of soluble lytic mediators.

There have been relatively few reports of in situ CTL in experimental neoplasms, although T cells are known to be present in a variety of tumour types (Sect. C.II) and there is circumstantial evidence for involvement at the tumour site (Kikuchi et al. 1976). Specific CTL have been recovered from both regressing and progressing MSV sarcomas, but from the latter only during the early phase of tumour growth (Holden et al. 1976; Gillespie et al. 1977). However, there appears little doubt that intratumour cytolytic T cells alone or in concert with other cells cause regression of Moloney sarcomas since the elimination of a tumour with an established blood supply was accomplished by remote intravenous infusion of syngeneic splenic effector cells with specificity for MSV tumour antigens (Fernandez-Cruz et al. 1979). Splenic cells were effective in vivo only after mixed lymphocyte tumour-cell culture in vitro. The specific effector cells were a subset of T blast cells W3/25$^+$ and W3/13$^+$ (Williams et al. 1977) as detected by monoclonal antibodies to rat T antigens and they apparently functioned as amplifier or helper cells in the tumour-bearing host. Interestingly, a W3/25$^-$ population, a melange of T cells, null cells, macrophages and B cells, was associated with enhancement of in vivo tumour growth (Fernandez-Cruz et al. 1980). Experiments of this degree of sophistication have yet to be applied to other tumour-host systems.

Chemically induced rat sarcomas of established immunogenicity failed to yield unequivocal evidence of resident cytotoxic T cells (Moore and Moore 1979) and in chemically induced murine tumours evidence for in situ CTL is also limited (Delustro and Haskill 1978): T-cell-enriched tumour-derived fractions and spleen cells from mice bearing progressive MCA-2 tumours were shown to be cytotoxic in vitro for cultured MCA-2 cells, but not for the antigenically unrelated SAD2 fibrosarcoma and T1699 mammary adenocarcinoma cells. Specific CTL have also been detected in ultraviolet light-induced murine tumours undergoing regression, but not in progressive neoplasms (Lill and Fortner 1978). UV-induced tumours differ from chemically induced murine and rat tumours in that they will grow progressively only in immunosuppressed mice (Kripke and Fisher 1976). The highly antigenic character and biological behaviour of these tumours is thus reminiscent of MSV-induced sarcomas wherein a distinction in the cytotoxic status of T-lymphocytes is apparent between progressors and regressors (Gillespie et al. 1977). In addition, this unusual tumour system has disclosed a complementary role for intratumour macrophages in the immune response (Woodward and Daynes 1978). UV-induced tumours consistently comprised about one-third of macrophages, which are critical for the in vitro generation of tumour-specific cytotoxicity by splenic lymphocytes.

Blazar et al. (1978 b) have reported that lymphoid cells isolated by isokinetic gradient centrifugation from mouse mammary tumours actually stimulate tumour-cell growth in a microcytotoxicity assay. The cell type responsible for the effect has not been definitively characterized, though there is evidence for the involvement of T cells (or a subpopulation thereof). Enhancement of tumour-cell growth by lymphoid cells has now been reported by several laboratories. Prehn (1977) has presented theories of immunostimulation to explain tumour growth in the presence of immune reactivity. The mechanism of the stimulation and its relation to the immune functions of lymphocytes remain active and controversial areas of research.

IV. Natural Killer Function

The detection of lymphoid cells which are capable of expressing other cytotoxic functions in tumours has been reported for several disparate tumour-host systems. Natural killer (NK) activity, monitored against NK-sensitive YAC (Moloney lymphoma) cells, systemic levels of which are genetically determined in the mouse (Herberman and Holden 1978), was detectable in lymphocytes isolated from MSV tumours in high NK-reactive CBA mice, but not in low NK-reactive A strain mice, in spite of regularly occurring regression in the latter strain

(BECKER and KLEIN 1976). It is not known whether autologous MSV tumours are NK sensitive.

NK cells with activity comparable with those from spleen have also been recovered from rat sarcomas (K. MOORE and M. MOORE 1979), indicating that these cells may extravasate and persist in tumour tissue. In this latter study, NK activity was detected by lysis of the xenogeneic cell line of erythroleukaemic origin, K562. The autologous tumour targets were also NK sensitive but to a much lesser degree, an observation which emphasizes the point that this effector function may be of limited biological significance for established neoplasms.

Lymphocytes recovered from another transplanted chemically induced sarcoma (MC7) were found to inhibit tumour growth in Winn assays (ROBINS et al. 1979), but their relationship to NK cells is unclear. The tests disclosed differences between spleen cells and TIL (the latter comprising about 50% T cells as determined by reactivity with the W3/13 monoclonal antibody (WILLIAMS et al. 1977), which could not have been predicted on the basis of in vitro cytotoxicity tests. Spleen cells were inactive under conditions where the TIL population was highly active, even at low effector-to-target cell ratios, regardless of whether the transfers were performed with in vivo-derived cells or cultured target cells. Further studies of this type should help to identify the most cytotoxic lymphocyte subpopulations, their mode and specificity of action, and eventually provide greater insight into the in situ requirements for more effective tumour restraint. In addition to the rat sarcoma, GERSON (1980) has provided evidence for in situ NK cells in spontaneous murine mammary carcinomas, the levels and activity of which were dependent on the age of the hosts and related to that found in peripheral blood and to the burden of disease.

There are several uncertainties about the basis of NK selectivity for different tumour targets in vitro and their biological relevance in vivo. Modulation of tumour susceptibility to NK cells occurs on explantation (BECKER et al. 1978), fresh non-cultured tumour cells being more resistant to lysis than those which have been adapted to tissue culture (the usual targets in in vitro tests). This distinction raises important questions about the efficacy of NK cells in vivo. Furthermore, in only a few instances has the extent to which tumours are sensitive to NK cells in vivo been properly evaluated (HALLER et al. 1977). Recently, this has extended to the use of radiolabelled tumour cells to monitor in vivo cell death attributable to NK cells in lethally irradiated mice of defined age and genetic constitution, from which the contribution of immune T cells has been eliminated (RICCARDI et al. 1979). NK cells are widely attributed with a role in the immunosurveillance of neoplasia, a hypothesis which draws support from the stimulatory effects on NK cells of a diversity of agents with antitumour properties such as bacillus Calmett-Guérin (BCG), *Corynebacterium parvum,* interferon and interferon inducers (WOLFE et al. 1976; TRACEY et al. 1977; OEHLER et al. 1978; POTTER and MOORE 1980).

V. Antibody-Dependent Cellular Cytotoxicity

The nature and functional diversity of host responses to experimental neoplasms is further illustrated by reference to the transplantable T1699 mammary carcinoma in DBA/2 mice (HASKILL et al. 1975b). Tumour cells propagated in tissue culture and transplanted to female mice show spontaneous immunologically mediated regression, or progression depending on the site of inoculation. This tumour elicits a delayed hypersensitivity response (HASKILL et al. 1976) and a strong tumour-specific antibody response of all classes and subclasses of immunoglobulin tested (HASKILL et al 1977). The IgG 2a subclass can cooperate with various monocyte-macrophage populations in an effective antibody-dependent cellular cytotoxicity (ADCC) reaction (HASKILL et al. 1977), which, like T-cell-mediated lysis, is an energy-requiring process, but independent of protein synthesis. Two distinct non-phagocytic effector-cell populations have been isolated from the T1699 tumours: a specific monocytoid adherent growth inhibitory cell with high levels of FcR (HASKILL 1977) and a smaller, blood-borne, bone-marrow-derived monocyte with low levels of FcR and capable of mediating ADCC. Their localization in tumour apparently depends solely neither on the evocation of an antibody response, nor on the evocation of an intact delayed hypersensitivity response.

E. Effector Functions of Intratumour Leucocytes: Human Neoplasms

I. Macrophage Function

In common with experimental tumours, more recent studies of inflammatory-cell infiltration of human neoplasms have incorporated a functional, as well as a descriptive, component (Table 4). Analyses of separated populations are subject to the same limitations as their experimental counterparts and suffer from the additional limitation of non-availability of replicate samples. Intratumour macrophages sometimes exhibit non-specific cytotoxicity against fresh and cultured tumour targets (VOSE 1978), analogous to that described for certain experimental tumours. That human macrophages from tissues other than tumour (BALKWILL and HOGG 1979) and peripheral blood monocytes (MANTOVANI et al. 1979) have a similar capacity to inhibit tumour-cell growth is well documented. KELLER (1978) and MANTOVANI et al. (1980) have reported that adherent, predominantly phagocytic mononuclear cells expressing spontaneous cytotoxicity against a diversity of targets in vitro are virtually ubiquitous in the organism, so that any differences in growth inhibitory effects between intratumour macrophages and those of other sites are likely to be quantitative rather than qualitative. Among the important questions is whether the activity of tumour macrophages is enhanced by an ongoing immune response, on the one hand, or compromised by hitherto ill-defined inhibitory factors in the tumour microenvironment, on the other, and few studies in man have yet addressed these questions (JAMES 1977).

Most of the functional data on the inflammatory cells of human neoplasms relate to tumour infiltrative lymphocytes (TIL).

II. T-Cell Function

The tumour cell of approximately one-third of all patients coming to surgery with solid neoplasms are capable of stimulating their own autologous peripheral blood

Table 4. Inflammatory cellular infiltrates of solid human neoplasms. II. Separation of infiltrative cells and delineation of in vitro function

Histological type (No. studied)	Composition of isolated population	In vitro function	References
Lung carcinoma (6), nasopharyngeal carcinoma (1), osteosarcoma (1), lung metastases from malignant melanoma and hypernephroma	37%–81% T (E^+) 10%–28% FcR^+	Natural killer activity (NK) weak or negative	E. KLEIN et al. (1980); VOSE and MOORE (1979); VOSE et al. (1977a)
Lung carcinoma, nasopharyngeal carcinoma (NPC) Sarcomas (3)	37%–81% T (E^+) 10%–21% FcR^+ 10%–16% B($SmIg^+$)	Depressed responses to phytohaemagglutinin (PHA) and to autologous tumour compared with PBL and LNC; autologous tumour kill (ATK) mainly a feature of NPC	E. KLEIN et al. (1980); VOSE et al. (1977b)
Lung carcinoma (18) Breast carcinoma (7)	13%–81% T (E^+) 6%–24% FcR^+	PHA response (↓) compared with PBL. NK-negative, ATK-negative, suppressor activity on PBL PHA response	VOSE and MOORE (1979)
Lung carcinoma (7), breast carcinoma (1), colon carcinoma (1)	64%–75% T (E^+)	PHA response variable; NK-negative; uninducible with interferon; no suppressor activity on PBL-NK	MOORE and VOSE (1981)
Various tumours (29) mainly carcinomas and neuroblastomas	Several procedures used to obtain enriched or pure lymphocyte populations	NK-weak or -negative; uninducible with interferon ?; suppressor activity	GERSON and HERBERMAN (1980) HERBERMAN et al. (1980)
Thyroid papillary carcinoma (3), breast carcinoma (1) ovarian papillary carcinoma (2), uterine carcinosarcoma (1), seminoma (3)	(For details of these populations see Table 2, HÄYRY and TÖTTERMAN (1978)	NK-negative ATK-negative	TÖTTERMAN et al. (1978)

Table 4 (Continued)

Histological type (No. studied)	Composition of isolated population	In vitro function	References
Nasopharyngeal carcinoma	72%–99% T (E^+)	NK-negative; T cells attach and kill EBV^+ targets	GALILI et al. (1980); E. KLEIN et al. (1980)
Breast carcinoma (12)	Lymphocyte-enriched	NK-weak or negative suppressor activity on PBL-NK	EREMIN (1980)
Lung (2), colon (2) and stomach (1) carcinomas	T cells cultured in T-cell growth factor (TCGF; Interleukin 2) for 14 days	Cytotoxicity versus autologous tumour targets	VOSE and MOORE (1981)
Lung (12), breast (10) and stomach (2) carcinomas	Macrophage	Non-specific cytotoxicity	VOSE (1978)
Colorectal carcinomas (60)	~59% T cells ~35% EAC-RFC	ATK in 30% of cases; associated with "cuffs" of lymphocytes at mesocolic or pararectal edge	WERKMEISTER et al. (1979)

lymphocytes (PBL) over a period of 5 days in tissue culture, as measured by the incorporation of radioactive nucleic precursors in the responding lymphocyte population (Vanky et al. 1974). These data provide evidence for the recognition by lymphocytes of specific antigens on the autologous stimulating tumour cells. This interpretation is corroborated by the fact that lymphocytes of the same patients frequently display a capacity to kill their own tumour cells in short-term cytotoxicity assays based on isotopic release. The killing is mediated by cells with the characteristics of T cells and is restricted to autologous tumour (Vose 1980). Increased frequency of cytotoxicity by PBL against autologous tumours can be generated in vitro by a period of cocultivation during which the cytotoxic effector cells are presumably amplified by stimulation with tumour cells (Vose et al. 1978).

Despite an often satisfactory recovery of T cells in TIL, relatively free of tumour-cell contaminants, their responsiveness to non-specific stimulae such as mitogens and in mixed lymphocyte culture is frequently depressed in comparison with PBL or lymph node cells (LNC) from the same tumour bearers (Vose et al. 1977b; Vose and Moore 1979). This depression appears to be attributable, at least in part, to the presence of suppressor T cells within the infiltrative populations, since TIL have the capacity to suppress the otherwise normal responses of PBL and LNC to mitogens and/or allogeneic lymphocytes. This generalized depression of TIL is reflected in other functions of T cells which are putatively tumour specific, as well as NK cells whose activity against targets such as K562 is greatly diminished.

Thus, TIL are less frequently stimulated by autologous tumour and also fail to effect autologous tumour cytotoxicity consistently (Vose and Moore 1979; Tötterman et al. 1978) with the exception of nasopharyngeal carcinoma (NPC) which may be unusually antigenic (Sect. C.III). The reasons for these functional deficits are clearly complex and may relate to the coexistence of suppressor cells, to lack of appropriate accessory cells for these functions, to a direct influence of tumour or tumour products and to a variety of other presently ill-defined factors. Presently, attempts are being made to amplify T cells reactive with autologous tumours by continuous culture in media containing T-cell growth factor (TCGF); interleukin 2 (Vose and Moore 1981).

III. Natural Killer Function

There is virtual unanimity that NK function is also markedly depressed in lymphocytes purified from a wide variety of tumours, in comparison with peripheral blood NK activity (Vose et al. 1977a; Tötterman et al. 1978; Eremin 1980; Gerson 1980). In this respect the distribution of human NK cells appears to differ from those of rodent tumours in which NK activity is frequently demonstrable. Whether the deficit in human tumours is intrinsic (due to failure of NK cells to extravasate), a failure of maturation (failure of non-cytolytic NK precursors to differentiate), is attributable to coexistent suppressor cells (Eremin 1980), or arises from contact with factors inhibitory of NK function in the microenvironment of the tumour (Droller et al. 1979) has not been finally settled and is likely to vary widely from tumour to tumour and as a function of stage of tumour growth.

F. Limitations of In Vitro Functional Data

Ironically, further analysis of the in vitro functions of purified subpopulations of intratumour lymphocytes and macrophages may be misleading; unless in experimental animals, the test systems can be designed in such a way that the in vitro milieu mimics the in vivo microenvironment. The efficacy with which such tumours as established MSV sarcomas in which the actual neoplasic component is in a minority can be eliminated by remote infusion of cytotoxic lymphocytes with enhanced activity against strong tumour antigens may be exceptional in tumour biology and paralleled only occasionally in other systems. A substantial proportion of experimental tumours are of only moderate or weak antigenicity and it is likely that human neoplasms are similar in this respect. In this situation other factors are likely to determine the balance between tumour progression and regression. It is clear from many studies that solid tumours differ from dissociated suspensions of cells in a variety of ways apart from obvious differences in geometry. For example, the concentration of critical metabolites such as oxygen and glucose (as well as toxic waste products) is diffusion limited in solid tumours, resulting in necrotic areas at distances sufficiently removed from the vascular supply. Also, the heterogeneity of the neoplastic compartment of solid tumours is such that cells are present in overlapping categories: undifferentiated and differentiated cells; cycling and non-cycling cells; cells in G_1-, S-, G_2-, and M-phases of the cell cycle; and cells subjected to differential physiological states of oxygen tension and pH. These and other factors are largely responsible for the variable response of solid tumours to experimental radiotherapy and chemotherapy and similar effects of microenvironment on immune responses might also be anticipated.

Attempts to develop in vitro systems which more accurately reflect the tumour microenvironment have concentrated on the establishment of three-dimensional colonies (or aggregates) of tumour cells in vitro (McDonald and Sordat 1980). A particularly interesting variant of this type involves the growth of tumour cells in vitro in the geometrical configuration of multicellular tumour spheroids. This system has a number of features in common with solid tumours, including considerable heterogeneity in the nutritional and cell cycle status of the tumour mour cells.

Application of this technique to the study of cells infiltrating the EMT6 tumour transplanted to immune and non-immune allogeneic recipients was based on experience of MTS in the study of immunological events in situ associated with allograft rejection. Destruction of the spheroids is accompanied by progressive infiltration of neutrophils, monocytes and some lymphocytes, the proportion varying with time after implantation. Functional analysis of the spheroid infiltrate in a short-term cytotoxicity assay revealed the presence of allospecific cytotoxic T-lymphocytes.

This system would appear to be well suited for quantitative studies of in situ immunity in syngeneic tumours and such experiments are now under way. Since it is also feasible to study dissemination and metastasis of tumour cells derived from individual spheroids, it is clear that MTS may be useful in unravelling the complex series of immunological and other events associated with growth and dissemination of solid tumours in vivo.

G. Implications for Therapy

Several experimental and clinical protocols have been based upon the observation that many tumours contain the whole spectrum of leucocytes found in the circulation and the various lymphoid organs. The rationale behind some forms of therapy, e.g. with BCG, *Corynebacterium parvum* or glucan injection, is to enhance cellular antitumour activity in situ and/or to mobilize certain putative effector cells such as lymphocytes and macrophages to the tumour site (for comprehensive review see WOODRUFF 1980). Likewise, compounds such as endotoxin, lipid A, double-stranded RNA and pyran copolymer may induce regressions, as well as, in common with the bacterial adjuvants, stimulating the appearance of cytotoxic peritoneal macrophages. Clinical, intralesional or subcutaneous administration of compounds such as glucan may result in tumour regression, and on the basis of histological sections it appears that macrophages are the main executors (MANSELL and DI LUZIO 1976). Against the background of this review, which has stressed the plethora of possible interactions which such intervention might generate, these forays in experimental immunotherapy appear empirical and premature. Virtually nothing is known about the kinetics of movement or accumulation of infiltrating cells at the tumour site, how long particular populations and their subsets remain there, whether the incumbent cells die in situ or move away, what is their relationship to the corresponding populations in the circulation from whence they were derived and whether in the case of the bacterial adjuvants stimulation of particular cell types is likely to result in preferential homing to the tumour mass. Nevertheless, despite the extent of this ignorance, intralesional injection of therapeutic agents has resulted in often dramatic tumour regression and this has been associated largely with the accumulation and/or activation of intratumour leucocytes, particularly macrophages. By contrast, when given systemically these agents frequently exhibit no antitumour effects, indicating the necessity for the stimulant at the site of growth and a concomitant failure to recruit more effector cells from the circulation.

There have been very few experiments on the effects of conventional therapy on tumour-infiltrating leucocytes and these are almost wholly confined to experimental systems. SZYMANIEC and JAMES (1976) found that the proportion of FcR^+ cells in a chemically induced murine sarcoma was increased by administration of cyclophosphamide to the host and occasionally by intraperitoneal injection of *C. parvum,* but that the antitumour effect of the latter, as ECCLES and ALEXANDER (1974) found for BCG, could be exerted without significantly increasing the macrophage content (phagocytic FcR^+ cells) of the tumours.

Experimental evidence suggests that radiation tumour control for immunogenic neoplasms depends both on radiation kill and the efficiency of the host rejection. Radiation response curves for immunogenic tumours are less steep than for non-immunogenic neoplasms such that even at low doses some tumours will be controlled. Some hosts reject more tumour cells than others; for these more competent hosts less radiation is needed to achieve tumour control. If the ability of each host to reject the tumour could be estimated, individuals requiring smaller amounts of irradiation (for the same control probability) could be identified. Given that for some experimental tumours the extent of host-cell infiltration principally by macrophages indicates the degree of host-tumour interaction, MENDIONDO et al. (1978) examined the macrophage infiltration of a strongly immunogenic fibrosarcoma and a weakly immunogenic mammary carcinoma in immune, immunosuppressed and immunostimulated hosts. A particular aspect of the investigation was the predictability of tumour control from the intensity of macrophage infiltration in immunogenic tumours. Macrophages were estimated in two ways: (a) by enumeration of phagocytic cells in tumour suspensions and (b) by measurement of serum and tumour lysozyme, levels of which correlate well with absolute numbers of macrophages and may reflect a macrophage-mediated host reaction to tumour (CURRIE and ECCLES 1976).

Serum lysozyme was found not to reflect changes occurring in a tumour accurately where the macrophage infiltrate was only moderate, and could not predict control probability for the fibrosarcoma after treatment by irradiation of intravenous *C. parvum*. The fibrosarcomas transplanted into immunosuppressed hosts contained $<1\%$ macrophages and this poor infiltrate was accompanied by a significantly lower control probability for a given radiation dose. The weakly immunogenic mammary carcinoma growing in normal mice contained virtually no macrophages. As with the fibrosarcoma in immunosuppressed mice, the incidence of distant metastases was significant and the TCD_{50}, relatively high.

Following intravenous injection of *C. parvum*, the sarcomas of some mice undergo complete regressions (SUIT et al. 1975). At a time when serum lysozyme levels are increasing, the proportion of macrophages in the tumours was not substantially greater; nor was the lysozyme concentration in the tumour itself more than marginally greater in the *C. parvum*-treated tumour-bearing mice than in the controls. These observations are reminiscent of those of SZYMANIEC and JAMES (1976) and suggest that the increase in serum lysozyme can be attributed to an increase in total body macrophages, but an increase in the number of macrophages in the tumour itself does not appear to be a necessary step prior to cell kill and tumour regression. Only in the fibrosarcomas undergoing regression was there an evident increase in the proportion of macrophages, which is probably accounted for by a decrease in the number of viable cells without change in the total number of macrophages. If minor variation in the macrophage content of fibrosarcoma treated with radiation or *C. parvum* expressed significant differences in the efficiency of the host reaction it might have been possible to identify a group with a higher probability of tumour control. However, in the event, cures or failures were scattered throughout different values of macrophage content or of lysozyme content per unit volume of tumour. It therefore seems that for a given host-tumour interaction variations occur among the individuals in each group, which are not of enough significance to serve as predictors of the probability of tumour control.

Present limitations on the exploitation of intratumour host cells to enhance the efficacy of therapeutic intervention are due to ignorance not only of the factors which regulate their ingress but also of their precise function in situ. In experiments with another syngeneic murine fibrosarcoma, which comprised a relatively high proportion of macrophages, it was shown that depletion of macrophages by either whole body irradiation or azathoprine treatment impaired the subsequent growth of the implanted cells (EVANS 1977a, b). Moreover, experiments designed to repopulate the tumours with macrophages resulted in normal tumour growth and suggested a requirement for bone-marrow-derived monocytes and macrophages.

In common with radiation therapy, there is evidence to suggest that some chemotherapeutic agents exert an antitumour effect best, or only, in the presence of established antitumour immunity (M. MOORE and WILLIAMS 1973; RADOV et al. 1976; STEELE and PIERCE 1974). The efficacy of such combined assaults varies, as might be expected from tumour to tumour, and it is not always clear whether the effects amount to total eradication, or partial regression. Again, the regression of immunogenic and non-immunogenic tumours with cyclophosphamide achieved by EVANS (1978) was not dependent on established immunity, total tumour eradication being achieved in the absence of overt immunity as long as the drug was given within a few days of tumour-cell implantation. This effect was almost certainly due (?exclusively) to the alkylating potential of the agent. However, partial regression was obtained with relatively large tumour burdens, and this was seen whether tumours were immunogenic or not, regardless of whether tumours were implanted into irradiated or control mice. Nevertheless eradication of large tumours was not achieved even when concomitant immunity could be demonstrated.

The obvious question to arise from experiments of this nature is why a challenge inoculum was rejected while in most cases there was a recrudescence of tumour growth. The problem of eradicating residual tumour is central to cancer therapy in general; thus any observations on changes (numerical and functional) that occur in cell populations within the tumour mass might contribute to our understanding of why neoplastic cells survive, even in the presence of a demonstrable systemic antitumour immunity. The possibility arises that this site, unlike that of the challenge, might have been refractory to infiltration by cells normally associated with graft rejection though it was later shown that the usual armamentarium – macrophages, T-lymphocytes, and granulocytes – appeared at the site particularly during regrowth after a period of remission (EVANS 1979). Whether these latter cells possessed cytotoxic or suppressor activity, whether they were actually stimulating recurrence and whether the re-emergent neoplastic population was phenotypically different from the parental population are all questions for future examination in a diversity of experimental systems. As has been stressed, very few studies have been reported at this particular level, but with increasing sophistication in the analysis of immune reactions at the tumour site and clearer notions about the cellular and molecular basis of tumour drug-resistance in general, the time has come for some convergence of these two important fields.

References

Abraham R, Barbolt TA (1978) Lysosomal enzymes in macrophages of colonic tumors induced in rats by 1,2-dimethylhydrazine dihydrochloride. Cancer Res 38:2763–2767

Apffel CA (1976) Non-immunological host defences. A review. Cancer Res 36:1527–1537

Balkwill FR, Hogg N (1979) Characterization of human breast milk macrophages cytostatic for human cell lines. J Immunol 123:1451–1456
Becker S (1980) Intratumour NK reactivity. In: Herberman R (ed) Natural cell-mediated immunity against tumours. Academic, London, p 985
Becker S, Haskill S (1981) Kinetics of inflammation and sarcoma cell development in primary Moloney sarcoma virus-induced tumours. Int J Cancer 27:229–234
Becker S, Klein E (1976) Decreased "natural killer" effect in tumour-bearing mice and its relation to the immunity against oncornavirus-determined cell surface antigens. Eur J Immunol 6:892–898
Becker S, Kiessling R, Lee N, Klein E (1978) Modulation of sensitivity to natural killer cell lysis after in vitro explantation of a mouse lymphoma. J Natl Cancer Inst 61:1495–1498
Berg JW (1971) Morphological evidence for immune response to breast cancer. Cancer 28:1453–1456
Blazar BA, Heppner GH (1978 a) In situ lymphoid cells of mouse mammary tumors. I. Development and evaluation of a method for the separation of lymphoid cells from mouse mammary tumors. J Immunol 120:1876–1880
Blazar JW, Heppner GH (1978 b) In situ lymphoid cells of mouse mammary tumors. II. The characterization of lymphoid cells separated from mouse mammary tumors. J Immunol 120:1881–1886
Boeryd B, Eriksson O, Knutson F, Lundin PM, Norrby K (1965) On the viability of tumour cells in artificially produced suspensions. Acta Pathol. Microbiol Scand 65:514–520
Carr I, Underwood JCE (1974) The ultrastructure of the local cellular reaction to neoplasia. Int Rev Cytol 37:329–347
Cerottini J-C, Brunner KT (1974) Cell-mediated cytotoxicity, allograft rejection, and tumor immunity. Adv Immunol 18:67
Champion HR, Wallace IW, Prescott RJ (1972) Histology in breast cancer prognosis. Br J Cancer 26:129–138
Currie GA, Eccles SA (1976) Serum lysozyme as a marker of host resistance. I. Production by macrophages resident in rat sarcomata. Br J Cancer 33:51–59
De Lustro F, Haskill JS (1978) In situ cytotoxic T cells in a methylcholanthrene induced tumor. J Immunol 121:1007–1009
Dexter DL, Kowalski HM, Blazar BA, Fligiel Z, Vogel R, Heppner GH (1978) Heterogeneity of tumor cells from a single mouse mammary tumor. Cancer Res 38:3174–3181
Droller MJ, Lindgren JA, Claessen H-E, Perlmann P (1979) Production of prostaglandin E_2 by bladder tumor cells in tissue culture and a possible mechanism of lymphocyte inhibition. Cell Immunol 47:261–273
Eccles SA (1978) Macrophages and cancer. In: Castro J (ed) Immunological aspects of cancer. MTP Press, Lancaster, p 123
Eccles SA, Alexander P (1974) Macrophage content of tumours in relation to metastatic spread and host immune reaction. Nature 250:667–669
Eccles SA, Alexander P (1975) Immunologically mediated restraint of latent tumour metastases. Nature 257:52–53
Eccles SA, Bandlow G, Alexander P (1976) Monocytosis associated with the growth of transplanted syngeneic rat sarcomata differing in immunogenicity. Br J Cancer 34:20–27
Eremin O (1980) NK cell activity in the blood, tumour-draining lymph nodes and primary tumours of women with mammary carcinoma. In: Herberman R (ed) Natural cell-mediated immunity against tumours. Academic, London, p 1011
Evans R (1972) Macrophages in syngeneic animal tumors. Transplantation 14:468–473
Evans R (1973) Macrophages and the tumour-bearing host. Br J Cancer 28 [Suppl 1]:19–25
Evans R (1976) Tumour macrophages in host immunity to malignancies. In: Fink M (ed) The macrophage in neoplasia. Academic, London, p 27
Evans R (1977 a) The effect of azathioprine on host cell infiltration and growth of a murine fibrosarcoma. Int J Cancer 20:120–128
Evans R (1977 b) The effect of X-irradiation on host cell infiltration and growth of a murine fibrosarcoma. Br J Cancer 35:557–566

Evans R (1977c) Macrophages in solid tumours. In: James K, McBride B, Stuart A (eds) Proceedings of the EURES symposium, Edinburgh 1977, pp 321–329
Evans R (1978) Failure to relate the anti-tumour action of cyclophosphamide with the immunogenicity of two murine fibrosarcomas. Int J Cancer 21:611–616
Evans R (1979) Host cells in transplanted murine tumours and their possible relevance to tumor growth. J Reticuloendothel Soc 26:427–437
Evans R (1980) Cellular basis for regulation of tumor growth. Contemp Top Immunobiol 10:255–266
Everson TC, Cole WH (1966) Spontaneous regression of cancer. Saunders, Philadelphia
Fernandez-Cruz E, Halliburtin B, Feldman JD (1979) In vivo elimination by specific effector cells of an established syngeneic rat Moloney virus-induced sarcoma. J Immunol 123:1772–1777
Fernandez-Cruz E, Woda BA, Feldman JD (1980) Elimination of syngeneic sarcomas in rats by a subset of T lymphocytes. J Exp Med 152:832–841
Fidler IJ (1974) Immune stimulation-inhibition of experimental cancer metastasis. Cancer Res 34:491–498
Fidler IJ (1978) Tumor heterogeneity and the biology of cancer invasion and metastasis. Cancer Res 38:2651–2660
Fidler IJ, Kripke ML (1977) Metastasis results from pre-existing variant cells within a malignant tumor. Science 197:893–895
Fidler IJ, Gersten DM, Kripke ML (1979) Influence of immune status on the metastasis of three murine fibrosarcomas of different immunogenicities. Cancer Res 39:3816–3821
Galili H, Vánky F, Rodriguez L, Klein E (1979) Activated T lymphocytes within solid tumours. Cancer Immunol Immunother 6:129–133
Galili H, Klein E, Klein G, Singh-Bal I (1980) Activated T lymphocytes in infiltrates and draining lymph nodes of nasopharyngeal carcinoma. Int J Cancer 25:85–89
Gauci CL, Alexander P (1975) The macrophage content of some human tumours. Cancer Lett 1:29–32
Gerson JM (1980) Systemic and in situ natural killer activity in tumour-bearing mice and patients with cancer. In: Herberman R (ed) Natural cell-mediated immunity against tumours. Academic, London, pp 1047–1062
Gillespie GY, Hansen CB, Hoskins RG, Russell SW (1977) Inflammatory cells in solid murine neoplasms. IV. Cytolytic T lymphocytes isolated from regressing and progressing Moloney sarcomas. J Immunol 119:564–570
Gillespie GY, Russell SW (1978) Development and persistence of cytolytic T lymphocytes in regressing and progressing Moloney sarcomas. Int J Cancer 21:94–99
Hakansson L, Tropé C (1974) Cell clones with different sensitivity to cytostatic drugs in methylcholanthrene-induced mouse sarcomas. Acta Pathol Microbiol Scand [A] 82:41–47
Haller O, Hansson M, Kiessling R, Wigzell H (1977) Role of non-conventional natural killer cells in resistance against syngeneic tumour cells. Nature 270:609–611
Haskill JS (1977) ADCC effector cells in a murine adeno-carcinoma. I. Evidence for blood-borne bone marrow-derived monocytes. Int J Cancer 20:432–440
Haskill JS, Fett JW (1976) Possible evidence for antibody-dependent macrophage-mediated cytotoxicity directed against murine adenocarcinoma cells in vivo. J Immunol 117:1992–1998
Haskill JS, Parthenais E (1978) Immunologic factors influencing the intratumor localization of ADCC effector cells. J Immunol 120:1813–1817
Haskill JS, Proctor JW, Yamamura Y (1975a) Host responses within solid tumours. I. Monocytic effector cells within rat sarcomas. J Natl Cancer Inst 54:387–393
Haskill JS, Yamamura Y, Radov L (1975b) Host responses within solid tumours. Non-thymus derived specific cytotoxic cells within a murine mammary adenocarcinoma. Int J Cancer 16:798–809
Haskill JS, Radov LA, Yamamura Y, Parthenais E, Korn JH, Ritter FL (1976) Experimental solid tumors. The role of macrophages and lymphocytes as effector cells. J Reticuloendothel Soc 20:233–241

Haskill JS, Radov LA, Fett JW, Parthenais E (1977) The antibody response to the T1699 murine adenocarcinoma: antibody class and subclass heterogeneity detected in serum and in situ. J Immunol 119:1000–1005

Häyry P, Tötterman TH (1978) Cytological and functional analysis of inflammatory infiltrates in human malignant tumours. I. Composition of the inflammatory infiltrates. Eur J Immunol 8:866–871

Henle W, Ho HC, Henle G, Kwan HC (1973) Antibodies to Epstein-Barr virus-related antigens in nasopharyngeal carcinoma. Comparison of active cases with long-term survivors. J Natl Cancer Inst 51:361–369

Herberman RB (1972) Cell-mediated immunity to tumor cells. Adv Cancer Res 19:207–263

Herberman RB, Holden HT (1978) Natural cell-mediated immunity. Adv Cancer Res 27:305–377

Herberman RB, Djeu JY, Kay HD, Ortaldo JR, Riccardi C, Bonnard GD, Holden HT, Fagnani R, Santoni A, Puccetti P (1979) Natural killer cells: characteristics and regulation of activity. Immunol Rev 44:43–70

Herberman RB, Holden HT, Varesio L, Taniyama T, Pucetti P, Kirchner H, Gerson J, White S, Keisari Y (1980) Immunologic reactivity of lymphoid cells in tumors. Contemp Top Immunobiol 10:61–78

Hewitt HB, Blake ER, Walder AS (1976) A critique of the evidence for active host defence against cancer, based on personal studies of 27 murine tumours of spontaneous origin. Br J Cancer 33:241–252

Hibbs JB (1976) The macrophage as a tumoricidal effector cell: a review of in vivo and in vitro studies on the mechanisms of the activated macrophage non-specific cytotoxic reaction. In: Fink M (ed) The macrophage and neoplasia. Academic, New York, p 83

Holden HT, Haskill JS, Kirchner H, Herberman RB (1976) Two functionally distinct antitumor effector cells isolated from primary murine sarcoma virus-induced tumors. J Immunol 117:440–446

Husby G, Hoagland PM, Strickland RG, Williams RC Jr (1976) Tissue T- and B-cell infiltration of primary and metastatic cancer. J Clin Invest 57:1471–1482

Ioachim HL (1976) The stromal reaction of tumours: an expression of immune surveillance. J Natl Cancer Inst 57:465–475

Ioachim HL (1980) Correlations between tumor antigenicity, malignant potential and local host immune response. Contemp Top Immunobiol 10:213–238

Ioachim HL, Dorsett B, Paluch E (1976) The immune response at the tumor site in lung carcinoma. Cancer 38:2296–2309

Ito E, Moore GE (1967) Characteristic differences in clones isolated from an S37 ascites tumor in vitro. Exp Cell Res 48:440–447

James K (1977) The influence of tumour cell products on macrophage function in vitro and in vivo. A Review. In: James K, McBride B, Stuart A (eds) The macrophage and cancer. University of Edinburgh, p 225

Jondal M, Klein G (1975) Classification of lymphocytes in nasopharyngeal carcinoma (NPC) biopsies. Biomedicine 23:163–165

Kaszubouski PA, Husby G, Tung KSK, Williams RC Jr (1980) T-Lymphocyte subpopulations in peripheral blood and tissues of cancer patients. Cancer Res 40:4648–4657

Keller R (1978) Macrophage-mediated natural cytotoxicity against various target cells in vitro. I. Macrophages from diverse anatomical sites and different strains of rats and mice. Br J Cancer 37:732–741

Kerbel RS, Davies AJS (1974) The possible biological significance of Fc receptors in mammalian lymphocytes and tumor cells. Cell 3:105–112

Kerbel RS, Pross HF (1976) Fc receptor-bearing cells as a reliable marker for quantitation of host lymphoreticular infiltration of progressively growing solid tumours. Int J Cancer 18:432–438

Kerbel RS, Pross HF, Elliot EV (1975) Origin and partial characterisation of Fc receptor-bearing cells found within experimental carcinomas and sarcomas. Int J Cancer 15:918–932

Kikuchi K, Ishii Y, Ueno H, Koshiba H (1976) Cell-mediated immunity involved in autochthonous tumor rejection in rats. Ann NY Acad Sci 276:188–206
Klein E, Vánky F, Galili U, Vose BM, Fopp M (1980) Separation and characteristics of tumor-infiltrating lymphocytes in man. Contemp Top Immunobiol 10:79–107
Klein G, Giovanella BC, Lindahl T, Fialkow PJ, Singh S, Stehlin J (1974) Direct evidence for the presence of Epstein-Barr virus DNA and nuclear antigen in malignant epithelial cells from patients with poorly differentated carcinoma of the nasopharynx. Proc Natl Acad Sci USA 71:4737–4741
Klimpel GR, Henney CS (1978) A comparison of the effects of T and macrophage-like suppressor cells on memory cell differentation in vitro. J Immunol 121:749–754
Kripke ML, Fisher MS (1976) Immunologic parameters of ultraviolet carcinogenesis. J Natl Cancer Inst 57:211–215
Lauder I, Aherne W, Stewart J, Sainsbury R (1977) Macrophage infiltration of breast tumours: a prospective study. J Clin Pathol 30:563–568
Levy JP, Leclerc JC (1977) The murine sarcoma virus-induced tumor. Exception or general model in tumor immunology? Adv Cancer Res 24:1–66
Lill PH, Fortner GW (1978) Identification and cytotoxic reactivity of inflammatory cells recovered from progressing or regressing syngeneic UV-induced murine tumors. J Immunol 121:1854–1860
Mansell PWA, Di Luzio NR (1976) The in vivo destruction of human tumor by glucan-activated macrophages. In: Fink M (ed) The macrophage and neoplasia. Academic, New York, p 227
Mantovani A, Jerrells TR, Dean JH, Herberman RB (1979) Cytolytic and cytostatic activity on tumour cells of circulating human monocytes. Int J Cancer 23:18–27
Mantovani A, Barshavit Z, Peri G, Polentarutti N, Bordignon C, Sessa C, Mangioni C (1980) Natural cytotoxicity on tumour cells of human macrophages obtained from diverse anatomical sites. Clin Exp Immunol 39:776–784
Massicot JG, Woods WA, Chirigos MA (1971) CEll line derived from a murine sarcoma virus (Moloney pseudotype)-induced tumor: cultural, antigenic and virological properties. Appl Microbiol 22:1119–1122
McDonald HR, Sordat B (1980) The multicellular tumor spheroid: a quantitative model for studies of in situ immunity. Contemp Top Immunobiol 10:317–342
Meltzer MJ, Stevenson MM, Leonard EJ (1977) Characterization of macrophage chemotaxis in tumor-cell cultures and comparison with lymphocyte-derived chemotactic factors. Cancer Res 37:721–725
Mendiondo O, Suit G, Fixler H (1978) Lysozyme levels and macrophage content of tumour tissue in C3H mice bearing fibrosarcoma transplants treated by radiation and *Corynebacterium parvum*. Int J Radiol Oncol Biol Phys 4:829–834
Mian N, Cowen DM, Nutman CA (1974) Glycosidases heterogeneity among dimethylhydrazine-induced rat colonic tumours. Br J Cancer 30:231–237
Mitelman F (1972) Predetermined sequential chromosomal changes in serial transplantation of Rous rat sarcomas. Acta Pathol Microbiol Scand [A] 80:313–328
Moore K, Moore M (1977) Intra-tumour host cells of transplanted rat neoplasms of different immunogenicity. Int J Cancer 19:803–813
Moore K, Moore M (1979) Systemic and in situ natural killer activity in tumour-bearing rats. Br J Cancer 39:636–647
Moore M, Moore K (1977) Kinetics of macrophage infiltration of experimental rat neoplasms. In: James K, McBride B, Stuart A (eds) The macrophage and cancer. Proceedings of EURES symposium, University of Edinburgh, p 330
Moore M, Moore K (1980) Intratumor host cells of experimental rat neoplasms: characterization and effector function. Contempt Top Immunobiol 10:109–142
Moore M, Vose BM (1981) Extravascular natural cytotoxicity in man: anti-K562 activity of lymph-node and tumour-infiltrating lymphocytes. Int J Cancer 27:265–272
Moore M, Williams DE (1973) Contribution of host immunity to cyclophosphamide therapy of a chemically induced murine sarcoma. Int J Cancer 11:358–368
Moore OS, Foote FW (1949) The relatively favorable prognosis of medullary carcinoma of the breast. Cancer 2:635–642
Morrison AS, Black MM, Lowe CL, McMahon B, Yuasa S (1973) Some international differences in histology and survival in breast cancer. Int J Cancer 11:261–267

Nathan CF, Hill VM, Terry WD (1976) Isolation of a subpopulation of adherent peritoneal cells with anti-tumour activity. Nature 260:146–148

Nowell PC (1976) The clonal evolution of tumor cell populations. Science 194:23–28

Oehler JR, Herberman RB (1978) Natural cell-mediated cytotoxicity in rats. III. Effects of immunopharmacologic treatments on natural reactivity and on reactivity augmented by polyinosinic-polycytidylic acid. Int J Cancer 21:221–229

Oehler JR, Lindsay LR, Numm ME, Holden HT, Herberman RB (1978) Natural cell-mediated cytotoxicity in rats. II. In vivo augmentation of NK-cell activity. Int J Cancer 21:210–220

Pályi I, Olah E, Sugar D (1977) Drug sensitivity studies on clonal cell lines isolated from heteroploid cell populations. I. Dose response of clones growing in monolayer cultures. Int J Cancer 19:859–865

Plata F, McDonald HR, Sordat B (1975) Studies on the distribution and origin of cytolytic T lymphocytes present in mice bearing Moloney murine sarcoma virus (MSV)-induced tumours. Bibl Haematologica 43:274

Pimm MV, Baldwin RW (1977) Antigenic differences between primary methylcholanthrene-induced rat sarcomas and post-surgical recurrences. Int J Cancer 20:37–43

Poste G, Fidler IJ (1980) The pathogenesis of cancer metastasis. Nature 283:139–146

Potter MR, Moore M (1980) The effect of BCG stimulation on natural cytotoxicity in the rat. Immunology 39:427–434

Prehn RT (1977) Immunostimulation of the lymphodependent phase of neoplastic growth. J Natl Cancer Inst 59:1043–1049

Pross HF, Kerbel KS (1976) An assessment of intra-tumour phagocytes and surface marker bearing cells in a series of autochthonous and early passaged chemically-induced murine sarcomas. J Natl Cancer Inst 57:1157–1167

Pucetti P, Holden HT (1979) Cytolytic and cytostatic anti-tumour activities of macrophages from mice injected with murine sarcoma virus. Int J Cancer 23:123–133

Radov LA, Haskill JS, Korn JH (1976) Host immune potentiation of drug responses to a murine mammary adenocarcinoma. Int J Cancer 17:773–779

Riccardi C, Pucetti P, Santoni A, Herberman RB (1979) Rapid in vivo assay of mouse NK cell activity. J Natl Cancer Inst 63:1041–1045

Robins RA, Flannery GR, Baldwin RW (1979) Tumour-derived lymphoid cells are able to prevent tumour growth in vivo. Br J Cancer 40:946–949

Rubin B, Hertel-Wulff B (1975) Biological significance of Fc receptor-bearing cells among activated T lymphocytes. Scand J Immunol 4:451–462

Russell SW, Cochrane CG (1974) The cellular events associated with regression and progression of murine (Moloney) sarcomas. Int J Cancer 13:54–63

Russell SW, Gillespie GY (1977) Nature, function and distribution of inflammatory cells in regressing and progressing Moloney sarcomas. J Reticuloendothel Soc 22:159–168

Russell SW, Doe WF, Hoskins RG, Cochrane CG (1976 a) Inflammatory cells in solid murine neoplasms. I. Tumour disaggregation and identification of constituent inflammatory cells. Int J Cancer 18:322–330

Russell SW, Gillespie GY, Hansen CB, Cochrane CG (1976 b) Inflammatory cells in solid murine neoplasma. II. Cell types found throughout the course of Moloney sarcoma regression or progression. Int J Cancer 18:331–338

Russell SW, Doe WF, McIntosh AT (1977) Functional characterization of a stable, noncytolytic stage of macrophage activation in tumors. J Exp Med 146:1511–1520

Russell SW, Witz IP, Herberman RB (1980 a) A review of data, problems and open questions pertaining to in situ immunity. Contemp Top Immunobiol 10:1–20

Russell SW, Gillespie GY, Pace JL (1980 b) Evidence for mononuclear phagocytes in solid neoplasms and appraisal of their non-specific cytotoxic capabilities. Contemp Top Immunobiol 10:143–166

Salmon SE (ed) (1980) Cloning of human tumor stem cells. Prog Clin Biol Res 48

Sauer HR, Burke EM (1949) Prognosis of testicular tumors. J Urol 62:69–74

Siegler R (1970) Pathogenesis of virus-induced murine sarcoma. I. Light microscopy. J Natl Cancer Inst 45:135–147

Simons PJ, McCully DJ (1970) Pathologic and virologic studies of tumours induced in mice by two strains of murine sarcoma virus. J Natl Cancer Inst 44:1289–1303

Snyderman R, Mergenhagen SE (1976) Chemotaxis of macrophages. In: Nelson DS (ed) Immunobiology of the macrophage. Academic, New York, p 323
Snyderman R, Pike MC (1976) An inhibitor of macrophage chemotaxis produced by neoplasms. Science 192:370–372
Snyderman R, Pike MC, Blaylock BL, Weinstein P (1976) Effects of neoplasms on inflammation: depression of macrophage accumulation after tumor implantation. J Immunol 116:585–589
Stanton MF, Law LW, Ting RC (1968) Some biologic, immunogenic and morphologic effects in mice after injection with a murine sarcoma virus. II. Morphologic studies. J Natl Cancer Inst 40:1113–1129
Steele G, Pierce GE (1974) Effects of cyclophosphamide on immunity against chemically induced syngeneic murine fibrosarcomas. Int J Cancer 13:572–578
Stewart CC, Beetham KL (1978) Cytocidal activity and proliferative ability of macrophages infiltrating the EMT6 tumour. Int J Cancer 22:152–159
Sugarbaker EV, Cohen AM (1972) Altered antigenicity in spontaneous pulmonary metastases from an antigenic murine sarcoma. Surgery 72:155–161
Suit HD, Sedlacek R, Wagner M, Orsi L (1975) Radiation response of C3H fibrosarcoma enhanced in mice stimulated by *Corynebacterium parvum*. Nature 255:493–494
Svennevig J-L (1980) T lymphocytes in malignant, non-lymphoid human tumours detected by esterase techniques. Scand J Immunol 12:513–517
Svennevig J-L, Svaar H (1979) Content and distribution of macrophages and lymphocytes in solid malignant human tumours. Int J Cancer 24:754–758
Svennevig J-L, Closs O, Harboe M, Svaar H (1978) Characterization of lymphocytes isolated from non-lymphoid human malignant tumours. Scand J Immunol 7:487–493
Svennevig J-L, Lovik M, Svaar H (1979) Isolation and characterization of lymphocytes and macrophages from solid, malignant human tumours. Int J Cancer 23:626–631
Szymaniec S, James K (1976) Studies on the Fc receptor bearing cells in a transplanted methylcholanthrene mouse fibrosarcoma. Br. J Cancer 33:36–50
Tanaka T, Cooper EH, Anderson CK (1970) Lymphocyte infiltration in bladder carcinoma. Rev Eur Etud Clin Biol 15:1081–1089
Taniyama T, Holden HT (1979) Cytolytic activity of macrophages isolated from primary murine sarcoma virus (MSV)-induced tumours. Int J Cancer 24:151–160
Thomson DMP, Steele K, Alexander P (1973) The presence of tumour-specific membrane antigen in the serum of rats with chemically-induced sarcomata. Br J Cancer 27:27–34
Tilney NL, Strom TB, Macpherson SG, Carpenter CB (1975) Surface porperties and functional characteristics of infiltrating cells harvested from acutely rejecting cardiac allografts in inbred rats. Transplantation 20:323–330
Tønder O, Krishnan EC, Morse PA Jr, Jewell WR, Humphrey LJ (1978) Localisation of Fc receptors in human and rat malignant tissues. Acta Pathol Microbiol Scand [C] 86:173
Tønder O, Matre R, Wesenberg F (1980) Mononuclear cells and IgG associated with human malignant tissue. Contemp Top Immunobiol 10:167–176
Tötterman TH, Häyry P, Saksela E, Timonen T, Eklund B (1978) Cytological and functional analysis of inflammatory infiltrates in human malignant tumours. II. Functional investigations of the infiltrating inflammatory cells. Eur J Immunol 8:872–875
Tracey DE, Wolfe SA, Durdick JM, Henney CS (1977) BCG-induced murine effector cells. I. Cytolytic activity in peritoneal exudates. An early response to BCG. J Immunol 119:1145–1151
Tropé C (1974) Selective elimination of sensitive cell clones in methylcholanthrene-induced sarcoma by vinblastine sulphate. Acta Pathol Microbiol Scand [A] 82:1–8
Ujházy V, Siracký J (1980) Heterogeneity of tumour cells. Antibiot Chemother 28:120–122
Umiel T, Trainin N (1974) Immunological enhancement of tumor growth by syngeneic thymus-derived lymphocytes. Transplantation 18:244–250
Underwood JCE (1974) Lymphoreticular infiltration in human tumours – prognostic and biological implications. A review. Br J Cancer 30:538–547
Underwood JCE, Carr I (1972) The ultrastructure of the lymphoreticular cell in non-lymphoid human neoplasms. Virchows Arch [Pathol Anat] 12:39

Vaage J (1978) A survey of the growth characteristics of, and the host reactions to, one hundred C3H/He mammary carcinomas. Cancer Res 38:331–338

Vanky F, Klein E, Stjernsward J, Nilsonne U (1974) Cellular immunity against tumour-associated antigens in humans: lymphocyte stimulation and skin reaction. Int J Cancer 14:277–288

Van Loveren H, Den Otter W (1974) Macrophages in solid tumours. I. Immunologically specific effector cells. J Natl Cancer Inst 53:1057–1060

Varesio L, Herberman RB, Gerson JM, Holden HT (1979) Suppression of lymphokine production of macrophages infiltrating murine virus-induced tumours. Int J Cancer 24:97–102

Vose BM (1978) Cytotoxicity of adherent cells associated with some human tumours and lung tissues. Cancer Immunol Immunother 5:173–179

Vose BM (1980) Specific T cell-mediated killing of autologous lung tumour cells. Cell Immunol 55:12–19

Vose BM, Moore M (1979) Suppressor cell activity of lymphocytes infiltrating human lung and breast tumours. Int J Cancer 24:579–585

Vose BM, Moore M (1981) Cultured human T cell lines kill autologous solid tumours. Immunol Lett 3:237–241

Vose BM, Vánky F, Argov S, Klein E (1977a) Natural cytotoxicity in man: activity of lymph node and tumour infiltrating lymphocytes. Eur J Immunol 7:753–757

Vose BM, Vánky F, Klein E (1977b) Human tumour-lymphocyte interaction in vitro. V. Comparison of the reactivity of tumour-infiltrating, blood and lymph node lymphocytes with autologous tumour cells. Int J Cancer 20:895–902

Vose BM, Vánky F, Fopp M, Klein E (1978) In vitro generation of cytotoxicity against autologous tumour biopsy cells. Int J Cancer 21:588–593

Werkmeister JA, Pihl E, Nind AAP, Flannery GR, Nairn RC (1979) Immunoreactivity by intrinsic lymphoid cells in colorectal carcinoma. Br J Cancer 40:839–847

Williams AF, Galfre G, Milstein C (1977) Analysis of cell surface by xenogeneic myeloma-hybrid antibodies: differentiation antigens of rat lymphocytes. Cell 12:663–673

Witz IP (1977) Tumor-bound immunoglobulins: in situ expression of humoral immunity. Adv Cancer Res 25:95–148

Wolfe SA, Tracey DE, Henney CS (1976) Induction of "natural killer" cells by BCG. Nature 262:584–586

Wood GW, Gillespie GY (1975) Studies on the role of macrophages in regulation of tumour growth and metastasis of murine chemically-induced tumours. Int J Cancer 16:1022–1029

Wood GW, Gollahon KA (1977) Detection and quantitation of macrophage infiltration into primary human tumours with the use of cell-surface markers. J Natl Cancer Inst 59:1081–1087

Wood GW, Gollahon KA (1978) T-lymphocytes and macrophages in primary murine fibrosarcomas at different stages in their progression. Cancer Res 38:1857–1865

Wood GW, Gillespie GY, Barth RF (1975) Receptor sites for antigen-antibody complexes on cells derived from solid tumors: detection by means of antibody-sensitized sheep erythrocytes labeled with technetium-99m. J Immunol 114:950–957

Woodruff MFA (1980) The interaction of cancer and host. Its therapeutic significance. Grune and Stratton, New York

Woods HE, Papadimitriou JM (1977) The effect of inflammatory stimuli on the stroma of neoplasms: the involvement of mononuclear phagocytes. J Pathol 123:163–174

Woodward JG, Daynes RA (1978) Cell-mediated immune response to syngeneic UV-induced tumors. I. The presence of tumor-associated macrophages and their possible role in the in vitro generation of cytotoxic lymphocytes. Cell Immunol 41:304–319

Yam LT, Li CY, Crosby WH (1971) Cytochemical identification of monocytes and granulocytes. Am J Clin Pathol 55:283

CHAPTER 8

Flow Cytometric Methods for Studying Enzyme Activity in Populations of Individual Cells

J. V. WATSON

A. Introduction

There are many possible classes of mechanism which may contribute to antitumour drug resistance. One such class involves cellular enzymes. An antitumour drug may produce an inhibition of a particular enzyme pathway but the cell may be able to overcome the lesion by inducing an alternative pathway for the conversion of substrate to product. Also, it is possible that enzymes may be induced which have the capacity to detoxicate an antitumour agent with the production of resistant clones. Most work describing a change in enzyme activity has been carried out with homogenized preparations. However, it has been reported by YOUDIM and WOODS (1975) that artefactual results may be generated by the disruption of cellular and subcellular permeability barriers in the preparation of the cell-free extracts. The review presented in this chapter describes methods for identifying different subsets of cells within a mixed population of cells and for studying both intracellular and plasma membrane enzyme reaction kinetics in intact cells using flow cytometric techniques. By such means it may be possible to obtain results that have greater relevance to the biological reality.

B. Principles of Flow Cytometry

Flow system instruments exhibit considerable diversity of form but the basic principles of operation are identical in each. Single cells are constrained to flow in fluid suspension so that one cell at a time passes through a high-intensity focused light flux which is frequently obtained from a laser source. Typically up to 5,000 cells can be analysed per second and a number of different measurements can be made simultaneously. These include narrow forward angle light scatter, which is directly proportional to cross-sectional area, as well as fluorescent light from suitably stained constituents and absorbed light. As each cell passes through the exciting beam a pulse of scattered and/or fluorescent light is rendered incident upon a light-sensitive detector which responds by giving an electrical pulse that is directly proportional to the quantity of light scattered or emitted from the cell. The electrical pulse is then digitized and stored electronically for computer analysis and display. A block diagram of a typical system for quantitating fluorescence emission is shown in Fig. 1.

Absorbed light can also be quantitated but this requires two sets of light-sensitive detectors as opposed to only one for scattered or fluorescent light (SUPER

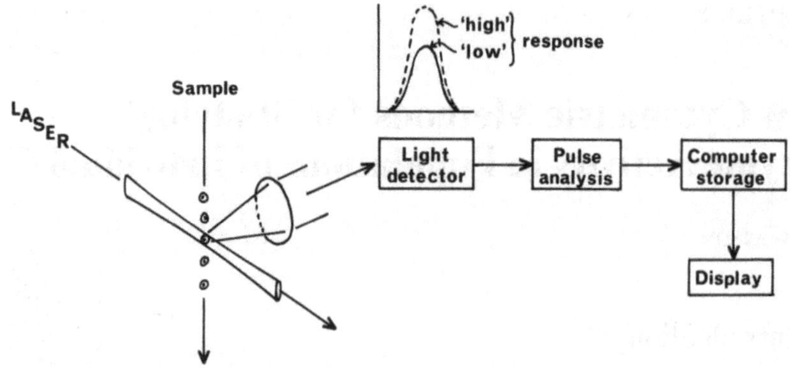

Fig. 1. Block diagram of a typical laser-based flow cytometer

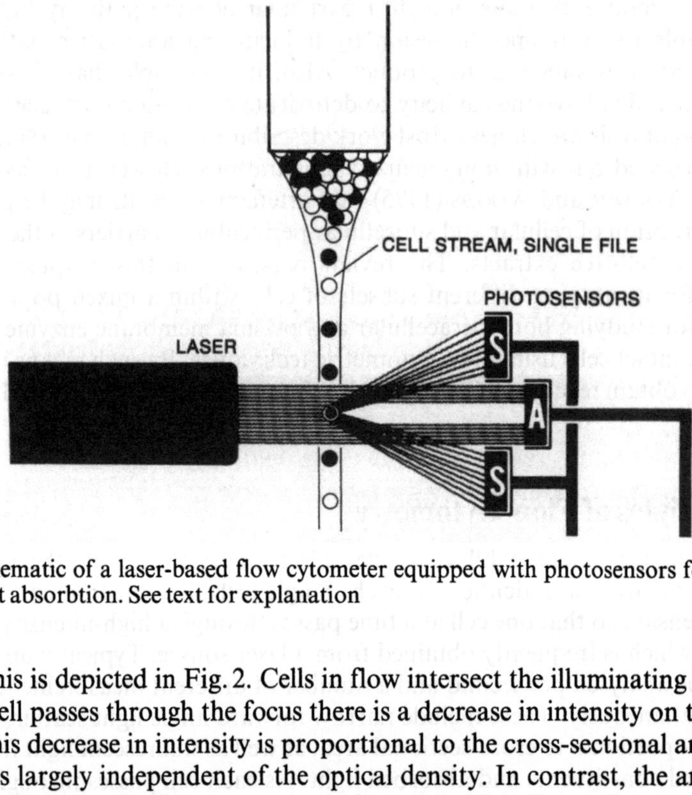

Fig. 2. Schematic of a laser-based flow cytometer equipped with photosensors for quantitating light absorbtion. See text for explanation

1979). This is depicted in Fig. 2. Cells in flow intersect the illuminating light and as each cell passes through the focus there is a decrease in intensity on the detector *A*. This decrease in intensity is proportional to the cross-sectional area of the cell and is largely independent of the optical density. In contrast, the amount of light scattered into the *S* detector is inversely proportional to optical density. The instrument is set up initially with an unstained sample so that the amplitudes of the pulses from the S and A detectors are adjusted to be approximately equal. When a sample containing cells stained with light-absorbing material is subsequently analysed there is a decrease in the amplitude of the S detector (but not of the A) whenever a stained cell passes through the light beam. Thus, by comparing the S-pulse with the A-pulse for each cell it is possible to define clusters which absorb light and hence to identify the stained cells in the population.

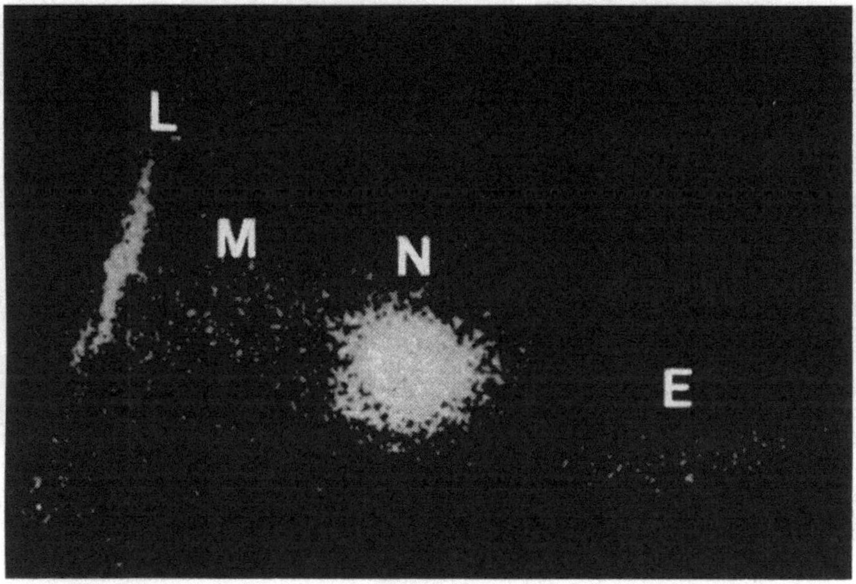

Fig. 3 Storage oscilloscope pattern of white blood cells stained for peroxidase activity. *L*, lymphocytes; *M*, monocytes; *N*, neutrophils; *E*, eosinophils

C. Enzyme Measurements Using Light Absorption

Many "classical" histochemical enzyme-staining procedures deposit insoluble light-absorbing products, which enables cells with the enzyme activity being studied to be identified. Some of these techniques have been adapted in flow technology. KAPLOW and EISENBERG (1975) have identified lymphocytes, monocytes, neutrophils and eosinophils in peripheral blood using peroxidase activity. The technique was based on the supravital benzidine dihydrochloride method of KAPLOW (1975), where zinc chloride was used as a stabilizer for the blue reaction product. The light source was a helium-neon laser emitting red light which was absorbed by the blue reaction product, and axial light loss was used as the measurement parameter. These data are reproduced in Fig. 3, in which scattered light (*ordinate*) is scored against axial light loss (*abscissa*). Each cell in the sample is represented by a single dot on the storage oscilloscope with x and y coordinates that are respectively proportional to axial light loss and scattered light intensity. This technique has also been applied to patients with various haematological disorders and the characteristic patterns of eosinophilia, lymphocytic leukaemia and chronic granulocytic leukaemia are reproduced in *panels a, b and c* respectively of Fig. 4 (KAPLOW 1979).

Monocyte esterase activity can also be determined using light-absorbing techniques developed for flow cytometry by KAPLOW et al. (1976). The method utilizes α-naphthol acetate as substrate which is coupled to fast blue salt BB. The final reaction product is grey-black which again absorbs the red laser light, and the activity is limited almost exclusively to monocytes. Figure 5 shows two samples

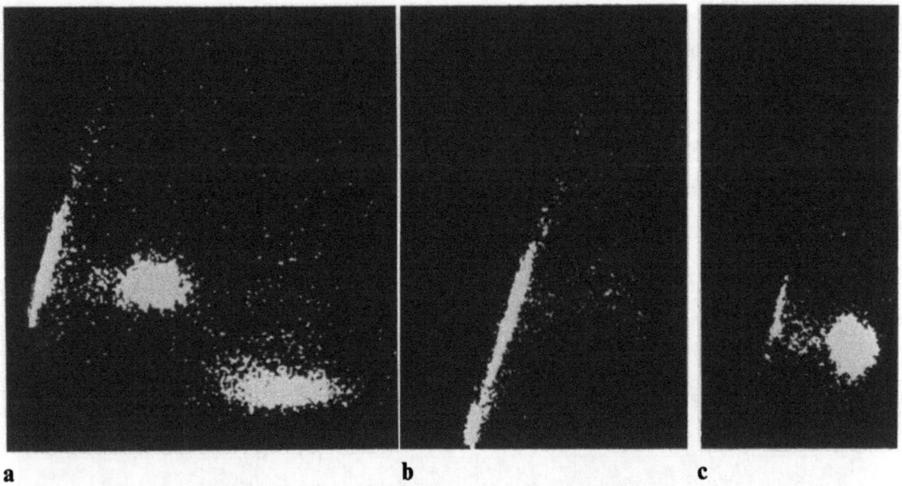

Fig. 4 a–c. Characteristic patterns of eosinophilia (**a**) lymphocytic leukaemia (**b**) and chronic granulocytic leukaemia (**c**) stained for peroxidase activity

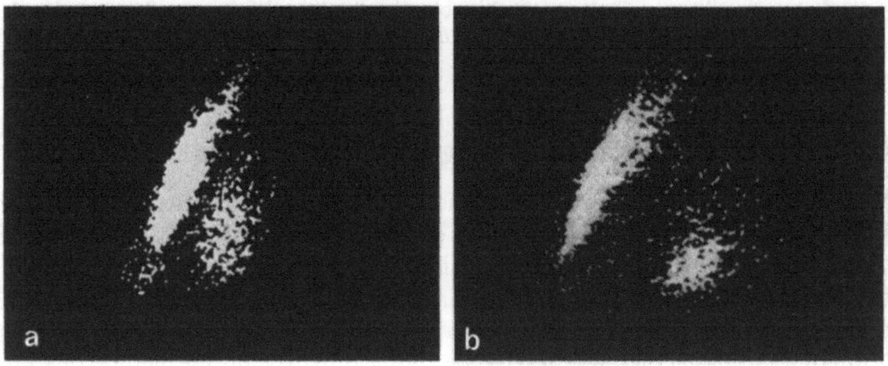

Fig. 5 a, b. Monocyte esterase activity. The clusters to the *bottom right* represent monocyte populations with low (**a**) and high (**b**) esterase acitivity

from peripheral blood, in which the monocyte clusters exhibited low (*panel a*) and high (*panel b*) esterase activity.

The methods developed by KAPLOW and collaborators are excellent for cellular identification in the systems for which the techniques were developed, but relatively "static" patterns are obtained. KAPLOW (1979) has investigated the influence of time of incubation of cells on monocyte esterase activity and has obtained increasing axial light loss with time, but these light-absorbing methods are relatively insensitive for dynamic studies. This is particularly true where enzyme progress curves are required in order to obtain the kinetic parameters of enzyme action. However, it will be shown later how these can be obtained for certain assays using fluorogenic substrates.

D. Enzyme Measurements Using Fluorogenic Substrates

I. Assays with Single Substrates

A large number of enzyme substrates based on methylumbelliferone, naphthol and fluorescein molecules as fluorochromic groups are available for studying a variety of enzymes. Essentially the principles involved with each class of molecule are the same in that the fluorochrome is released from the fluorochrome-conjugate complex by enzyme action. With increasing time a greater amount of fluorochrome is released in each cell and this can be quantitated by the flow system to distinguish between cell types with different enzyme reaction rates and to generate enzyme progress curves (WATSON et al. 1977; MARTIN and SCHWARTZENDRUBER 1980). In general the fluorescein-based substrate conjugates are nonfluorescent. In contrast, the 4-methylumbelliferone conjugates are generally fluorescent but the excitation and emission wavelengths are much shorter than those of the released product 4-methylumbelliferone and with correct optical design any "overlap" can be eliminated. Flow system techniques with the naphthol derivatives involve "trapping" of the released product within the cell by coupling with 5-nitrosalicylaldehyde which forms an insoluble fluorescent complex with an emission spectrum that is shifted into the red (DOLBEARE and SMITH 1977).

Both static and dynamic flow cytometry techniques have been developed for studying enzyme activity in populations of individual cells using these fluorogenic substrates. Static techniques, which may be defined as methods involving incubation for a single length of time before analysis, have been used fairly extensively to distinguish between many different cell types. PALLAVICHINI et al. (1977) have not only distinguished between intestinal crypt and villus cells, but have also sorted these subpopulations based on leucine-amino peptidase activity. The differentiated villus cells contain considerably higher activity of this enzyme than the non-differentiated cells of the crypt.

DOLBEARE and SMITH (1979) have used a combination of forward light scatter and β-glucuronidase activity to distinguish lymphocytes, monocytes and macrophages in washings from the peritoneal cavity of the rat. These data are reproduced in Fig. 6, which shows the two-dimensional histogram of frequency on the vertical axis versus light scatter and fluorescence on the two horizontal axes. VANDERLAAN et al. (1979) have shown that γ-glutamyl transpeptidase activity is considerably higher in hepatocytes following carcinogen exposure than in control populations. However, VANDERLAAN (1979) has shown that in mixed populations it can be difficult to identify positively the transformed cells, as the reaction product can diffuse from cells with enzyme activity into those with little or no activity. This problem can be partially overcome by short incubation times with two fluorogenic substrates used simultaneously. Recently, WATSON et al. (in preparation) have been able to discriminate between normal and malignant liver-cell lines by measuring a combination of esterase and γ-glutamyl transpeptidase activity using fluorescein diacetate and γ-glutamyl-7-amino-4-methyl-coumarin simultaneously as substrates. This technique requires a twin-laser instrument to excite the reaction product from γ-glutamyl transpeptidase activity (4-methylumbelliferone, krypton UV excitation) and esterase activity (fluorescein, 488-nm argon

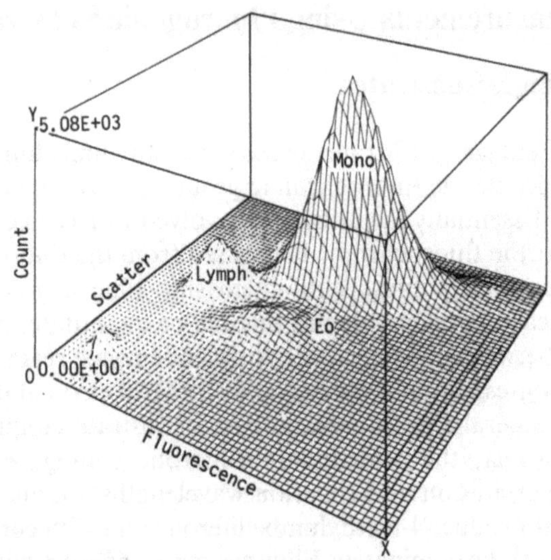

Fig. 6. Three-dimensional histogram of frequency (*vertical axis*) versus light scatter and β-glucuronidase activity (fluorescence) on the two *horizontal axes*. Peritoneal washings from the rat containing lymphocytes, monocytes and eosinophils

excitation). Esterase and γ-glutamyl transpeptidase activities were both greater in the aflatoxin-transformed malignant cells which enabled an excellent discrimination to be made between the two cell types.

Dolbeare et al. (1980) have shown that alkaline phosphatase and an arylamidase can be used as markers for normal and transformed WI-38 cells. Their results demonstrated that the transformed cell enzymes differed by not only a qualitative but also a quantitative change in alkaline phosphatase and a quantitative loss of an arylamidase.

Dynamic enzyme measurements in cell populations can not only be used to identify different subsets of cells but they can also be used to extract enzyme kinetic information. These techniques involve the measurement of rates of change for which flow cytometry is ideally suited. Watson et al. (1977) described a method for measuring enzyme reaction kinetics in intact cells where the population was automatically sampled for predetermined periods at discrete time intervals after mixing the cell sample with fluorescein diacetate, which is a non-specific esterase substrate. The outputs from the photomultipliers of the instrument were directed through to an AR/11 analog-to-digital converter on the front end of a PDP 11/40 computer. The latter was instructed to record for 5 s, then to wait for 10 s sequentially for up to 3 min. As the reaction proceeded there was a build up of fluorescence in the cells of the population which was recorded as an increase in the median of the fluorescence distribution with time. Thus, by analysing the population sequentially it was possible to generate enzyme progress curves. This technique has two major disadvantages. Firstly, cells are continuing in flow in the intervals between recordings; thus much of the sample is wasted. Secondly, the fluorescence will be increasing during the recording interval and will result in a tendency for the distribution records to be skewed to the right, giving an overestimate of the median. The artefact produced will not be very great for "slow" reactions but is likely to be significant for "fast" reactions. Some compensation can be achieved for the latter by increasing the sample throughput and simultaneously decreasing the recording period, but this has limitations. These problems have now been overcome very elegantly by MARTIN and SCHWARTZENDRUBER (1980) by incorporating time as an additional flow cytometry parameter. Each cell analysed will have not only its specific fluorescence intensity recorded but also the time in relation to the start of the reaction at which the fluorescence was analysed. Thus, by plotting fluorescence intensity on the ordinate versus time on the abscissa an enzyme progress curve is generated directly.

In spite of the relative lack of elegance of the method described by WATSON et al. (1977) they were able to show that a series of enzyme progress curves for EMT 6 mouse mammary tumour cells could be generated at different substrate concentrations. The resulting substrate-dependent initial velocity plots showed abnormal Michaelis-Menten kinetic behaviour, with the double reciprocal derivative plots (LINEWEAVER and BURK 1934) of these data departing from linearity. It was also noted that the coefficient of variation (CV, relative standard deviation) of the enzyme activity within the population increased from about 30% at 45 s to about 50% at 180 s and this increasing CV with time suggested population heterogeneity. These studies were carried out during the early plateau phase of growth of EMT 6 cells in tissue culture when about 60% of the population was in a non-cycling state (TWENTYMAN et al. 1975; WATSON 1977). Thus, from a cell kinetic standpoint the population was far from homogeneous. As it has been shown that enzymes can exhibit cyclical changes through the cell cycle (KLEVECZ and KAPP 1973) it is highly likely that some of the increase in CV at 180 s was due to a mixture of cells with different enzyme content.

Using this same technique it was later shown that late plateau phase EMT 6 cells, when more than 95% of the population was arrested in a $G1/G_0$ state, had considerable higher esterase activity than exponentially growing cells (WATSON et al. 1978). The progress curves are shown in Fig. 7, with the data from the exponentially growing population in Fig. 7a and the plateau phase data depicted in Fig. 7b. The concentrations of substrate in micromolar concentrations are shown against each progress curve. Figure 8 shows the substrate-dependent velocity plots associated with these data, which should theoretically follow the Michaelis-Menten rectangular hyperbola. There is a highly abnormal "double-sigmoid" pattern for the plateau phase cells but the exponentially growing cells exhibit less abnormal kinetic behaviour. However, the latter population, unlike the plateau phase cells, is very heterogeneous and the DNA histogram obtained with propidium iodide staining (KRISHAN 1975) was compatible with a cell population consisting of 40% in G1, 50% in S-phase and 10% in G2+M. Because of this heterogeneity the assay was repeated with cells synchronized by mitotic selection (TERESIMA and TOLMACH 1963; WATSON and TAYLOR 1977). Substrate-dependent velocity plots for cells in early G1, mid- to late G1, early S-phase, mid- to late S-phase and mitosis are shown in Fig. 9. As can be seen there was a reappearance of the double-sigmoid pattern when relatively homogeneous populations of expo-

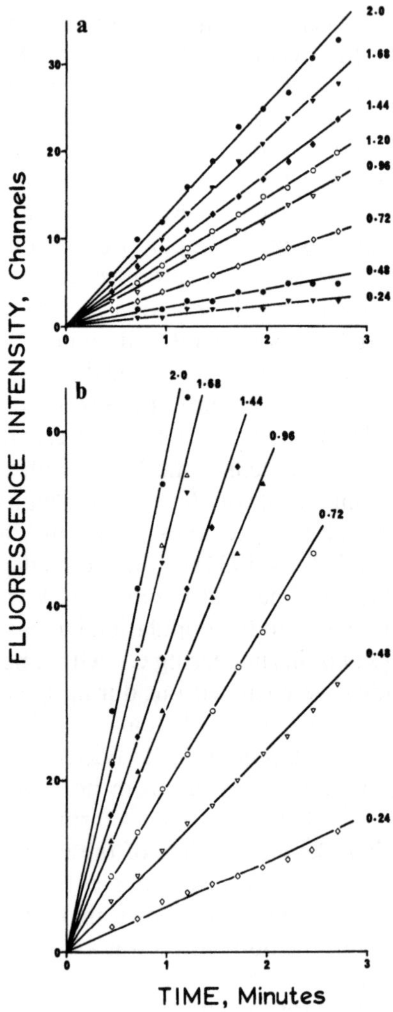

Fig. 7 a, b. Enzyme progress curves for the conversion of fluorescein diacetate to fluorescein in EMT6 mouse mammary tumour cells growing in tissue culture. **a** Exponentially growing cells. **b** Late plateau phase cells 28 days after seeding the monolayers. The medians of the distributions are represented by the *points* and the substrate concentrations (μ*M*) are shown against each progress curve

nentially growing cells were analysed. It is highly probable that at least two enzymes are hydrolysing fluorescein diacetate to give this type of abnormal kinetic behaviour, and further evidence for this hypothesis is presented later.

In an attempt to elucidate the abnormal pattern of substrate-dependent reaction velocity a series of experiments was carried out with homogenized preparations in the cuvette of a standard spectrofluorimeter. The substrate-dependent velocity plots for exponentially growing and plateau phase cells are presented in Fig. 10, where it is apparent that normal Michaelis-Menten kinetics were ob-

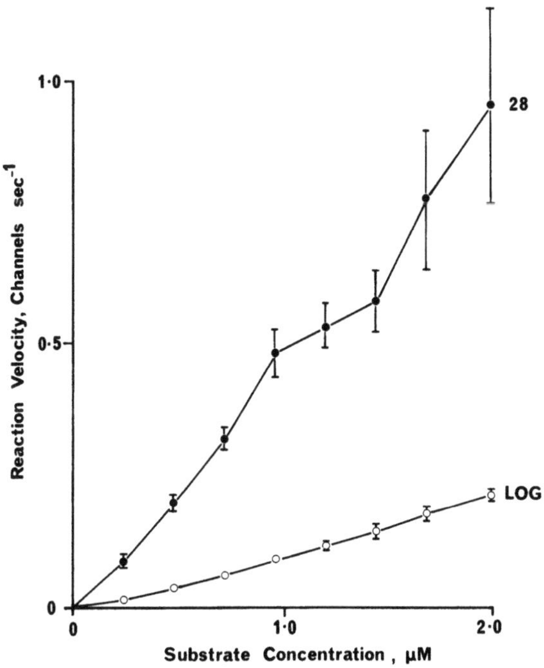

Fig. 8. Substrate-dependent initial velocity plots obtained by regression analysis of the data shown in Fig. 7. The *error bars* represent the 95% confidence limits where these are greater than the diameter of the symbol

served. Furthermore, when the reaction velocity was compared in whole cells and homogenates, both in the cuvette of the spectrofluorimeter, it was found that the intact cells were between four and five times more efficient per milligram of protein at converting substrate than were the homogenates (WATSON 1980a).

Calculation of the kinetics parameters (K_m and V_{max}) for esterase activity assayed with fluorescein diacetate in EMT 6 cells has not yet been possible for the intact-cell preparations. This has been partly due to the probable presence of more than one esterase as suggested by the abnormal kinetic behaviour, and indeed GUIBAULT and KRAMER (1966) have shown that fluorescein diacetate hydrolysis is catalysed by a number of enzymes including α- and γ-chymotrypsin, lipase and achylase. However, further factors must also be considered for the abnormal kinetic behaviour shown in Figs. 8 and 9. Firstly, cellular and subcellular permeability barriers may exist in the intact cell which could limit the availability of substrate at the enzyme site. Secondly, there could be active transport mechanisms for the substrate with intracellular accumulation. Each of these factors would result in a difference between the substrate concentration external to the cell and at the site of enzyme action.

KRISCH (1971) has reported abnormal kinetic behaviour in certain esterase preparations and it has been suggested that the reaction mechanism may need two or more interacting catalytic sites. Substrate activation, where the reaction proceeds most rapidly when more than one substrate molecule is bound to a single

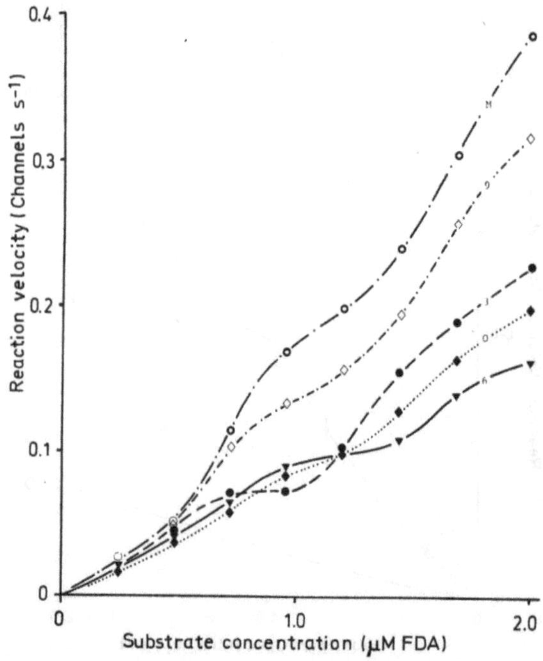

Fig. 9. Substrate-dependent initial velocity plots for fluorescein diacetate conversion, in synchronized EMT6 mouse mammary tumour cells. Early G1 (··○··◆··), mid→late G1 (--3-●-), early S-phase (—6—▼—), mid-late S-phase (-·-9-·◇·-) and mitotic cells (—·—M—·0—)

enzyme molecule, may also be involved. These last factors could account for the upward concavity ("lag kinetics") in the plateau phase cells (Fig. 8) and all of the data in Fig. 9.

The problem of calculating K_m and V_{max} is further compounded by the observation that normal kinetics occurred in homogenized preparations (Fig. 10) but that these homogenates were four to five times less efficient per milligram protein at converting substrate than intact cells. This loss of activity in homogenates could be due to the release of esterase inhibitors that are not normally exposed to enzyme in an uncontrolled manner, or to the disruption of an ordered spatial arrangement of enzyme molecules. This last suggestion is compatible with the change from lag kinetics in whole cells to normal kinetics in homogenates as well as with the drop in activity which could be related to the possible disruption of multiple interacting catalytic sites by the homogenization. Although values for K_m and V_{max} have been obtained from the data given in Fig. 10 these are not presented, as they would seem to have little relevance to the biological reality.

An automated fluorimetric method for assaying alkaline phosphatase using 3-*O*-methyl fluorescein phosphate was developed by HILL et al. (1968). An adaptation of this technique has been applied to intact cells using flow cytometry by WATSON et al. (1979). The discrete sequential sampling method described above was used in the assay to obtain enzyme progress curves at different sub-

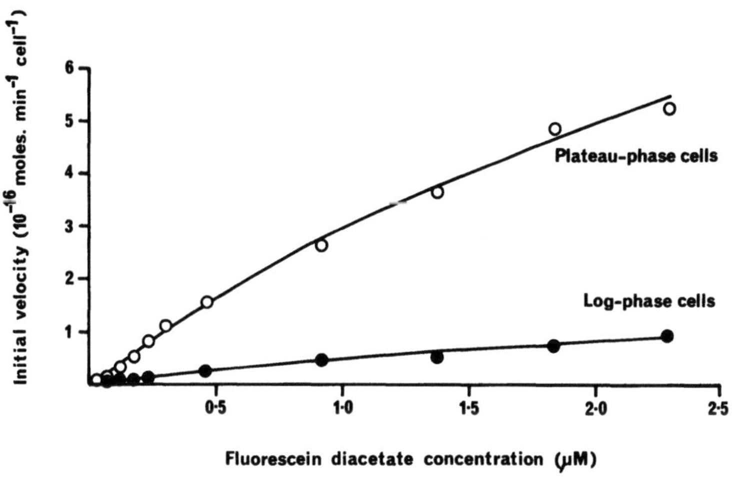

Fig. 10. Initial reaction velocities plotted against substrate concentration for fluorescein diacetate hydrolysis in cell-free esterase extracts of log and 28-day plateau phase EMT6/M/CC cells

strate concentrations. The results for plateau phase EMT 6 cells are shown in Fig. 11. These results are obviously very different from those shown in Fig. 7 and they presented a considerable interpretative problem which was not resolved until a sample was viewed under the fluorescence microsope. It was then seen that the fluorescence was due to "halos" at the external cell membranes with no fluorescence from the interior of the cells. Subsequent incubation of cells with product, 3-*O*-methyl fluorescein, failed to demonstrate entry into intact cells. The viability of EMT 6 cells decreases considerably after 3 h of incubation with protein-free phosphate-buffered saline (PBS). In a sample of cells so treated it was found that the fluorescence from 3-*O*-methyl fluorescein was no longer located at the cell surface but was being emitted from granular structures surrounding the nucleus. This fluorescence was considerably more intense than that emitted from the cell surface, so much so that the latter could no longer be seen. These various data suggested that substrate hydrolysis in intact viable cells takes place at or in the cell surface by phosphatases located in the plasma membrane and that the product was lost from the immediate vicinity of the cells by diffusion and consequently was not "seen" by the instrument, which only responded to fluorescence from a preset size distribution. Thus, a steady state would be reached in which the rate of production of fluorescent product would equal the rate of loss, giving rise to asymptotic fluorescence responses from the population at each substrate concentration. On the assumption that this hypothesis was correct WATSON et al. (1979) were able to show that the progress curve at a given substrate concentration, S, should be described by the equation:

$$P(t) = P_{\infty}\left(\frac{S}{S+\mathrm{K_m}}\right) \times (1.0 - EXP(-k \times t)), \qquad (1)$$

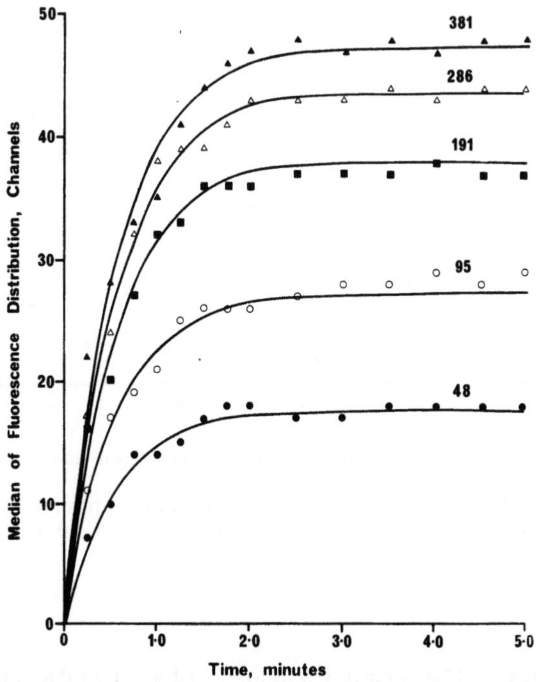

Fig. 11. Reaction progress curves of the increase in median fluorescence intensity with time for the hydrolysis of 3-*O*-methyl fluorescein phosphate in 14-day plateau phase EMT6/M/CC cells. The substrate concentrations (μ*M*) are shown against each curve

where $P(t)$ is the fluorescence response at time t, P_∞ is the theoretical maximum asymptotic response at infinite substrate concentration, $\mathrm{K_m}$ is the Michaelis constant and k is the rate constant for product loss assuming a first order kinetic process. When a steady state exists (i.e. beyond 2.5–3 min in Fig. 11) the term $EXP(-k\times t)$ in Eq. (1) will tend to zero and the asymptotic fluorescence response will be given by the expression $P_\infty(S/(S+\mathrm{K_m}))$ and will vary with substrate concentration. P_∞ can be eliminated from the expression by taking ratios, thus:

$$\frac{P_2(t_\infty)}{P_1(t_\infty)}=\frac{S_2}{S_1}\times\frac{(S_1+\mathrm{K_m})}{(S_2+\mathrm{K_m})}=R_{12}, \tag{2}$$

where $P_1(t_\infty)$ and $P_2(t_\infty)$ are the asymptotic fluorescence values associated with substrate concentrations S_1 and S_2 and where R_{12} is the ratio of $P_2(t_\infty)$ to $P_1(t_\infty)$. Equation (2) can be rearranged to give:

$$R_{ij}=\mathrm{K_m}\left(\frac{1}{S_i}-\frac{R_{ij}}{S_j}\right)+1,$$

where for n substrate concentrations i varies from 1 to (n-1) and j varies from $(i+1)$ to n to give a triangular matrix for the ratios containing $n(n\text{-}1)/2$ values. Thus, by plotting R_{ij} against $[(1/S_i)-(R_{ij}/S_j)]$ a line with slope K_m is obtained which intersects the ordinate at unity. In three separate analyses, values of $110.0 \pm 23\ \mu M$, $122.3 \pm 31\ \mu M$ and $120.5 \pm 24\ \mu M$ were obtained, where the limits were calculated at two standard errors and in all cases the ordinate intercept did not differ from unity, $p > 0.1$. It can be seen from Eq. (2) that if P_∞ is the asymptotic fluorescence response at infinite substrate concentration, S_∞, then:

$$\frac{P_\infty}{P_n} = \frac{S_\infty}{S_n} \times \frac{(S_n + K_m)}{(S_\infty + K_m)},$$

where P_n is the asymptotic response at S_n. The term $S_\infty/(S_\infty + K_m)$ is unity; therefore, $P_n(S_n + K_m) = P_\infty S_n$. By plotting $P_n(S_n + K_m)$ against S_n a line of slope P_∞ is obtained which intersects the origin. Thus P_∞ can be obtained after a value for K_m is found. It was also shown previously (WATSON et al. 1979) that the maximum reaction velocity, V_{max}, is equal to the product $P_\infty \times k$. As Eq. (1) is an inverted exponential a value of k can be found from the time taken for the curves to reach half their maximum height. Thus, V_{max} can be defined in the arbitrary units of channels min^{-1}. The three analyses gave maximum reaction velocities of 107.0, 110.0, and 109.2 channels per minute.

It would seem that the hydrolysis of 3-*O*-methyl fluorescein phosphate at the cell membrane in EMT 6 cells follows "classical" Michaelis-Menten kinetics. This result is at variance with those from fluorescein diacetate hydrolysis by intracellular esterases, and two major differences between these fluorogenic substrates should be considered. Firstly, 3-*O*-methyl fluorescein, the reaction product of 3-*O*-methyl fluorescein phosphate, is considerably less polar than fluorescein, the reaction product of fluorescein diacetate (ROTMAN and PAPERMASTER 1966). Thus, if 3-*O*-methyl fluorescein enters the cell we would expect the rate constant for leakage from the cell to be greater than that for fluorescein. Previous studies indicated that fluorescein leaks out of EMT 6 cells with a half-time of 7–8 min (WATSON et al. 1977). This compares with between 20 and 25 s for 3-*O*-methyl fluorescein (WATSON et al. 1979; WATSON 1980a), thus the leakage rate constant is about 20 times greater than that for fluorescein. Secondly, fluorescein diacetate is lipophilic and will penetrate the cell membrane rapidly. In contrast, 3-*O*-methyl fluorescein phosphate is lipophobic as well as ionized at physiological pH and would not be expected to penetrate the cell without prior dephosphorylation by membrane phosphatases. The direct observations made with the fluorescence microscope suggest that the product of 3-*O*-methyl fluorescein phosphate hydrolysis either does not enter the cell or it diffuses out of the cell very rapidly although some remains associated with the external membrane. Both possibilities are compatible with the magnitude of the loss rate constant whatever the mechanism and this is interesting as it suggests that dephosphorylation at the cell membrane does not necessarily lead to appreciable uptake or accumulation in the cytoplasm.

A number of inactive antitumour agents have been designed to be activated specifically by phosphatases. These include estramustine phosphate, which releases oestradiol and normustine following cleavage of a carbamate linkage and loss of the phosphate moiety. This compound is activated by phosphatase-rich tissues including gut, liver and prostate carcinoma. Honvan is also activated by phosphatase-rich tissues to release a synthetic oestrogen. Both agents were synthesized for the treatment of prostatic carcinoma, which exhibits high acid phosphatase activity. However, it is not known if intracellular or external cell membrane phosphatases are primarily responsible for release of the active agents. If the latter are primarily responsible it is distinctly possible that prostate carcinoma cells resistant to these agents might be "deficient" in plasma membrane phosphatases. It would, therefore, be useless to test for efficacy on homogenates as the intracellular enzymes would also be included and would give rise to totally artefactual results.

II. Assays Using Two Substrates Simultaneously

The substrate-dependent initial velocity plots shown in Figs. 8 and 9 suggested the possibility that two or more enzymes were hydrolysing fluorescein diacetate in EMT 6 cells. As this is a non-specific esterase substrate it was not unreasonable to expect that a second non-specific esterase substrate with a different molecular structure might show different reaction rate characteristics. Furthermore, it was also not unreasonable to postulate that two different cell types would contain either different esterases or if the same enzymes were present they were unlikely to be present at the same concentration. Thus, by assaying with two different non-specific esterase substrates (fluorescein diacetate and 4-methylumbelliferyl acetate) simultaneously in a mixture of two different cell types it should be possible to distinguish between the populations. The results of one such assay are shown in Fig. 12, where the green (fluorescein diacetate) fluorescence for each cell is scored on the *ordinate* against the violet (4-methyl umbelliferyl acetate) fluorescence on the *abscissa* and two distinct populations are apparent. The cluster to the *upper left* represents the EMT 6 mouse mammary tumour (90% of the mixed population) and that to the *lower right* represents the human colonic adenocarcinoma HT 29. These two cell lines were chosen for the first analysis using this type of assay for two main reasons. Firstly, the cell types were sufficiently different to stand a reasonable chance of obtaining a discrimination and, secondly, the plating efficiencies and culture characteristics were well documented and understood. Apart from the primary objective of distinguishing between different cell types these assays are being developed with a view to maintaining cell viability. This has largely been achieved in these two cell types with a plating efficiency of about 90% being obtained for a 6-h exposure to maximum concentrations of the substrate mixture. Also, a slope of 1.077 was obtained for the regression analysis of known versus instrument-counted percentages of HT 29 in mixtures of the two cell types (WATSON 1980a). It has also been reported that a discrimination can be made between fibroblasts, a lung tumour and a second colon carcinoma, all of human origin, using this combined esterase assay (CHAMBERS and WATSON 1980; WATSON 1980b). These results were sufficiently encouraging to attempt to discriminate between the different subsets to be found in the much more complex system of bone marrow. Using a combination of six simultaneous measurements on each cell (UV and blue light both scattered at 90° and at narrow forward angles coupled with the two non-specific esterase substrates, fluorescein diacetate and 4-methyl umbelliferyl acetate) it has been possible to identify between 10 and 16

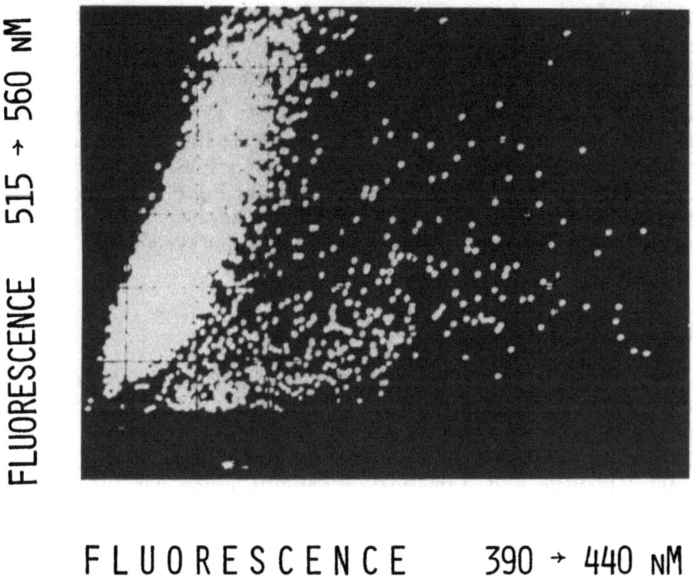

Fig. 12. Combined enzyme assay using fluorescein diacetate (1.6 μ*M*) and 4-methyl umbelliferyl acetate (460 μ*M*) with EMT6 (1.5×10^6 cells/ml, *top left*) and HT 29 (1.7×10^5 cells/ml, *bottom right*)

different subsets in mouse bone marrow (WATSON and CHAMBERS 1980; WATSON 1980b). However, positive morphological identification of these subsets must await the upgrading of the instrument to cell sorting.

E. Conclusions

Assays for assessing enzymtic activity in populations of individual cells using flow cytometry are a very recent development but already techniques are available for peroxidases, esterases/lipase, leucine amino petidase, alkaline phosphatase, arylamidase, β-glucuronidase, membrane phosphatases and γ-glutamyl transpeptidase. It has been demonstrated that the kinetic parameters of enzyme action (K_m and V_{max}) can be obtained for some assays (membrane phosphatases) but not yet for others (esterases). Furthermore, it has been shown that results obtained from cell-free extracts are not necessarily related to those obtained from intact cells. This simple fact must necessarily focus attention on the requirement to study "enzyme biochemistry" under as near physiological conditions as possible in order to obtain biologically relevant data. Although most, if not all, of the assays developed so far have little or no direct relevance to antitumour drug resistance it will not be very long, judging from the current rate of progress, before such assays are forthcoming. Flow cytometry is a very powerful research tool with limitations that appear to be imposed only by the inventiveness of the users and although the instruments incorporate very sophisticated technology it must never be forgotten that the function of these instruments is for biologists to ask biological questions.

This chapter has been written with the express purpose of exposing the potential and hopefully of stimulating those primarily concerned with enzymatic drug resistance mechnisms to think in terms of flow cytometric assays.

Acknowledgements. I would like to express my thanks to the following for permission to reproduce their data and figures. Bernard Super, Ortho Instruments for Fig. 2; Leonard Kaplow and the editors of *Flow Cytometry and Sorting* for Figs. 3, 4, and 5; and Frank Dolbeare and the editors of *Flow Cytometry and Sorting* for Fig. 6. I am also very grateful for the contribution of my scientific colleagues Stephen Chambers and Paul Workman, and the excellent technical assistance of Paula Rayner and Karen Wright.

References

Chambers SH, Watson JV (1980) Identification of different cell types using two enzyme reactions measured simultaneously in single cells with a multi-parameter flow cytometer. Br J Cancer 42:184 (abstract)

Dolbeare FA, Smith RE (1977) Flow cytometric measurement of peptidases with use of 5-nitrosalicylaldehyde and 4-methoxy β-naphthylamine derivatives. J Clin Chem 23:1485–1491

Dolbeare FA, Smith RA (1979) Flow cytoenzymology; rapid enzyme analysis of single cells. In: Melamed MR, Mullaney PF, Mendelsohn ML (eds) Flow cytometry and sorting. Wiley, New York, chap 17, pp 317–333

Dolbeare FA, Vanderlaan M, Phares W (1980) Alkaline phosphatase and an acid arylamidase as marker enzymes for normal and transformed WI-38 cells. J Histochem Cytochem 28:419–423

Guibault GG, Kramer DN (1966) Lipolysis of fluorescein and eosin esters. Kinetics of hydrolysis. Anal Biochem 14:28–32

Hill HD, Summer GK, Waters MD (1968) An automated fluorimetric assay for alkaline phosphatase using 3-O-methyl fluorescein phosphate. Anal Biochem 24:9–14

Kaplow LS (1975) Substitute for benzidine in myeloperoxidase stains. Am J Clin Pathol 63:451–454

Kaplow LS (1979) Leucocyte peroxidase and non-specific esterase. In: Melamed MR, Mullaney PF, Mendelsohn ML (eds) Flow cytometry and sorting. Wiley, New York, chap 29, pp 531–545

Kaplow LS, Eisenberg M (1975) Leukocyte differentiation and enumeration by cytochemical-cytographic analysis. In: Haanen CAM, Hellen HFP, Wessels JHC (eds) First international symposium on pulse-cytophotometry. European Press Medicon, Ghent, pp 262–274

Kaplow LS, Dauber H, Lerner E (1976) Assessment of monocyte esterase activity by flow cytophotometry. J Histochem Cytochem 24:363–372

Klevecz RR, Kapp LN (1973) Intermittent DNA synthesis and periodic expression of enzyme activity in the cell cycle of WI-38 cells. J Cell Biol 58:564–570

Krisch K (1971) Carboxylic ester hydrolases. In: Boyer PD (ed) The enzymes, vol 5. Academic, New York, p 43–69

Krishan A (1975) Rapid flow cytofluorimetric analysis of mammalian cell cycle by propidium iodide staining. J Cell Biol 66:188–192

Lineweaver H, Burk D (1934) The determination of enzyme dissociation constants. J Am Chem Soc 56:658–661

Martin JC, Swartzendruber DE (1980) Time: a new parameter for kinetic measurements in flow cytometry. Science 207:199–200

Pallavicini MG, Dolbeare FA, Gray JW, Cohen AM, Dethlefsen LA (1977) Separation of crypt and villus cell populations by flow cytometry. 3rd International symposium of pulse cytophotometry, Vienna

Rotman B, Papermaster BW (1966) Membrane properties of living mammalian cells as studies by enzymatic hydrolysis of fluorogenic esters. Proc Natl Acad Sci USA 55:134–141

Super BS (1979) The ortho cytofluorograf. In: Melamed MR, Mullaney PF, Mendelsohn ML (eds) Flow cytometry and sorting. Wiley, New York, chap 36, pp 639–652

Teresima T, Tolmach LJ (1963) Growth and nucleic acid synthesis in synchronously dividing populations of HeLa cells. Exp Cell Res 30:344–358

Twentyman PR, Watson JV, Bleehen NM, Rowles PM (1975) Changes in cell proliferation kinetics occurring during the life history of monolayer cultures of a mouse mammary tumour cell line. Cell Tissue Kinet 8:41–47

Vanderlaan M (1979) Adaptation of dialysis membrane techniques to fluorescent cytoenzymology. Automated cytology conference III, Asilomar, California

Vanderlaan M, Cutter C, Dolbeare FA (1979) Flow microfluorimetric identification of hepatocytes with elevated γ-glutamyl transpeptidase activity following carcinogen exposure. J Histochem Cytochem 27:114–119

Watson JV (1977) The application of age distribution theory in the analysis of cytofluorimetric DNA histogram data. Cell Tissue Kinet 10:157–169

Watson JV (1980 a) Enzyme kinetic studies in cell populations using fluorogenic substrates and flow cytometric techniques. Cytometry 1:143–151

Watson JV (1980 b) Cellular identification using light scatter and two esterase substrates simultaneously. 5th International conference of flow cytometry, Rome

Watson JV, Chambers SH (1980) Physico-biochemical properties of subpopulations in mouse bone marrow. Br J Cancer 42:184 (abstract)

Watson JV, Taylor IW (1977) Cell cycle analysis in vitro using flow cytofluorimetry following synchronization. Br J Cancer 36:281–285

Watson JV, Chambers SH, Workman P, Horsnell TS (1977) A flow cytofluorimetric method for measuring enzyme reaction kinetics in intact cells. FEBS Lett 81:179–182

Watson JV, Workman P, Chambers SH (1978) Differences in esterase activity between exponential and plateau growth phases of EMT6/M/CC cells monitored by flow cytofluorimetry. Br J Cancer 37:397–402

Watson JV, Workman P, Chambers SH (1979) An assay for plasma membrane phosphatase activity in populations of individual cells. Biochem Pharmacol 28:821–828

Watson JV, Neal GE, Chambers SH, Legg RF (in preparation) Flow cytometric discrimination between aflotoxin transformed and normal hepatocytes using fluorogenic substrates for γ-glutamyl transpeptidase and esterase activity assayed simultaneously

Youdim MBE, Woods HF (1975) The influence of tissue environment on the rates of metabolic processes and the properties of enzymes. Biochem Pharmacol 24:317–323

CHAPTER 9

Chromosome Studies

D. SCOTT

A. Introduction

This chapter will be devoted to two main themes. The first will be to show that the acquisition of resistance to antitumour drugs may be accompanied by specific chromosome changes which occur spontaneously or are drug induced. The second will be to show that many antitumour drugs induce chromosome damage lethal to cells and that the development of resistance to these drugs may be accompanied by a reduction in such damage. In both contexts consideration will be given only to those chromosome changes which are visible at the level of the light microscope.

B. Chromosome Constitution and Resistance

I. Derivation of Drug-Resistant Cells

Most of the information on the relationship between chromosome constitution and sensitivity to antitumour agents has been derived from studies on mammalian cell lines of tumour or non-tumour origin in which comparisons have been made between karyotypes of wild-type cell lines and drug-resistant lines derived from them after treatment with antitumour drugs in vitro or after treatment of animal tumours in vivo (Table 1). The value of the information derived from such studies has been variable, the most useful arising from investigations which satisfy the following four criteria.

One requirement of such a study is for parallel observation of the control and treated population to be made throughout the investigation. In too many studies the chromosome constitution of the wild-type population has only been examined prior to treatment with an antitumour agent to derive a resistant line, but untreated wild-type cells have not been passaged alongside the treated cells under identical conditions to monitor spontaneous chromosome changes. The necessity for such careful control studies stems from the fact that most of the cell systems used for these investigations have a heterogeneous and unstable chromosome constitution, a situation which is often found in human tumours (SANDBERG 1980).

Ideal control studies are difficult, if not impossible, to achieve since, for example, treatment with an antitumour agent almost inevitably results in some cell killing and consequent population depletion, which means that treated cells are usually less frequently passaged or do not spend as much time in a stationary,

Table 1. Selected examples of chromosome studies in antitumour drug-resistant cells compared with more sensitive wild-type cells

Class of drug	Drug	Cell type	Chromosome observations	Derivation of resistant cells	Comments	References
Purine analogues	6-Thioguanine (6-TG)	Human fibroblasts in vitro	Up to 40% of R clones had structural changes of X chr; banding used	Induced by ionising radiation, then 6-TG for 1–2 weeks	See Figs. 1, 2 and text (Sect. B. II. 1. a.)	COX and MASSON (1978)
		Human lymphoblastoid cell lines in vitro	Wild-type (WT) and R are aneuploid and heterogeneous with markers; no systematic difference between WT and R; banding	Induced by MNNG or ethylmethane sulphonate (EMS), then 6-TG for 4 weeks	Almost totally deficient in HPRT	DUNCAN (1977)
		Human lymphoblastoid cell line (Raji) in vitro	Considerable deviation from normal human karyotype; some differences between WT and R but both have one normal X chr; banding	EMS-induced. Increasing concentrations of 6-TG		YOSHIDA and KODAMA (1977)
		Chinese hamster (DON) in vitro	Unstable karyotypes cf. WT; no banding	Low-dose 6-TG	Gene dosage effect, not true mutants. See text (Sect. B. II. 1. a)	TERZI (1974)
		Chinese hamster (V79) in vitro	A resistant clone had pericentric inversion of X chr; banding	α-Particle induced, then 6-TG for 2 weeks	See Fig. 3 and text (Sect. B. II. 1. a)	THACKER (1981)
		Mouse neuroblastoma (C1300) in vitro	Four parental and four R clones; in three R clones modal no. less than WT; in fourth, modal no. more; change in markers in three R clones cf. WT; no banding	Induced by nitrosoguanidine, then 5–6 gen'ns in 0.3 μg/ml 6-TG and 8-azaguanine	No consistent change in chr. constitution	CIESIELSKI-TRESKA et al. (1975)

	6-Mercaptopurine	Rat ovarian tumour (OJ) in vivo	WT stemline 48–49; R stemline 46–47, same markers as WT; no banding	In vivo, 19 generations		VOITOVITSKII et al. (1970)
Pyrimidine analogues	5-Fluorodeoxyuridine (FUdR)	Mouse lymphocytic leukaemia in vitro (P388)	WT mode 49 incl. biarmed chrs. (mode 14); R mode 40 with biarmed chrs. (mode 21); no banding	In vitro, continuous treatment	Suggest that chr. changes in R cells are induced by FUdR	YOSHIDA et al. (1968)
		Chinese hamster (DON) in vitro	WT mode 22. Step 1^R mutant, mode 22. Step 2^R mutant, mode 22, more structural changes than WT but no consistent differences after banding	In vitro. Two steps. Step 1, EMS treatment,selection in 0.1 µg/ml FUdR. Step 2, no mutagen, selection in 1 µg/ml FUdR	See text (Sect. B. II. 2)	SLACK et al. (1976)
	Cytosine arabinoside (araC)	Mouse lymphoma (L5178Y)	Majority cells with 40 chrs in WT and R, some with 39 and some tets; no clear chr. diff. between WT and R. No banding	In vitro. 12 days	Larger pool of deoxycytidine nucleotides in R	MOMPARLER et al. (1968)
Antifolates	Methotrexate or methasquin	Chinese hamster (DC-3F) in vitro	HSR on chrs. 2 or 4 or on a marker (see Fig. 4)	In vitro. Increasing drug concn	Excess DHFR	BIEDLER and SPENGLER (1976)
		Chinese hamster (DC-3F) in vitro	Abnormal banding or HSR in R cells, preferentially on chr. 2 but not exclusively. Loss of R assoc. with decrease HSR	In vitro. Increasing drug concn	See Table 2 and Figs. 12–14	BIEDLER et al. (1980a)

Table 1 (continued)

Class of drug	Drug	Cell type	Chromosome observations	Derivation of resistant cells	Comments	References
Antifolates (continued)	Methotrexate (MTX)	Chinese hamster (CHO) in vitro	HSR on chr. 2 (see Fig. 6)	In vitro. Increasing drug concn	200X DHFR cf. WT	Nunberg et al. (1978)
		Mouse lymphoma (L5178Y) in vitro	Large HSR on chr. 2 (see Fig. 7)	In vitro. Increasing drug concn	300X DHFR cf. WT	Dolnick et al. (1979)
		Mouse melanoma (PG19) in vitro	WT near tetraploid; R, large marker chrs. with HSRs; one clone had five large markers with HSRs representing about 20% of chr. complement by length (see Fig. 5)	In vitro. Increasing drug concn., nine steps >3 weeks each step. 15 clones selected	Up to 1000X DHFR in R clones cf. WT. Stable R in absence of MTX	Bostock et al. (1979)
		Mouse sarcoma (S-180) in vitro	Higher freq. of DMs in unstable R line cf. stable R line or WT	In vitro	Unstable R → stable R assoc. with loss of DMs (see Table 4)	Kaufman et al. (1979)
		Mouse lymphoma (L5178Y) in vitro	Higher freq. DMs in unstable R line cf. stable R line or WT	In vitro. Unstable line by incr. drug concn. over 10 weeks. Stable line, no info. given	See Table 4	Kaufman et al. (1979)
		Mouse embryo and fibroblasts (3T6) in vitro	Higher freq. DMs in unstable R line, cf. WT	In vitro. Increasing drug concn	See Table 4	Kaufman et al. (1979)

Alkylating agents	Nitrogen mustard (HN2)	Mouse lymphoma (L5178Y) in vitro	Increase in tetraploidy with increasing resistance; no banding	In vitro. Increasing doses over many months	Poor correlation between tetraploidy and resistance when grown in vivo	GOLDENBERG (1969)
		Yoshida sarcoma, rat, in vivo	WT mode 40; R mode 39; no obvious diffs. in markers in WT and R cells; no banding	In vivo. Single-dose MDMS	Cross-resistant to MDMS, SM and busulphan. WT more susceptible to induced chromosome damage (see text)	SCOTT et al. (1974)
	HN3	Yoshida sarcoma, rat, in vivo	WT mode 39, large subtel. marker; three R lines have mode 39, large telo. marker in all three lines but not in WT; banding	In vivo. Incr. drug concn. for >six passages. Three R lines developed	Repeatability of R marker suggestive of causal relationship with resistance (see Sect. B. II. 1. e)	UJHAZY (1974)
	Nitrogen mustard N-oxide	Yoshida sarcoma (rat) in vivo	WT mode 38–39, marker in 36% cells; R mode 37, 33% of cells with the marker; no banding	In vivo, "consecutive injections"	No clear chr. diff. between WT and R	HIRONO and YOKOYAMA (1955)
	Melphalan	Human melanoma in vitro	WT mode 53; R mode 72; no banding	In vitro. Increasing concns. of drug, 14 months	Difference in freq. of drug-induced chr. aberrations between WT and R cells	PARSONS and MORRISON (1978)
		Mouse leukaemia (L1210) in vitro	WT mode 41, two markers; R mode 40, same markers as WT; no banding	In vivo. Repeated low-dose exposure	WT sustain more chr. damage than R line after melphalan	SCHUETTE et al. (1980)
	Cyclophosphamide	Mouse L1210 leukaemia, in vivo	WT with three main stemlines. R tumours different from each other and WT; wider spread of chr. nos. than WT; unstable; no banding	In vivo. Single high dose. Four R tumours at 30 days after tr.	Suggest that chr. changes in R tumours are induced	JOHNSON and HARDY (1965)

Table 1 (continued)

Class of drug	Drug	Cell type	Chromosome observations	Derivation of resistant cells	Comments	References
Alkylating agents (continued)	Thio-tepa	Rat ovarian tumour (OJ) in vivo	WT stemline 48–49; R stemline 46–47, same markers as WT; no banding	In vivo, 12 generations		VOITOVITSKII et al. (1970)
	Sarcolysine	Rat ovarian tumour (OJ) in vivo	WT mode 48–49, 9% polyploid (60–95), three markers; R mode 46–47, 5% polyploid, subtelo marker of WT not present, additional dicentric and metacentric markers; no banding	In vivo, low-dose 12 generations	In mixed WT and R tumours those with WT karyotype eliminated by sarcolysine treatment	VOITOVITSKII et al. (1971)
	Dibromodulcitol	Yoshida tumour, rat ascites in vivo	WT mode 39, 65% cells with large marker; R mode 36, 9% with the large marker, other diffs. from WT; revertant mode 39; no banding	In vivo. Increasing doses over 26–28 passages. Reverted to WT after 30 passages without treatment	Suggest that chr. changes in R line caused by selection and induction	GATI (1979)
Platinum compound	*cis*-PAD	Mouse lymphoma (L5178Y) in vitro	WT mode 40, unstable; R mode 39; no banding	Spontaneous transformation of WT line to R line in vitro	R line cross-R to UV but more sensitive than WT to ionising radiation	SZUMIEL (1979a)
Antibiotics	Actinomycin D	Mouse sarcoma in vitro	Modal no. sim. in WT and R; more metacentrics in R than WT; modal no. reduced after drug removed, markers not lost; no banding	In vitro. Low-dose 22 days	No clear chr. diff. in WT and R	BELEHRADEK et al. (1974)

		Chinese hamster fibroblasts in vitro (DC-3F and CLM-7)	No consistent diff. in chr. no. or structure between WT and R lines; no banding	In vitro. Stepwise increase in drug concn. Several R lines produced	Greater structural abnormality with higher selective concns. of drug	BIEDLER and RIEHM (1970)
		Chinese hamster hybrid cells by fusion (in vitro)	Marker freq. in clones positively correlated with degree of resistance; no banding	One of parental cells made drug resistant by exposure to incr. drug concns. in vitro		IMBERT et al. (1975)
	Daunomycin	Ehrlich ascites, mouse (EHR 2)	WT near tet. with two markers; R hyperdip, with three different markers; banding	In vivo. Approx. 25 weeks treatment	Cross-R to Adriamycin (ADM), Vincristine (VCR) and Vinblastine (VLB)	HASHOLT and DANØ (1974)
	Adriamycin	Ehrlich ascites mouse (EHR 2)	WT near tet. with two markers; R with four different markers; banding	In vivo. Approx. 25 weeks treatment	Cross-R to daunorubicin (DNR), VCR and VLB	HASHOLT and DANØ (1974)
Vinca alkaloids	Vincristine	Ehrlich ascites mouse (EHR 2)	WT near tet. with two markers; R near tet. with two markers as in WT, + one additional marker; banding	In vivo. Approx. 25 weeks treatment	Cross-R to ADM, DNR and VLB	HASHOLT and DANØ (1974)
		Chinese hamster in vitro	HSR at different location to MTX^R HSR (see Sect. B.II.5.c); banding	In vitro. Other details not given	Reduced drug uptake. Cross-R to DNR, actinomycin D, etc. Suggests membrane mutant	BIEDLER et al. (1980c)
	Vinblastine	Ehrlich ascites mouse (EHR 2)	WT near tet. with two markers; R hyperdip with three different markers; banding	In vivo. Approx. 25 weeks treatment	Cross-R to ADM, DNR and VCR	HASHOLT and DANØ (1974)

Table 1 (continued)

Class of drug	Drug	Cell type	Chromosome observations	Derivation of resistant cells	Comments	References
Miscel-laneous	Asparaginase	Mouse leukaemia (EARAD1) in vivo	WT and R tumours studied for eight passages in vivo; modal no. 39 in WT and R; a marker chr. in a higher propn. of WT than R cells; no banding	In vivo. Repeat passages in mice treated with suboptimal doses	Asparagine synthetase higher in R tumour	Banerjee and Banerjee (1972)
	6-Diazo-5-oxo-L-nor-leucine (DONV)	Mouse mast cell tumour (P815)	WT mode 40–41; R1, mode 40, two markers; R2 mode 40–41, no diff. markers to WT; no banding	Not given. Two R lines produced	Markers not causally related to R since only present in one R line	Hauschka (1958)
	Cortisone	Mouse lymphosarcoma (P1798) in vivo	WT, 89% cells near tet. (about 28 chr). R, 88.6% near diploid, mode 41	In vivo. Intermittent treatment (six times). Stable R in absence of cortisone		Hauschka (1958)

chr, chromosome; R, resistant; sim, similar; subtelo, subtelocentric; telo, telocentric; tet, tetraploid; tr, treatment confluent or non-cycling phase as wild-type cells. Such a difference will inevitably lead to different selection pressures on treated and control populations which may be reflected in the chromosome constitution.

Many chromosome comparisons between wild-type and drug-resistant cells have been made at long intervals, sometimes many years after the original isolation of the drug-resistant line. Any specific chromosome changes initially associated with resistance may well, by this time, be obscured by subsequent evolution of the karyotype.

In view of the above and other considerations, a second requirement of studies which claim to show specific chromosome changes associated with the development of drug resistance is that such changes must be observed consistently in repeated studies. This is particularly important in cases where antitumour drugs are known to *induce* chromosome changes which are not lethal to the cells (Table 5) since in these circumstances there is a high probability that chromosome changes in resistant cells will not be causally related to the resistant phenotype.

A third requirement is for the use of chromosome-banding techniques which allow for greater resolution of the chromosome constitution. Their usefulness has been particularly well demonstrated in the case of antifolate resistance (Sect. B.II.3).

The fourth and most stringent requirement is for biochemical differences related to drug susceptibility, between wild-type and drug-resistant cells, to be consistently associated with specific chromosome differences.

II. Resistance to Various Classes of Antitumour Drugs

In considering the association, if any, of chromosome changes with the acquisition of resistance to different classes of drug, I will begin with those agents for which there is most information available on the biochemical basis of resistance and progress to those for which there is less information.

1. Purine Analogues

The only commonly used purine analogue for which there is any detailed information relating cytogenetic changes with drug resistance is 6-thioguanine (6-TG) and this information derives from in vitro studies in which 6-TG has been used as a selective agent in somatic-cell genetics.

6-TG is lethal to cells by virtue of its incorporation, via the purine salvage pathway, into DNA, a process which involves the enzyme hypoxanthine-guanine phosphoribosyl transferase (HPRT) (see Caskey and Kruh 1979). The HPRT locus is located on the X chromosome in mammals and is therefore in the hemizygous condition in both normal male (XY) and female (XX) cells, in the latter because of the inactivation of one of the two X chromosomes.

It has been recognised that there is a considerable diversity in 6-TG-resistant phenotypes (see Fox and Radacic 1978) and the relationship between chromosome constitution and resistance is different for the different classes of resistant phenotype.

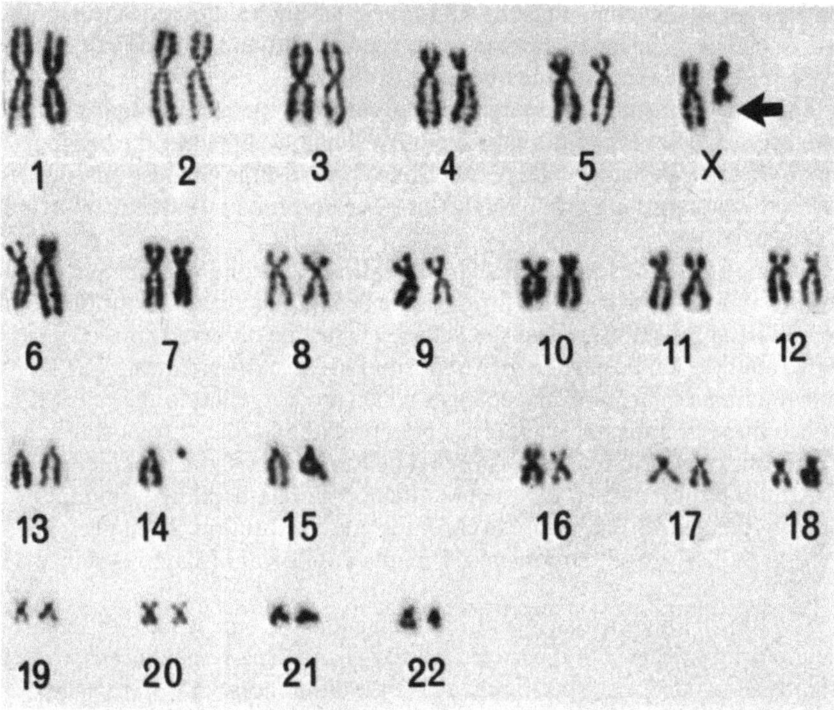

Fig. 1. G-banded karyotoype of a 6-TG-resistant human fibroblast clone induced by ionising radiation. The cell shows a deletion of the long arm of an X chromosome where the HPRT locus is located. A translocation involving chromosomes 6 and 14 is also present (Cox and Masson 1979; courtesy authors and Taylor and Francis, London)

a) Stable 6-Thioguanine-Resistant Cell Lines

The best understood class are those derived by a single exposure to a high dose of 6-TG. These have generally been regarded as true gene mutants ($HPRT^+ \rightarrow HPRT^-$) and are characterised by little or no HPRT activity, stable resistance in the absence of the drug and low reversion freqency (to $HPRT^+$) (Fox and Radacic 1978). However, Cox and Masson (1978) have now shown that up to 40% of such "mutants" induced by ionising radiation in human fibroblasts involve visible deletions (Fig. 1) or rearrangements (Fig. 2) affecting the terminal region of the long arm of the X chromosome where the HPRT locus is located (J. A. Brown et al. 1976).

Cox and Mason argue that the 6-TG resistance of deletion mutants probably arises from complete loss of the HPRT gene whereas loss of HPRT in the exchange mutants could result from gene inactivation as a consequence of "position effect" (Baker 1968) or loss of the gene during the exchange process. Two out of 25 HPRT-deficient mutants in human fibroblasts induced by MNNG (*N*-methyl-*N'*-nitro-*n*-nitrosoguanidine) also carried X-chromosome structural changes (Cox 1980) and a proportion of X-ray-induced 6-TG-resistant mutants in Chinese hamster cells also involve X-chromosome changes (Brown and Thacker 1980; Thacker 1981, Fig. 3). Both MNNG (Kelly and Legator 1970)

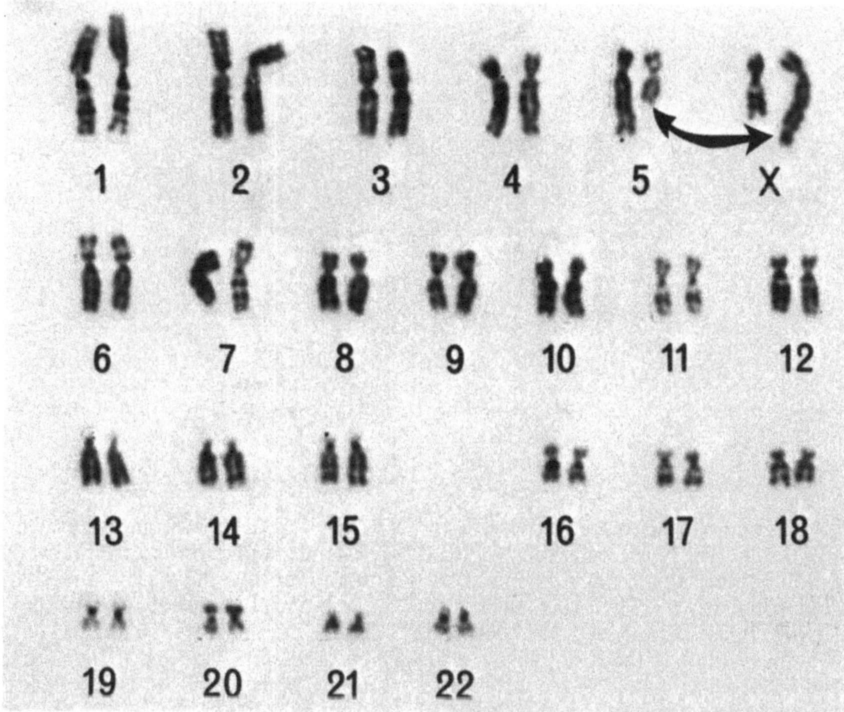

Fig. 2. Legend as for Fig. 1, except that cell shows translocation between long arm of an X chromosome and a chromosome 5

and ionising radiation (EVANS 1962) are known to be potent inducers of chromosome structural change.

The proportion of spontaneous stable 6-TG-resistant mutants which are manifested at the chromosome level is not yet clear since many cytogenetic studies of 6-TG resistance have been performed without banding techniques and/or before the location of the HPRT gene on the X chromosome was known.

It has been shown that cells with more than one active X chromosome mutate less readily to 6-TG resistance than cells with only one active X. This is true of both spontaneous (MORROW et al. 1978) and induced (CHASIN and URLAUB 1975; RASKIND and GARTLER 1978; MORRY and TS'O 1980) mutation and is attributable to the recessive nature of the $HPRT^-$ mutation. Such mutants probably arise by a combination of gene mutation and X-chromosome loss (see MORRY and TS'O 1980).

b) Unstable 6-Thioguanine-Resistant Cell Lines

Another class of 6-TG-resistant mammalian cells can be generated by low-dose treatment over long periods. Such cells have reduced HPRT activity but are unstable in the absence of the drug and their level of resistance declines. TERZI (1974) has shown that this type of resistance is associated with instability of the karyotype in Chinese hamster cells and argues that in chromosomally heterogeneous

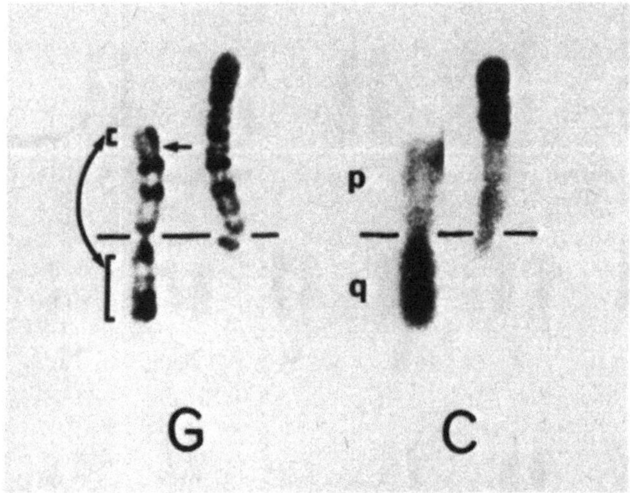

Fig. 3. G- and C-banded X chromosomes of WT (*left*) and 6-TG resistant (*right*) Chinese hamster cells. The X chromosome of the 6-TG-resistant cell line shows a reciprocal translocation between the terminal region of the p arm and most of the q arm (see G-banded chromosome of WT). This brings the heterochromatin (darkly stained with C-banding) of the q arm in association with the euchromatin (lightly staining with C-banding) of the p arm at the position of the HPRT locus (*arrow*) giving a possible "position effect" (see text). (Modified from THACKER 1981; courtesy author and S. Karger AG, Basel, Switzerland)

populations the genes determining drug sensitivity may be represented in different numbers, or "doses", in different cells. In the case of 6-TG resistance, cells with a low dose of HPRT genes (e.g. one copy) would be expected to survive better than those with multiple copies which, on average, would tend to favour cells with low chromosome numbers. However, clones of cells isolated by TERZI after a low dose of 6-TG did not consistently have lower chromosome numbers than wild-type cells.

c) The Prediction of 6-Thioguanine Resistance

The foregoing information suggests the potential usefulness of X-chromosome identification in predicting 6-TG resistance of malignant cells. Increase in numbers of X chromosomes or X-chromosome regions carrying the HPRT locus may well be associated not only with increasing drug sensitivity but with a reduced likelihood of mutation to 6-TG resistance. On the other hand X-chromosome loss (total or partial) or translocation could be a valuable marker of drug resistance. In this connection, it is of interest to note that, of all malignancies investigated, X loss is most frequently associated with acute myeloblastic leukaemia (SANDBERG 1980) against which 6-TG is frequently used.

2. Pyrimidine Analogues

Chromosome studies on cells resistant to pyrimidine analogues in clinical use are limited and have not usually involved parallel biochemical studies or chromosome-banding analyses. A comprehensive study of two 5-fluorodeoxyuridine (FUdR)-resistant lines of Chinese hamster cells was, however, performed by SLACK et al. (1976). They found that both resistant lines had very low thymidine kinase activity, this being the enzyme normally involved in pyrimidine salvage but which can also phosphorylate FUdR to FdUMP (5-fluoro-2′-deoxyuridine 5′-mono-phosphate), which inhibits thymidylate synthetase activity, thus blocking DNA synthesis (Chap. 19).

Unlike the HPRT locus the chromosomal location of the thymidine kinase (TK) locus is not known in Chinese hamster cells but experience with cells exhibiting stable 6-TG resistance (Sect. B.II.1.a) suggests that chromosome studies on FUdR-resistant mutants might reveal the location of this gene, particularly if the cells are hemizygous for this locus (SIMINOVITCH 1976). The modal chromosome number of both FUdR-resistant lines compared with the parent revealed no consistent chromosome differences that could be associated with the resistance. It should be borne in mind, however, that it is only a minority of 6-TG-resistant mutants that are associated with visible chromosome changes so further studies of FUdR-resistant lines would be worthwhile and may be of value in gene mapping.

The TK locus is on the long (q) arm of chromosome 17 in human cells so screening of tumour cells for the number of copies of this chromosome (loss or gain) or for structural changes involving 17 q could be useful, perhaps in conjunction with TK assays, in predicting response to FUdR (see Sect. B.II.1.c).

3. Antifolates

The most exciting recent discovery in the cytogenetics of antitumour drug resistance, which also has much wider implications in cellular genetics, relates to the induction of antifolate resistance by chronic exposure of cells to these drugs. This induced resistance is often accompanied by dramatic and consistent chromosome changes. BIEDLER and SPENGLER (1976) first described a "homogeneously staining region" (HSR) in trypsin-Giemsa-banded karyotypes of several Chinese hamster cell lines (Fig. 4) which had been subjected to increasing concentrations of methotrexate (MTX) or methasquin (a quinazoline antifolate). Cells with this HSR were highly resistant to antifolates and had more than a 100-fold increase in the enzyme dihydrofolate reductase (DHFR) compared with wild-type cells. DHFR catalyses a central step in one-carbon metabolism and is inhibited by antifolate drugs such as MTX. Increasing levels of DHFR, the target enzyme, are associated with increasing MTX resistance. An obvious implication of this observation is that HSRs contain multiple copies of the genes coding for DHFR (see Sect. B.II.3.e).

Since the original cytogenetic observation of BIEDLER and SPENGLER there has been an explosion of interest in this phenomenon, the main aspects of which are considered below:

a) HSRs in Different Cell Types

HSRs have now been observed in different Chinese hamster cell lines and in cultured mouse cells of tumour or non-tumour origin after exposure to a stepwise increase in MTX concentration (Table 1, Figs. 4–10, 12, 14).

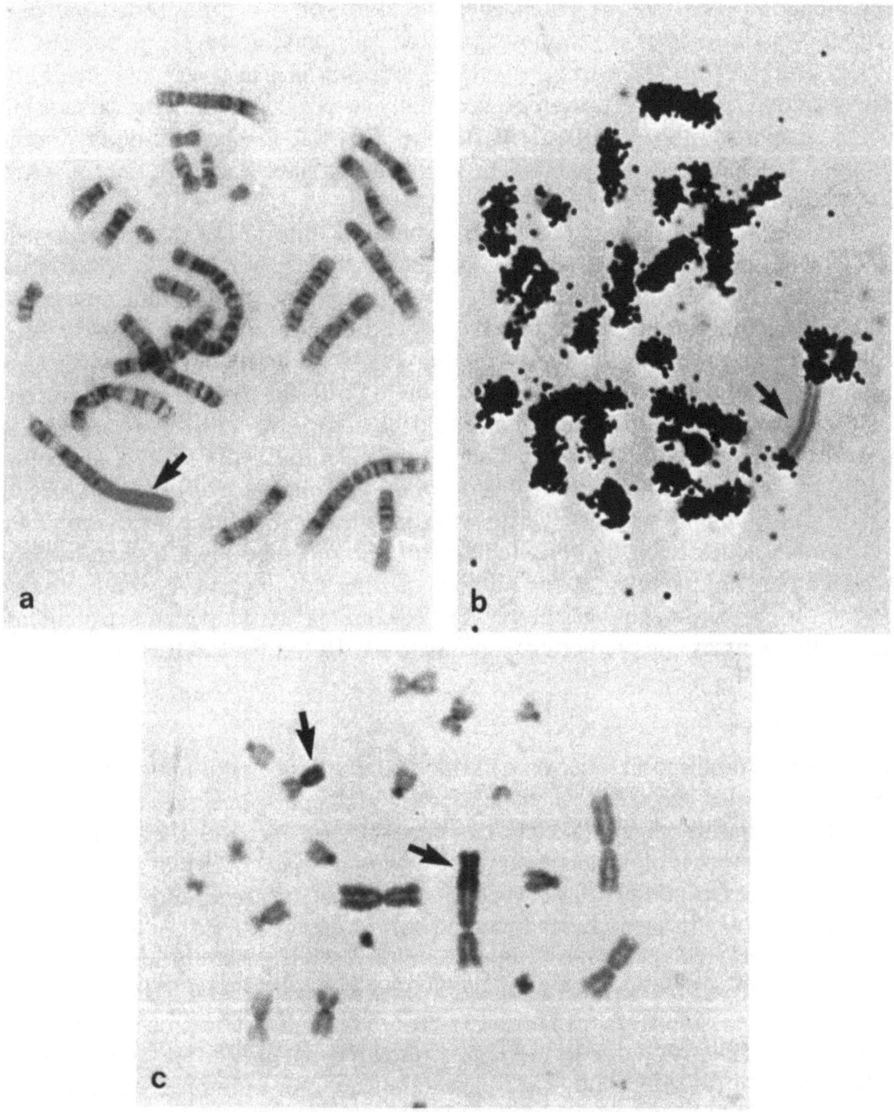

Fig. 4. a–c. HSRs in antifolate-resistant Chinese hamster cells. **a** HSR on chromosome 2. Cells have 170-fold increase in DHFR (see BIEDLER et al. 1980 a). **b** Unlabelled HSR in cell treated with tritiated thymidine during third quarter of the S-phase. **c** HSR of chromosome 2 after C-banding (*centre arrow*). Long arm of an X chromosome (*arrow*) also C-banded. (BIEDLER and SPENGLER 1976; courtesy authors and copyright, 1981, by the American Association for the Advancement of Science)

b) Number, Size, and Location of HSRs

There is usually only one HSR per cell but BOSTOCK et al. (1979) have generated several MTX-resistant mouse melanoma lines with four or five large marker chromosomes with extensive HSR regions (Fig. 5). These cells contain up to 1,000 times the level of DHFR activity of the parental line.

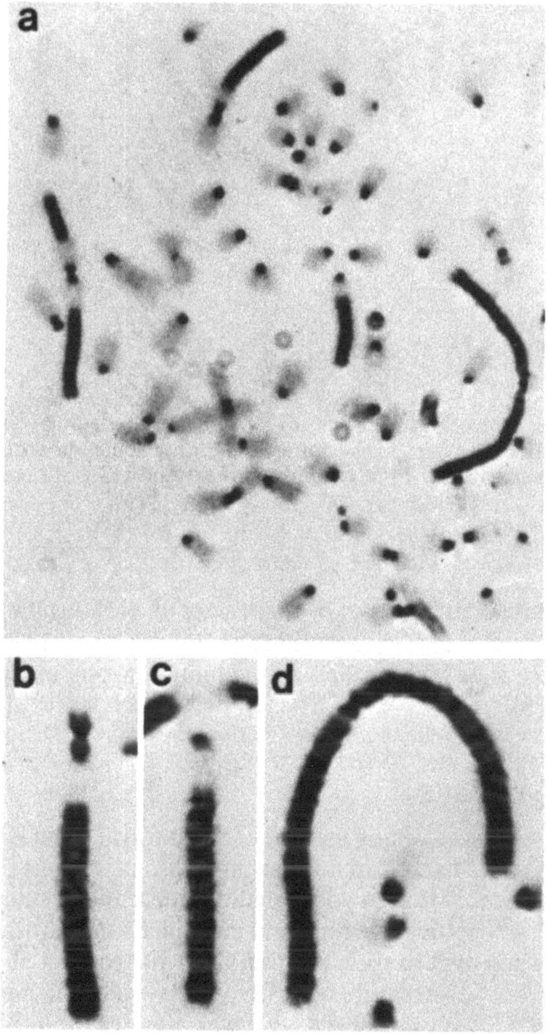

Fig. 5. a–d. C-banded chromosomes of methotrexate-resistant mouse melanoma cells. **a** Complete metaphase spread showing dense staining of centromeric heterochromatin of normal and marker chromosomes and dense staining of HSRs of four marker chromosomes. **b** Marker chromosome R3. **c** Marker chromosome R5. **d** Marker chromosome R1. (BOSTOCK and CLARK 1980; courtesy authors and MIT Press, Bedford, England)

In an MTX-resistant line of Chinese hamster (CHO) cells (NUNBERG et al. 1978) and in an MTX-resistant L5178Y mouse lymphoma line (DOLNICK et al. 1979) there is a single HSR located, in both cases, interstitially on a chromosome number 2 (Fig. 6, 7). Although a single HSR is characteristic of the antifolate-resistant Chinese hamster (DC-3F) cell lines of BIEDLER and colleagues its location is not consistent in all lines; there is a preferential localisation to chromosome 2, usually terminally, but in one line the HSR is terminal on a chromosome 4 and, in another, on an X chromosome (Table 2; BIEDLER et al. 1980 a).

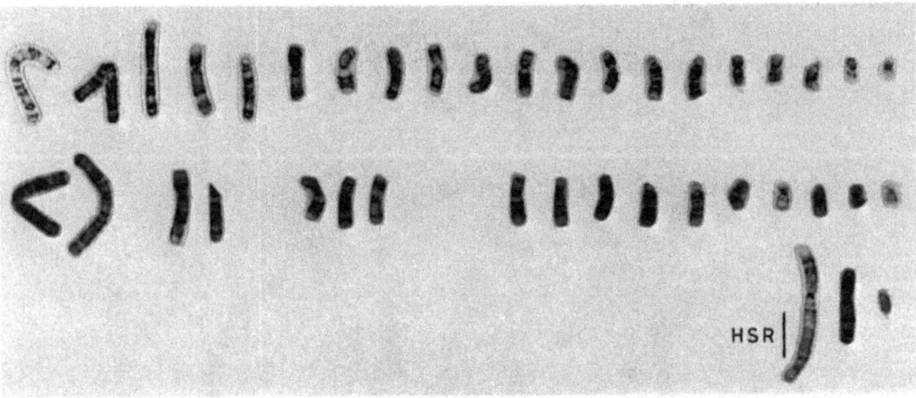

Fig. 6. Karyotypes of methotrexate-sensitive (*top*) and -resistant (*middle and bottom*) Chinese hamster cells. The *bottom row* shows the chromosome abnormalities in the resistant cell line. (Nunberg et al. 1978; courtesy authors and US National Academy of Sciences)

In the antifolate-resistant lines of Biedler et al. (1980a) the HSRs comprise 2%–5% of the length of the metaphase chromosome complement (Table 2) whereas this value is as high as 20% in the mouse melanoma lines of Bostock et al. (1979) (Fig. 5).

c) HSR-Staining Properties

With the trypsin/Giemsa staining method of Seabright (1972) HSRs do not have the cross-striations or "bands" of normal chromosome regions (Figs. 4–7). Biedler et al. (1980a) report that in good quality preparations subjected to this G-banding technique "very narrow, faint and indistinct bands are discernible within the HSR and are constant in their location" and Bostock et al. (1979) have occasionally seen some substructure of HSRs which "gives the impression of a repeating structure".

Using a C-banding technique (Hsu and Arrighi 1971), Biedler and Spengler (1976) found that the HSR in Chinese hamster cells stained intensely, to the same extent as the heterochromatin of the X chromosome (Fig. 4c). Bostock et al. (1979) and Bostock and Clark (1980) also found that HSRs in their MTX-resistant melanoma cells stain intensely (Fig. 5) and fluoresce brightly (Fig. 8) with a C-banding technique (Sumner 1972) and with Hoechst 33258 stain (Latt 1973), respectively, these being characteristic staining properties of centromeric regions of normal mouse chromosomes where highly repetitious "satellite" DNA is located (Jones 1970). The HSRs of these melanoma cells are, in fact, not homogeneously stained but consist of many fine C-bands linked closely together (Fig. 5). If cells which have incorporated bromodeoxyuridine (BrdUrd) into their DNA during one S-phase are stained by the fluorescence plus Giemsa (FPG) staining technique (Perry and Wolff 1974) then those chromosome regions which normally are intensely stained by C-banding show asymmetrical staining

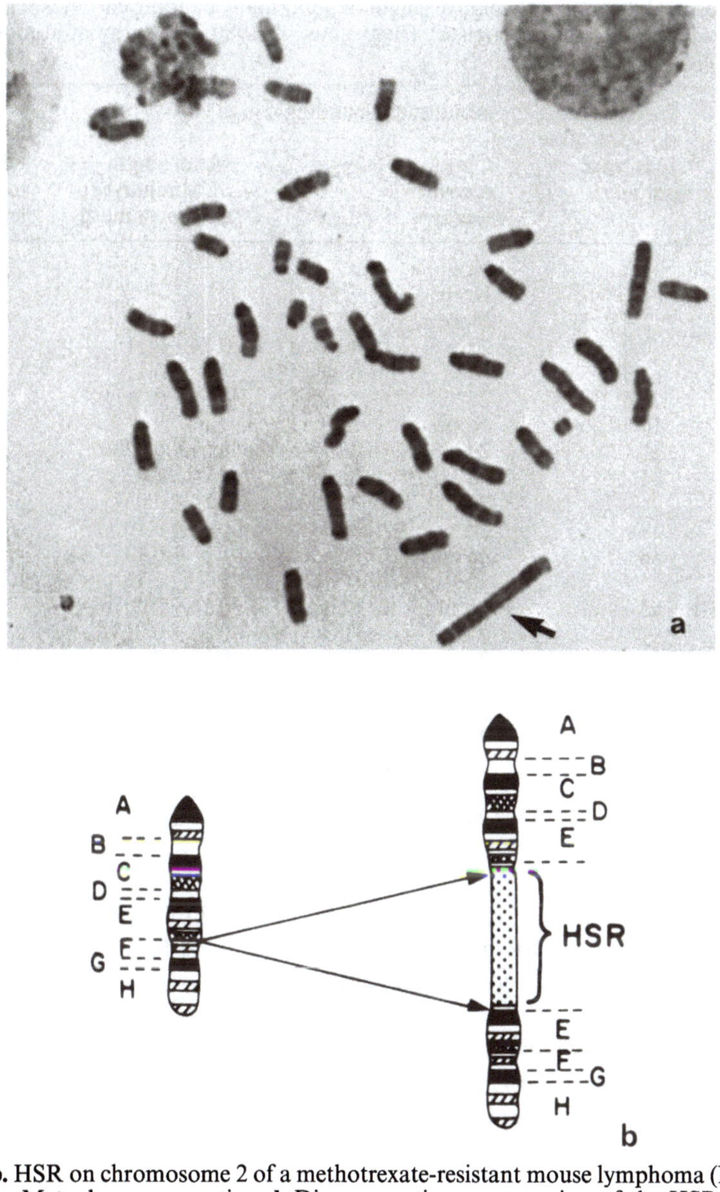

Fig. 7 a, b. HSR on chromosome 2 of a methotrexate-resistant mouse lymphoma (L5178Y) cell line. **a** Metaphase preparation. **b** Diagrammatic representation of the HSR; normal homologue on *left*, homologue with HSR on *right*. (DOLNICK et al. 1979; courtesy authors and Rockefeller University Press, NY)

(see BOSTOCK and CHRISTIE 1976). This is thought to be because these C-banding regions contain "satellite" DNA with a bias in the distribution of thymidine between complementary DNA strands. When BOSTOCK and CLARK (1980) used this procedure on their MTX-resistant cells they found complex asymmetries within HSR regions (Fig. 9) and additional evidence for the presence of satellite DNA

Table 2. Chromosomal location and relative length of abnormally banding chromosome regions in antifolate-resistant cell lines of chinese hamster. (BIEDLER et al. 1980a; courtesy of authors and Elsevier-North Holland, New York)

Cell line	Increase in dihydrofolate reductase activity	Abnormally banding region			
		Chromosomal location	Type	Mean length ± SEM relative to chromosome 2p	Percent ± SEM of total chromosome length per cell
DC-3F	1	None			
DC-3F8	1	None			
DC-3F/A XXI	1.4	None			
DC-3F/MQ10	2.9	2q	Banded	0.74 ± 0.11	
DC-3F/MQ31	3.9	2q	Banded	2.2 ± 0.11	
DC-3F8/A55	4.6	2q	Banded	0.62 ± 0.011	
DC-3F8/A50	10	None			
DC-3F/A1	21	2q	Banded	0.61 ± 0.028	
DC-3F8/A40	35	4q or	Banded	0.74 ± 0.023	
		9p	Banded	0.54 ± 0.057	
DC-3F/MQ20	49	2q	Banded	2.0 ± 0.10	
DC-3F/MQ21	86	9p or	Banded	1.3 ± 0.13	
		2q	HSR	1.3 ± 0.16	4.7 ± 0.58
DC-3F/A XXVIII	95	9q and	Banded	0.16 ± 0.0076	
		Xp	HSR	0.51 ± 0.015	2.2 ± 0.030
DC-3F8/A75	121	2q	HSR	0.79 ± 0.018	3.4 ± 0.093
DC-3F/MQ29	122	4q	HSR	1.3 ± 0.046	4.8 ± 0.17
DC-3F/MQ25	129	2q	HSR	0.71 ± 0.022	2.8 ± 0.11
DC-3F/MQ8	144	2q	HSR	0.92 ± 0.074	4.7 ± 0.44
DC-3F/MQ19	151	2q	HSR	1.1 ± 0.029	4.9 ± 0.23
DC-3F/A3	170	2q	HSR	0.97 ± 0.025	3.9 ± 0.11
DC-3F/Ab-17	281	2q	HSR	1.0 ± 0.029	4.3 ± 0.17

within HSRs. It is not yet clear whether the satellite DNA plays a positive role in amplification of DHFR genes or has been amplified fortuitously along with these genes in the acquisition of MTX resistance.

d) DNA Synthesis in HSRs

BIEDLER and SPENGLER (1976) have shown that the HSR in their MTX-resistant Chinese hamster cells completes DNA replication rapidly during the first half of the S-phase (Fig. 4b).

e) Gene Amplification Demonstrated Cytogenetically

The formal demonstration that HSRs do indeed contain multiple copies of DHFR genes has been made by in situ molecular hybridisation of tritiated DNA which is complementary to the mRNA of DHFR. Specific clustering of grains over HSRs is seen in autoradiographs (DOLNICK et al. 1979; NUNBERG et al. 1978; Fig. 10).

f) Formation of HSRs

BOSTOCK et al. (1979) made a detailed study of the karyotype changes occurring during the acquisition of MTX resistance in mouse melanoma cells. There is an

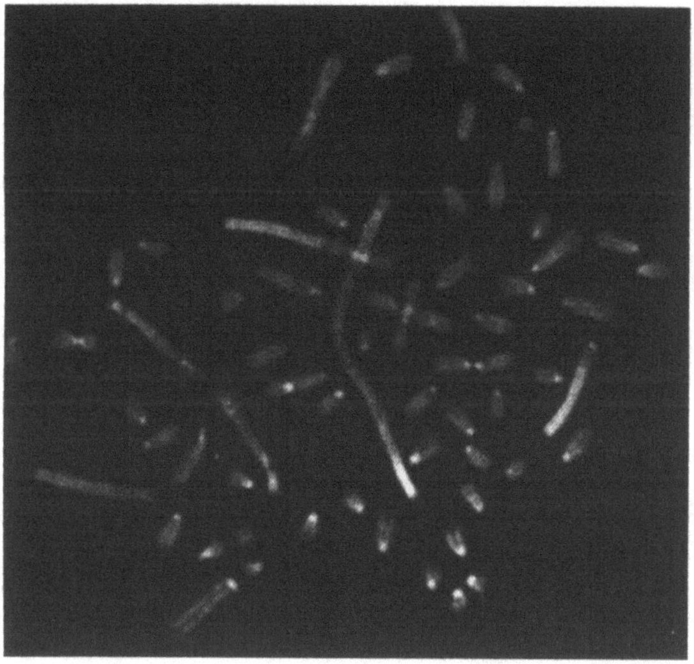

Fig. 8. Fluorescence of HSRs in a methotrexate-resistant mouse melanoma cell stained with Hoechst 33258 stain. (BOSTOCK et al. 1979; courtesy authors and Springer-Verlag, Heidelberg)

initial increase in chromosome length, the formation of ring chromosomes and an increase in the size of HSRs and the number of HSR-containing chromosomes. The observations suggest that the five marker chromosomes (Fig. 5) are derived from a common precursor chromosome as a result of exchange and duplication events. The FPG-staining technique (Fig. 9) demonstrates repetitive units within the HSRs, suggesting sequential duplication.

The formation of HSRs may not be entirely dependent on the selection of spontaneously occurring exchange/duplication events since MTX has been found to *induce* not only chromosomal breaks which may be cell lethal (Table 5) but a significant frequency of chromosomal exchanges (STEVENSON 1978; JENSEN and NYFORS 1979) some of which may be compatible with continued cell viability. This observation also provides a possible explanation for the occurrence in MTX-resistant cells of chromosome changes other than those associated with increased DHFR (e.g. NUNBERG et al. 1978; Fig. 6).

g) Stability of HSRs

BIEDLER et al. (1980a) have made detailed studies of HSR size, extent of antifolate resistance and DHFR activity in two cloned antifolate-resistant Chinese hamster lines after removal from selective medium. A progressive reduction in all these end points was observed over a period of several months (Table 3). In contrast, BOSTOCK et al. (1979) observed no decrease in DHFR levels, and therefore presumably no decrease in size of HSRs in their MTX-resistant mouse melanoma

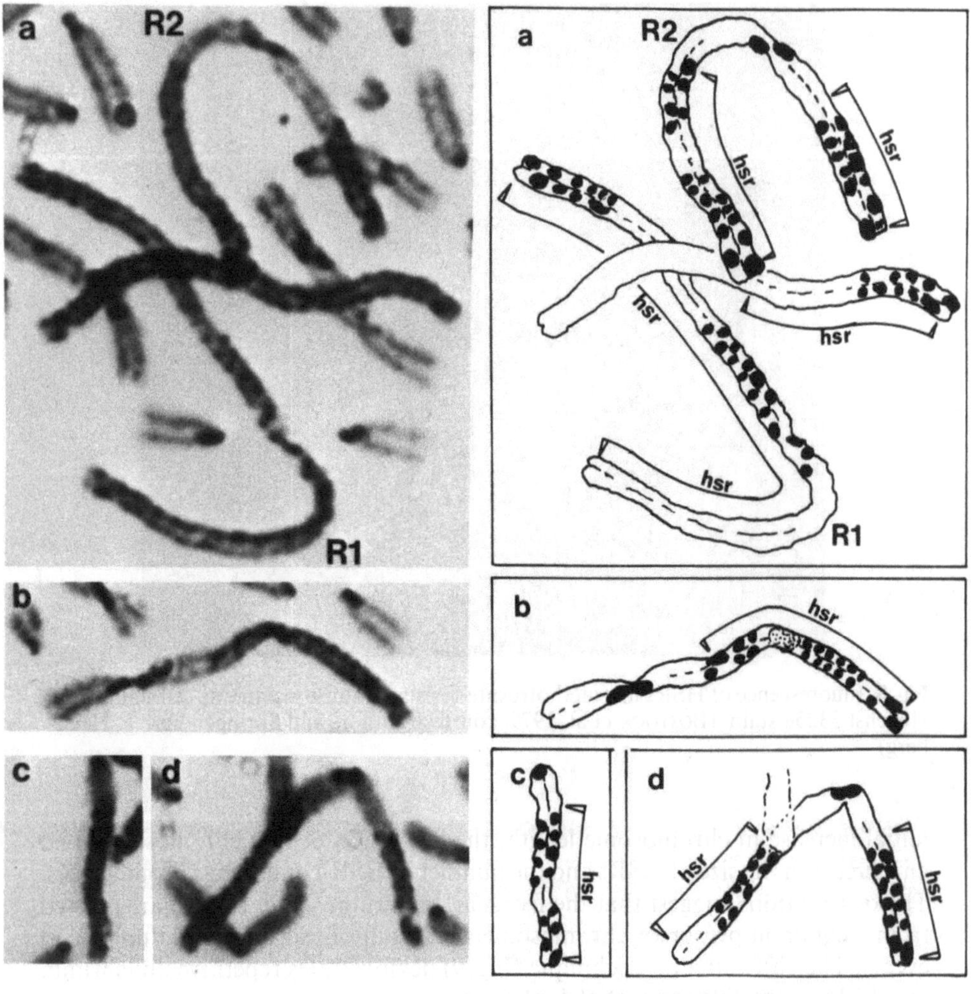

Fig. 9 a–d. Asymmetry in HSRs of marker chromosomes of methotrexate-resistant mouse melanoma cells after BrdUdr treatment and FPG staining (Sect. B.II.3.c). **a** Marker chromosomes R1, R2, and R4. **b** Marker chromosome R3. **c** Marker chromosome R5. **d** Marker chromosome R2. On the *right* are diagrams showing the principal areas of asymmetrical staining. (Bostock and Clark 1980; courtesy authors and MIT Press, Bedford, England)

cells over a period of 150 days after removal from MTX. They suggest that the predominantly interstitial location of HSRs in their cells may confer more stability on these regions than a terminal location as in Chinese hamster cells.

h) Double Minute Chromosomes

Kaufman et al. (1979) have found small paired chromosomal elements, called "double minutes" (Fig. 11), in MTX-resistant cell lines which lose their resistance when MTX is removed, i.e. are unstable. They present convincing evidence that

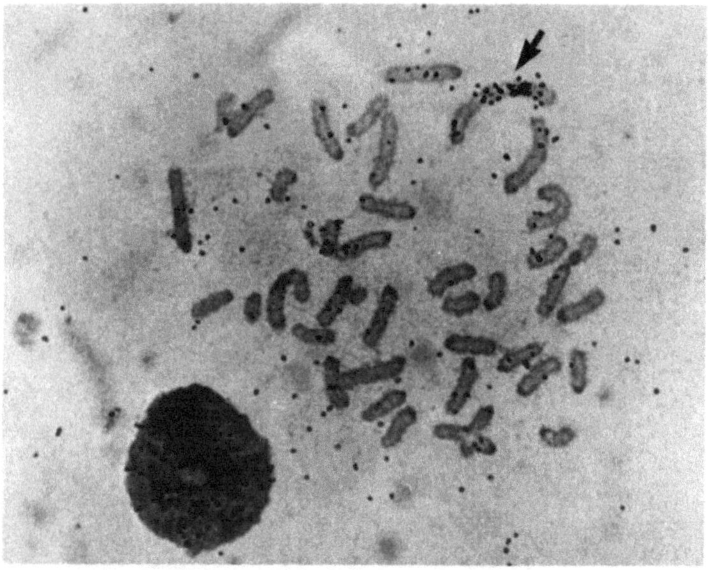

Fig. 10. In situ molecular hybridization of a methotrexate-resistant mouse lymphoma cell. A tritiated DNA probe complementary to DHFR-specific RNA hybridises exclusively at the HSR on chromosome 2 (*arrow*, see Fig. 7). (Acknowledgements as for Fig. 7)

Table 3. Drug resistance, dihydrofolate reductase and HSR length characteristics of revertant Chinese hamster clones grown in antifolate-free medium. (Biedler et al. 1980 a; courtesy of authors and Elsevier-North Holland, New York)

Clone	Number of weeks in drug-free medium	Relative resistance to selective agent	Relative dihydrofolate reductase activity	Length of HSR relative to chromosome arm (%)	Apparent molecular weight of dihydrofolate reductase
MQ19-D-U	2	1,700	157	50.3	20,000
	7	233	64		
	12			24.0	
	22	27	21		
	39	6	10		
	43			7.2	
	92	6	11		
	101				20,000
A2-P-U	2	254,000	222	61.9	21,000
	7	254,000	244		
	11			58.2	
	31	46,300		39.2	
	33		95		
	70	284	23	6.3	
	91	179	18	0	21,000
	100				

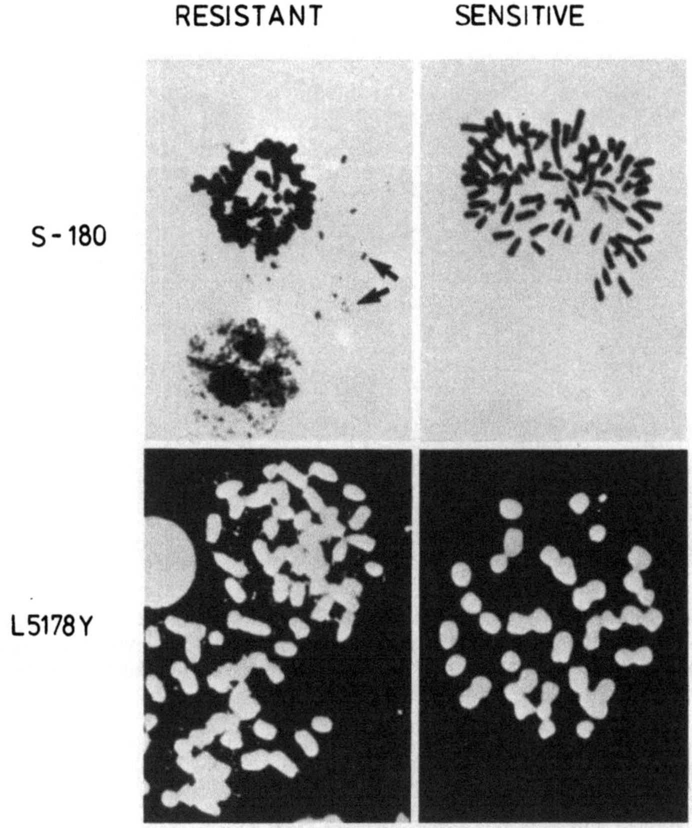

Fig. 11. Double minutes (*arrowed*) in unstably methotrexate-resistant cells compared with sensitive parental cells. S-180 mouse cells prepared without Colcemid or hypotonic treatment. L5178Y mouse lymphoma cells after Colcemid prefixation treatment and ethidium bromide staining. (KAUFMAN et al. 1979; courtesy authors and the US National Academy of Sciences)

amplified DHFR DNA sequences are associated with these double minutes (DMs). The higher frequency of DMs in unstable MTX-resistant cells as opposed to stable or parental cells is shown in Table 4. DMs appear during the development of unstable resistance, may reach over 300/cell and are lost as the MTX resistance of cells declines in the absence of the drug. Since DMs do not aggregate on the mitotic spindle it is likely that the segregation between daughter cells at mitosis is unequal, resulting in heterogeneity of DM numbers between cells. KAUFMAN et al. (1979) have observed a faster growth rate of cells with least numbers of DMs in MTX-free medium which would account for the progresive loss of DMs.

The origin of DMs and their possible relationship with HSRs is unknown, but various suggestions have been made. KAUFMAN et al. (1979) have suggested that DMs may represent the incorporation of DNA from lysed cells followed by selective replication, in the presence of MTX, of DNA which contains DHFR se-

Table 4. Unstable MTX-resistant murine cell lines contain minute chromosomes. (KAUFMAN et al. 1979; courtesy of authors and US National Academy of Sciences)

Cell line	DHFR gene copy no. relative to sensitive	Double minutes (mean ± SD)	Mean chromosome no.
S-180:			
Stably resistant (R_1C)	60	5.5 ± 2.8	77
Unstably resistant (R_1A)	70	26 ± 35	68
Unstably resistant (R_2)	50	22 ± 17	83
Parental sensitive (S_3)	1	1 ± 0.8	74
L5178Y:			
Stably resistant	400	0.1 ± 0.3	40
Unstably resistant	ND	41 ± 33	49
Parental sensitive	1	1.3 ± 1.4	42
3T6:			
Unstably resistant	35	59 ± 23	75
Parental sensitive	1	3 ± 3.0	82
CHO:			
Stably resistant	150	0.5 ± 1.4	20

ND, not determined

quences. As an alternative, DMs may be derived from unstable HSRs (SCHIMKE et al. 1979). BIEDLER et al. (1980b) have suggested that the DHFR gene, possibly with associated DNA sequences, may be excised and amplified extrachromosomally as DMs and then reinserted as HSRs, usually but not always, in the place of origin. The ability of MTX to induce chromosome breakage and reunion (Sect. B.II.3.f and Table 5) may assist in these processes.

i) Abnormal Band Patterns

BIEDLER and SPENGLER (1976) reported that HSRs are only found in antifolate-resistant cells if the DHFR level increases by more than 100-fold. Recently, however, BIEDLER et al. (1980a) have observed "abnormal banding patterns" in antifolate-resistant Chinese hamster lines in which DHFR levels are between 2.9 and 95 times the level in wild-type cells (Figs. 13, 14; Table 2). Some part of each of these abnormally banding regions has alternating dark and medium-dark bands. As with HSRs, these abnormal banding regions are preferentially but not exclusively localised to the long arm of chromosome number 2.

This recent observation suggests that it may be worthwhile examining banded chromosomes of patients who have received MTX therapy because BERTINO et al. (1963) have reported 5- to 25-fold increases in DHFR in cells of such patients. Cytogenetic studies of the malignant cells of such patients may provide an indication of acquired drug resistance.

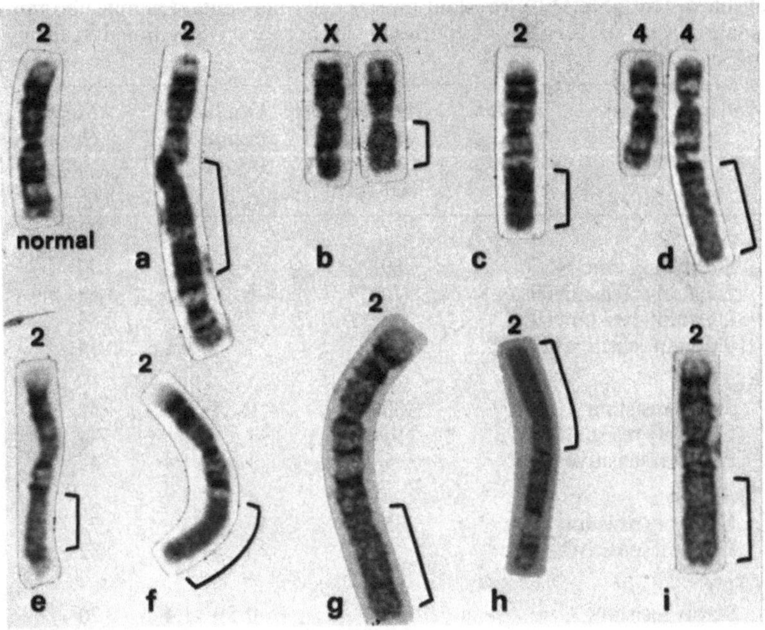

Fig. 12. Examples of HSR-bearing chromosomes in Chinese hamster sublines with high dihydrofolate reductase levels. Chromosomes are arranged in order of increasing enzyme activity of sublines (Table 2). HSR is demarcated by a *bracket*. *a*, DC-3F/MQ21; *b*, DC-3F/A XXVIII (normal X chromosome is *on left*); *c*, DC-3F8/A75; *d*, DC-3F/MQ29 (normal 4 is shown for comparison); *e*, DC-3F/MQ25; *f*, DC-3F/MQ8; *g* DC-3F/MQ19; *h* DC-3F/A3; *i*, DC-3F/Ab-17. (BIEDLER et al. 1980a; but see *Erratum, Cancer Genetics and Cytogenetics* 2: 381, 1980; courtesy authors and Elsevier/North Holland, New York)

4. Alkylating Agents

These agents are cell lethal by virtue of their direct interaction with DNA (Chap. 15). Resistance to alkylating agents is usually associated with decreased drug uptake or increased repair of damage to the DNA (Chap. 12). The biochemistry of these processes and the identification of enzymes involved in the determination of resistance is less well understood than in the case of resistance to purine/pyrimidine analogues or antifolates. The chromosomal location of the genes involved is not known and has not been revealed by comparative cytogenetic studies of wild-type and resistant cells which normally have different chromosome constitutions but, in general, with no clear specificity or consistency (Table 1).

If specific chromosome changes are sometimes present in alkylating agent-resistant cells, as we have seen in other cases of drug resistance, they are likely to be less easily recognised because of the high frequency of non-specific chromosome changes which alkylating agents are known to induce (Table 5). The best example of specificity of chromosome change associated with the development of resistance to an alkylating agent is presented by UJHAZY (1974), who found the

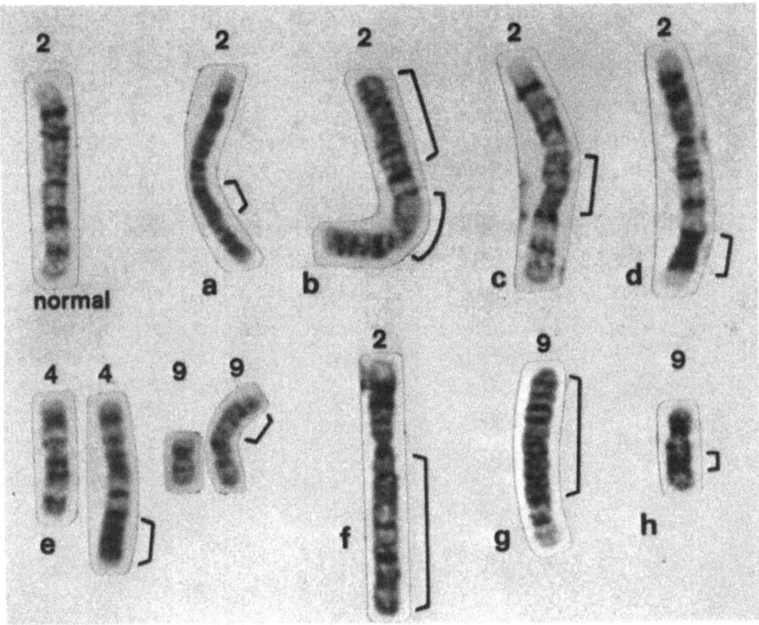

Fig. 13. Examples of chromosomes with specific, abnormally banding regions in Chinese hamster sublines with 3- to 86 fold increases in dihydrofolate reductase activity. Abnormal region is demarcated by a *bracket*. *a*, DC-3F/MQ10; *b*, DC-3F/MQ31; *c*, DC-3F/A55; *d*, DC-3F/A1; *e*, DC-3F8/A40 (normal homologue is *on left*); *f*, DC-3F/MQ20; *g*, DC-3F/MQ21; *h*, DC-3F/A XXVIII. (Acknowledgements as for Fig. 12)

same large subtelocentric marker chromosome, not present in the parental line, in three independently derived tris-(chlorethyl)-amine hydrochloride (HN3)-resistant lines of the Yoshida sarcoma of the rat. Banding studies did not reveal any obvious HSR in this chromosome.

A clear example of differential sensitivity to alkylating agents which is associated with gene mutation and not with visible karyotype differences is seen in the case of individuals with the autosomal recessive disease Fanconi's anaemia. Cells from such individuals are highly sensitive to cross-linking alkylating agents (Sasaki 1978) by virtue of a defect in DNA repair (Chap. 12) but have a normal chromosome constitution.

5. Platinum Compounds

The *cis*-platinum compounds are believed to be cell-lethal by virtue of their ability to cross-link DNA (Chap. 12). Resistance of these agents has been shown to be associated with increased ability of cells to tolerate, in their DNA, the presence of platinum-induced lesions which produce a block to DNA synthesis in sensitive cells (Chap. 12). The genes/enzymes involved in the determination of resistance are not known.

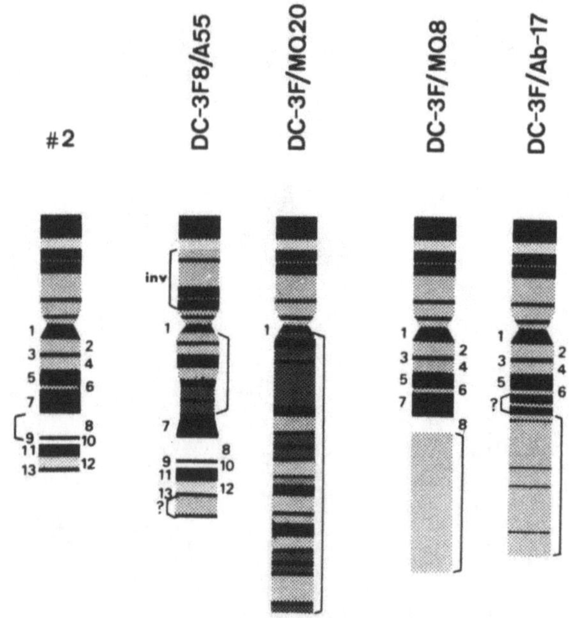

Fig. 14. Diagrammatic representation of the G-band pattern of normal Chinese hamster chromosome #2 and abnormal #2 chromosomes of several antifolate-resistant sublines. A normal chromosome #2 is depicted *on left*. Only normal bands of the q arm are numbered. Abnormally banding regions are demarcated by *brackets to the right of each chromosome*. Examples of the two types of specifically altered regions are shown: DC-3F8/A55 and DC-3F/MQ20 have strongly banded segments with an abnormal band pattern; DC-3F/MQ8 and DC-3F/Ab-17 have HSRs. (Acknowledgements as for Fig. 12)

SZUMIEL (1979a) studied a pair of mouse lymphoma cell lines with a differential sensitivity to *cis*-dichlorobis (cyclopentylamine) platinum (II) (*cis*-PAD), the resistant line having arisen spontaneously from the wild-type line. Wild-type cells were chromosomally unstable and prone to changes in ploidy. No difference in sensitivity to *cis*-PAD was observed between near tetraploid and near-diploid derivatives of the parental line. The model chromosome number of the near-diploid parental line (mode = 40) was higher than that of the resistant line (mode = 39) but changes in chromosome number in the resistant line did not appear to influence the response to *cis*-PAD.

6. Antibiotics

The modes of action and mechanisms of resistance vary with the different antitumour antibiotics but in most cases the biochemical basis of resistance is not clearly understood. In general the chromosome constitutions of antibiotic-resistant cells, selected by chronic exposure of wild-type cells to the drug, are different to the parental line (Table 1), possibly because the antibiotics can induce chromosome changes (Table 5), but specific chromosome changes which can be directly related to the acquisition of resistance are lacking. The most suggestive

Table 5. Antitumour drugs which produce chromosome changes

Class of drug	Drug	Cells treated	Chromosome changes	Reference
Purine analogues	6-Mercaptopurine	Human lymphocytes in vivo	Structural and numerical (polyploidy)	NASJLETI and SPENCER (1966)
Pyrimidine analogues	5-Fluorouracil	Human colonic tumour xenograft	Structural	SOKOVA and VOLGAREVA (1977)
	Cytosine arabinoside	Normal and leukaemic bone marrow cells of man in vivo	Structural	BELL et al. (1966) BENEDICT and JONES (1979) review
Antifolates	Methotrexate	Human bone marrow in vivo	Structural	JENSEN and NYFORS (1979)
		Early embryos of mouse	Structural and numerical	HANSMANN (1973)
Alkylating agents	Nitrogen mustard	Human lymphocytes in vivo	Structural and numerical	FOX and SCOTT (1980) review
	Melphalan	Human lymphocytes in vivo	Structural	SHARPE (1971)
	Cyclophos-phamide	Human lymphocytes in vivo	Structural and numerical (polyploidy)	MOHN and ELLENBERGER (1976) review
		Mouse germ cells in vivo	Non-lethal structural Numerical	MOHN and ELLENBERGER (1976) review
	Thio-tepa	Human lymphocytes in vivo	Structural	SELEZNEVA and KORMAN (1973)
		Mouse germ cells in vivo	Non-lethal structural	GENEROSO et al. (1980) review
	Chlorambucil	Human lymophyctes in vivo	Structural	DOBOS et al. (1977)
	Busulphan	Human lymphocytes in vivo	Structural	GEBHART et al. (1974) HONEYCOMBE (1981)
	1,3-Bis(2-chloro-ethyl)-1-nitro-sourea (BCNU)	Human lymphocytes in vitro	Structural	HARROD and CORTNER (1968)
	1-(2-Chloroethyl)-3-cyclohexyl-1-nitrosourea (CCNU)	Chinese hamster cells in vitro	Structural	RAO and RAO (1976)
	Procarbazine	Human lymphocytes and bone marrow in vivo	Structural	LEE and DIXON (1978) review
		Mouse germ cells in vivo	Non-lethal structural	GENEROSO et al. (1980) review
Platinum compounds	*cis*-dichloro-diammine platinum (II)	Human lymphocytes in vivo	Structural	SCOTT and STALKER (unpublished)
Antibiotics	Actinomycin D	Human lymphocytes in vivo	Structural	VIG (1979), review
	Daunomycin	Human lymphocytes in vivo	Structural and numerical	VIG (1979), review

Table 5. (continued)

Class of drug	Drug	Cells treated	Chromosome changes	Reference
	Adriamycin	Human lymphocytes in vivo	Structural and numerical	VIG (1979), review
		Mouse germ cells in vivo	Non-lethal structural	AU and HSU (1980)
	Bleomycin	Human lymphocytes in vivo	Structural	VIG (1979), review
	Bleomycin	Mouse germ cells in vivo	Non-lethal structural	VAN BUUL and GOUDZWAARD (1980)
	Mitomycin C	Human lymphocytes in vivo	Structural	VIG (1979), review
		Mouse germ cells in vivo	Non-lethal structural	GENEROSO et al. (1980), review
Vinca alkaloids	Vincristine	Human lymphocytes in vivo	Numerical (structural?)	DEGREAVE (1978), review
	Vinblastine	Human lymphocytes in vivo	Numerical	DEGREAVE (1978), review
		Chinese hamster in vitro	Structural	SEGAWA et al. (1979)
Steroid hormones	Diethystilbestrol-diphosphate	Mouse bone marrow in vivo	Numerical	CHRISMAN and HINKLE (1974)
	Estradiol	Human synovial cells in vitro	Numerical	LYCETTE et al. (1970)
Miscel-laneous	Hydroxyurea	Human lymphocytes in vivo	Structural	TIMSON (1975), review

When there are human in vivo data for a particular end point (structural, structural non-lethal or numerical changes) additional references, e.g. non-human in vivo or human in vitro references, are not given

association was found by IMBERT et al. (1975), who observed a positive correlation between the degree of actinomycin-D resistance and the proportion of cells with a marker chromosome in different clones of Chinese hamster cells.

An increased sensitivity to mitomycin C and bleomycin, with no associated karyotype change, is seen, respectively, in cells of patients with Fanconi's anaemia (FUJIWARA et al. 1977) and ataxia-telangiectasia (TAYLOR et al. 1979), which are both autosomal recessive diseases.

7. *Vinca* Alkaloids

These drugs interfere with the function of microtubules but little is known about mechanisms of resistance to these drugs. There have been few cytogenetic investigations of alkaloid-resistant cells (Table 1) but one such recent study is of considerable significance. BIEDLER et al. (1980c) have found an HSR in vincristine-resistant Chinese hamster cells. This has similar properties to HSRs in their anti-

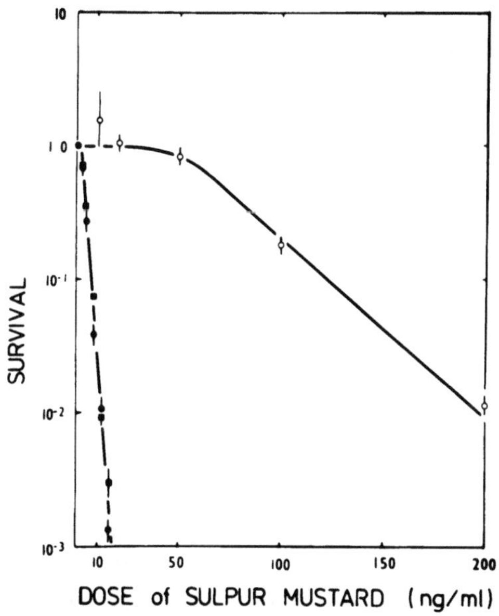

Fig. 15. Survival curves of cultured cells of the Yoshida sarcoma of the rat which are sensitive (*solid symbols*) or resistant (*open symbols*) to bifunctional alkylating agents (see text). (SCOTT et al. 1974; courtesy Elsevier/North-Holland)

folate-resistant cell but has a different chromosomal location. The cells are cross-resistant to other drugs (e.g. daunorubicin and actinomycin D), have a reduced capacity for drug uptake and differ in their membrane glycoproteins compared with wild-type cells, suggesting an altered membrane and/or cytoskeleton in the resistant cells.

The search for HSRs in cells resistant to other classes of antitumour drugs is clearly made more worthwhile by this recent observation.

C. Resistance to Induced Chromosome Damage

Many of the antitumour agents in current use have been found to induce chromosome structural damage in mammalian, and often in human, cells (Table 5). In the case of ionising radiation this appears to be the principal mechanism of cell killing (see SCOTT et al. 1976). The contribution of such damage to cell death after treatment with antitumour drugs is unknown, since both end points are rarely studied simultaneously, but SCOTT (1977) has found that the proportion of Yoshida sarcoma cells carrying chromosomal aberrations which lead to loss of chromosome material at mitosis is similar to the proportion of cells which are killed by the alkylating agent, sulphur mustard. This suggests a causal relationship. When the frequency of chromosome aberrations (CAs) and cell death is positively correlated, the possibility arises of using CA frequencies as an indicator of cellular sensitivity. A limited number of studies, primarily with alkylating agents, have revealed differences in CA induction in wild-type and drug-resistant cells.

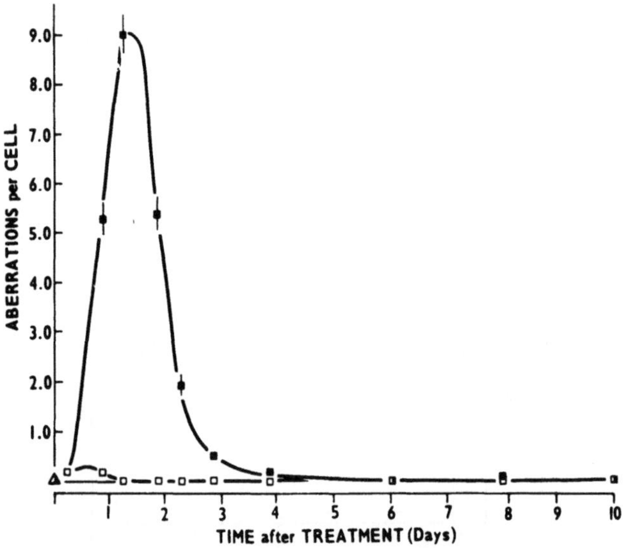

Fig. 16. Yields of chromosome structural aberrations in alkylating-agent-sensitive (■) and -resistant (□) Yoshida sarcoma cells treated in vitro with 20 ng/ml sulphur mustard. (Acknowledgements as for Fig. 15)

A pronounced difference in CA frequencies in wild-type Yoshida sarcoma cells compared with alkylating agent-resistant cells derived from them has been observed after treatment with sulphur mustard (SCOTT et al. 1974; Figs. 15–17), methylene dimethane sulphonate (SCOTT et al. 1978) or busulphan (BEDFORD and FOX 1980). The differential sensitivity of these two cell lines can be attributed to differences in their capacity to repair and/or tolerate DNA damage (FOX, Chap. 12). The DNA damage can lead to the production of CAs at the time of DNA synthesis and result in cell death (SCOTT 1977). Similar observations and interpretations were made by SZUMIEL (1979 b) in a pair of mouse lymphoma cells with a differential sensitivity to the platinum compound *cis*-PAD (Sect. B.II.5).

Higher frequencies of CAs induced by melphalan have been found in wild-type human melanoma (PARSONS and MORRISON 1978) and mouse leukaemia (SCHUETTE et al. 1980) cells than in derived melphalan-resistant cells although the biochemical basis of differential sensitivity of these cells was not known.

Other examples of an association between CA frequencies and sensitivity to antitumour agents are found in some of the rare, inherited, cancer-prone conditions in man. Cells of patients with Fanconi's anaemia are not only sensitive to the lethal effects of cross-linking agents such as mitomycin C (FUJIWARA et al. 1977; Sect. B.II.4) but sustain more chromosome damage than cells of normal individuals exposed to these agents (SASAKI and TONOMURA 1973). Similarly cells of patients with ataxia-telangiectasia are sensitive to both the lethal and chromosome-damaging effects of bleomycin (TAYLOR et al. 1979).

D. Summary

When the acquisition of resistance of cells to antitumour drugs has a genetic basis it is not always by simple gene, or point, mutation, but may result from specific,

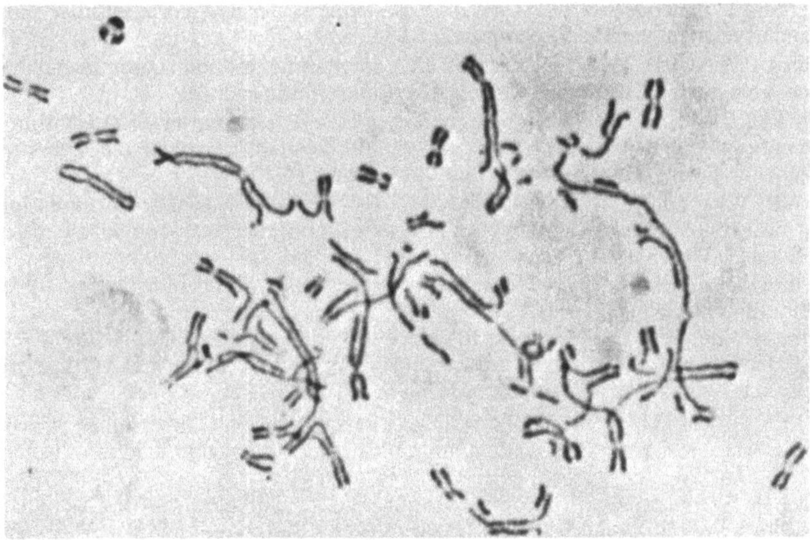

Fig. 17. Metaphase preparation of extensively damaged chromosomes of the alkylating-agent-sensitive line of Yoshida sarcoma cells after treatment with 20 ng/ml sulphur mustard in vitro. This dose produces very little chromosome damage in cells of the resistant line (see Fig. 16). (Acknowledgements as for Fig. 15)

non-cell-lethal changes in chromosome constitution which are visible at the level of the light microscope. These changes may occur spontaneously or be drug induced. Those drugs which are capable of inducing such chromosome changes will also induce other alterations in chromosome constitution which are unrelated to drug resistance and may mask the specific events.

In some cases specific resistance-related chromosome changes are clearly associated with the loss, gain or amplification of particular gene products. Where the chromosomal location of determinants of drug resistance is known, cytogenetic analyses of malignant cells may be of value in predicting their sensitivity or resistance to particular drugs. Where the location is not known, chromosome studies of drug-resistant cells can be useful in gene mapping.

Many antitumour drugs also induce cell-lethal chromosome damage, the amount of which can provide an indication of the sensitivity or resistance of cells to killing by these drugs.

Acknowledgements. The author wishes to thank Mr. Nigel Barron for his expert assistance in preparing the figures, Ms. Eileen Waters of the Environmental Mutagen Information Centre (U.K. Office, Swansea) for her literature searches and Ms. Deborah J. G. Stevens for her help in preparing Table 5. The author is supported by the Cancer Research Campaign.

References

Au WW, Hsu TC (1980) The genotoxic effects of adriamycin in somatic and germinal cells of the mouse. Mutat Res 79:351–361

Baker WK (1968) Position effect variegation. Adv Genet 14:133–169

Banerjee AT, Banerjee SP (1972) Chromosomal pattern of asparaginase sensitive leukemia and its resistant variant. Experientia 28:1236–1237

Bedford P, Fox BW (1982) Repair of DNA interstrand crosslinks after Busulphan. A possible mode of resistance. Cancer Chenother Pharmacol 8:3–7

Belehradek J, Biedler JL, Thonier M, Barski G (1974) Actinomycin-D-resistant in vitro mouse cell line derived from a methylcholanthrene-induced sarcoma: decrease of malignancy and antigenic characteristics. Int J Cancer 14:779–788

Bell WR, Whang JJ, Carbone PP, Brecher G, Block JB (1966) Cytogenetic and morphological abnormalities in human bone marrow cells during cytosine arabinoside therapy. Blood 27:771–781

Benedict WF, Jones PA (1979) Mutagenic, clastogenic and oncogenic effects of 1-β-D-arabinofuranosylcytosine. Mutat Res 65:1–20

Bertino JR, Donohue DM, Simmons B, Gabrio BW, Silber R, Huennekens FM (1963) The "induction" of dihydrofolic reductase activity in leukocytes and erythrocytes of patients treated with amethopterin. J Clin Invest 42:466–475

Biedler JL, Riehm H (1970) Cellular resistance to actinomycin D in Chinese hamster cells in vitro: cross-resistance, radioautographic and cytogenetic studies. Cancer Res 30:1174–1184

Biedler JL, Spengler BA (1976) Metaphase chromosome anomaly. Association of drug resistance and cell specific products. Science 191:185–187

Biedler JL, Melera PW, Spengler BA (1980a) Specifically altered metaphase chromosomes in antifolate-resistant Chinese hamster cells that overproduce dihydrofolate reductase. Cancer Genet Cytogenet 2:47–60

Biedler JL, Ross RA, Shanske S, Spengler BA (1980b) Human neuroblastoma cytogenetics: search for significance of homogeneously staining regions and double minute chromosomes. In: Evans AE (ed) Program in cancer research and therapy, vol 12. Raven, New York, pp 81–96

Biedler JL, Meyers MB, Peterson RH, Spengler BA (1980c) Marker chromosome with a homogeneously staining region (HSR) in vincristine-resistant cells (meeting abstract). Proc Am Assoc Cancer Res 21:292

Bostock CJ, Christie S (1976) Analysis of the frequency of sister chromatid exchange in different regions of chromosomes of the kangaroo rat (*Dipodomys ordii*). Chromosoma 56:275–287

Bostock CJ, Clark EM (1980) Satellite DNA in large marker chromosomes of methotrexate resistant mouse cells. Cell 19:709–715

Bostock CJ, Clark EM, Harding NGL, Mounts PM, Tyler-Smith C, Heyningen V van, Walker PMB (1979) The development of resistance to methotrexate in a mouse melanoma cell line. I. Characterisation of the dihydrofolate reductases and chromosomes in sensitive and resistant cells. Chromosoma 74:153–177

Brown JA, Goss S, Klinger HP, Miller OJ, Ohno S, Siniscalco M (1976) Genetic constitution of the X and Y chromosomes. Cytogenet Cell Genet 16:54–59

Brown R, Thacker J (1980) Characterisation of radiation-induced mutants of cultured mammalian cells (meeting abstract). Radiat Environ Biophs 17:341

Caskey CT, Kruh GD (1979) The HPRT locus. Cell 16:1–9

Chasin LA, Urlaub G (1975) Chromosome-wide event accompanies the expression of recessive mutations in tetraploid cells. Science 187:1091–1093

Chrisman CL, Hinkle LL (1974) Induction of aneuploidy in mouse bone marrow cells with diethylstilbestrol-diphosphate. Can J Genet Cytol 16:831–835

Ciesielski-Treska J, Warter S, Mandel P (1975) Morphological, histochemical and chromosomal patterns of neuroblastoma parental and purine resistant lines. Neurobiology 5:382–392

Cox R (1980) Comparative mutagenesis in cultured mammalian cells. In: Alacevic M (ed) Progress in environmental mutagenesis. Elsevier/North Holland, pp 33–46

Cox R, Masson WK (1978) Do radiation-induced thioguanine-resistant mutants in cultured mammalian cells arise by HGPRT gene mutation or X-chromosome rearrangement. Nature 276:629–630

Cox R, Masson WK (1979) Mutation and inactivation of cultured mammalian cells exposed to beams of accelerated heavy ions. III. Human diploid fibroblasts. Int J Radiat Biol 36:149–160

Degreave N (1978) Genetic and related effects of Vinca rosea alkaloids. Mutat Res 55:31–42

Dobos M, Fekete G, Schuler D, Szakmary E (1977) Chromosome aberrations produced in vivo by chemicals (meeting abstract). Mutat Res 46:216

Dolnick BJ, Berenson RJ, Bertino JR, Kaufman RJ, Nunberg JH, Schimke RT (1979) Correlation of dihydrofolate reductase elevation with gene amplification in a homogeneously staining chromosomal region in L5178Y cells. J Cell Biol 83:394–402

Duncan ME (1977) Isolation and preliminary characterisation of drug resistant mutants of human lymphoblastoid cells. Cytobios 19:45–66

Evans HJ (1962) Chromosome aberrations induced by ionising radiation. Int Rev Cytol 13:221–321

Fox M, Radacic M (1978) Adaptational origin of some purine-analogue resistant phenotypes in cultured mammalian cells. Mutat Res 49:275–296

Fox M, Scott D (1980) The genetic toxicology of nitrogen and sulphur mustard. Mutat Res 75:131–168

Fujiwara Y, Tatsumi M, Sasaki MS (1977) Cross-link repair in human cells and its possible defect in Fanconi's anaemia cells. J Mol Biol 113:635–649

Gati E (1979) Chromosomal analysis on Yoshida tumor cells sensitive and resistant to dibromodulcitol. Neoplasma 26:79–83

Gebhart E, Schwanitz G, Hartwich G (1974) Chromosomenaberrationen bei Busulfanbehandlung. Dtsch Med Wochenschr 99:52–56

Generoso WM, Bishop JB, Gosslee DG, Newell GW, Sheu C-J, von Halle E (1980) Heritable translocation test in mice. Mutat Res 76:191–215

Goldenberg GJ (1969) Properties of L5178Y lymphoblasts highly resistant to nitrogen mustard. Symposium on biological effects of alkylating agents. Ann NY Acad Sci 163:936–953

Hansmann I (1973) Induced chromosomal aberrations in pronuclei, 2 cell stages and morulae of mice. Mutat Res 20:353–367

Harrod EK, Cortner JA (1968) Prolonged survival of lymphocytes with chromosomal defects in children treated with 1,3-bis(2-chlorethyl)-1-nitrosourea. J Natl Cancer Inst 40:269–279

Hasholt L, Danø K (1974) Cytogenetic investigations on an Ehrlich ascites tumor, and four sublines resistant to daunomycin, adriamycin, vincristine and vinblastine. Hereditas 77:303–310

Hauschka TS (1958) Correlation of chromosomal and physiologic changes in tumours. J Cell Comp Physiol 52 (Suppl 1):197–233

Hirono I, Yokoyama C (1955) Chromosomal features in the original and resistant sublines of Yoshida sarcoma. Cytologia 20:84–88

Honeycombe JR (1981) The cytogenetic effects of busulphan therapy on the Ph[1]-positive cells and lymphocytes from patients with chronic myeloid leukaemia. Mutat Res 81:81–102

Hsu TC, Arrighi FE (1971) Distribution of constitutive heterochromatin in mammalian chromosomes. Chromosoma 34:243–253

Imbert I, Barra Y, Berebbi M (1975) Correlation between resistance to actinomycin D, karyology, agglutination by concanavalin A and tumorigenicity in Chinese hamster hybrid cells. J Cell Sci 18:67–77

Jensen MK, Nyfors A (1979) Cytogenetic effect of methotrexate on human cells in vivo. Comparison between results obtained by chromosome studies on bone marrow cells and blood lymphocytes by the micronucleus test. Mutat Res 64:339–343

Johnson RE, Hardy WG (1965) Chemotherapeutic effects on mammalian tumor cells II. Biologic and chromosomal instability of a cyclophosphamide treated murine leukaemia. Cancer Res 25:604–608

Jones KW (1970) Chromosomal and nuclear location of mouse satellite DNA in individual cells. Nature 225:912–915

Kaufman RJ, Brown PC, Schimke RT (1979) Amplified dihydrofolate reductase genes in unstably methotrexate-resistant cells are associated with double-minute chromosomes. Proc Natl Acad Sci USA 76:5669–5673

Kelly F, Legator M (1970) Effect of *n*-methyl-*n'*-nitrosoguanidine on the cell cycle and chromosomes of human embryonic lung cells. Mutat Res 10:237–246

Latt SA (1973) Microfluorimetric detection of DNA synthesis in human chromosomes. Proc Natl Acad Sci USA 70:3395–3399

Lee IP, Dixon RL (1978) Mutagenicity, carcinogenicity and teratogenicity of procarbazine. Mutat Res 55:1–14

Lycette RR, Whyte S, Chapman CJ (1970) Aneuploid effect of estradiol on cultured synovial cells. NZ Med J 74:114–117

Mohn GR, Ellenberger J (1976) Genetic effects of cyclophosphamide, ifosfamide and trofosfamide. Mutat Res 32:331–360

Momparler RL, Chu MY, Fischer GA (1968) Studies on a new mechanism of resistance of L5178Y murine leukemia cells to cytosine arabinoside. Biochim Biophys Acta 23:481–493

Morrow J, Stocco D, Barron E (1978) Spontaneous mutation rate to thioguanine resistance is decreased in polyploid hamster cells. J Cell Physiol 96:81–86

Morry DW, Ts'o PO (1980) Ploidy dependence of induced mutation frequency in transformed Syrian hamster cells. Mutat Res 70:221–229

Nasjleti CE, Spencer HH (1966) Chromosome damage and polyploidisation induced in human peripheral leukocytes in vivo and in vitro with nitrogen mustard, 6-mercaptopurine, and A649. Cancer Res 26:2437–2443

Nunberg JH, Kaufman RJ, Schimke RT, Urlaub G, Chasin LA (1978) Amplified dihydrofolate reductase genes are localised to a homogeneously stained region of a single chromosome in a methotrexate-resistant Chinese hamster ovary cell line. Proc Natl Acad Sci USA 75:5553–5556

Parsons PG, Morrison L (1978) Melphalan-induced chromosome damage in sensitive and resistant human melanoma cell lines. Int J Cancer 21:438–443

Perry P, Wolff S (1974) New Giemsa method for the differential staining of sister chromatids. Nature 251:156–158

Rao AP, Rao PN (1976) The cause of G_2 arrest in Chinese hamster ovary cells treated with anticancer drugs. J Natl Cancer Inst 57:1139–1143

Raskind WH, Gartler SM (1978) The relationship between induced mutation frequency and chromosome dosage in established mouse fibroblast lines. Somatic Cell Genet 4:491–506

Sandberg AA (1980) The chromosomes of human cancer and leukemia. Elsevier, New York

Sasaki MS (1978) Fanconi's anaemia. A condition possibly associated with a defective DNA repair. In: Hanawalt PC, Friedberg EC, Fox CF (eds) DNA repair mechanisms. ICN-ULCA Symposia on molecular and cellular biology, vol 9. Academic, New York, pp 675–684

Sasaki MS, Tonomura A (1973) A high susceptibility of Fanconi's anaemia to chromosome breakage by DNA cross-linking agents. Cancer Res 33:1829–1836

Schimke RT, Kaufman RJ, Nunberg JH, Dana SL (1979) Studies on the amplification of dihydrofolate reductase genes in methotrexate-resistant cultured mouse cells. Cold Spring Harbor Symp Quant Biol 43:1297–1303

Schuette BP, Rabinovitz M, Vistica DT (1980) A comparative cytogenetic study of melphalan-sensitive and resistant murine L1210 leukemia cells. Cancer Lett 8:335–341

Scott D (1977) Chromosome aberrations, DNA post-replication repair and lethality in tumour cells with a differential sensitivity to alkylating agents. In: de la Chapelle A, Sorsa M (eds) Chromosomes today, vol 16. Elsevier, Amsterdam, pp 391–401

Scott D, Fox M, Fox BW (1974) The relationship between chromosomal aberrations, survival and DNA repair in tumour cells of differential sensitivity to X-rays and sulphur mustard. Mutat Res 22:207–221

Scott D, Craig AW, Iype PT (1976) Effects of ionising radiation on mammalian cells. In: Symington T, Carter RL (eds) Scientific foundations of oncology. Heinemann, London, pp 427–443

Scott D, Radacic M, Fox M (1978) Enhancement of lethality and chromosome damage by caffeine in Yoshida sarcoma cells treated with sulphur mustard or MDMS. Annual report 1977–1978, Paterson Laboratories and Medical Oncology, Christie Hospital and Holt Radium Institute, Manchester, pp 74–76

Seabright M (1972) The use of proteolytic enzymes for the mapping of structural rearrangements in the chromosomes of man. Chromosoma 36:204–210

Segawa M, Nadamitsu S, Kondo K, Yoshizaka I (1979) Chromosomal aberrations of DON lung cells of Chinese hamster after exposure to vinblastine in vitro. Mutat Res 66:99–102

Selezneva TG, Korman NP (1973) Analysis of chromosomes of somatic cells in patients treated with antitumor drugs. Sov Genet 9:1575–1579

Sharpe HBA (1971) Observations on the effect of therapy with nitrogen mustard or a derivative on chromosomes of human peripheral blood lymphocytes. Cell Tissue Kinet 4:501–504

Siminovitch L (1976) On the nature of heritable variations in cultured somatic cells. Cell 7:1–11

Slack C, Morgan RH, Carritt B, Goldfarb PS, Hooper ML (1976) Isolation and characterisation of Chinese hamster cells resistant to 5-fluorodeoxyuridine. Exp Cell Res 98:1–14

Sokova OI, Volgareva GM (1977) The effect of fluorafur and 5-fluoruracil on chromosomes of normal and tumor cells in vivo. Vopr Onkol 23:94–97

Stevenson AC (1978) Effects of twelve folate analogues on human lymphocytes in vitro. In: Evans HJ, Lloyd DC (eds) Mutagen-induced chromosome damage in man. Edinburgh University Press, Edinburgh, pp 227–238

Sumner AT (1972) A simple technique for demonstrating centromeric heterochromatin. Exp Cell Res 75:304–306

Szumiel I (1979a) Response of two strains of L5178Y cells to *cis*-dichorobis-(cyclopentylamine) platinum(II) I. Cross-sensitivity to *cis*-PAD and UV light. Chem Biol Interact 24:51–72

Szumiel I (1979b) Response of two strains of L5178Y cells to *cis*-dichlorobis-(cyclopentylamine) platinum(II) II. Differential effects of caffeine. Chem Biol Interact 24:73–82

Taylor AMR, Rosney CM, Campbell JB (1979) Unusual sensitivity of ataxia telangiectasia to bleomycin. Cancer Res 39:1046–1050

Terzi M (1972) On the selection for the model chromosome number in Chinese hamster cells. J Cell Physiol 80:359–366

Terzi M (1974) Chromosomal variation and the origin of drug-resistant mutants in mammalian cell lines. Proc Natl Acad Sci USA 71:5027–5031

Thacker J (1981) The chromosomes of a V79 Chinese hamster line and a mutant subline lacking HPRT activity. Cytogenet Cell Genet 29:16–25

Timson J (1975) Hydroxyurea. Mutat Res 32:115–132

Ujhazy V (1974) Identical karyotypes in acquired drug-resistant sublines of Yoshida sarcoma. Neoplasma 21:665–669

Van Buul PPW, Goudzwaard JH (1980) Bleomycin-induced structural chromosomal aberrations in spermatogonia and bone marrow cells of mice. Mutat Res 69:319–324

Vig BK (1979) Mutagenic effects of some anticancer Antibiotics. Cancer Chemother Pharmacol 3:143–160

Voitovitskii VK, Edygenova AK, Kabiev OK (1970) Cytogenetic analysis of rat ovarian tumor variants resistant to 6-mercaptopurine and thio-tepa. Vopr Onkol 16:87–92

Voitovitskii VK, Edygenova AK, Kabiev OK (1971) Comparative cytogenetic study of the resistance of tumor cells to sarcolysine. Sov Genet 7:766–769

Yoshida MC, Kodama Y (1977) Karyological characterisation of a human lymphoblastoid cell resistant to 6-thioguanine. Hum Genet 35:201–208

Yoshida TH, Ohara H, Roosa RA (1968) Chromosomal alteration and development of tumors XVIII. Karyotypes of a 5-fluorodeoxyuridine resistant subline in vitro. Jinrui Idengaku Zasshi 43:49

CHAPTER 10

Alterations of Drug Transport

G. J. GOLDENBERG and A. BEGLEITER

A. Introduction

Twenty years ago, defective transport of the antimetabolite methotrexate was recognized as a specific cause of resistance to that drug in a mutant line of murine L5178Y leukemia (FISCHER 1962). Since that time numerous reports of antitumor drug resistance based on defective drug transport have appeared involving several different groups of antitumor agents. In order to achieve a more complete understanding of this type of drug resistance, the basic mechanisms of drug uptake by mammalian cells will first be reviewed followed by a more detailed description of specific examples of drug resistance due to deficient transport. Next we will consider attempts that have been made to circumvent this type of resistance by increasing drug uptake in resistant transport mutants. The review will conclude with a brief discussion of the possible direction of future studies of this area of investigation.

B. Mechanism of Drug Transport

I. Characteristics of Passive Diffusion and Mediated Transport

Drug uptake by mammalian cells may occur by at least three different mechanisms: (1) passive diffusion, in which drug influx is directly proportional to substrate concentration and the drug enters the cell presumably through pores in the cell membrane by a process that does not involve interaction between the transport substrate and a specific site on the cell membrane; (2) facilitated diffusion, in which drug influx is a process that involves a specific interaction between drug and a transport site in the membrane that follows saturation kinetics, exhibits chemical specificity, and is temperature dependent, but the intracellular drug concentration does not exceed the extracellular level; and (3) active transport in which drug transport is similar to facilitated diffusion except uptake is energy dependent and proceeds "uphill" against a concentration gradient. For drugs which are electrolytes at physiological pH, the distribution ratio observed at the steady state will also reflect differences in cell membrane potential. Since the inner surface of the cell membrane is negatively charged, a drug bearing a negative charge will have a cell/medium distribution ratio of less than one for an equilibrating process at the steady state, and a positively charged drug will have a distribution ratio greater than one. An analysis of "uphill" transport will require comparison of the measured distribution ratio with that expected for an equilibrating system.

It is possible to attempt quantitative predictions of the ability of a cell to take up a compound of unknown chemical structure by simple passive diffusion. To make such a prediction, the analysis of LIEB and STEIN (1969, 1971) of the permeability behavior of a number of different cell membranes may be used, provided the molecular weight of the test substance and its partition coefficient between a solvent which mimics the cell membrane and water are known. Where the partition coefficient of a compound is not known, this can be estimated from the chemical structure using predictive techniques pioneered by LEO et al. (1971). The predicted permeability coefficient can then be compared with experimental data. If the predicted rate is of the same order of magnitude as the observed one, then passive diffusion may account for transport. However, it is also essential to show that not only is influx consistent with passive diffusion, but the steady-state level of substrate reached and the influx characteristics are those expected for simple diffusion.

LIEB and STEIN (1969, 1971) suggested that the permeability of a membrane toward a particular substance depends on three factors: (a) the molecular weight M of the permeant relative to that of methanol and the ability of the membrane to discriminate between permeance by virtue of size (the mass selectivity coefficient s_m); (b) the partition coefficient K for the distribution of the permeant between a model solvent and water, and the accuracy with which the model solvent describes the solvent properties of the membrane under consideration (the selectivity index s_k); and (c) the overall tightness of the membrane, the parameter P_o. The permeability coefficient for a given substance, P_s, is given by the formula:

$$P_s = P_o M^{-s_m} K^{s_k}.$$

The parameters P_o, s_m, and s_k can be determined by a multivariate regression analysis of the measured permeabilities of a large number of different substances entering a particular cell. With these parameters available the above equation allows the permeability of an unknown substance to be estimated. Having calculated the predicted permeability coefficient P_s for a compound then the predicted half-time ($t_{1/2}$) for entry of that compound may be calculated by simple integration of Fick's law of diffusion (TROSHIN 1966). When rapid rates of entry of a compound are predicted then the need to postulate a mediated transport system for such a compound may not be necessary.

II. Kinetics of Membrane Transport

The kinetic analysis of influx of a particular drug should begin with a simple time course of drug uptake. To ensure an accurate determination of the influx K_m subsequent kinetic studies must be performed at a sufficiently short time interval so that only unidirectional drug influx is being measured. This condition is satisfied by conducting experiments along the initial linear region of the time course so that initial uptake velocity is determined. Uptake studies performed at later portions of the time course when uptake is no longer linear may be complicated by drug efflux, metabolism, or binding.

Drug uptake must often be corrected for rapid association of drug to the cell membrane. This represents drug that rapidly binds to the cell membrane through covalent or noncovalent interactions, and/or drug "trapped" between cells or between folds on the cell surface which is not washed away or totally corrected for by the extracellular marker. This component may be determined by measuring the cell/medium distribution ratio of drug at 4 °C with as short an incubation period as is technically feasible since it is temperature independent. This value for cell/medium distribution ratio should approximate that obtained by extrapolation of the time course for drug uptake at 37 °C back to the *y*-intercept. The cell/medium ratio due to surface adsorption should remain constant over a wide range of drug concentrations. This value should be routinely subtracted from the observed cell/medium distribution ratio at each experimental point in order to measure drug which enters the cell.

Kinetic analysis of drug influx is performed by measuring initial uptake velocity over a wide range of substrate concentrations. Drug uptake by simple diffusion follows a first-order kinetic reaction, in which velocity of drug uptake v is directly proportional to extracellular drug or substrate concentration S and may be expressed by the equation:

$$v = k[S]\,, \qquad (1)$$

where k is the first-order rate constant, signifying that a fixed fraction of drug is transported per unit of time.

Influx of drug by a carrier-mediated system, which may be either by facilitated diffusion or active transport, obeys saturation kinetics as described by the Michaelis-Menten equation:

$$v = \frac{V_{max}[S]}{K_m + [S]}\,, \qquad (2)$$

where v is velocity of unidirectional drug influx, $[S]$ is the extracellular drug concentration, V_{max} is the maximum transport capacity, which is a measure of the number and mobility of transport carriers, and K_m, the Michaelis constant, is the drug concentration at which influx is one-half the V_{max} and is an index of the affinity of the carrier for the drug. Since the extracellular volume is extremely large compared with the intracellular volume in these influx studies, extracellular drug concentration remains essentially constant during the incubation period.

From an examination of Eqs. (1) and (2) it is apparent that under conditions where drug concentration is very low (e.g. $[S] < 0.01\ K_m$), Eq. (2) is reduced to the form:

$$v = \frac{V_{max}}{K_m}[S]\,, \qquad (3)$$

which is identical to Eq. (1), in which the first-order rate constant $k = (V_{max}/K_m)$. In practical terms this means that at drug concentrations much lower than the K_m for a carrier-mediated influx system, it is impossible by kinetic analysis to distinguish between simple diffusion and a carrier-mediated process.

Under conditions where drug concentration is very high (e.g. $[S] > 100\ K_m$) Eq. (2) reduces to the term:

$$v = V_{max}, \tag{4}$$

where velocity of drug influx is constant and independent of drug concentration and the reaction follows zero-order kinetics.

If influx follows saturation kinetics, the Lineweaver-Burk plot of reciprocal uptake velocity against reciprocal substrate concentration should be linear; such a finding is strong evidence that influx is carrier mediated. The kinetic parameters K_m and V_{max} may be derived from a linear regression analysis of the Lineweaver-Burk plot; the slope represents K_m/V_{max}, the y-intercept is $1/V_{max}$, and the x-intercept is $-1/K_m$.

III. Drug Uptake by Multiple Mechanisms

Drug influx may occur by two mechanisms, passive diffusion and a carrier-mediated process. In such cases velocity of influx is described by the equation:

$$v = \frac{V_{max}[S]}{K_m + [S]} + k[S], \tag{5}$$

which includes a diffusion component identical to Eq. (1) and a carrier-mediated component as in Eq. (2), both terms using extracellular drug concentration or drug on the same side of the membrane from which the flux is directed. This equation is probably an oversimplification since there is considerable evidence that oneway fluxes depend on the *trans* concentration of substrate, that is drug on the side toward which the flux is directed, as well as on the *cis* concentration (JACQUEZ 1975).

Drug influx may also be mediated by two or more carrier-mediated systems which may be described mathematically as the sum of two or more Michaelis-Menten equations, each with different kinetic parameters (CHRISTENSEN 1966, 1969; SCRIVER and MOHYUDDIN 1968, SCRIVER and HECHTMAN 1970; SEGAL et al. 1967; GOLDENBERG et al. 1974). A Lineweaver-Burk plot of such data would be biphasic or multiphasic, and an Eadie-Augustinsson plot likely would accentuate the observed heterogeneity (GOLDENBERG et al. 1974, 1979; BEGLEITER et al. 1979). The kinetic parameters of biphasic influx systems may be corrected for two component interactions using the formulae derived by NEAL (1972).

Studies with competitive inhibitors serve not only to establish chemical specificity of the transport system (GOLDENBERG and BEGLEITER 1980) but also to provide information as to whether or not uptake involves a single system. If a single transport carrier is involved the reciprocal experiments may be performed where uptake of the inhibitor, serving as substrate, is competitively blocked by the addition of the drug now acting as inhibitor. If both the drug and inhibitor share a single common transport pathway then the K_m for either compound acting as substrate should approximate the K_i of that same compound acting as inhibitor (AHMED and SCHOLEFIELD 1962).

IV. Evaluation of Drug Efflux

In evaluating the role of membrane transport in the development of resistance to antitumor agents drug efflux from the cell must also be considered. Drug efflux is particularly important for agents that are not readily metabolized and for those that bind to intracellular sites but can still accumulate within the cell in an exchangeable form as free intact drug. Far fewer studies have appeared on drug efflux than influx; efflux studies are technically more difficult and prone to greater error. Unlike influx experiments the efflux rate is calculated from the difference between two determinations of intracellular drug concentration; furthermore, intracellular substrate concentration must be measured experimentally.

A large volume of suspending medium must be used in measuring unidirectional efflux to avoid the problem of drug re-entry (CHRISTENSEN and HANDLOGTEN 1968; SIROTNAK 1980). Due to the imprecise technology available to study efflux, it has not been feasible to establish with any confidence kinetic parameters for drug efflux. At times, it is impossible to distinguish between efflux by passive diffusion or a technically nonsaturable carrier-mediated process. A semilogarithmic plot of the time course of exchangeable drug remaining within the cell will yield a linear plot from which a first-order rate constant (K) for efflux may be derived from the negative slope of the regression line. The $t_{1/2}$, or half-life, for drug efflux may also be calculated from the equation:

$$t_{1/2}=\frac{\log_e 2}{K} \tag{6}$$

Efflux by passive diffusion will be characterized by first-order kinetics as will carrier-mediated efflux in systems in which the efflux K_m is much greater than the intracellular drug concentration to which cells may be loaded. If the intracellular drug concentration approximates the K_m, efflux will exhibit saturation kinetics.

By using model substrates and inhibitors almost completely specific to known transport systems, CHRISTENSEN and HANDLOGTEN (1968) demonstrated similarities between the modes of entry and exodus of various amino acids. Within the limited accuracy available, estimates of V_{max} for the mediated exodus of four amino acids were similar to the V_{max} for entry of the same substrates. It was concluded that concentrative accumulation, when it occurs, may be accounted for by differences in K_m for entry and for exodus.

C. Antitumor Drug Resistance Due to Defects in Membrane Transport

I. Alkylating Agents

1. Nitrogen Mustard

a) Historical Review

A review of the literature discloses that several studies have compared uptake of radiolabeled alkylating agents by drug-sensitive and -resistant tumors. WHEELER and ALEXANDER (1964) found no difference in uptake of ^{14}C-labeled nitrogen mustard (HN2), thio-triethylenephosphoramide (TEPA), or cyclophosphamide (ring- and ethyl-labeled) by cyclophosphamide-sensitive and -resistant plasmacytomas growing bilaterally in the same hamster. The distribution of ^{14}C among the subcellular fractions was similar in both tumors and there was no correlation between the extent of fixation of ^{14}C and the tumor-inhibitory activities of the agents. Several deficiencies in this study are apparent. The experimental design tacitly assumes that uptake of three different alkylating agents is by the same mechanisms; although varying degrees of cross-resistance may be demonstrated by tumors against many alkylating agents (GOLDENBERG 1975) there is conclusive evidence that uptake is mediated by independent transport processes (GOLDENBERG et al. 1970, 1974, 1977). Furthermore, the HN2 used was labeled in the CH_3 group; this raises serious concerns about the nature of the radiolabeled compounds and the interpretation of the experimental findings. This study did not attempt to answer the question as to whether transport or metabolism is rate limiting and whether metabolites, if formed, are retained within the cell.

Several investigators have reported reduced uptake of nitrogen mustard by resistant cells or that reduced permeability may be a factor in the development of resistance (HIRONO et al. 1962; MIURA and MORIYAMA 1961; YAMADA et al. 1963). RUTMAN's group (RUTMAN et al. 1968; CHUN et al. 1969) reported decreased uptake of [^{14}C]HN2 by resistant sublines of Lettre-Ehrlich ascites tumor cells, but permeability changes were insufficient to account for the magnitude of resistance observed. KLATT et al. (1969) confirmed the finding of reduced HN2-uptake by resistant Ehrlich tumor cells and also showed that uptake of phenylalanine mustard did not differ in HN2-sensitive and -resistant cells; the authors suggested that sensitivity or resistance to alkylating agents was chemically specific.

WOLPERT and RUDDON (1969) also demonstrated reduced uptake of [^{14}C] HN2 by HN2-resistant Ehrlich ascites cells and suggested that not only permeability changes but also the superior capacity of sensitive cells to bind and retain the drug might explain the findings. They indicated that although the uptake process had many characteristics of a mediated transport system, the apparent concentration of drug within the cell could be accounted for by diffusion and binding to the cell membrane or intracellular sites. KESSEL et al. (1969) found apparent concentrative accumulation of [^{14}C] HN2 by L1210 leukemia cells incubated at 37 °C but also attributed this to extensive binding of drug to cell components, even though an examination of their data reveals that approximately 50% of the radioactivity was not "bound" and could be eluted with fresh medium or 5% trichloroacetic acid.

A major defect in most if not all of the above studies of HN2 uptake is the use of HN2, an active alkylating agent, as substrate, making it extremely difficult to separate simple uptake from alkylation reactions. The latter could result in drug binding to nucleophilic groups within the cell or on the cell membrane, with the formation of apparent concentration gradients.

b) Mechanism of Nitrogen Mustard Transport

We first demonstrated that uptake of HN2 by L5178Y lymphoblasts was by an active carrier-mediated process (GOLDENBERG et al. 1970). The finding that the hydrolyzed derivative HN2–OH, which is inactive as an alkylating agent, served as a mutual and reciprocal competitive inhibitor of HN2 uptake, enabled us to examine the HN2 transport system without the complication of alkylation reactions. Uptake of HN2 and HN2–OH by L5178Y lymphoblasts proceeded "uphill" against a concentration gradient of approximately 35-fold, was almost completely inhibited at 4 °C, and was partially inhibited by ouabain and 2,4-dinitrophenol, all of which suggested an active process. Evidence for a carrier mechanism was that influx obeyed simple Michaelis-Menten kinetics and demonstrated chemical specificity. A 20-fold excess of structural analogs of HN2 such as cyclophosphamide, melphalan, and chlorambucil did not inhibit drug influx, suggesting that uptake of these other alkylating agents was by an independent process.

The nature and identity of the transport carrier for HN2 was investigated, since the existence of a specific carrier solely for a toxic compound not found under physiological conditions was considered unlikely. Evidence indicated that transport of HN2 by L5178Y lymphoblasts was mediated by the transport carrier for choline (GOLDENBERG et al. 1971 a). Choline influx was an active process proceeding "uphill" against a concentration gradient of at least 45-fold and was competitively inhibited by HN2, HN2–OH, ethanolamine, and hemocholinium-3, a specific inhibitor of choline transport in other tissues (POTTER 1968; DIAMOND and KENNEDY 1969). The K_m (mean $\pm$SD) for choline influx was 25 ± 9 μM and the V_{max} was $3.08 \pm 0.70 \times 10^{-17}$ mol/cell per min; choline was a competitive inhibitor of HN2–OH influx with a K_i of 36 μM. The K_m for HN2–OH influx was 69 ± 13 μM, which approximated the K_i of 54 μM for that agent acting as inhibitor of choline influx. This similarity of K_m and K_i for choline and HN2–OH suggested that both compounds were transported on the same carrier. The K_m for intact HN2 as substrate was 135 μM; thus the relative affinity for the transport carrier was choline > HN2–OH > HN2, suggesting that choline was the preferred transport substrate.

The observation that a toxic compound HN2 enters the cell on the transport carrier for a natural substrate, choline, appeared to be another example of a general pattern of drug transport. Similar interactions include active transport of 5-fluoro- and 5-bromouracil on the pyrimidine carrier in rat intestine (SCHANKER and JEFFREY 1961), transport of 8-mercapto- and 8-bromoadenine on the purine carrier in polymorphonuclear leukocytes (HAWKINS and BERLIN 1969), methotrexate transport on the carrier for reduced folates in L1210 leukemia cells (GOLDMAN et al. 1968), and shared transport of ouabain and steroid in rat liver slices (KUPFERBERG 1969). In each case the drug was a close structural analog of the natural substrate.

The relative affinity for the transport carriers was choline > HN2–OH > HN2. This may be due, in part, to differences in the affinities of the transport carrier for protonated versus nonprotonated forms of these compounds. Both HN2 and HN2–OH exist in two forms, one protonated the other unprotonated, the relative amount of each depending on the pH. The *pKa* for HN2 is 6.1 while that for HN2–OH is 8.3 (HANBY et al. 1947). Thus under physiological conditions the major portion of HN2 will exist in the unprotonated form while the major portion of the hydrolyzed drug will be in the protonated form, which more closely resembles the structure of choline. The monofunctional analog of HN2, dimethyl

2-chloroethylamine (HN1) also served as a competitive inhibitor of HN2 transport (GOLDENBERG et al. 1970).

c) Nitrogen Mustard Transport in Human Lymphoid Cells

Transport of HN2–OH and choline by lymphoid cells from normal individuals and patients with chronic lymphocytic leukemia or acute lymphoblastic leukemia was also studied (LYONS and GOLDENBERG 1972). Transport of [^{14}C] HN2–OH and [^{14}C]choline into normal and leukemic cells proceeded "uphill" against a concentration gradient, was temperature-dependent, followed Michaelis-Menten kinetics, and demonstrated chemical specificity, thus suggesting that transport was an active, carrier-mediated process. The influx K_m for both substrates was lowest in acute lymphoblastic leukemia lymphoblasts, suggesting that carrier sites in those cells have the greatest affinity for these substrates. Transport capacity as measured by V_{max} was also greatest in acute lymphoblastic leukemia lymphoblasts, indicating a larger number of transport sites and/or more rapid carrier mobility.

Certain inconsistencies in HN2–OH and choline transport suggested that more than a single common transport system was involved in HN2 transport by human cells. Discrepancies between K_m and K_i suggested that HN2–OH appeared to be a more efficient inhibitor of choline transport and, conversely, that choline appeared to be a less efficient inhibitor of HN2–OH transport than would be expected from their K_m values. HN2–OH acting as inhibitor completely blocked transport of choline; however, in the reciprocal experiment, choline, even at concentrations 500-fold greater than that of HN2–OH, failed to eliminate drug transport. HN2–OH influx examined over a 100-fold range in drug concentration was clearly biphasic. From these findings, at least two components of HN2–OH transport were identified for human lymphoid cells: a low-affinity, high-capacity system that is operative at "high" drug concentrations and a high-affinity, low-capacity system that is shared with choline at "low" drug concentrations.

d) Resistance to Nitrogen Mustard Due to Diminished Drug Uptake

A comparative study of HN2 uptake was undertaken in HN2-sensitive and -resistant L5178Y lymphoblasts in vitro (GOLDENBERG et al. 1970). Cells were rendered resistant to HN2 by repeated exposure to increasing concentrations of drug in vitro over a period of several months (GOLDENBERG 1969). A comparison of D_o (the dose of drug reducing survival to $1/e$, i.e. 37% of the initial cell population) revealed that the resistant cell line was 30-fold more resistant to HN2 than the sensitive parent line. In a preliminary experiment uptake of radioactivity in cells treated with 10 μM [^{14}C]HN2 was three fold greater in sensitive than in resistant cells (GOLDENBERG et al. 1970); this difference in uptake was observed not only for whole cells but also for cell sap and membrane fractions. In cells treated with 200 μM [^{14}C]HN2 uptake of radioactivity was only 1.6- to 2-fold greater in sensitive than in resistant cells. From this early study it was apparent that, firstly, drug resistance was, at least, in part due to reduced membrane permeability to the drug and, secondly, that differences between sensitive and resistant cells appeared to be drug concentration dependent.

Accordingly a more detailed investigation of the mechanism of drug influx was undertaken in sensitive and resistant L5178Y lymphoblasts (GOLDENBERG et al. 1970). A time course of drug influx was more rapid in sensitive cells. A kinetic analysis demonstrated that the K_m (mean $\pm$SE) for HN2 influx in sensitive cells was 144 ± 5 μM and that in resistant cells was 187 ± 8 μM and the difference was highly significant ($P<0.001$); this suggested that in resistant cells HN2 influx was characterized by a reduced affinity of the transport carrier for drug. The V_{max} (mean $\pm$SE) for resistant cells was $3.76 \pm 0.20 \times 10^{-17}$ mol/cell per min and that in sensitive cells was $4.78 \pm 0.16 \times 10^{-17}$ mol/cell per min and this difference was also statistically significant ($P<0.001$); this suggested that there was a reduction in the number of transport sites and/or slower carrier mobility in resistant cells. Part of this difference may be due to differences in cell size, resistant cells being smaller than sensitive cells (GOLDENBERG 1969); however, interpretation of changes in V_{max} are futile since critical information on the density and distribution of transport carriers is not available. Similar changes in kinetic parameters were reported in HN2-resistant Yoshida sarcoma cells (INABA 1973).

e) Sensitivity to Nitrogen Mustard as a Function of Transport Activity and Proliferative Rate of the Target Cells

The sensitivity of L5178Y lymphoblasts to the cytocidal action of HN2 was found to be a function of the proliferative state of the cells (GOLDENBERG et al. 1971b). The D_o for log-phase cells was 6.52 ng/ml, and that for stationary-phase cells was 17.17 ng/ml, indicating that log-phase cells were 2.6-fold more sensitive to HN2 than resting cells and the difference was highly significant ($P<0.001$). Carrier-mediated transport of ^{14}C-labeled HN2, hydrolyzed HN2, and the native substrate choline was also a function of the proliferative state of the cells. Transport was more efficient in log-phase cells than in resting cells; the transport K_m for each of the three substrates was lower in log-phase cells, suggesting that the more efficient transport was due to a higher binding affinity between carrier and drug. In addition transport capacity, as measured by V_{max}, for HN2–OH and choline was significantly higher in log-phase cells than in resting cells, suggesting that dividing cells had a greater number of transport sites and/or more rapid carrier mobility. The greater sensitivity of log-phase cells to HN2 to a large extent could be accounted for by these differences in drug transport.

Similarly sensitivity of mouse bone marrow and spleen colony-forming cells to HN2 was found to be a function of the proliferative state of the cells (VAN PUTTEN and LELIEVELD 1971). Rapidly repopulating mouse spleen or marrow cells were approximately two fold more sensitive than normal resting bone marrow cells; however, transport studies were not reported. Transport of physiological substrates such as cystine (STATES and SEGAL 1968), valine (REISER et al. 1970), and basic amino acids (PALL 1970) have also been noted to be more rapid in proliferating than resting cells. The activity of the HN2-choline transport system may be dependent upon proliferative rate, transport being more active in rapidly dividing cells.

f) The Interrelationship of Drug Transport and Cross-Resistance to Alkylating Agents

An investigation was undertaken of the mechanism of resistance to HN2 and other alkylating agents, with particular emphasis on the relationship between cross-resistance and drug transport (GOLDENBERG 1975). HN2-sensitive L5178Y cells were 18.5-fold more responsive to HN2 than were resistant cells. Dose-survival curves were obtained for chlorambucil, melphalan, 1,3-bis(2-chloroethyl)-1-nitrosourea (BCNU), mitomycin C, and trenimon for both the HN2-sensitive and -resistant cell lines. HN2-resistant cells were, in part, cross-resistant to each of these compounds and the degree of cross-resistance was remarkably similar; HN2-resistant cells were approximately two- to three fold more resistant than sensitive cells to the cytocidal effect of each of these drugs. However, a major portion of resistance to HN2 was not shared by these alkylating agents. Furthermore transport of HN2, HN2–OH, and choline was not competitively inhibited by any of these compounds, suggesting that transport of these other alkylating agents was by an independent mechanism. These findings suggested that a major portion of resistance to HN2 may be circumvented by drugs using independent transport mechanisms, and that nontransport factors may explain the partial cross-resistance demonstrated by HN2-resistant cells toward other alkylating agents. Resistance unrelated to transport, such as elevated thiol groups and differences in cross-linking and/or DNA repair, may be relatively nonspecific, since they appear capable of protecting cells to the same degree against a wide range of alkylating agents. Conversely, transport of alkylating agents would appear to be a highly specific process (GOLDENBERG et al. 1970, 1971 a, 1974; GOLDENBERG 1975).

2. Melphalan

a) Historical Review

Melphalan, the phenylalanine derivative of nitrogen mustard, was synthesized with the aim of increasing specificity of action of the mustards; the expectation was that the presence of the amino acid phenylalanine would promote incorporation of the alkylating agent into proteins (BERGEL and STOCK 1953, 1954). BALL et al. (1966) found no difference in uptake of [^{3}H]melphalan by HN2-sensitive and -resistant Yoshida sarcoma cells; however, the experimental design was faulty since it was based on the erroneous assumption that melphalan and HN2 share the same transport system. Uptake of melphalan by sensitive and resistant lines of Yoshida ascites sarcoma was also investigated by HARRAP and HILL (1970). The pattern of uptake and subsequent hydrolysis of melphalan was identical in both sensitive and resistant cells. However, this study was restricted to a time course of melphalan uptake; accordingly a detailed investigation of the mechanism of drug transport by L5178Y cells in vitro was undertaken (GOLDENBERG et al. 1977).

b) Mechanism of Melphalan Transport

In studies of HN2 transport referred to above, hydrolyzed drug was preferred to the intact compound in that transport could be studied without the complication of alkylation reactions (GOLDENBERG et al. 1970, 1971 a). However, with melphalan transport evidence was obtained that uptake of the parent compound and of its hydrolyzed derivative was by independent mechanisms so that it was necessary to utilize intact drug in order to study the transport mechanism. Thin layer chromatography was used to distinguish between free drug and that which had become bound or hydrolyzed.

A time course of melphalan influx by L5178Y lymphoblasts in vitro was approximately linear for 5–10 min and thereafter entered a plateau region (GOLDENBERG et al. 1977). Evidence that influx of melphalan was carrier mediated was that uptake obeyed Michaelis-Menten kinetics and demonstrated chemical specificity. Other alkylating agents including HN2, hydrolyzed HN2, hydrolyzed chlorambucil, and cyclophosphamide had no effect on melphalan uptake, confirming earlier studies that transport of several different alkylating agents occurs by independent systems (GOLDENBERG et al. 1970, 1974).

VISTICA et al. (1976) reported that the amino acids L-leucine and L-glutamine protected L1210 cells against the cytocidal effect of melphalan in vitro. They attributed this protective action to inhibition of [^{14}C]melphalan transport by leucine and glutamine (VISTICA et al. 1976, 1977, 1978 a) and published preliminary evidence that melphalan and leucine share a common transport system in L1210 leukemia cells (VISTICA et al. 1977, 1978 a).

We investigated the mechanism of melphalan uptake in murine LPC-1 plasmacytoma cells in vitro (GOLDENBERG et al. 1978, 1979). Plasmacytoma cells, rather than leukemia cells, were selected using the rationale that such cells were a more appropriate model of human multiple myeloma, a disease which has been treated effectively with melphalan for many years (HOOGSTRATEN et al. 1967; BERGSAGEL et al. 1967; ALEXANIAN et al. 1968). Evidence was obtained that in LPC-1 cells melphalan is actively transported by a carrier mechanism that is mediated by two distinct amino acid transport systems (GOLDENBERG et al. 1978, 1979). A time course of uptake of 100 μM [^{14}C]melphalan was approximately linear for 2 min and thereafter entered a plateau phase. Accordingly, subsequent kinetic experiments were terminated at 2 min in order to approximate initial uptake velocity conditions. Melphalan uptake proceeded "uphill" against a cell/medium concentration ratio (mean $\pm$SD) of 11.0 ± 3.1 at a substrate concentration of 20 μM. Thin layer chromatography of cell sap constituents confirmed that 80%–85% of the radioactivity migrated as a single prominent peak with an R_f value identical to that of free intact drug.

Kinetic analysis of melphalan uptake by plasmacytoma cells over a substrate concentration range of 2–100 μM was biphasic. Kinetic parameters were calculated after correction for rapid binding and application of the Neal analysis for interaction of two-component transport (NEAL 1972). The K_m (mean $\pm$SE) for transport at the low concentration range was 25 ± 6 μM and the V_{max} (mean $\pm$SE) was 0.20 ± 0.06 fmol/cell per min; at the high concentration range the K_m was 95 ± 24 μM and the V_{max} was 0.21 ± 0.04 fmol/cell per min. Since negative cooperativity may produce biphasic kinetic plots (GLOVER et al. 1975), additional evidence for involvement of two or more transport systems for melphalan uptake was sought.

An extensive evaluation of the chemical specificity of melphalan transport by LPC-1 plasmacytoma cells was undertaken. Several amino acids significantly inhibited melphalan transport and the degree of inhibition, with a 50-fold excess of amino acid, ranged from approximately 20% for serine to 75% for leucine. The amino acids included some transported predominantly by system L, system A, or the ASC system, all of which have been described and studied in detail in other cells (CHRISTENSEN and LIANG 1965; CHRISTENSEN et al. 1967; EAVENSON and CHRISTENSEN 1967; GARCIA-SANCHO et al. 1977; OXENDER and CHRISTENSEN 1963; OXENDER et al. 1977; THOMAS and CHRISTENSEN 1971; WINTER and CHRISTENSEN 1965).

To determine the applicability of the L-A-ASC classification of amino acid transport for LPC-1 plasmacytoma cells, influx of glutamine and leucine in the presence of near saturating levels of BCH (D,L-β-2-aminobicyclo[2.2.1]heptane-2-carboxylic acid), AIB (2-aminoisobutyric acid) and serine was examined. Assuming that system L is specifically inhibited by BCH and that system A is inhibited by AIB as in other mammalian (CHRISTENSEN et al. 1967; EAVENSON and CHRISTENSEN 1967; GARCIA-SANCHO et al. 1977; THOMAS and CHRISTENSEN 1971; WINTER and CHRISTENSEN 1965), active transport of glutamine by LPC-1 cells appeared to be mediated by system L, system A, and a third system that may correspond to ASC. Leucine transport was mediated predominantly by system L, and to a lesser extent by system A and a third, unassigned, system which may represent ASC.

The biphasic kinetic plots for melphalan influx and the effects of amino acid inhibitors suggested that a least two transport systems are involved. Melphalan uptake by one component was inhibited by BCH, but was unaffected by Na^+ depletion. Since BCH sensitivity and Na^+ independence are properties of the L system described for other cells (CHRISTENSEN et al. 1967; GARCIA-SANCHO et al. 1967; OXENDER et al. 1977) we have identified this component as system L. Melphalan uptake by the other component was Na^+ dependent, unaffected by BCH, AIB, or Me-AIB [2-(methylamino)isobutyric acid] and was inhibited by at least six amino acids, with the following order of activity: leucine > glutamine > phenylalanine > alanine = serine = cysteine. In other cells, system ASC demonstrates total Na^+ dependence and insensitivity to AIB and Me-AIB and mediates the uptake of several amino acids including alanine, serine, and cysteine (CHRISTENSEN et al. 1967; EAVENSON and CHRISTENSEN 1967; GARCIA-SANCHO et al. 1977; THOMAS and CHRISTENSEN 1971; WINTER and CHRISTENSEN 1965). However, the sequence of reactivity of the amino acids tested in LPC-1 cells differs from what has been observed previously for ASC, especially by the high activity of leucine and phenylalanine (CHRISTENSEN et al. 1967; EAVENSON and CHRISTENSEN 1967; THOMAS and CHRISTENSEN 1971).

There are at least three possible interpretations of these findings. The second melphalan transport component may be: (a) an ASC system more readily inhibited by leucine and phenylalanine than that described previously; (b) a mixture of two or more systems, probably including ASC and one more reactive with leucine and phenylalanine; (c) a heretofore undescribed transport system. The data do not permit a clear choice of one of these options.

At low concentrations of melphalan ranging from 2 to 20 μM, approximately 25% of drug uptake was mediated by system L and 65% by the second component. At higher drug concentrations uptake by system L increased dramatically and that by the second system decreased so that at 100 μ*M* melphalan uptake by both systems was nearly equal. The shift in transport to system L at higher drug concentrations may be due to saturation of the other system, suggesting that the latter may have a lower K_m for melphalan transport.

In view of our findings in LPC-1 plasmacytoma cells that melphalan uptake is an active process, mediated by two separate amino acid transport systems (GOLDENBERG et al. 1979), and the preliminary reports by VISTICA et al. (1977, 1978 a) that melphalan and leucine shared a common transport carrier in L1210 leukemia cells, we reinvestigated in detail the mechanism of melphalan uptake by L5178Y lymphoblasts with particular emphasis on the chemical specificity of the transport process (BEGLEITER et al. 1979). The study produced results qualitatively similar to those described above for LPC-1 plasmacytoma cells.

VISTICA and RABINOVITZ have suggested that the protective activity of amino acids against melphalan cytotoxicity is related to their affinity for the leucine carrier (VISTICA et al. 1978 c; VISTICA 1979). They have also demonstrated that basic amino acids block leucine-conferred protection against melphalan cytotoxicity of L1210 cells in vitro (VISTICA et al. 1978 b). The ability of basic amino acids to abrogate leucine protection appeared to increase with decreasing carbon chain length of the arginine homologous series so that the relative activities were α-amino-γ-guanidinobutyric acid > arginine > homoarginine. However, the lowest arginine homolog, α-amino-β-guanidinopropionic acid, was ineffective. Although cationic amino acids have been shown to stimulate uptake of system L amino acids by exchange diffusion in other cells, the exact mechanism whereby basic amino acids enhance melphalan uptake and cytotoxicity of L1210 cells in the presence of leucine requires further study (VISTICA et al. 1978 b). Recently, the basic amino acids have been shown to raise cellular levels of melphalan in the presence of leucine by acting on the monovalent cation-dependent, high-affinity melphalan influx system and also possibly by antagonizing drug efflux (VISTICA and SCHUETTE 1981).

c) Melphalan Transport by Sensitive and Resistant Cells

REDWOOD and COLVIN studied melphalan transport in melphalan-sensitive and -resistant L1210 cells (REDWOOD and COLVIN 1980). A time course study demonstrated both a lower initial velocity of uptake and a lower intracellular drug concentration at the steady state in resistant cells. At high concentrations of melphalan (14–80 μ*M*), a kinetic analysis of drug uptake showed a three fold increase in the apparent K_m with no significant change in V_{max}; this suggested that resistant cells were characterized by a reduced binding affinity between the system L carrier and drug. At low melphalan concentrations (3–10 μ*M*), the K_m for melphalan influx was four fold higher and the V_{max} approximately 2.5-fold greater in resistant than sensitive cells; this finding suggested a reduced binding affinity between drug and the carrier of the Na^+-dependent ASC-like system. Furthermore, the authors argued that since the transport difference between sensitive and resistant cells at low drug concentrations was eliminated by BCH, a specific inhibitor of system L, the alteration in melphalan transport in resistant cells may represent a specific mutation of system L.

In this study the authors focused attention on the difference in drug influx at low melphalan concentrations, where the Na^+-dependent ASC-like system dominates. The ability of BCH to eliminate transport differences between sensitive and resistant cells at high drug concentrations, where the BCH-sensitive system L is more dominant, was not evaluated.

In a similar but preliminary report, a leucine-transport mutant of Chinese hamster ovary (CHO) cells was isolated on the basis of its inability to grow at a low leucine concentration (DANTZIG et al. 1981). The mutant (CHY-2) exhibited a 50% reduction in the initial uptake rate of leucine, when transport was measured in sodium-free medium in which influx would be restricted to system L. The cytocidal activity of melphalan was evaluated and the CHY-2 mutant was 100 times more resistant to drug than was the parent line. The findings suggested that resistance to melphalan may be due to a specific transport mutant of CHO cells which affects system L.

VISTICA reported differences in melphalan transport between murine bone marrow CFU-C cells and L1210 leukemia cells (VISTICA 1980). Transport activity was evaluated indirectly by measuring the ability of leucine and the synthetic amino acids BCH and AIB to protect cells against melphalan cytotoxicity. Melphalan cytotoxicity against L1210 cells was reduced 50% by BCH; and leucine, but not AIB, completely eliminated the remaining 50%. This suggested that melphalan cytotoxicity to L1210 cells is dependent on drug uptake by two separate amino acid transport systems; one system is BCH sensitive and corresponds to system L, the other is insensitive to BCH and AIB but is sensitive to leucine. However, BCH failed to block melphalan cytotoxicity against bone marrow progenitor cells (CFU-C), although leucine was effective, this signified that CFU-C cells lack the BCH-sensitive system L. VISTICA suggested that synthesis of nitrogen mustard analogs that are transported by the BCH-sensitive system L may result in chemotherapeutic agents with an improved therapeutic index, by exploiting this putative difference in drug transport between tumor cells and host bone marrow stem cells.

Melphalan transport was also investigated in Chinese hamster ovary (CHO) cell mutants resistant to melphalan (ELLIOTT and LING 1981). A colchicine-resistant clone (CH^RC5), isolated previously (LING and THOMPSON 1974), is cross-resistant to a wide variety of drugs including melphalan, chlorambucil, nitrogen mustard, adriamycin, and puromycin. The resistance of this mutant to colchicine and other drugs has been attributed to decreased membrane permeability to those compounds (LING and THOMPSON 1974; SEE et al. 1974). The phenotype of CH^RC5 appears to be correlated quantitatively with the presence of a high molecular weight glycoprotein, called the P-glycoprotein, in the plasma membrane (CARLSEN et al. 1977; JULIANO and LING 1976; RIORDAN and LING 1979). Accumulation of melphalan by whole cells at steady-state conditions was significantly lower in CH^RC5 cells than in the parental line. The mechanism of resistance in CH^RC5 cells was attributed to reduced drug accumulation due to a plasma membrane alteration that also confers resistance to other drugs.

Although the above study reported a correlation between membrane transport and sensitivity to melphalan, no difference in melphalan transport was found in human melanoma cell lines that were sensitive (MM253) or resistant (MM253-

12M) to the drug (PARSONS et al. 1981). The cytocidal activity of melphalan was attributed to comparatively rare DNA cross-linking events and drug resistance was associated with decreased susceptibility of DNA to this damage.

Stably resistant clones of melphalan-resistant cells were also isolated by a single exposure of CHO cells to melphalan (ELLIOTT and LING 1981). The objective was to obtain clones exhibiting the minimal number of changes to give a melphalan-resistant phenotype; the method of selection is presumed to yield clones arising from a single mutation. In two clones of melphalan-resistant CHO cells, Mel^R1 and Mel^R6, uptake of [^{14}C]melphalan was not significantly different from that observed in the parental line, leading the authors to conclude that the Mel^R clones were not membrane-altered mutants of the CH^RC5 type. Analysis of drug uptake into the nuclear and cytoplasmic fractions revealed no difference in drug uptake in the cytoplasmic fraction but decreased drug accumulation in the nuclear fraction of both Mel^R clones. The mechanism of resistance proposed for Mel^R cells was a nuclear alteration of drug processing that might include a mechanism for exclusion of specific drugs from the nucleus or a mechanism by which the interaction of certain drugs with DNA is recognized and cleared rapidly.

3. Cyclophosphamide

As indicated previously, transport studies of alkylating agents may be obscured by covalent binding of drug to cellular constituents through alkylation reactions. However, cyclophosphamide is inactive as an alkylating agent as long as the cyclic phosphamide ester ring structure remains intact (CONNORS et al. 1970; FOLEY et al. 1961; SLADEK 1971), thereby providing an opportunity for studying drug transport without the complication of alkylation reactions.

A time course of cyclophosphamide uptake by L5178Y lymphoblasts showed an initial component of rapid association that was temperature and sodium independent (GOLDENBERG et al. 1974). At time points up to 1 min, a cell/medium ratio of 0.14 ± 0.02 was observed at cyclophosphamide concentrations ranging from 0.1 to 10 mM. This value of 0.14, which presumably represents rapid drug binding to the cell membrane, noted by others for other substances (CHRISTENSEN and LIANG 1965, 1966; GOLDMAN et al. 1968; KESSEL 1971), was routinely subtracted from the observed cell/medium ratio. Subsequent influx into the cells appeared to be carrier mediated and consisted of two components.

Analysis of drug influx over a 40-fold range of drug concentration from 0.25 to 10 mM showed biphasic kinetics with evidence of saturation only at low drug concentrations whereas, at high drug levels, influx occurred by a second transport system that deviated from first-order kinetics but technically could not be saturated. After correction for rapid association and the interaction of two transport components (NEAL 1972), kinetic parameters for the higher affinity transport route were a K_m (mean $\pm$SE) of 0.39 ± 0.03 mM and a transport capacity, V_{max}, of $0.49 \pm 0.07 \times 10^{-17}$ mol/cell per min; the apparent transport K_m for the lower-affinity route was 75 ± 29 mM, and the V_{max} was $49 \pm 14 \times 10^{-17}$ mol/cell per min. Cell/medium distribution ratios of drug did not exceed unity over a drug concentration range of 0.1–10 mM.

In an evaluation of chemical specificity of cyclophosphamide transport, equimolar concentrations of other alkylating agents including HN2, chlorambucil, melphalan, enzyme-activated cyclophosphamide, and isophosphamide failed to inhibit cyclophosphamide influx in L5178Y lymphoblasts. This finding was consistent with studies of transport of other alkylating agents and supported the concept that transport of several alkylating agents proceeds by independent transport mechanisms.

Several naturally occurring substrates were studied in an attempt to identify a native substrate for the cyclophosphamide carrier. However, a wide range of amino acids and several components of nucleic acids had no effect on cyclophosphamide uptake. Thus a native substrate has not yet been identified for the cyclophosphamide carrier. To our knowledge, comparative studies of cyclophosphamide transport in drug-sensitive and drug-resistant cells have not been reported.

4. Nitrosoureas

a) Mechanism of Nitrosourea Transport

The mechanism of uptake of the nitrosoureas BCNU and 1-(2-chloroethyl)-3-cyclohexyl-1-nitrosourea (CCNU) was investigated in L5178Y lymphoblasts in vitro (BEGLEITER et al. 1977). Using thin layer chromatography to separate intact drug from decomposition products evidence was obtained that uptake of [^{14}C] BCNU was by passive diffusion. Drug uptake was temperature independent and reached equilibrium in less than 1 min with a cell/medium distribution ratio of 0.2–0.6. Uptake did not appear to be a saturable process in that neither unlabeled BCNU nor CCNU inhibited uptake of labeled BCNU.

Transport studies of intact CCNU appeared to be more complex. Uptake of either ethylene- or ring-labeled CCNU reached steady-state rapidly, was temperature independent, but unlike BCNU cell/medium distribution ratios were greater than unity. Since it was not possible to examine uptake of intact CCNU under initial uptake velocity conditions, other types of experiments were performed to determine whether there was any evidence that drug uptake was carrier mediated. Evidence against a carrier-mediated process was that uptake of intact CCNU was independent of Na^+ concentration; was unaffected by the metabolic inhibitors, sodium fluoride, sodium cyanide, and DNP; and was not inhibited by CCNU and BCNU. Thus all the evidence obtained except for the cell/medium ratios supported the concept that uptake of intact CCNU was by passive diffusion. The borderline elevation of cell/medium ratio could represent technical variation or non-covalent drug interaction with cell components, allowing further diffusion of drug into the cell. Subsequently, dissociation of the loose binding of intact CCNU from cell constituents during the extraction and/or thin layer chromatographic procedures might artificially increase the cell/medium distribution ratio of intact drug.

Uptake of the glucose-containing nitrosourea, chlorozotocin, was also studied in L5178Y cells (LAM et al. 1980). Thin layer chromatographic analysis showed that uptake of intact drug was not a saturable process, was Na^+ independent, and was not inhibited by several metabolic inhibitors or by the structural analogs glucose or glucosamine. These findings, together with the relatively low temperature quotient for the uptake process, suggested that chlorozotocin uptake also occurs by passive diffusion.

b) Investigation of Resistance and Cross-Resistance to Nitrosoureas and Other Alkylating Agents

An evaluation of resistance and cross-resistance to alkylating agents was performed on three sublines of L1210 leukemia, one resistant to cyclophosphamide (L1210/CPA), one resistant to BCNU (L1210/BCNU), and one resistant to melphalan (L1210/L-PAM); the sublines were stable after 50–400 serial passages (SCHABEL et al. 1978). The L1210/CPA line was "totally resistant" to cyclophosphamide, was partly cross-resistant to melphalan and thio-TEPA, but retained full sensitivity to BCNU, CCNU, methylCCNU (MeCCNU), chlorozotocin, and *cis*-diamminedichloro(DD) platinum. The L1210/BCNU line demonstrated full sensitivity to cyclophosphamide and melphalan. The L1210/L-PAM cell line was fully sensitive to BCNU, CCNU, and MeCCNU; demonstrated partial cross-resistance to chlorozotocin, cyclophosphamide, and melphalan; and complete cross-resistance to *cis*-DD platinum. These studies clearly illustrate that tumor cells selected for resistance to one alkylating agent are not predictably cross-resistant to other alkylating agents.

Unfortunately, a systematic evaluation of drug transport by each of the three resistant sublines was not undertaken by the SCHABEL group. However, REDWOOD and COLVIN (1980) described differences in melphalan transport between the L1210/L-PAM line and the drug-sensitive L1210 parent, as discussed previously (see Sect. C.I.2.c).

5. Chlorambucil

Chlorambucil uptake by Yoshida ascites sarcoma cells was reported to be identical in drug-sensitive and drug-resistant cell lines (HARRAP and HILL 1970). Drug uptake occurred over the first 5 min of the incubation period, during which time there was no significant hydrolysis of the mustard groups. Alkylating activity of the drug declined at a rate 2.5 times faster in resistant than in sensitive cells. Degradation of the aromatic ring of the drug was also reported to be faster in resistant cells (HARRAP and HILL 1970). The enhanced ability of resistant cells to metabolize chlorambucil was associated with lower levels of binding to DNA, RNA, and protein than those observed in sensitive cells (HILL 1972).

The mechanism of chlorambucil uptake by Yoshida ascites sarcoma cells was subsequently reinvestigated by the same group using [^{3}H]chlorambucil (HILL et al. 1971; HILL 1972). Uptake was directly proportional to the drug concentration in the suspending medium suggesting that uptake was by passive diffusion (HARRAP and HILL 1970). Additional evidence for passive diffusion was that chlorambucil uptake was temperature independent, did not proceed against a concentration gradient, and was unaffected by ouabain or metabolic inhibitors such as fluoride, cyanide, 2,4-dinitrophenol (DNP), and iodoacetate (HILL 1972).

A comparison of chlorambucil uptake by sensitive and resistant cells revealed that uptake by sensitive cells at a concentration of 10^6 cell/ml was approximately 50% greater than that of resistant cells, while at 10^8 cell/ml both cell lines contained comparable amounts of drug (HILL et al. 1971). The explanation given for this finding was that sensitive cells might contain a greater number of drug-binding sites than resistant cells and that access to these sites was limited by increasingly close physical contact of cells as their concentration was increased. This report of greater drug uptake by sensitive cells and the accompanying explanation require further evaluation for two reasons: (a) in two other studies by the same group (HARRAP and HILL 1970; HILL 1972) no difference was noted in the extent of drug uptake between sensitive and resistant cells and (b) evidence is presented that chlorambucil uptake occurs by passive diffusion, thus eliminating the need to invoke "drug-binding sites" in the uptake mechanism.

6. Busulfan

Uptake of [^{3}H] busulfan by L1210 cells in vitro was found to be rapid, equilibrium being reached in 1 min, and temperature independent; and the cell/medium distribution ratio did not exceed unity (KESSEL et al. 1969). These findings suggested that busulfan uptake was by passive diffusion. Using either a colorimetric method to measure drug (HARRAP and HILL 1969) or ^{3}H-labeled busulfan (HILL et al. 1971) no difference in drug uptake was detected between sensitive and resistant cells. Furthermore, the rate of disappearance of active drug was comparable in sensitive and resistant cells (HARRAP and HILL 1970).

7. Procarbazine

Uptake of total radioactivity and of free intact procarbazine (PCZ) showed little difference in L5178Y lymphoblasts; in each case uptake reached a plateau within 1 s, showed little, if any, temperature dependence, and the cell/medium distribution ratio never exceeded 0.7 (LAM et al. 1978). The presence of cold PCZ, up to concentrations of 1 m*M*, did not inhibit uptake of 50 μ*M* [^{14}C]PCZ. This indicated that uptake of PCZ was first-order from 50 μ*M* to 1.05 m*M*. Uptake of [^{14}C]PCZ by L5178Y lymphoblasts was not impeded by a wide range of metabolic inhibitors including iodoacetate, *N*-ethylmaleimide (NEM), *p*-hydroxymecuribenzoate (POMB), sodium cyanide, oligomycin, DNP, and *m*-chlorophenyl carbonyl cyanide hydrazone (CCCP). Finally, PCZ uptake was independent of sodium ion concentration.

The findings that the rate of PCZ uptake was of the order of magnitude expected for a simple diffusion system, demonstrated little temperature dependence, was not saturable, was unaffected by several metabolic inhibitors, was sodium insensitive, and that the cell/medium distribution ratio of free intact drug was less than unity all suggested that uptake of PCZ by L5178Y lymphoblasts in vitro occurs by simple diffusion. Drug uptake by sensitive and resistant cell lines has not been described.

8. Hexamethylmelamine and Pentamethylmelamine

Uptake of hexamethylmelamine (HMM) and pentamethylmelamine (PMM) by L5178Y lymphoblasts was studied using both theoretical and experimental approaches (BEGLEITER et al. 1980). Using the analysis of LIEB and STEIN (1969), it was predicted that, if these two drugs enter cells by simple diffusion, uptake would be essentially complete in less than 10 s. Experimentally, uptake of intact HMM and PMM reached a steady state within 10 s, and the cell/medium distribution ratio for HMM was approximately 0.4 and that for PMM did not exceed 0.1. Additional evidence that uptake of both drugs was by simple diffusion was that uptake of intact HMM and PMM showed little temperature dependence and was not inhibited by a variety of metabolic inhibitors. A comparative study of drug uptake in sensitive and resistant cells has not been reported.

II. Antimetabolites

1. Methotrexate

The folic acid antagonist, methotrexate (4-amino-10-methylpteroyl glutamic acid), has probably been studied more extensively than any other cancer chemotherapeutic agent. Detailed reviews of the mechanism of transport of methotrexate and correlates of transport with drug responsiveness have been published (GOLDMAN 1971 a; HARRAP and JACKSON 1978; SIROTNAK 1980; BERTINO 1980). Accordingly this review will present only some of the main features of the transport mechanism and will concentrate on those studies correlating drug responsiveness with transport activity and on attempts that have been made to circumvent resistance due to impaired transport.

a) Mechanism of Methotrexate Transport

Methotrexate (MTX) transport in L1210 leukemia and other murine tumor cells appears to be both a carrier-mediated and an active process (GOLDMAN et al. 1968; GOLDMAN 1971 a; SIROTNAK et al. 1968; SIROTNAK 1980; BERTINO 1980). Drug influx follows Michaelis-Menten kinetics and is chemically specific, being competitively inhibited by folic acid, 5-formyltetrahydrofolate (5-CHO–FH_4) and 5-methyltetrahydrofolate (5-CH_3–FH_4) although the affinity for inhibition by folate is two orders of magnitude lower than that of the reduced folates (GOLDMAN 1971 a). The system is characterized by a high affinity for MTX, with a K_m in the range of 3–10 μM, and a low transport capacity, with a V_{max} of 3–15 mμmol/min per gram dry weight. Additional evidence for a carrier mechanism is that in cells loaded with folic acid, 5-CHO–FH_4, or 5-CH_3–FH_4, methotrexate influx is stimulated, a transconcentration effect known as heterologous exchange diffusion or transstimulation (GOLDMAN 1971 a, 1971 b). More recently, homologous exchange diffusion of [^{3}H] MTX by unlabeled drug has been demonstrated in Ehrlich ascites cells suspended in a high K^+, low Na^+ medium (FRY et al. 1980 a).

Evidence that MTX transport is an active process is that influx is highly temperature sensitive, with a Q_{10} of 6–8 between 27 °C and 37 °C, and also appears to be concentrative, proceeding "uphill" against an electrochemical potential gradient for "free" drug (GOLDMAN et al. 1968; GOLDMAN 1971 a; SIROTNAK and DONSBACH 1976; SIROTNAK 1980; BERTINO 1980). The energy requirements of the system are complex; the presence of a cell/medium gradient for "free" drug would suggest that transport is energy dependent and that the steady-state level of "free" drug should be reduced by metabolic inhibitors (GOLDMAN 1969, 1971 a; FRY et al. 1980 a, 1980 b). However, metabolic antagonists such as azide and DNP increased the steady-state level of MTX. This apparent paradox was explained by preferential inhibition of MTX efflux relative to influx (GOLDMAN 1971 a; FRY et al. 1980a). In the proposed model, MTX influx, which is linked by countertransport to a large gradient of organic phosphates moving out of the cell, is not immediately affected by metabolic inhibitors; however, MTX efflux, which actively drives drug out of the cell, is markedly inhibited by metabolic antagonists. HAKALA (1965) also proposed an active, energy-dependent mechanism for MTX efflux from sarcoma 180 cells.

Influx of MTX and the reduced folates, but not folic acid, are inhibited by sulfhydryl-binding agents, suggesting the importance of sulfhydryl groups in the MTX-tetrahydrofolate carrier (GOLDMAN et al. 1968; RADER et al. 1974). This observation was also interpreted as evidence for a separate carrier for folic acid not shared by MTX or reduced folates (RADER et al. 1974). Additional evidence for a separate carrier for folic acid was the finding that MTX-resistant W1–L2 human lymphoblastoid cells exhibited reduced uptake of MTX and 5-CH_3–FH_4 but not of folic acid (NIETHAMMER and JACKSON 1975).

An asymmetrical model for folate analog transport has also been proposed in which MTX influx and efflux are mediated by separate carriers (DEMBO and SIROTNAK 1976; SIROTNAK 1980). MTX influx into CEM human lymphoblastoid cells was reported to occur by two distinct routes (WARREN et al. 1978). At low-drug doses (1–20 μM), influx was mediated by a temperature-sensitive, high-affinity, saturable process with a K_m of 5.94 μM. At high drug concentrations (20–100 μM), transport was by a second process in which it was not possible to establish if influx was by passive diffusion or a technically nonsaturable carrier-mediated process. The presence of a second route of MTX transport at high drug concentrations may explain the clinical effectiveness of high-dose MTX regimens against MTX-resistant tumors.

b) Resistance to Methotrexate Due to Decreased Drug Transport

Resistance to MTX may arise as a result of: (a) an elevation of the enzyme dihydrofolate reductase (FISCHER 1961); (b) an alteration affecting the membrane permeability of the drug (FISCHER 1962); or (c) a structural alteration of the enzyme dihydrofolate reductase (FLINTOFF and SAYA 1978). Only resistance due to altered membrane permeability will be considered in this review.

The concept of resistance to antitumor agents being due to defective drug transport began with the classical paper by FISCHER (1962), in which defective transport of MTX was the mechanism of resistance established in "second-step" mutants of L5178Y leukemia highly resistant to the drug. At equivalent extracellular concentrations of MTX, drug uptake by sensitive cells was 14 times more rapid than in resistant cells and after equilibration the cell/medium distribution ratio was 2–3 in sensitive cells and only 0.1–0.2 in resistant cells. The activity of folic acid reductase was equal in both cell lines.

MTX uptake was evaluated in ten transplantable mouse leukemias including cell lines with varying degrees of natural resistance, as well as two lines with acquired resistance and one with collateral sensitivity (KESSEL et al. 1965). A highly significant correlation was found between sensitivity of the leukemias to MTX therapy in vivo and drug uptake by each cell line in vitro. These studies were extended to an evaluation of MTX uptake by normal and leukemic human leukocytes in vitro (KESSEL et al. 1968). Drug uptake was significantly greater in patients with either acute lymphoblastic or myeloblastic leukemia who subsequently responded clinically to MTX therapy, compared with unresponsive patients. MTX uptake was not significantly different in a smaller number of sensitive and resistant patients with chronic granulocytic leukemia.

SIROTNAK et al. (1968) investigated the kinetic properties of MTX uptake in a transport mutant of L1210 leukemia. The rate of drug transport in the mutant was reduced four fold and the transport K_m was increased four fold with little change in V_{max}. The authors suggested that resistance to MTX was due primarily to alteration of the binding properties of the MTX carrier. Difficult to explain was the finding that in a second drug-resistant cell line characterized by elevated levels of dihydrofolate reductase and an unaltered rate of drug uptake, the transport K_m for MTX influx was increased threefold and the V_{max} 2.5-fold relative to the parent line.

In a more complete study from the same laboratory the kinetic parameters for MTX transport were compared in five murine tumors exhibiting different drug responsiveness in vivo (SIROTNAK and DONSBACH 1976). Therapeutic responsiveness of the tumors correlated inversely with influx K_m and directly with the steady-state level of drug; no such correlation was noted with either influx V_{max} or efflux rate constant.

Conflicting results were obtained in a study of MTX transport in drug-sensitive and -resistant W1–L2 human lymphoblastoid cell lines (NIETHAMMER and JACKSON 1975). Resistant mutants with elevated levels of dihydrofolate reductase and impaired transport of MTX were isolated. Kinetic analysis of MTX transport in resistant cells was characterized by at least a 17-fold reduction of V_{max} with no significant change in K_m.

Transport properties of MTX, aminopterin, 5-CH_3–FH_4, and folate were evaluated in two L5178Y cell lines, one with impaired transport of MTX (HILL et al. 1979). Transport in the resistant line differed from that in the sensitive line by showing evidence of transport by more than one pathway. Evidence for transport heterogeneity included: (a) only partial inhibition of MTX influx in resistant cells by a sulfhydryl-binding agent that markedly inhibited the MTX-FH_4 carrier in sensitive cells; (b) only partial inhibition of MTX influx by the competitive inhibitor 5-CHO–FH_4 in resistant cells at concentrations that markedly inhibited carrier-mediated influx in sensitive cells; and (c) marked differences in temperature sensitivity with a Q_{10} for drug influx of 6.4 in sensitive cells and only 1.4 in resistant cells. It was estimated that only 25% of MTX influx in resistant cells was mediated by the MTX-FH_4 cofactor carrier. Low transport rates, relatively high surface binding, and the presence of transport heterogeneity with only a small component of MTX influx mediated by the MTX-FH_4 carrier precluded a kinetic analysis of drug influx in resistant cells. Thus, it was impossible to establish if the transport defect in resistant cells was due to an alteration of binding affinity or to a reduction in number and/or mobility of transport carriers.

MTX transport and metabolism was investigated in Reuber H35 rat hepatoma cells sensitive and resistant to MTX (GALIVAN 1979, 1981). Cells resistant to 1 μM MTX, or less, demonstrated defective transport of MTX; cells resistant to higher levels of drug also showed elevated levels of dihydrofolate reductase. Active transport of MTX by a carrier mechanism shared with reduced folates was demonstrated in sensitive cells. The following evidence suggested that the MTX-FH_4 carrier was lost in resistant cells: (a) mutual and reciprocal competitive inhibition of transport of MTX and 5-CH_3–FH_4 was observed in sensitive but not in resistant cells; (b) uptake of MTX and 5-CH_3–FH_4 was temperature dependent in sensitive but not from in resistant cells; (c) the rate of efflux of 5-CH_3–FH_4 was accelerated from sensitive but not from resistant cells, by the presence of MTX in the transport medium; and (d) trans-stimulation of 5-CH_3–FH_4 was noted only in sensitive cells. Although these findings are consistent with the concept of a loss of carrier, MTX influx at higher drug levels continues in resistant cells by a nonsaturable, temperature-insensitive passive diffusion process.

c) Interaction of Methotrexate and Vincristine

The net uptake of MTX in several animal and human cell lines is augmented by vincristine, as described in detail below (see Sect. C.IV.1.c).

d) Circumvention of Methotrexate Resistance Due to Impaired Drug Transport

Several reports have appeared in recent years using a variety of approaches to circumvent MTX resistance resulting from impaired drug transport. NIETHAMMER and JACKSON (1975) showed that W1–L2 human lymphoblastoid cells have a transport pathway for folic acid that is separate from that for MTX, and suggested that antifolate drugs, which enter cells by the folic acid pathway, might circumvent MTX resistance resulting from transport mutations.

ROSOWSKY et al. (1980) offered three approaches for overcoming MTX resistance due to impaired transport: (a) the use of high-dose MTX schedules to permit MTX to enter cells by passive diffusion; (b) the use of “small molecule” antifolates such as triazinate (Baker’s antifol), which lack the negatively charged glutamate side chain, enabling compounds to enter cells more readily by passive diffusion; and (c) the use of “hybrid antifolates” such as mono- and dibutyl esters of MTX, in which the glutamate side chain is modified, rendering the drug more lipophilic and thereby more permeable by diffusion. This group showed that CEM human lymphoblasts 120-fold more resistant to MTX than the parent line as a result of a transport defect were completely sensitive to the mono-butyl ester of MTX and demonstrated collateral sensitivity to the dibutyl ester, as well as to two “small molecule” antifolates. The results supported the concept that MTX-resistant human lymphoblasts, which have impaired carrier-mediated transport of drug, appeared responsive to chemotherapy with lipophilic antifolates that enter cells by passive diffusion.

GALIVAN (1981) postulated that H35 hepatoma cells resistant to MTX lacked a functional transport carrier, and as such could serve as a test system for the evaluation of modified or carrier-bound types of MTX designed to overcome drug resistance. Triazinate, a “small molecule” antifolate, which inhibits dihydrofolate reductase and enters cells by a different pathway than MTX, inhibited growth of transport-resistant H35 hepatoma cells and sensitive cells to the same extent.

Another approach to circumvent transport resistance has been the use of MTX-poly(L-lysine) conjugates, which are transported more effectively by both MTX-sensitive and -resistant Chinese hamster ovary cells in vitro (RYSSER and

SHEN 1978, 1980; SHEN and RYSSER 1979). MTX was conjugated through a carbodiimide-catalyzed reaction to poly(L-lysine) at a ratio approximating one molecule/27 lysyl residues; conjugates of molecular weight ranging from 3,100 to 130,000 had comparable activity.

The ID_{50} for growth inhibition of a MTX-resistant transport mutant was reduced 100-fold if MTX was used as the poly(L-lysine) conjugate rather than as the free drug (RYSER and SHEN 1980). The poly(L-lysine) conjugates failed to inhibit dihydrofolate reductase in vitro and conjugates using poly(D-lysine) had no cytocidal activity, even though cellular uptake of both D and L forms were identical. These findings suggested that two steps are involved in the activity of the conjugates: (a) cellular uptake probably by endocytosis and (b) intracellular breakdown of the conjugate probably by hydrolysis of the polymeric backbone by lysosomal enzymes, leading to release of free MTX. Poly-D lysine is not susceptible to hydrolysis by common proteolytic enzymes and this would explain the absence of growth inhibitory activity of the D isomer.

More recently, the activity of MTX conjugated to bovine serum albumin (BSA) has been compared with that of free drug against MTX-resistant, transport and enzyme mutants of L1210 leukemia (CHU et al. 1981). Transport mutants were more sensitive to MTX-BSA conjugate than enzyme mutants both by growth inhibition and by incorporation of [^{3}H]uridine into DNA. By contrast, transport and enzyme mutants demonstrated comparable resistance to free drug. This suggested that impairment of the normal MTX-FH_4 carrier in transport mutants affected influx of MTX but not uptake of MTX-BSA, confirming previous reports that MTX and MTX-BSA are transported by different mechanisms (CHU and WHITELEY 1980). In vivo, MTX-BSA was equally effective against the sensitive parent line and the resistant transport mutant, whereas MTX was active only against the sensitive parent tumor. Thus, the MTX-BSA conjugate was able to circumvent resistance to MTX in the transport mutant in vivo.

2. 6-Mercaptopurine and 6-Thioguanine

6-Mercaptopurine (6-MP) and 6-thioguanine (6-TG) are purine antimetabolites that are activated by the enzyme hypoxanthine-guanine phosphoribosyl transferase (HGPRTase) to the nucleotide form (BROCKMAN 1961, 1963a). The mechanism of action of 6-MP is probably inhibition of conversion of inosinic acid to adenylic and guanylic acids (DAVIDSON 1960; SALSER et al. 1960), whereas 6-TG is incorporated into DNA and thereby inhibits DNA replication (LEPAGE 1960; LEPAGE and JONES 1961; BROCKMAN 1963a). In addition both agents may act by inhibition of de novo purine biosynthesis (BROCKMAN 1963b, 1965; SARTORELLI and LEPAGE 1958).

a) Mechanism of Purine Antimetabolite Transport

Uptake of 6-MP by normal human leukocytes was rapid, reaching near steady-state conditions in less than 2 min (KESSEL and HALL 1967). Uptake was temperature insensitive and nonsaturable, and cell/medium distribution ratios approximated unity over the concentration range from 100 μM to 5 mM; however, these studies were performed at the steady state rather than at initial uptake velocity conditions. Drug efflux was rapid, reaching a plateau after 10 min with greater than 80% of the drug leaving the cell. A later study with murine leukemia cells demonstrated that the cell/medium distribution ratio approximated unity for extracellular concentrations of 6-MP ranging from 50 μ*M* to 1 m*M* (KESSEL and HALL 1969b). Based on these findings KESSEL and HALL concluded that 6-MP uptake was by a passive diffusion mechanism. A study by BIEBER and SARTORELLI (1964) of 6-TG uptake in sarcoma 180 cells showed that the cell/medium distribution ratio for drug also approximated unity at the steady state.

Conflicting evidence has been obtained suggesting that influx of purine antimetabolites is mediated by a facilitated diffusion mechanism. The uptake of adenine and xanthine in rabbit neutrophils appeared to be mediated by distinct facilitated diffusion mechanisms; excess 6-MP inhibited cellular uptake of xanthine by greater than 80% (HAWKINS and BERLIN 1969). In addition uptake of [^{14}C]6-MP by mouse neuroblastoma cells was significantly inhibited by adenine or unlabeled drug (BASKIN and ROSENBERG 1975). A more detailed study of the transport mechanism of these agents would be of interest.

b) Resistance to Purine Antimetabolites Due to Impaired Drug Permeability

Although the most common mechanism of resistance to 6-MP is reduced activation of the drug due to low levels of HGPRTase (BROCKMAN 1961, 1963a, 1963b, 1965), several examples of resistance due to decreased drug permeability have been reported. PATERSON (PATERSON 1962; PATERSON and HORI 1962) studied the synthesis of thioinosinate from 6-MP in intact cells and extracts of Ehrlich ascites carcinoma sensitive and resistant to the drug. Sensitive cells accumulated substantial amounts of thioinosinate in the presence of 6-MP, whereas resistant cells contained only low levels of this nucleotide. However, the capacity of extracts from both cell lines to synthesize thioinosinate was similar; furthermore, no difference in purine nucleotide metabolism was noted in the two cell lines. It was concluded that the failure of intact resistant cells to synthesis thioinosinate was due to reduced permeability to 6-MP.

In a study of two mouse neuroblastoma cell lines 110- and 575-fold resistant to 6-MP, the resistant cells showed considerably less accumulation of [^{14}C]6-MP when compared with sensitive cells (BASKIN and ROSENBERG 1975). The drug accumul lation rates and plateau concentration of 6-MP correlated with the degree of resistance. In addition both resistant cell lines appeared to have normal HGPRTase activity, suggesting that decreased drug uptake was the primary cause of resistance in these cells. By contrast several studies with L1210 leukemia and sarcoma 180 have revealed no significant differences in uptake of either 6-MP or 6-TG by sensitive and resistant cells (DAVIDSON 1958; BIEBER and SARTORELLI 1964).

Other mechanisms of resistance to 6-MP include an increased capacity for de novo purine synthesis (BALIS et al. 1958) and altered affinity of the pyrophosphorylase enzyme for 6-MP (BROCKMAN et al. 1961). Mechanisms of resistance to 6-TG appear to be more varied (BROCKMAN 1961, 1963a, 1963b, 1965). They include decreased pyrophosphorylase activity (STUTTS and BROCKMAN 1963), greater capacity to degrade 6-TG (SARTORELLI et al. 1958), enhanced breakdown of the active nucleotide form of 6-TG by alkaline phosphohydrolase (WOLPERT et al. 1971; LEE et al. 1978), and increased conversion of 6-TG to the nucleoside level and subsequent efflux from the cell (LEE and SARTORELLI 1981).

c) Circumvention of Resistance to Purine Antimetabolites

Several limited attempts have been made to overcome resistance to the purine antimetabolites. LEPAGE used 2′-deoxythioguanosine instead of 6-TG to overcome resistance to 6-TG in two resistant cell lines; in one, resistance was due to decreased activity of HGPRTase and in the other, to decreased conversion of ribonucleotides to deoxyribonucleotides (LEPAGE et al. 1964). Although the deoxyribonucleoside showed some activity in these cells, other cell lines were unresponsive (NELSON et al. 1975). Other studies have used metallo complexes of 6-MP (SKINNER and LEWIS 1977) and encapsulation of 6-MP into liposomes (KANO and FENDLER 1977). Circumvention of resistance due to reduced drug transport has not been studied.

3. Fluorouracil

The transport of 5-fluorouracil (5-FU) in isolated cells was thought to take place by a passive diffusion mechanism (JACQUEZ 1962; KESSEL and HALL 1967); however more recent work has shown that uracil and its derivatives enter cells and tissues on a membrane carrier system that is shared with other purine and pyrimidine bases (HAWKINS and BERLIN 1969; BERLIN and OLIVER 1975; WOHLHUETER et al. 1980). In several cell lines uptake appears to be a facilitated diffusion process, although an additional diffusional process operates at high concentrations of the bases (BERLIN and OLIVER 1975). By contrast influx of 5-FU across the intestinal epithelium was shown to be mediated by an active transport mechanism (SCHANKER and JEFFREY 1961).

The mechanism of action of 5-FU is believed to involve formation of 5-fluoro-2′-deoxyuridine-5′-monophosphate which inhibits the activity of thymidylate synthetase. In addition 5-FU is converted to the triphosphate and incorporated into RNA (LASKIN et al. 1979; HEIDELBERGER 1965).

The mechanism of resistance of cells to 5-FU has been studied extensively (LASKIN et al. 1979; ARDALAN et al. 1980; KASBEKAR and GREENBERG 1963; KESSEL et al. 1966). Reduced uptake of label by resistant cells treated with radiolabeled 5-FU has been reported by some workers (LASKIN et al. 1979); however, more careful study revealed that the decreased incorporation of radioactivity resulted from reduced drug metabolism and that the kinetics of transport (ARDALAN et al. 1980) and the intracellular levels of free intact drug were unchanged in resistant cells (LASKIN et al. 1979). The primary mechanism of resistance to 5-FU appears to result from reduced conversion of the drug to its active nucleotides as a result of reduced enzyme activity (LASKIN et al. 1979; ARDALAN et al. 1980; KASBEKAR and GREENBERG 1963; REICHARD et al. 1959, 1962). Another mechanism of resistance that has been described involves an altered thymidylate synthetase that is not inhibited by 5-fluoro-2′-deoxyuridine-5′-monophosphate (HEIDELBERGER et al. 1960).

Ribose donors such as glucose and inosine were found to stimulate the action of 5-FU (KESSEL and HALL 1969a; GOTTO et al. 1969; KUNG et al. 1963) and this was accompanied by increased drug uptake. However, the increased uptake was unrelated to transport since the intracellular levels of parent drug remained unchanged although metabolism and incorporation of the resulting nucleotide into RNA was potentiated (KESSEL and HALL 1969a; GOTTO et al. 1969).

4. Arabinosylcytosine and Arabinosyladenine

1-β-D-Arabinofuranosylcytosine (araC) transport was studied in a resistant subline of L1210 murine leukemia which is unable to metabolize the nucleoside (KESSEL and SHURIN 1968). Uptake was strongly temperature dependent but the cell/medium distribution ratio over a broad range of external nucleoside levels was approximately unity at 37 °C. However, at 0 °C, where uptake was considerably slower and could be measured more accurately, drug influx was clearly saturable and uptake of araC was inhibited by purine and pyrimidine nucleosides but not by free bases, arabinose, or metabolic inhibitors. These findings suggested that araC transport was by a facilitated diffusion mechanism. Efflux of araC was also a rapid temperature-dependent, saturable process that was inhibited by pyrimidine but not by purine nucleosides (KESSEL and SHURIN 1968).

Studies with Yoshida sarcoma cells and L1210 and L5178Y leukemic cells demonstrated the existence of two facilitated diffusion systems for uptake of araC, a high-affinity system with a K_m of 400 μM and V_{max} of 100–130 nmol/min per 10^9 cells and a high-capacity system with a K_m of 2 mM and V_{max} of 200–300 nmol/min per 10^9 cells at 19 °C (MULDER and HARRAP 1975). By contrast PLAGEMANN reported the existence of only one facilitated diffusion system for this drug in cultured Novikoff rat hepatoma cells (PLAGEMANN et al. 1978). A kinetic study of araC transport in rat fibroblasts revealed a carrier-mediated mechanism displaying a K_m of approximately 500 μM and a V_{max} of approximately 300 pmol/min per 10^6 cells at 20 °C (KOREN et al. 1979). CASS and PATERSON demonstrated that 9-β-D-arabinosyladenine (araA) accelerated the exchange diffusional efflux of uridine by a "trans" membrane effect in human erythrocytes (CASS and PATERSON 1973). The uptake of araA by human and mouse erythrocytes can be inhibited by nitrobenzylthioinosine, a potent inhibitor of nucleoside transport (CASS and PATERSON 1975). These studies show that araC and araA enter a variety of animal and human cells by a facilitated diffusion mechanism which they share with other nucleosides (BERLIN and OLIVER 1975).

Both araC and araA are readily converted to their 5′-triphosphates (BRINK and LEPAGE 1964; SCHRECKER 1970), which may act as competitive inhibitors of DNA polymerase (BRINK and LEPAGE 1964; YORK and LEPAGE 1966; FURTH and COHEN 1968; DICIOCCIO and SRIVASTAVA 1977; MULLER et al. 1975, 1977). In addition they may be incorporated into DNA and at high concentrations may cause chromosome breakage (MULLER et al. 1975; NICHOLS 1964) or they may be incorporated into RNA (CHU and FISCHER 1968).

No evidence has been obtained for the involvement of transport in resistance to araC and araA. In fact, several studies with two lines of L5178Y cells resistant to araC showed no difference in incorporation of this drug into resistant cells compared with sensitive cells (CHU and FISCHER 1965; MOMPARLER et al. 1968). Resistance to both araC and araA in a number of cell lines has been shown to be due to reduced kinase activity resulting in decreased formation of the active nucleoside triphosphates (CHU and FISCHER 1965; SCHRECKER 1970; UCHIDA and KREIS 1969). In addition, resistance to these two agents may result from the presence of elevated levels of specific deaminases which inactivate the drugs (KOSHIURA and LAPAGE 1968; HO and FREI 1971). Some success has been reported for the use of adenosine deaminase inhibitors in overcoming resistance resulting from deamination (CASS 1979).

III. Antibiotics

1. Actinomycin D

The antibiotic, actinomycin D, which is obtained from a culture broth of *Streptomyces,* has been particularly useful in the treatment of choriocarcinoma in women and of Wilm's tumor and rhabdomyosarcoma in children (CALABRESI and PARKS 1980). The drug binds to DNA, by intercalation between adjacent guanine-cytosine base pairs, resulting in inhibition of DNA-dependent RNA polymerase. The formation of the DNA-actinomycin D complex introduces a complication into studies of the mechanism of drug uptake, in that uptake of radiolabeled drug is dependent on drug binding to DNA, dissociation of drug from the complex, as well as transport considerations.

a) Mechanism of Actinomycin D Transport

From a review of the literature, it is apparent that a well-defined mechanism of influx of actinomycin D has not been established. In a preliminary report, uptake of [^{3}H]actinomycin D by lens epithelial cells was temperature sensitive and was also inhibited by dinitrophenol (SONNEBORN and ROTHSTEIN 1966). These findings suggested that actinomycin D uptake might be carrier mediated; however, it was recognized that drug binding to DNA complicated this interpretation.

KESSEL and WODINSKY (1968) also noted that uptake of actinomycin D by L1210 cells was temperature sensitive. A cell/medium distribution ratio of 2 was obtained after 5–10 min of uptake at 37 °C. However, the contribution of drug binding was not evaluated, nor was a Q_{10} for drug influx measured to determine whether temperature sensitivity was of such a level so as to invoke a carrier-mediated process. In a subsequent report from this same laboratory, the implication was made that a temperature-sensitive facilitated uptake process for actinomycin D was present in drug-sensitive L5178Y cells but supporting evidence was not presented (KESSEL and BOSMANN 1970).

Influx of actinomycin D in Ehrlich ascites cells was first-order over a broad concentration range, a finding against a high-affinity transport carrier (BOWEN and GOLDMAN 1975). Influx of actinomycin D was temperature dependent with a Q_{10} of 4.5 between 27° and 37 °C; however, this was attributed in part to the high thermal energy required to break hydrogen bonds, to permit drug penetration of the lipid membrane. Neither drug influx nor binding was inhibited by metabolic antagonists and the apparent chemical gradient for exchangeable actinomycin D was accounted for by loose binding of drug within the cell. BOWEN and GOLDMAN (1975) were unable to distinguish whether drug transport was by diffusion or by a low-affinity carrier mechanism.

b) Drug Uptake in Sensitive and Resistant Cells

SLOTNICK and SELLS (1964) working with drug-sensitive and resistant strains of the bacteria B subtilis were the first to report that resistance to actinomycin D was due to a difference in drug uptake. Incorporation of [^{14}C]uracil into cellular RNA was completely inhibited by actinomycin D in sensitive whole cells but only partially blocked in drug-resistant cells. However, incorporation of uracil into RNA of protoplasts was completely inhibited in preparations from both sensitive and resistant cells. Since other studies had shown that actinomycin D was not degraded in resistant cells, resistance was considered to result from a change in cell permeability.

Hela cells were rendered resistant to actinomycin D by intermittent exposure to increasing concentrations of the antibiotic (GOLDSTEIN et al. 1960). Uptake of [^{3}H]actinomycin D was 100-fold greater in drug-sensitive than in resistant cells and radioautographic studies showed that only the nuclei of sensitive cells incorporated the tritium (GOLDSTEIN et al. 1966). Thus resistance of mammalian cells to actinomycin D was also attributable to changes in membrane permeability.

KESSEL and WODINSKY (1968) examined uptake of actinomycin D in vitro and in vivo in six mouse leukemia cell lines, which varied in sensitivity to the drug from complete resistance to "cures." Drug uptake in vitro was similar for all six cell lines tested. However, uptake of [^{3}H]actinomycin D by cells in vivo, in mice with ascitic tumors, appeared to be directly proportional to the sensitivity of the cell lines to the drug. The reason for the different uptake behaviour of cells in vitro and in vivo was stated to be unknown.

In a later publication by the same group, uptake of actinomycin D by L5178Y cells was reduced in resistant cells both in vivo and in culture (KESSEL and BOSMANN 1970). The cell/medium distribution ratio of drug was 10 in sensitive cells and approximately 0.5 in resistant cells 30 min after treatment in vivo. The authors acknowledged that because of drug binding to cell components these findings could not be interpreted solely in terms of transport. The transport medium was critical for the in vitro studies; drug uptake was identical in sensitive and resistant L5178Y cells cultured in Tris-buffered medium; however, drug uptake by resistant cells was markedly reduced in Fischer's medium. Although this influence of the transport medium was attributed to growth requirements of drug-resistant L5178Y cells, it may reflect the presence of a glucose-dependent active efflux mechanism for actinomycin D, operative only in glucose-containing medium such as Fischer's, and analogous, if not identical to, the efflux system for anthracycline antibiotics (see Sect. C.III.2.b, below).

In a study of SV-40 transformed Syrian hamster cell lines, resistance to actinomycin D was not related to changes in drug uptake; differences in membrane permeability between sensitive and resistant cells were less than 20%, a value considered inadequate to explain the level of resistance (SIMARD and CASSINGENA 1969). However, in a subsequent report from the same laboratory using the same cell lines, uptake of [^{3}H]actinomycin D was 100-fold greater in sensitive cells than in resistant cells and permeability differences were considered the major factor in the development of resistance (LANGELIER et al. 1974). No difference was noted between sensitive and resistant cells in either the capacity of chromatin to bind actinomycin D or in the sensitivity of RNA polymerase to the drug.

The reduced permeability to actinomycin D in resistant cells might be due to changes in the glycoprotein content of the cell membrane (KESSEL and BOSMANN 1970). Assays for carbohydrates in protein released by papain revealed that membranes from resistant cells contained more carbohydrate, fucose, and sialic acid, in papain-sensitive linkages, than did the parent L5178Y line. Enzymes responsible for glycoprotein formation and degradation were also measured. The activity of degradative glycosidases, especially α-glucosidase and β-*N*-acetylglucosaminidase, was lower in resistant cells; the finding that acid phosphatase activity was identical in sensitive and resistant cells suggested that the decreased glycosidase activity was not simply due to a general decrease of lysosomal enzyme activity. The resistant cells also had a higher activity of membrane and secreted glycoprotein transferases; the most striking increases were noted for the endogenous transfer of glucose (collagen : glucosyl assay) and the exogenous transfer of fucose onto fetuin and porcine submaxillary glycoprotein (KESSEL and BOSMANN 1970).

c) Cross-resistance of Actinomycin D-Resistant Cells to Other Chemotherapeutic Agents

Chinese hamster fibroblast cell lines up to 2,500-fold more resistant than the parent cell line to actinomycin D were obtained by exposing cells stepwise to increasing concentrations of drug in vitro (BIEDLER and RIEHM 1970). Dose-response studies of sensitive and resistant cells showed that actinomycin D-resistant cells were cross-resistant to mithramycin, vinblastine, and mitomycin C in decreasing order. In general, the greater the molecular weight of a drug, the greater was the degree of cross-resistance observed, although the relationship was imperfect. In a series of resistant sublines, as resistance to actinomycin D increased there was a decrease in sensitivity to both daunorubicin (DNR) and vincristine (VCR). A log plot of the ED_{50} values (the concentration of drug that kills 50% of the cells) for actinomycin D against similar values for DNR and VCR followed a linear relationship.

Autoradiographs of sensitive cells and of several resistant sublines following treatment with [^{3}H]actinomycin D showed an inverse relationship between the degree of drug resistance and the extent of nuclear labeling. Similarly, radioautography of cells exposed to [^{3}H]uridine and unlabeled drug demonstrated an inverse relationship between drug resistance and inhibition of uridine incorporation.

In a reciprocal study daunorubicin-resistant Chinese hamster cells were also shown to be cross-resistant to actinomycin D. This phenomenon is discussed in greater detail below (see Sect. C.III.2). These studies supported the hypothesis that resistance to actinomycin D in Chinese hamster cells is due to qualitative differences in the cell membrane resulting in decreased permeability to actinomycin D and other drugs.

SV-40 transformed Syrian hamster cell lines resistant to actinomycin D were also shown to be cross-resistant to puromycin but not to cytosine arabinoside (LANGELIER et al. 1974). Furthermore, the resistant hamster cell lines were cross-resistant to two other chemically unrelated antibiotics, nogalamycin and chromomycin, although both agents also inhibit DNA-dependent RNA polymerase (SIMARD and CASSINGENA 1969).

d) Circumvention of Resistance to Actinomycin D by Drug-Containing Vesicles

Chinese hamster cells 250-fold more resistant to actinomycin D than the parent sensitive line were treated in vitro with either free actinomycin D or actinomycin D entrapped within lipid vesicles (POSTE and PAPAHADJOPOULOS 1976). The dose of antibiotic required to inhibit RNA synthesis in resistant cells was reduced 200-fold and that needed for inhibition of cell growth was lowered 100-fold, if the drug was delivered in lipid vesicles rather than in the free form. Cells exposed to [^{3}H] actinomycin D in vesicles incorporated five to six times more drug than cells treated with identical concentrations of free actinomycin D. The finding that vesicle-mediated delivery of actinomycin D increased drug uptake only five- to six fold, but reduced the dose of drug required to inhibit cell growth and RNA synthesis by 100- to 200-fold, suggested that the vesicles may deliver drug to a particularly sensitive site of drug action within the cell.

The actinomycin D-resistant phenotype results from a lower capacity to incorporate actinomycin D, produced by a lower permeability of the cell membrane to drug. Vesicle-mediated delivery of drug into resistant tumor cells appears to be a method of circumventing drug resistance. This approach might be applicable in vivo, especially if "recognition ligands" could be incorporated into the vesicle membrane to induce preferential uptake of vesicles by tumor cells.

2. Daunorubicin and Doxorubicin

Daunorubicin (DNR) and doxorubicin (Adriamycin) are antibiotics produced by the fungus *Streptomyces peucetius* (CALABRESI and PARKS 1980). These agents are anthracyclines with a tetracyclic ring structure and an unusual sugar, daunosamine, attached by a glycosidic linkage. Their chemical structures differ by a single hydroxyl group at position 14.

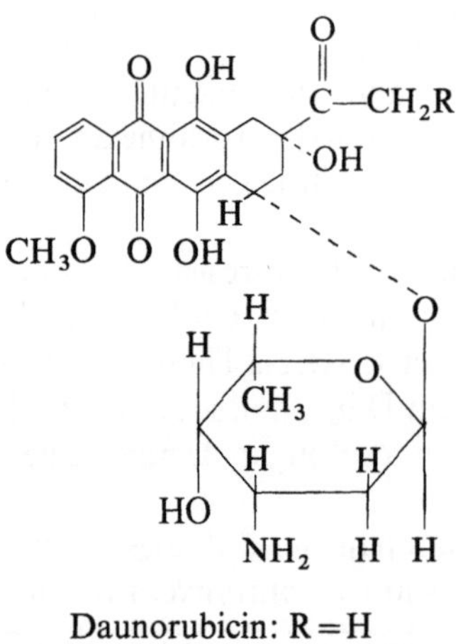

Daunorubicin: R = H

Doxorubicin: R = OH

DNR is useful in the treatment of acute leukemias, and doxorubicin is active against a wide range of solid tumors, as well as the acute leukemias and non-Hodgkin's lymphoma.

a) Mechanism of Daunorubicin and Doxorubicin Transport

Although general agreement exists in the literature that efflux of anthracycline antibiotics is mediated by an active carrier-mediated process (DANO 1973; SKOVSGAARD 1978a, b, c, 1980; INABA et al. 1979; DI MARCO 1978), the evidence is less conclusive with respect to drug influx. In an early study, uptake of DNR was linear with increasing drug concentration but it was not possible to determine whether uptake was by passive diffusion or a nonsaturable carrier-mediated mechanism (DANO 1973). A decrease in the steady-state level of DNR with temperature, combined with the finding of carrier-mediated efflux, suggested that influx was also carrier mediated and more temperature dependent than efflux. The finding that adriamycin (ADR) reduced accumulation of daunorubicin also supported the concept that DNR influx was carrier mediated (DANO 1973).

Subsequently SKOVSGAARD (1978a) presented evidence that influx of DNR and ADR was carrier mediated. Influx of both drugs demonstrated chemical specificity and obeyed simple saturation kinetics. Furthermore influx of DNR was highly temperature sensitive ($Q_{10} = 2.9$), and evidence of countertransport of DNR was also obtained.

The K_m for DNR acting as substrate was similar to the K_i for the drug serving as inhibitor (SKOVSGAARD 1978a). However, the inhibitory activity of ADR on DNR influx was five fold less effective than would have been expected from the K_m of ADR acting as transport substrate. This finding suggested that DNR influx might be mediated by more than one transport system. However, the monophasic Lineweaver-Burk plot of DNR influx was evidence against the involvement of more than one system.

There was no evidence that DNR influx was an active process (SKOVSGAARD 1978a, b). Although the mean intracellular drug concentration very rapidly exceeded the extracellular concentration, this was not a result of influx against an electrochemical gradient but represented drug binding to DNA. Based on the binding affinity for cell homogenate, the cell/medium distribution ratio of free DNR at the steady state in Ehrlich ascites cells was 0.6–1.0 (SKOVSGAARD 1978b). The initial rate of uptake of DNR was increased by the metabolic inhibitor sodium azide and this was attributed to inhibition of the active efflux mechanism. Indeed the component of active efflux is detectable so early in the uptake process that determination of unidirectional influx is not possible in standard medium (SKOVSGAARD 1978c).

b) Drug Resistance Secondary to Alterations of Membrane Transport

Chinese hamster cell lines highly resistant to DNR were obtained by treating sensitive cells with various time-dose schedules of drug in vitro (RIEHM and BIEDLER 1971). Cell lines almost 900-fold more resistant to DNR were obtained, and these demonstrated complete cross-resistance to ADR and considerable cross-resistance to actinomycin D. Radioautographic studies with [^{3}H]DNR showed a decrease in grain counts over the nuclei of resistant cells, leading the authors to suggest that resistance to DNR is due primarily to differences in the cell membrane, resulting in decreased permeability to the drug.

DANO (1973), using spectrofluorometric and isotopic techniques, compared the uptake of DNR by sensitive and resistant Ehrlich ascites cells and isolated nuclei. Little difference was noted in drug binding to isolated nuclei of the two cell types, but uptake by resistant whole cells was markedly reduced (DANO et al. 1972; DANO 1973). Furthermore accumulation of DNR in resistant cells was enhanced by structural analogs (*N*-acetyldaunorubicin and daunorubicinol) and by metabolic inhibitors (2-deoxyglucose and iodoacetate). The lower rate of DNR uptake in resistant cells was attributed to a higher rate of active drug efflux and a lower rate of drug influx.

Vincristine (VCR) and vinblastine (VLB) also increased the intracellular accumulation of DNR in resistant cells. This finding, together with the observation that DNR-resistant cells are cross-resistant to the *Vinca* alkaloids, suggested that these drugs share a common extrusion mechanism with DNR (DANO 1973). An active efflux system for DNR was also present in sensitive cells but operated at a lower level of activity than that found in resistant cells.

Uptake and binding of DNR were evaluated in Ehrlich ascites cells sensitive and resistant to the drug (SKOVSGAARD 1978 b). At the steady state the cell/medium distribution ratio was about ten times higher in sensitive than in resistant cells. Furthermore, cell homogenates of sensitive cells bound significantly more daunorubicin than homogenates of resistant cells. Based on the binding affinity for cell homogenates, the cytoplasm/medium ratio for DNR in sensitive cells was 0.6–1.0 and that in resistant cells was below 0.15.

In both DNR-sensitive and -resistant cells drug uptake in glucose-free medium containing azide was increased; however, this effect was three times greater in resistant than in sensitive cells. Influx followed saturation kinetics with a K_m of 35 μg/ml and a V_{max} of 1.27 μg/μl of packed cells/min in sensitive cells, compared with a K_m of 21.9 μg/ml and a V_{max} of 0.54 μg/μl of packed cells/min in resistant cells. Thus the lower drug influx in resistant cells was due primarily to a lower V_{max}, signifying either a lower number of reactive sites or reduced carrier mobility (SKOVSGAARD 1978 b).

DNR efflux was also studied in drug-sensitive and -resistant Ehrlich ascites cells (SKOVSGAARD 1978 a, b, c). In both cell types efflux was biphasic, consisting of an initial rapid phase, probably due to exodus of free drug or drug weakly bound to intracellular components, and a second slower phase, which may represent efflux of drug more firmly bound to DNA in the nucleus (SKOVSGAARD 1978 b). The initial rapid phase of efflux was significantly greater in resistant cells than in wild-type cells; however, the second slower phase was nearly equal for both cell lines. DNR efflux from cells suspended in glucose-free medium containing either sodium azide or iodoacetic acid was markedly enhanced by the addition of glucose (SKOVSGAARD 1978 b, c); this effect was more pronounced in resistant cells than in sensitive cells (SKOVSGAARD 1980).

At higher drug concentrations the homogenate of wild-type Ehrlich ascites cells bound significantly more DNR than did that of resistant cells. Therefore, the lower drug uptake observed in resistant cells was attributed to at least three different mechanisms: (a) decreased drug influx, (b) increased active drug efflux, and (c) reduced affinity for intracellular binding sites (SKOVSGAARD 1978 b).

Uptake of DNR and ADR was also studied in P388 leukemia cells sensitive and resistant to ADR (INABA and SAKURAI 1979; INABA et al. 1979). Net uptake of both anthracyclines was markedly enhanced in sensitive and resistant cells by metabolic inhibitors in the absence of glucose, apparently due to inhibition of an active drug efflux system. Under these conditions, unidirectional drug influx was examined and no difference was detected in the uptake of either DNR or ADR by sensitive and resistant P388 cells (INABA et al. 1979). Influx was reported to be by simple diffusion but efflux was an active process. Binding of DNR to the nuclei of ADR-sensitive and -resistant P388 cells was similar (INABA and JOHNSON 1978). Thus resistance to ADR was attributed solely to a more active drug efflux mechanism in resistant cells (INABA et al. 1979).

Somewhat different results were obtained in a study of DNR and ADR uptake by L1210 cells sensitive or resistant to DNR (L1210/DNR) or to ADR (L1210/ADR). In sensitive cells uptake of DNR was considerably greater than that of ADR (CHERVINSKY and WANG 1976). Although a kinetic analysis of uptake of each drug appeared to follow saturation kinetics, no apparent attempt was made to distinguish between drug influx and binding to intracellular sites. Using a fluorescent technique no evidence of efflux of either drug was detected from sensitive cells.

Uptake of DNR was markedly reduced in L1210/DNR cells relative to that observed in L1210/S cells, both in vitro and in vivo, but no difference in ADR uptake was found between L1210/S and L1210/ADR cells. Uptake of DNR was also not significantly different in L1210/S and L1210/ADR cells, but uptake of ADR was 30% lower in DNR-resistant cells than in sensitive cells. Using a fluorescent technique no evidence of efflux of either drug was detected from sensitive cells; similar studies were not described for drug-resistant cells.

Uptake of DNR and ADR by human leukemia cells in vitro was also studied in five patients, one with AML and four with ALL (CHERVINSKY and WANG 1976). Uptake of DNR ranged from 1.8–3.5 $\mu g/10^7$ cells and that of ADR from 0.3–1.2 $\mu g/10^7$ cells. It was not possible to correlate any differences in drug uptake with differences in clinical response.

c) The Interrelationship of Drug Transport and Cross-Resistance to Anthracycline Antibiotics and *Vinca* Alkaloids

In several studies cross-resistance between anthracycline antibiotics and *Vinca* alkaloids has been demonstrated (BIEDLER and RIEHM 1970; DANO 1972; INABA and SAKURAI 1979; SKOVSGAARD 1978c). An investigation of the mechanism of cross-resistance of Ehrlich ascites cells to DNR and VCR was undertaken as a model of cross-resistance to anthracycline antibiotics and *Vinca* alkaloids (SKOVSGAARD 1978c). No significant difference was detected in a time course of [^{3}H] VCR uptake in cells resistant to DNR (EHR2/DNR) and in cells resistant to VCR (EHR2/VCR); however, wild-type cells (EHR2) accumulated nearly six fold more drug at steady state. Uptake of [^{3}H]VCR and of DNR was decreased in both resistant cell lines; if the cells were treated with metabolic inhibitors in glucose-free medium, uptake of [^{3}H]VCR and of DNR was markedly augmented in both resistant cell types. The study demonstrated active extrusion of DNR and VCR from cells resistant either to DNR or VCR; these findings suggested that an energy-dependent efflux process was the common mechanism of resistance to DNR and VCR.

No obvious similarity in chemical structure exists between DNR and VCR: DNR is a glycoside consisting of a tetracyclic aglycone, daunomycinone, and an amino sugar, daunosamine; whereas VCR is a dimeric periwinkle alkaloid. In order to share a common active efflux pathway portions of the two molecules may have a similar configuration but this is not apparent from the structural formulae (SKOVSGAARD 1978c).

Influx of DNR and VCR was also reduced in both EHR2/DNR and EHR2/VCR cell lines, compared with wild-type cells. Thus reduced drug influx as well as enhanced drug efflux contribute to VCR and DNR resistance. The lower influx in resistant cells could reflect a change in a common carrier system; however, a 50-fold excess of VCR had no effect on DNR influx, a finding which does not suggest a chemically specific transport mechanism. The reduced influx of the drugs in resistant cells may represent nonspecific changes in membrane structure (SKOVSGAARD 1978c).

A stable ADR-resistant subline (P388/ADR) of mouse leukemia P388 (P388/S) was obtained by repeated treatment of the latter in vivo (INABA and SAKURAI 1979). The subline was 69-fold more resistant to ADR than the wild-type line; cross-resistance of the subline to other drugs was also observed, amounting to 223-fold against actinomycin D, 64-fold against VCR, and 44-fold against VLB, compared with the sensitivity of P388/S cells. Decreased uptake of [^{3}H] VLB, [^{3}H] VCR, and [^{3}H]actinomycin D was found in ADR-resistant cells. Uptake of the three drugs was augmented by the metabolic inhibitor 2,4-dinitrophenol (DNP) in both sensitive and resistant cells but the effect was more marked in resistant cells; the increase in uptake was attributed to inhibition of drug efflux. These findings suggested that P388/ADR cells have an enhanced capacity for outward transport not only of anthracycline antibiotics but also of the non-anthracycline antibiotic actinomycin D and the *Vinca* alkaloids VCR and VLB (INABA and SAKURAI 1979).

d) Circumvention of Resistance to Daunorubicin

As noted previously, resistance to DNR is associated with decreased net drug uptake (RIEHM and BIEDLER 1972; DANO 1973; SKOVSGAARD 1978b). Decreased membrane permeability to DNR was considered the main factor in the development of drug resistance in Chinese hamster cells exposed to the drug (RIEHM and BIEDLER 1971). Tween 80 and some other nonionic and ionic surface-active detergents appeared capable of increasing permeability of the cell membrane and of enhancing uptake of dyes and proteins (RIEHM and BIEDLER 1972). YAMADA et al. (1963) demonstrated that treatment of rat ascites hepatoma cells with Tween 80 rendered them more sensitive to nitrogen mustard *N*-oxide, presumably by increasing drug uptake. Accordingly RIEHM and BIEDLER (1972) evaluated the effect of Tween 80 on the uptake and cytocidal activity of DNR in drug-sensitive and resistant Chinese hamster cells. Tween 80 caused a marked potentiation of the growth inhibitory activity of the antibiotic, as well as an increased uptake of [^{3}H]

DNR, and both effects were more marked in resistant cells. These findings supported the concept that resistance to DNR is due to an acquired alteration of the cellular membrane, and potentiation of drug uptake by Tween 80 resulted in circumvention of such resistance.

The inhibitory activity of DNR on the growth of Landschutz ascites tumor in organs of the chick embryo was enhanced by the nonionic detergent Triton WR 1339 and related analogs (EASTY et al. 1972). The greatest enhancement found was with a dimeric analog Gem 30; none of the detergents alone inhibited tumor growth. Several mechanisms were proposed to explain this effect of nonionic detergents, including increased uptake of DNR by detergents of the linear Triton type.

Another method of overcoming resistance to DNR involved the administration of drug in the form of a complex with DNA (TROUET et al. 1972). Thus intracellular concentration of free drug was dependent on uptake of the DNA-daunorubicin complex by pinocytosis and release of free drug by hydrolytic enzymes in cellular lysosomes. Treatment of mice with L1210 leukemia using high drug doses yielded better results with the complex than with free drug; the superior survival result was attributed to lower toxicity of the complex. Four patients with DNR-resistant leukemia were reported to show "dramatic hematologic responses" to the complex and were entirely resistant to the free drug. Unfortunately, follow-up studies of this interesting report have not been forthcoming.

As noted previously, resistance to DNR is due primarily to a more active drug efflux system in resistant cells, although other factors, such as reduced drug influx and reduced drug binding to DNA, have also been described (DANO 1973; SKOVSGAARD 1978b). DANO observed that uptake of [^{3}H] DNR at the steady state by resistant Ehrlich ascites cells was increased by VLB, *N*-acetyldaunorubicin, VCR, and daunorubicinol in decreasing order of activity (DANO 1973). DANO considered these effects were not only compatible with competitive inhibition of an active outward transport system for DNR, but also supported the concept that anthracycline antibiotics and *Vinca* alkaloids share the same efflux system.

SKOVSGAARD demonstrated that *N*-acetyldaunorubicin inhibited both active efflux and unidirectional influx of DNR in Ehrlich ascites cells, resulting in a net increase in drug uptake at the steady state (SKOVSGAARD 1980). This effect on net drug uptake was much more pronounced in DNR-resistant cells than in sensitive cells.

Administration of *N*-acetyldaunorubicin to mice receiving DNR had no effect on DNR-induced toxicity. Combination therapy with DNR and *N*-acetyldaunorubicin was synergistic in the treatment of mice with DNR-resistant Ehrlich ascites tumor; however, the same combination was no more effective than DNR alone in the treatment of mice with drug-sensitive tumor. These findings indicated that *N*-acetyldaunorubicin, or related analogs, are able to circumvent acquired resistance to DNR. The mechanism of this effect is probably due to competitive inhibition of active efflux of DNR, by the structural analog *N*-acetyldaunorubicin.

3. Bleomycin

To our knowledge, a definitive study of the mechanism of uptake of bleomycin by mammalian cells has not been reported. Response of a tumor to bleomycin may correlate with the level of inactivation enzyme of the drug in the tumor (UMEZAWA 1975), or with the degree of membrane permeability to the antibiotic, as described in bacteria (YAMAGAMI et al. 1974).

A radioautographic study indicated that [^{14}C] bleomycin was adsorbed to the surface of the cell membrane of mouse ascites tumor cells 2 h after treatment of tumor-bearing mice in vivo (FUJIMOTO 1974). By 4 h drug was incorporated into the cells and radioactivity was localized primarily to the nuclear membrane. It was concluded that the concentration of drug at the nuclear membrane was closely related to cell injury.

A comparison was made of the uptake and binding of [^{14}C] bleomycin to bleomycin-sensitive (AH-66) and -resistant (AH-66F) rat ascites hepatoma cells (MIYAKI et al. 1975). Uptake of radioactivity by sensitive cells was 1.02- to 1.44-fold greater than in resistant cells but this difference was not considered significant. The level of bleomycin-inactivating enzyme in resistant cells was 3.5 times higher than in sensitive cells. Binding of [^{14}C] bleomycin to DNA was 8.7 times higher in sensitive cells than in resistant cells, and the number of single-strand scissions of DNA was also eight fold greater in sensitive cells. The similar ratio of activity of drug-binding to DNA and of strand breaks in sensitive and resistant cells suggested that both phenomena occur at the same locus. These observations suggested that sensitivity to bleomycin was dependent on bleomycin-inactivating enzyme, which determined the amount of free drug available to the cell.

The influence of polyene antibiotics on bleomycin uptake was investigated in polyene-sensitive Chinese hamster V79 cells and in a polyene-resistant subline AMB^R-1 (AKIYAMA et al. 1979). Three polyene antibiotics, filipin, pentamycin, and pimaricin, enhanced the action of bleomycin A_2 but amphotericin B and nystatin were inactive. The combination of filipin and bleomycin was synergistic with respect to inhibition of DNA synthesis and by clonogenic activity of polyene-sensitive V79 cells but had little effect on polyene-resistant AMB^R-1 cells. The cellular uptake of [^{14}C] bleomycin A_2 was augmented two- to four fold by pentamycin or filipin. Thus the synergy observed may be due to the effects of certain polyene antibiotics on bleomycin permeation.

Polyene antibiotics have been classified into two groups: firstly, those that cause K^+ leakage and cell death (or hemolysis) at the same dose of antibiotic and, secondly, those that cause K^+ leakage at low doses and cell death at high antibiotic doses (KOTLER-BRAJTBURG et al. 1979). Group 1 drugs include pimaricin, a tetraene, and filipin, a pentaene, whereas group 2 drugs include amphotericin B, a heptaene, and nystatin, a degenerated heptaene. Thus the activity of bleomycin A_2 appears to be potentiated by group 1 polyenes and it would appear that bleomycin A_2 may be unable to permeate the pore formed by group 2 polyenes such as amphotericin B (AKIYAMA et al. 1979).

4. Mitomycin C

The cytocidal activity of the antibiotic mitomycin C is usually attributed to its ability to function as an alkylating agent (CROOKE and BRADNER 1976). The uptake and intracellular distribution of [^{3}H]mitomycin C has been studied in mouse P388 cells in vitro (ORSTAVIK 1974). Cellular uptake of radioactivity was proportional to extracellular drug concentration over the range of 0.5–50 μg/ml; approximately 60% of the intracellular radioactivity was trichloroacetic acid (TCA) soluble, and among the cell fractions RNA had the highest activity. However, no attempt has been made to study uptake of the free drug using thin-layer chromatography or high-pressure liquid chromatography, so that no information is available on the nature of the uptake mechanism; nor is there information on relative uptake by sensitive and resistant cells.

IV. Alkaloids

1. *Vinca* Alkaloids

The *Vinca* alkaloids vincristine (VCR) and vinblastine (VLB) have been used extensively either as single agents or in combination with other agents in the treatment of a variety of human neoplasms (CARTER 1974; BONADONNA et al. 1975; EINHORN and DONOHUE 1977; MAUER and SIMONE 1976; SAWITSKY et al. 1970). Both VCR and VLB arrest cell mitosis at the metaphase stage (PALMER et al. 1960; CARDINALI et al. 1963) by interfering with assembly of spindle fiber proteins (JOURNEY et al. 1968; GEORGE et al. 1965) and causing dissolution of existing tubules (MALAWISTA et al. 1968). Both drugs bind rapidly to tubulin, the soluble protein component of microtubules (OWELLEN et al. 1972, 1974, 1976).

a) Mechanism of Vincristine and Vinblastine Transport

Several reports of rapid uptake and reversible binding of VCR and VLB by rat platelets (HEBDEN et al. 1970; SECRET et al. 1972), Ehrlich ascites carcinoma (CREASEY and MARKIW 1968), and sarcoma 180 cells (CREASEY 1968) have appeared. However, it was not until a detailed study by BLEYER et al. (1975) that a precise transport mechanism for these agents was established.

A time course of uptake of [^{3}H]VCR by L1210 leukemia cells in vitro appeared to be biphasic with an early linear component between 1 and 4 min. Kinetic studies of the early component showed that influx was saturable and followed Michaelis-Menten kinetics having a V_{max} of 143 nmol/min per gram dry weight and a K_m of 9.2 μ*M*. VCR uptake was chemical type specific, being competitively inhibited by VLB. Furthermore, VCR uptake was markedly temperature dependent, with a Q_{10} of 6.3 between 27 °C and 37 °C, and strongly energy dependent, being inhibited by metabolic antagonists such as sodium fluoride, *p*-chloromercuribenzoate, and ouabain. Binding of the drug to cell components accounted for approximately 20% of total uptake and cell/medium distribution ratios for free drug ranged from 5.2 to 18.7. These findings provided strong evidence that transport of VCR by L1210 cells was by an active, carrier-mediated process; similar results were obtained with P388 cells.

Efflux studies showed that [^{3}H]VCR could be washed out of cells very rapidly at 37 °C reaching a plateau level in approximately 10 min; efflux was totally inhibited at 4 °C. The plateau was considered to represent bound drug; however, [^{3}H]VCR could be released from binding sites by resuspending the cells in medium containing unlabeled drug. The amount of bound drug increased with increasing length of cell exposure to VCR in the medium. During the early linear component of uptake, bound drug accumulated more slowly than did total drug, while during the second uptake component total and bound VCR increased in a parallel fashion.

A more recent study of VCR transport in human lymphoblasts revealed a similar transport mechanism (BENDER and NICHOLS 1978). Uptake was rapid for 40 min, reaching a steady state by 60 min with cell/medium distribution ratios for free drug of 16–45 being observed. Influx appeared to follow saturation kinetics, with a V_{max} of 65.6 nmol/min per gram dry weight and a K_m of 6.45 μM, was temperature sensitive with a Q_{10} of 4, and was strongly energy dependent, being inhibited by azide, iodoacetate, and fluoride. The amount of bound intracellular VCR increased linearly with time, reaching a maximum by 60 min.

b) Resistance to Vincristine and Vinblastine Due to Decreased Drug Transport

Decreased drug uptake has been well documented as one cause of resistance to the *Vinca* alkaloids. CREASEY (1968) reported that VLB influx and binding were diminished in drug-resistant Ehrlich ascites cells. In a more detailed transport study BLEYER et al. (1975) compared VCR influx and efflux in sensitive and resistant P388 murine leukemia cells. Both VCR influx and binding were significantly greater in drug-sensitive cells than in resistant cells. The initial uptake component in both cell lines was saturable, temperature dependent, and inhibited by metabolic antagonists; however, a quantitative comparison of the influx kinetics in the two cell lines was not determined.

SKOVSGAARD (1978c) found that Ehrlich ascites tumor cells resistant to VCR showed decreased drug uptake. Both the rate of net uptake and the steady state were considerably higher in the sensitive tumor than in the resistant line; at the steady state the cell/medium ratios were 10 and 1.8 respectively. Inhibition of oxidative phosphorylation by sodium azide had no effect on VCR uptake whereas inhibition of glycolysis by iodoacetic acid resulted in a moderate increase in drug uptake. However, the presence of both inhibitors in cell suspensions resulted in a synergistic increase in drug uptake and this effect was more pronounced in resistant cells. In cells loaded with VCR to steady-state levels in medium containing sodium azide without glucose, the addition of glucose resulted in a loss of drug from the cells; again this effect was more pronounced in resistant cells. To compare VCR influx in the two cell lines, incubations were performed in glucose-free medium containing sodium azide in order to suppress drug efflux. Under these conditions the rate of drug influx was significantly higher in sensitive cells. Thus resistance to VCR in Ehrlich ascites tumor cells is a result of both reduced drug influx and enhanced efflux.

Similar results were obtained by INABA and SAKURAI (1979) in an adriamycin-resistant P388 leukemia cell line cross-resistant to VCR. In Hank's balanced salt solution the resistant cells showed reduced net uptake of VCR. However, in glucose-free Hank's balanced salt solution containing dinitrophenol both cell lines showed enhanced and nearly equal drug uptake. Addition of glucose to the incubation medium resulted in decreased intracellular drug levels as a result of drug efflux and this effect was more marked in resistant cells. Thus the lower levels of net drug uptake in resistant cells were due primarily to more active drug efflux.

In another study VCR uptake by sensitive P388 leukemia cells was three times greater than that in resistant cells (CSUKA et al. 1980). In addition, the plasma membrane and tubulin fractions of sensitive cells bound 1.6 and 3.1 times more VCR respectively than corresponding fractions from resistant cells.

In a study by BECK et al. (1979), in an established line of human lymphoblasts, VLB resistance correlated with the presence of a membrane glycoprotein with a molecular weight of 170,000–190,000. The level of glycoprotein correlated with resistance in cells up to 269 times more resistant to drug than sensitive cells. In cells with a greater degree of resistance, no further increment in glycoprotein was noted, suggesting the presence of an additional mechanism of resistance. Since the primary mechanism of resistance to *Vinca* alkaloids for these resistant cells appeared to be diminished uptake and retention of drug (BECK et al. 1979), a correlation may exist between the presence of the glycoprotein and reduced transport. Such a correlation has been suggested for colchicine-resistant Chinese hamster ovary cells (Sect. C.IV.2.b).

A VCR-resistant subline of Chinese hamster cells contained an abnormal chromosome with a well-defined homogeneously staining region; it has been suggested that this might lead to an overproduction of a specific protein as a result of gene amplification (MEYER and BIEDLER 1981). An acidic protein with a molecular weight of 19,000 was synthesized in relatively large amounts by VCR-resistant Chinese hamster cells; reduced amounts of this protein were present in a revertant line and only trace amounts were detected in sensitive cells. A similar protein was found in a VCR-resistant mouse line and two drug-resistant human neuroblastoma cell lines.

Although both VCR and VLB are believed to have similar modes of action their chemotherapeutic effectiveness for different types of malignant cells varies greatly. The uptake and binding of these two agents has been compared in rat platelets, rat lymphoma cells, and murine L5178Y lymphoblasts; VLB uptake was more rapid than that of VCR but VLB efflux was also more rapid (GOUT et al. 1978). The amount of VCR retained by the cells eventually exceeded the amount of VLB retained. Since it has been shown that both alkaloids have nearly identical association constants for tubulin in vitro and also interact comparably with preformed microtubules (HIMES et al. 1976), the difference in uptake and binding may reflect a difference in transport.

c) Interaction of Vincristine and Vinblastine with Other Chemotherapeutic Agents

An interesting aspect of tumor-cell resistance to the *Vinca* alkaloids is the observation of cross-resistance to anthracycline antibiotics and to actinomycin D (see Sect. C.III.2.c).

The *Vinca* alkaloids have been shown to increase the net uptake of MTX in a number of animal (ZAGER et al. 1973; FYFE and GOLDMAN 1973) and human cell lines (BENDER et al. 1975; WARREN et al. 1977) at both conventional (ZAGER et al. 1973; FYFE and GOLDMAN 1973; CHELLO et al. 1979) and "high-dose" extracellular MTX concentrations (GOLDMAN et al. 1976; WARREN et al. 1977; BENDER et al. 1978). This effect was shown to be due to noncompetitive inhibition of the energy-dependent efflux system for MTX by VCR in L1210 leukemia cells (FYFE and GOLDMAN 1973; GOLDMAN et al. 1976) and in human myeloblasts (BENDER et al. 1975), the increased levels of MTX represented higher levels of exchangeable drug (FYFE and GOLDMAN 1973; GOLDMAN et al. 1976; BENDER et al. 1975).

The clinical relevance of VCR stimulation of MTX uptake has been studied. Clinically attainable concentrations of VCR had no effect on MTX uptake in two human lymphoblastoid cell lines; however, higher concentrations of VCR increased net MTX uptake (WARREN et al. 1977). ZAGER et al. (1973) found that combination chemotherapy with VCR and MTX increased the survival time of mice with L1210 leukemia compared with that obtained with single-agent therapy. However, attempts to repeat these results both at conventional and "high-dose" methotrexate concentrations showed no therapeutic synergism for the two drug combination when the VCR was given up to 2.5 h prior to MTX treatment (BENDER et al. 1978; CHELLO et al. 1979). Only when VCR was given 24 h after MTX was synergism observed (CHELLO et al. 1979), and the question of whether the mechanism of synergism was related to the interaction between the two drugs was raised. The effect of MTX on transport of the *Vinca* alkaloids has not been investigated.

d) Attempts to Increase Therapeutic Effectiveness of Vincristine and Vinblastine

Several attempts have been made to overcome resistance to the *Vinca* alkaloids and to increase their therapeutic index. Verapamil, an inhibitor of the slow channel of Ca^{2+} transport across membranes, has been shown to enhance the cytotoxicity of VCR and VLB in both sensitive and resistant P388 leukemia cells in vitro (TSURUO et al. 1981 b). Cytotoxicity in resistant cells was increased more than in sensitive cells so that resistance appeared to be entirely eliminated. Verapamil increased the intracellular level of VCR in sensitive cells approximately two fold and in resistant cells approximately ten fold; thus the four fold difference in intracellular drug concentration between the two cell lines was eliminated. Verapamil had no effect on drug binding to tubulin and appeared to increase the intracellular levels of VCR by inhibiting the active efflux system. In vivo verapamil partially circumvented resistance to both VCR and VLB in mice with P388 leukemia (TSURUO et al. 1981 b).

Several other attempts have been made to improve the effectiveness of the *Vinca* alkaloids by decreasing their toxicity. CASS et al. (1981) found that treatment of L1210 leukemia-bearing mice with lithium resulted in modest protection against the myelosuppressive effects of VLB without effecting the tumoricidal activity of the drug. Ruthenium red, an inorganic dye, prevents VLB-induced cytotoxicity in cultured KB cells by inhibiting drug uptake with no effect on drug efflux (TSURUO et al. 1981 a). Finally liposomal encapsulation of VCR provided no increase of therapeutic index compared with free drug in the treatment of mice with P388 leukemia (LAYTON and TROUET 1980).

2. Colchicine

Although colchicine is not used clinically in the chemotherapy of malignant disease it has a similar mechanism of action to the *Vinca* alkaloids, and cross-resistance to colchicine and other antitumor agents has been reported (CRICHLEY et al. 1980; BECH-HANSEN et al. 1976; LING and THOMPSON 1974). Accordingly we have included this agent in the present review.

a) Mechanism of Colchicine Transport

E. W. TAYLOR (1965) studied the uptake of ^{3}H-labeled colchicine by human KB cells. Total cell-associated radioactivity increased rapidly during the first 10 min and more slowly thereafter. The initial rapid increase was attributed to drug permeation up to equilibrium conditions and subsequent increments to drug binding within the cell. The cell/medium ratio for free colchicine was not considered to be significantly greater than unity. The rate of colchicine penetration was more rapid than the rate of binding.

A kinetic analysis of colchicine uptake by Chinese hamster ovary (CHO) cells was consistent with a simple diffusion process in the concentration range from 1 to 100 μM (CARLSEN et al. 1976). A 100-fold excess of Colcemid, a close structural analog of colchicine, and several metabolic inhibitors did not inhibit colchicine uptake. However, the activation energy for colchicine uptake was 19 kcal/mol.

In the absence of glucose, metabolic inhibitors stimulated colchicine uptake by CHO cells; this effect was abrogated by glucose or ribose and correlated inversely with cellular ATP levels (SEE et al. 1974). A similar effect was noted on uptake of actinomycin D and puromycin. From these findings Ling postulated the presence of an energy-dependent permeability barrier to drugs in these cells. Local anesthetics, nonionic detergents, and drugs such as VCR, VLB, DNR, and antinomycin D also increased the rate of colchicine uptake in CHO cells (CARLSEN et al. 1976). Unlike metabolic inhibitors, these compounds did not alter cellular ATP; however, they are capable of interacting with cell membranes and may also modify membrane permeability.

The stimulation of colchicine uptake into CHO cells may be similar to the augmentation of net uptake of VCR and DNR by metabolic inhibitors reported by others (SKOVSGAARD 1978c; DANO 1973; INABA and SAKURAI 1979). This effect was attributed to inhibition of an energy-dependent, carrier-mediated, drug-efflux system. Thus re-examination of colchicine transport with particular emphasis on drug efflux appears warranted.

b) Resistance to Colchicine Due to Decreased Drug Transport

Colchicine-resistant mutants of Friend erythroleukemia cells showing reduced membrane permeability to drug have been reported; these cells were also cross-resistant to daunorubicin, actinomycin D, emetine, and puromycin (CRICHLEY et al. 1980). LING has also isolated a series of CHO cell lines resistant to colchicine (LING and THOMPSON 1974). All clones demonstrated reduced drug permeability, but the ability to bind and inactivate drug was unchanged; the reduction in colchicine uptake correlated strongly with resistance. The resistant cell lines were also cross-resistant to other drugs such as actinomycin D, VLB and, Colcemid (BECH-HANSEN et al. 1976).

A membrane glycoprotein with a molecular weight of 165,000 was present in resistant CHO cells, absent from sensitive cells and at a reduced level in revertant cells (LING 1975; JULIANO and LING 1976; JULIANO et al. 1976). The relative amount of this surface glycoprotein correlated with the degree of drug resistance. Highly resistant mutants showed enhanced phosphorylation of high molecular weight membrane proteins (CARLSEN et al. 1977). LING proposed that in resistant cells conformational changes in certain membrane glycoproteins can modulate membrane fluidity and thereby alter drug permeability (LING 1975). The conformation of these glycoproteins may in turn be modulated by an ATP-dependent, phosphorylation-dephosphorylation process.

V. Hormones

1. Glucocorticoids

Prednisone and dexamethasone synthetic analogs of cortisol have been used clinically in the treatment of acute and chronic leukemia (EZDINLI et al. 1969; DEBUSSCHER and STRYCKMANS 1978) and lymphomas (HALL et al. 1967). Like other antineoplastic hormones, a hormone-receptor complex formed in the cytoplasm is translocated into the nucleus, with subsequent dissociation liberating hormone to interact with nuclear components (BAXTER et al. 1971; MUNCK et al. 1972; LIPPMAN et al. 1974, 1978; THOMPSON and LIPPMAN 1974). This interaction results in inhibition of various metabolic functions – including synthesis of proteins and nucleic acids, transport of amino acids and nucleosides, and uptake and utilization of glucose – and eventually in cell lysis (NICHOLSON and YOUNG 1978).

a) Mechanism of Glucocorticoid Transport

Early studies suggested a simple diffusion mechanism for cortisol uptake (BELLAMY et al. 1962; WIRA and MUNCK 1974). However, cortisol uptake by rat liver cells was rapid, temperature dependent and accumulated against a concentration gradient (RAO et al. 1974, 1976a, b). Kinetic studies demonstrated carrier-mediated influx of cortisol by two saturable systems in addition to simple diffusion, with diffusion becoming increasingly important at hormone concentrations above 600 nM. One carrier system had a K_m of 90 nM and V_{max} of 4 pmol/min per milligram protein while the second system had a K_m of 600 nM and V_{max} of 17 pmol/min per milligram protein. Influx was sodium independent but was inhibited by metabolic inhibitors and sulfhydryl-binding reagents. Cortisol influx showed chemical specificity being inhibited competitively by the cortisol analogs cortisone and corticosterone; other steroid hormones such as dexamethasone, estrone, estradiol, and testosterone inhibited cortisol uptake noncompetitively. Considerable care was taken to distinguish between cortisol uptake and receptor binding. Hormone uptake and binding differed in saturability and in sensitivity to temperature and metabolic inhibitors.

GROSS et al. (1968, 1970) described an energy-dependent carrier-mediated transport system for efflux of cortisol, dexamethasone, and other glucocorticoids in fibroblasts, lymphoblasts, and adrenal cells. Other steroids, including deoxycorticosterone, corticosterone, cortisone, and progesterone inhibited the efflux mechanism but did not serve as substrates.

b) Resistance to Glucocorticoids

No examples of glucocorticoid resistance due to altered transport have been reported. The major causes of hormone resistance appear to be absence or defects of the cytoplasmic hormone receptors (STEVENS et al. 1978; NICHOLSON et al. 1981), impaired translocation of hormone-receptor complexes into the nucleus (YAMAMOTO et al. 1974), changes in the cell membrane which reduce susceptibility to lysis (BEHRENS et al. 1974; BEHRENS and HOLLANDER 1976), and changes in protein synthesis (NICHOLSON et al. 1981).

2. Estrogens

There are two classes of estrogenic hormones: steroidal compounds such as estradiols, which are naturally occurring, and synthetic, nonsteroidal compounds such as diethylstilbestrol. Both the steroidal and nonsteroidal agents have been used in the treatment of carcinoma of the breast and prostate (TAYLOR 1959; CROWLEY and DUWE 1969; KAPLAN 1968). As with glucocorticoids (see Sect. C.V.1) estrogens form a cytoplasmic hormone-receptor complex which is translocated into the nucleus; estrogens modulate cell growth by altering synthesis of macromolecules (HILF and WITTLIFF 1975).

a) Mechanism of Estrogen Transport

Uptake of estradiol by rat uterus and diaphragm was reported to be by passive diffusion (PECK et al. 1973). By contrast, MILGROM et al. (1973) reported that estradiol and diethylstilbtestrol share a saturable, chemically specific, carrier-mediated transport system in rat uterine cells. Estradiol uptake was highly temperature dependent, inhibited by sulfhydryl-blocking reagents, but unaffected by potassium cyanide and 2,4-dinitrophenol.

A kinetic analysis of estradiol and estrone uptake by rat liver cells followed Michaelis-Menten kinetics with a K_m of 0.5 μM and V_{max} of 46 pmol/5 s per milligram protein for estradiol and a K_m of 2.2 μM and V_{max} of 210 pmol/5 s per milligram protein for estrone (BREUER et al. 1974; RAO et al. 1977). Uptake of both estrogens was concentrative, with cell/medium distribution ratios of 12–23, and was inhibited by metabolic inhibitors and sulfhydryl reagents. These results suggested the involvement of an active carrier-mediated process for uptake of estrogens in rat liver cells.

b) Resistance to Estrogens

Resistance to estrogens resulting from decreased transport has not been described. The major cause of resistance to estrogens results from the absence of an estrogen receptor in the cell (GUSTAFSSON et al. 1978; KIANG et al. 1978).

3. Androgens and Progestins

Androgens are steroidal derivatives of testosterone which have been used in the treatment of breast cancer (THOMAS et al. 1962; BRODSKY 1973; RIGBERG and BRODSKY 1975), while progestins are steroidal compounds related to progesterone which have been used to treat carcinoma of the breast and endometrium and hypernephroma (KELLEY and BAKER 1960, 1970; KENNEDY 1968; KNEALE and EVANS 1969; STOLL 1969).

Several studies of androgen uptake in human and canine prostatic tissue indicated the possible involvement of a carrier (GIORGI et al. 1973, 1974). Testosterone influx in rat liver cells followed Michaelis-Menten kinetics, with a K_m of 1.6 μM and a V_{max} of 76 pmol/5 s per milligram protein (RAO et al. 1977). The cell/medium distribution ratio for testosterone was 9–10 and uptake was inhibited by 2,4-dinitrophenol and antimycin A but not by sulfhydryl reagents. Thus testosterone appears to be transported into rat liver cells by an energy-dependent, carrier-mediated mechanism. Transport studies of progestins have not been reported nor have studies dealing with hormone resistance due to altered uptake.

D. Future Considerations

The mechanism of transport of several chemotherapeutic agents remains to be elucidated and in those cases further studies will be required to determine whether a correlation exists between drug resistance and defective transport. The application of knowledge of established mechanisms of transport has and will be used in attempts to circumvent resistance due to impaired drug permeability. One of the earliest examples of this approach was the report by YAMADA et al. (1963) in which treatment of rat ascites hepatoma cells with the detergent Tween 80 resulted in greater sensitivity to the alkylating agent nitrogen mustard, N-oxide, presumably due to enhanced drug uptake. RIEHM and BIEDLER (1972) evaluated the effect of Tween 80 on the uptake and cytocidal activity of daunorubicin in drug-sensitive and -resistant Chinese hamster cells. Tween 80 markedly augmented the growth inhibitory activity of the antibiotic and increased uptake of [^{3}H]DNR; both effects were more marked in resistant cells. Although the use of Tween 80 is not feasible clinically, these observations clearly established that transport could be modified so as to overcome drug resistance.

The use of alternate drug pathways has been recommended in cases of drug resistance linked to faulty or defective drug transport. For example, evidence has been presented that MTX influx is mediated by a carrier system that transports reduced folates and is separate from the pathway that transports folic acid (RADER et al. 1974; NIETHAMMER and JACKSON 1975). Accordingly it was suggested that antifolate drugs, which enter cells by the folic acid pathway, might circumvent MTX resistance due to impaired drug transport (NIETHAMMER and JACKSON 1975). ROSOWSKY et al. (1980) offered three different approaches for overcoming MTX resistance due to impaired transport: (a) the use of high-dose MTX schedules to permit MTX to enter cells by passive diffusion; (b) the use of "small molecule" antifolates such as triazinate, which lack the negatively charged glutamate side chain, enabling compounds to enter cells more readily by passive diffusion; and (c) the use of "hybrid antifolates" such as mono- and dibutyl esters of MTX, in which the glutamate side chain is modified, rendering the drug more lipophilic and thereby more permeable. This group showed that CEM human lymphoblasts, resistant to MTX as a result of a transport defect, were completely sensitive to the monobutyl ester of MTX and demonstrated collateral sensitivity to the dibutyl ester as well as to two "small molecule" antifolates. These findings suggested that MTX-resistant human lymphoblasts with defective drug transport are responsive to lipophilic antifolates which enter cells by passive diffusion. GALIVAN (1981) claimed that H35 rat hepatoma cells resistant to MTX lacked a functional transport carrier for the drug. Triazinate, a "small molecule" antifolate, which enters cells by a different pathway than MTX, inhibited growth of the transport-resistant hepatoma cells.

Another approach to circumvent transport resistance has been the use of drug conjugates. For example, a complex of the antibiotic DNR with DNA was used to overcome DNR resistance (TROUET et al. 1972). Treatment of mice with L1210 leukemia using high drug doses yielded better results with the complex than with free drug; the superior result was attributed to lower toxicity of the complex. Four patients with DNR-resistant leukemia were reported to show dramatic responses to the complex although being entirely resistant to the free drug.

The antimetabolite MTX has been conjugated to poly-L-lysine in order to circumvent transport resistance (RYSSER and SHEN 1978, 1980; SHEN and RYSSER 1979). The dose of drug required to inhibit a MTX-resistant transport mutant of CHO cells was reduced 100-fold if MTX was given as the conjugate rather than as free drug; uptake of the conjugate was believed to take place by endocytosis (RYSSER and SHEN 1980). More recently. MTX has been conjugated to bovine serum albumin (BSA) and MTX-resistant transport and enzyme mutants of L1210 leukemia have been treated with the conjugate and free drug (CHU et al. 1981). Transport mutants were more sensitive to MTX-BSA conjugate than enzyme mutants, whereas both mutants demonstrated similar sensitivity to free drug. This suggested that impairment of the normal MTX-FH_4 carrier in transport mutants affected MTX influx but not uptake of MTX-BSA. In vivo, MTX-BSA was equally effective against the sensitive parent line and the resistant transport mutant, whereas MTX was active only against the sensitive L1210 cell line. Thus, the MTX-BSA conjugate was able to circumvent resistance to MTX in the transport mutant in vivo (CHU and WHITELEY 1980).

Another approach that has been used to overcome resistance due to faulty transport has been the development of drug-encapsulated liposomes. Chinese hamster cells markedly resistant to actinomycin D responded to a 100-fold lower concentration of antibiotic if the drug was delivered in lipid vesicles rather than in the free form (POSTE and PAPAHADJOPOULOUS 1976). The actinomycin D-resistant phenotype resulted from a lower capacity to incorporate actinomycin D, produced by a lower permeability of the cell membrane to drug. Vesicle-mediated delivery of drug into resistant tumor cells appeared to be a method of bypassing drug resistance. Such an approach might be applicable clinically, particularly if "recognition ligands" could be incorporated into the vesicle membrane to induce preferential uptake of vesicles by tumor cells.

Application of knowledge of drug transport mechanisms should provide the clinician with a more rational approach to the development and design of combination chemotherapy programs. For example, the *Vinca* alkaloids have been shown to increase the net uptake of MTX in a number of animal and human cell lines (ZAGER et al. 1973; FYFE and GOLDMAN 1973; BENDER et al. 1975; WARREN et al. 1977). This effect was shown to be due to noncompetitive inhibition of the energy-dependent efflux system for MTX by VCR in L1210 leukemia cells (FYFE and GOLDMAN 1973; GOLDMAN et al. 1976) and in human myeloblasts (BENDER et al. 1975). Combination chemotherapy of mice with L1210 leukemia using VCR and MTX increased survival time relative to that observed with single-agent therapy (ZAGER et al. 1973), and indeed this combination has been used with success clinically in the treatment of acute lymphoblastic leukemia (NACHMAN et al. 1981).

The observation that anthracycline antibiotics and *Vinca* alkaloids share a common active efflux system (DANO 1973; SKOVSGAARD 1978c) suggests the possibility that combination chemotherapy regimes employing drugs from each class might be particularly effective. Apparent selective inhibition of DNR efflux was also achieved by administration of the close structural analog *N*-acetyl daunorubicin (SKOVSGAARD 1980). Combination therapy with DNR and *N*-acetyl daunorubicin was synergistic in the treatment of mice with DNR-resistant Ehrlich ascites tumor. These findings indicated that *N*-acetyl daunorubicin, or related analogs, are able to overcome acquired resistance to DNR. Thus, the use of structural analogs of chemotherapeutic agents with little or no cytocidal activity may result in synergistic activity through such transport interactions.

References

Ahmed K, Scholefield PG (1962) Biochemical studies on 1-aminocyclopentane carboxylic acid. Can J Biochem Physiol 40:1101–1110

Akiyama S, Hidaka K, Komiyama S, Kuwano M (1979) Control of permeation of bleomycin A_2 by polyene antibiotics in cultured Chinese hamster cells. Cancer Res 39:5150–5154

Alexanian R, Bergsagel DE, Migliore PJ, Vaughn WK, Howe CD (1968) Melphalan therapy for plasma cell myeloma. Blood 31:1–10

Ardalan B, Cooney DA, Jayaram HM, Carrico CK, Glazer RI, MacDonald J, Schein PS (1980) Mechanism of sensitivity and resistance of murine tumors to 5-fluorouracil. Cancer Res 40:1431–1437

Balis ME, Hylin V, Coultas MK, Hutchison DJ (1958) Metabolism of resistant mutants of *Streptococcus faecalis*. II. Incorporation of exogenous purines. Cancer Res 18:220–225

Ball CR, Connors TA, Double JA, Ujhazy V, Whisson ME (1966) Comparison of nitrogen mustard-sensitive and -resistant Yoshida sarcoma. Int J Cancer 1:319–327

Baskin F, Rosenberg RN (1975) Decreased 6-mercaptopurine retention by two resistant variants of mouse neuroblastoma with normal hypoxanthine-guanine-phosphoribosyltransferase activity. J Pharmacol Exp Ther 193:293–300

Baxter JD, Harris AW, Tomkins GM, Cohn M (1971) Glucocorticoid receptors in lymphoma cells in culture: relationship to glucocorticoid killing activity. Science 171:189–191

Bech-Hansen NT, Till JE, Ling V (1976) Pleiotropic phenotype of colchicine-resistant CHO cells: cross-resistance and collateral sensitivity. J Cell Physiol 88:23–32

Beck WT, Mueller TJ, Tanzer LR (1979) Altered surface membrane glycoproteins in *Vinca* alkaloid-resistant human leukemia lymphoblasts. Cancer Res 39:2070–2076

Begleiter A, Lam HYP, Goldenberg GJ (1977) Mechanism of uptake of nitrosoureas by L5178Y lymphoblasts in vitro. Cancer Res 37:1022–1027

Begleiter A, Lam HYP, Grover J, Froese E, Goldenberg GJ (1979) Evidence for active transport of melphalan by amino acid carriers in L5178Y lymphoblasts in vitro. Cancer Res 39:353–359

Begleiter A, Grover J, Goldenberg GJ (1980) Uptake and metabolism of hexamethylmelamine and pentamethylmelamine by L5178Y lymphoblasts in vitro. Cancer Res 40:4489–4494

Behrens UJ, Hollander VP (1976) Cell membrane sialoglycopeptides of corticoid-sensitive and -resistant lymphosarcoma P1798. Cancer Res 36:172–180

Behrens UJ, Mashburn LT, Stevens J, Hollander VP, Lampen N (1974) Differences in cell surface characteristics between glucocorticoid-sensitive and -resistant mouse lymphomas. Cancer Res 34:2926–2932

Bellamy D, Phillips JG, Jones IC, Leonard RA (1962) The uptake of cortisol in rat tissues. Biochem J 85:537–545
Bender RA, Nichols AP (1978) Membrane transport of vincristine (VCR) in human lymphoblasts. Proc Am Assoc Cancer Res 19:35
Bender RA, Bleyer WA, Frisby SA, Oliverio VT (1975) Alteration of methotrexate uptake in human leukemia cells by other agents. Cancer Res 35:1305–1308
Bender RA, Nichols AP, Norton L, Simon RM (1978) Lack of therapeutic synergism between vincristine and methotrexate in L1210 murine leukemia in vitro. Cancer Treat Rep 62:997–1003
Bergel F, Stock JA (1953) Cytotoxic alpha amino acids and peptides. Br Emp Cancer Campaign Annu Rep 31:6–7
Bergel F, Stock JA (1954) Cytoactive amino acids and derivatives. I. Substituted phenylalanines. J Chem Soc 2409–2417
Bergsagel DE, Griffith KM, Haut A, Stuckey WJ Jr (1967) The treatment of plasma cell myeloma. Adv Cancer Res 10:311–359
Berlin RD, Oliver JM (1975) Membrane transport of purine and pyrimidine bases and nucleosides in animal cells. Int Rev Cytol 42:287–336
Bertino JR (1980) Approaches to drug selectivity in cancer therapy on the basis of differences between membranes of normal vs. neoplastic cells. Adv Pathobiol 7:377–386
Bieber AL, Sartorelli AC (1964) The metabolism of thioguanine in purine analog-resistant cells. Cancer Res 24:1210–1215
Biedler JL, Riehm H (1970) Cellular resistance to actinomycin-D in Chinese hamster cells in vitro, in cross-resistance, radioautographic and cytogenetic studies. Cancer Res 30:1174–1184
Bleyer WA, Frisby SA, Oliverio VT (1975) Uptake and binding of vincristine by murine leukemia cells. Biochem Pharmacol 24:633–639
Bonadonna G, Zucadi R, Monfardini S (1975) Combination chemotherapy of Hodgkin's disease with adriamycin, bleomycin, vinblastine and imidazole carboximide versus MOPP. Cancer 36:252–259
Bowen D, Goldman ID (1975) The relationship among transport, intracellular binding, and inhibition of RNA synthesis by actinomycin-D in Ehrlich ascites tumor cells in vitro. Cancer Res 35:3054–3060
Breuer H, Rao ML, Rao GS (1974) Uptake of steroid hormones by isolated rat liver cells. J Steroid Biochem 5:359
Brink JJ, LePage GA (1964) Metabolic effects of 9-D-arabinosylpurines in ascites tumor cells. Cancer Res 24:312–318
Brockman RW (1961) Symposium on the experimental pharmacology and clinical use of antimetabolites. VI. Mechanisms of resistance to metabolite analogues with anticancer activity. Clin Pharmacol Ther 2:237–261
Brockman RW (1963a) Mechanism of resistance to anticancer agents. Adv Cancer Res 7:129–234
Brockman RW (1963b) Biochemical aspects of mercaptopurine inhibition and resistance. Cancer Res 23:1191–1201
Brockman RW (1965) Resistance to purine antagonists in experimental leukemia systems. Cancer Res 25:1596–1605
Brockman RW, Debavadi CS, Stutts P, Hutchison DJ (1961) Purine ribonucleotide pyrophosphorylases and resistance to purine analogues in *Streptococcus faecalis*. J Biol Chem 236:1471–1479
Brodsky I (1973) The role of androgens and anabolic steroids in the treatment of cancer. Semin Drug Treat 3:15–25
Calabresi P, Parks RE Jr (1980) Chemotherapy of neoplastic diseases. In: Gilman AG, Goddman LS, Gilman A (eds) The pharmacologic basis of therapeutics, 6th edn. MacMillan, New York, pp 1290–1297
Cardinali G, Cardinali G, Enein MA (1963) Studies on the antimitotic activity of leurocristine (vincristine). Blood 21:102–110
Carlsen SA, Till JE, Ling V (1976) Modulation of membrane drug permeability in Chinese hamster ovary cells. Biochim Biophys Acta 455:900–912

Carlsen SA, Till JE, Ling V (1977) Modulation of drug permeability in Chinese hamster ovary cells. Possible role for phosphorylation of surface glycoproteins. Biochim Biophys Acta 467:238–250

Carter SK (1974) The chemical therapy of breast cancer. Semin Oncol 1:131–141

Cass CE (1979) 9-β-D-Arabinofuranosyladenine. In: Hahn FE (ed) Antibiotics, mechanism of action, vol 5. Springer, Berlin Heidelberg New York

Cass CE, Paterson ARP (1973) Mediated transport of nucleosides by human erythrocytes. Specificity toward purine nucleosides as permeants. Biochim Biophys Acta 291:734–746

Cass CE, Paterson ARP (1975) Inhibition by nitrobenzylthioinosine of uptake of adenosine, 2′-deoxyadenosine and 9-β-D-arabinosyladenine by human and mouse erythrocytes. Biochem Pharmacol 24:1989–1993

Cass CE, Turner AR, Selner M, Allalunis MJ, Tan TH (1981) Effect of lithium on the myelosuppressive and chemotherapeutic activities of vinblastine. Cancer Res 41:1000–1005

Chello PL, Sirotnak FM, Douck DM (1979) Different effects of vincristine on methotrexate uptake by L1210 cells and mouse intestinal epithelia in vitro and in vivo. Cancer Res 39:2106–2112

Chervinsky DS, Wang JJ (1976) Uptake of adriamycin and daunomycin in L1210 and human leukemia cells: a comparative study. J Med 7:63–79

Christensen HN (1966) Methods for distinguishing amino acid transport systems of a given cell or tissue. Fed Proc 25:850–853

Christensen HN (1969) Some special kinetic problems of transport. Adv Enzymol 32:1–20

Christensen HN, Handlogten ME (1968) Modes of mediated exodus of amino acids from the Ehrlich ascites tumor cell. J Biol Chem 243:5428–5438

Christensen HN, Liang M (1965) An amino acid transport system of unassigned function in the Ehrlich ascites tumor cell. J Biol Chem 240:3601–3608

Christensen HN, Liang M (1966) Modes of uptake of benzylamine by the Ehrlich cell. J Biol Chem 241:5552–5556

Christensen HN, Liang M, Archer EG (1967) A distinct Na^+-requiring transport system for alanine, serine, cysteine, and similar amino acids. J Biol Chem 242:5237–5246

Chu MY, Fischer GA (1965) Comparative studies of leukemia cells sensitive and resistant to cytosine arabinoside. Biochem Pharmacol 14:333–341

Chu MY, Fischer GA (1968) The incorporation of ^{3}H-cytosine arabinoside and its effect on murine leukemic cells (L5178Y). Biochem Pharmacol 17:753–767

Chu BC, Whiteley JM (1980) The interaction of carrier-bound methotrexate with L1210 cells. Mol Pharmacol 17:382–387

Chu BCF, Fan CC, Howell SB (1981) Activity of free and carrier-bound methotrexate against transport-deficient and high dihydrofolate dehydrogenase-containing methotrexate-resistant L1210 cells. J Natl Cancer Inst 66:121–124

Chun EHL, Gonzales L, Lewis FS, Jones J, Rutman RJ (1969) Differences in the in vivo alkylation and cross-linking of nitrogen mustard-sensitive and -resistant lines of Lettre-Ehrlich ascites tumors. Cancer Res 29:1184–1194

Connors TA, Grover PL, McLoughlin AM (1970) Microsomal activation of cyclophosphamide in vivo. Biochem Pharmacol 19:1533–1535

Creasey WA (1968) Modifications in biochemical pathways produced by the vinca alkaloids. Cancer Chemother Rep 52:501–507

Creasey WA, Markiw ME (1968) Uptake of vinblastine (VLB) by Ehrlich ascites carcinoma cells in vitro. Fed Proc 25:733

Crichley V, Mager D, Bernstein A (1980) Colchicine resistant Friend cells: application to the study of actinomycin D induced erythroid differentiation. J Cell Physiol 102:63–70

Crooke ST, Bradner WT (1976) Mitomycin-C: a review. Cancer Treat Rev 3:121–139

Crowley ZG, Duwe SA (1969) Current status of the management of patients with endocrine-sensitive tumors. Calif Med 110:139–150

Csuka O, Sugar J, Palyi I, Somfai-Relle S (1980) The mode of action of *Vinca* alkaloids. Oncology 37:83–87

Dano K (1972) Cross-resistance between *Vinca* alkaloids and anthracyclines in Ehrlich ascites tumor in vivo. Cancer Chemother Rep 56:701–708

Dano K (1973) Active outward transport of daunomycin in resistant Ehrlich ascites tumor cells. Biochim Biophys Acta 323:466–483

Dano K, Frederiksen S, Hellung-Larsen P (1972) Inhibition of DNA and RNA synthesis by daunorubicin in sensitive and resistant Ehrlich ascites tumor cells in vitro. Cancer Res 32:1307–1314

Dantzig AH, Slayman CW, Adelberg EA (1981) An amino acid transport mutant of Chinese hamster ovary cells resistant to the chemotherapeutic agent melphalan. Fed Proc 40:1894

Davidson JD (1958) Permeability of resistant L1210 leukemia cells to 8-azaguanine and 6-mercaptopurine. Proc Am Assoc Cancer Res 2:290–291

Davidson JD (1960) Studies on the mechanism of action of 6-marcaptopurine in sensitive and resistant L1210 leukemia in vitro. Cancer Res 20:225–232

Debusscher L, Stryckmans PA (1978) Non-lymphocytic leukemia. In: Staquet MJ (ed) Randomized trials in cancer: a critical review by sites. Raven, New York, pp 25–54

Dembo M, Sirotnak FM (1976) Antifolate transport in L1210 leukemia cells. Kinetic evidence for the non-identity of carriers for influx and efflux. Biochim Biophys Acta 448:505–516

Diamond I, Kennedy EP (1969) Carrier-mediated transport of choline into synaptic nerve endings. J Biol Chem 244:3258–3263

Dicioccio RA, Srivastava BIS (1977) Kinetics of inhibition of deoxynucleotide-polymerizing enzyme activities from normal and leukemic human cells by 9-β-D-arabinofuranosyladenine 5′-triphosphate and 1-β-D-arabinofuranosylcytosone 5′-triphosphate. Eur J Biochem 79:411–418

Di Marco A (1978) Mechanism of action and mechanism of resistance to antineoplastic agents that bind to DNA. Antibiot Chemother 23:216–227

Easty GC, Stock JA, Ukleja-Bortkiewicz A (1972) Potentiation of the antitumor effect of rubidomycin by non-ionic detergents. Eur J Cancer 8:633–640

Eavenson E, Christensen HN (1967) Transport systems for neutral amino acids in the pigeon erythrocyte. J Biol Chem 242:5386–5396

Einhorn LH, Donohue J (1977) *cis*-Diamminedichloroplatinum, vinblastine and bleomycin combination chemotherapy in disseminated testicular cancer. Ann Intern Med 87:293–298

Elliott EM, Ling V (1981) Selection and characterization of Chinese hamster ovary cell mutants resistant to melphalan (L-phenylalanine mustard). Cancer Res 41:393–400

Ezdinli EZ, Stutzman L, Aungst WC, Firat D (1969) Corticosteroid therapy for lymphomas and chronic lymphocytic leukemia. Cancer 23:900–909

Fischer GA (1961) Increased levels of folic acid reductase as a mechanism of resistance to amethopterin in leukemia cells. Biochem Pharmacol 7:75–80

Fischer GA (1962) Defective transport of amethopterin (methotrexate) as a mechanism of resistance to the antimetabolite in L5178Y leukemia cells. Biochem Pharmacol 11:1233–1234

Flintoff W, Saya L (1978) The selection of wild-type revertants from methotrexate permeability mutants. Somatic Cell Gen 4:143–156

Foley GE, Friedman OM, Drolet BP (1961) Studies of the mechanism of action of cytoxan. Evidence of activation in vivo and in vitro. Cancer Res 21:57–63

Fry DW, Cybulski RL, Goldman ID (1980a) K^+-induced alterations of energetics and exchange diffusion in the carrier-mediated transport of the folic acid analog, methotrexate, in Ehrlich ascites tumor cells. Biochim Biophys Acta 603:157–170

Fry DW, White JC, Goldman ID (1980b) Effects of 2,4-dinitrophenol and other metabolic inhibitors on the bidirectional carrier fluxes, net transport, and intracellular binding of methotrexate in Ehrlich ascites tumor cells. Cancer Res 40:3669–3673

Fujimoto J (1974) Radioautographic studies on the intracellular distribution of bleomycin-^{14}C in mouse tumor cells. Cancer Res 34:2969–2974

Furth JJ, Cohen SS (1968) Inhibition of mammalian DNA polymerase by the 5′-triphosphate of 1-β-D-arabinofuransylcytosine and the 5′-triphosphate of 9-β-D-arabinofuranosyladenine. Cancer Res 28:2061–2067

Fyfe MJ, Goldman ID (1973) Characteristics of the vincristine-induced augmentation of methotrexate uptake in Ehrlich ascites tumor cells. J Biol Chem 248:5067–5073

Galivan J (1979) Transport and metabolism of methotrexate in normal and resistant cultured rat hepatoma cells. Cancer Res 39:735–743

Galivan J (1981) 5-Methyltetrahydrofolate transport by hepatoma cells and methotrexate-resistant sublines in culture. Cancer Res 41:1757–1762

Garcia-Sancho J, Sanchez A, Christensen HN (1977) Role of proton dissociation in the transport of acidic amino acids by the Ehrlich ascites tumor cell. Biochim Biophys Acta 464:295–312

George P, Journey LJ, Goldstein MN (1965) Effects of vincristine on the fine structure of HeLa cells during mitosis. J Natl Cancer Inst 35:355–375

Giorgi EP, Shirley IM, Grant JK, Stewart JC (1973) Androgen dynamics in vitro in the human prostate gland. Biochem J 132:465–474

Giorgi EP, Moses TF, Grant JK, Scott R, Sinclair J (1974) In vitro studies of the regulation of androgen-tissue relationship in normal canine and hyperplastic human prostate. Mol Cell Endocrinol 1:271–284

Glover GI, D'Ambrosio SM, Jensen RA (1975) Versatile properties of a non-saturable homogeneous transport system in *Bacillus subtilis*: genetic, kinetic, and affinity labeling studies. Proc Natl Acad Sci USA 72:814–818

Goldenberg GJ (1969) Properties of L5178Y lymphoblasts highly resistant to nitrogen mustard. Ann NY Acad Sci 163:936–953

Goldenberg GJ (1975) The role of drug transport in resistance to nitrogen mustard and other alkylating agents in L5178Y lymphoblasts. Cancer Res 35:1687–1692

Goldenberg GJ, Begleiter A (1980) Membrane transport of alkylating agents. Pharmacol Ther 8:237–274

Goldenberg GJ, Vanstone CL, Israels LG, Ilse D, Bihler I (1970) Evidence for a transport carrier of nitrogen mustard in nitrogen mustard-sensitive and -resistant L5178Y lymphoblasts. Cancer Res 30:2285–2291

Goldenberg GJ, Vanstone CL, Bihler I (1971 a) Transport of nitrogen mustard on the transport carrier for choline in L5178Y lymphoblasts. Science 172:1148–1149

Goldenberg GJ, Lyons RM, Lepp JA, Vanstone CL (1971 b) Sensitivity to nitrogen mustard as a function of transport activity and proliferative rate in L5178Y lymphoblasts. Cancer Res 31:1616–1619

Goldenberg GJ, Land HB, Cormack DV (1974) Mechanism of cyclophosphamide transport by L5178Y lymphoblasts in vitro. Cancer Res 34:3274–3282

Goldenberg GJ, Lee M, Lam HYP, Begleiter A (1977) Evidence for carrier-mediated transport of melphalan by L5178Y lymphoblasts in vitro. Cancer Res 37:755–760

Goldenberg GJ, Lam HYP, Begleiter A (1978) Active carrier-mediated transport of melphalan by two separate amino acid transport systems in LPC-1 plasmacytoma cells in vitro. Clin Res 26:874A

Goldenberg GJ, Lam HYP, Begleiter A (1979) Active carrier-mediated transport of melphalan by two separate amino acid transport systems in LPC-1 plasmacytoma cells in vitro. J Biol Chem 254:1057–1064

Goldman ID (1969) Transport energetics of the folic acid analogue, methotrexate, in L1210 leukemia cells. J Biol Chem 244:3779–3785

Goldman ID (1971 a) The characteristics of the membrane transport of amethopterin and the naturally occurring folates. Ann NY Acad Sci 186:400–422

Goldman ID (1971 b) A model system for the study of heteroexchange diffusion: methotrexate-folate interactions in L1210 leukemia and Ehrlich ascites tumor cells. Biochim Biophys Acta 233:624–634

Goldman ID, Lichtenstein NS, Oliverio VT (1968) Carrier-mediated transport of the folic acid analogue methotrexate, in the L1210 leukemia cell. J Biol Chem 243:5007–5017

Goldman ID, Gupta V, White JC, Loftfield S (1976) Exchangeable intracellular methotrexate levels in the presence and absence of vincristine at extracellular drug concentrations relevant to those achieved in high-dose methotrexate-folinic acid "rescue" protocols. Cancer Res 36:276–279

Goldstein MN, Slotnick IJ, Journey LJ (1960) In vitro studies with Hela cell lines sensitive and resistant to actinomycin-D. Ann NY Acad Sci 89:474–483

Goldstein MN, Hamm K, Amrod E (1966) Incorporation of tritiated actinomycin-D into drug-sensitive and drug-resistant Hela cells. Science 151:1555–1556

Gotto AM, Belkhode ML, Touster O (1969) Stimulatory effects of inosine and deoxyinosine on the incorporation of uracil-2-^{14}C, 5-fluorouracil-2-^{14}C, and 5-bromouracil-2-^{14}C into nucleic acids by Ehrlich ascites tumor cells in vitro. Cancer Res 29:807–811

Gout PW, Wijcik LL, Beer CT (1978) Differences between vinblastine and vincristine in distribution in the blood of rats and binding by platelets and malignant cells. Eur J Cancer 14:1167–1178

Gross SR, Aronow L, Pratt WB (1968) The active transport of cortisol by mouse fibroblasts growing in vitro. Biochem Biophys Res Commun 32:66–72

Gross SR, Aronow L, Pratt WB (1970) The outward transport of cortisol by mammalian cells in vitro. J Cell Biol 44:103–114

Gustafsson JA, Ekman P, Snochowski M, Zetterberg A, Pousette A, Hogberg B (1978) Correlation between clinical response to hormone therapy and steroid receptor content in prostatic cancer. Cancer Res 38:4345–4358

Hakala MT (1965) On the nature of permeability of sarcoma-180 cells to amethopterin in vitro. Biochim Biophys Acta 102:210–225

Hall TC, Choi OS, Abadi A, Krant MJ (1967) High-dose corticoid therapy in Hodgkin's disease and other lymphomas. Ann Intern Med 66:1144–1153

Hanby WE, Hartley GS, Powell EO, Rydon HN (1947) The chemistry of 2-chloroalkylamines. Part II. Reactions of tertiary 2-chloroalkylamines in water. J Chem Soc 519–533

Harrap KR, Hill BT (1969) The selectivity of action of akylating agents and drug resistance. 1. Biochemical changes occurring in sensitive and resistant strains of the Yoshida ascites sarcoma following chemotherapy. Br J Cancer 23:210–226

Harrap KR, Hill BT (1970) The selectivity of action of alkylating agents and drug resistance. 3. The uptake and degradation of alkylating drugs by Yoshida ascites sarcoma cells in vitro. Biochem Pharmacol 19:209–217

Harrap KR, Jackson RC (1978) Biochemical mechanisms of resistance to antimetabolites. Antibiot Chemother 23:228–237

Hawkins RA, Berlin RD (1969) Purine transport in polymorphonuclear leukocytes. Biochim Biophys Acta 173:324–337

Hebden HF, Hadfield JR, Beer CT (1970) The binding of vinblastine by platelets in the rat. Cancer Res 30:1417–1424

Heidelberger C (1965) Fluorinated pyrimidines. Prog Nucleic Acid Res Mol Biol 4:1–50

Heidelberger C, Kaldor G, Mukherjee KL, Danneberg PB (1960) Studies on fluorinated pyrimidines XI. In vitro studies on tumor resistance. Cancer Res 20:903–909

Hilf R, Wittliff JL (1975) Mechanisms of action of estrogens. In: Sartorelli AC, Johns DG (eds) Antineoplastic and immunosuppressive agents II. Springer, Berlin Heidelberg New York

Hill BT (1972) Studies on the transport and cellular distribution of chlorambucil in the Yoshida ascites sarcoma. Biochem Pharmacol 21:495–502

Hill BT, Jarman M, Harrap KR (1971) Selectivity of action of alkylating agents and drug resistance. 4. Synthesis of tritium-labeled chlorambucil and a study of its cellular uptake by drug-sensitive and drug-resistant strains of the Yoshida ascites sarcoma in vitro. J Med Chem 14:614–618

Hill BT, Bailey BD, White JC, Goldman ID (1979) Characteristics of transport of 4-amino antifolates and folate compounds by two lines of L5178Y lymphoblasts, one with impaired transport of methotrexate. Cancer Res 39:2440–2446

Himes RH, Kersey RN, Heller-Bettinger I, Samson FE (1976) Action of the *Vinca* alkaloids vincristine, vinblastine and desacetyl vinblastine amide on microtubules in vitro. Cancer Res 36:3798–3802

Hirono I, Kachi H, Ohashi H (1962) Mechanism of natural and acquired resistance to methyl-bis(2-chloroethyl)amine *N*-oxide in ascites tumors. II. Permeability of tumor cells to alkylating agents. Gan 53:73–80

Ho DHW, Frei E (1971) Clinical pharmacology of 1-β-D-arabinofuranosyl cytosine. Clin Pharmacol Ther 12:944–954

Hoogstraten B, Sheehe PR, Cuttner J, Cooper T, Kyle RA, Oberfield RA, Townsend SR, Harley JB, Hayes DB, Costa G, Holland JF (1967) Melphalan and multiple myeloma. Blood 30:74–83

Inaba M (1973) Mechanism of resistance of Yoshida sarcoma to nitrogen mustard. III. Mechanism of suppressed transport of nitrogen mustard. Int J Cancer 11:231–236

Inaba M, Johnson RK (1978) Uptake and retention of adriamycin and daunorubicin by sensitive and anthracycline-resistant sublines of P388 leukemia. Biochem Pharmacol 27:2123–2130

Inaba M, Sakurai Y (1979) Enhanced efflux of actinomycin-D, vincristine, and vinblastine in adriamycin-resistant subline of P388 leukemia. Cancer Lett 8:111–115

Inaba M, Kobayashi H, Sakurai Y, Johnson RK (1979) Active efflux of daunorubicin and adriamycin in sensitive and resistant sublines of P388 leukemia. Cancer Res 39:2200–2203

Jacquez JA (1962) Permeability of Ehrlich cells to uracil, thymine, and fluorouracil. Proc Soc Exp Biol Med 109:132–135

Jacquez JA (1975) One-way fluxes of α-amino-isobutyric acid in Ehrlich ascites tumor cells. J Gen Physiol 65:57–83

Journey LG, Burdman J, George P (1968) Ultrastructural studies on tissue culture cells treated with vincristine. Cancer Chemother Rep 52:509–517

Juliano RL, Ling V (1976) A surface glycoprotein modulating drug permeability in Chinese hamster ovary cell mutants. Biochim Biophys Acta 455:152–162

Juliano R, Ling V, Graves J (1976) Drug-resistant mutants of Chinese hamster ovary cells possess an altered cell surface carbohydrate component. J Supramol Struct 4:521–526

Kano K, Fendler JH (1977) Enhanced uptake of drugs in liposomes: use of labile vitamin B_{12} complexes of 6-mercaptopurine and 8-azaguanine. Life Sci 20:1729–1734

Kaplan L (1968) Cancer of the prostate: estrogen therapy. Natural conjugated estrogen vs. stilboestrol. Rev Surg 25:323–329

Kasbekar DK, Greenberg DM (1963) Studies in tumor resistance to 5-fluorouracil. Cancer Res 23:818–824

Kelley RM, Baker WH (1960) Clinical observations on the effect of progesterone in the treatment of metastatic endometrial carcinoma. In: Pincus G, Vollmer E (eds) Biological activities of steroids in relation to cancer. Academic, New York, pp 447–455

Kelley RM, Baker WH (1970) Progestational agents in the treatment of carcinoma of the genitourinary tract. In: Sturgis S, Taymore M (eds) Progress in gynecology. Grune and Stratton, New York, pp 362–375

Kennedy BJ (1968) Progestogens in the treatment of carcinoma of the endometrium. Surg Gynecol Obstet 127:103–114

Kessel D (1971) Determinants of camptothecin responsiveness in leukemia L1210 cells. Cancer Res 31:1883–1887

Kessel D, Bosmann HB (1970) On the characteristics of actinomycin D resistance in L5178Y cells. Cancer Res 30:2695–2701

Kessel D, Hall TC (1967) Studies on drug transport by normal human leukocytes. Biochem Pharmacol 16:2395–2403

Kessel D, Hall TC (1969 a) Influence of ribose donors on the action of 5-fluorouracil. Cancer Res 29:1749–1754

Kessel D, Hall TC (1969 b) Retention of 6-mercaptopurine derivatives by intact cells as an index of drug response in human and murine leukemias. Cancer Res 29:2116–2119

Kessel D, Shurin SB (1968) Transport of two non-metabolized nucleosides, deoxycytidine and cytosine arabinoside in a subline of L1210 murine leukemia. Biochim Biophys Acta 163:179–187
Kessel D, Wodinsky I (1968) Uptake in vivo and in vitro of actinomycin D by mouse leukemias as factors in survival. Biochem Pharmacol 17:161–164
Kessel D, Hall TC, Roberts D (1965) Uptake as a determinant of methotrexate response in mouse leukemias. Science 150:752–753
Kessel D, Hall TC, Wodinsky I (1966) Nucleotide formation as a determinant of 5-fluorouracil response in mouse leukemias. Science 154:911–913
Kessel D, Hall TC, Roberts D (1968) Modes of uptake of methotrexate by normal and leukemic human leukocytes in vitro and their relation to drug response. Cancer Res 28:564–570
Kessel D, Meyers M, Wodinsky I (1969) Accumulation of two alkylating agents, nitrogen mustard and busulfan, by murine leukemia cells in vitro. Biochem Pharmacol 18:1229–1234
Kiang DT, Frenning DH, Goldman AI, Ascensao VF, Kennedy BJ (1978) Estrogen receptors and responses to chemotherapy and hormonal therapy in advanced breast cancer. N Engl J Med 299:1330–1334
Klatt O, Stechlin JS Jr, McBride C, Griffin AC (1969) The effect of nitrogen mustard treatment on the deoxyribonucleic acid of sensitive and resistant Ehrlich tumor cells. Cancer Res 29:286–290
Kneale B, Evans J (1969) Progestogen therapy for advanced carcinoma of the endometrium. Med J Aust 2:1101–1104
Koren R, Shohami E, Yeroushalmi S (1979) A kinetic analysis of the uptake of cytosine-β-D-arabinoside by rat-B77 cells. Eur J Biochem 95:333–339
Koshiura R, LePage GA (1968) Some inhibitors of deamination of 9-β-D-arabinofuranosyladenine and 9-β-D-xylofuranosyladenine by blood of neoplasms of experimental animals and humans. Cancer Res 28:1014–1020
Kotler-Brajtburg J, Medoff G, Kobayashi GS, Boggs S, Schlessinger D, Pandey RC, Rinehalt KL Jr (1979) Classification of polyene antibiotics according to chemical structure and biological effects. Antimicrob Agents Chemother 15:716–722
Kung S, Goldberg ND, Dahl JL, Parks RE Jr (1963) Potentiation of 5-fluorouracil inhibition of Flexner-Jobling carcinoma by glucose. Science 141:627–628
Kupferberg HJ (1969) Inhibition of ouabain-H^3 uptake by liver slices and its excretion into the bile by compounds having a steroid nucleus. Life Sci 8:1179–1185
Lam HYP, Begleiter A, Stein WD, Goldenberg GJ (1978) On the mechanism of uptake of procarbazine by L5178Y lymphoblasts in vitro. Biochem Pharmacol 27:1883–1885
Lam HYP, Talgoy MM, Goldenberg GJ (1980) Uptake and decomposition of chlorozotocin in L5178Y lymphoblasts in vitro. Cancer Res 40:3950–3955
Langelier Y, Simard R, Brailovsky C (1974) Mechanism of actinomycin resistance in SV40-transformed hamster cells. Differentiation 2:261–267
Laskin JD, Evans RM, Slocum HK, Burke D, Hakala MT (1979) Basis for natural variation in sensitivity to 5-fluorouracil in mouse and human cells in culture. Cancer Res 39:383–390
Layton D, Trouet A (1980) A comparison of the therapeutic effects of free and liposomally encapsulated vincristine in leukemic mice. Eur J Cancer 16:945–950
Lee SH, Sartorelli AC (1981) Conversion of 6-thioguanine to the nucleoside level by purine nucleoside phosphorylase of sarcoma 180 and sarcome 180/TG ascites cells. Cancer Res 41:1086–1090
Lee ML, Huang YM, Sartorelli AC (1978) Alkaline phosphatase activities of 6-thiopurine-sensitive and -resistant sublines of sarcoma 180. Cancer Res 38:2413–2418
Leo A, Hansch C, Elkins D (1971) Partition coefficients and their uses. Chem Rev 71:525–616
LePage GA (1960) Incorporation of 6-thioguanine in nucleic acids. Cancer Res 20:403–408
LePage GA, Jones M (1961) Further studies on the mechanism of action of 6-thioguanine. Cancer Res 21:1590–1594
LePage GA, Junga IG, Bowman B (1964) Biochemical and carcinostatic effects of 2′-deoxythioguanosine. Cancer Res 24:835–840

Lieb WR, Stein WD (1969) Biological membranes behave as non-porous polymeric sheets with respect to the diffusion of non-electrolytes. Nature 224:240–243
Lieb WR, Stein WD (1971) The molecular basis of simple diffusion within biological membranes. In: Koeinzeller A, Bronner FR (eds) Current topics in membranes and transport, vol 2. Academic, New York, pp 1–39
Ling V (1975) Drug resistance and membrane alteration in mutants of mammalian cells. Can J Genet Cytol 17:503–515
Ling V, Thompson LH (1974) Reduced permeability in CHO cells as a mechanism of resistance to colchicine. J Cell Physiol 83:103–116
Lippman ME, Perry S, Thompson EB (1974) Cytoplasmic glucocorticoid-binding proteins in glucocorticoid-unresponsive human and mouse leukemic cell lines. Cancer Res 34:1572–1576
Lippman ME, Yarbro GK, Leventhal BG (1978) Clinical implications of glucocorticoid receptors in human leukemia. Cancer Res 38:4251–4256
Lyons RM, Goldenberg GJ (1972) Active transport of nitrogen mustard and choline by normal and leukemic human lymphoid cells. Cancer Res 32:1679–1685
Malawista SE, Sato H, Bensch KG (1968) Vinblastine and griseofulvin reversibly disrupt the living mitotic spindle. Science 160:770–772
Mauer AM, Simone JV (1976) The current status of the treatment of childhood acute lymphoblastic leukemia. Cancer Treat Rev 3:17–41
Meyers MB, Biedler JL (1981) Increased synthesis of a low-molecular-weight protein in vincristine-resistant cells. Biochem Biophys Res Commun 99:228–235
Milgrom E, Atger M, Baulieu EE (1973) Studies on estrogen entry into uterine cells and on estradiol-receptor complex attachment to the nucleus. Is the entry of estrogen into uterine cells a protein-mediated process? Biochim Biophys Acta 320:267–283
Miura Y, Moriyama A (1961) Studies on the metabolism of rat ascites tumor with nitrogen mustard sensitive and resistant strains. VI. Inhibition of the in vitro incorporation of C^{14}-orotic acid into nucleic acids by nitrogen mustard. J Biochem (Tokyo) 50:362–366
Miyaki M, Ono T, Hori S, Umezawa H (1975) Binding of bleomycin to DNA in bleomycin-sensitive and -resistant rat ascites hepatoma cells. Cancer Res 35:2015–2019
Momparler RL, Chu MY, Fischer GA (1968) Studies on a new mechanism of resistance of L5178Y murine leukemia cells to cytosine arabinoside. Biochim Biophys Acta 161:481–493
Mulder JA, Harrap KR (1975) Cytosine arabinoside uptake by tumor cells in vitro. Eur J Cancer 11:373–379
Muller WEG, Rohde HJ, Beyer R, Maidhof A, Lachmann M, Taschner H, Zahn RK (1975) Mode of action of 9-β-D-arabinofuranosyladenine on the synthesis of DNA, RNA and protein in vivo and in vitro. Cancer Res 35:2160–2168
Muller WEG, Maidhof A, Zahn RK, Shannon WM (1977) Effect of 9-β-D-arabinofuranosyladenine on DNA synthesis in vivo. Cancer Res 37:2282–2290
Munck A, Wira C, Young DA, Mosher KM, Hallahan C, Bell PA (1972) Glucocorticoid-receptor complexes and the earliest steps in the actions of glucocorticoids on thymus cells. J Steroid Biochem 3:567–578
Nachman J, Baum E, Norris D, Ramsay N, Weetman R, Neerhout R, Griffin T, Littman P, Sather H, Chard R, Hammond D (1981) Prolonged remission after bone marrow (BM) relapse in childhood acute lymphocytic leukemia (ALL). Proc Am Soc Clin Oncol 22:476
Neal JL (1972) Analysis of Michaelis kinetics for two independent saturable membrane transport functions. J Theor Biol 35:113–118
Nelson JA, Kuhns JN, Carpenter JW (1975) Lack of activity of β-2′-deoxythioguanosine against two tumors resistant to 6-thioguanine. Cancer Res 35:1372–1374
Nichols WW (1964) In vitro chromosome breakage induced by arbinosyladenine in human leukocytes. Cancer Res 24:1502–1505
Nicholson ML, Young DA (1978) Effect of glucocorticoid hormones in vitro on the structural integrity of nuclei in corticosteroid-sensitive and -resistant lines of lymphosarcoma P1798. Cancer Res 38:3673–3680

Nicholson ML, Voris BP, Young DA (1981) Proteins associated with emergence of the resistance to lethal glucocorticoid actions in P1798 mouse lymphosarcoma cells. Cancer Res 41:3530–3537

Niethammer D, Jackson RC (1975) Changes of molecular properties associated with the development of resistance against methotrexate in human lymphoblastoid cells. Eur J Cancer 11:845–854

Orstavik J (1974) Uptake and release of ^{3}H-mitomycin-C in mouse P388 cell cultures. Acta Pathol Microbiol Scand [B] 82:270–276

Owellen RJ, Owens AH Jr, Donigian DW (1972) The binding of vincristine, vinblastine and colchicine to tubulin. Biochem Biophys Res Common 47:685–691

Owellen RJ, Donigian DW, Hartke CA, Dickerson RM, Kuhar MJ (1974) The binding of vinblastine to tubulin and to particulate fractions of mammalian brain. Cancer Res 34:3180–3186

Owellen RJ, Hartke CA, Dickerson RM, Hains FO (1976) Inhibition of tubulin-microtubule polymerization of drugs of the *Vinca* alkaloid class. Cancer Res 36:1499–1502

Oxender DL, Christensen HN (1963) Distinct mediating systems for the transport of neutral amino acids by the Ehrlich cell. J Biol Chem 238:3686–3699

Oxender DL, Lee M, Moore PA, Cecchini G (1977) Neutral amino acid transport systems of tissue culture cells. J Biol Chem 252:2675–2679

Pall ML (1970) Amino acid transport activity in *Neurospora crassa*. II. Properties of a basic amino acid transport system. Biochim Biophys Acta 203:139–140

Palmer CG, Livengood D, Warren AK, Simpson PJ, Johnson IS (1960) The action of vincaleukoblastine on mitosis in vitro. Exp Cell Res 20:198–201

Parsons PG, Carter FB, Morrison L, SR Regius Mary (1981) Mechanism of melphalan resistance developed in vitro in human melanoma cells. Cancer Res 41:1525–1534

Paterson ARP (1962) Resistance to 6-mercaptopurine. II. The synthesis of thioinosinate in a 6-mercaptopurine-resistant subline of the Ehrlich ascites carcinoma. Can J Biochem Physiol 40:195–206

Paterson ARP, Hori A (1962) Resistance to 6-mercaptopurine. I. Biochemical differences between the Ehrlich ascites carcinoma and a 6-mercaptopurine-resistant subline. Can J Biochem Physiol 40:181–194

Peck EJ Jr, Burgner J, Clark JH (1973) Estrophilic binding sites of the uterus. Relation to uptake and retention of estradiol in vitro. Biochemistry 12:4596–4603

Plagemann PGW, Marz R, Wohlhueter RM (1978) Transport and metabolism of deoxycytidine and 1-β-D-arabinofuranosylcytosine into cultured Novikoff rat hepatoma cells, relationship to phosphorylation and regulation of triphosphate synthesis. Cancer Res 38:978–989

Poste G, Papahadjopoulos D (1976) Drug-containing lipid vesicles render drug-resistant tumor cells sensitive to actinomycin-D. Nature 261:699–701

Potter LT (1968) Uptake of choline by nerve endings isolated from the rat cerebral cortex. In: Campbell PN (ed) Interaction of drugs and subcellular components. Churchill, London, pp 293–304

Rader JF, Niethammer D, Huennekens FM (1974) Effects of sulphydryl inhibitors upon transport of folate compounds into L1210 cells. Biochem Pharmacol 23:2057–2059

Rao ML, Rao GS, Holler M, Breuer H (1974) Uptake of cortisol by isolated rat liver cells. Hoppe Seylers Z Physiol Chem 355:1239–1240

Rao GS, Schulze-Hagen K, Rao ML, Breuer H (1976a) Kinetics of steroid transport through cell membranes: comparison of the uptake of cortisol by isolated rat liver cells with binding of cortisol to rat liver cytosol. J Steroid Biochem 7:1123–1129

Rao ML, Rao GS, Holler M, Breuer H, Schattenberg PJ, Stein WD (1976b) Uptake of cortisol by isolated rat liver cells. A phenomenon indicative of carrier-mediated and simple diffusion. Hoppe Seylers Z Physiol Chem 357:573–584

Rao ML, Rao GS, Breuer H (1977) Uptake of estrone, estradiol-17β and testosterone by isolated rat liver cells. Biochem Biophys Res Commun 77:566–573

Redwood WR, Colvin M (1980) Transport of melphalan by sensitive and resistant L1210 cells. Cancer Res 40:1144–1149

Reichard P, Sköld O, Klein G (1959) Possible enzymic mechanism for the development of resistance against fluorouracil in ascites tumors. Nature 183:939–941
Reichard P, Sköld O, Klein G, Renesz L, Magnusson P (1962) Studies on resistance against 5-fluorouracil. I. Enzymes of the uracil pathway during development of resistance. Cancer Res 22:235–243
Reiser S, Fitzgerald JF, Christensen PA (1970) Kinetics of the accelerated intestinal valine transport in 2-day-old rats. Biochim Biophys Acta 203:351–353
Riehm H, Biedler JL (1971) Cellular resistance to daunomycin in Chinese hamster cells in vitro. Cancer Res 31:409–412
Riehm H, Biedler JL (1972) Potentiation of drug effect by Tween 80 in Chinese hamster cells resistant to actinomycin-D and daunomycin. Cancer Res 32:1195–1200
Rigberg SV, Brodsky I (1975) Potential roles of androgens and the anabolic steroids in the treatment of cancer – a review. J Med 6:271–290
Riordan JR, Ling V (1979) Purification of P-glycoprotein from plasma membrane vesicles of Chinese hamster ovary cell mutants with reduced colchicine permeability. J Biol Chem 254:12701–12705
Rosowsky A, Lazarus H, Yuan GC, Beltz WR, Mangini L, Abelson HT, Modest EJ, Frei E (1980) Effects of methotrexate esters and other lipophilic antifolates on methotrexate-resistant human leukemic lymphoblasts. Biochem Pharmacol 29:648–652
Rutman RJ, Chun EHL, Lewis FS (1968) Permeability differences as a source of resistance to alkylating agents in Ehrlich tumor cells. Biochem Biophys Res Commun 32:650–657
Rysser HJP, Shen WC (1978) Conjugation of methotrexate to poly (L-lysine) increases drug transport and overcomes drug resistance in cultured cells. Proc Natl Acad Sci USA 75:3867–3870
Rysser HJP, Shen WC (1980) Conjugation of methotrexate to poly (L-lysine) as a potential way to overcome drug resistance. Cancer 45:1207–1211
Salser JS, Hutchison DJ, Balis ME (1960) Studies on the mechanism of action of 6-mercaptopurine in cell-free preparations. J Biol Chem 235:429–432
Sartorelli AC, LePage GA (1958) Metabolic effects of 6-thioguanine. II. Biosynthesis of nucleic acid purines in vivo and in vitro. Cancer Res 18:1329–1335
Sartorelli AC, LePage GA, Moore EC (1958) Metabolic effects of 6-thioguanine. I. Studies on thioguanine-resistant and -sensitive Ehrlich ascites cells. Cancer Res 18:1232–1239
Sawitsky A, Desposito F, Treat C (1970) Vincristine and cyclophosphamide therapy in generalized neuroblastoma: a collaborative study. Am J Dis Child 119:308–313
Schabel FM, Trader MW, Laster WR, Wheeler GP, Witt MH (1978) Patterns of resistance and therapeutic synergism among alkylating agents. Antibiot Chemother 23:200–215
Schanker LS, Jeffrey JJ (1961) Active transport of foreign pyrimidines across the intestinal epithelium. Nature 190:727–728
Schrecker AW (1970) Metabolism of 1-β-D-arabinofuranosylcytosine in leukemia L1210: nucleoside and nucleotide kinases in cell-free extracts. Cancer Res 30:632–641
Scriver CR, Hechtman P (1970) Human genetics of membrane transport with emphasis on amino acids. Adv Hum Genet 1:211–274
Scriver CR, Mohyuddin S (1968) Amino acid transport in kidney: heterogeneity of α-aminoisobutyric acid uptake. J Biol Chem 243:3207–3213
Secret CJ, Hadfield JR, Beer CT (1972) Studies on the binding of ^{3}H-vinblastine by rat blood platelets in vitro. Biochem Pharmacol 21:1609–1624
See YP, Carlsen SA, Till JE, Ling V (1974) Increased drug permeability in Chinese hamster ovary cells in the presence of cyanide. Biochim Biophys Acta 373:242–252
Segal S, Schwartzman L, Blair A, Bertoli D (1967) Dibasic amino acid transport in rat kidney cortex slices. Biochim Biophys Acta 135:127–135
Shen WC, Rysser HJP (1979) Poly(L-lysine) and poly(D-lysine) conjugates of methotrexate: different inhibitory effect on drug-resistant cells. Mol Pharmacol 16:614–622
Simard R, Cassingena R (1969) Actinomycin resistance in cultured hamster cells. Cancer Res 29:1590–1597
Sirotnak FM (1980) Correlates of folate analog transport, pharmacokinetics and selective antitumor action. Pharmacol Ther 8:71–103

Sirotnak FM, Donsbach RC (1976) Kinetic correlates of methotrexate transport and therapeutic responsiveness in murine tumors. Cancer Res 36:1151–1158
Sirotnak FM, Kurita S, Hutchison DJ (1968) On the nature of a transport alteration determining resistance to amethopterin in the L1210 leukemia. Cancer Res 28:75–80
Skinner SM, Lewis RW (1977) Anti-leukemic activity (L1210) of 6-mercaptopurine and its metallo complexes in mice. Res Commun Chem Pathol Pharmacol 16:183–186
Skovsgaard T (1978a) Carrier-mediated transport of daunorubicin, adriamycin, and rubidazone in Ehrlich ascites tumor cells. Biochem Pharmacol 27:1221–1227
Skovsgaard T (1978b) Mechanisms of resistance to daunorubicin in Ehrlich ascites tumor cells. Cancer Res 38:1785–1791
Skovsgaard T (1978c) Mechanism of cross-resistance between vincristine and daunorubicin in Ehrlich ascites tumor cells. Cancer Res 38:4722–4727
Skovsgaard T (1980) Circumvention of resistance to daunorubicin by *N*-acetyldaunorubicin in Ehrlich ascites tumor. Cancer Res 40:1077–1083
Sladek NE (1971) Metabolism of cyclophosphamide by rat hepatic microsomes. Cancer Res 31:901–908
Slotnick IJ, Sells BH (1964) Actinomycin resistance in *Bacillus subtilis*. Science 146:407–408
Sonneborn D, Rothstein H (1966) Tritiated actinomycin-D uptake by amphibian lens epithelial cells. J Cell Biol 31:163a
States B, Segal S (1968) Developmental aspects of cystine transport in rat intestinal segments. Biochim Biophys Acta 163:154–162
Stevens J, Stevens YW, Rhodes J, Steiner G (1978) Differences in nuclear glucocorticoid binding between corticoid-sensitive and corticoid-resistant lymphocytes of mouse lymphoma P1798 and stabilization of nuclear hormone receptor complexes with carbobenzoxy-L-phenylalanine. J Natl Cancer Inst 61:1477–1485
Stoll BA (1969) Hormone management of advanced breast cancer. Br Med J 2:293–297
Stutts P, Brockman RW (1963) A biochemical basis for resistance of L1210 mouse leukemia to 6-thioguanine. Biochem Pharmacol 12:97–104
Taylor EW (1965) The mechanism of colchicine inhibition of mitosis. J Cell Biol 25:145–160
Taylor JR (1959) Intravenous and oral trial of stilbestrol diphosphate in prostatic cancer. Can Med Assoc J 80:880–882
Thomas AN, Gordan GS, Goldman L, Lowe R (1962) Antitumor efficacy of 2-α-methyl dihydrotestosterone propionate in advanced breast cancer. Cancer 15:176–178
Thomas EL, Christensen HN (1971) Nature of the cosubstrate action of Na^+ and neutral amino acids in a transport system. J Biol Chem 246:1682–1688
Thompson EB, Lippman ME (1974) The mechanism of action of glucocorticoids. Metabolism 23:159–202
Troshin AS (1966) Problems of cell permeability. Pergamon, Oxford, pp 16–20
Trouet A, Deprez-De, Campeneere D, DeDuve C (1972) Chemotherapy through lysosomes with a DNA-daunorubicin complex. Nature New Biol 239:110–112
Tsuruo T, Iida H, Tsukagoshi S, Sakurai Y (1981a) Prevention of vinblastine-induced cytotoxicity by ruthenium red. Biochem Pharmacol 30:213–216
Tsuruo T, Iida H, Tsukagoshi S, Sakurai Y (1981b) Overcoming of vincristine resistance in P388 leukemia in vivo and in vitro through enhanced cytotoxicity of vincristine and vinblastine by verapamil. Cancer Res 41:1967–1972
Uchida K, Kreis W (1969) Studies on drug resistance. I. Distribution of 1-β-D-arabinofuranosylcytosine, cytidine and deoxycytidine in mice bearing ara-C-sensitive and -resistant P815 neoplasms. Biochem Pharmacol 18:1115–1128
Umezawa H (1975) Bleomycin. In: Corcoran JW, Hahn FE (eds) Antibiotics, vol 3. Springer, Berlin Heidelberg New York, pp 21–33
van Putten LM, Lelieveld P (1971) Factors determining cell kill by chemotherapeutic agents in vivo. II. Melphalan, chlorambucil, and nitrogen mustard. Eur J Cancer 7:11–16
Vistica DT (1979) Cytotoxicity as an indicator for transport mechanism: evidence that melphalan is transported by two leucine-preferring carrier systems in the L1210 murine leukemia cell. Biochim Biophys Acta 550:309–317

Vistica DT (1980) Cytotoxicity as an indicator for transport mechanism: evidence that murine bone marrow progenitor cells lack a high-affinity leucine carrier that transports melphalan in murine L1210 leukemia cells. Blood 56:427–429
Vistica DT, Schuette BP (1981) Carrier mechanism and specificity accounting for the increase in intracellular melphalan by the basic amino acids. Mol Pharmacol 19:92–96
Vistica DT, Toal JN, Rabinovitz M (1976) Amino acid-conferred resistance to melphalan. I. Structure-activity relationship in cultured L1210 leukemia cells. Cancer Treat Rep 60:1363–1367
Vistica DT, Toal JN, Rabinovitz M (1977) Amino acids affecting melphalan transport and cytotoxicity in cultured L1210 cells. Proc Am Assoc Cancer Res 18:26
Vistica DT, Rabon A, Rabinovitz M (1978a) Interference with melphalan transport and therapy in the L1210 murine leukemia system, its significance and prevention. Proc Am Assoc Cancer Res 19:44
Vistica DT, Rabon A, Rabinovitz M (1978b) Enhancement of melphalan therapy with glutaminase: asparaginase. Res Commun Chem Pathol Pharmacol 22:83–92
Vistica DT, Toal JN, Rabinovitz M (1978c) Amino acid-conferred protection against melphalan: characterization of melphalan transport and correlation of uptake with cytotoxicity in cultured L1210 murine leukemia cells. Biochem Pharmacol 27:2865–2870
Warren RD, Nichols AP, Bender RA (1977) The effect of vincristine on methotrexate uptake and inhibition of DNA synthesis by human lymphoblastoid cells. Cancer Res 37:2993–2997
Warren R, Nichols AP, Bender RA (1978) Membrane transport of methotrexate in human lymphoblastoid cells. Cancer Res 38:668–671
Wheeler GP, Alexander JA (1964) Studies with mustards. V. In vivo fixation of C^{14} of labeled alkylating agents by bilaterally grown sensitive and resistant tumors. Cancer Res 24:1331–1337
Winter CG, Christensen HN (1965) Contrasts in neutral amino acid transport by rabbit erythrocytes and reticulocytes. J Biol Chem 240:3594–3600
Wira CR, Munck A (1974) Glucocorticoid-receptor complexes in rat thymus cells. J Biol Chem 249:5328–5336
Wohlhueter RM, McIvor RS, Plagemann PGW (1980) Facilitated transport of uracil and 5-fluorouracil and permeation of orotic acid in cultured mammalian cells. J Cell Physiol 104:309–319
Wolpert MK, Ruddon RW (1969) A study on the mechanism of resistance to nitrogen mustard (HN2) in Ehrlich ascites tumor cells; comparison of uptake of HN2-^{14}C into sensitive and resistant cells. Cancer Res 29:873–879
Wolpert MK, Damle SP, Brown JE, Sznycer E, Agrawal KC, Sartorelli AC (1971) The role of phosphohydrolases in the mechanism of resistance of neoplastic cells to 6-thiopurines. Cancer Res 31:1620–1626
Yamada T, Iwanami Y, Baba T (1963) The transport of ^{14}C-labeled nitrogen mustard N-oxide through cellular membrane treated with Tween 80 in vitro. Gann 54:171–176
Yamagami H, Ishizawa M, Endo H (1974) Phenotypic and genetic characteristics of bleomycin sensitive mutants of *Escherichia coli*. Gann 65:61–67
Yamamoto KR, Stampfer MR, Tomkins GM (1974) Receptors from glucocorticoid-sensitive lymphoma cells and two classes of insensitive clones: physical and DNA-binding properties. Proc Natl Acad Sci USA 71:3901–3905
York JL, LePage GA (1966) A proposed mechanism for the action of 9-β-D-arabinofuranosyladenine as an inhibitor of the growth of some ascites cells. Can J Biochem 44:19–26
Zager RF, Frisby SA, Oliverio VT (1973) The effects of antibiotics and cancer chemotherapeutic agents on the cellular transport and antitumor activity of methotrexate in L1210 murine leukemia. Cancer Res 33:1670–1676

CHAPTER 11

Cell Hybridisation

J. M. BOYLE

A. Introduction

It has been suggested that cell fusion could be an early event in the neoplastic process (MILLER 1974). In this chapter we examine the evidence for the occurrence of cell fusion in vivo, and explore the possibility that drug resistance can derive from mutations that accumulate in the enlarged gene pool of the hybrid cell. Since there is little direct information concerning the expression of drug resistance in hybrid cells in vivo, we shall discuss the implications for chemotherapy of the lessons learnt from the study of drug resistance in hybrid cells in vitro. The fusion of two cells is but one means of increasing cell ploidy (review, BRODSKY and URYVAEVA 1977), so much of this discussion may be applicable to polyploid cells in general. Emphasis is placed on resistance to antitumour agents which exclusively involve nuclear genes. Mutants deficient in mitochondrial protein synthesis and respiratory functions coded by both nuclear and mitochondrial DNA are providing interesting insights into nuclear/cytoplasmic relationships, but to date none of these have involved antitumour drug resistance and will not be discussed. The interested reader can find information on this topic reviewed by WRIGHT et al. (1980) and background reading on somatic-cell genetics in HARRIS (1970), EPHRUSSI (1972), DAVIDSON and DE LA CRUZ (1974), RINGERTZ and SAVAGE (1976) and SHOWS and SAKAGUCHI (1980).

The initial product of cell fusion (Fig. 1) is a bi- or multinucleate cell that is either a heterokaryon if the parental cells were genetically different (Fig. 2) or a homokaryon if they were similar. In vivo, cells resulting from genetically programmed fusions often remain as multinucleate homokaryons. In vitro, the fused cells will be in cycle and will attempt to divide. At mitosis chromosomes from different nuclei come to share a common spindle apparatus and are drawn to the poles at anaphase to form two hybrid nuclei at telophase (Fig. 3). Clonogenic hybrids usually result from the fusion of two or three cells, since fusions of four or more cells run into mechanical difficulties at mitosis or are liable to contain a mixture of mitotic and interphase nuclei that are subject to premature chromosome condensation (Sect. D.V). The genetic redundancy in a hybrid nucleus permits the cell to accumulate recessive mutations and to undergo chromosomal rearrangements and loss of chromosomes without loss of viability. If these changes are beneficial, permitting the cell to divide faster or allowing it to occupy a new niche, then they will be selected for and persist. We now examine the evidence that supports the idea that drug resistance in vivo could result from such processes.

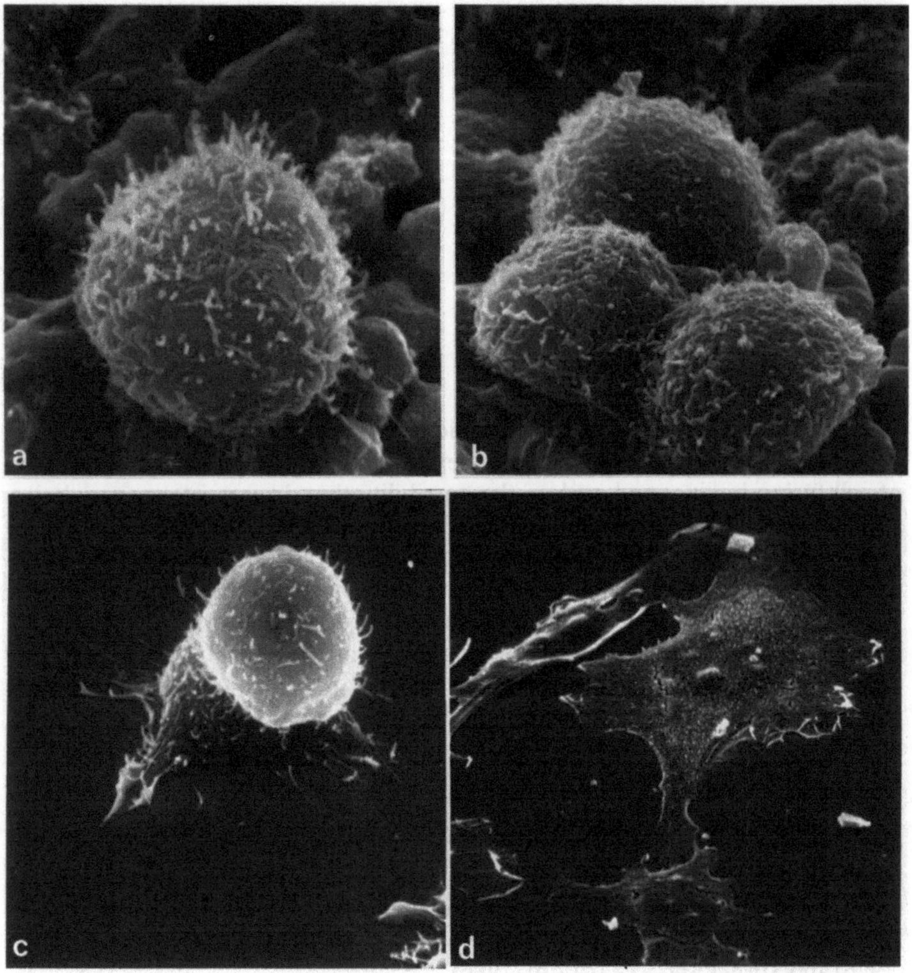

Fig. 1 a–d. In vitro fusion of Chinese hamster fibroblasts observed by scanning electron microscopy. **a** A Chinese hamster fibroblast observed prior to fusion showing a typical spherical morphology and microvillous topography of a cell in suspension. × 10,000. **b** Sendai virus, inactivated by treatment with β-propiolactone, has been added at 0 °C to a suspension of cells, causing agglutination. This clump of cells may be indicative of an early step in fusion with the microvilli of adjacent cells in intimate contact. × 7,000. **c** After adsorption of the virus the fusion mixture was incubated for 15 min at 37 °C before diluting into growth medium and incubating for a further 4 h. At this stage cells are resettling onto the substratum: the upper member of this pair still retains its spherical morphology. × 5,000. **d** 24 h postfusion, all cells are now attached to the substratum. The large cell, *upper right,* is approximately twice the size of the adjacent cells indicative of a heterokaryon. × 1,200. (P. J. Smith, T. D. Allen and J. M. Boyle, unpublished)

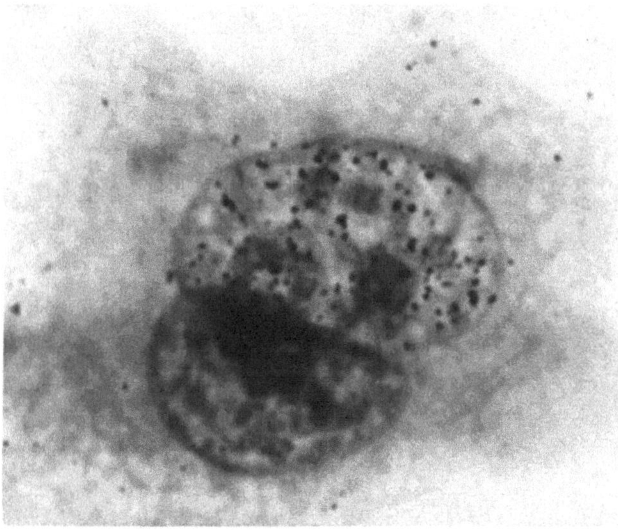

Fig. 2. A binucleate heterokaryon. Radioautogram of a heterokaryon containing one unlabelled and one labelled nucleus, resulting from fusion of two populations of Chinese hamster fibroblasts, one of which had been grown in the presence of [^{3}H]thymidine. (J. M. Boyle, unpublished)

B. Cell Fusion In Vivo

I. Occurrence of Multinucleate Cells

Bi- and multinucleate cells have been observed in a wide range of normal and pathological tissues (Table 1, and review by CHAMBERS 1978). In principle the presence of more than one nucleus could result from a mitotic division without cytokinesis. In many cases, however, multinucleation results from cell fusions that are a genetically programmed part of differentiation and can be observed to occur in tissue cultures. This is particularly important in haemopoietic tissues where macrophage-like cells fuse to form multinucleated giant cells and osteoclasts (TESTA et al. 1981). In vivo fusion of mononuclear cells to form giant cells may be in response to the presence of foreign bodies (SILVERMAN and SHORTER 1963) and occur in tuberculous lesions as Langhans cells (W. H. LEWIS 1927) and as frequent constituents of solid tumours (EVANS 1956). Fusions of macrophages to form multinucleated giant cells (M. R. LEWIS and W. H. LEWIS 1926; SUTTON and WEISS 1966), myoblasts (HOLTZER et al. 1958; KONIGSBERG et al. 1960; KONIGSBERG 1963; CAPERS 1960; YAFFE and FELDMAN 1965) and trophoblasts (PRIEST et al. 1980) have all been observed in vitro. In most cases where fusion is part of differentiation and the expression of specialised functions, there is little evidence that such cells divide and multiply (STOCKDALE and HOLTZER 1961), although synchronous DNA synthesis (RYAN and SPECTOR 1970) and both synchronous and asynchronous mitoses of multinucleated macrophages have been observed in vivo (MARIANO and SPECTOR 1974).

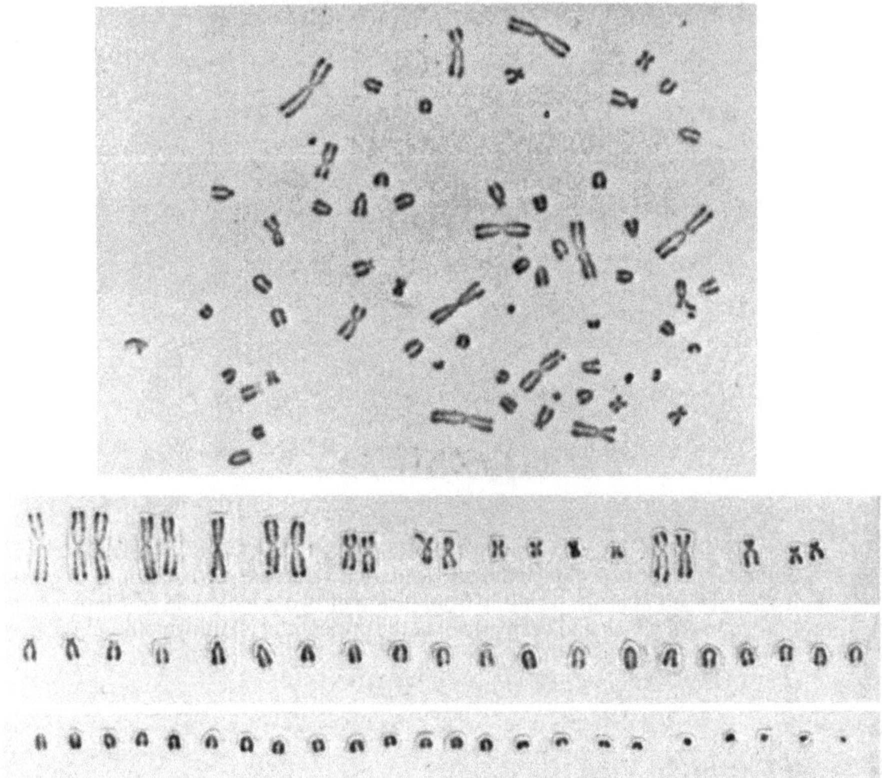

Fig. 3. Karyotype of a Chinese hamster V79 × mouse L1210 hybrid. *Upper*, metaphase figure stained with aceto-orcein. *Lower*, chromosomes of some metaphase chromosomes arranged in order of size, *top line* containing meta- and submetacentric chromosomes typical of Chinese hamster, *bottom line* containing telocentric chromosomes typical of mouse. (L. G. Durrant and J. M. Boyle, unpublished)

Two groups of viruses that frequently produce lesions containing fused cells are herpesvirus, which causes syncytia in skin lesions of patients with varicella (Tyzzer 1906) and the paramyxoviruses, which include mumps, measles, respiratory syncytial virus and Sendai or haemagglutinating virus of Japan (HJV). Sendai virus is of interest as the agent used to produce the first intespecies hybrid cells between human and mouse (Harris and Watkins 1965). Roizman (1962a) discussed evidence that polykaryocytosis occurred mainly following low-level infection insufficient to allow virus multiplication and was enhanced by viral antibodies that prevented the spread of free viral particles. Viruses from other taxonomic groups (Table 1) have also been observed to cause fusion of cell cultures. This does not necessarily mean that such viruses cause fusion in vivo, since Cascardo and Karzon (1965) showed that, although many epithelial cell lines were susceptible to fusion by measles virus, neither diploid human fibroblasts nor primary human epithelial cultures were susceptible. The Togavirus causing Western equine encephalomyelitis, apparently caused the production of hybrid erythrocytes when injected into chimeric chickens (Karakoz et al. 1969), al-

Table 1. Multinucleate cells in vivo

Occurrence	Reference
A. Normal tissues	
Binucleate cells of liver	LE BOUTON (1976)
Multinucleate cells of bladder epithelium	MARTIN (1972)
Myoblast fusion to give myotubules	MINTZ and BAKER (1967)
Megakaryocyte formation:	
Foreign body giant cells	CHAMBERS (1978)
Langhans giant cells	MARIANO and SPECTOR (1974)
Formation of osteoclasts	HAM (1974)
	TESTA et al. (1981)
Syncytiotrophoblast fusion during implantation	ENDERS and SCHLAFKE (1971)
Erythroid cell fusion in chimeric cattle	STONE et al. (1964)
Leucocyte fusion following transfusion *in utero*	TURNER et al. (1973)
B. Infected tissues	
Giant cells in tuberculous lesions	LEWIS (1927)
Viral infections:	
a) Paramyxoviruses	
Mumps	HENLE et al. (1954)
Measles	WARTHIN (1931)
Respiratory syncytial virus	MORRIS et al. (1956)
Sendai virus (HVJ)	OKADA (1962)
Newcastle disease virus	KOHN (1965)
b) Herpesviruses	
Varicella/zoster	TYZZER (1906)
	WELLER et al. (1958)
Herpes simplex	HOGGAN and ROIZMAN (1959)
	SCHERER (1953)
c) Leukoviruses	
Rous sarcoma virus	MOSES and KOHN (1963)
Visna virus	HARTER and CHOPPIN (1967)
d) Poxviruses	
Vaccinia	MCCLAIN (1965)
e) Togaviruses	
Dengue	SUITTER and PAUL (1969)
Western equine encephalomyelitis	KARAKOZ et al. (1969)
f) Bungaviruses	
Germiston	
Wesselsbron	DJINAWI and OLSEN (1973)
g) Coronavirus	
Avian infectious bronchitis virus	AKERS and CUNNINGHAM (1968)
C. Malignant tissues	
Giant cells in malignant tissues	LUDFORD and SMILES (1952)
Warren sarcoma	LEWIS (1927)
Reed-Sternberg binucleate cells in Hodgkins lymphoma	JACKSON and PARKER (1944)

though other cases of hybrid blood cells did not involve (known) viruses (STONE et al. 1964; TURNER et al. 1973).

Multinucleate cells are frequently observed in tumours (ROIZMAN 1962 b), and CHAMBERS (1978) distinguished between multinucleated tumour cells capable of division and "tumour-associated giant cells" that are rarely mitotic and have nuclei that are uniform in size and shape. These cells resemble foreign body giant cells and are thought to have a similar stem-cell origin. Examples cited are giant-cell tumour of soft parts (villonodular tenosynovitis), malignant giant-cell tumour of soft parts, osteoclastoma and malignant fibrous histiocytoma. Multinucleated tumour cells also occur. SHEEHY et al. (1974) found the frequency of bi- and multinucleated cells among malignant cells of ovarian carcinoma to be 7% and 65% respectively. Both DNA synthesis and mitosis were observed occurring asynchronously among nuclei of a single cell. Since multinucleate tumour cells are cycling, they will generate mononucleate hybrid cells that will contribute to the polyploidy of tumours. Some examples from an abundant literature on the incidence of polyploidy in tumours will illustrate the principles that the incidence and degree of polyploidy vary widely with the type of cancer and the stage of malignancy. MORARU and FADEI (1974) distinguished giant and multinucleated cells in eight cases of ovarian papillary adenocarcinomas. Frequencies varied from 0%–31% for giant cells to 0%–24% for multinucleated cells, the most invasive tumours having the highest proportion of both cell types. Mean chromosome numbers of the eight tumours showed variations from near diploid to hypotetraploid. In one tumour approximately 6% of metaphases had over 100 chromosomes. Comparison of tumour morphology and karyotype distinguished three stages of malignancy: stage I, mainly diploid, papilliform; stage II, mainly diploid with some heteroploid, proliferating malignant epithelium, covering papilli; stage III, heteroploid with marker chromosomes, invasive malignant epithelium. Ploidy can be more rapidly determined by microdensitometry of the DNA content of Feulgen-stained cells. A study of 23 ovarian carcinomas showed a good correlation between the DNA content measured in this way and the ploidy determined by chromosome counting (ATKIN 1971). A large study of the DNA contents of 1,465 malignant tumours of many different types was made by ATKIN and KAY (1979). Ploidy values were analysed in terms of 2.5-year survival data, and it was shown that most tumours except those of testis showed both low (near diploid) and high (triploid-tetraploid) groups, with prognosis being better for patients in the low group for all sites except carcinoma of the cervix uteri.

II. Experimental Production of Hybrids In Vivo

Support for the inference that cell fusion is involved in the production of polyploidy among tumour cells comes from studies with animal tumour-cell lines. There is strong evidence for fusion occurring in vivo between different tumour cell lines (JANZEN et al. 1971) and between tumour cells and normals cells of the host animal (Table 2). Definitive proof of hybridisation requires the demonstration that a cell possesses chromosomes, antigenic determinants or isozymes characteristic of both cell types involved in the fusion. To facilitate these measurements biopsy material is cultured in vitro to obtain hybrid clones, a necessity which led to the criticism that the hybrid clones isolated could have arisen from fusions occurring during culture in vitro. To overcome the objection as far as possible, BER et al. (1978) used tumour-cell lines of the universal fuser type (Sect. C), which allowed biopsy material to be cultured in a selective medium that rapidly killed both the tumour-cell line and normal host cells, but permitted the growth of hybrid cells.

Table 2. Hybridisation involving tumour cells in vivo

Tumour cells	Host	Reference
A. Tumour × tumour hybrids		
Mouse L5178Y lymphoma × mouse sarcoma 180	C3H mice	JANZEN et al. (1971)
B. Tumour × host hybrids		
Human gastric stem-cell lymphoma	Golden hamster (*Mesocricetus auratus*)	GOLDENBERG et al. (1971, 1974)
Mouse cell lines:		
A9HT	C3H × CBA mice	
	C3H × C57B1	
	C3H × ACA	
	CBA T6T6	
B82HT	C3H × CBA	
	C3H × C57B1	
	C3H × ACA	WIENER et al. (1972)
SEWA (polyoma-induced sarcoma, ascitic form)	$(A \times A.SW)F_1$; $(A \times DBA/2)F_1$ CBA/H T_6	FENYO et al. (1973)
SEYF (polyoma-induced fibrosarcoma)	$(A \times A.BY)F_1$; $(A.BY \times C3H)F_1$ $(A.BY \times A.SW)F_1$	
MSWBS (methylcholanthrene-induced ascites sarcoma)	$(A.SW \times C3H)F_1$	
TA3Ha (ascitic form, spontaneous mammary adenocarcinoma)	$(C3H \times C57B1)F_1$ $(C3H \times DBA/2)F_1$	WIENER et al. (1974a)
A9HT(*HGPRT⁻ OUA*ʳ)	C3H; C3H × C57B1	
	C3H × A.SW: C3H × A CA	
501-1(*HGPRT⁻ OUAʳCAPʳ*)	C3H × A.CA: C3H × C57B1	BER et al. (1978)
Ehrlich ascites	CBA/H T_6 mice	LALA et al. (1980)
Ehrlich ascites	Swiss mice	AGNISH and FEDEROFF (1968)
C1.1D (L cell)	C3H	
	C3H × DBA/2 mice	AVILES et al. (1977)
PAZG (non-pigmented 8 AzGʳ P/51 melanoma derived from B16 melanoma in C57B1/6 mice)	C57B1/6 mice	HU and PASZTOR (1975)
Cloudman (*HGPRT⁻*) melanoma	C57B1 DBA/2 mice	HALABAN et al. (1980)

The same group found that hybridisation in vivo occurs within 24 h of tumour-cell injection, a conclusion shared by LALA et al. (1980) for Ehrlich ascites cells grown subcutaneously in CBA/H T_6 mice. In the latter study the proportion of cells carrying the host marker chromosome T_6 increased to about 18% after 60 weekly passages of the tumour and subsequently stayed at this level. However, after only 16 weekly passages, all cells that had the sum of Ehrlich ascites plus host-cell chromosome numbers carried the T_6 marker. Examination of tumour smears showed that up to 5.6% of the cells of old tumours (13 days after injection) were multinucleate of which the majority were tumour × tumour homokaryons. The remainder were tumour × host heterokaryons in which the host nuclei had the morphology of macrophages or lymphocytes but not granulocytes, and host × host homokaryons. WIENER et al. (1974b) also obtained evidence that ascites tumour cells fuse in vivo with haemopoietic cells. Tumour cells were injected into radiation chimeras that had been repopulated with donor cells carrying T_6 chromosomal and H-2 antigenic markers. Ascites tumours formed hybrids with the repopulating haemopoietic cells whereas solid tumours fused with cells of the irradiated host. Subsequent experiments established that the host-cell component of ascites tumour hybrids was non-thymus derived (WIENER et al. 1976).

III. Modified Phenotypes of Hybrids Induced In Vivo

Apart from the use of $HGPRT^-$ (hypoxanthine guanine phosphoribosyl transferase) and ouabain resistance in the selection of hybrids, there appear to have been no studies of drug resistance in hybrids formed in vivo. However, some observations have been made on factors that may affect the fitness of hybrid cells to grow in vivo, and thereby contribute indirectly to drug resistance.

There appear to be no clear rules about the expression of malignancy in hybrids made in vivo. Malignancy was increased in hybrids of human tumours grown in golden hamsters (GOLDENBERG et al. 1971, 1974), was similar to that of the tumour-cell line (WIENER et al. 1974c; AVILES et al. 1977; HALABAN et al. 1980), or was suppressed (HU and PASZTOR 1975). When Ehrlich ascites tumour cells were injected subcutaneously into mice, their malignancy was related to the haplotype expressed, which changed according to the strain of mouse in which the tumour was passed (LALA et al. 1980). The authors interpreted this observation as the result of tumour × host fusion followed by extensive chromosome loss giving rise to "isoantigenic variants" (WIENER et al. 1974a) that were insensitive to immune attack at the subcutaneous site of injection. The malignancy of Ehrlich cells passed as ascites showed no such haplotype dependency.

Occasionally an unexpected phenotype has been observed in hybrids produced in vivo. Thus hybrids between host cells and B16 (HU and PASZTOR 1975) or Cloudman (HALABAN et al. 1980) melanomas showed increased melanogenesis in contrast to the usual observation that melanin synthesis is a differentiated function that is extinguished in hybrids produced in vitro (DAVIDSON et al. 1966; SILAGI 1967). It was suggested that this difference might result from gene dosage, or from differences in the cell type with which the melanomas fused in vitro and in vivo.

C. Use of Drug Resistance for the Selection of Hybrid Clones In Vitro

Table 3 gives a selected list of cytotoxic drugs which have been used in cell hybridisation studies. Not all are antitumour agents, but their cellular targets include those important for antitumour agents, and therefore information on the expression of resistance to these agents in hybrid cells should provide insights into the principle modes of expression of antitumour drug resistance in hybrids.

The selection of resistance in many instances is multistep through a series of increasing drug concentrations, in line with clinical experience. Many of the

Table 3 Selectable drug resistance markers used in cell hybridisation studies

Marker designation	Drug selection	Molecular target	Expression in hybrids	Reference
AzaG^r	8-Azaguanine, single-step	HGPRT (hypoxanthine guanine phosphoribosyl transferase)	Recessive	SZYBALSKI and SMITH (1959) LITTLEFIELD (1963)
TG^r	6-Thioguanine, single-step	HGPRT	Recessive	STUTTS and BROCKMAN (1963)
AzaA^r	8-Azaadenine, multistep	APRT (adenine phosphoribosyl transferase)	Recessive	JONES and SERGENT (1974)
FA^r	2-Fluoroadenine, multistep, 0.05–40 μg ml^{-1}	APRT	Recessive	BENNETT et al. (1966)
DAP^r	2,6-Diaminopurine, multistep, 2.5–100 μg ml^{-1}	APRT	Recessive	LIEBERMAN and OVE (1960) HARRIS and RUDDLE (1961) ATKINS and GARTLER (1968) CHASIN (1974)
FAR^r	2-Fluoroadenosine, multistep, up to 10 μg ml^{-1}	ADK (adenosine kinase)	Recessive	CHAN et al. (1978)
Toy^r	Toyocamycin, single-step, 0.02–0.10 μg ml^{-1}	ADK (for *Toy*^{r}, *Tub*^{r}, *MeMPR*)	Recessive	GUPTA and SIMINOVITCH (1978d)
Tub^r	Tubericidin single-step, 0.1–1.0 μg ml^{-1}			
MeMPR	6-Methyl thiopurine ribonucleoside, single-step, 2–20 μg ml^{-1}			
AraC^r	Cytosine arabinoside, multistep, 0.5 (low) to 5 μg ml^{-1} (high)	Complex dCTP pools (low^r) deoxycytidine kinase (high)	Codominant recessive	DE SAINT VINCENT and BUTTIN (1979) DESCHAMPS et al. (1974)
	0.2–2.4 μg ml^{-1} plus 0.2 μg ml^{-1} thymidine	Ribonucleotide reductase	Codominant (*araC*^{r}, *TdR*^{r}) TdR auxotrophy, recessive	MEUTH et al. (1979)
BudR^r	Bromodeoxyuridine, multistep	TK (thymidine kinase)	Recessive	KIT et al. (1963) CLIVE et al. (1972)
IUdR^r	Iododeoxyuridine, multistep	TK	Recessive	FOX (1971)

Table 3 (continued)

Marker designation	Drug selection	Molecular target	Expression in hybrids	Reference
FUdR^r	Fluorodeoxyuridine, multistep	TK	Recessive	MORSE and POTTER (1965) SLACK et al. (1976)
emt^r	Emetine, multistep *emt*^{rI}, 0.1–0.2 μ*M* *emt*^{rII}, 3–5 μ*M*	40S ribosome subunit	Recessive emt^{rII} recessive to emt^{rI}	GUPTA and SIMINOVITCH (1978 a)
tri^r	Trichodermin, single-step $10^{-6}M$	60S ribosome subunit	Recessive	GUPTA and SIMINOVITCH (1978 b)
oua^r	Ouabain, single step $10^{-6}M$ (human) $3\times10^{-3}M$ (rodent)	Na/K ATPase transport system	Codominant	BAKER et al. (1974) CORSARO and MIGEON (1978)
CH^r	Colchicine, multistep 0.1–5 μg ml^{-1}	High mol. wt. membrane glycoprotein P	Codominant	LING and BAKER (1978)
Dip^r	Diphtheria toxin, single-step 0.01–20 flocullating units	I. membrane receptor II a. elongation factor 2 II b. unidentified protein synthesis factor	Recessive	MOEHRING and MOEHRING (1977) GUPTA and SIMINOVITCH (1978 c) GUPTA and SIMINOVITCH (1980)
Dex^r	Dexamethasone, single-step $10^{-6}M$	Steroid receptor	Recessive	VENETIANER et al. (1978) PFAHL and BOURGEOIS (1980)
Polyene, antibiotic resistance				
Amphotericin B		Sterols	Dominant	FISHER et al. (1979)
Amphotericin B methyl ester				GOLDSTEIN and FISHER (1978)
Fungizone				
Filipin				FISHER et al. (1979)
Primaricin				
Nystatin methyl ester				FISHER et al. (1978)
CL^r	Cyclo-leucine, single-step 4–8 mg ml^{-1}	MAT (methionine adenosine transferase)	Codominant	CABOCHET and MULSANT (1978)

Table 4. Systems for the selection of hybrid clones

Acronym	Selective components	Phenotype selected	Reference
HAT	Hypoxanthine, aminopterin (methotrexate), thymidine	*HGPRT*$^{+}$ *TK*$^{+}$	Szybalski et al. (1962) Littlefield (1964)
HAM	Hypoxanthine, aminopterin (methotrexate), 5-methydeoxycytidine	*Deoxycytidine deaminase*$^{+}$ *HGPRT*$^{+}$ *TK*$^{+}$	Chan et al. (1975)
HAT dC	Hypoxanthine, aminopterin, thymidine, deoxycytidine	*Deoxycytidine kinase*$^{+}$ *HGPRT*$^{+}$ *TK*$^{+}$	Deschamps et al. (1974)
AA	Alanosine, adenine	*APRT*$^{+}$	Kusano et al. (1971)
GAMA	Guanine, adenine, mycophenolic acid, azaserine	*HGPRT*$^{+}$ *APRT*$^{+}$	Liskay and Patterson (1979)
AAU	Alanosine, adenosine, uridine	*ADK*$^{+}$	Chan et al. (1978)
ArUr	Adenosine, uridine	*Uridine kinase*$^{+}$	Medrano and Green (1974)
Systems for use with "universal fusers"			
HOT	HAT + ouabain	*HGPRT*$^{+}$ *oua*^{r} or *TK*$^{+}$ *oua*^{r}	Corsaro and Migeon (1978) Weissman and Stanbridge (1980)
–	HAT polyene antibiotics	*HGPRT*$^{+}$ *antibiotic*^{r} or *TK*$^{+}$ *antibitiotic*^{r}	Fisher et al. (1978, 1979) Goldstein and Fisher (1978)

markers involve the purine and pyrimidine salvage pathways. Mutants can be selected that are resistant to toxic analogues because they are deficient in target enzymes required for the incorporation of exogeneously supplied purines and pyrimidines into DNA and RNA. If such mutants are grown in the presence of methotrexate (amethopterin) then de novo synthesis of purine and pyrimidines is prevented and the mutants die. Complementation between different mutants can be demonstrated by the rescue of hybrid clones from methotrexate toxicity by salvage of normal nucleotide precursors. Thus LITTLEFIELD (1964) demonstrated intergenic complementation between mutants resistant to 8-azaguanine ($HGPRT^- TK^+$) and bromodeoxyuridine ($HGPRT^+ TK^-$) by selection in medium containing hypoxanthine, aminopterin and thymidine (HAT medium). A number of other selective systems have been devised based on this principle (Table 4). Cell lines called "universal fusers" have used in situations where it is desirable to produce hybrids with wild-type cell lines or primary cultures. Such cells carry two mutations, one recessive, the other dominant. On fusion with a wild-type cell, the hybrid phenotype expresses the dominant wild-type allele that complements the recessive mutation, as well as the dominant mutation of the universal fuser (Table 4).

The use of these selection systems has yielded information concerning gene expression in hybrids, which will now be discussed.

D. Expression of Drug Resistance in Hybrid Cells

I. Dominance and Complementation

The HAT system of Littlefield described above is an example of intergenic complementation in which one parent contributes an active enzyme for which the other parent is deficient. The active allele is thus dominant over the inactive, recessive allele. Recessive mutations may be due to deletion of a gene (no product) or alteration of the coding sequence resulting in an altered product that may be inactive or partially active. If the gene product is a protein consisting of several identical subunit polypeptides, then occasionally the subunits of two altered proteins may interact to produce an active protein. Such intragenic complementation has been observed in rare *HGPRT* mutants having altered electrophoretic mobilities (CHASIN and URLAUB 1976). Since it requires the interaction of two different mutants of the same gene, intragenic complementation is unlikely to occur in vivo. Enzyme deficiency in mutants might also result from repression of mRNA synthesis, and KADOURI et al. (1978) produced evidence for a transacting dominant repressor of HGPRT. Such a mechanism is clearly important since it would permit the spread of TG^r in tumour-host hybrids formed in vivo. However, we have been unable to confirm this observation (BOYLE and FOX 1980).

Dominant gene expression implies the production of an altered gene product or an increase in the amount of gene product. In hybrids, wild-type and resistant alleles may be expressed together and result in resistance intermediate between that of the wild-type (sensitive) parent and the resistant mutant. This incomplete dominance, or codominance, is observed for resistance to ouabain (BAKER et al. 1974; ROBBINS and BAKER 1977) due to modification of the membrane-bound

Na^+/K^+-dependent ATPase; to colchicine (LING and BAKER 1978) due to increased production of a high molecular weight membrane glycoprotein; and to cycloleucine (CABOCHET and MULSANT 1978) due to increased levels of methionine adenosyl transferase. Resistance to several polyene macrolide antibiotics which affect sterol binding has also been shown to be dominant, but the membrane target of this resistance has not been defined (FISHER et al. 1979). Other chemotherapeutic agents to which resistance is codominant are α-amanitin (LOBBAN and SIMINOVITCH 1975), hydroxyurea (LEWIS and WRIGHT 1979) and some classes of methotrexate resistance (FLINTOFF et al. 1976).

The selection of mutants resistant to different concentrations of a drug can result in a series of mutants whose alleles show markedly different expression in hybrids. Thus Chinese hamster cells selected in 0.5 μg/ml araC (class I) were cross-resistant to excess thymidine (TdR) and had an expanded pool of deoxycytidine-5′-triphosphate (dCTP). When selected in 5 μg/ml araC only class II mutants were obtained which exhibited resistance to high levels of araC (50 μg/ml) and were deficient in deoxycytidine kinase. In hybrids with wild-type, araC-sensitive cells, class I mutants were recessive and class II mutants were codominant (DE SAINT VINCENT and BUTTIN 1979). A third class of *araC*^{r} mutant has been described (MEUTH et al. 1979) which is resistant to 0.2–2.4 μg/ml araC when grown in the presence of 0.2 μg/ml TdR. These mutants require TdR for growth, and in hybrids TdR auxotrophy is recessive whereas resistance to araC and TdR is dominantly expressed. Reversion to TdR prototrophy is accompanied by reversion to araC and TdR sensitivity, suggesting that a single mutation controls both auxotrophy and resistance and the authors favour an altered ribonucleotide reductase.

Low and high levels of resistance to emetine, which is a potent inhibitor of protein synthesis through its action on 40S ribosome subunits, are expressed by mutant classes *rI* and *rII* that are both recessive to emetine sensitivity. High-level *rII* mutants are also recessive to *rI* in hybrids (GUPTA and SIMINOVITCH 1978a). Although hybrid cells produce both *em*^{s} and *em*^{r} 40S subunits the dominance of sensitivity in this case is due to the mode of action of emetine which blocks the passage of ribosomes along the mRNA (GUPTA and SIMINOVITCH 1978b).

II. Gene Dosage and Functional Hemizygosity

When resistance results from a recessive mutation of an autosome-linked gene, mutation of only one homologue often results in partial resistance. Such is the case with resistance to pyrimidine analogues (CLIVE et al. 1972), purine analogues (RAPPAPORT and DEMARS 1973; JONES and SERGENT 1974) and dexamethasone (BOURGEOIS and NEWBY 1977; PFAHL et al. 1978; PFAHL and BOURGEOIS 1980). The phenomenon arises because the cellular concentration of the target macromolecules is dependent on the number and proportion of recessive and dominant alleles that a cell inherits.

Gene dosage can also affect the phenotype of cells when resistance results from a dominant autosomal mutation, as with class IIb resistance to diphtheria toxin. Subunit B of the toxin binds to specific membrane receptors that are altered or deficient in class I mutants, whereas subunit A causes ADP ribosylation of elongation factor 2, thus interfering with translation of mRNA. Class IIa mutants possess altered elongation factor 2 which is insensitive to ADP ribosylation. In hybrids class I mutations are recessive whereas class IIa mutations of Chinese hamster ovary (CHO)-K1 cells are codominant (MOEHRING and MOEHRING 1977), although apparently similar mutations in Chinese hamster V79 cells behave recessively (GUPTA and SIMINOVITCH 1980). A second class of mutant (IIb) with altered protein synthesis was described by GUPTA and SIMINOVITCH (1978c) which showed 50% inhibition of protein synthesis in the presence of toxin, implying that only one of a pair of homologous chromosomes carried the mutant allele, and that both wild-type and mutant alleles were being expressed equally. In these mutants the resistant allele (*R*) was codominant with the wild-type allele (*S*). However, when the mutant (*R*/*S*) was fused with a wild-type cell (*S*/*S*) the resulting hybrids were sensitive, indicating that three sensitive alleles were dominant over one resistant allele. Class IIb mutants are apparently affected in an unidentified protein synthesis factor since these mutants complement those of class IIa (GUPTA and SIMINOVITCH 1980).

The interpretation of gene dose relationships is clearly dependent on a knowledge of the number of gene copies per cell, their distribution among chromosomes and what proportion are functional. The question of functional ploidy was raised by DEAVAN and PETERSON (1973) and reviewed by SIMINOVITCH (1976), who argued that the relatively high frequently with which recessive mutations arise in CHO cells might be due to the production of functionally hemizygous portions of chromosomes as a result of extensive chromosomal rearrangements. This idea was substantiated by GUPTA (1980), who showed that hemizygosity was not restricted to one or a few chromosomal regions. SICILIANO et al. (1978), who examined the isoenzyme patterns of electrophoretic shift variants from 11 different loci and found that the majority expressed both wild-type and mutant isozymes, concluded that CHO cells are only as functionally hemizygous as would be expected of a slightly hypodiploid cell line.

III. Multifunctional Enzymes

During the past 5 years evidence has been accumulating that, as in prokaryotes, one mechanism of coordinate regulation in mammalian cells is the association of related enzymic activities in a single multifunctional structure (reviewed KIRSCHNER and BISSWANGER 1976). Such complex enzymes are known for tetrahydrofolate metabolism (PAUKERT et al. 1976; TAN et al. 1977) where formyltetrahydrofolate synthetase, methenyltetrahydrofolate cyclohydrolase and methylene tetrahydrofolate dehydrogenase reside in a protein of one (pig liver) or two (sheep liver) identical subunits. Pig liver also contains formiminoglutamate-tetrahydrofolate formiminotransferase and formiminotetrahydrofolate cyclodeaminase activities, in a protein of probably eight identical polypeptides (DRURY et al. 1975).

The elegant analyses of pyrimidine biosynthesis by groups led by PATTERSON and STARK have revealed three complementation groups, urd A, B and C (Fig. 4). *urd* A^- mutants selected as uridine auxotrophs simultaneously lose carbamyl phosphatase, aspartate transcarbamylase and dihydroorotase activites, which are regained simultaneously in revertants (PATTERSON and CARNRIGHT 1977). These observations are consistent with an active enzyme of molecular weight 600,000

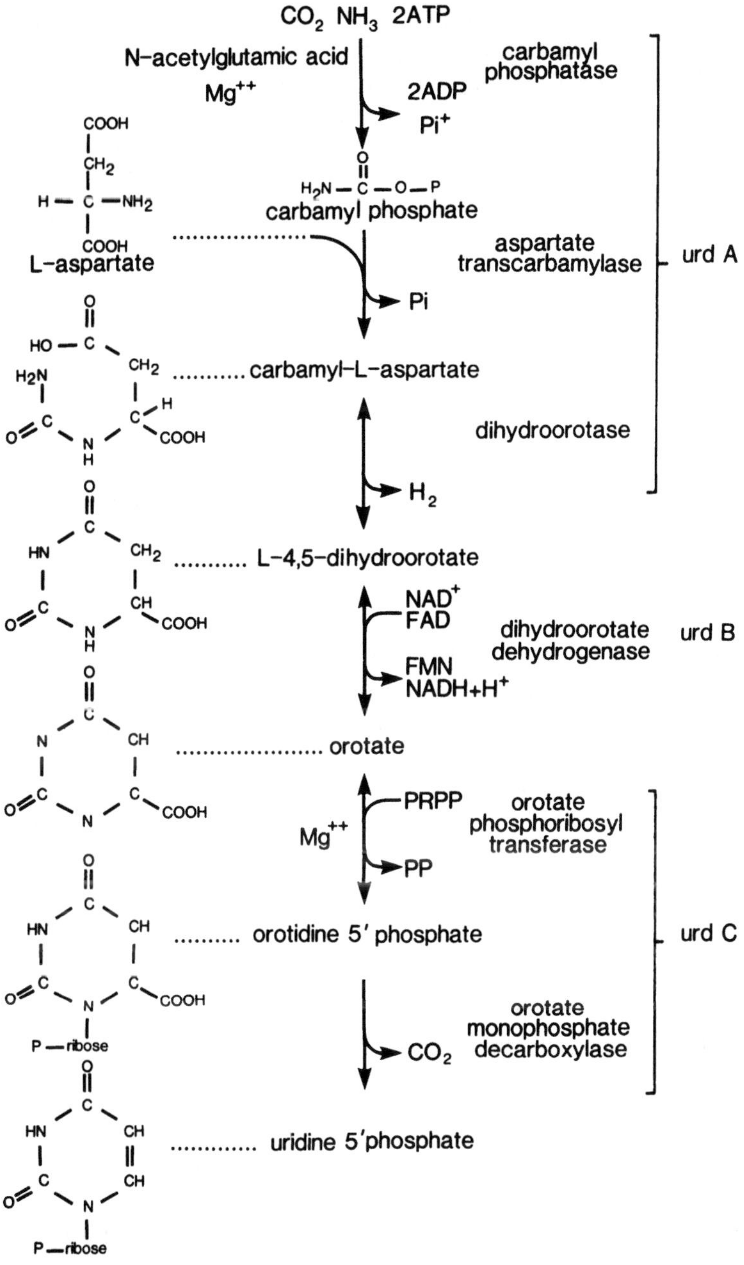

Fig. 4. Pathway of de novo synthesis of pyrimidines, showing the relationships between the biochemical pathway, genetic complementation groups urd A, B and C, and the steps catalysed by multifunctional enzymes (*bracketed*)

consisting of a trimer of identical polypeptides (Coleman et al. 1977; Davidson et al. 1979). All three activites are overproduced in mutants resistant to *N*-(phosphonacetyl)-L-aspartate (PALA), which inhibits aspartate transcarbamylase (Kempe et al. 1976). *urd* B^- is represented by a mutant of the fourth enzyme in the pathway, dihydro-orotate dehydrogenase (STAMATO and PATTERSON 1979). Unlike all the other enzymes of pyrimidine synthesis, which are found in the cytosol, this one is located in mitochondria although coded by the nucleus (CHEN and JONES 1976). *urd* C^- mutants show a simultaneous deficiency in the last two enzymes of pyrimidine synthesis, orotate phosphoribosyltransferase (OPRT) and orotate monophosphate decarboxylase (ODCase). In CHO cells which lack uracil phosphoribosyl transferase, the conversion of 5-fluorouracil (FU) to the nucleotide is dependent on OPRT, and hence OPRT-deficient mutants can be isolated that are resistant to the toxic effects of FU (PATTERSON 1980). Patients with orotic acid uria are similarly deficient in both OPRT and ODCase (KROOTH 1964). In order to grow most *urd* C^- mutants need to salvage uridine. However, some do not and these are most probably partially defective in OPRT and ODCase since there is no complementation between uridine-requiring and non-requiring mutants (PATTERSON 1980). Mutants of all three complementation groups have mutations that are recessive to wild-type alleles, and since *urd* A^- and *urd* C^- mutants complement each other, the multifunctional activites of these two classes exist on separate polypeptides.

IV. Steroid Resistance and Enzymic Induction by Hormones

Many lymphoid cell lines are killed by high concentrations of glucocorticoid sterols. This results from a chain of events starting with the binding of glucocorticoid to a specific membrane-bound receptor that is activated and transports the glucocorticoid to the nucleus (nuclear transfer). Here the hormone-receptor complex binds to DNA and initiates an as yet poorly understood mechanism which finally leads to cell death. Mutants resistant to high concentrations of dexamethasone have been classified into four classes distinguishable biochemically and genetically as being affected at different stages of hormone interaction (GEHRING 1980). Mutants resistant to killing can either lack the receptor (r^-) or have normal receptors but fail to perform nuclear transfer (nt^-) of the receptor-hormone complex. In a study of dexamethasone resistance in mouse S49 lymphoma and WEHI 7 thymoma PFAHL and BOURGEOIS (1980) found no complementation between r^- and nt^- mutants, supporting the idea that both r^- and nt^- are alleles of r^+. Fusions between wild-type Dex^s (r^+) and Dex^r (r^-) cells resulted in Dex^s hybrid cells, indicating dominance of r^+, accompanied by the synthesis of widely differing numbers of receptor sites in different hybrid clones.

A third phenotype (nt^i) of S49 lymphoma cells, reported by YAMAMOTO et al. (1976), was characterised by increased affinity of the receptor-steroid complex for DNA that was due to abonormal nt^i receptors of molecular weight 50,000 compared with molecular weight 90,000 for wild-type receptors. In wild-type $\times\, nt^i$ hybrids synthesis of both types of receptors occurred (codominance), and sensitivity of dexamethasone was codominant when cloning ability was measured: $nt^i \times r^-$ failed to complement. Thus in each case involving mutant receptors sensitivity to dexamethasone was dominant.

A fourth class of Dex^r mutant has been described in mouse L cells which apparently has normal steroid receptors (VENETIANER et al. 1978). Most Dex^r (r^+)

mutants were cross-resistant to the glucocorticoids dexamethasone (9-α-fluoro-16-α-methyl prednisolone), prednisolone, cortisolone, corticosterone, aldosterone and also non-glucocorticoids 17-α-methyl testosterone, progesterone and 17-β-esteradiol when inhibition of [^{3}H]-thymidine uptake was the end point measured. Fusions of $Dex^r(r^+) \times Dex^s(r^+)$ fibroblasts showed sensitivity to be dominant, as was also observed in hybrids between $Dex^r(r^+)$ mouse lymphoma and $Dex^s(r^+)$ mouse myeloma (GEHRING et al. 1972). Other reports of $Dex^r(r^+)$ mutants have been made in other murine and human cell lines (YAMAMOTO et al. 1976; LIPPMANN et al. 1974) although HUET (1979) reported that only $Dex^r(r^-)$ or $Dex^r(nt^-)$ mutants could be isolated from WEHI 7 thymoma after a variety of treatments inducing point mutations, deletions, chromosome rearrangements and chromosome loss. YAMAMOTO et al. (1976) coined the term "deathless" (d^-) for their mutants, implying that resistance was due to some defect in cell killing after nuclear transfer had occurred. There has been no study of complementation between d^- mutants and the other three classes (GEHRING 1980).

In contrast to the dominant lethal effects of glucocorticoids in lymphoid cells the ability of glucocorticoids to induce enzymes in hepatoma cells is a recessive phenotype. Thus in rat hepatoma cells tyrosine aminotransferase (TAT) and alanine amino transferase can be modulated from low constitutive levels to high induced levels by exposure of cells to dexamethasone (SCHNEIDER and WEISS 1971; WEISS and CHAPLAIN 1971; SPARKES and WEISS 1973), a property that is lost (extinguished) upon hybridisation with mouse fibroblasts or rat epithelial cells. Subclones isolated some time after hybridisation show loss of some chromosomes (Sect. D.V) and the reappearance of inducibility. In some subclones inducibility of alanine aminotransferase was re-expressed in the absence of inducibility of tyrosine aminotransferase, indicating that steroid induction of these enzymes may have some steps that are independent. Rat hepatoma hybrids also show extinction of enzymes that are not inducible (BERTOLOTTI and WEISS 1972a, b). On the other hand, inducible enzymes are not always extinguished. Thus BENEDICT et al. (1972) made hybrids between mouse 3T3 fibroblasts, which have arylhydrocarbon hydroxylase inducible by benz(*a*)anthracene, and rat hepatoma cells with TAT inducible by dexamethasone. The hybrids produced inducible hydroxlase at levels the same as, to 20-fold greater than, the 3T3 parent, while TAT was not inducible, even though most hybrids contained nearly complete sets of chromosomes from both parents. Hydroxlase induction is therefore a dominant trait in hybrids and involves a mechanism that is different to induction of TAT.

V. Segregation of Resistance

The conversion of polykaryons into hybrid cells occurs at mitosis when two or more genomes become aligned on a common spindle apparatus, and is followed by the subsequent formation of hybrid nuclei at telophase. The probability that a fusion event will give rise to a viable hybrid cell capable of producing a clone is very low. Even under optimal experimental conditions where more than 50% of nuclei are in heterokaryons, the frequency of hybrid clones is rarely more than one per hundred cells fused (BOYLE and FOX 1980; BOYLE et al. 1977; RECHSTEINER and PARSONS 1976; DAVIDSON 1969). By the use of interspecies fusions involving cells with morphologically distinct nuclei, or by labelling the nuclei of one parent with [^{3}H]-thymidine prior to fusion, it is possible to follow the fate of parental chromosomes during the first four divisions after fusion. In human × mouse fusions (Rechsteiner and Parsons 1976) and human × rat kangaroo (*Potorous tridactylis*) (Peterson and Berns 1979) the chromosomes from different nuclei tended to remain separate during the initial mitosis after fusion, mingling in subsequent mitoses, although separation of human and mouse chromosomes was still seen in some hybrid colonies containing eight cells. In half the human × rat kangaroo metaphases, chromosomes were left at the metaphase plate at anaphase and became trapped by the constricting mid-body during cytokinesis. In polykaryons containing nuclei of different ages, interphase nuclei that were in close proximity to mitotic nuclei were observed to go into mitosis before completion of the cell cycle (Peterson and Berns 1979). The interphase chromosomes went through a process of premature chromosome condensation (PCC, Johnson and Rao 1970; Johnson et al. 1970) and presented different morphologies depending on the phase of the cycle they were in before condensation. Prematurely condensed G1 and G2 chromosomes were entire and had one or two chromatids respectively, whilst condensed S-phase chromosomes appeared pulverised. Rao and Johnson (1972) demonstrated a correlation between PCC involving S-phase nuclei and a reduced chromosome complement in derived hybrid clones. PCC appears largely confined to the first mitosis after fusion (Rechsteiner and Parsons 1976), since the chromosomes in homokaryons rapidly become synchronised at mitosis and at the initiation of DNA synthesis (Graves 1972). Trapping of chromosomes and PCC provide two mechanisms that contribute to the phenomenon of chromosome loss in hybrid cells.

Loss of human chromosomes from human × rodent hybrids can be extensive, and the concordant loss of a biochemical phenotype with a specific chromosome has been a fruitful method for assigning genes to chromosomes (Migeon and Miller 1968; Matsuya and Green 1969; Kao and Puck 1970). (For recent reviews of human gene mapping the reader is directed to McKusick and Ruddle 1977 and Human Gene Mapping 1978, 1979). The method for assigning genes to chromosomes assumes that chromosome segregation occurs randomly *in a population*. However, it is worth pointing out that *within a cell* chromosome loss may not be entirely random, the loss of one chromsome influencing the loss of others, an observation that may result from the compartmentalisation of chromosomes at mitosis described above (Marin and Pugliatti-Crippa 1972; Rushton 1976).

In general, intraspecies hybrids tend to be more stable than interspecies hybrids (Siniscalco et al. 1969; Nadler et al. 1970; Sobel et al. 1971; Handmaker 1973; Spurna and Nebola 1973; Worton et al. 1977) although some exceptions have been described (Engel et al. 1969a, b, 1971). It is possible that this observation is more apparent than real, being governed by the rodent and human cell types available for fusion. If, instead of fusing primary human cells with heteroploid rodent cells, one fuses heteroploid human cells with primary rodent cells then rodent chromosomes are preferentially lost instead of human (Minna and Coon 1974; Croce 1976). Although the factors controlling chromosome loss are obscure, there may be some relationship between these observations and those of

RUSSELL et al. (1979), who demonstrated an initially rapid segregation of chromosomes in mouse hybrids between heteroploid and euploid cells as compared with heteroploid × heteroploid hybrids or euploid × euploid human cells (MIGEON et al. 1974; HOEHN et al. 1975). Some progress towards understanding the genetic control of segregation, at least in rodent × human hybrids, has come from the intriguing observation that transcription of rRNA genes is suppressed from the chromosomes of the species that will show preferential chromosome loss in human × rodent hybrids (PERRY et al. 1979; DEV et al. 1979), whereas the rRNA genes of both parents are transcribed in rodent × rodent hybrids (MILLER et al. 1978; WEIDE et al. 1979). Mouse-human hybrids also appear to lose the mitochondrial DNA of the parent whose chromosomes are preferentially lost (ATTARDI and CROCE 1980). Because of the implications for gene mapping, attempts to influence the direction and extent of chromosome loss have also been made by the selective production of damage in the chromsomes whose loss was desired (PONTECORVO 1971, 1974; GOSS and HARRIS 1977; LAW and KAO 1978; GRAVES 1980) (see also Sect. E.II).

Chromosome segregation appears to be the main cause of re-expression of recessive alleles in hybrid cells, although recombination (WORTON et al. 1980) and epigenetic events (HARRIS 1975) have also been suggested as possible mechanisms. RUSSELL et al. (1977) inferred that segregation chiefly accounts for chromosome loss, while recombination, i.e. translocations, accounted for chromosome heterogeneity. Loss of the X chromosomes was correlated with segregation of X-linked markers from intraspecies hybrids of human (BENGTSSON et al. 1975), mouse (HASHMI and MILLER 1976) and Chinese hamster (FARRELL and WORTON 1977). The application of selective pressure can cause preferential loss of chromosomes from the parent complement carrying the allele selected against. Thus growth of Chinese hamster (*HGPRT*$^-$) × mouse (*TK*$^-$) hybrids with 6-thioguanine or bromodeoxyuridine resulted in loss of many mouse or hamster chromosomes respectively (MARIN and PUGLIATTI-CRIPPA 1972). Similarly chromosomal segregants can be selected by immune mechanisms (KNOWLES and SWIFT 1975; COLLINS et al. 1975) which may be significant in producing hemizygosity in vivo. Chromosome loss may also be important in the expression of recessive drug resistance mutations occuring in autosomes (see Sect. D.II), causing the "unmasking" of a recessive mutation by removal of the wild-type allele upon loss of the homologous chromosome (CHASIN and URLAUB 1975).

The frequency with which recessive alleles are re-expressed in hybrid populations can vary widely. In hamster × mouse hybrids the frequencies of resistance to 6-thioguanine and bromodeoxyuridine (BUdR) varied from $<10^{-5}$ to 3×10^{-2} and from $<10^{-5}$ to 7×10^{-3} respectively (MARIN and MANDUCA 1972). The greater stability of intraspecies hybrids may be reflected by lower segregation frequencies, as in mouse hybrids where segregation of 8-azaguanine (8-AZG) was 5×10^{-6}–5.2×10^{-4} (SPURNA and NEBOLA 1973). In quasi-tetraploid Chinese hamster hybrids the *rate* of segregation for membrane-defective *8-AZG*^{r}*ts* and phytohaemaglutinin resistance was 5×10^{-5} and 10^{-5} events/cell per generation, and these values increased 40- and 200-fold respectively in quasi-hexaploid hybrids in which the resistance alleles were present at twice the gene dosage (2*r* : 1*s*) but decreased to 0.04×10^{-5} when the sensitive alleles were present at twice the dosage ($1r:2s$) (HARRIS and WHITMORE 1977). Similarly PFAHL and BOURGEOIS (1980) found the frequency of *Dex*^{r} segregants from mouse hybrids ($3r:1s$) was about 10^3–10^4 times more frequent than from heterozygous diploid cells ($1r:1s$).

VI. Gene Activation

Occasionally hybrid clones are isolated that unexpectedly show a phenotype expressed by neither parent, as with fusion of rat hepatoma cells and mouse fibroblasts or lymphocytes which resulted in the production of mouse serum albumin (PETERSON and WEISS 1972; MALAWISTA and WEISS 1974). Fusion of rat × mouse cells also resulted in hybrids that were unexpectedly resistant to ionising radiations (LITTLE et al. 1972, see Sect. E.I). Such examples presumably reflect changes in regulatory control. Two further examples indicate that activation can be locus specific and can apparently operate against very strong repression mechanisms. Female cells are functionally hemizygous for the X chromosomes, one X chromosome becoming inactive early in embryogenesis (LYON 1971). In hybrid cells, active X chromosomes usually remain active and inactive chromosomes remain inactive (SINISCALCO et al. 1969; SILAGI et al. 1969; MIGEON et al. 1974). However, exceptional human × mouse hybrid clones have been isolated carrying an active gene on an otherwise inactive X chromosome (KAHAN and DEMARS 1975; HELLKUHL and GRZESCHIK 1978). Localised derepression occurred at a rate of 10^{-6} per inactive X chromosome per cell generation and was maintained in the absence of any other human chromosome (KAHAN and DEMARS 1980). There have also been a number of reports of *HGPRT*$^+$ human × *HGPRT*$^-$ rodent hybrids which expressed rodent HGPRT, despite the fact that the rodent parent cells were previously thought to contain HGPRT deletions due to the extremely low frequency or absence of reversion at this locus (WATSON et al. 1972; CROCE et al. 1973; BAKAY et al. 1973, 1978). In the light of KAHAN and DEMARS' observations it is possible that some HGPRT "deletions" may represent locally inactive regions on the X chromosome that can be occasionally reactivated by the conditions used for cell hybridisation (SHIN et al. 1973), through a mechanism involving DNA methylation.

The pattern of methylation of DNA at the 5-position carbon atom of cytosine appears to be an important epigenetic mechanism controlling tissue differentiation (review, RAZIN and RIGGS 1980), lack of methylation of critical cytosine residues being correlated with transcriptional activity. Hypomethylation can be induced experimentally by growing cells with 5-azacytidine, which replaces cytosine in DNA, but cannot be methylated because of a nitrogen atom at position 5. The pattern of methylation is inherited in daughter cells in the absence of more 5-azacytidine, supposedly because the critical sites are in palindromic sequences which are monitored by a maintenance methylase that methylates daughter strands in half-methylated palindromes. Using 5-azacytidine to induce hypomethylation in a human × mouse hybrid MOHANDAS et al. (1981) were able to reactivate the human *HGPRT* gene on an inactive X chromosome. BOEHM and DRAHOVSKY (1981) reported that MNU (1-methyl-1-nitrosourea) caused hypomethylation of the DNA of human Raji cells, thus suggesting the possibility of an epigenetic origin for some dominant "mutations" induced by alkylating agents. The converse, i.e. hypermethylation, might explain some forms of recessive "mutation".

E. Radiation Responses of Hybrid Cells

I. Sensitivity to Ionising Radiation and Ultraviolet Light

Studies of the radiation sensitivity of hybrid cells were stimulated by reports that mouse and rat hybrids were unexpectedly twofold more resistant to X-rays (ratio of Do values) than their parent cell lines (LITTLE et al. 1972) and were cross-resistant to α-particles (ROBERTSON and RAJU 1980) and also to actinomycin D and cordycepin, suggesting that X-ray resistance might involve some aspect of RNA metabolism (ROBERTSON et al. 1977). Resistance was not associated with enhancement of the repair of either sublethal or potentially lethal damage.

Later reports on a range of inter- and intraspecies hybrids showed that the resistance of rat × mouse hybrids was exceptional. The sensitivities of hybrids showed the same range as that previously observed with tetraploid cell lines (LIMBOSCH et al. 1974; ZAMPETTI-BOSSELER et al. 1976; BOYLE et al. 1979). From the fusion of a pair of cell lines, hybrid clones can be selected with sensitivities ranging from similar or intermediate to the parent cells, to marginally more resistant. Resistance appears to be a dominant phenotype and is unstable, its loss being associated with loss of chromosomes in some but not all cases (BOYLE et al. 1979; ROBERTSON and RAJU 1980).

Similar results have been obtained for hybrids exposed to ultraviolet light. Hybrid sensitivity was similar to (ROMMELAERE and ERRERA 1972; ROBERTSON et al. 1977) or less than (BOYLE et al. 1979; ZAMPETTI-BOSSELER et al. 1980) the parental cell lines, and the resistant phenotype was unstable (PETROVA 1977; BOYLE et al. 1979).

The variable sensitivity of hybrid cells probably reflects the polygenic control of DNA repair and cellular recovery mechanisms. These observations may be significant for adjuvent therapy and perhaps give a clue to the likely responses of hybrids to chemotherapeutic agents that damage DNA.

Mouse L5178Y lymphoma cells (LS) are relatively radiation sensitive with reported Do values of 40–60 rads (ZAMPETTI-BOSSELER et al. 1976; DALE 1979) compared with 100–200 rads for the majority of mammalian cells. Complementation of the sensitive phenotype was achieved after hybridisation with a radiation-resistant L5178Y variant (LR) or with Chinese hamster fibroblasts and mouse L cells (DALE 1979; ZAMPETTI-BOSSELER et al. 1976). FOX (1979) showed that resistance to UV and ethyl methane sulphate (EMS) was also dominant in LS × LR hybrids. The sensitivity of LS cells reflects their lymphocyte origin; hence these results suggest that hybridisation in vivo of lymphoid tumours with cells of other tissues could markedly affect the response of the tumour to DNA-damaging agents.

II. Rescue of Genes from Lethally Irradiated Cells

As described earlier, hybrid clones resulting from the fusion of TG^r and $BUdR^r$ cell lines can be selected in HAT medium because the respective genotypes $HGPRT^- TK^+$ and $HGPRT^+ TK^-$ are complementary for the enzymes that salvage exogenous hypoxanthine and thymidine. HARRIS (1972) demonstrated that even if one of the fusion partners was lethally irradiated it was still capable of contributing the complementary allele for hybrid selection. These experiments paral-

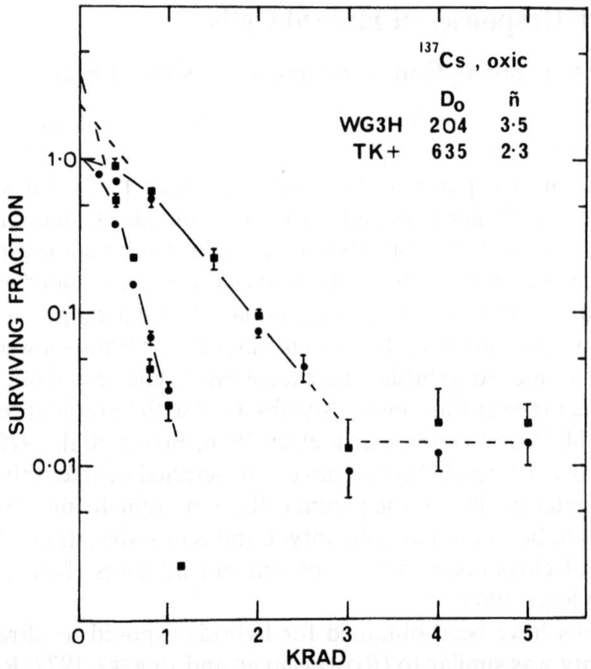

Fig. 5. Cell survival, and rescue of TK^+ by cell fusion following γ-irradiation. Chinese hamster wg3h cells (TK^+, $HGPRT^-$) were irradiated in oxic suspensions with the indicated doses of γ-radiation from a ^{137}Cs source and cell survival measured by colony formation in growth medium. Cell samples from each radiation treatment were also fused with unirradiated Chinese hamster a23 cells ($TK^- HGPRT^+$) and the frequency of hybrid clones expressing TK^+ derived from irradiated wg3h cells was measured by colony formation in HAT-selective medium. *Circles* and *squares* represent two separate experiments. *Left curve*, survival of wg3h; *right curve*, survival of TK^+ hybrids. [Boyle (1979), reproduced by kind permission of Taylor and Francis Ltd]

leled those of Pontecorvo (1971, 1974), who demonstrated that irradiation of either mouse or Chinese hamster cells prior to fusion led to the preferential loss of the irradiated chromosomes from the resulting hybrids (Sect. D.V). However, irradiation of mouse cells prior to fusion with human cells did not reverse the genetically controlled preference for loss of human chromosomes.

Another way of expressing Harris' observations is that the unirradiated fusion partner is able to rescue a functional salvage enzyme gene from the irradiated genome. Since hybrid clones are produced in inverse proportion to the radiation dose, the Do value (^{1}/slope) is an index of the sensitivity of those processes leading to the rescue of the marker gene. When compared with the radiation sensitivity of the colony-forming ability of cells irradiated, marker rescue was approximately two to eight times more resistant for fusions involving different markers and different cell lines (Kinsella et al. 1976; Boyle et al. 1977; Jullien et al. 1978). For hybridisation between a given pair of cell lines the ratio Do marker rescue: Do cell survival was fairly constant between 3 and 4 for cells irradiated with X-rays, ^{137}Cs and 14-MeV neutrons, and in air or under hypoxic conditions (Boyle 1979)

(Fig. 5). Marker rescue data from high-LET (linear energy transfer) radiations (14 MeV neutrons) have been analysed by target theory and resulted in a target volume that was equivalent to 0.54%–0.91% of the DNA of a Chinese hamster cell (BOYLE 1979). Since this is orders of magnitude larger than a gene, the implication is that genes are inactivated largely by events occurring outside their coding sequences.

At X-ray doses above 2–3 krad there is an abrupt change in slope of the marker rescue curve at about 1% survival, the curve now becoming infinitely more resistant to further radiation (JULLIEN et al. 1978; BOYLE 1979). Indeed, hybrids have been isolated even after doses to one partner of 20 krad (MEGUMI 1976). It has been suggested (BOYLE 1979) that for doses up to the inflexion point marker gene inactivation may result from loss of markers in acentric fragments produced by chromosome breaks occurring between the centromere and the marker. With increasing dose further breaks will reduce the acentric fragments to a size that can readily undergo recombination with intact chromosomes. At doses above the inflexion point further marker inactivation may be the result of damage sustained within the marker gene. One implication of this interpretation is that the frequency with which genes syntenic with the marker allele will be retained in hybrids will be largely dependent on their linkage to the selected marker. This has been born out in practice and developed into a radiological method of gene mapping by GOSS and HARRIS (1977).

Marker rescue has also been demonstrated after exposure of one parent to other agents that damage DNA, e.g. ultraviolet light (BOYLE et al. 1977) and methyl nitrosourea (J. M. Boyle, unpublished results), but not after exposure to acute thermal shock (HARRIS 1972).

When both partners were irradiated prior to fusion the dose response for hybrid colony formation was either intermediate between the two parents (JULLIEN et al. 1978) or marginally more resistant by virtue of an increased shoulder on the survival curve (BOYLE et al. 1977).

F. Conclusions: Possible Therapeutic Implications of Cell Hybridisation

In considering the possible implications of these genetic studies we are concerned primarily with drug resistance in tumour cells. We have seen that in animals tumour cells can fuse with each other and with host cells to produce clonogenic mononucleate hybrid cells. The frequency with which this occurs is apparently high, since hybrids can be detected as early as 24 h after tumour inoculation (BER et al. 1978; LALA et al. 1980). An approximate estimate of the proportion of hybrids in tumours was 10^{-5}–10^{-6} (see discussion following WIENER et al. 1974b). If fusion occurs at similar frequencies in humans then hybrid clones may be well established by the time clinical diagnosis is made and therapy started. Because malignancy is a recessive character (HARRIS et al. 1969) tumour × tumour hybrids will be at an advantage over tumour × host hybrids until the latter have segregated the wild-type alleles that suppress malignancy. However, the animal studies clearly demonstrate that tumour × host hybrids do proliferate.

Within the hybrid populations drug-resistance mutations can accumulate prior to therapy, although presumably they will not usually confer any advantage on the cells possessing them until challenged by therapy. Recessive mutations will be masked by wild-type alleles and dominant mutations may be subject to gene dose effects which only allow partial expression. The enlarged gene pool may also favour the generation of dominant resistance by gene amplification (Biedler et al. 1974) and recessive resistance by gene inactivation which has been postulated to result from translocation of euchromatin adjacent to heterochromatin (Morrow 1977) or by changes to the pattern of DNA methylation (Sect. D.VI).

The full expression of resistance in hybrid cells may require the unmasking of the mutation by removal of the wild-type allele in cases where resistance is autosomally linked. Segregation by loss of the homologous chromosome carrying the wild-type allele is probably the most important means whereby unmasking occurs and has been demonstrated in vitro for X-linked 6-thioguanine resistance in intraspecies Chinese hamster hybrids (Chasin and Urlaub 1975). The frequency of segregation of intraspecies hybrids in vitro is about 10^{-5} and is affected by a number of variables including the ratio of sensitive to resistant alleles and the cell types involved (Sect. D.V). The segregation rate in vivo is unknown. Presumably it may be at least as high as in vitro and could be higher due to immune selection of segregants and the clastogenic effects of some drugs once therapy has started.

The frequent observation of tumours with karyotypes in the triploid-hypotetraploid range is consistent with segregation from a tetraploid origin. If the general concept that polyploidy, whether derived by hybridisation or not, is a means of harbouring mutations has any validity, then tumours from patients resistant to therapy might be expected to show higher ploidy than tumours from a similar group of patients before therapy. Leistenschneider and Nagel (1979) reported such a situation in a group of 26 patients with prostatic carcinoma. Ten patients had received no treatment and had tumours with ploidies ranging from diploid to tetraploid. Sixteen patients had received treatment and their tumours were resistant to either cyproterone acetate (an antiandrogen) or estracyte (estramustine phosphate). Of these the karyotypes of three were mainly tetraploid, seven were 2n–6n and six were 2n–8n. The bases of resistance were not explored, nor is it known whether resistance to these agents is dominant or recessive; hence it is not possible to assess the importance of gene dosage in this context. Clearly it would be useful to have more data relating karyotype and drug resistance in tumours where polyploidy is a feature. The current use of combination therapy in humans makes experimental tumours in animals attractive, particularly where such studies can be augmented by the in vitro manipulation of cell lines with suitable genotype.

References

Agnish ND, Federoff S (1968) Tumour cell populations of the Ehrlich ascites tumours. Can J Genet Cytol 10:723–745

Akers TG, Cunningham CH (1968) Replication and cytopathogenicity of avian infectious bronchitis virus in chicken embryo kidney cells. Arch Ges Virusforsch 25:30–37

Atkin NB (1971) Modal DNA value and chromosome number in ovarian neoplasia: a clinical and histological assessment. Cancer 27:1064–1073

Atkin NB, Kay R (1979) Prognostic significance of modal DNA values and other factors in malignant tumours, based on 1465 cases. Br J Cancer 40:210–221

Atkins JH, Gartler SM (1968) Development of a non-selective technique for studying 2,6-diaminopurine resistance in an established murine cell line. Genetics 60:781–792

Attardi FL, Croce CM (1980) Uniparental propagation of mitochondrial DNA in mouse-human cell hybrids. Proc Natl Acad Sci USA 77:4079–4083

Aviles D, Jami J, Rousset J-P, Ritz E (1977) Tumor × host cell hybrids in the mouse: chromosomes from the normal cell parent maintained in malignant hybrid tumors. JNCI 58:1391–1399

Bakay B, Croce CM, Koprowski H, Nyhan WL (1973) Restoration of hypoxanthine phosphoribosyl transferase activity in mouse 1 R cells after fusion with chick-embryo fibroblasts. Proc Natl Acad Sci USA 70:1998–2002

Bakay B, Graf M, Carey S, Nissinen E, Nyhan WL (1978) Re-expression of HPRT activity following cell fusion with polyethylene glycol. Biochem Genet 16:227–237

Baker RM, Brunette DM, Mankovitz R, Thompson LH, Whitmore GF, Siminovitch L, Till JE (1974) Ouabain-resistant mutants of mouse and hamster cells in culture. Cell 1:9–21

Benedict WF, Nebert DW, Thompson EB (1972) Expression of aryl hydrocarbon hydroxylase induction and suppression of tyrosine aminotransferase induction in somatic cell hybrids. Proc Natl Acad Sci USA 69:2179–2183

Bengstsson BO, Nabholz M, Kennett R, Bodmer WF, Povey S, Swallow D (1975) Human intraspecific somatic cell hybrids: a genetic and karyotypic analysis of crosses between lymphocytes and D98/AH-2. Somatic Cell Genet 1:41–64

Bennett LL, Vail MH, Chumley S, Montgomery JA (1966) Activity of adenosine analogs against a cell culture, line resistant to 2-fluoroadenine. Biochem Pharmacol 15:1719–1728

Ber R, Weiner F, Fenyo E-M (1978) Proof of in vivo fusion of murine tumor cells with host cells by universal fusers. JNCI 60:931–933

Bertolotti R, Weiss MC (1972a) Expression of differentiated functions in hepatoma cell hybrids II. Aldolase. J Cell Physiol 79:211–224

Bertolotti R, Weiss MC (1972b) Expression of differentiated functions in hepatoma cell hybrids. VI. Extinction and re-expression of liver alcohol dehydrogenase. Biochimie 54:195–201

Biedler JL, Albrecht AM, Spengler BA (1974) Non-banding (homogeneous) chromosome regions in cells with very high dihydrofolate reductase levels. Genetics 77:s4–5

Boehm TLJ, Drahovsky D (1981) Hypomethylation of DNA in Raji cells after treatment with *N*-methyl-*N*-nitrosourea. Carcinogenesis 2:39–42

Bourgeois S, Newby RF (1977) Diploid and haploid states of the glucocorticoid receptor gene of mouse lymphoid cell lines. Cell 11:423–430

Boyle JM (1979) Rescue of marker phenotypes: effects of BUdR sensitisation, hypoxia and high LET. Int J Radiat Biol 35:509–520

Boyle JM, Fox M (1980) A genetic complementation study of purine analogue resistance in Chinese hamster fibroblasts. Mutat Res 73:419–423

Boyle JM, Kinsella AR, Smith PJ (1977) Rescue of marker phenotypes mediated by somatic cell hybridisation. Int J Radiat Biol 31:45–58

Boyle JM, Kinsella AR, Smith PJ (1979) Changes in sensitivity to X-rays and ultraviolet radiation during passage of mammalian cell hybrids. In: Edwards HE, Navaratnam S, Parsons BJ, Phillips GO (eds) "Radiation biology and chemistry: research developments" Elsevier, Amsterdam, pp 273–281

Brodsky WY, Uryvaeva IV (1977) Cell ploidy: its relation to tissue growth and function. Int Rev Cytol 50:275–232

Cabochet M, Mulsant P (1978) Selection and preliminary characterization of cycloleucine-resistant CHO cells affected in methionine metabolism. Somatic Cell Genet 4:407–421

Capers CR (1960) Multinucleation of skeletal muscle in vitro. J Biophys Biochem Cytol (J Cell Biol) 7:559–566

Cascardo MR, Karzon DT (1965) Measles virus giant cells inducing factor (fusion factor). Virology 26:311–325

Chambers TJ (1978) Multinucleate giant cells. J Pathol 126:125–148
Chan T, Long C, Green H (1975) A human-mouse somatic hybrid line selected for human deoxycytidine deaminase. Somatic Cell Genet 1:81–90
Chan T, Creagan RP, Reardon MP (1978) Adenosine kinase as a new selective marker in somatic cell genetics: isolation of adenosine kinase-deficient mouse cell lines and human-mouse hybrid cell lines containing adenosine kinase. Somatic Cell Genet 4:1–12
Chasin LA (1974) Mutations affecting adenine phosphoribosyl transferase activity in Chinese hamster cells. Cell 2:37–41
Chasin LA, Urlaub G (1975) Chromosome-wide event accompanies the expression of recessive mutations in tetraploid cells. Science 187:1091–1093
Chasin LA, Urlaub G (1976) Mutant alleles for hypoxanthine phosphoribosyl transferase: codominant expression, complementation, and segregation in hybrid Chinese hamster cells. Somatic Cell Genet 2:453–467
Chen JJ, Jones ME (1976) The cellular location of dihydroorotate dehydrogenase: relation to de novo biosynthesis of pyrimidines. Arch Biochem Biophys 176:82–90
Clive D, Flamm WG, Machesko MR, Bernheim NJ (1972) A mutational assay system using the thymidine kinase locus in mouse lymphoma cells. Mutat Res 16:77–87
Coleman PF, Suttle DP, Stark GR (1977) Purification from hamster cells of the multi-functional protein that initiates de novo synthesis of pyrimidine nucleotides. J Biol Chem 252:6379–6385
Collins JJ, Destree AT, Marshall CJ, Macpherson IA (1975) Selective depletion of chromosomes in a stable mouse-Chinese hamster cell line using antisera directed against species-specific cell-surface antigens. J Cell Physiol 86:605–620
Corsaro CM, Migeon BR (1978) Gene expression in euploid human hybrid cells: ouabain resistance is codominant. Somatic Cell Genet 4:531–540
Croce CM (1976) Loss of mouse chromosomes in somatic cell hybrids between HT-1080 human fibrosarcoma cells and mouse peritoneal macrophages. Proc Natl Acad Sci USA 73:3248–3252
Croce CM, Bakay B, Nyhan WL, Koprowski H (1973) Re-expression of the rat hypoxanthine phosphoribosyl transferase gene in rat-human hybrids. Proc Natl Acad Sci USA 70:2590–2594
Dale B (1979) Radiation response of an intraspecific somatic cell hybrid (L5178Y, X-ray resistant line × L5178Y, X-ray sensitive line). Radiat Res 79:338–348
Davidson JN, Carnright DV, Patterson D (1979) Biochemical genetic analysis of pyrimidine biosynthesis in mammalian cells III. Association of carbamyl phosphate synthetase, aspartate transcarbamylase and dihydroorotase in mutants of cultured Chinese hamster cells. Somatic Cell Genet 5:175–191
Davidson R (1969) Regulation of melanin synthesis in mammalian cells as studied by somatic hybridization. III. A method of increasing frequency of cell fusion. Exp Cell Res 55:424–427
Davidson RL, De La Cruz FF (eds) (1974) Somatic cell hybridisation. Raven, New York
Davidson RL, Ephrussi B, Yamamoto K (1966) Regulation of pigment synthesis in mammalian cells as studied by somatic hybridization. Proc Natl Acad Sci USA 56:1437–1440
Deavan LL, Peterson DF (1973) The chromosomes of CHO, an aneuploid Chinese hamster cell line: G-band, C-band, and autoradiographic analysis. Chromosoma 41:129–144
De Saint Vincent R, Buttin G (1979) Studies on 1-β-D-arabinofuranosyl cytosine-resistant mutant of Chinese hamster fibroblasts III. Joint resistance to arabinofuranosyl cytosine and to excess thymidine – a semi-dominant manifestation of deoxycytidine triphosphate pool expansion. Somatic Cell Genet 5:67–82
Deschamps M, De Saint Vincent R, Evrard C, Sassi M, Buttin G (1974) Studies on 1-β-D-arabinofuranosyl-cytosine (ara-C) resistant mutants of Chinese hamster fibroblasts II. High resistance to ara-C as a genetic marker for cellular hybridisation. Exp Cell Res 86:269–279
Dev VG, Miller DA, Rechsteiner M, Miller OJ (1979) Time of suppression of human rRNA genes in mouse-human hybrid cells. Exp Cell Res 123:47–54

Djinawi NK, Olsen LC (1973) Cell fusion induced by Germiston and Wesselsbron viruses. Arch Gesamte Virusforsch 43:144–151
Drury EJ, Bazar LS, Mackenzie RE (1975) Formiminotransferase-cyclodeaminase from Porcine liver. Purification and physical properties of the enzyme complex. Arch Biochem Biophys 169:662–668
Enders AC, Schlafke S (1971) Penetration of the uterine epithelium during implantation in the rabbit. Am J Anat 132:219–240
Engel E, Macgee BJ, Harris H (1969a) Cytogenetic and nuclease studies on A9 and B82 fused together by Sendai virus: the early phase. J Cell Sci 5:93–120
Engel E, Mcgee BJ, Harris H (1969b) Recombination and segregation in somatic cell hybrids. Nature 223:152–155
Engel E, Empson J, Harris H (1971) Isolation and karyotypic characterization of segregants of intraspecific hybrid somatic cells. Exp Cell Res 68:231–234
Ephrussi B (1972) Hybridization of somatic cells. Princeton University Press, Princeton
Evans RW (1956) Histological appearances of tumours. Livingstone, Edinburgh
Farrell SA, Worton RG (1977) Chromosome loss is responsible for segregation at the HPRT locus in Chinese hamster cell hybrids. Somatic Cell Genet 3:539–551
Fenyo EM, Wiener F, Klein G, Harris H (1973) Selection of tumour-host cell hybrids from polyoma virus- and methyl cholanthrene-induced sarcomas. JNCI 51:1863–1872
Fisher PB, Sisskin EE, Goldstein NI (1978) Selecting somatic cell hybrids with HAT media and nystatin methyl ester. J Cell Sci 32:433–439
Fisher PB, Bryson V, Shaffner CP (1979) Polyene macrolide antibiotic cytotoxicity and membrane permeability alterations II. Phenotypic expression in intraspecific and interspecific somatic cell hybrids. J Cell Physiol 100:335–341
Flintoff W, Spindler SM, Siminovitch L (1976) Genetic characterization of methotrexate-resistant hamster ovary cells. In Vitro 12:749–757
Fox M (1971) Spontaneous and X-ray induced genotypic and phenotypic resistance to 5-iodo-2-deoxyuridine in lymphoma cells in vitro. Mutation Res 23:403–419
Fox M (1979) Dominance of a repair function for X-ray, UV and alkylating agent induced damage in hybrids between mouse lymphoma cells of different sensitivity. Int J Radiat Biol 36:335–348
Gehring U (1980) Cell genetics of glucocorticoid responsiveness. Biochem Actions Horm 7:205–232
Gehring U, Mohit B, Tomkin GM (1972) Glucocorticoid action on hybrid clones derived from cultured myeloma and lymphoma cell lines. Proc Natl Acad Sci USA 69:3124–3127
Goldenberg DM, Bhan RD, Pavia RA (1971) In vivo human-hamster somatic cell fusion indicated by glucose-6-phosphate dehydrogenase and lactate dehydrogenase profiles. Cancer Res 31:1148–1152
Goldenberg DM, Pavia RA, Tsao M (1974) In vivo hybridisation of human tumour and normal hamster cells. Nature 250:649–651
Goldstein NI, Fisher PB (1978) Selection of mouse × hamster hybrids using HAT media and a polyene antibiotic. In Vitro 14:200–206
Goss SJ, Harris H (1977) Gene transfer by means of cell fusion. 1. Statistical mapping of the human X-chromosome by analysis of radiation-induced gene segregation. J Cell Sci 25:17–37
Graves JAM (1972) Cell cycles and chromosome replication patterns in interspecific somatic hybrids. Exp Cell Res 73:81–94
Graves JAM (1980) Evidence for an indirect effect of radiation on mammalian chromosomes. 1. Indirectly-induced chromosome loss from somatic cell hybrids. Exp Cell Res 125:483–486
Gupta RS (1980) Random segregation of multiple genetic markers from CHO-CHO hybrids: evidence for random distribution of functional hemizygosity in the genome. Somatic Cell Genet 6:115–125
Gupta RS, Siminovitch L (1978a) Mutants of CHO cells resistant to the protein synthesis inhibitor emetine: genetic and biochemical characterization of second-step mutants. Somatic Cell Genet 4:77–93

Gupta RS, Siminovitch L (1978 b) Genetic and biochemical characterization of mutants of CHO cells resistant to the protein synthesis inhibitor trichodermin. Somatic Cell Genet 4:355–374

Gupta RS, Siminovitch L (1978 c) Diphtheria-toxin-resistant mutants of CHO cells affected in protein synthesis: a novel phenotype. Somatic Cell Genet 4:553–571

Gupta RS, Siminovitch L (1978 d) Genetic and biochemical studies with the adenosine analogs toyocamycin and tubericidin: mutation at the adenosine kinase locus in Chinese hamster cells. Somatic Cell Genet 4:715–735

Gupta RS, Siminovitch L (1980) Diphtheria toxin resistance in Chinese hamster cells: genetic and biochemical characteristics of the mutants affected in protein synthesis. Somatic Cell Genet 6:361–379

Halaban R, Norlund J, Francke U, Moellmann G, Eisenstadt JM (1980) Supermelanotic hybrids derived from mouse melanomas and normal mouse cells. Somatic Cell Genet 6:29–44

Ham AW (1974) Histology, 7th edn. Lippincott, Philadelphia

Handmaker SD (1973) Hybridization of eukaryotic cells. Annu Rev Microbiol 27:189–204

Harris H (1970) Cell fusion, the Dunham lectures. Oxford University Press, London

Harris H, Watkins JF (1965) Hybrid cells derived from mouse and man: artificial heterokaryons of mammalian cells from different species. Nature 205:640–646

Harris H, Miller OJ, Klein G, Worst P, Tachibana T (1969) Suppression of malignancy by cell fusion. Nature 223:363–368

Harris JF, Whitmore GF (1977) Segregation studies in CHO hybrid cells: I spontaneous and mutagen-induced segregation events of two recessive drug resistance loci. Somatic Cell Genet 3:173–193

Harris M (1972) Effect of X-irradiation of one partner on hybrid frequency in fusions between Chinese hamster cells. J Cell Physiol 80:119–126

Harris M (1975) Non-Mendelian segregation in hybrids between Chinese hamster cells. J Cell Physiol 86:413–430

Harris M, Ruddle FH (1961) Cloned strains of pig kidney cells with drug resistance and chromosomal markers. J Natl Cancer Inst 26:1405–1411

Harter DH, Choppin PW (1967) Cell-fusing activity of visna virus particles. Virology 31:279–288

Hashmi S, Miller OJ (1976) Further evidence of X-linkage of hypoxanthine phosphoribosyl transferase in the mouse. Cytogenet Cell Genet 17:35–41

Hellkuhl B, Grzeschik K-H (1978) Partial reactivation of a human inactive X chromosome in human-mouse somatic cell hybrids. Cytogenet Cell Genet 22:527–530

Henle G, Deinhardt F, Girardi A (1954) Cytogenetic effects of mumps virus in tissue cultures of epithelial cells. Proc Soc Exp Biol Med 87:386–393

Hoehn H, Bryant EM, Johnston P, Norwood TH, Martin GM (1975) Non-selective isolation, stability and longevity of hybrids between normal human somatic cells. Nature 258:608–610

Hoggan MD, Roizman B (1959) The isolation and properties of a variant of herpes simplex producing multinucleated giant cells in monolayer cultures in the presence of antibody. Am J Hyg 70:208–219

Holtzer H, Abbott J, Lash J (1958) The formation of multinucleate myotubes. Anat Rec 131:537 (abstract)

Hu F, Pasztor LM (1975) In vivo hybridisation of cultured melanoma cells and isogenic normal mouse cells. Differentiation 4:93–97

Huet MD (1979) Induction of glucocorticoid resistance by various mutagens in a murine lymphoid cell line. Cancer Treat Rep 63:1172 (abstract)

Human Gene Mapping 4 (1978) Fourth international workshop on human gene mapping, Birth defects: original article series XIV, 4. The National Foundation, New York; also in Cytogenet Cell Genet 22 (1–6)

Human Gene Mapping 5 (1979) Fifth international workshop on human gene mapping. Birth defects: original article series XV, 11. The National Foundation, New York; also in Cytogenet Cell Genet 25 (1–4)

Jackson H, Parker E (1944) Hodgkins disease II. Pathology. New Engl J Med 231:35–44

Janzen HW, Millman PA, Thurston OG (1971) Hybrid cells in solid tumors. Cancer 27:455–459

Johnson RT, Rao PN (1970) Mammalian cell fusion: induction of premature chromosome condensation in interphase nuclei. Nature 226:717–722

Johnson RT, Rao PN, Hughes SD (1970) Mammalian cell fusion III. A HeLa cell inducer of premature chromosome condensation active in cells from a variety of animal species. J Cell Physiol 77:151–158

Jones GE, Sergent PA (1974) Mutants of cultured Chinese hamster cells deficient in adenine phosphoribosyl transferase. Cell 2:43–54

Jullien P, Bornecque D, Szafarz D (1978) Effect of X-irradiation on the ability of mammalian cells to form viable hybrids. Radiat Res 75:217–229

Kadouri A, Kunce JJ, Lark KG (1978) Evidence for dominant mutations reducing HGPRT activity. Nature 274:256–259

Kahan B, Demars R (1975) Localized derepression on the human inactive X-chromosome in mouse-human cell hybrids. Proc Natl Acad Sci USA 72:1510–1514

Kahan B, Demars R (1980) Autonomous gene expression on the human inactive X-chromosome. Somatic Cell Genet 6:309–323

Kao FT, Puck TT (1970) Genetics of somatic mammalian cells: linkage studies with human-Chinese hamster cell hybrids. Nature 228:329–332

Karakoz I, Gresikova M, Hala K, Hasek M (1969) Attempts to induce recombinant and somatic cells in chicken erythrocyte chimeras by repeated injection of western equine encephalomyelitis virus. Folia Biol (Prague) 15:81–86

Kempe TD, Swyryd EA, Bruist M, Stark GR (1976) Stable mutants of mammalian cells that overproduce the first three enzymes of pyrimidine nucleotide biosynthesis. Cell 9:541–550

Kinsella AR, Smith PJ, Boyle JM (1976) Recovery from radiation damage mediated by somatic cell hybridisation. In: Kiefer J (ed) Radiation and cellular control processses. Springer, Berlin Heidelberg New York, pp 170–177

Kirschner K, Bisswanger H (1976) Multifunctional proteins. Annu Rev Biochem 45:143–166

Kit S, Dubbs DR, Piekarski LJ, Hsu TC (1963) Deletion of thymidine kinase activity from L cells resistant to bromodeoxyuridine. Exp Cell Res 31:297–312

Knowles BB, Swift K (1975) Cell-mediated immunoselection against cell-surface antigens of somatic cell hybrids. Somatic Cell Genet 1:123–135

Kohn A (1965) Polykaryocytosis induced by Newcastle disease virus in monolayers of animal cells. Virology 26:228–245

Konigsberg IR (1963) Clonal analysis of myogenesis. Science 140:1272–1284

Konigsberg IR, McIlvain N, Tootle M, Hermann H (1960) The dissociability of deoxyribonucleic acid synthesis from the development of multinuclearity of mouse cells in culture. J Biophys Biochem Cytol 8:333–343

Krooth RS (1964) Properties of diploid cell strains developed from patients with an inherited abnormality of uridine biosynthesis. Cold Spring Harbor Symp Quant Biol 29:189–212

Kusano T, Long C, Green H (1971) A new reduced human-mouse somatic cell hybrid containing the human gene for adenine phosphoribosyl transferase. Proc Natl Acad Sci USA 68:82–86

Lala PK, Santer V, Rahil KS (1980) Spontaneous fusion between Ehrlich ascites tumour cells and host cells in vivo: kinetics of hybridisation and concurrent changes in the histocompatibility profile of the tumour after propagation in different host strains. Eur J Cancer 16:487–510

Law ML, Kao F-T (1978) Induced segregation of human syntenic genes by 5-bromodeoxyuridine and near-visible light. Somatic Cell Genet 4:465–476

Le Bouton AV (1976) DNA synthesis and cell proliferation in the simple liver acinus of 10- to 20-day old rats: evidence for cell fusion. Anat Record 184:679–688

Leistenschneider W, Nagel R (1979) Nuclear DNA analysis by scanning single cell photometry in prostatic carcinoma (in German). Aktuel Urol 10:353–358

Lewis MR, Lewis WH (1926) Transformation of mononuclear blood cells into macrophages, epthelial cells and giant cells in hanging drop cultures of lower vertebrates. Carnegie Institute of Washington, publ no 96. Contrib Embryol 18:95–120

Lewis WH (1927) The formation of giant cells in tissue culture and their similarity to those in tuberculous lesion. Am Rev Tuberc 15:616–628

Lewis WH, Wright JH (1979) Isolation of hydroxyurea-resistant CHO cells with altered levels of ribonucleotide reductase. Somatic Cell Genet 5:83–96

Lieberman I, Ove P (1960) Enzyme studies with mutant mammalian cells. J Biol Chem 235:1765–1768

Limbosch S, Heilporn V, Lievens A, Decoen JL, Zampetti-Bosseler F (1974) Radiation response of a somatic cell hybrid. Int J Radiat Biol 26:197–201

Ling V, Baker RM (1978) Dominance of colchicine resistance in hybrid CHO cells. Somatic Cell Genet 4:193–200

Lippman ME, Perry S, Thompson EB (1974) Cytoplasmic glucocorticoid-binding proteins in glucocorticoid-unresponsive human and mouse leukemic cell lines. Cancer Res 34:1572–1576

Liskay RM, Patterson D (1979) A selective medium (GAMA) for the isolation of somatic cell hybrids from $HPRT^-$ and $APRT^-$ mutant cells. Cytogenet Cell Genet 23:61–69

Little JB, Richardson UI, Tashijian AH (1972) Unexpected resistance to X-irradiation in a strain of hybrid mammalian cells. Proc Natl Acad Sci USA 69:1363–1365

Littlefield JW (1963) The inosinic acid pyrophosphorylase activity of mouse fibroblasts partially resistant to 8-azaguanine. Proc Natl Acad Sci USA 50:568–576

Littlefield JW (1964) Selection of hybrids from matings of fibroblasts in vitro and their presumed recombinants. Science 145:709–710

Lobban PE, Siminovitch L (1975) α-Amanitin resistance: a dominant mutation in CHO cells. Cell 4:167–172

Ludford H, Smiles E (1952) Malignant cell polymorphism studied by phase-contrast microscopy. Proc R Microsc Soc 72:149–154

Lyon MF (1971) Possible mechanisms of X-chromosome inactivation. Nature New Biol 232:229–232

Malawista SE, Weiss MC (1974) Expression of differentiated functions in hepatoma cell hybrids. High frequency of induction of mouse albumin production in rat hepatoma × mouse lymphoblast hybrids. Proc Natl Acad Sci USA 71:333–361

Mariano M, Spector WG (1974) The formation and properties of macrophage polykaryons (inflammatory giant cells). J Pathol 113:1–19

Marin G, Manduca P (1972) Synchronous replication of the parental chromosomes in a Chinese hamster-mouse somatic hybrid. Exp Cell Res 75:290–293

Marin G, Pugliatti-Crippa L (1972) Preferential segregation of homospecific groups of chromosomes in heterospecific somatic cell hybrids. Exp Cell Res 70:253–256

Martin BF (1972) Cell replacement and differentiation in transitional epithelium: a histological and autoradiographic study of the guinea-pig bladder and ureter. J Anat 112:433–455

Matsuya Y, Green H (1969) Somatic cell hybrid between the established human line D98 (presumptive HeLa) and 3T3. Science 163:697–698

McClain ME (1965) The host range and plaque morphology of rabbit pox virus (*R.Pu*$^+$) and its *U* mutants on chick fibroblasts PK-2a and L929 cells. Aust J Exp Biol Med Sci 43:31–44

McKusick VA, Ruddle EH (1977) The status of the gene map of the human chromosomes. Science 196:390–405

Medrano L, Green H (1974) A uridine kinase-deficient mutant of 3T3 and a selective method for cells containing the enzyme. Cell 1:23–26

Megumi T (1976) Recovery of colony-forming ability of X-irradiated L cells by cell fusion. Radiat Res 67:178–183

Melera PW, Lewis JA, Biedler JL, Hession C (1980) Antifolate-resistant Chinese hamster cells. Evidence for dihydrofolate reductase gene amplification among independently derived sublines overproducing different dihydrofolate reductases. J Biol Chem 255:7024–7028

Meuth M, Trudel M, Siminovitch L (1979) Selection of Chinese hamster cells auxotrophic for thymidine by 1-β-D-arabinofuranosyl cytosine. Somatic Cell Genet 5:303–318

Migeon BR, Miller CS (1968) Human-mouse somatic cell hybrids with single human chromosome (group E): linked with thymidine kinase activity. Science 162:1005–1006

Migeon BR, Norum RA, Corsaro CM (1974) Isolation and analysis of somatic hybrids derived from two human diploid cells. Proc Natl Acad Sci USA 71:937–941

Miller OJ (1974) Cell hybridisation in the study of the malignant process including cytogenetic aspects. In: German J (ed) Chromosomes and cancer. Wiley, New York, pp 521–563

Miller OJ, Dev VG, Miller DA, Tantravahi R, Eliceiri GL (1978) Transcription and processing of both mouse and Syrian hamster ribosomal RNA genes in individual somatic cell hybrids. Exp Cell Res 115:457–460

Minna JD, Coon HG (1974) Human × mouse hybrid cells segregating mouse chromosomes and isozymes. Nature 252:401–404

Mintz B, Baker WW (1967) Normal mammalian muscle differentiation and gene control of isocitrate dehydrogenase. Proc Natl Acad Sci USA 58:592–598

Moehring TJ, Moehring JM (1977) Selection and characterisation of cells resistant to diphtheria toxin and Pseudomonas exotoxin A: presumptive translational mutants. Cell 11:447–454

Mohandas T, Sparkes RS, Shapiro LJ (1981) Reactivation of an inactive human X chromosome: evidence for X inactivation by DNA methylation. Science 211:393–396

Moraru I, Fadei L (1974) Comparative morphological and cytogenetical studies on human ovarian papillary adenocarcinomas. Oncology 30:113–124

Morris JA, Blount RF, Savage RE (1956) Recovery of a cytopathogenic agent from chimpanzees with coryza. Proc Soc Exp Biol Med 92:544–549

Morrow J (1977) Gene inactivation as a mechanism for the generation of variability in somatic cells cultivated in vitro. Mutation Res 44:391–400

Morse PA, Potter VR (1965) Pyrimidine metabolism in tissue culture cells derived from rat hepatomas. 1. Suspension cell cultures derived from the Novikoff hepatoma. Cancer Res 25:499–508

Moses E, Kohn A (1963) Polykaryocytosis induced by Rous sarcoma virus in chick fibroblasts. Exp Cell Res 32:182–186

Nadler HL, Chacko CM, Rachmeler M (1970) Interallelic complementation in hybrid cells derived from human diploid strains deficient in galactose-1-phosphate uridyl transferase activity. Proc Natl Acad Sci USA 67:976–982

Okada Y (1962) Analysis of giant polynuclear cell formation caused by HVJ virus from Ehrlich's ascites tumour cells. 1. Microscopic observation of giant polynuclear cell formation. Exp Cell Res 62:98–107

Patterson D (1980) Isolation and characterization of 5-fluorouracil-resistant mutants of Chinese hamster ovary cells deficient in the activities of orotate phosphoribosyl transferase and orotidine 5'monophosphate decarboxylase. Somatic Cell Genet 6:101–114

Patterson D, Carnright D (1977) Biochemical genetic analysis of pyrimidine biosynthesis in mammalian cells. I. Isolation of a mutant defective in the early steps of de novo pyrimidine synthesis. Somatic Cell Genet 3:483–495

Paukert JL, Strauss LDA, Rabinowitz JC (1976) Formyl-methenyl-methylene tetrahydrofolate synthetase (combined) J Biol Chem 251:5104–5111

Perry RP, Kelley DE, Schibler U, Huebner K, Croce CM (1979) Selective suppression of the transcription of ribosomal genes in mouse-human hybrid cells. J Cell Physiol 98:553–560

Peterson JA, Weiss MC (1972) Expression of differentiated functions in hepatoma cell hybrids: induction of mouse albumin production in rat hepatoma-mouse fibroblast hybrids. Proc Natl Acad Sci USA 69:571–575

Peterson SP, Berns MW (1979) Mitosis in flat PTK_2-human hybrid cells. Exp Cell Res 120:223–236

Petrova ON, Manuilova ES, Shapiro NI (1977) Hybridisation of cultures of Chinese hamster cells, sensitive to UV-light (in Russian). Genetika 13:637–645

Pfahl M, Bourgeois S (1980) Analysis of steroid resistance in lymphoid cell hybrids. Somatic Cell Genet 6:63–74
Pfahl M, Kelleher RJ, Bourgeois S (1978) General features of steroid resistance in lymphoma cell lines. Mol Cell Endocrinol 10:193–208
Pontecorvo G (1971) Induction of directional chromosomal elimination in somatic cell hybrids. Nature 230:367–369
Pontecorvo G (1974) Induced chromosome elimination in hybrid cells. In: Davidson RL, de la Cruz F (eds) Somatic cell hybridization. Academic, New York, pp 65–69
Priest RE, Priest JH, Laundon CH, Snider PW (1980) Multinucleate cells in cultures of human amniotic fluid form by fusion. Lab Invest 43:140–144
Rao PN, Johnson RT (1972) Premature chromosome condensation: a mechanism for the elimination of chromosomes in virus-fused cells. J Cell Sci 10:495–513
Rappaport H, Demars R (1973) Diaminopurine-resistant mutants of cultured diploid human fibroblasts. Genetics 75:335–345
Razin A, Riggs AD (1980) DNA methylation and gene function. Science 210:604–610
Rechsteiner M, Parsons B (1976) Studies on the intranuclear distribution of human and mouse genomes and formation of human-mouse hybrid cells. J Cell Physiol 88:167–180
Ringertz NL, Savage RE (1976) Cell hybrids. Academic, New York
Robbins MR, Baker RM (1977) (Na,K)ATPase activity in membrane preparations of ouabain-resistant HeLa cells. Biochemistry 16:5163–5168
Robertson JB, Raju MR (1980) Sudden reversion to normal radiosensitivity to the effects of X-irradiation and plutonium-238 α particles by a radio-resistant rat-mouse hybrid cell line. Radiat Res 83:197–204
Robertson JB, Williams JR, Little JB (1977) Relative responses of an X-ray resistant hybrid cell line and its parent line to X-irradiation, ultra-violet light, actinomycin-D and cordycepin. Int J Radiat Res 31:529–539
Roizman B (1962a) A polykaryocytosis induced by viruses. Proc Natl Acad Sci USA 48:228–234
Roizman B (1962b) Polykaryocytosis. Cold Spring Harbor Symp Quant Biol 27:327–340
Rommelaere J, Errera M (1972) The effect of caffeine on the survival of UV-irradiated diploid and tetraploid Chinese hamster cells. Int J Radiat Biol 22:285–291
Rushton AR (1976) Quantitative analysis of human chromosome segregation in man-mouse cell hybrids. Cytogenet Cell Genet 17:243–253
Russell MH, Engel E, Vaughn WK, McGee BJ (1977) Karyotypic analysis of parental and hybrid intraspecific mouse cells A9/B82, by Giemsa and centromeric banding. J Cell Sci 25:59–71
Russell MH, McGee BJ, Engel E (1979) Extent and rate of chromosome segregation in two intraspecific mouse cell hybrids: A9 × diploid foetal erythrocyte and A9 × B82. J Cell Sci 36:215–221
Ryan GB, Spector WG (1970) Macrophage turnover in inflamed connective tissue. Proc R Soc Lond [Biol] 175:269–292
Scherer WF (1953) The utilization of a pure strain of mammalian cells (Earle) for the cultivation of viruses in vitro. I. Multiplication of pseudorabies and herpes simplex viruses. Am J Pathol 29:113–137
Schneider JA, Weiss MC (1971) Expression of differentiated functions in hepatoma cell hybrids, I. Tyrosine aminotransferase in hepatoma-fibroblast hybrids. Proc Natl Acad Sci USA 68:127–131
Shows TB, Sakaguchi AY (1980) Gene transfer and gene mapping in mammalian cells in culture. In Vitro 16:55–76
Sheehy PF, Wakunig-Vaartuja T, Winn R, Clarkson BD (1974) Asynchronous DNA-synthesis and asynchronous mitoses in multinuclear ovarian cancer cells. Cancer Res. 34:991–996
Shin S, Caneva R, Schildkraut CL, Klinger HP, Siniscalo M (1973) Cells with phosphoribosyl transferase activity recovered from mouse cells resistant to 8-azaguanine. Nature 241:194–196

Siciliano MJ, Siciliano J, Humphrey RM (1978) Electrophoretic shift mutants in Chinese hamster ovary cells: evidence for genetic diploidy. Proc Natl Acad Sci USA 75:1919–1923

Silagi SG (1967) Hybridization of a malignant melanoma cell line with L cells in vitro. Cancer Res 27:1953–1960

Silagi S, Darlington G, Bruce SA (1969) Hybridization of two biochemically marked human cell lines. Proc Natl Acad Sci USA 69:1085–1092

Silverman L, Shorter RG (1963) Histogenesis of the multinucleated giant cell. Lab Invest 12:985–990

Siminovitch L (1976) On the nature of hereditable variation in cultured somatic cells. Cell 7:1–11

Siniscalco M, Klinger HP, Eagle H, Koprowski H, Fujimoto WY, Seegmiller JE (1969) Evidence for intergenic complementation in hybrid cells derived from two human diploid strains each carrying an X-linked mutation. Proc Natl Acad Sci USA 62:793–799

Slack C, Morgan RHM, Carr HB, Goldfarb PSG, Hooper M (1976) Isolation and characterization of Chinese hamster cells resistant to 5-fluorodeoxyuridine. Exp Cell Res 98:1–14

Sobel JS, Albrecht AM, Riehm H, Biedler JL (1971) Hybridization of actinomycin-D and methotrexate resistant Chinese hamster cells in vitro. Cancer Res 31:297–307

Sparkes RS, Weiss MC (1973) Expression of differentiated functions in hepatoma cell hybrids: alanine aminotransferase. Proc Natl Acad Sci USA 70:377–381

Spurna V, Nebola M (1973) Segregation of hybrids derived from mouse lymphosarcoma cells and biochemically marked L cells. Folia Biol (Prague) 19:424–432

Stamato TD, Patterson D (1979) Biochemical genetic analysis of pyrimidine biosynthesis in mammalian cells. II. Isolation and characterization of a mutant of Chinese hamster ovary cells with defective dihydroorotate dehydrogenase (E. C. 1. 3. 3. 1) activity. J Cell Physiol 98:459–468

Stockdale FE, Holtzer H (1961) DNA synthesis and myogenesis. Exp Cell Res 24:508–520

Stone WH, Friedman J, Fregin A (1964) Possible somatic cell mating in twin cattle with erythrocyte mosaicism. Proc Natl Acad Sci USA 51:1036–1044

Stutts P, Brockman RW (1963) A biochemical basis for resistance of L1210 mouse leukaemia to 6-thioguanine. Biochem Pharmacol 12:97–104

Suiter EC, Paul FJ (1969) Syncytia formation of mosquito cell cultures mediated by type-2 Dengue virus. Virology 38:482–485

Sutton JS, Weiss L (1966) Transformation of monocytes in tissue cultures into macrophage epithelioid cells and multinucleate cells, an electron microscope study. J Cell Biol 28:303–332

Szybalski W, Smith MJ (1959) Genetics of human cell lines. I. 8-Azaguanine resistance, a selective "single step" marker. Proc Soc Exp Biol Med 101:662–666

Szybalski W, Szybalska EH, Ragni G (1962) Genetic studies with human cell lines. Cancer Inst Monogr 7:75–89

Tan LVL, Drury EJ, Mackenzie RE (1977) Methylene tetrahydrofolate dehydrogenase-methylene tetrahydrofolate cyclohydrolase-formyltetrahydrofolate synthetase. A multifunctional protein from porcine liver. J Biol Chem 252:1117–1122

Testa NG, Allen TD, Lajtha LG, Onions D, Jarrett O (1981) Generation of osteoclasts in vitro. J Cell Sci 47:127–137

Turner JH, Hutchinson DL, Petricciani JC (1973) Chimerism following foetal transfusion: report of leucocytic hybridisation and infant with acute lymphocytic leukaemia. Scand J Haematol 10:358–366

Tyzzer EE (1906) The histology of the skin lesions in varicella. J Med Res NS 9:361–392

Venetianer A, Bajnoczky K, Gal A, Thompson EB (1978) Isolation and characterization of L-cell variants with altered sensitivity to glucocorticoids. Somatic Cell Genet 4:513–530

Warthin AS (1931) Occurrence of numerous large giant cells in the tonsils and pharyngial mucosa in the prodromal stages of measles. AMA Arch Pathol 11:864–874

Watson B, Gormley IP, Gardiner SE, Evans HJ, Harris H (1972) Reappearance of murine hypoxanthine guanine phosphoribosyl transferase acitivity in mouse A9 cells after attempted hybridization with human cell lines. Exp Cell Res 75:401–409
Weide LG, Dev VG, Rupert CS (1979) Activity of both mouse and Chinese hamster ribosomal RNA genes in somatic cell hybrids. Exp Cell Res 123:424–429
Weiss MC, Chaplain M (1971) Expression of differentiated functions in hepatoma cell hybrids: reappearance of tyrosine aminotransferase inducibility after the loss of chromosomes. Proc Natl Acad Sci USA 68:3026–3030
Weissman B, Stanbridge EJ (1980) Characterisation of ouabain resistant, hypoxanthine phosphoribosyl transferase deficient human cells and their usefulness as a general method for the production of human cell hybrids. Cytogenet Cell Genet 28:227–239
Weller TH, Witton MH, Bell EJ (1958) The etiologic agents of varicella and herpes zoster; isolation, propagation and cultural characteristics in vitro. J Exp Med 108:843–868
Wiener F, Fenyo EM, Klein G, Harris H (1972) Fusion of tumour cells with host cells. Nature 238:155–159
Wiener F, Fenyo EM, Klein G (1974a) Tumor-host cell hybrids in radiochimeras. Proc Natl Acad Sci USA 71:148–152
Wiener F, Fenyo EM, Klein G, Harris H (1974b) Fusion of tumor cells with host cells. In: Davidson RL, de la Cruz F (eds) Somatic cell hybridization. Academic, New York, pp 105–118
Wiener F, Dalianis T, Klein G, Harris H (1974c) Cytogenetic studies on the mechanism of formation of isoantigenic variant sublines derived from the fusion of TA3 Ha carcinoma with MSWBS sarcoma cells. J Natl Cancer Inst 52:1779–1796
Wiener F, Fenyo EM, Klein G, Davies AJS (1976) Tumor-host cell hybrids in radiochimeras reconstructed with bone marrow and thymus grafts. Somatic Cell Genet 2:81–92
Worton RG, Ho CC, Duff C (1977) Chromosome stability in CHO cells. Somatic Cell Genet 3:27–45
Worton RG, Duff C, Campbell CE (1980) Marker segregation without chromosome loss at the *emt* locus in Chinese hamster cell hybrids. Somatic Cell Genet 6:199–213
Wright JA, Lewis WH, Parfett CLJ (1980) Somatic cell genetics: a review of drug resistance, lectin resistance and gene transfer in mammalian cells in culture. Canad J Genet Cytol 22:443–496
Yaffe D, Feldman M (1965) The formation of hybrid multinucleated muscle fibers from myoblasts of different genetic origin. Dev Biol 11:300–317
Yamamoto KR, Gehring V, Stampfer MR, Sibley CH (1976) Genetic approaches to steroid hormone action. Recent Prog Hormone Res 32:3–32
Zampetti-Bosseler F, Heilporn V, Lieven A, Limbosch S (1976) X-ray sensitivity of somatic cell hybrids. Radiat Res 68:292–299
Zampetti-Bosseler F, Delhaisse P, Limbosch S (1980) UV survival and sensitizing effect of caffeine in mouse cell hybrids. Radiat Res 84:77–86

Section IV:
Modification of Tumor Biochemistry

CHAPTER 12

Drug Resistance and DNA Repair

M. Fox

A. Introduction

In discussing the role of DNA repair in resistance to cytotoxic drugs used in cancer chemotherapy, several important facts should initially be emphasised. Firstly, a significant number of drugs at present in current use in cancer chemotherapy exert their cytotoxic effect by mechanisms other than direct interaction with DNA; thus the role of DNA repair in development of resistance to such drugs will be minimal. Thus, I exclude from consideration resistance to antimetabolites, the *Vinca* alkaloids and many of the antitumour antibotics whose mode of action is unknown or for which there is little evidence implicating DNA as the critical intracellular target.

There are, however, several important classes of anticancer drugs, the cytotoxic effects of which are attributable to the ability of the drug to interact directly with DNA either by intercalation or by covalent reaction at various sites on the DNA molecule. These drugs include the bi- and polyfunctional alkylating agents, *cis*-platinum compounds, the antitumour nitrosoureas 1,3- bis -2-chlorethylnitrosourea (BCNU) and 1-(2-chloroethyl)3-cycohexyl-1-nitrosourea (CCNU), adriamycin, daunorubicin and bleomycin and some related antibotics. The evidence that DNA is the critical target for the cytotoxic action of these drugs rests mainly on the following types of observations:

1. Inhibition of DNA synthesis in cultured cells by doses of the drugs which have little or no effect on DNA, RNA and protein synthesis.
2. The demonstration of DNA single-strand breaks and DNA-DNA or DNA-protein cross-links at doses of drugs which allow for measurable survival of exposed cells.
3. The direct demonstration of reaction of drug with DNA either in vitro (isolated DNA) or in cultured cells by use of labelled drugs or by changes in base-stacking properties of DNA in the case of intercalating agents.
4. The demonstration of the ability of drugs to induce chromosome damage of the exchange aberration type. Chromosome-shattering effects can be induced by many of the antimetabolites if given in high doses and probably result from effects other than direct interaction of the drug with DNA.

In the following discussion, reference will frequently be made to observations on cells treated with chemicals (mostly carcinogens) which are not used in cancer chemotherapy. These compounds (e.g. sulphur mustard) have been used as prototype compounds in elucidating the mode of action of particular classes of drugs.

Their derivatives and related compounds, e.g. nitrogen mustard, chlorambucil and L-phenylalanine mustard, are used extensively in cancer chemotherapy. Thus, there are many overlaps between the fields of experimental cancer chemotherapy and experimental carcinogenesis not the least of which is the important fact that many of the drugs which are used as cytotoxic agents are also mutagens and carcinogens by virtue of their ability to interact directly with DNA.

In the following discussion I shall therefore first review our knowledge of how mammalian cells repair damage in their DNA. Much information about DNA repair processes has been gleaned from the study of UV-light-induced DNA damage often in prokaryotic cells; this will be referred to where appropriate. Secondly, I will examine the evidence for the role of DNA repair in resistance to DNA-damaging drugs in mammalian cells.

B. Mechanisms of DNA Repair

DNA repair in its strictest sense is defined as the reversal or removal of damage in DNA and/or the restoration of the correct complementary sequence at sites of base loss (HANAWALT et al. 1979). This process, which involves a number of different enzymes in recognition of base damage, its incision, excision and the subsequent replacement of damaged bases, is generally known as excision repair. The classification and enzymology of the various known excision repair pathways will be discussed in more detail. Under conditions where such excision repair processes are inoperative, for whatever reason, and DNA lesions are not completely removed prior to the first postinsult round of DNA synthesis, other cellular responses occur. These responses have in the past been variously termed postreplication repair, bypass repair, tolerance repair or just replication repair. The use of the word repair in these terms is a misnomer, because the lesions involved are never actually removed from the DNA and what is really observed is the cell's attempt, sometimes abortive, to complete a round of DNA synthesis on a DNA template containing unexcised DNA lesions. Such lesions interfere in a variety of ways (to be discussed later) with replicon initiation and strand elongation.

I. Excision Repair

Until relatively recently excision repair implied a single enzymatic mechanism for removal of damaged bases from DNA typified by the excision of pyrimidine dimers from the DNA of UV-irradiated bacteria. It is now clear, largely from studies of the enzymology of DNA repair, that the situation is far more complex than this and that damaged bases can be removed from DNA by two distinct processes: (a) base excision repair, in which the damage is removed from DNA as the free base and (b) nucleotide excision repair, in which damaged bases are removed as mono- or oligonucleotides. A classification of DNA repair has been proposed by FRIEDBURG et al. (1980) and is shown in Table 1.

Enzymatic photoreactivation of base damage is known to occur only in response to pyrimidine dimers in DNA and hence to be relevant only to UV irradiation and therefore will not be discussed further.

Table 1. Proposed classification of DNA repair

A. Reversal of base damage
   1. Enzymatic photoreactivation (the enzyme-catalysed monomerisation of pyrimidine dimers in DNA)
   2. Base modification (the enzyme-catalysed removal of specific chemical groups, thereby restoring modified bases to their normal chemistry)

B. Removal of base damage
   1. Nucleotide excision (the enzyme-catalysed excision of bases from DNA as mono- or oligonucleotides)
   2. Base excision (the enzyme-catalysed excision of bases from the DNA as free base)

C. Base restoration
   1. Repair synthesis (the enzyme-catalysed insertion of one or more nucleotides at sites of pre-existing base damage)
   2. Base insertion (enzyme-catalysed covalent linkage of a base to the deoxyribose phosphate backbone of DNA at sites of base loss)

1. Base Modification

This repair process, listed as a theoretical possibility by FRIEDBURG et al. (1980), has now been established as a practical reality. The recent studies of KARREN and GRIFFIN (1979), GRIFFIN et al. (1980) and OLSSON and LINDAHL (1980) have demonstrated the specific enzymatic removal of the methyl groups from the O-atom position of guanine leaving the base intact in "adapted" *Escherichia coli* cells. The methyl group appears to be transferred to *S*-methyl cysteine, the methyltransferase activity appears to be associated with a protein of mol. wt. 16,000 and the molecule itself is expended in the reaction. This response has so far been demonstrated only in prokaryotes. Attempts to mimic the adaptive response in *E. coli* in mammalian cells will be discussed later in this chapter.

2. Enzymatic Excision of Base Damage

A class of DNA repair enzymes called the DNA glycosylases, which can specifically catalyse the hydrolysis of the *N*-glycosylic bond, linking certain bases to the deoxyribose-phosphate backbone of DNA, is now recognised. A number of these enzymes have been isolated and characterised from pro- and eukaryotic systems (LINDAHL et al. 1969, 1977; LINDAHL 1979; CONE et al. 1977, LAVAL 1977). Each enzyme appears to be highly specific for a particular damaged or inappropriate base and this class of enzymes as a whole has the following properties: (a) all are relatively small proteins, with a mol. wt. of 20,000–30,000 (b) none requires any cofactors, (c) all are active in the presence of EDTA, (d) all are DNA specific, i.e. do not catalyse the excision of bases from RNA, and (e) the product of the reaction is an apurinic or apyrimidinic site in DNA and repair is effected by base restoration mechanisms such as repair synthesis or base insertion.

3. Repair of Base Damage

The repair of sites from which damaged bases have been removed appears to involve at least two steps: firstly, the hydrolysis of the phosphodiester bonds at or near the sites of base loss and, secondly, the exonucleolytic degradation of DNA at these sites to remove the apurinic or apyrimidinic residues. Several enzymes which have this activity have now been isolated and are collectively termed the apurinic/apyrimidinic endonucleases (AP endonucleases). These enzymes have been most studied in *E. coli* and several have been identified which have different substrate specificities and some which have other associated acitivities (LINDAHL et al. 1977; CONE et al. 1977; LAVAL 1977; GATES and LINN 1977a, b; LIVINGSTON and RICHARDSON 1975). AP endonucleases have also been isolated from eukaryotic cells (LINN et al. 1978; GROSSMAN et al. 1978; KUNNLEIN et al. 1978; NES 1980).

Following incision by AP endonucleases, excision of the deoxyribose phosphate residue and endonucleolytic degradation is dependent on the polarity of the incision event. Incision 5′ with respect to the site of base loss requires 5′-3′ endonuclease activity and vice versa. Excision of the damaged base is usually accompanied by loss of undamaged nucleotides. At least four exonucleases have been identified in *E. coli* which are capable of degrading DNA in the 5′→3′ direction. One of these, *E. coli* DNA polymerase I, has both excision and polymerising activities (KLETT et al. 1968). Several preparations which have 5′-exonuclease activity have also been purified from mammalian cells, the activities of some of which are listed below:

1. A 5′-exonuclease activity from human lymphoblasts which has associated AP endonuclease activity (STRAUSS et al. 1978).
2. DNAse IV from rabbit shows a preference for double-stranded DNA and can excise pyrimidine dimers from UV-irradiated DNA in the 5′→3′ direction if DNA is previously treated with *Micrococcus luteus* UV-specific endonuclease (LINDAHL et al. 1969).
3. Three different exonucleases have been purified from human KB cells (COOK and FRIEDBURG 1978a, b).
4. An exonuclease has been prepared from placenta and tissue culture cells which hydrolyses single-stranded DNA from both the 3′ and 5′ ends, releasing 5′-phosphorylated oligonucleotides averaging four residues from DNA randomly nicked or specifically incised with *M. luteus* UV endonuclease leaving gaps ~40 nucleotides in length (DONINGER and GROSSMAN 1976).

An activity capable of promoting the direct insertion of a free purine base or deoxynucleoside into DNA which has no requirement for a high-energy donor molecule has recently been isolated from human fibroblasts and has been termed DNA insertase (DEUTSCH and LINN 1979). An enzyme with similar activity but different requirement has been isolated from *E. coli* (LIVENEH et al. 1979). Sealing of the excision repair gap is then completed by DNA ligase.

4. Nucleotide Excision and Repair

DNA incision in prokaryotes is an extraordinarily complex process and is even more so in eukaryotes (FRIEDBURG et al. 1980; DEMPLE and LINN 1980). The precise molecular mechanisms involved in dimer excision even in *E. coli* are still matters for considerable debate. Studies on XP cells suggest that many or all of them are deficient in incision capacity and not excision as previously thought (TANAKA et al. 1975, 1977). The excision of pyrimidine dimers and/or other bulky lesions in DNA, repair synthesis of the resulting gap and DNA ligation are thought to be effected by the same enzymes as described above for base excision repair. The ability of mammalian cells to excise a variety of chemically induced lesions in DNA has been clearly established. Many of these studies have been reviewed by ROBERTS (1978) and several general features emerge:

1. Loss or excision of DNA lesions occurs in all cases; however, the rate of loss depends on the type of lesion induced and the cell line studied.
2. Some cell lines, e.g. Chinese hamster V79 cells (WARREN et al. 1979; FOX and BRENNAND 1980), Chinese hamster ovary (CHO) cells (GOTH-GOLDSTEIN 1980) and XP cells, are unable to remove some lesions, e.g. O^6-methyl and O^6-ethylguanine, which are removed by normal human cells (ALTAMIRANO-DIMAS 1979).
3. Excision repair capacity appears to saturate when high concentrations of DNA-damaging agents are used.
4. Excision of chemical lesions from mammalian cell DNA is slow, taking hours or days, and rarely goes to completion even when total replication of cellular DNA can be demonstrated and viable cells result.

Two pathways for repair synthesis have been identified in mammalian cells, which have been termed "short-" and "long-patch" pathways (REGAN and SELTOW 1974). The short-patch pathway operates on the major damage caused by some alkylating agents and by X-rays and is largely completed by 1–2 h. The size of the patch inserted has been estimated to be three to four nucleotides after X-irradiation (PAINTER and YOUNG 1972; FOX and FOX 1973 b). In making these estimates however, the number of repair events was assumed to be equal to the number of single-strand breaks sealed, and the numbers of bases inserted may thus be an overestimate. It is possible therefore that this short-patch repair can be equated to base excision repair, initiated by AP endonuclease, but this is not proven.

Long-patch repair operates after exposure to agents which produce "bulky" substituents in DNA, e.g. UV dimers. The frequency of incision breaks is low after this type of damage and continues for many hours. The patch size for repair of UV-damaged DNA in human cells has been estimated by various techniques to be between 35 and 100 nucleotides long (EDENBURG and HANAWALT 1972; REGAN et al. 1971). Patch sizes ranging from 30 to 120 have been reported for a number of mutagens (REGAN and SETLOW 1974). The biological significance of these different patch sizes in mammalian cells is currently unknown, but may be related to the spectrum of lesions produced by any given agent. Some DNA-damaging agents apparently produce damage repaired by both long and short patches, e.g. 4NQO and X-rays (REGAN and SETLOW 1974). Long and short patches may therefore reflect the activities of nucleotide excision and base excision repair modes respectively. For more detailed discussion of the enzymology and methodology involved in studies of excision repair of DNA the reader is referred to several excellent recent reviews on the topic (ROBERTS 1978; HANAWALT et al. 1979; FRIEDBURG et al. 1980; DEMPLE and LINN 1980). Figure 1 illustrates schematically the various repair pathways discussed.

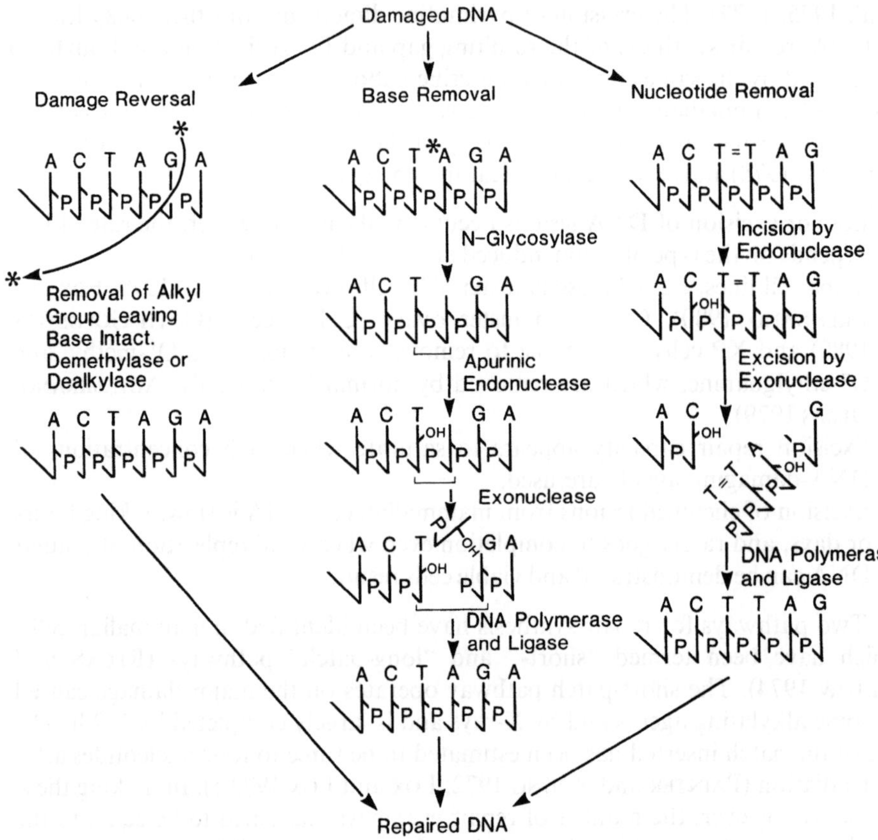

Fig. 1. Summary of possible pathways for DNA excision repair in mammalian cells

5. Influence of Chromatin Structure on DNA Excision Repair

Chromatin in eukaryotic cells is a complex structure consisting of nucleoprotein core units, nucleosomes which consist of well-defined lengths of DNA ~200 base pairs complexed with an octomer of histones made up of equimolor amounts of four types, two lysine-rich histones H2A und H2B and two arginine-rich histones H3 and H4. Separating the nucleosome cores is linker DNA which is generally more sensitive to digestion with staphylococcal nuclease. The length of this linker DNA is variable (15–100 base pairs) from one cell type to another, but in its native state appears to be coiled or folded in the normal state of chromatin. Superimposed on this basic subunit structure are several higher orders of supercoiling to allow packaging of DNA into the chromosome. For further details and experimental evidence in support of this proposed structure the reader is referred to several excellent reviews on the topic (Kornberg 1978; Felsenfeld 1978).

Several recent studies have measured the relative numbers of DNA lesions produced in "core" and linker DNA in mammalian cells and their relative rates of repair. Variations in the reactivity of chromatin subfractions with alkylating agents have been demonstrated (Cox 1979; Galbraith et al. 1979; Feldman et al. 1980; Smulson et al. 1979) and it was originally suggested that there was preferential repair of DNA damage in linker regions (Cleaver 1977; Smerdon et al. 1978; Williams and Friedberg 1979). However, this interpretation is now less favoured; Bodell and Cleaver (1981) measured the nuclease sensitivity of DNA labelled for 15 min after UV irradiation and always found, even with this short pulse time, that 30% of the repair label was nuclease resistant, whereas if the repair label were only in the linker region it should be completely nuclease sensitive. They argue that since the estimated size of the repair patch is generally larger than the linker region and there are no detectable differences in dimer excision between core and linker regions (Williams and Friedberg 1979) the immediate nuclease sensitivity of the label is the result of a transient structural change in chromatin configuration and not the result of preferential repair in linker regions. After alkylation damage, however, repair does appear to be preferentially located in linker regions as repair patches were still nuclease sensitive even after a 2-h labelling period (Bodell 1977; Bodell and Cleaver 1979).

Distribution of DNA damage after exposure to 7-bromomethyl-benz(a)anthracene has been found to be non-random in confluent human fibroblasts. More total damage occurred in nucleosome core than in linker DNA. Over a 24-h period damage was removed at approximately the same rate from both regions. Immediately after 7-BMBA damage almost all the repair-incorporated nucleotides were nuclease sensitive, the sensitivity of repair patches declined rapidly with time and by 1.5 h 85% of incorporated nucleotides had become nuclease resistant, indicating redistribution into core DNA. There was, however, still some residual nuclease sensitivity at 24 h. Even when repair synthesis occured late after treatment, repair patches were initially nuclease sensitive then rapidly became resistant. On the basis of this and other data the authors suggest that the repair process itself induces a conformational change in the DNA which results in dissociation of DNA from nucleosome cores, so that *all* repair incorporation is initially nuclease sensitive i.e. nuclease sensitivity cannot be equated with linker DNA (Oleson et al. 1979).

It has also been suggested that a number of cofactors may be necessary to dissociate histone from DNA before repair can occur (Cleaver 1977). This step may be common to repair of most kinds of damage and may be the one defective in XP cells (Mortelmans et al. 1976). Obviously, given this degree of complexity of chromatin, many factors influence the distribution and accessibility of DNA damage, and from the results discussed above it is evident that the situation is not a static one. Further indications of the potential importance of chromatin structure in determining the response of cells to DNA damage have come from detailed studies of the effects of caffeine on DNA synthesis in irradiated and unirradiated cells (Painter 1980). Caffeine has been repeatedly shown to reverse the inhibition of DNA synthesis normally caused by irradiation and exposure to cytotoxic drugs (Painter 1980; Roberts 1978; Murname et al. 1980). The inhibitory effect of many such DNA-damaging agents has been shown to be largely due to inhibition of replicon initiation (Painter 1977, 1978a b, 1980). In untreated cells, caffeine has been shown to increase the number of replication origins used within the same replicon cluster and in irradiated cells to reverse the inhibition of replicon initiation which is a normal cellular response to DNA damage. Paint-

ER (1980) has argued on the basis of these and other data that such effects are the results of a change in chromatin configuration caused by caffeine in both irradiated and unirradiated cells causing more and smaller replicons to become active. In irradiated or drug-treated cells post-treated with caffeine, DNA replication may thus occur in regions of the chromatin which still contain unrepaired DNA damage or where the chromatin is not in its normal configuration. Such replication may lead to fixation of damage which subsequently leads to enhancement of chromosome aberrations and cell death (SCOTT 1977, 1980). If these interpretations are correct, the reported differences between different cell lines of different inherent drug sensitivity in their response to caffeine post-treatment (FUJIWARA and TATSUMI 1976; ROBERTS 1978; SCOTT 1977, 1980) more closely reflect differences in chromatin structure in the different cell lines than differences in repair capacity. The possible role of differences in chromatin structure in resistance and/or sensitivity of normal and tumour cells to the cytotoxic effects of various drugs is only just beginning to be explored, as is the possible role of alterations in chromatin structure in responses to chronic drug administration, adaptive responses (see later) and the development of resistance.

II. DNA Synthesis on a Template Containing Unexcised DNA Lesions

If the various excision repair mechanisms discussed above fail to remove or modify the various types of DNA lesions induced, then the cell is faced with the problem of replicating its DNA on a template containing lesions which may slow down or block DNA synthesis completely. The number of lesions with which the cell is left to cope will depend on:

1. The numbers of lesions initially induced
2. The efficiency of the excision repair process, which will depend on the time available for excision repair and also on numbers of lesions
3. The accessibility of the lesions within the complex structure of mammalian chromatin
4. The type of lesion induced.

Obviously therefore this process is extremely complex and its complexity has led to considerable confusion in the past as to the precise way in which lesions are circumvented.

Much of the data pertaining to DNA synthesis on a damaged template has been obtained from the study of UV-irradiated cells. Even here, however, the situation is confused and the precise responses observed appear to depend upon the cell line used. UV irradiation inhibits DNA synthesis as measured by [^{3}H]-thymidine uptake in a dose-dependent manner (CLEAVER 1977; FOX and FOX 1973a).

Results using fibre autoradiography to distinguish between inhibition of DNA synthesis as a result of inhibition of replicon initiation or strand elongation in V79 cells (EDENBURG 1978; DONINGER 1978) indicated that inhibition of strand elongation was primarily responsible. However, in HeLa cells, DNA synthesis appeared to be completely blocked by thymine dimers (EDENBURG 1979).

The current situation can be summarised as follows [for more detailed discussion see CLEAVER (1978), LEHMAN (1978), PARK and CLEAVER (1979) and

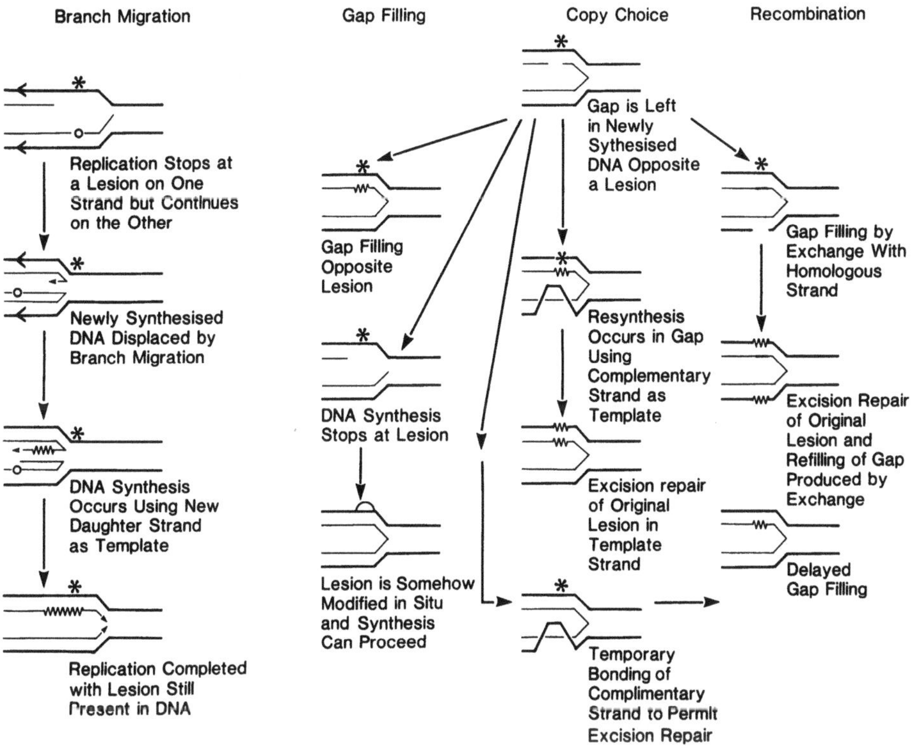

Fig. 2. Possible mechanisms for tolerating DNA lesions not excised before the first post-treatment S-phase. Schemes modified and redrawn from those presented by ROBERTS (1978)

EDENBURG (1978)]: UV irradiation may block replicon initation, or strand elongation or both. In functioning replicons, when the fork reaches a dimer on the parental strand, it may be blocked permanently, delayed for a short or long period or not delayed at all. Subsequent to the block, the replication fork may reinitiate beyond the lesion or it may reinitiate in an entirely new position. These possibilities are not mutually exclusive, and even in one cell line some forks may be delayed for a long time and then proceed past the lesions, whilst others may be delayed only for a short time and reinitiate beyond lesions, leaving a gap. Eventually, whether actual gaps are left or not, DNA of control molecular weight is eventually made.

It has recently been emphasised that we are still ignorant of many of the details of DNA replication and chromatin structure, even in undamaged cells, and therefore it is not surprising that many of the interpretations of the responses in damaged cells appear contradictory (HANAWALT et al. (1979). An additional complication of these studies is that dimers which initially apparently caused blocks to DNA synthesis fail to do so at later times after irradiation (MENEGHINI and MEUCK 1976). This implies some alteration in either the dimer or the replication machinery which allows synthesis past the lesion. The mechanisms involved are completely unknown. A number of mechanisms have been proposed for toleration of unexcised DNA lesions and these are presented in Figure 2.

Given this complexity of response to a single lesion it is therefore not surprising that the responses of different cell lines from different species to the many possible chemically induced DNA lesions are even less well understood. Treatment of rodent and human cells with HN2 has been shown to result in the synthesis of DNA of lower molecular weight for several hours after treatment; eventually DNA of normal molecular weight was synthesised (MURNAME et al. 1980) DNA-DNA interstrand cross-links are thought to produce a complete block to DNA synthesis, but the precise effects of DNA-DNA intrastrand and DNA protein cross-links known to be formed after exposure of cells to a variety of anticancer drugs including adriamycin, busulfan, BCNU and CCNU are largely unknown (KOHN 1977, 1979; ROSS et al. 1978; ERIKSON et al. 1977, 1978, 1980a, b, c; EWIG and KOHN 1977, 1978; TONG and LUDLUM 1980).

Adriamycin intercalates into DNA but does not induce detectable repair replication (PAINTER 1978b) although it appears to induce strand breaks which are localised with respect to DNA-protein cross-links also produced by the drug (KOHN 1979). It has been proposed that the protein may be bound to one end of the break and that it may be the enzyme which generated the break. Adriamycin inhibits replicon initiation but this effect is a minor one relative to the inhibition of chain elongation (PAINTER 1978b). Other intercalating agents such as daunomycin, ellipticine and actinomycin also produce similar effects, i.e. DNA protein cross-links occur at a frequency approximately similar to the number of strand breaks induced.

Ethylenimine, a polyfunctional alkylating agent, produces lesions in parental DNA which result in strand breaks when cells are exposed to alkali. This compound also produces a strong block to replicon initiation and the lesions induced initially block nascent DNA synthesis (PAINTER 1978b). Subsequently nascent DNA synthesis proceeds beyond the lesions and the rate of DNA synthesis returns towards normal. Methyl methane sulphonate (MMS) and X-rays also appear to block initiation of replicons (PAINTER and YOUNG 1975, 1976; PAINTER 1977). At later times chain elongation is inhibited by all these agents. The relative efficiency with which different classes of DNA-damaging agents produce the different types of DNA lesions that produce such effects is largely unknown as is the identity of the chemical lesion which produces the effect. A common mechanism for many of the above effects may be that a single "hit" within a large subunit of chromosomal DNA, mol. wt. $\sim 10^9$, may relax the supercoiling to the extent that replicon initiation is inhibited. The nature of this lesion is not known, but strand breaks may well be involved, produced either directly or as a result of the activity of repair enzymes. Again until more is known of the organisation and control of mammalian cell DNA replication it is difficult to interpret the many different perturbations caused in this highly organised system by a multitude of chemically and physically induced lesions (PAINTER and YOUNG 1976; PORVIRK and PAINTER 1976; PAINTER 1978a, b).

Given the degree of complexity of mammalian DNA repair processes described above, the possibilities for variations in repair capacity are considerable. Because of the multiplicity of enzymes and pathways involved in DNA repair there are many possible ways in which changes in DNA repair mechanisms could be involved in differences in both intrinsic and acquired resistance to anticancer drugs. Some of these are listed below; however, it should be emphasised that the majority of these are theoretical possibilities:

1. Increased rate of excision of a particular lesion
2. Alteration in the spectrum of lesions excised and/or excision of a lesion not previously excised
3. Increased capacity to bypass or circumvent DNA lesions
4. Decrease in susceptibility of replicon initiation sites to inactivation
5. Decreased susceptibility of repair enzymes to inhibition
6. Alteration in chromatin packing, making available sites not previously accessible to repair enzymes.

The direct correlation of changes in DNA repair capacity with differential resistance to anticancer drugs requires if possible closely isogenic cell lines, which exhibit a large differential sensitivity to the cytotoxic effects of the drug, and the demonstration that with equal doses of agent there is equal reaction of the drug with DNA, thus eliminating possible differences in drug permeability. It also requires the identification of all the DNA reaction products, measurement of repair replication over a significant period at different doses and correlation of this with measurements of the rates of loss of individual DNA lesions at a number of different doses as excision repair processes are known to show saturation. There are few studies in the literature which even approach these ideals.

C. The Relationship Between DNA Repair and Cellular Sensitivity

I. Alkylating Agents

Early studies in the field (Ball and Roberts 1970, 1972) measured the overall loss of alkylation products from the DNA of sensitive and resistant Yoshida sarcoma cells treated in vitro with sulphur mustard (SM). There was no demonstrable difference in the rate of loss of total alkylation products and the authors concluded that the differential cellular sensitivity was most likely due to the operation of another repair process which was operating in the resistant but not the sensitive cells. Reid and Walker (1969), however, apparently were able to correlate cellular resistance to SM with increased rate of loss of overall alkylation roducts. In the sensitive parent L-cell line, the half-time was 16 h as compared with 5–7 h in the resistant line. However, as Roberts (1978) has pointed out, no allowance was made in this study for differences in rates of post-treatment DNA synthesis, and resistant cells may well have been able to synthesise more DNA in a given time than sensitive cells, thus diluting the label to a greater extent and causing an artefactually increased loss rate. Studies in mouse cells with differential sensitivity to nitrogen mustard confirmed the ability of rodent cells to excise alkylation products (Yin et al. 1973). The apparent rates of loss of bi- and monoalkylation products were similar in the two cell lines; however, the sensitive cells apparently showed rapid and uncoordinated nicking of DNA after alkylation. By contrast, resistant cells showed a coordinated process of excision and repair. A deficiency in the ligase which forms segments of newly synthesised DNA was indicated in subsequent studies (Goldstein and Rutman 1974). However, the level of cell killing in the two cell lines was vastly different and it is not clear how much of the "uncoordinated" synthesis represented the death throes of sensitive cells. From these data therefore the role of excision repair in survival of treated cells is far from clear, since in none of these experiments was a clear difference in overall rate of removal of cross-links demonstrable. However, it does appear that the rate of loss of the diguanyl cross-links, whether they be inter- or intrastrand, is faster than the loss of total alkylation products. More recently Zwelling et al. (1981) have described the isolation of an L1210 cell line resistant to L-phenylalanine mustard (L-PAM). The dose modification factor, i.e. ratio of doses required to produce equitoxic effects on the parental and resistant cell lines, was 1.8 for phenylalanine mustard. The same cell line was also cross-resistant to *cis*-diaminedichloroplatinum(II), dose modification factor 2.4. When DNA cross-linking after L-PAM treatment was assayed by alkaline elution techniques without proteinase (total cross-links DNA-DNA and DNA-protein) and with proteinase (DNA-DNA interstrand cross-links), no differences in the rate of formation or removal of either type of cross-links could be detected. However, when the relative cross-linking frequencies were measured as a function of drug concentration in the two cell lines the ratio of the slopes of the cross-linking coefficients plotted against dose differed by a factor approximately equal to the drug sensitivity difference as determined by reduction in survival of colony-forming ability.

The degree of cross-linking by L-PAM was also measured in a line of L1210 leukaemia cells made resistant to L-PAM in vivo and compared with that in the sensitive parental cells. Again, a reduction in the amount of cross-linking was seen in the resistant cell line.

Since no difference in the rates of removal of DNA-DNA cross-links were detectable in the two cell lines, the authors suggest that the resistant cells may more rapidly remove monoadducts before these convert to DNA-DNA cross-links (Fig. 3). They may also remove monoadducts not destined to form cross-links more rapidly. Such monoadducts which constitute 75% of total DNA lesions in the case of sulphur mustard (Fox and Scott 1980) may contribute significantly to the cytotoxic effects of L-PAM but would be undetectable by the alkaline elution techniques used. Thus, although differences in DNA repair mechanisms are implicated in the resistance of this cell line to L-PAM, the precise contribution of DNA repair to the decreased sensitivity has not been fully elucidated. Indeed, it may be difficult to define precisely since the difference in sensitivity in this pair of cell lines is relatively small.

Other recent studies have provided better evidence that different cell lines differ in their capacity to remove particular DNA lesions and that repair capacity is related to intrinsic cellular sensitivity to the cytotoxic effects of these agents.

A number of human tumour cell strains and cell lines derived from SV40 transformed human fibroblasts have been shown to exhibit a mer$^-$ phenotype (Day et al. 1980a, b). This phenotype is characterised by increased sensitivity to inactivation of colony-forming ability, increased sensitivity to sister chromatid exchange (SCE) induction by *N*-methyl-*N'*-nitro-*N*-nitrosoguanidine (MNNG),

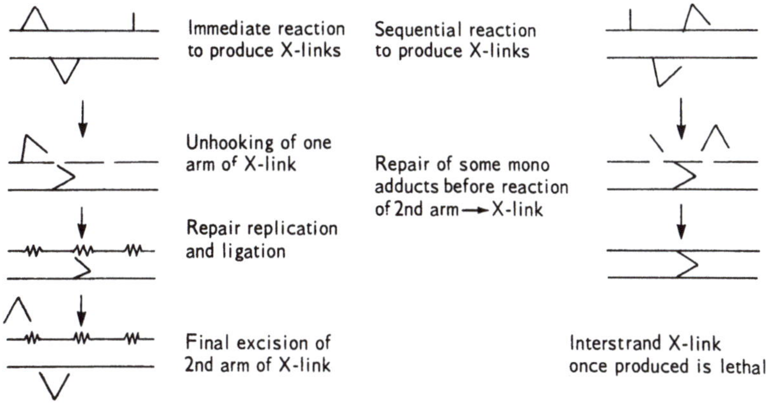

Fig. 3. Possible schemes for production and repair of DNA cross-links in mammalian cells

increased MNNG-induced repair synthesis and deficient repair of MNNG-damaged adenovirus 5, compared with mer$^+$ cell strains (Day et al. 1980a). Mer$^+$ cell strains were subsequently shown to be able to remove both O^6-methylguanine and *N*^{7}-methylguanine from their DNA. Mer$^-$ strains lack the ability to excise O^6-alkylguanine, but lose *N*^{7}-methylguanine at a rate similar to that observed in mer$^+$ strains. Similar findings have also been recently reported by Sklar and Strauss (1981). In a survey of excision capacity of 26 lines of human lymphoblasts from normal individuals XP homozygotes (complementation groups A, C, D) and parental heterozygotes, they found seven lines which lacked the capacity to excise O^6-methylguanine. There was no correlation between the XP phenotype and inability to excise O^6-methylguanine. Two of the cell lines derived from normal patients lacked excision ability. In excision-proficient lines (mex$^+$ phenotype) excision was rapid, with half-time approximately 1 h after doses of MNNG which reduced the survival of treated cells to approximately 20%. After higher doses, saturation of capacity to remove O^6-alkylguanine was evident. Mex$^-$ cells (those lacking excision capacity for O^6-methylguanine) were more sensitive than mex$^+$ cells to growth inhibition. Both the above sets of data suggest that O^6-methylguanine is a potentially cytotoxic lesion in human cells. A similar conclusion can also be drawn from a comparison of the cytotoxic effects of MNU, MNNG and MMS at an equal level of DNA reaction in HeLa cells (Roberts et al. 1971). MNU and MNNG, which produce significantly higher levels of O^6-alkylguanine than does MMS, were considerably more cytotoxic. HeLa cells thus appear to lack the capacity to excise O^6-alkylguanine (Day et al. 1980b). The role of this particular lesion in determining cytotoxic effects on mammalian cells is, however, far from clear. Several V79 cell lines have been shown to be unable to excise this lesion (Roberts et al. 1978; Warren et al. 1979; Fox and Brennand 1980) but a comparison of the sensitivity of V79 cells to the cytotoxic effects at equal binding levels of the same three methylating agents revealed no differences comparable to those observed in HeLa cells (Roberts et al. 1971, 1978). Similar observations have been made by Fox and Brennand (1980) and Fox (1981) for

MNU, *N*-ethyl-*N*-nitrosourea (ENU), ethyl methane sulphonate (EMS) and MMS, also in V79 cells.

ROBERTS (1978) has suggested that the greater resistance of V79 cells to inactivation by these agents is the result of their greater facility to replicate DNA on a template containing DNA lesions. FRIEDMAN and HUBERMAN (1980) have recently provided some evidence that a V79 (VR43) cell line isolated for its resistance to the cytotoxic effects of MNNG has enhanced postreplication repair (PRR) capacity as manifested by more rapid ligation of nascent DNA.

The ability to excise N^7- and O^6-alkylguanine after MNU treatment has been compared in V79 and V79/79 cells; the latter show increased sensitivity to inactivation of colony-forming ability by MNU. After similar overall levels of alkylation N^7-alkylguanine was lost at similar rates from both cell lines, O^6-alkylguanine was *not* lost from V79 cells, but V79/79 cells, the more sensitive line, lost O^6-alkylguanine with a half-life of approximately 24 h (DURRANT et al. 1981). Thus, although there appears to be a correlation between cellular sensitivity and lack of ability to excise O^6-alkylguanine in human cells, this correlation does not hold for hamster cells.

Some recent studies have indicated that the repair function which removes O^6-alkylguanine from DNA is involved in the removal of chloroethyladducts produced in DNA by the 1-(2-chloroethyl) nitrosoureas which are potent anticancer drugs (ERIKSON et al. 1980 a, b, c). Human-cell strains which have a mer^- phenotype were consistently shown to have higher levels of DNA interstrand cross-links after CCNU exposure than did those with mer^+ phenotypes. Assays for total cross-links, including DNA protein cross-links, showed no difference between the two lines. Mer^- cell strains were more sensitive to the growth inhibitory effects of CCNU. The authors suggest that the delay in forming cross-links when cells are treated with CCNU allows time for the removal of the chloroethyl monoadduct in mer^+ cells before the reaction of the second arm of the cross-link, thus conferring resistance to the cytotoxic effects of this compound (Fig. 3).

The relationship between repair of damage induced by cytotoxic drugs as measured by "repair replication" non-semi-conservative DNA synthesis and increased drug resistance is also far from clear. In SM-sensitive and -resistant Yoshida rat sarcoma cells, no difference in the amount of induced repair replication could be demonstrated either by BALL and ROBERTS (1972) or by SCOTT et al. (1974). In the latter experiments equal levels of DNA reaction were demonstrated in the two cell lines, which differed considerably in their cellular sensitivity. However, repair replication was measured only at 3 h after treatment and after high doses of SM, which, as discussed above, could have totally saturated excision repair capacity in both cell lines, saturated repair capacity differentially in the two cell lines, or saturated the repair capacity for particular lesions differentially. There is obviously a need for detailed time course studies of the rate of removal of cross-links and monofunctional adducts in these cell lines. The same two Yoshida cell lines which showed differential SM sensitivities also showed differential cellular sensitivity to methylene dimethanesulphonate (MDMS) and induced repair replication which appeared to be greater in the resistant cell line than in the sensitive at a given dose (FOX and FOX 1973c). This compound is highly effective in curing Yoshida sarcoma in vivo and the above observation represents one of the few instances in which apparently increased capacity to perform excision repair as manifested by induced repair replication correlated with reduced drug sensitivity. However, other manifestations of repair, e.g. loss of lesions and ligase activity, were not measured at this time.

The possibility that the different levels of repair replication observed could be due to a somewhat trivial difference in either endogenous thymidine pools or to a differential affinity of thymidine kinase for thymidine in the two lines was excluded to a large extent by the demonstration that equal amounts of repair replication were induced after a given dose of MMS to which the two cell lines do not show differential sensitivity (Fox and Fox 1973c). However, the possibilities discussed above, i.e. that the differences in incorporation could be due to differential saturation of excision capacities in the two cell lines, were not excluded. Subsequently, attempts have been made to demonstrate covalent binding of MDMS to DNA using ^{14}C-labelled drug. No covalent binding could be demonstrated but equal amounts of ^{14}C-labelled drug were found to be associated with the nucleic acid fraction in the two cell lines (Carr 1979). The differences in repair capacity of these two cell lines were subsequently further analysed after exposure to MDMS and SM.

In Yoshida S and R lines increasing doses of MDMS produced increasing inhibition of DNA synthesis. Inhibition was initially more rapid and recovered more rapidly in resistant than in sensitive cells. The dose of MDMS required to produce an equal degree of inhibition of DNA synthesis was greater by a factor of 4 in resistant cells than in sensitive cells. Equitoxic doses were not compared but from the survival data these differ by a factor of 6 at a surviving fraction of 0.05 (Carr and Fox 1981b). The size of nascent DNA was measured after a dose of 50 μg/ml to both cell lines, and after correction for differential inhibition of DNA synthesis was slightly smaller in the sensitive than in the resistant cell line. At equal doses of drug there was more transient inhibition of DNA synthesis in resistant cells and nascent DNA of slightly higher molecular weight was synthesised. These data suggest that resistant cells can bypass some lesions which produce blocks to DNA synthesis in sensitive cells. Evidence that equal numbers of lesions are induced by equal doses of MDMS comes from the observation that equal numbers of alkali-labile sites are initially induced in the two cell lines (Carr and Fox 1981 a). The rate of disappearance of such sites (strand breaks) was apparently more rapid in resistant than in sensitive cells but very high doses (100 μg/ml) were used in this study. The previously reported difference in MDMS-induced repair synthesis (Fox and Fox 1973) was confirmed by this study (Carr and Fox 1981a). However, very high doses of MDMS were again used. The two cell lines appear to have equal capacities for incision as evidenced by the similar accumulation of incision repair gaps in the presence of araC. The more rapid disappearance of strand breaks in resistant cells may be a reflection of more efficient ligation in resistant cells; however, the possibility of non-specific effects at these very high doses cannot be overlooked. Similarly, the rather small difference in repair replication observed may simply be the result of differential repair saturation at these high doses.

Thus, a major difference between the two cell lines in their response to MDMS may relate to a differential ability to bypass unexcised DNA lesions. This idea is

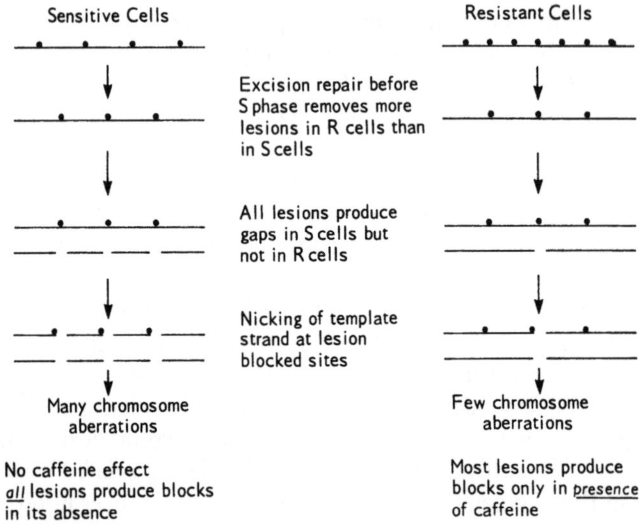

Fig. 4. One possible model to explain the differential drug sensitivity and differential sensitivity to caffeine-induced potentiation of cell lethality in Yoshida sarcoma cells exposed to MDMS

supported by the observations that caffeine consistently potentiated induced cell lethality to a greater extent in resistant than in sensitive cells (CARR and FOX 1981 a). Caffeine also potentiated MDMS-induced chromosome damage more effectively in resistant cells (Radacic, Fox and Scott, unpublished data).

DNA synthesis inhibition after SM exposure to which the two lines also exhibit differential sensitivity (SCOTT et al. 1974) was also measured. Again, after equal doses, inhibition of DNA synthesis was more extensive in the sensitive cell line (CARR and FOX 1981 a). Analysis of nascent DNA synthesis in the two cell lines indicated that SM had little effect on synthesis of higher mol. wt. DNA. The authors therefore suggest that inhibition of replicon initiation alone is responsible for inhibition of DNA synthesis by SM. The differential effects of SM on DNA synthesis in the two Yoshida cell lines, their differential susceptibility to induced chromosome damage (SCOTT et al. 1974), their differential susceptibility to caffeine potentiation of SM-induced cell lethality and chromosome damage (SCOTT 1977) are in line with the interpretation proposed above to explain the differential MDMS sensitivity, i.e. resistant cells possess some mechanism for modifying or bypassing lesions lacking in sensitive cells. In the presence of caffeine this mechanisms is inhibited, so that lesions in the resistant cells which do not produce blocks in the absence of caffeine do so in its presence (Fig. 4). A model relating these different obervations to differences in susceptibility to induced chromosome damage has recently been presented (SCOTT 1980).

Alternatively, since little difference in excision capacity and only marginal differences in effects on molecular weight of nascent DNA are demonstrable, the differences may lie at the level of chromatin structure. Caffeine markedly potentiates both MDMS- and SM-induced cell lethality and chromosome damage in resistant but not in sensitive cells, and PAINTER (1980) has proposed that such lethal potentiation may be the result of replication of DNA in unrepaired regions due to the increase in number of replication origins caused by caffeine. The MDMS concentration required to produce, for example, 90% cell kill differs by a factor of 8–10 and since equal doses of MDMS produce equal numbers of alkali-labile sites (CARR and FOX 1981 b) there must be eight to ten times as many lesions/unit DNA in the resistant than in the sensitive cells. If some or all of these lesions cause inhibition of initiation then reversal of the inhibition by caffeine at some or all of these sites may cause a greater proportion of the genome to be replicated in unrepaired regions in resistant than in sensitive cells and hence a greater caffeine effect.

These two cell lines, therefore, appear to differ in the way in which they handle DNA lesions which escape the excision repair process rather than in their overall excision capacity. Although it remains possible that the observed difference in repair incorporation in the resistant line after MDMS exposure is due to the excision of particular DNA lesions, which when not excised in the sensitive line produce lethal blocks to DNA synthesis. There is, however, no direct experimental evidence to support this hypothesis to date.

Repair replication induced by MNNG was measured in several mer$^-$ and mer$^+$ human cell lines by DAY et al. (1980a). Paradoxically, cells with mer$^-$ phenotype apparently incorporated more [^{3}H]thymidine after exposure to a given dose of MNNG than did those with a mer$^+$ phenotype, which were shown to be excision proficient for N^7- and O^6-methylguanine. However, "repair incorporation" was only studied over a 1-h period after exposure to increasing doses of MNNG (DAY et al. 1980a). In view of the relatively slow loss of some DNA lesions, a detailed study of repair incorporation with time after treatment is obviously necessary before the significance of the reported differences can be assessed.

The precise relationships between the levels of repair replication and cellular sensitivity are further confused by the observations of HIGGINS and STRAUSS (1979). Six Burkitt's lymphoma cell lines were found to be generally more resistant to cellular inactivation by methyl methanesulphonate than were six lymphoblastoid lines. Raji, the most resistant strain, showed greater than 20% survival when exposed to 0.4 m*M* MMS whereas in the most sensitive line, L-33-6-1, survival was ~0.5% after exposure to a similar concentration. The differences in survival were shown not to be due to different initial levels of reaction of MMS with DNA. Excision repair activity was measured after exposure of all cell lines to a single concentration of MMS, 2.0 m*M*, and considerable differences in maximum repair incorporation were evident between the two cell lines. However, there was no direct correlation between the maximum level of repair incorporation and cellular sensitivity. However, in these assays of repair incorporation, as in many previous ones, very high doses of drug were used. It is thus difficult to know the precise contribution of the observed differences in repair incorporation to cell survival.

Thus many of the observed differences in repair replication cannot be unequivocally related to differences in repair capacity defined in its strictest sense. However, these observations point to the importance of mechanisms for circumventing unexcised DNA lesions and their role in determining absolute cellular sensitivity.

There are a number of other observations in pairs of rodent tumour lines which show differences in sensitivity to melphalan, chloroambucil and cyclophosphamide which may be associated with differences in DNA repair capacity, but the associations between the phenomena observed and DNA repair is even further from being proven.

Strains of both Walker carcinosarcoma and Yoshida sarcoma which are sensitive to the cytotoxic effects of melphalan, chloroambucil and cyclophosphamide have been reported to show loss of condensed chromatin, increased phosphorylation of nuclear proteins and increased DNA cross-linking after exposure to alkylating agents at doses which killed 90% of cells (WILKINSON et al. 1979). When tumour lines which had acquired resistance to these alkylating agents were studied, after exposure to the same doses of alkylating agents (no cell kill?), no such changes in chromatin, condensation or phosphorylation patterns were observed. The addition of prednisolone after alkylating-agent exposure enhanced cell killing in resistant lines and also resulted in enhanced nuclear protein phosphorylation and DNA cross-linking.

It is not possible to deduce from these data the actual amount of reaction of the drugs with DNA or the actual numbers of cross-links induced although the percentage of cross-linked DNA in the two cell lines was similar at equal doses as was the kinetics of loss of cross-linked material over the first 24 h post-treatment. This implies that both sensitive and resistant cells were able to remove cross-links. The late increase in amount of cross-linked DNA in sensitive cells is difficult to explain as being diretly drug induced and may be an artefact arising during the isolation of DNA from severely damaged cells. The increase in phosphorylation in sensitive but not resistant cells appears to be associated with their lethal response, and phosphorylation of nuclear histone proteins is known to be associated with control of gene activity. It has been suggested that polyADP ribose may be involved in extending and condensing chromatin, and inhibition of poly ADP ribose polymerase results in enhanced alkylating agent sensitivity (DURKACZ et al. 1980). Thus phosphorylation and ADP ribosylation are of obvious importance in cellular responses to and recovery from DNA damage. Whether these responses are related to the observed changes in chromatin condensation remains to be determined.

II. Platinum Compounds

Another important class of cytotoxic drugs widely used in cancer chemotherapy include the platinum coordination complexes. Two important drugs of this type are *cis*-dichlorodiaminoplatinum (*cis*PtII) and *cis-trans*-dichlorodihydroxy-bis-(isopropylamine)platinum I (CHIP). The precise mechanism whereby these platinum complexes kill cells is not completely understood; however, their ability to produce cross-links in DNA appears to be crucial to their cytotoxic potential, as platinum complexes structurally incapable of cross-linking (*trans* isomers) are considerably less cytotoxic than their bifunctional counterparts (PASCOE and ROBERTS 1974a, b).

Studies with purified DNA and in whole cells have indicated that bifunctional binding of cisplatin forms intrastrand cross-links between guanines (ROSS 1977), interstrand cross-links and DNA-protein cross-links (ZWELLING et al. 1979a, b). At first, the degree of cross-linking was thought to be inadequate to account for cytotoxicity; however, it was later found that the degree of cross-linking increases severalfold over a period of hours after the drug is removed.

In L1210 cells total cross-linking as measured by alkaline elution assay (KOHN 1979) was evident immediately on removal of the drug and increased by a factor of 5 over the next 12 h (ZWELLING et al. 1979a, b). The frequency of cross-links fell subsequently but was still measurable by 24 h. Treatment of cells with proteinase K (EWIG and KOHN 1978) eliminated the rapidly formed cross-links and reduced overall numbers, but cross-link frequency still rose over a 12-h post-treatment period; again the cross-links disappeared between 12 and 24 h. Similar kinetics have been observed in V79 Chinese hamster cells (ZWELLING et al. 1979b). Evidence that interstrand DNA cross-links are important cytotoxic lesions has been obtained from a comparison of the effects of *cis* and *trans* isomers. The *trans* isomer exhibits much higher total cross-linking activity for a given level of kill but this is largely of the DNA-protein type and is less toxic than the *cis* isomer. After removal of DNA-protein cross-links a comparison of DNA-DNA cross-links at equitoxic doses of the two compounds indicated similar levels (ZWELLING et al. 1979a, 1981).

Using different methods to those described above, i.e. direct assay of the Pt content of DNA isolated from treated cells, a correlation has been established between the extent of Pt bound to DNA and cell survival in HeLa, V79 Chinese hamster (FLAVEL and ROBERTS 1978a), human fibroblasts and XP cells deficient in UV repair (FLAVEL et al. 1978b); and Pt adducts have been shown to be removed from DNA of both cells by an excision repair process, the half-time of loss being ~28 h for exponentially growing cells and slower, half-time 2–3 days, for stationary phase cells which were considerably more sensitive to the drug (ROBERTS and FLAVEL 1980). The difference in sensitivity thus appears to be directly related to the slower excision of Pt DNA adducts and not to a difference in uptake of the drug. These and other data therefore indicate that cell killing after exposure to *cis*PtII is the result of unexcised damage in DNA and that cellular resistance to these compounds is related to excision repair capacity. XP cells are cross-sensitive to *cis*PtII but this cross-sensitivity is not due to lack of a UV endonuclease as the *M. luteus* enzyme fails to recognise *cis*PtII-induced DNA damage (ROBERTS and FLAVEL 1980). Thus both normal human and rodent cells are able to excise *cis*PtII-induced damage. Theoretically therefore, increased resistance to the cytotoxic effects could result from (a) an increased ability to repair interstrand DNA cross-links, (b) an increased ability to repair monoadducts destined to become cross-links or (c) increased cellular thiol concentrations, since addition of thiourea has been shown to reduce the cytotoxic effects of *cis*PtII (ZWELLING et al. 1979b), indicating a possible protective effect of elevated intracellular thiol concentration. Other evidence has been presented which indicates that removal of *cis*PtII adducts is drug specific in human cells, e.g. an SV40 transformed human-cell line (VA-13) which was more sensitive to chloroethylnitrosoureas (ERICKSON et al. 1978) than a normal untransformed cell line was more resistant to *cis*PtII than the normal human line (ERICKSON et al. 1980c).

Chinese hamster cells are inherently more resistant to *cis*PtII than are HeLa cells in spite of the fact that higher amounts of Pt are bound to the DNA of the latter in both G1- and S-phases of the cell cycle (ROBERTS and FLAVEL 1980). V79 cells have been shown to differ from HeLa cells in their response to other cytotoxic drugs, e.g. sulphur mustard and MNU (ROBERTS 1978). The difference in response appears to be related to the way in which these two cell lines synthesise DNA on damaged templates. In both HeLa and hamster cells treated with equitoxic doses of sulphur mustard and *cis*PtII in G1, DNA synthesis is inhibited in the first post-treatment S-phase. However, in hamster cells both the apparent time of onset of DNA synthesis and the time of attainment of the peak rate of DNA synthesis are delayed relative to the control whereas in HeLa cells no displacement of the peak rate of DNA synthesis was observed. In hamster cells which are sensitised to the cytotoxic effect of *cis*PtII by caffeine post-treatment, this delay in onset of DNA synthesis was reversed on caffeine exposure. These data together with detailed studies on the effects of *cis*PtII on nascent DNA synthesis in the two cell lines and the effects of caffeine on this process led to the proposal that V79 cells posses a replication repair process which is caffeine sensitive and inducible (FLAVEL and ROBERTS 1978 a, b).

The two cell lines have essentially similar excision repair capacities for SM-induced lesions and similar overall sensitivities to SM-induced cell killing. Similar excision capacity for *cis*PtII-induced lesions has been inferred. Thus the difference in number of Pt molecules bound in hamster and HeLa cells together with the higher survival found in the former cell line indicates that V79 cells have a significantly higher tolerance capacity for Pt-induced lesions compared with HeLa cells.

The relationship between DNA cross-linking and cytotoxicity was studied by ZWELLING et al. (1981) in paris of L1210 cell lines showing sensitivity and resistance to *cis*-diaminedichloroplatinumII (*cis*-DDP). A line of L1210 cells resistant to *cis*-DDP was developed in vitro after repeated exposure to the drug. This cell line, which showed a dose modification factor of 2.8 for induced cytotoxicity, was also cross-resistant to L-phenylalanine mustard (see earlier). In the resistant line interstrand DNA cross-linking and DNA-protein cross-linking were reduced relative to that in the sensitive line by a factor similar to that observed for cytotoxicity. An L1210 line which had developed resistance to *cis*-DDP in vivo also exhibited a marked reduction in both types of cross-linking after exposure to *cis*-DDP when compared with the sensitive line. This line was not cross-resistant to L-PAM and no differences in levels of DNA cross-links after exposure to this drug were detected. Another cell line made resistant to L-PAM in vivo was cross-resistant to *cis*-DDP. This line showed a reduced cross-linking after exposure to L-PAM; however, little reduction in *cis*-DDP cross-linking was demonstrable in vitro, a result not in line with its lack of in vivo sensitivity. The possibility of population heterogeneity in this latter case was largely discounted and the reasons for the differences observed are not clear. A good correlation between initial level of cross-linking and sensitivity to induced cytotoxicity was, however, established in three of the four situations exmained. No differences were detected however, in the rates of removal of DNA cross-links. Formation of DNA-DNA cross-links is time dependent for both drugs (maximum frequency occurring arround 6 h) and the authors suggest reduction in numbers of DNA interstrand cross-links by removal of monoadducts prior to interstrand cross-link formation as a possible mechanism for resistance. They point out, however, that this hypothesis cannot account for the reduced formation of DNA-protein cross-links in *cis*-DDP-treated resistant cells since the latter appear to be formed very rapidly. It is possible that DNA-protein cross-links are not cytotoxic lesions and therefore not subject to repair, the observed fall in frequency being largely due to removal of DNA-DNA cross-links, and the reason for the observed differences lies in differences in chromatin configuration in the two cell lines.

If monoadduct removal is a major determinant of the differential sensitivities observed, then as the authors suggest it must be lesion specific. Evidence for the specificity of enzymes which remove DNA lesions has been presented earlier in this chapter. An L5178Y cell line which was UV resistant but X-ray sensitive was shown to be more resistant to the cytotoxic effects of *cis*PtII than a related UV-sensitive line (Szumiel 1979a, b). A correlation was also observed between the amount of *cis*PtII-induced chromosome damage and cell lethality in the two lines. In resistant cells, caffeine post-treatment potentiated cell lethality but no lethal potentiation was observed in the *cis*PtII-sensitive line; division delay and DNA synthesis were not differentially affected. Evidence indicating similar uptake of *cis*PtII in the two cell lines was also presented, but no measurements of rates of loss of lesions are available. The difference in sensitivity appears to be most closely associated with a difference in the ability of the resistant line to replicate on a damaged template by a caffeine-sensitive mechanism but this has not been characterised biochemically. In summary therefore, the major cytotoxic effects of the *cis*-acting platinum complexes appear to be associated with the ability of these compounds to produce DNA interstrand cross-links. DNA-protein cross-links and monoadducts appear to be less important, as such lesions are produced in considerable numbers by *trans* isomers of these compounds which are consider-able numbers by *trans* isomers of these compounds which are considerably less cytotoxic. There is no substantial evidence to indicate that differences in the rates of removal of DNA-DNA cross-links contribute to resistance to *cis*-platinum compounds but there is circumstantial evidence for the more efficient removal of monoadducts, thus preventing the formation of DNA-DNA cross-links in some resistant cell lines. Increased resistance to the cytotoxic effects of these drugs is also in some cases associated with an increased ability to replicate on templates containing unexcised DNA lesions, a process which is caffeine sensitive in mouse and hamster cell lines.

III. Mitomycin C

Mitomycin C is an antitumour antibiotic which is known to exert its cytotoxic action as a result of its ability to cross-link complementary DNA strands in a manner similar to nitrogen and sulphur mustard (Szybalski and Iyer 1967). Its similarity to mustards also extends to the fact that it is a preferential inhibitor of DNA synthesis, probably as a consequence of its ability to cross-link DNA (Kersten 1975). The degree of cross-linking achieved is dependent on the G-C content of the DNA and it has been suggested that alkylation of guanine takes place at some position other than N^7. Reaction with O^6-position is considered the most likely. The compound apparantly requires activation before reaction which is achieved by enzymatic reduction of the quinone group. The cross-linking takes place in a stepwise fashion with sequential alkylation first at the aziridine and then at the carbamate region. As for the mustards, the majority of reactions with DNA, however, is in the form of monofunctional alkylations. Other aspects of the chemistry of interaction of mitomycin C with DNA have been recently reviewed (LOWN 1979) Although it has been stated that resistance to mitomycin C develops rapidly (CARTER 1979) there are to my knowledge no good examples of pairs of tumour-cell lines sensitive and resistant to this drug in which the role of DNA repair in drug resistance has been evaluated. The involvement of DNA repair in resistance is indicated, however, from studies on fibroblasts (FA cells) from patients suffering from the autosomal recessive disease Fanconi's anaemia. These cells show extreme sensitivity to the cytotoxic and chromosome-breaking effects of mitomycin C, to HN2 and to busulphan when compared with normal human fibroblasts (SAZAKI 1978). This obervation points to the fact that FA cells are defective in their ability to repair interstrand DNA cross-links. Evidence that this is indeed the case is now available, and it would appear that FA cells are defective in their ability to unhook the first arm of the cross-link, a process which appears to be independent of repair of thymine dimers, as XP cells are proficient in this process (FUJIWARA and TATSUMI 1975; FUJIWARA et al. 1977). It has been proposed that further repair of DNA-DNA cross-links or overlapping monofunctional damage can only proceed if there is also recombination between sister strand duplexes (SAZAKI 1978). However, experimental evidence for this hypothesis is not available. Theoretically, resistance to mitomycin C could also result from a loss of the enzyme or enzymes which activate the drug, but to the best of my knowledge this mechanism has not been demonstrated to occur.

IV. Bleomycin

Bleomycin is thought to exert its cytotoxicity by induction of DNA-strand breaks which occur in vivo only after activation of the bleomycin molecule by mechanisms at present unclear. The ultimate damage appears to be fragmentation of the DNA by the cleavage of thymine *N*-glycosidic bonds, leading to the liberation of thymine and deoxyribose (CAPUTO 1976; MUELLER and ZAHN 1977). DNA synthesis in L cells is inhibited by doses of bleomycin which have little effect on protein and RNA synthesis, and their inhibition appears to be a consequence of DNA damage and not due to direct interaction of the antibiotic with DNA (WATANABE et al. 1973). In this respect bleomycin appears to resemble the alkylating agents. The sensitivity or resistance of a cell to bleomycin, however, is correlated at least partially with the presence or absence of an enzyme which disrupts the active site of the molecule, and the presence of an intact and unmodified bleomycin molecule is necessary for biological activity (UMEZAWA 1976).

The detailed study of the cytotoxic effects of bleomycin in cultured mammalian cells has revealed several features which distinguish bleomycin from other agents interacting directly with DNA. In the majority of mammalian cell lines studied, including mouse fibroblast L5 (TERASIMA et al. 1972), HeLa S3 (TER-

ASIMA et al. 1976), CHO cells (BARRANCO and HUMPHREY 1971 b), dose-response curves are initially exponential, then show a much less sensitive final slope, i.e. the dose-response curves are markedly biphasic. Several hypotheses have been offered to explain this phenomenon (CAPUTO 1976).

Firstly, all cultured cell lines may contain a fraction of cells inherently resistant to bleomycin. This is an unlikely explanation on two counts. Firstly, it is unlikely that all cultured cell lines do have a similar proportion of inherently resistant cell, and second clones isolated from the survival curve tail show the same sensitivity as the original untreated population (TERASIMA et al. 1972). Secondly, the resistance may be associated with a particular phase of the cell cycle. Data on cell-cycle phase sensitivity to bleomycin are, however, conflicting in different cell lines. In HeLa S3 cells maximum resistance was observed in late S-phase cells (TERASIMA and UMEZAWA 1970). In CHO cells, mitotic cells were most sensitive and resistance was greatest in G1 and S (BARRANCO and HUMPREY 1971 b). Dose survival curves for both plateau and exponentially growing Chinese hamster cells (MAURO et al. 1974) also show this biphasic response as do those of mouse EMT6 tumour in vitro (TWENTYMAN and BLEEHAN 1973). These data all suggest that there is no consistent relationship between cell-cycle phase and bleomycin sensitivity. Thirdly, it has been postulated that resistance can be induced by the antibiotic. This hypothesis is supported by several studies which indicate that resistance decays rapidly when the bleomycin is removed (MAURO et al. 1974). This interpretation is supported by the biochemical evidence mentioned earlier which indicates the existence of a bleomycin-inactivating enzyme (UMEZAWA 1976). If this last hypothesis is true, then the role of DNA repair in cellular resistance to this drug may be minimal.

Several reports have indicated that bleomycin can produce single-strand breaks in DNA and that these breaks are rapidly repaired. These breaks are similarly rapidly repaired in ataxia telangiectasia (AT) cells which are X-ray sensitive and more sensitive than normal human fibroblasts to cellular inactivation by bleomycin although showing the same biphasic dose-response curves shown by normal fibroblasts (TAYLOR et al. 1979). AT cells show a higher level of induced chromosome aberrations after exposure to both bleomycin and X-rays than do normal human fibroblasts (NHF) and an elevated level of chromatid gaps and breaks. A moderate increase in dicentrics has been demonstrated in lymphocytes from some AT patients after bleomycin exposure. On the basis of these observations, the involvement of a similar repair defect in sensitivity of cells to bleomycin and to X-rays has been inferred. However, the repair defect in AT cells exposed to ionising radiation has not been unequivocally identified. No differences in the induction or repair of single – or double-strand breaks have been demonstrated after X-ray or bleomycin treatment (TAYLOR et al. 1975; LEHMANN and STEVANS 1977, 1979). The studies on AT cells which do suggest a repair defect were performed at such high doses that inhibition or saturation of repair processes could have occurred (PATERSON et al. 1976). The biphasic dose-response curves for bleomycin in contrast to the shoulder and exponential type curves for X-rays strongly suggest a completely different mechanism of cell killing for bleomycin and ionising radiation. Thus even though bleomycin does apparently produce strand breaks in DNA and chromosome damage in ataxia cells which is qualitatively similar to that produced by X-rays, these phenomena are not necessarily quantitatively and/or causally related to cellular sensitivity. The existence of a bleomycin-inactivating enzyme also casts doubt on the hypothesis that bleomycin sensitivity or resistance is directly related to DNA repair capacity. Ataxia cells could be non- or minimally inducible for this enzyme. In addition, there are to my knowledge no data to indicate similar levels of reaction of bleomycin with DNA in cells of sensitive and resistant lines and in view of the size and complexity of the molecule, differential permeability of bleomycin into different cells seems a highly likely explanation for some of the observed differences in cellular sensitivity. Thus, although there are several reports of differential cellular sensitivity to this drug the role of DNA repair in these differences may be minimal.

D. Cell-Cycle Perturbations and Their Possible Relationships to DNA Repair

Treatment of synchronised HeLa cells in the G1-phase of the cell cycle with a variety of cytotoxic agents including sulphur mustard, *cis*PtII and cyclophosphamide has an immediate effects on the rate of progress of the cells through the subsequent S- and G2-phases, resulting in a mitotic delay (ROBERTS 1978). These effects are dose dependent, demonstrable at doses of drugs which allow a high level of survival of the exposed cell populations and appear to be directly associated with inhibition of DNA synthesis by the drugs. In contrast, exposure of HeLa cells in G1 to similarly toxic doses of methylating agents did not result in inhibition of DNA synthesis during the immediately sequential S-phase, neither did G1 exposure result in mitotic delay (ROBERTS 1978). However, de novo DNA synthesis was inhibited in the subsequent S-phase with the production of secondary damage and this secondary inhibition was followed by mitotic delay. V79 Chinese hamster fibroblasts, on the other hand, responded to exposure to methylating agents by exhibiting a delay in the first post-treatment S-phase and a mitotic delay during the first cycle after treatment with equitoxic doses of the same methylating agents. V79 cells were much more resistant to the toxic effects of these compounds. Exposure of G1 human lymphoblastoid cells to a variety of cytotoxic drugs including actinomycin D, L-phenylalanine mustard, Yoshi 864 and VP 16 has also been shown to affect cell-cycle traverse through S and G2 (DREWINKO and BARLOGIE 1976; BARLOGIE and DREWINKO 1978). A number of other cytotoxic drugs, e.g. BCNU, and related compounds (WHEELER et al. 1970; BARRANCO and HUMPHREY 1971c; NOMURA et al. 1978) have been shown in a variety of cell lines to produce delays in progression of cells from G1 to S, to prolong S-phase and to delay progress of G2 cells into mitosis. A detailed discussion of the different effects of the many different drugs in the different cell lines is presented in Chap. 6 of this volume.

Although the precise relationships between dose, length of S- or G2-phase delay and cellular sensitivity, as measured by loss of colony-forming ability, are not readily discernible for all drugs, it is apparent that a large number of anticancer drugs produce cell-cycle delays in a number of different cell lines. It has been proposed, on the basis of studies using premature chromosome condensation (PCC) analysis (RAO and RAO 1976), the degree of G2 arrest (TOBEY 1975) and the spectrum of proteins produced in G2-arrested cells compared with those in cells progressing normally (RAO and RAO 1976) that chromosome damage, mainly gene deletion, is responsible for G2 arrest. Gene deletions results in the loss of ability of cells to synthesise certain proteins necessary for their normal progress through G2. Although this is an attractive hypothesis, much more information about dose-response relationships is necessary before firm conclusions can be drawn.

More important, however, in the relationship between effects on cell-cycle progression and cellular sensitivity is the apparent correlation between cellular ability to recognise damage and respond with an inhibition of replicon initiation, depression in DNA synthesis and delay in subsequent mitosis, e.g. hamster cells exposed to MNU compared with HeLa cells (ROBERTS 1978) and normal fibroblasts compared with AT cells after exposure to X-rays (PAINTER 1980; FORD and LAVIN 1981). These observations suggest that an immediate S-phase prolongation as a result of inhibition of replicon initiation and DNA synthesis and the consequent mitotic delay are positive cellular responses to damage, and inhibition of replicon initiation and its recovery reflect a repair process (PAINTER 1980). In support of this view are the observations that AT cells fail to synthesise polyADP-ribose in response to X-ray-induced DNA damage (EDWARDS and TAYLOR 1980) and that inhibition of polyADP-ribose synthesis can be correlated with an increase in sensitivity to the cytotoxic effects of a number of DNA-damaging agents in some cell lines (DURKACZ et al. 1980). In practical terms, however, if it can be shown that drug-resistant cells regularly respond to induction of DNA damage with S-phase elongation which can be readily and rapidly measured by cytofluorimetry, i.e. are DRP (damage-recognition proficient) whereas drug-sensitive cells do not respond in this way, i.e. are damage-recognition deficient (DRD), then a rapid method of monitoring development of drug resistance in treated tumours would be available.

E. Attempts to Develop Resistance to DNA-Damaging Drugs in Cultured Cell Lines In Vitro

There are few reported successful attempts to induce drug resistance in cultured mammalian cells by repeated exposure to high concentrations and none where the increased cellular resistance has been directly related to increased DNA repair capacity. An HN2-resistant L5178Y cell line was developed by GOLDENBERG (1969) after multiple exposures to HN2. The cell line was stably resistant to further challenge with HN2, but resistance was subsequently shown to be due to altered transport kinetics for the drug and not increased DNA repair capacity. Attempts to induce resistance to dimethyl myleran also in L5178Y cells in vitro using a similar repeated dosage schedule proved negative (GOLDENBERG and ALEXANDER 1965). Exposure of P388 cells to MMS and retreatment of survivors with the same dose of MMS after an appropriate recovery interval eventually induced a transient increase in resistance (FOX and NIAS 1968). The loss of resistant cells from the population may well have been due to selective overgrowth by sensitive cells as the population was not cloned. In these examples the initial dose-response curve of the sensitive population was characterised by a shoulder and an exponential decline with no evidence for heterogeneity in sensitivity within the population. From studies of this nature it has been generally concluded that development of resistance to cytotoxic alkylating agents is a multistep process requiring the concurrent or sequential mutation of many genes. If this is so, then it is surprising that resistance to alkylating agents in vivo develops quite readily.

In an attempt to shed some light on this problem, studies were carried out using Yoshida sarcoma of rats, which is very sensitive to the cytotoxic effects of a number of alkylating agents, e.g. MDMS. Resistance readily develops in vivo (Fox 1969) apparently in a single step, in contrast to the difficulties of selecting single-step resistant lines in vitro as described above.

Cloned cell lines developed in vitro from these sensitive and resistant tumours also showed a large differential sensitivity to MDMS and were cross-resistant to SM and HN2 (Fox and Fox 1972). The probable role of DNA repair in their differential sensitivity has been discussed in detail earlier. When the sensitive line was exposed in increasing concentrations of MDMS in vitro, the dose-response curve showed a concave shape, suggesting the presence of resistant cells or the induction of resistance to the drug in a fraction of the population (SZENDE and FOX 1973). Survivors from high doses of MDMS were repeatedly rechallenged, cloned and retested for sensitivity to MDMS. On retesting, a progressive increase in the resistant fraction was evident. The lack of development of resistance in a single step in vitro may simply be due to the fact that at least 10^4 more cells are exposed in vivo than in vitro; thus the probability of selecting or inducing a resistant variant is much enhanced in the former situation.

The existence of heterogeneity in the population with respect to initial drug sensitivity is of interest in this respect, as biphasic survival curves have been reported for many different mammalian cell lines in vitro after exposure to bleomycin (TERASIMA et al. 1976), after exposure of CHO cells to MNNG (BARRANCO and HUMPHREY 1971 a) and after exposure of human lymphoblasts to MNU and MNNG (SLAPIKOFF et al. 1980) The concave shape of these curves may be due to the induction of resistance to the drug by the drug itself as has been postulated for bleomycin. However, bleomycin resistance appears to be due to induction of a bleomycin-inactivating enzyme rather than to alterations in DNA repair capacity.

Recently, induction of resistance to simple alkylating agents in mammalian cells by chronic exposure to low doses of alkylating agents has undergone a revival of interest as a result of the discovery and characterisation of an adaptive response in *E. coli* (SAMSON and CAIRNS 1977; JEGGO et al. 1977, 1978; SCHENDEL and ROBBINS 1978; ROBBINS and CAIRNS 1979; CAIRNS 1980). Growth of cells in very low concentrations of MNNG results in increased resistance to the cytotoxic effects of subsequent challenge with higher doses and reduced mutability, although the two responses are not of equal magnitude. The induction of enzymes which specifically remove the methyl group from O^6-alkylated guanine has been implicated (KARREN and GRIFFIN 1979).

Induction of resistance to MNNG and MNU by prior exposure of CHO and human skin fibroblasts cells to chronic low doses has recently been reported (SAMSON and SCHWARTZ 1980); the pretreatment did not increase cellular thiol concentrations known to be important in modulating MNNG cytotoxicity and did not appreciably alter cell-cycle progression. A concomitant reduction in SCEs was observed, implicating induction of a repair process. However, in V79 cells exposed to MNU, although a transient increase in survival could be induced by a non-toxic pretreatment regime, no alterations in the rate or extent of loss of DNA lesions could be detected (DURRANT et al. 1981). Thus the involvement of repair processes in these transient changes in resistance is far from clear. Whether adaptive responses are important in the development of drug resistance in tumours in vivo remains to be explored as does the precise nature of such responses in vitro. The high frequency of attainment of drug resistance in vivo compared with that in vitro may be related to such adaptive responses, in that tumour cells in vivo may be in a more favourable environment for adaptation to occur. The nature of the adaptive response may explain the many failures to induce resistance to alkylating agents previously. High initial doses of alkylating agents were used which necessitated long periods of post-treatment growth before sufficient survivors were available for rechallenge. The adaptive response in surviving cells may be inhibited by such high doses, and is known to fade with time. A re-examination of the situation using low initial doses and different treatment regimes (the precise treatment regime appears to be very critical in inducing resistance to cytotoxicity) may well indicate that adaptive responses are important in development of resistance to DNA-damaging drugs in general. Indeed, the doses of drugs reaching tumour cells in vivo may well be in the "adaptive" range, and certainly most treatment regimes involve multiple exposures. Multiple exposures may fix or select for highly adapted cells, thus accounting for the refractory nature of tumours in vivo. Many of these questions remain to be explored but they open up a number of interesting possibilities.

F. Conclusions

Although much is now known regarding the detailed mechanisms of DNA repair in mammalian cells after their exposure to a variety of DNA-damaging agents, there are few instances in which a specific defect in DNA repair has been directly correlated with increased cellular sensitivity to a DNA-damaging drug or increased repair capacity related to cellular resistance. With respect to the DNA-damaging drugs used clinically in cancer chemotherapy, there are to the best of my knowledge no good examples where the involvement of DNA repair in cellular resistance has been unequivocally demonstrated in human cells. Indeed, there is a paucity of data indicating that human tumour cells do indeed acquire intrinsic cellular resistance to DNA-damaging anticancer drugs, although there are several examples of lack of responsiveness of human tumour cells to DNA-damaging agents. The development of improved methods for culturing human tumour cells, the use of xenografted human tumours, the discovery of adaptive responses in bacteria and our increasing overall knowledge of DNA repair processes in mammalian cells should, however, allow detailed analysis of the role of DNA repair, both constitutive and induced, in human tumour drug resistance in the foreseeable future.

References

Altimirano-Dimas M, Sklar R, Strauss B (1979) Selectivity of the excision of alkylation products in a Xeroderma pigmentosum-derived lymphoblast line. Mutat Res 60:197–206

Ball CR, Roberts JJ (1970) DNA repair after mustard gas alkylation by sensitive and resistant Yoshida sarcoma cells in vitro. Chem Biol Int 7:321–329

Ball CR, Roberts JJ (1972) Estimation of interstrand DNA cross-linking resulting from mustard gas alkylation of HeLa cells. Chem Biol Interact 4:297–303

Barlogie B, Drewinko B (1978) Cell cycle stage-dependent induction of G2 phase arrest by different antitumour agents. Eur J Cancer Clin Oncol 14:741–745

Barranco SC, Humphrey RM (1971 a) The response of Chinese hamster cells to *N*-methyl-*N*-nitrosoguanidine. Mutat Res 11:424–429

Barranco SC, Humphrey RM (1971 b) Effects of bleomycin on survival and cell progression in Chinese hamster cells in vitro. Cancer Res 31:1218–1223

Barranco SC, Humphrey RM (1971 c) The effects of 1,3-bis(2.chloroethyl)-1-nitrosourea on survival and cell progression in Chinese hamster cells. Cancer Res 31:1919–1924

Barranco SC, Haenelt BR, Gee EL (1978) Differential sensitivities of five rat hepatoma cell lines to anticancer drugs. Cancer Res 38:656–661

Bodell WJ (1977) Non-uniform distribution of DNA repair in chromatin after treatment with methyl methanesulphonate. Nucleic Acids Res 4:2619–2628

Bodell WJ, Cleaver JE (1981) Transient conformation changes in chromatin during excision repair of ultraviolet damage to DNA. Nucleic Acids Res 9:203–213

Cairns J (1980) Efficiency of the adaptive response of E. coli to alkylating agents. Nature 286:176–178

Caputo A (1976) Importance of experimental data for the improvement of the therapeutical effect of bleomycin. Prog Biochem Pharmacol 11:2–17

Carr F (1979) Temporal studies of mammalian DNA repair processes and DNA synthesis following anti-tumour agents. PhD Thesis, University of Manchester

Carr FJ, Fox BW (1981 a) DNA strand breaks and repair synthesis on Yoshida sarcoma cells with differential sensitivities to bifunctional alkylating agents and UV light. Mutat Res 83:233–249

Carr F, Fox BW (1982) The effects of bifunctional alkylating agents on DNA synthesis in sensitive and resistant Yoshida cells. Mutat Res 95:441–456

Carrocchi G, Linn S (1978) Cell-free assay measuring repair DNA synthesis in human fibroblasts. Proc Natl Acad Sci USA 75:1887–1891

Carter SK (1979) Preface in mitomycin C current status and new developments. In: Carter SK, Cooke ST (eds) Academic, New York

Chase JW, Richardson CC (1974) Exonuclease VII of *Escherichia coli* mechanism of action. J Biol Chem 249:4545–4552

Cleaver JE (1977) DNA repair processes and their impairment in some human diseases. In: Scott D, Bridges B, Sobels FH (eds) Progress in genetic toxicology. Elsevier North Holland, Amsterdam, pp 29–39

Cleaver JE (1978) DNA repair and its coupling to DNA replication in eukaryotic cells. Biochem Biophys Acta 516:489–502

Cone R, Duncan J, Hamilton L, Friedburg EC (1977) Partial purification and characterisation of a uracil DNA *N*-glycosidase from *Bacillus subtilis*. Biochemistry 16:3194–3201

Cook KH, Friedburg EC (1978) Multiple thymine dimer excising nuclease activities in extracts of human KB cells. Biochemistry 17:850–857

Cox R (1979) Differences in removal of *N*-methyl-*N*-nitrosourea methylated products in DNase I sensitive and resistant regions of rat brain DNA. Cancer Res 39:2675–2678

Day RS III, Chuc H, Ziolkowski CHJ, Scudiero DA, Meyer SA, Mattern MA (1980 a) Human tumour cell strains defective in repair of alkylation damage. Carcinogenesis 1:21–32

Day RS III, Ziolkowski CHJ, Scudiero DA, Meyer SA, Lubinieki AS, Girdi AJ, Galloway SM, Bynum GD (1980 b) Defective repair of alkylated DNA by human tumour and SV 40 transformed human cell strains. Nature 288:724–727

Demple B, Linn S (1980) DNA *N*-glycosylases and UV repair. Nature 287:203–207
Deutsch WA, Linn S (1979) DNA binding activity from cultured human fibroblasts that is specific for partially depurinated DNA that inserts purines into apurinic sites. Proc Natl Acad Sci USA 76:141–144
Doninger J (1978) DNA replication in ultraviolet irradiated Chinese hamster cells. The nature of replicon inhibition and post-replication repair. J Mol Biol 120:433–447
Doninger L, Grossman L (1976) Human corexonuclease. Purification and properties of a DNA repair exonuclease from placenta. J Biol Chem 251:4579–4587
Drewinko B, Barlogie B (1976) Age-dependent survival and cell-cycle progression of cultured cells exposed to chemotherapeutic drugs. Cancer Treat Rep 60:1707–1715
Durkacz BW, Omidiji O, Gray DA, Shall S (1980) (ADP-ribose) particpates in excision repair. Nature 283:593–596
Durrant L, Margison GP, Boyle JM (1981) Pretreatment of Chinese hamster cells with MNU increases survival withouth affecting DNA repair or mutagenicity. Carcinogenesis 2:55–61
Edenburg HJ (1976) Inhibition of DNA replication by ultraviolet light. Biophys J 16:849–860
Edenburg HJ (1978) DNA replication in ultraviolet-irradiated mammalian cells. In: Hanawalt PC, Friedburg EC, Fox CF (eds) DNA repair mechanisms. ICN-UCLA symposia in molecular and cellular biology. Academic New York
Edenberg H, Hanawalt P (1972) Size of repair patches in the DNA of ultraviolet irradiated HeLa cells. Biochem Biophys Acta 272:361–372
Edwards MJ, Taylor AMR (1980) Unusual levels of (ADP-ribose) and DNA synthesis in ataxia telangiectasia cells following γ-irradiation. Nature 287:745–747
Erikson LC, Bradley MO, Kohn KW (1977) Strand breaks in DNA from normal and transformed human cells treated with 1.3 bis (2-chloroethyl)1-nitrosourea. Cancer Res 37:3744–3751
Erikson LC, Osieka R, Kohn KW (1978) Differential repair of 1-(2.chloroethyl)3-(4-methylcyclohexyl)-1-nitrosourea induced damage in two human colon tumor cell lines. Cancer Res 38:802–809
Erikson LC, Mathews OB, Ducore JM, Ewig RAG, Kohn KW (1980 a) DNA cross-linking and cytotoxicity in normal and transformed human cells by antitumor nitrosoureas. Proc Natl Acad Sci USA 77:467–472
Erikson LC, Laurent G, Sharkey NA, Kohn KW (1980 b) DNA cross-linking and monoadduct repair in nitrosourea treated human cells. Nature 228:727–729
Erikson LC, Zwelling L, Kohn KW (1980 c) Differential cytotoxicity and DNA cross-linking in normal and transformed human fibroblasts treated with cisplatin in vitro. Proc Am Assoc Cancer Res 21:267 A
Ewig R, Kohn KW (1977) DNA damage and repair in mouse leukemia cells treated with nitrogen mustard, 1,3bis(2-chloroethyl)-1-nitrosurea and other nitrosoureas. Cancer Res 37:2114–2122
Ewig RAG, Kohn KW (1978) DNA-protein cross-linking and DNA-interstrand cross-linking by holoethylnitrosoureas in L1210 cells. Cancer Res 38:3198–3203
Feldman G, Remsen J, Wang TV, Cerutti P (1980) Formation and excision of covalent deoxyribonucleic acid adducts of benzo[a]pyrene 4;5-epoxide and benz[a]pyrenediol epoxide 1 in human lung cells A549. Biochemistry 19:1095–1101
Felsenfeld G (1978) Chromatin. Nature 271:115–122
Flavel HNA, Roberts JJ (1978 a) Effects of cisplatin(II) diaminedichloride on survival and the rate of DNA synthesis in synchronously growing Chinese hamster V79.379A cells in the absence and presence of caffeine. Evidence for an inducible repair mechanism. Chem Biol Interact 23:99–110
Flavel HNA, Roberts JJ (1978 b) Effects of cisPlatinumII diaminedichloride on survival and the rate of DNA synthesis in synchronously growing HeLa cells in the absence and presence of caffeine. Chem Biol Interact 23:111–119
Ford MD, Lavin MF (1981) Ataxia telangiectasia: an anomaly in DNA replication after irradiation. Nucleic Acids Res 9:1395–1404

Fox BW (1969) The sensitivity of Yoshida sarcoma to methylene dimethanesulphonate. Int J Cancer 4:54–60

Fox M (1981) Some quantitative aspects of mammalian cell mutagenesis. In: Marchalonis JJ, Hanna MG (eds) Cancer biology reviews vol 3. Marcel Decker, pp 23–63

Fox M, Brennand J (1980) Evidence for the involvement of lesions other than O^6-alkylguanine in mammalian cell mutagenesis. Carcinogenesis 1:795–800

Fox M, Fox BW (1972) The establishment of cloned cell lines from Yoshida sarcomas having differential sensitivities to methylene dimethanesulphonate in vivo and their cross-sensitivity to X-rays, UV and other alkylating agents. Chem Biol Interact 4:363–375

Fox M, Fox BW (1973 a) Repair replication after UV-irradiation in rodent cell lines of different sensitivity. Int J Radiat Biol 23:359–376

Fox M, Fox BW (1973 b) Repair replication in X-irradiated lymphoma cells in vitro, Int J Radiat Biol 23:333–358

Fox M, Fox BW (1973 c) Repair replication and unscheduled DNA synthesis in mammalian cells showing differential sensitivity to alkylating agents. Mutation Res 19:119–128

Fox M, Nias AHW (1968) A modification of the sensitivity of mammalian cells surviving treatment with methyl methanesulphonate. Eur J Cancer Clin Oncol 4:325–335

Fox M, Scott D (1980) The genetic toxicology of nitrogen and sulphur mustard. Mutation Res 75:131–168

Friedburg EC, Bonura T, Reynolds RJ, Rodney EH (1980) Some aspects of the enzymology of DNA repair. In: Alecevic M (ed) Progress in environmental mutagenesis. Elsevier/North Holland Amsterdam, p 175–188

Friedman J, Huberman E (1980) Post-replication repair and susceptibility of Chinese hamster cells to cytotoxic and mutagenic effects of alkylating agents. Proc Natl Acad Sci USA 77:6072–6076

Fujiwara Y, Tatsumi M (1975) Repair of mitomycin C damage to DNA in mammalian cells and its impairment in Fanconi's anemia cells. Biochem Biophys Res Commun 66:592–597

Fujiwara Y, Tatsumi M (1976) Replicative bypass repair of ultraviolet damage to DNA of mammalian cells, caffeine-sensitive and caffeine-resistant mechanism. Mutat Res 37:91–110

Fujiwara Y, Tatsumi M, Sasaki MS (1977) Cross-link repair in human cells and its possible defect in Fanconi's anaemia cells. J Mol Biol 11:635–649

Galbraith AI, Barker M, Itzhaki RF (1979) Methylation of DNase-digestible DNA and RNA in chromatin from rats treated with dimethylnitrosamine. Biochem Biophys Acta 561:334–344

Gates FT, Linn S (1977 a) Endonuclease V or *Escherichia coli*. J Biol Chem 252:1647–1653

Gates FT, Linn S (1977 b) Endonuclease from *Escherichia coli* that acts specifically upon duplex DNA damage by ultraviolet light, Osmium tetroxide acid or X-rays. J Biol Chem 252:2802–2809

Goldenberg GJ (1969) Properties of L5178Y lymphoblasts highly resistant to nitrogen mustard. Symposium on biological effects of alkylating agents. Ann NY Acad Sci 163:936–951

Goldenberg GJ, Alexander P (1965) The effect of nitrogen mustard and dimethylmyleran on murine leukemia cell lines of different radiosensitivity in vitro. Cancer Res 25:1401–1409

Goldstein NO, Rutman RJ (1974) The abortive synthesis of new DNA chains in Erlich ascites tumor cells treated with nitrogen mustard (HN_2). Chem Biol Interact 8:1–9

Goth-Goldstein R (1980) Inability of Chinese hamster ovary cells to excise O^6-alkylguanine. Cancer Res 40:2623–2642

Grossman L, Riazuddin S (1978) Enzymatic pathways of damaged nucleotide excision. In: Hanawalt PC, Friedberg EC, Foc CF (eds) DNA repair mechanisms. ICN-UCLA symposia in molecular cell biology. Academic, New York, pp 205 215

Hanawalt PC, Cooper PK, Ganesan AK, Smith CA (1979) DNA repair in bacteria and mammalian cells. Annu Rev Biochem 48:783–836

Higgins NP, Strauss BS (1979) Differences in the ability of human lymphoblastoid lines to exclude bromodeoxyuridine and in their sensitivity to methyl methanesulphonate and to incorporated [^{3}H]-thymidine. Cancer Res 39:312–320

Ishikawa T, Matsuda A, Miyamato K, Tsubosaki M, Kaihava T, Sakamoto K, Umezawa H (1967) Biological studies on bleomycin A. J Antibiot (Tokyo) 20:149–155

Jeggo P, Defais M, Samson I, Schendel P (1977) Adaptive response of *E. coli* to low levels of alkylating agent; comparison with previously characterised DNA repair pathways. MGG 157:1–11

Jeggo P, Defais M, Samson L, Schendel P (1978) Adaptive response of *E. coli* to low levels of alkylating agent – role of polA in killing adaptation. MGG 162:299–307

Karren P, Griffin B (1979) Adaptive response to alkylating agents involves alterations *in situ* of O(6)methylguanine residues in DNA. Nature 280:76–77

Karren P, Lindahl T, Griffin B (1980) Adaptive response to alkylating agents involves alterations *in situ* of O^6-methylguanine residues in DNA. Nature 280:76–77

Kersten H (1975) Mechanisms of action of mitomycins. In. Sartorelli AC, Johns DG (eds) Antineoplastic and immunosuppressive agents, part 2. Springer, Berlin Heidelberg New York, pp 47–61

Kirtikar DM, Goldthwait DA (1974) The enzymatic release of O^6-methylguanine and 3-methyladenine from DNA reacted with the carcinogen *N*-methyl-*N*-nitrosourea. Proc Natl Acad Sci USA 71:2022–2026

Klett RP, Cerami A, Reich E (1968) Endonuclease VI. A new nuclease activity associated with *E. coli* DNA polymerase. Proc Natl Acad Sci USA 60:943–950

Kohn KW (1977) Interstrand cross-linking of DNA by 1,3-Bis(2.chloroethyl)-1-nitrosurea and other 1-(-2-haloethyl)-1-nitrosoureas. Cancer Res 37:1450–1454

Kohn KW (1979) DNA as a target in cancer chemotherapy measurement of macromolecular damage produced in mammalian cells by anticancer agents. Methods Cancer Res 16:291 345

Kornberg RD (1978) Structure of chromatin. Annu Rev Biochem 931–954

Kunnlein U, Lee B, Linn S (1978) Human uracil DNA-*N*-glycosidase: Studies in normal and repair-defective cultured fibroblasts. Nucleic Acids Res 5:117-127

Laval J (1977) Two enzymes are required for strand incision in repair of alkylated DNA. Nature 269:829–833

Lehmann AR (1978) Replicative bypass mechanisms in mammalian cells. In: Hanawalt PC, Friedburg EC, Fox CF (eds) DNA repair mechanisms. ICN-UCLA symposia in cellular and molecular biology. Academic, New York pp 485–488

Lehmann AR, Stevans S (1977) Production and repair of double strand breaks in cells from normal humans and from patients with ataxia telangiectasia. Biochem Biophys Acta 474:49–60

Lehmann AR, Stevans S (1979) The response of ataxia-telangiectasia cells to bleomycin. Nucleic Acid Res 6:1953–1960

Lindahl T (1979) DNA glycosylases, endonucleases for apurinic/apyrimidinic sites and base excision repair. Prog Nucleic Acid Res Mol Biol 22:135–192

Lindahl T, Gally JA, Edelman GM (1969) Deoxyribonuclease IV: A new exonuclease from mammalian tissues. Proc Natl Acad Sci USA 62:597–603

Lindahl T, Ljundquist S, Siegert M, Nyberg B, Sperens B (1977) DNA *N*-glycosidases. Properties of uracil-DNA glycosidase from *Escherichia coli*. J Biol Chem 252:3286–3294

Linn S, Kuhnlein U, Deutsch WA (1978) Enzymes from human fibroblasts for the repair of AP DNA. In: Hanawalt PC, Friedburg EC, Fox CF (eds) DNA repair mechanisms. ICN-UCLA symposia in molecular biology. Academic, New York, pp 199–203

Liveneh Z, Elad D, Sperling J (1979) Enzymatic insertion of purine bases into depurinated DNA in vitro. Proc Natl Acad Sci USA 76:1089–1093

Livingston DM, Richardson CC (1975) Deoxyribonucleic acid polymerase III of *Escherichia coli*. Characterization of associated exonuclease activities. J Biol Chem 250:370–478

Ljunquist S (1977) A new endonuclease from *E. coli* acting at apurinic sites in DNA. J Biol Chem 252:2808–2814

Lown JW (1979) The molecular mechanism of antitumor action of the mitomycins in mytomycin C. In: Carter SK, Crooke ST (eds) Current status and new developments. Academic, New York, pp 5–26

Lown JW, Begleiter A, Johnson D, Morgan R (1976) Studies related to antitumour antibiotics V. Reactions of mitomycin C with DNA examined by ethidium bromide fluorescence assay. Can J Biochem 54:110–119

Mattern MR, Hariharan PV, Cerutti PA (1976) Selective excision of γ-ray damaged thymine from the DNA of cultured mammalian cells. Biochem Biophys Acta 395:49–55

Mauro F, Falpo B, Briganti G, Eilli R, Zupi G (1974) Effects of antineoplastic drugs on plateau-phase cultures of mammalian cells. II. Bleomycin and hydroxyurea. J Natl Canc Inst 52:715–723

Meneghini R, Meuck CFM (1978) Pyrimidine dimers in DNA strands of mammalian cells synthesised after UV irradiation. In: Hanawalt PC, Friedberg EC, Fox F (eds) DNA repair mechanism. Academic, New York, pp 493–499

Mortelmans K, Friedberg EC, Slor H, Thomas GH, Cleaver JE (1976) Defective thymine dimer excision by cell-free extracts of xeroderma pigmentosum cells. Proc Natl Acad Sci USA 73:2757–2761

Müller WEG, Zahn RK (1977) Bleomycin, an antibiotic that removes thymine from double-stranded DNA. In: Cohn WE (ed) Prog Nucl Acid Res and Mol Biol Academic New York, pp 21–57

Murname JP, Byfield JE, Ward JF, Calabro-Jones P (1980) Effects of methylated xanthines on mammalian cells treated with bifunctional alkylating agents. Nature 285:326–329

Nes IF (1980) Purification and characterisation of an endonuclease specific for apurinic sites in DNA from a permanently established mouse plasmacytoma cell line. Nucleic Acids Res 8:1575–1591

Nomura K, Hoshino T, Knebel K, Deen D, Barker M (1978) BCNU-induced perturbations in the cell cycle of 9L rat brain tumor cells. Cancer Treat Rep 62:747–754

Oleson FB, Mitchell BL, Dipple A, Lieberman MW (1979) Distribution of DNA damage in chromatin and its relationship to repair in human cells treated with 7-bromomethylbenz(a)anthracene. Nucleic Acids Res 7:1343–1360

Olsson M, Lindahl T (1980) Repair of alkylated DNA in *E. coli*, methyl group transfer from O^6-methylguanine to a protein cysteine residue. J Biol Chem 255:10569–10572

Painter RB (1977) inhibition of initiation of HeLa cell replicons by methyl methanesulphonate. Mutat Res 42:299–304

Painter RB (1978a) Inhibition of DNA replicon initiation by 4-nitroquinoline-1-oxide adriamycin and ethyleneimine. Cancer Res 38:4445–4449

Painter RB (1978b) action of three mutagens on HeLa DNA replication. In: Hanawalt PC, Friedberg EC, Fox CF (eds) DNA repair mechanisms. ICN-UCLA symposia in molecular and cellular biology. Academic, New York, pp 789–791

Painter RB (1980) Effect of caffeine on DNA synthesis in irradiated and unirradiated mammalian cells. J Mol Biol 143:389–301

Painter RB, Young BR (1972) Repair replication in mammalian cells after X-irradiation. Mutat Res 14:225–235

Painter RB, Young BR (1975) Y-ray-induced inhibition of DNA synthesis in Chinese hamster overay human HeLa, and mouse L cells. Radiat Res 64:648–656

Painter RB, Young BR (1976) Formation of nascent DNA molecules during inhibition of replication initiation in mammalian cells. Biochem Biophys Acta 418:146–154

Painter RB, Young BR (1980) Radiosensitivity in ataxia telangiectasia. A new explanation. Proc Natl Acad Sci USA 77:7315–7317

Park SD, Cleaver JE (1979) Post replication repair, questions of its definition and possible alteration in xeroderma pigmentosum cell strains. Proc Natl Acad Sci USA 76:3927–3932

Pascoe JM, Roberts JJ (1974a) Interactions between mammalian cell DNA and inorganic platinum compounds. I. DNA interstrand cross-linking and cytotoxic properties of platinum (II) compounds. Biochem Pharmacol 23:1345–1357

Pascoe JM, Roberts JJ (1974b) Interactions between mammalian cell DNA and inorganic platinum compounds. II. Interstrand cross-linking of isolated and cellular DNA by platinum(IV) compounds. Biochem Pharmacol 23:1359–1365

Paterson MC, Smith BP, Lohman PHM, Anderson AK, Fishman L (1976) Defective excision repair of γ-ray-damaged DNA in human (ataxia telangiectasia) fibroblasts. Nature 260:444–447

Porvirk L, Painter RB (1976) The effect of 313 nanometer light on initiation of replicons in mammalian DNA containing bromodeoxyuridine. Biochem Biophys Acta 432:267–272

Rao PN (1979) G2 Arrest induced by anticancer drugs. In: Busch H, Crooke ST, Daskal Y (eds) Effects of drugs on the cell nucleus. Academic, New York, pp 475–490

Rao AP, Rao PN (1976) The cause of G2 arrest in Chinese hamster ovary cells treated with anticancer drugs. J Natl Cancer Inst 57:1139–1146

Regan JE, Setlow RB (1974) Two forms of DNA repair in the DNA of human cells damaged by chemical carcinogens and mutagens. Cancer Res 34:3318-3325

Regan JD, Setlow RB, Ley RD (1971) Normal and defective repair of damaged DNA in human cells: A sensitive assay utilizing photolysis of bromodeoxyuridine. Proc Natl Acad Sci USA 68:708–712

Reid BD, Walker IG (1969) The response of mammalian cells to alkylating agents. II. On the mechanism of the removal of sulphur mustard-induced cross-links. Biochem Biophys Acta 179:179–188

Robbins P, Cairns J (1979) Quantitation of the adaptive response to alkylating agents. Nature 280:74–76

Roberts JJ (1975) Inactivation of the DNA template in HeLa cells treated with chlorambucil. Int J Cancer 16:91–103

Roberts JJ (1978) The repair of DNA modified by cytotoxic mutagenic and carcinogenic chemicals Adv Radiat Biol 7:211–436

Roberts JJ, Flavel HA (1980) Repair of *cis*-platinum(II)diaminedichloride-induced DNA damage and cell sensitivity. In: Prestayko AW, Crooke ST, Carter SK (eds) Cisplatin. Current status and new developments. Academic, New York, pp 53–77

Roberts JJ, Pascoe JM, Plant JE, Sturrock JE, Crathorn AR (1971) Quantitative aspects of the repair of alkylated DNA in cultured mammalian cells. 1. The effect on Hela and Chinese hamster cell survival of alkylation of cellular macromolecules. Chem Biol Interact 3:29–47

Ross LAG (1977) The interaction of an anti-tumour platinum complex with DNA. Chem Biol Interact 16:39–55

Ross WE, Ewig RA, Kohn KW (1978) Differences between melphalan and nitrogen mustard in formation and removal of cross-links from DNA. Cancer Res 38:1502–1507

Rudé JM, Friedberg EC (1977) Semi-conservative DNA synthesis in unirradiated and UV-irradiated xeroderma pigmentosum and normal human skin fibroblasts. Mutat Res 42:433–442

Samson L, Cairns J (1977) A new pathway for DNA repair in *E. coli.* Nature 267:281–283

Samson L, Schwartz JL (1980) Evidence for an adaptive DNA repair pathway in CHO and human fibroblast cell lines. Nature 287:861–863

Sazaki MS (1978) Fanconi's anaemia. A condition possibly associated with defective DNA repair. In: Hanawalt PC, Friedburg EC, Fox CF (eds) DNA repair mechanisms. ICN-UCLA symposia in molecular and cellular biology. Academic, New York, pp 675–683

Schendel PF, Robins PE (1978) Repair of O^6-methylguanine in adapted *E. coli* Proc Natl Acad Sci USA 75:6017–6020

Scott D (1977) Chromosome aberrations, DNA post-replication repair and lethality in tumour cells with a differential sensitivity to alkylating agents. In: De la Chapell A, Sorsa M (eds) Chromosomes today vol 6. Elsevier/North Holland, Amsterdam, pp 391–401

Scott D (1980) Molecular mechanisms of chromosome structural changes. In: Alâcévic M (ed) Progress in environmental mutagenesis. Elsevier/North Holland, Amsterdam, pp 101–113

Scott D, Zampetti-Bosseler F (1980) The relationship between cell killing, chromosome aberrations, spindle defects and mitotic delay in mouse lymphoma cells of differential sensitivity to X-rays. Int J Radiat Biol 37:33–47

Scott D, Fox M, Fox BW (1974) The relationship between chromosomal aberrations survival and DNA repair in tumor cell lines of differential sensitivity to X-rays and sulphur mustard. Mutat Res 22:207–221

Shatkin AH, Reich E, Franklin RM, Tatum EL (1962) Effect of mitomycin C on mammalian cells in culture. Biochem Biophys Acta 55:277–28

Sklar R, Strauss B (1981) Removal of O^6-methylguanine from DNA of normal and xeroderma pigmentosum-derived lymphoblastoid lines. Nature 289:417–420

Slapikoff SA, Andon BW, Thilly WG (1980) Comparison of toxicity and mutagenicity of methylnitrosourea, methylnitrosoguanidine and ICR 191 among human lymphoblast cell lines. Mutat Res 70:365–371

Smerdon MJ, Tisty TD, Lieberman MW (1978) Distribution of ultraviolet-induced DNA repair synthesis in nuclease-sensitive and -resistant regions of human chromatin. Biochemistry 17:2377–2386

Smith PJ, Paterson MC (1980) Defective DNA repair and increased lethality in ataxia telangiectasia cells exposed to 4-nitroquinoline-1-oxide. Nature 287:747–749

Smulson ME, Sudhakar S, Tew KD, Butt TR, Jump DB (1979) The influence of nitrosoureas an chromatin nucleosomal structure and function. In: Busch H, Crooke ST, Daskal Y (eds) Effects of drugs on the cell nucleus. Academic, New York, pp 333–357

Strauss B, Bose K, Altamirano-Dimas, Sklar R, Tatsumi K (1978) Response of mammalian cells to chemial damage. In: Hanawalt PC, Friedburg EC, Fox CF (eds) DNA repair mechanisms. ICN-UCLA symposia in molecular and cellular biology. Academic, New York, pp 621–624

Suzuki H, Nagai K, Yamaki H, Tanaka B, Umezawa H (1969) On the mechanism of action of bleomycin, scission of DNA strands in vitro and in vivo. J Antibiot (Tokyo) 22:446–468

Szende B, Fox M (1973) The establishment of MDMS-resistant cloned cell lines from in vitro-cultured MDMS-sensitive Yoshida sarcoma cells. Chem Biol Interact 6:19–25

Szumiel I (1979a) Response of two trains of L5178Y cells to *cis*-dichlorobis-(cyclopentylamine)platinum(II). II. Differential effects of caffeine. Chem Biol Interact 24:73–82

Szumiel I (1979b) Response of two strains of L5178Y cells to *cis*-dichlorobis-(cyclopentylamine)platinum(II). I. Cross-sensitivity to *cis*-PAD and UV light. Chem Biol Interact 24:51–72

Szybalski W, Iyer VN (1967) The mitomycins and porfiromycins. In: Gottleib DG, Shaw PD (eds) Antibiotics I, mechanism of action. Springer, Berlin Heidelberg New York, pp 211–245

Tanaka K, Sekiguchi M, Okada Y (1975) Restoration of ultraviolet induced unscheduled DNA synthesis of xeroderma pigmentosum cells by concomitant treatment with bacteriophage T4 endonuclease V and HVJ (Sendai virus) Proc Natl Acad Sci USA 72:4071–4075

Tanaka K, Hayakawa H, Sekiguichi M, Okada Y (1977) Specific action of T4 endonuclease V on damaged DNA in xeroderma pigmentosum cells in vivo. Proc Natl Acad Sci USA 74:2958–2962

Taylor AMR, Harnden DG, Arlett CF, Harcourt SA, Lehmann AR, Stevens S, Bridges BA (1975) Ataxia telangiectasia: a human mutation with abnormal radiation sensitivity. Nature 258:427–429

Taylor AMR, Metcalf JA, Oxford JM, Harnden DG (1976) Is chromatid-type damage in ataxia telangiectasia after irrdiation at Go a consequence of defective repair? Nature 260:441–443

Taylor AMR, Rosney CM, Campbell JB (1979) Unusual sensitivity of ataxia telangiectasia cells to bleomycin. Cancer Res 39:1046–1052

Terasima T, Umezawa H (1970) Lethal effect of bleomycin on cultured mammalian cells. J Antibiot (Tokyo) A23:300–304

Terasima T, Takebe Y, Katsumata T, Watanabe M, Horikawa (1972) Effect of bleomycin on mammalian cell survival. J Natl Cancer Inst 49:1093–1102

Terasima T, Takebe Y, Watanabe M, Katsumata T (1976) Effect of bleomycin on cell survival and some implications for tumour therapy. Prog Biochem Pharmacol 11:67–77
Tobey RA (1975) Different drugs arrest cells at different stages in G2. Nature 254:245–248
Tomaz M (1970) Novel assay of 7-alkylation of guanine residues in DNA. Application to nitrogen mustard, triethyleneamelamine and mitomycin C. Biochem Biophys Acta 213:288
Tong WP, Ludlum DB (1980) Cross-linking of DNA by busulphan formation of diguanyl derivations. Biochem Biophys Acta 608:174–181
Twentyman PR, Bleehan NM (1973) The sensitivity of cells in exponential and stationary phases of growth to bleomycin and to 1,3.bis(2-chloroethyl)-1-nitrosourea. Br J Cancer 28:500–507
Umezawa H (1976) Structure and action of bleomycins. Prog Biochem Pharmacol 11:18–27
Warren W, Crathorn AR, Shooter KV (1979) The stability of methylated purines and of methylphosphototriesters in the DNA of V79 cells after treatment with *N*-methyl-*N*-nitrosourea. Biochem Biophys Acta 563:82–88
Watanabe M, Takebe Y, Katsumata T, Terasima T, Umezawa H (1973) Response of macromolecular synthesis of mouse L cells to bleomycin with special reference to cell antibiotic interaction. J Antibiot (Tokyo) 26:417–425
Watanabe M, Takebe Y, Katsumata T, Terasima T (1974) Effects of bleomycin on progression through the cell cycle of mouse cells. Cancer Res 34:878–881
Weisbach A, Lisco A (1965) Alkylation of nucleic acid by mitomycin C and porfiromycin. Biochemistry 4:196–212
Wheeler GP, Bowde BJ, Adamson DJ (1970) Effect of 1,3-bis(2-chloromethyl)-1-nitrosourea and some chemically related compounds upon the progression of cultured H.Ep.2. cells through the cell cycle. Cancer Res 30:1817–1827
Williams JI, Friedberg EC (1979) Deoxyribonucleic acid excision repair in chromatin after ultraviolet irradiation of human fibroblast in culture. Biochemistry 18:3965–3972
Wilkinson R, Birbeck MSC, Harrap KR (1979) Enhancement of nuclear reactivity of alkylating agents by prednisolone. Cancer Res 39:4256–4262
Yin L, Chun EHL, Rutman RJ (1973) A comparison of the effects of alkylation on the DNA of sensitive and resistant Lettre-Erlich cells following in vivo exposure to nitrogen mustards. Biochem Biophys Acta 324:472–481
Zwelling LA (1979) Mutagenicity cytotoxicity and DNA cross-linking in V79 Chinese hamster cells treated with *cis*- and *trans*-Pt(II)diamminedichloride. Mutat Res 67:271–386
Zwelling LA, Kohn KW (1979) The effcts of cisplatin on DNA and the possible relationships to cytotoxicity and mutagenicity in mammalian cells. In: Prestayko AW, Crooke St, Carter SK (eds) Cisplatin, current status and new developments. Academic New York, pp 21–35
Zwelling LA, Kohn KW, Rosa WE, Ewig RAG, Anderson Y (1978) Kinetics of formation and disappearance of a cross-linking effect in mouse leukemia L1210 cells treated with *cis*- and *trans*-diaminedichloroplatinum(II). Cancer Res 38:1762–1768
Zwelling LA, Anderson T, Kohn KW (1979a) DNA-protein and DNA interstrand cross-linking by *cis*- and transplatinum(II) diaminedichloride in L210 mouse cells and relation to cytotoxicity. Cancer Res 39:365–369
Zwelling LA, Filipski J, Kohn KW (1979b) Effect of thiourea on survival and DNA cross-link formation in cells treated with platinum(II) complexes, L-phenylalanine mustard and bis(2-chloroethyl)methylamine. Cancer Res 39:4989–4995
Zwelling LA, Michaels S, Schwartz H, Dobson PP, Kohn KW (1981) DNA cross-linking as an indicator of sensitivity and resistance of mouse L1210 leukemia to *cis*-diaminedichloroplatinum(II) and L-phenylalanine mustard. Cancer Res 41:640–649

CHAPTER 13

Cyclic AMP and Prostaglandins

M. J. TISDALE

A. Cyclic AMP

Adenosine 3′,5′-monophosphate (cyclic AMP) is a ubiquitous nucleotide, having a myriad of biological effects. Tissue specificity of cyclic AMP actions is provided by the hormone-sensitive adenylate cyclase, located on the inner side of the plasma membrane which converts ATP to cyclic AMP. Binding of the hormone to its receptor causes a conformational change resulting in activation of the cyclase. Most of the biological effects of cyclic AMP are mediated via protein phosphorylation; the newly synthesized cyclic AMP binds to the regulatory subunit of an inactive protein kinase holoenzyme, causing dissociation of the latter into active catalytic subunits. This provides another source of specificity for cyclic AMP action since only those cells possessing the requisite substrates for phosphorylation will experience modifying effects. Free cytosolic cyclic AMP is rapidly degraded to 5′AMP by a specific phosphodiesterase which exists in several isoenzymic forms and may show tissue selectivity.

I. Cyclic AMP and Neoplasia

The intracellular level of cyclic AMP has been shown to be altered in many tissues after neoplastic transformation. However, studies of malignant tissues have not revealed any uniform pattern in the derangement of the cyclic nucleotide system. While early in vitro studies suggested a lower level of cyclic AMP in tumours an elevated level of both cyclic AMP and guanosine 3′,5′ monophosphate (cyclic GMP) and increased activities of both adenylate and guanylate cyclase have often been observed in vivo.

II. Tumour Growth Inhibition by Cyclic AMP and Derivatives

Cyclic AMP can influence division of a number of cell types both in vitro and in vivo. Increasing the cellular cyclic AMP concentration is generally associated with an inhibition of cell growth. On the other hand a decrease in intracellular cyclic AMP may be associated with stimulation of cell division. Addition of serum which is followed by an increase in DNA synthesis and mitotic activity is accompanied by a decreased cellular cyclic AMP (OTTEN et al. 1972). Mitogenic stimulation of mouse lymphocytes is associated with a sharp rise and then fall in cyclic AMP levels preceding DNA synthesis (WANG et al. 1978). Initiation of cell division in fibroblast cultures by pronase can be blocked by the addition of $N^6,O^{2'}$-dibutyryl cyclic AMP, an analogue of cyclic AMP (BOMBIK and BURGER 1973).

Some cells are particularly sensitive to the effects of cyclic AMP. When exposed to dibutyryl cyclic AMP or agents which increase the intracellular level of cyclic AMP, S 49 mouse lymphosarcoma cells show not only inhibition of growth, but also die (BOURNE et al. 1975).

In contrast to these results studies with lymphocytes (WHITFIELD et al 1976), hepatocytes (MACMANUS et al. 1973), kidney tubule cells and parotid gland acinar cells (DURHAM et al. 1974) show substantial surges of cyclic AMP at the beginning of prereplicative development, suggesting that cyclic AMP may have a positive effect on growth. It is possible that different cells respond to cyclic nucleotides in fundamentally different ways, such dissimilarities resulting from different embryonic origins (PASTAN and WILLINGHAM 1979). Another possibility arises from the proposal (RUSSEL 1978) that the stimulatory and inhibitory effects of cyclic AMP on growth are conveyed by protein kinase type I and type II respectively. Although there is little experimental evidence to validate such a scheme it raises interesting possibilities since differences arise in the complement of type I and type II protein kinase in normal and neoplastic tissues (RIOU et al. 1977; HANDSCHIN and EPPENBERGER 1979).

An exogenous supply of dibutyryl cyclic AMP produces regression of the Walker carcinoma in vivo. Two cell populations can be distinguished, one regressing (dibutyryl cyclic AMP responsive) and the other growing (dibutyryl cyclic AMP unresponsive) under dibutyryl cyclic AMP treatment (CHO-CHUNG and GULLINO 1974a). The unresponsive tumour has been shown to have a decreased binding of cyclic AMP compared with the responsive tumour, and a higher apparent dissociation constant, K_d, for cyclic AMP binding and unsaturability of cyclic AMP binding in response to elevated cyclic AMP levels in vivo (CHO-CHUNG and CLAIR 1975). There is also a decreased stimulation of cyclic-AMP-dependent protein kinase in the unresponsive tumour. Whereas protein kinase acitivity in the cytosol of the responsive tumour is stimulated about fivefold by cyclic AMP, the enzyme in the unresponsive tumour is stimulated only twofold (CHO-CHUNG et al. 1977a). Cyclic AMP also causes a decrease in the K_m for ATP in the enzyme from the responsive tumour, but has no effect on the affinity of the enzyme for ATP in the unresponsive tumour.

Total nuclear cyclic AMP binding in the responsive tumour is increased threefold within 1 day of dibutyryl cyclic AMP treatment. This increase in nuclear binding is accompanied by a 50% decrease in total cytoplasmic cyclic AMP binding (CHO-CHUNG et al. 1977b). The same treatment produces no change in the binding by unresponsive tumour cytosol or nuclei. Using a cell-free system it has been shown (CHO-CHUNG et al. 1977c) that cytoplasmic cyclic-AMP-binding protein-cyclic AMP complex from responsive tumour binds to isolated nuclei from both responsive and unresponsive tumours, whereas the complex from the unresponsive tumour binds neither nuclei. This suggests that the lack of nuclear accumulation of cyclic-AMP-binding proteins and protein kinase observed in unresponsive Walker tumour could have been due to a defect in cytoplasmic cyclic-AMP-binding proteins which fail to interact with nuclear components.

Resistance to dibutyryl cyclic AMP is also accompanied by shifts in the molecular weights of cyclic-AMP-binding proteins and protein kinase. Cytosol from the responsive tumour exhibits three major peaks of cyclic-AMP-binding activity sedimenting at 4.3S, 5.6S and 6.9S (CHO-CHUNG et al. 1977b). The cytosol also contains cyclic-AMP-independent and -dependent forms of protein kinase sedimenting at 3.3S, 5.6S and 6.9S. In the unresponsive tumour cytosol, the binding component of 4.3S and the protein kinase fraction of 3.3S decrease while the higher molecular weight forms of these proteins (> 7S) increase. Treatment with dibutyryl cyclic AMP results in a shifting of the heavier binding and kinase fractions to their respective lighter components in the responsive, but not in the unresponsive, tumour (CHO-CHUNG et al. 1977b). The major cyclic-AMP-binding components of the responsive tumour cytosol show electrophoretic mobilities distinctive from those in the unresponsive tumour cytosol.

These data suggest that the nuclear accumulation of cyclic-AMP-binding proteins and protein kinase may play an important role in the cyclic-AMP-mediated control of growth and that a molecular lesion in cyclic-AMP-binding proteins could be a cause of dibutyryl cyclic AMP unresponsiveness.

III. Role of Cyclic AMP in Regression of Hormone-Dependent Mammary Tumours

Growth of two hormone-dependent rat mammary tumours in vivo is arrested by treatment of the animals with dibutyryl cyclic AMP (CHO-CHUNG and GULLINO 1974b). While the oestrogen content does not change, acid ribonuclease activity and synthesis increase twofold during treatment with dibutyryl cyclic AMP, as shown during tumour regression due to hormonal deprivation. Growth arrest thus appears to derive from enhanced tissue catabolism.

Most 7,12-dimethylbenz(a)anthracene (DMBA)-induced mammary tumours regress after ovariectomy of the host, indicating a dependence of tumour growth on ovarian steroids (HUGGINS et al. 1969). Ovarian-dependent tumours have been shown to contain specific oestrogen-binding proteins in the tumour cytosol and oestrogen-binding activity decreases in regressing tumour cytosols following ovariectomy and also treatment with dibutyryl cyclic AMP (BODWIN and CHO-CHUNG 1977). This suggests that dibutyryl cyclic AMP treatment mimics oestrogen deprivation in the growth control of a hormone-dependent mammary tumour. This is strengthened by the observation that cyclic AMP levels are significantly elevated in regressing DMBA-induced tumours after ovariectomy (MATUSIK and HILF 1976). In addition to the increase in cyclic AMP content the cyclic-AMP-binding activity as well as the activities of adenylate cyclase and cyclic-AMP phosphodiesterase increase in regressing tumours after either ovariectomy or dibutyryl cyclic AMP treatment (BODWIN et al. 1977). The increase in intracellular cyclic AMP and adenylate cyclase and phosphodiesterase activities subside in those tumours resuming growth following the injection of oestradiol valerate or cessation of dibutyryl cyclic AMP treatment. When DMBA-induced tumours fail to regress after ovariectomy the change in activities binding cyclic AMP and oestrogen does not occur. Concomitant with the increase of cyclic-AMP-binding activity the activity of type II isoenzyme of protein kinase also increases (CHO-CHUNG et al. 1978). This suggests that the type II protein kinase is involved in the regression of hormone-dependent mammary tumours.

Regression of DMBA-induced mammary carcinoma of rats by either ovariectomy or treatment with dibutyryl cyclic AMP is associated with a new non-histone protein species becoming the predominant endogenous substrate of cyclic-AMP-dependent protein kinase in tumour nuclei (CHO-CHUNG and REDLER 1977). Phosphorylation of this regression-associated protein ceases when resumption of tumour growth is induced either by the injection of 17β-oestradiol or cessation of dibutyryl cyclic AMP treatment.

An inverse relationship appears to exist between oestrogen and cyclic-AMP-binding activities in DMBA-induced tumours, i.e. as the oestrogen-binding activity decreases the cyclic-AMP-binding activity increases. These reciprocal changes in cyclic AMP and oestrogen-binding activities are detectable within 1 day of either ovariectomy or dibutyryl cyclic AMP treatment. The mechanism of growth inhibition probably involves nuclear protein phosphorylation. It also appears that cyclic AMP levels are low in oestrogen target tissues that are under a physiological concentration of oestrogen and high under supraphysiological and subphysiological concentrations of oestrogen. Increased levels of cyclic AMP have also been found in DMBA-induced tumours that are regressing due to inhibition of prolactin secretion or insulin deficiency (MATUSIK and HILF 1976).

Treatment with dibutyryl cyclic AMP may be useful in those patients having oestrogen receptor (ER) negative mammary tumours who do not respond to antioestrogens, since dibutyryl cyclic-AMP-induced regression appears neither to be related to hormone dependency nor restricted to mammary carcinomas (CHO-CHUNG 1974). Also the relative concentrations of ER- and cyclic-AMP-binding protein (CR) in tumour cytosol may be a more sensitive indicator of hormone dependency than measurement of ER alone. In a study of 70 rat mammary tumours 95% of hormone-dependent tumours had an ER/CR ratio of 35×10^{-3} or more, whereas 97% of hormone-independent tumours had ratios of less that 35×10^{-3} (BODWIN et al. 1980). When ER alone was measured hormone dependency could only be predicted in 60% of the tumours. Whether the correlation of these two binding activities with hormone dependency is applicable to human carcinomas has still to be determined.

IV. Role of Cyclic AMP in Growth Inhibition by the Antitumour Alkylating Agents

The cytotoxic effects of the bifunctional alkylating agents have been attributed to an interaction with the DNA of the target cells (LAWLEY 1966), resulting in both inter- and intrastrand cross-linking (WALKER 1971). All alkylating antitumour agents cause a time-dependent inhibition of the incorporation of labelled thymidine into DNA, which has been largely interpreted as indicating an inhibition of DNA synthesis by these agents.

Resistance to anticancer drugs has often proved useful in establishing the biochemical mechanism of growth inhibition. The high chemical reactivity of the alkylating agents enables reaction with a variety of cellular nucleophiles, which makes it difficult to establish the important reaction in growth inhibition. If the mechanism of the antitumour activity of the alkylating agents solely involved interaction with DNA then differences in binding or extent of excision of alkylated bases might be expected between sensitive and resistant cells. However, nitrogen-mustard-sensitive and – resistant Yoshida sarcomas have a similar chromosome number, growth rate, nucleic acid, protein and free thiol content (BALL et al. 1966). Also, while *Escherichia coli* cells resistant to bifunctional alkylating agents can excise the bifunctional alkylated guanine moieties from their DNA (LAWLEY and BROOKS 1965), there appears to be no difference between sensitive and resistant Yoshida sarcoma cells in the level of alkylation of their DNA, the rate of excision of alkylated moieties or in their ability to carry out non-semi-conservative DNA synthesis following treatment with mustard gas (BALL and ROBERTS 1970). The repair inhibitors chloroquine and caffeine are effective in rendering cyclophosphamide-resistant plasmacytomas sensitive to the action of cyclophosphamide, nitrogen mustard and X-rays (GAUDIN and YIELDING 1969). However, these results do not provide direct evidence that repair capacity is implicated in tumour resistance.

Evidence that mitotic inhibition by nitrogen mustard is more complex than simple inhibition of DNA synthesis and action by cross-linkage is suggested by the in vivo protection against bone marrow (WEISSBERG et al. 1978) and intestinal mucosa damage (LIEBERMAN et al. 1970) by cycloheximide. Protection of the suppressive effect of nitrogen mustard on bone marrow DNA synthesis is achieved with concentrations of cycloheximide having no effect on protein synthesis. DETKE et al. (1980) have shown that chlorambucil inhibits the replication of DNA indirectly as well as inhibiting the appearance of newly synthesized histones and non-histone proteins on chromatin.

There is a similarity in some of the biochemical effects produced by cyclophosphamide and those produced by cyclic AMP. Both agents cause growth arrest in the G_2-phase of the cell cycle (BARLOGIE and DREWINKO 1978; STAMBROOK and VELEZ 1976). Cyclophosphamide injected into rats bearing Jensen sarcomas produces a hyperglycaemia which last up to 72 h (SCHMIDT 1970) and reduces the total amounts of both lipid and phospholipid (DINESCU and TAUTU 1965). This is equivalent to the well-known glycogenolytic and lipolytic effects of cyclic AMP (ROBISON et al. 1971). Cyclophosphamide lowers plasma and erythrocyte cholesterol in rats (PROKES and APPAWU 1970). This effect could also be mediated by cyclic AMP since the latter has been shown to inhibit the conversion of acetate to cholesterol in broken cell preparations from liver (ROBISON et al. 1971). Cyclophosphamide causes a rise in tyrosine transaminase in the livers of rats (POPOV et al. 1972), in ornithine decarboxylase in plasmacytomas of hamsters (TOMISEK et al. 1972) and in alkaline phosphatase activity (LEE et al. 1973). These enzymes are thought to be induced by cyclic AMP (CHONG-CHENG and OLIVER 1972; BYUS and RUSSELL 1975, KOYAMA et al. 1972). Interferon production in response to Sendai virus in mice is inhibited during the early stages of the disease with cyclophosphamide (ROBINSON and HEATH 1968). Production of interferon is also prevented by exposure of activated lymphocytes to substances which elevate cyclic AMP (BOURNE et al. 1974). The metabolite of cyclophosphamide, 4-hydroxycyclophosphamide, which is thought to be responsible for the antitumour effects, competes with cyclic AMP for binding to both cyclic AMP phosphodiesterase and the regulatory subunit of the cyclic-AMP-dependent protein kinase holoenzyme (TISDALE 1977 a). Binding to the latter causes an activation of the kinase and results in a dissociation into regulatory and catalytic subunits.

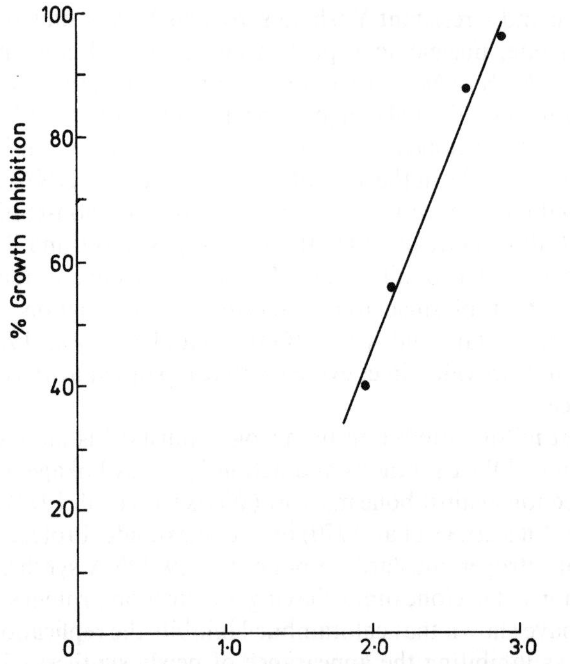

Fig. 1. Relationship between the percentage inhibition of growth of Walker carcinoma in tissue culture by chlorambucil and the intracellular level of cyclic AMP

1. Effect on Cyclic AMP Phosphodiesterase

The bifunctional alkylating agents have been shown to cause an elevation of the intracellular level of cyclic AMP in sensitive tumour cells which is linearly related to the dose required to produce growth inhibition (TISDALE and PHILLIPS 1975, a, c) (Fig. 1). Such an effect is not produced by monofunctional analogues and is not observed in cells resistant to the cytotoxic effect of these drugs. The increase in cyclic AMP appears to be due, at least in part, to the inhibition of the low-K_m form of the cyclic nucleotide phosphodiesterase, since only this form of the enzyme is inhibited and only in sensitive cells when an effect on cell growth and cyclic AMP content is observed (TISDALE and PHILLIPS 1975 a). Enzyme kinetic studies show that chlorambucil inhibits the low-K_m form of the phosphodiesterase with a velocity constant for inactivation three times that for inhibition of the high-K_m form (TISDALE 1974), while the monofunctional *N*-ethyl analogue of chlorambucil is ineffective as an inhibitor of either form of the enzyme. The greater sensitivity of the low-K_m form of the enzyme to the inhibitory effects of bifunctional alkylating agents may be due to linking of subunits or parts of the tertiary structure which would leave the enzyme permanently in its inactive form. The high-K_m form of the enzyme obeys Michaelis-Menten kinetics and might be expected to have a simpler tertiary structure which does not require a conformational change for activity.

The cyclic AMP phosphodiesterase of most tissues behaves kinetically as if two separate activities exist, one with a low affinity and the other with a high af-

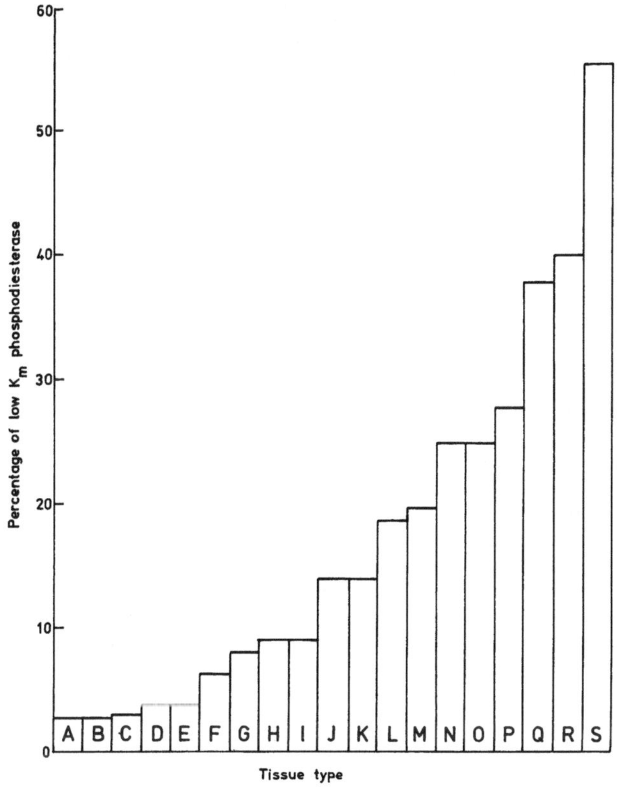

Fig. 2. Contribution of the high-affinity form of the phosphodiesterase to the total activity in: *A*, adipose tissue; *B*, muscle; *C*, HeLa cells; *D*, liver: *E*, mouse fibroblasts A9; *F*, sarcoma 180; *G*, W_{CHL3}; *H*, W_{CHL2}; *I*, NK lymphoma; *J*, W_{CHL1}; *K*, pancreas; *L*, gastrointestinal mucosa; *M*, platelets; *N*, PC6 plasmacytoma; *O*, hepatoma 3924A; *P*, bone marrow; *Q*, Walker carcinoma sensitive; *R*, Novikoff N151–67; *S*, lymphocytes

finity for the substrate. In Walker carcinoma and PC6 plasmacytoma, tumours which are sensitive to alkylating agents, the apparent V_{max} of the high-affinity forms represents 38% and 25% respectively of the total activity (Tisdale and Phillips 1975b). Similarly bone marrow and intestinal mucosa, tissues which are also sensitive to alkylating agent cytotoxicity, have a high contribution of the high-affinity form of the phosphodiesterase to the total activity (28% and 20% respectively) (Fig. 2). In those tumours which are naturally resistant to the alkylating agents such as NK lymphoma and Sarcoma 180, as well as normal tissues not suspectible to alkylating agent cytotoxicity such as muscle and liver, the high-affinity form contributes less than 10% of the total activity (Fig. 2). In Walker carcinoma showing a 20-fold resistance to chlorambucil, the V_{max} of the low-K_m form is decreased to 15% of the total, while in a 70-fold-resistant line the contribution of the low-K_m form is further decreased to 9% (Fig. 2, Table 1). This decrease in the activity of the high-affinity form of the enzyme in resistant tumours does not appear to be due to the presence of an endogenous inhibitor. Thus a correlation appears to exist between sensitivity of tissues to alkylating agents

Table 1. Sensitivity of Walker cell lines to chlorambucil and dibutyryl cyclic AMP, specific cyclic-AMP-binding activity at pH 4.0, apparent K_a values for activation of protein kinase, K_m and V_{max} of the low-K_m form of the cyclic AMP phosphodiesterase and inhibition constant for dibutyryl cyclic AMP[a]

Cell line	LD_{50} μg/ml		Binding activity pmol/mg protein	Apparent $K_a \times 10^{-7} M$	K_m μM	V_{max} nmol/min/mg protein	K_i μM
	Chlorambucil	Dibutyryl cyclic AMP					
WS	0.045	32	13.3	1.8	0.7	0.27	42.0
WCHL 1	1.9	48	7.8	3.0	2.2	0.13	13.2
WCHL 2	4.6	100	7.5	7.5	1.7	0.12	21.8
WCHL 3	9.0	150	6.9	20	4.5	0.09	52.0

[a] Cell lines with increasing resistance to chlorambucil were developed as described (TISDALE and PHILLIPS 1976a). Drug sensitivity was determined by daily recording of cell number, which was then used to construct dose-response curves. Chlorambucil was dissolved in dimethyl sulphoxide and dibutyryl cyclic AMP in Dulbecco's modified Eagle medium. Cyclic-AMP binding was determined by the filtration method on cytosolic extracts of cell lines in 50 mM sodium acetate, pH 4.0, using 80 nM 8-[^{3}H]cyclic AMP. The K_a value is the concentration of cyclic AMP producing half maximal stimulation of protein kinase determined by the method of TISDALE and PHILLIPS (1976b). Cyclic AMP phosphodiesterase was determined as described (TISDALE and PHILLIPS 1975b). Incubations were carried out at 35 °C for a time interval which gave less than 10% hydrolysis of the substrate and 8-[^{3}H]5'AMP was separated from 8-[^{3}H]cyclic AMP by thin-layer chromatography. Lineweaver-Burk plots were constructed from initial rate measurements and the K_m and K_i values determined from the slopes of the lines in the absence and presence of dibutyryl cyclic AMP

and the cytoplasmic concentration of the high-affinity form of the cyclic AMP phosphodiesterase.

Using Sepharose 6B gel filtration the cyclic AMP phosphodiesterase of Walker carcinoma can be separated into four active forms with apparent molecular weights of >1000000, 430000, 350000 and 225000 when assayed at low substrate concentration (TISDALE 1975). The loss of enzyme activity with the acquisition of resistance appears to be due to a reduction in the specific activity of the forms with molecular weights 430000 and 350000 (Fig. 3) rather than to a general loss of enzyme activity. This suggests that these forms are important in binding of the bifunctional alkylating agents.

There is also an alteration of the pH optimum of the high-affinity form of the phosphodiesterase in resistant tumours. The pH optima of the enzymes with both high and low affinity for the substrate is pH 8.0 in the sensitive Walker carcinoma (TISDALE 1975). In the resistant tumour the pH optimum of the high-affinity form is shifted to pH 8.4 while the low-affinity form remains at pH 8.0. These results provide evidence for a change in the tertiary structure of the high-affinity form of the phosphodiesterase in resistant tumours.

The high-affinity forms of the phosphodiesterase from sensitive and resistant Walker carcinoma can further be distinguished by their response to inhibition by the methyl-xanthine, theophylline. In both cases inhibition is of the competitive type, but K_i values were calculated to be 2.35 and 0.32 mM for the enzyme from sensitive and resistant tumours respectively. The lower inhibition constant for the resistant tumour correlates with its greater sensitivity to theophylline (LD_{50}

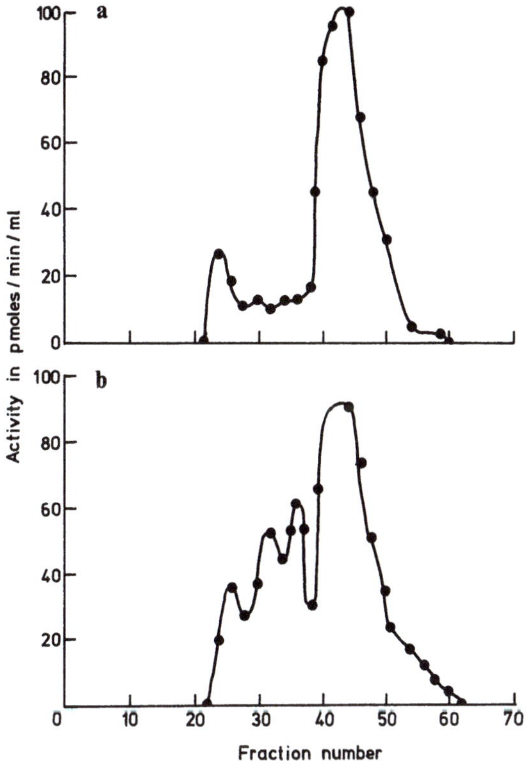

Fig. 3a, b. Sepharose 6B gel filtration of resistant (**a**) and sensitive (**b**) Walker carcinoma $100\,000 \times g$ supernatant fraction in 40 m*M* Tris-HCl, pH 7.5, containing 10 m*M* $MgCl_2$ and 10 m*M* 2-mercaptoethanol. A volume of 2.5 ml total supernatant containing 27.5 mg protein was applied to a column (110×1.8 cm) and elution was performed with Tris-$MgCl_2$-mercaptoethanol buffer. Flow rate was 0.5 ml/min. Fractions of 3 ml were collected and phosphodiesterase activity was determined at a cyclic AMP concentration of 5 μ*M* using the method of TISDALE (1975)

150 μg/ml) compared with the sensitive line (LD_{50} 250 μg/ml) (TISDALE and PHILLIPS 1975a). These results further suggest an alteration of the primary structure of the catalytic site of the enzyme in the resistant tumour.

2. Effect on Specific Cyclic-AMP-Binding Proteins

When compared with sensitive cells alkylating-agent-resistant Walker carcinomas show a loss of specific cyclic-AMP-binding activity with increasing resistance (Table 1) (TISDALE and PHILLIPS 1976a). A similar decrease in specific cytosolic binding of cyclic GMP has also been observed with increasing resistance of Walker cells to alkylating agents (TISDALE and PHILLIPS 1977). This suggests that both cyclic AMP and cyclic GMP bind with the same proteins, as suggested previously for neuroblastoma cells in culture (PRASAD et al. 1975). Since cyclic AMP is believed to exert its biological effects by binding to a specific cytosolic protein, it might be expected that resistance to alkylating agents might be accompanied by resistance to growth inhibition by cyclic AMP. The results in Table 1 show that resistance to dibutyryl cyclic AMP increases with increasing resistance to chlorambucil. Mouse lymphosarcoma cells resistant to the cytotoxic effect of

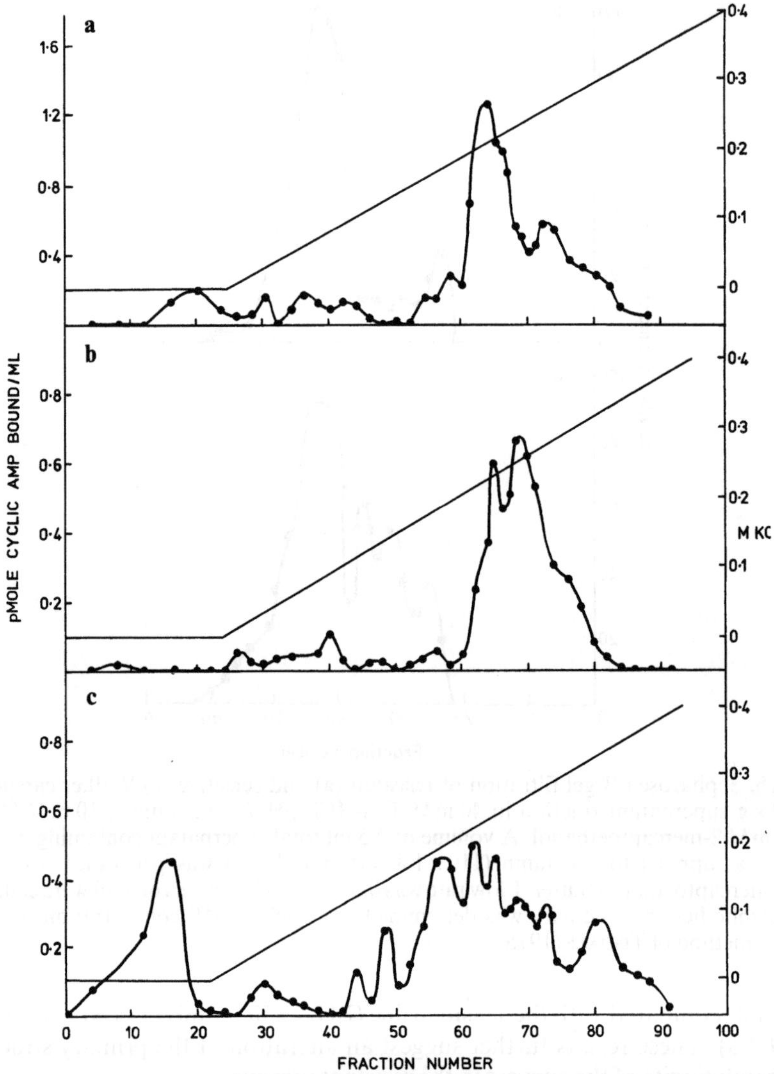

Fig. 4 a–c. DEAE cellulose chromatography of cyclic-AMP-binding protein from sensitive Walker cells (**a**) and those with a 32-fold (**b**) and 16000-fold (**c**) resistance to CB 1954. For each cell line 4.3 mg total cell protein in 1 ml 100 m*M* Tris-HCl, pH 8.1, was applied to the column and fractions of 1 ml were collected. When 24 ml had been eluted from the column and linear salt gradient from 0 to 0.4 *M* KCl was applied so that the total volume eluted from the column was 100 ml

dibutyryl cyclic AMP also contain less cytoplasmic cyclic-AMP-binding proteins and decreased cyclic-AMP-stimulated protein kinase activity compared with the sensitive line (Daniel et al. 1973).

In addition to differences in inhibition of the low-K_m form of the cyclic-AMP phosphodiesterase in chlorambucil-resistant Walker cell lines differences are also apparent in the K_i values towards N^6-monobutyryl cyclic AMP (Table 1). In each case Lineweaver-Burk plots indicate that inhibition at low substrate concentrations is of the non-competitive type, while at high substrate concentrations it is of the competitive type. Dibutyryl cyclic AMP is believed to mediate its growth inhibitory effect by deacylation to N^6-monobutyryl cyclic AMP, which then acts as an inhibitor of cyclic AMP phosphodiesterase. Thus the differences in K_i values of monobutyryl cyclic AMP to the phosphodiesterases in each of the cell lines will affect the LD_{50} values for growth inhibition, particularly since the K_i values are increased in two of the resistant cell lines. If the K_i values in Table 1 are taken into account the cross-resistance of each of the cell lines resistant to chlorambucil is about fivefold. Differences in extent of inhibition at high substrate concentrations need not be taken into account since the K_m value (80 μM) of this form of the enzyme is much higher than the intracellular level of cyclic AMP (2 μM) and would not be expected to play a major role in the regulation of cyclic AMP levels under normal conditions.

The binding proteins from alkylating-agent-resistant cells are also more sensitive to temperature than those from sensitive cells, suggesting a difference in conformation of the receptor (TISDALE and PHILLIPS 1978). Both 2-mercaptoethanol and 5′,5′ dithiobis (2-nitrobenzoic acid) increase the temperature sensitivity, with 2-mercaptoethanol producing a greater effect on the proteins from the resistant lines. The binding proteins from neuroblastoma cells resistant to the cytotoxic effect of dibutyryl cyclic AMP have also been shown to be more sensitive to temperature than the binding proteins from sensitive cells (SIMANTOV and SACHS 1975). However, 2-mercaptoethanol was reported to decrease the temperature sensitivity of the binding proteins from neuroblastoma cells.

Diethylaminoethyl (DEAE) cellulose chromatography of cyclic-AMP-binding proteins from Walker cells sensitive to 5(1-aziridinyl)2,-4-dinitrobenzamide (CB 1954) or those with a 32-fold or 16000-fold resistance is shown in Fig. 4. Since both sensitive and resistance cells contain the same amount of protein per cell the specific activities can be compared directly. In addition to the decrease in concentration of specific binding proteins with increasing resistance, the peaks of activity for the individual cell lines differ in the salt concentration at which they elute, suggesting that they differ in ionic charge.

3. Alterations in Protein Kinase Acitivty

The major cyclic-AMP-binding protein is believed to be the regulatory subunit of the cyclic-AMP-dependent protein kinase. Treatment of sensitive Walker carcinoma with chlorambucil (5 μg/ml) causes an activation of a cyclic-AMP-dependent protein kinase with a time-course paralleling the effect on cyclic AMP levels (TISDALE and PHILLIPS 1976b). Activation of kinase after chlorambucil treatment also occurs in resistant cells, though much higher levels of the drug are required (100 μg/ml). The degree of stimulation of cytosolic protein kinase by saturating concentrations of cyclic AMP and the apparent dissociation constant for cyclic AMP bound to protein kinase decrease with increasing resistance of the cell lines to alkylating agents (Table 1). There is a progressive decrease in the activity of type I protein kinase with increasing resistance of Walker carcinoma to the alkylating agents (TISDALE and PHILLIPS 1978). Heterogeneous reconstituted holoenzymes using separated subunits from sensitive and resistant cells show defects in both regulatory and catalytic subunits of protein kinase in resistant cells. Mutant S49 mouse lymphoma cells which exhibit a tenfold resistance to the biological effects of cyclic AMP also show an altered regulatory component of the protein kinase holoenzyme, which leads to an apparent K_a' for activation by cyclic AMP which is tenfold greater than for the wild type (HOCKMAN et al. 1975).

The reduction of binding protein per cell, as well as alterations in the molecular structure of the regulatory and catalytic components of the protein kinase holoenzyme, explain the cross-resistance of the alkylating-agent-resistant cell lines to dibutyryl cyclic AMP and suggest a fundamental role for cyclic AMP in the mechanism of action of the cytotoxic alkylating agents.

4. Possible Role of Cyclic AMP in the Cytotoxic Action of Alkylating Agents

One possible role for the elevation of cyclic AMP in response to an alkylating agent in sensitive, but not in resistant cells, could be inhibition of repair of DNA damage. The methyl-xanthines, caffeine and theophylline, both inhibitors of cyclic AMP phosphodiesterase, inhibit postreplication repair of DNA in mammalian cells. This raises the possibility that there may be some connection between the intracellular level of cyclic AMP and postreplication repair. Cyclic AMP has been shown to modify the postirradiation survival of mammalian cells (LEHNERT 1975), protecting against low doses of radiation, but increasing the radiosensitivity at high doses of radiation. However, experiments using a cyclic-AMP-resistant mouse lymphoma cell mutant and its wild-type counterpart show no connection between cellular cyclic AMP concentrations and the rate of postreplication repair (EHMANN et al. 1976). Similarly, Walker carcinoma, which is sensitive to the inhibitory effect of caffeine on postreplication repair of DNA damage after treatment with chlorambucil, is unaffected by analogues of either cyclic AMP or cyclic GMP. This is, perhaps, surprising, since cyclic AMP has been shown to inhibit DNA polymerase (TISDALE 1980), and it seems likely that postreplication repair and normal DNA synthesis work by closely related mechanisms (LEHMANN 1974).

Another possible role for the increased cyclic AMP in alkylating-agent-sensitive cell lines could be related to nuclear protein phosphorylation. Chlorambucil, melphalan and cyclophosphamide have been shown to induce nuclear protein phosphorylation after in vivo treatment of Yoshida sarcoma sensitive to alkylating agents, but not in resistant tumour cells (RICHES et al. 1977; WILKINSON et al. 1979). Such nuclear protein phosphorylation may modify transcriptional activity, DNA-protein cross-linking or the ability to repair alkylated DNA.

V. Effect of Other Antitumour Agents on the Cyclic Nucleotide System

In addition to the bifunctional alkylating agents the antitumor agent 5-(3,3-dimethyl-1-triazeno)imidazole-4-carboxamide (DTIC), which also has alkylating properties, has been shown to inhibit the low-K_m form of cyclic AMP phosphodiesterase from rat liver (LARSSON et al. 1979). Treatment of intact isolated hepatocytes and cultured hepatoma cells with DTIC causes an increase in both basal and hormone-stimulated cyclic AMP.

Cyclic AMP phosphodiesterase may be an important target for other antineoplastic agents with alkylating activity. Two antitumour diazoketones have been shown to cause a greater inhibition of cyclic AMP phosphodiesterase than of other cytoplasmic enzymes (JULLIEN and KALOFOUTIS 1976).

Both vincristine and vinblastine have been shown to increase cyclic AMP levels in lymphoma cells (KOTANI et al. 1978). Although there is a depression of cyclic AMP phosphodiesterase activity, this is probably insufficient to explain the increase in intracellular cyclic AMP and it is possible that *Vinca* alkaloids elevate cyclic AMP concentration in lymphoma cells by interacting with a specific receptor in the plasma membrane.

Methotrexate has also been shown to increase cyclic AMP concentrations 1.65-fold in L5178Y murine lymphoma cells after 1 h of treatment (KREML et al. 1979). Since methotrexate does not inhibit cyclic AMP phosphodiesterase the increase in cyclic AMP was attributed to accumulation of cells in the G_1-phase of the cell cycle.

Quercetin, a flavenoid known to cause inhibition of ATPase activity and cell growth in vitro, increases cyclic AMP levels in Ehrlich ascites tumour cells (GRAZIANI and CHAYOTH 1977). The level of cyclic AMP was also found to increase in cells treated with ouabain, a specific inhibitor of $(Na^+ + K^+)$-ATPase. This suggests a relationship between ATPase activity and cyclic AMP levels. This result is interesting in view of the recent finding of inhibition of cell membrane ATPase by bifunctional, but not monofunctional, nitrogen mustard (SPURGIN and HICKMAN 1979).

The relationship between the elevation of intracellular cyclic AMP and the antitumour activity of these agents is not known.

B. Prostaglandins

The prostaglandins are a group of essential unsaturated fatty acids which are biosynthesized from polyunsaturated fatty acids in response to a variety of stimuli. The prostaglandins have a large number of actions that vary according to the particular prostaglandin series and the tissue upon which they are acting (KADOWITZ et al. 1975). Generally the prostaglandin E (PGE) and prostaglandin F (PGF) series elicit opposite effects.

Prostaglandins appear to be involved in the control of cell proliferation. Endogenous PGE_2 synthesis has been found to inhibit the growth of virally transformed cells (LINDGREN et al. 1979) and Walker tumour cells in vitro (TISDALE, unpublished results). An inverse relationship has been established between the amount of PGE produced and the proliferation rate of cells (THOMAS et al. 1974). There is evidence of enhanced prostaglandin content and synthetic capacity in a variety of human tumours (EASTY and EASTY 1976). However, the importance and mode of action of the increased tumour prostaglandin levels in modifying tumour growth has yet to be determined, although PGE_2 may restrict cell proliferation by raising the intracellular level of cyclic AMP (THOMAS et al. 1974).

Recently POWLES et al. (1978) have suggested that prostaglandins may be involved in the mechanism of in vivo tumour resistance to antitumour cytotoxic drugs. Concurrent treatment of the host with the prostaglandin synthetase inhibitors indomethacin and flurbiprofen was shown to enhance the sensitivity of a chemoresistant line of Walker carcinoma to the alkylating agent chlorambucil.

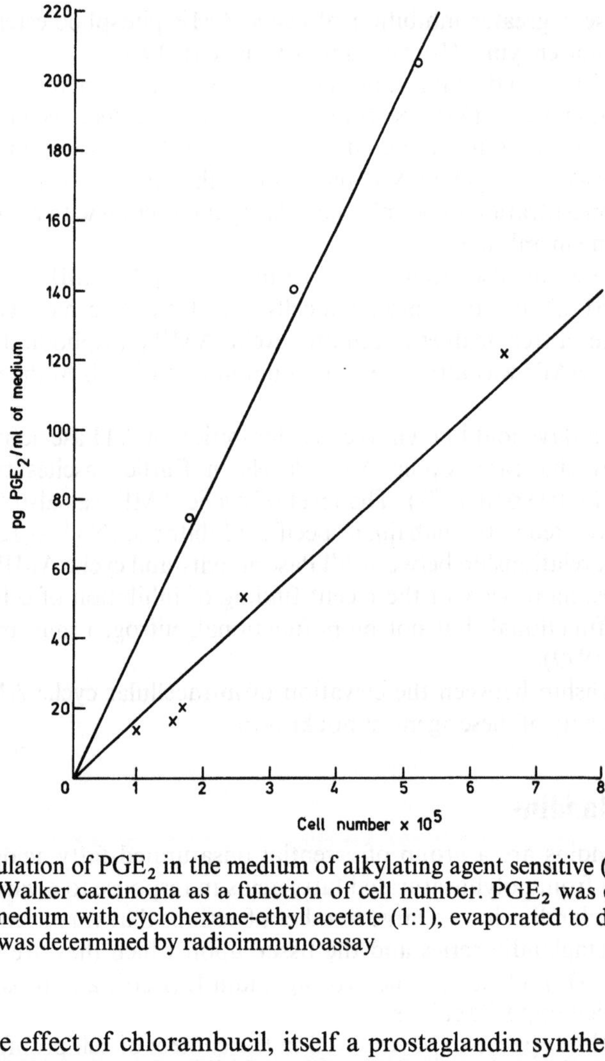

Fig. 5. Accumulation of PGE_2 in the medium of alkylating agent sensitive (×–×) and resistant (o–o) Walker carcinoma as a function of cell number. PGE_2 was extracted from the acidified medium with cyclohexane-ethyl acetate (1:1), evaporated to dryness and the level of PGE_2 was determined by radioimmunoassay

Although the effect of chlorambucil, itself a prostaglandin synthetase inhibitor (TISDALE 1977 b), on growth inhibition of the Walker carcinoma was enhanced by indomethacin, other tissues susceptible to the action of chlorambucil (e.g. bone marrow and gut mucosa) appeared to recover more quickly (POWLES et al. 1978). Combination of flurbiprofen with melphalan and methotrexate also prolongs the survival time of mice (BERSTOCK et al. 1979).

Prostaglandin E_2 (PGE_2) has been found to be an inhibitor of the growth of the Walker carcinoma. At equimolar concentrations PGE_2 causes greater inhibition of chlorambucil-resistant Walker carcinoma (LD_{50} 1.8 μg/ml) than of the sensitive line (LD_{50} 3.4 μg/ml). This may be related to the enhanced production of PGE_2 by the resistant cell line (Fig. 5) (40 pg PGE_2/ml medium/10^5 cells for the resistant tumour and 17 pg PGE_2/ml medium/10^5 cells for sensitive tumour). Indomethacin alone causes growth inhibition of both sensitive and resistant Walker carcinoma in vitro and causes a reduction in PGE_2 production. At low concentrations, chlorambucil also inhibits secretion of both PGE_2 and $PGF_{2\alpha}$ by

Walker carcinoma, though at high concentrations (>0.25 μg/ml) an enhancement of prostaglandin synthesis occurs.

Recent evidence (De Mello et al. 1980) suggests that prostaglandins do not have a role in the cytostatic action of anti-inflammatory drugs since the prostaglandins and arachidonic acid do not reverse the effects of indomethacin and in high concentrations also inhibit growth. Also it seems unlikely that prostaglandins secreted by tumour cells protect against growth inhibition by chlorambucil since the combination of chlorambucil and indomethacin acts subadditively to control growth.

C. Conclusion

Resistance to anticancer drugs, whether natural or acquired, is one of the major limitations to cancer chemotherapy. Investigations into the mode of action of cytotoxic agents as well as the mechanism of resistance may give insight into improvement of current therapeutic regimens. Thus concurrent treatment of alkylating-agent-resistant neoplasms with a cyclic AMP analogue in addition to the alkylating agent may produce synergism if the inability to raise cyclic AMP levels is important in the mechanism of resistance. Likewise oestrogen-receptor-negative mammary tumours may respond to dibutyryl cyclic AMP in a manner similar to hormone-dependent tumours after either ovariectomy or high-oestrogen therapy. Further research at the clinical level needs to be carried out to investigate the role of cyclic AMP in the mechanism of drug resistance.

References

Ball CR, Roberts JJ (1970) DNA repair after mustard gas alkylation by sensitive and resistant Yoshida sarcoma cells in vitro. Chem Biol Interact 2:321–329

Ball CR, Connors TA, Double JA, Uzhazy V, Whisson ME (1966) Comparison of nitrogen mustard-sensitive and -resistant Yoshida sarcomas. Int J Cancer 1:319–327

Barlogie B, Drewinko B (1978) Cell cycle stage-dependent induction of G_2 phase arrest by different antitumour agents. Eur J Cancer 14:741–745

Berstock DA, Houghton J, Bennett A (1979) Improved anticancer effect by combining cytotoxic drugs with an inhibitor of prostaglandin synthesis. Cancer Treat Rev 6 (Suppl):69–71

Bodwin JS, Cho-Chung YS (1977) Decreased estrogen binding in hormone-dependent mammary carcinoma following ovariectomy or dibutyryl cyclic AMP treatment. Cancer Lett 3:289–294

Bodwin JS, Clair T, Cho-Chung YS (1977) Role of estrogen receptor and cyclic AMP-binding protein in the growth control of hormone-dependent mammary carcinoma. Proc Am Assoc Cancer Res 18:117

Bodwin JS, Clair T, Cho-Chung YS (1980) Relationship of hormone dependency to estrogen receptor and adenosine 3′,5′-cyclic monophosphate-binding proteins in rat mammary tumours. J Natl Cancer Inst 64:395–398

Bombik BM, Burger MM (1973) cAMP and the cell cycle: inhibition of growth stimulation. Exp Cell Res 88:88–94

Bourne HR, Lichtenstein LM, Melmon KL, Henney S, Weinstein Y, Shearer GM (1974) Modulation of inflammation and immunity by cyclic AMP. Science 184:19–28

Bourne HR, Coffino P, Melmon KL. Tomkins GM, Weinstein Y (1975) Genetic analysis of cyclic AMP in a mammalian cell. In: Drummond GI, Greengard P, Robison GA (eds) Advances in cyclic nucleotide research, vol 5. Raven, New York, p 771

Byus CV, Russell DH (1975) Ornithine decarboxylase activity: control by cyclic nucleotides. Science 187:650–652

Cho-Chung YS (1974) In vivo inhibition of tumor growth by cyclic adenosine 3′,5′-monophosphate derivatives. Cancer Res 34:3492–3496

Cho-Chung YS, Clair T (1975) The role of cAMP in neoplastic cell growth and regression. III. Altered cAMP-binding in DB cAMP-unresponsive Walker 256 mammary carcinoma. Biochem Biophys Res Commun 64:768–772

Cho-Chung YS, Gullino PM (1974a) Effect of dibutyryl cyclic adenosine 3′,5′-monophosphate on in vivo growth of Walker 256 carcinoma: isolation of responsive and unresponsive cell population. J Natl Cancer Inst 52:995–996

Cho-Chung YS, Gullino PM (1974b) In vivo inhibition of growth of two hormone-dependent mammary tumours by dibutyryl cyclic AMP. Science 183:87–88

Cho-Chung YS, Redler BH (1977) Dibutyryl cyclic AMP mimics ovariectomy: nuclear protein phosphorylation in mammary tumor regression. Science 192:272–275

Cho-Chung YS, Clair T, Yi PN, Parkinson C (1977a) Comparative studies on cyclic AMP binding and protein kinase in cyclic AMP-responsive and -unresponsive Walker 256 mammary carcinomas. J Biol Chem 252:6335–6341

Cho-Chung YS, Clair T, Porper R (1977b) Cyclic AMP-binding proteins and protein kinase during regression of Walker 256 mammary carcinoma. J Biol Chem 252:6342–6348

Cho-Chung YS, Clair T, Huffman P (1977c) Loss of nuclear cyclic AMP binding in cyclic AMP-unresponsive Walker 256 mammary carcinoma. J Biol Chem 252:6349–6355

Cho-Chung YS, Clair T, Zubialde JP (1978) Increase of cyclic AMP-dependent protein kinase type II as an early event in hormone-dependent mammary tumor regression. Biochem Biophys Res Commun 85:1150–1155

Chong-Cheng C, Oliver IT (1972) A translational control mechanism in mammalian protein synthesis modulated by cyclic adenosine monophosphate. Biochemistry 11:2547–2553

Daniel V, Litwack G, Tomkins GM (1973) Induction of cytolysis of cultured lymphoma cells by adenosine 3′,5′ cyclic monophosphate and the isolation of resistant variants. Proc Natl Acad Sci USA 70:76–79

De Mello MCF, Bayer BM, Beaven MA (1980) Evidence that prostaglandins do not have a role in the cytostatic action of anti-inflammatory drugs. Biochem Pharmacol 29:311–318

Detke S, Stein JL, Stein GS (1980) Influence of chlorambucil, a bifunctional alkylating agent on DNA replication and histone gene expression in HeLa S_3 cells. Cancer Res 40:967–974

Dinescu G, Tautu P (1965) Reduction of lipid content of Jensen sarcoma by cyclophosphamide. Studii Cercet Biochim 8:187–190

Durham JP, Baserga R, Butcher FR (1974) The effect of isoproterenol and its analogs upon adenosine 3′,5′-monophosphate and guanosine 3′,5′-monophosphate levels in mouse parotid gland in vivo. Biochim Biophys Acta 372:196–217

Easty G, Easty D (1976) Prostaglandins and cancer. Cancer Treat Rev 3: 217–225

Ehmann UK, Gehring U, Tomkins GM (1976) Caffeine, cyclic AMP and postreplication repair of mammalian cell DNA. Biochim Biophys Acta 447:133–138

Gaudin D, Yielding KL (1969) Response of a resistant plasmacytoma to alkylating agents and X-ray in combination with the excision repair inhibitors caffeine and chloroquinine. Proc Soc Exp Biol Med 131:1413–1416

Graziani Y, Chayoth R (1977) Elevation of cyclic AMP level in Ehrlich ascites tumour cells by quercetin. Biochem Pharmacol 26:1259–1261

Handschin JC, Eppenberger U (1979) Altered cellular ratio of type I and type II cyclic AMP-dependent protein kinase in human mammary tumours. FEBS Lett 106:301–304

Hockman J, Insel PA, Bourne HR, Coffino P, Tomkins GM (1975) A structural gene mutation affecting the regulatory subunit of cyclic AMP-dependent protein kinase in mouse lymphoma cells. Proc Natl Acad Sci USA 72:5051–5055

Huggins C, Brizarelli G, Sutton H (1969) Rapid induction of mammary carcinoma in the rat and the influence of hormones on the tumors. J Exp Med 109:25–41

Jullien GL, Kalofoutis AT (1976) The action of two alkylating agents on the cyclic AMP system. In: Deutsch E, Moser K, Rainer H, Stacher A (eds) Molecular basis of malignancy. Thieme, Stuttgart, p 97

Kadowitz PJ, Joiner PD, Hyman AL (1975) Physiological and pharmacological roles of prostaglandins. Annu Rev Pharmacol Toxicol 15:285–306

Kotani M, Koizumi Y, Yamada T, Kawasaki A, Akabane T (1978) Increase of cyclic adenosine 3′,5′monophosphate concentration in transplantable lymphoma cells by *Vinca* alkaloids. Cancer Res 38:3094–3099

Koyama H, Kato R, Ono T (1972) Induction of alkaline phosphatase by cyclic AMP or its dibutyryl derivative in a hybrid line between mouse and Chinese hamster in culture. Biochem Biophys Res Commun 46:305–311

Kreml JA, Hryniuk WM, Yamada EW (1979) Effect of methotrexate on cyclic AMP levels in cultured L 5 178Y cells. Biochem Med 22:43–49

Larsson PG, Haffner F, Brønstad GO, Christoffersen T (1979) The antitumour agent 5-(3,3-dimethyl-1-triazone) imidazole-4-carboxamide (DTIC) inhibits rat liver cyclic AMP phosphodiesterase and amplifies hormone effects in hepatocytes and hepatoma cells. Br J Cancer 40:768–773

Lawley PD (1966) Effects of some chemical mutagens and carcinogens on nucleic acids. Prog Nulceic Acid Res Mol Biol 5:89–131

Lawley PD, Brookes P (1965) Molecular mechanism of the cytotoxic action of difunctional alkylating agents and of resistance to this action. Nature 206:480–483

Lee CC, Castles TR, Kinter LD (1973) Single-dose toxicity of cyclophosphamide in dogs and monkeys. Cancer Chemother Rep 4:51–76

Lehmann AR (1974) Postreplication repair of DNA in mammalian cells. Life Sci 15:2005–2016

Lehnert S (1975) Modification of postirradiation survival of mammalian cells by intracellular cyclic AMP. Radiat Res 62:107–116

Lieberman MN, Verbin RS, Landay M, Liang H, Farber E, Lee TN, Starr R (1970) A probable role for protein synthesis in intestinal epithelial cell damage induced in vivo by cytosine arabinoside, nitrogen mustard or X-irradiation. Cancer Res 30:942–951

Lindgren J, Glaesson H, Hammarstrom S (1979) Endogenous prostaglandin E_2 synthesis inhibits growth of polyoma virus-transformed 3T3 fibroblasts. Exp Cell Res 124:1–5

MacManus JP, Braceland BM, Youdale T, Whitfield JF (1973) Adrenergic antagonists and a possible link between the increase in cyclic adenosine 3′,5′-monophosphate and DNA synthesis during liver regeneration. J Cell Physiol 82:157–164

Matusik RJ, Hilf R (1976) Relationship of adenosine 3′,5′-cyclic monophosphate to growth of dimethylbenz (α) anthracene-induced mammary tumours in rats. J Natl Cancer Inst. 56:659–661

Otten J, Johnson GS, Pastan I (1972) Regulation of cell growth by adenosine 3′,5′-monophosphate. J Biol Chem 247:7082–7087

Pastan I, Willingham M (1979) Cellular transformation and the morphologic phenotype of transformed cells. Nature 274:645–650

Popov PG, Kaurakirova SV, Belokonski IS, Golovinski E (1972) The effect of some cytostatics on tyrosine aminotransferase activity in rat liver. Acta Biol Med Ger 29:751–755

Powles TJ, Alexander P, Millar JL (1978) Enhancement of anticancer activity of cytotoxic chemotherapy with protection of normal tissues by inhibition of prostaglandin synthesis. Biochem Pharmacol 27:1389–1392

Prasad KN, Sinha PK, Sahu SK, Brown JL (1975) Binding of cyclic nucleotides with soluble proteins. Biochem Biophys Res Commun 66:131–138

Prokes J, Appawu F (1970) The influence of endoxan on cholesterol and its esters in the blood of rats (in Czech). Cesk Farm 19:21–28

Riches PG, Sellwood SM and Harrap KR (1977) Some effects of chlorambucil in nuclear protein phosphorylation in the Yoshida ascites sarcoma. Chem Biol Interact 18:11–22

Riou JP, Evian D, Perrin F, Saez JM (1977) Adenosine 3′,5′-cyclic monophosphate-dependent protein kinase in human adrenocortical tumours. J Clin Endocrinol Metab 44:413–419

Robinson TWE, Heath RB (1968) Effect of cyclophosphamide on the production of interferon. Nature 217:178–179
Robison GA, Butcher RW, Sutherland EW (1971) In: Cyclic AMP. Academic, New York, p 183
Russell DH (1978) Type I cyclic AMP-dependent protein kinase as a positive effector of growth. In. George WJ, Ignarro LJ (eds) Advances in cyclic nucleotide research, vol 4. Raven, New York, p 493
Schmidt GC (1970) Cancerostatic effects of alkylating agents with reference to the glycolysis of tumour cells in vivo. 2 Krebsforsh 73:223–238
Simantov R, Sachs L (1975) Temperature sensitivity of cyclic adenosine 3′,5′-monophosphate binding proteins in the regulation of growth and differentiation in neuroblastoma cells. J Biol Chem 250:3236–3242
Spurgin GE, Hickman JA (1979) Studies on the mode of action of the antitumour drug nitrogen mustard (mustine) J Pharm Pharmacol 31 (Suppl.):68
Stambrook PJ, Velez C (1976) Reversible arrest of Chinese hamster V79 cells in G_2 by dibutyryl cyclic AMP. Exp Cell Res 99:57–62
Thomas P, Philpott G, Jaffe B (1974) The relationship between concentrations of prostaglandin E and rates of cell replication. Exp Cell Res 84:40–46
Tisdale MJ (1974) The reaction of alkylating agents with cyclic 3′,5′-nucleotide phosphodiesterase. Chem Biol Interact 9:145–153
Tisdale MJ (1975) Characterisation of cyclic adenosine 3′,5′-monophosphate phosphodiesterase from Walker carcinoma sensitive and resistant to bifunctional alkylating agents. Biochim Biophys Acta 397:134–143
Tisdale MJ (1977 a) Interaction of cyclophosphamide and its metabolites with adenosine 3′,5′-monophosphate binding proteins. Biochem Pharmacol 28:1469–1474
Tisdale MJ (1977 b) Inhibition of prostaglandin synthetase by anti-tumour agents. Chem Biol Interact 18:91–100
Tisdale MJ (1980) The effect of cyclic nucleotides on DNA polymerase, thymidylate synthetase, thymidine kinase and deoxynucleoside levels of Walker carcinoma. Chem Biol Interact 30:115–124
Tisdale MJ, Phillips BJ (1975 a) inhibition of cyclic 3′,5′-nucleotide phosphodiesterase – a possible mechanism of action of bifunctional alkylating agents. Biochem Pharmacol 24:211–217
Tisdale MJ, Phillips BJ (1975 b) Adenosine 3′,5′-monophosphate phosphodiesterase activity in experimental animal tumours which are either sensitive or resistant to bifunctional alkylating agents. Biochem Pharmacol 24:205–210
Tisdale MJ, Phillips BJ (1975 c) Comparative effects of alkylating agents and other antitumour agents on the intracellular level of adenosine 3′,5′-monophosphate in Walker carcinoma. Biochem Pharmacol 24:1271–1276
Tisdale MJ, Phillips BJ (1976 a) Alterations in adenosine 3′,5′-monophosphate-binding protein in Walker carcinoma cells sensitive or resistant to alkylating agents. Biochem Pharmacol 25:1831–1836
Tisdale MJ, Phillips BJ (1976 b) The effect of alkylating agents on the activity of adenosine 3′,5′-monophosphate dependent protein kinase in Walker carcinoma cells. Biochem Pharmacol 25:2365–2370
Tisdale MJ, Phillips BJ (1977) Guanosine 3′,5′-monophosphate and the action of alkylating agents. Chem Biol Interact 19:375–381
Tisdale MJ, Phillips BJ (1978) Cyclic nucleotide metabolism in Walker carcinoma cells resistant to alkylating agents. Biochem Pharmacol 27:947–952
Tomisek AJ, Allan PW, Chesnutt F, Johnson BT (1972) Some early effects of cyclophosphamide therapy on Fortner plasmacytoma. Chem Biol Interact 4:175–184
Walker IG (1971) Intrastrand bifunctional alkylation of DNA in mammalian cells treated with mustard gas. Can J Biochem 49:332–336
Wang T, Sheppard JR and Foker JE (1978) Rise and fall of cyclic AMP required for onset of lymphocyte DNA synthesis. Science 201:155–157
Weissberg JB, Herion JC, Walker RI, Palmer JG (1978) Effect of cycloheximide on the bone marrow toxicity of nitrogen mustard. Cancer Res 38:1523–1527

Whitfield JF, MacManus JP, Rixon RH, Boynton AL, Youdale T, Swierenga S (1976) The positive control of cell proliferation by the interplay of calcium ions and cyclic nucleotides. In Vitro 12:1–18
Wilkinson R, Birbeck MSC, Harrap KR (1979) Enhancement of the nuclear reactivity of alkylating agents by prednisolone. Cancer Res 39:4256–4262

CHAPTER 14

Properties of Mitochondria

A. K. BELOUSOVA

A. Introduction

Recently it has become evident that antitumor drug resistance is associated with some features of target enzymes and those enzyme systems which participate in drug transport, activation and catabolism (BROCKMAN 1974; BELOUSOVA 1978; BELOUSOVA and GERASIMOVA 1980).

Among the effective antitumor drugs used in the management of clinical cancers, alkylating agents are still of primary importance (ZUBROD 1972; CARTER and SLAVIK 1977). General features of these cytostatics include their ability to alkylate cellular DNA, RNA and proteins, to form DNA-DNA and DNA-protein crosslinks, and to induce the formation of single-strand and double-strand breaks in DNA molecules (LAWLEY and BROOKES 1967; ROSS 1962; ROSS et al. 1978).

Damage to cellular genetic material leads, in turn, to disturbances in DNA replication, transcription and protein synthesis, and to lethal and mutagenic effects (LOVELESS 1966; MITSKEVITSH et al. 1972; KLAMERTH 1973; VEROVSKY and GORBATCHEVA 1979).

The initial degree of DNA alkylation may be the same in cells sensitive and resistant to cytostatics, but in resistant cells defects in DNA structure are effectively eliminated by repair enzymes. Therefore the presence of a potent enzyme system for DNA repair is generally accepted as an appropriate criterion of cell resistance to alkylating agents (ROBERTS 1980).

However, cytotoxic effects of antitumor alkylating agents are not limited to damage to the structure and template functions of DNA and chromatin alone.

B. Damage of Mitochondrial Membranes by Alkylating Agents

It was first shown by BELOUSOVA and colleagues (BELOUSOVA 1965; BELOUSOVA et al. 1964, 1966) that some chloroethylamines with aromatic and more complex carriers (sarcolysine, its dipeptides, and other analogs) are able to uncouple respiration and oxidative phosphorylation in isolated mitochondria of tumor and normal cells.

The detailed study of these effects by ROMANOVA (1971, 1972) suggested that sarcolysine is similar to classic uncouplers of the dinitrophenol type. The uncoupling effect is manifested by (a) the inhibition of ATP synthesis, (b) activation of the latent mitochondrial ATPase and (c) releasing of the respiratory control. Like 2,4-dinitrophenol (DNP), sarcolysine uncouples respiration and phosphorylation at all three points. Similar effects were also shown for chlorophenacyl (GUDZ et al. 1974; YAGUZHINSKY et al. 1976).

The dipeptides of sarcolysine are more potent inhibitors of oxidative phosphorylation than the parental compound. They exhibit a rather strong inhibitory effect on respiration, being in this respect similar to oligomycin (ROMANOVA 1972; BELOUSOVA 1978).

It was found that tumor mitochondria are much more sensitive to the uncoupling action of alkylating agents than those of the liver (BELOUSOVA et al. 1964; BELOUSOVA and ROMANOVA 1971)

During the investigation of in vivo effects of sarcolysine and its dipeptides on oxidative phosphorylation in mitochondria of animal tumors and normal tissues, a correlation between energetics impairment and cytotoxicity was shown (SPASSKAJA et al. 1968; ROMANOVA and SOFÍNA 1969; BELOUSOVA and ROMANOVA 1971).

Among normal tissue spleen and thymus were the most vulnerable to cytostatics, while liver was much less sensitive. The uncoupling effect of cytostatics was maximal in thymus and spleen mitochondria and minimal in those of the liver.

Tumor mitochondria were highly sensitive to uncoupling effects of alkylating agents. Thus in these investigations a positive correlation between uncoupling effects and cytotoxicity of antitumor alkylating agents was found.

C. The Structure and Functions of Energy-Coupling Complexes in Mitochondria

The enzymes of respiration and oxidative phosphorylation are known to be built up into the inner membrane of mitochondria as repeated multienzyme complexes (GREEN 1974) (Fig. 1). Each complex contains, in its basal part, three units of the respiratory electron transfer chain and a transhydrogenase. At the inner side of this complex there is an energy-transforming unit, which, in turn, is composed of two subunits: the headpiece (factor F_1) and the basepiece (factor F_0). Both subunits form an ATPase complex, which accomplishes the transformation of substrate oxidation energy into the high-energy phosphoanhydride bond of ATP.

The molecular mechanism of coupling is not yet understood. Several different hypotheses exist concerning the nature of the primary intermediate which acquires energy directly from the substrate oxidation and which is used as an energy donor for ATP synthesis (RACKER 1976).

The "chemical" hypothesis (SLATER 1966; RACKER 1976) suggests the hypothetical unphosphorylated high-energy compound $X \sim I$ as the first intermediate of energy transformation.

In the "conformational" hypothesis it is assumed that the transformation of oxidoreductive energy occurs in some energized conformations of membraneous proteins (GREEN 1974; BOYER 1975; GOMEZ-PUYOU et al. 1978). The "chemio-osmotic" hypothesis of MITCHELL (1977) postulates the establishment of an electrochemical potential gradient of protons and transmembrane potential during substrate oxidation as a direct mechanism of ATP synthesis.

But whatever the mechanism of coupling of biological oxidation energy with ATP synthesis consists of, experimental data suggest that in intact mitochondria the multienzyme complex involved in this process is working as ATP synthetase.

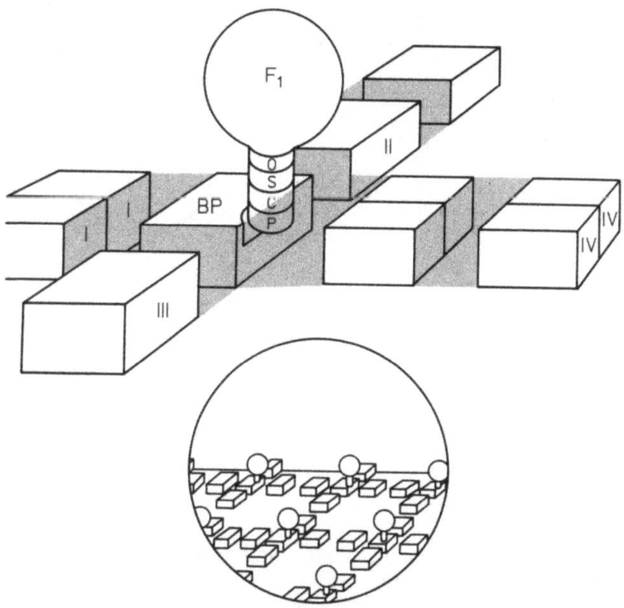

Fig. 1. Diagram of supermolecular complexes of the inner mitochondrial membrane carrying out electron transport and energy transformation (according to GREEN 1974). The complexes are separated from one another by bilayer phospholipid. The headpiece – F_1ATPase – and the stalk – oligomycin-sensitivity-conferring protein (*OSCP*) – are assumed to be linked laterally to the basepiece (*BP*). Complexes *I–IV* are the components of the electron transport system

ATP synthesis from ADP and inorganic phosphate (P_i) is localized in headpieces of an ATPase complex, factor F_1.

However, under the action of uncouplers, F_1 begins to function as ATPase. This activation of latent ATPase is blocked by oligomycin (TSAGALOFF 1971; GLASER et al. 1980).

Evidently, the key to the discovery of the coupling mechanism and the mode of uncoupler action lies in the study of the structure and functions of the ATPase complex. Recently there has been some progress in this field.

It was shown that the basepiece of the ATPase complex (factor F_0) responsible for its oligomycin sensitivity is composed of several hydrophobic proteins which form proton- and cation-conducting channels. Some proteins of the basepiece interact directly with the electron transport chain and play the primary role in the coupling of oxidative reactions with ATP synthesis (WILSON and FAIRS 1974; GUDZ et al. 1974; GLASER et al. 1980).

The headpiece (factor F_1) is also a complex supermolecule, composed of three pairs of large subunits. Each subunit has hydrophobic and polar sites necessary for binding of ADP and ATP, as well as separate catalytic sites (PEDERSEN 1975; KOZLOV 1975; RECKTENWALD and HESS 1980).

Data about the specific binding of uncouplers with proteins of basepiece and headpiece of ATPase complexes have been obtained (HANSTEIN 1976; KOZLOV

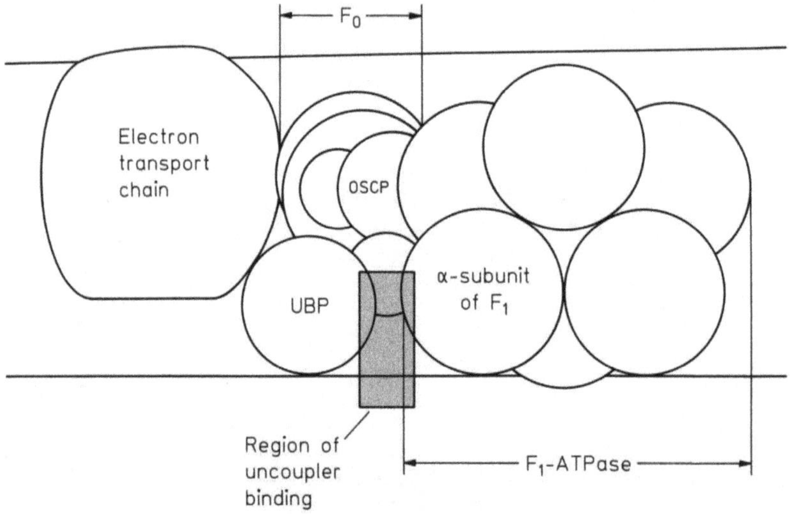

Fig. 2. Hypothetical structure of the uncoupler-binding site (according to HANSTEIN 1976). Uncoupler-binding protein (*UBP*) and α-subunit of the F_1 ATPase are two peptides interacting specifically with the uncoupler. Other proteins of the ATPase complex bind the uncoupler nonspecifically. The UBP is assumed to be close to the electron transport system

and MILGROM 1980) (Fig. 2). Activation of the latent ATPase is the first consequence of such binding.

A greater extent of uncoupling leads to loosening of bonds between the basepieces and heads of the ATPase complex, resulting in a progressive activation of latent ATPase which becomes Mg^{2+} dependent and less activated by uncouplers. As the heads finally break away from the basepieces, complete loss of enzyme sensitivity to oligomycin and the appearance of absolute Mg^{2+} dependence occurs.

Thus, as a result of the study on the mechanism of uncoupler interaction with the mitochondrial ATPase the evaluation of different stages of uncoupling between respiration and ATP synthesis has become possible.

D. Search for Correlations Between Cell Sensitivity or Resistance to Alkylating Agents and Functional State of Mitochondrial Membranes

When a positive correlation between the sensitivity of some normal tissues and tumors to alkylating agents and an impairment of their energetics was found, it became possible to search for causes of cell sensitivity or resistance to these drugs in the structural and functional characteristics of the mitochondrial membranes.

The first efforts in this field were made by BIRK (1967), who compared the functional stability of isolated mitochondria from normal animal tissues and tumors with different sensitivity to alkylating agents. As normal tissues, liver and

Table 1. Effects of ageing and intensive functioning on the tightness of coupling between respiration and oxidative phosphorylation in the mitochondria of rat liver and spleen

Mitochondria	Time in ice bath (min)	First ADP addition		Second ADP addition		Third ADP addition	
		ADP/O	RCR [a]	ADP/O	RCR	ADP/O	RCR
Liver	0	2.6 ± 0.2	5.4 ± 1.5	2.7 ± 0.5	3.0 ± 1.0	2.2 ± 0.3	1.5
	40–60	2.4 ± 0.3	4.1 ± 1.5	–	–	–	–
Spleen	0	1.6 ± 0.2	2.6	1.3	1.4	–	–
	30–60	1.1 ± 0.3	1.6	1.2	1.2	–	–

The incubation medium contains 85 m*M* KCl, 6 m*M* $MgCl_2$, 3 m*M* KH_2PO_4, 13 m*M* Na_2HPO_4, 12 m*M* NaF, pyruvate and malate potassium salts (15 m*M* each), and 0.2 m*M* ADP. Incubation at 26 °C. The oxygen consumption was measured polarographically with a platinum electrode

[a] RCR, respiratory control ratio, the quotient of the respiratory rates in the presence of oxidizable substrate, oxygen, ADP and phosphate (active state 3), and in the presence of substrate and oxygen but in the absence of either ADP or phosphate (controlled state 4) (CHANCE and WILLIAMS 1955)

spleen were studied. Among the tumors under study, Jensen sarcoma and sarcoma 45 are highly sensitive to alkylating agents, while sarcoma 180 and Ehrlich ascites tumor are much less sensitive.

The author has used the phosphorylation efficiency (ADP/O) and respiratory control ratio (RCR) as criteria of coupling in freshly isolated mitochondria as well as their changes after ageing in an icebath or during intensive functional activity.

The results of experiments with mitochondria of normal cells are presented in Table 1 and Fig. 3a, from which it is evident that liver mitochondria are distinguished by very tight coupling of oxidative phosphorylation. The 60-min maintenance of mitochondria in an icebath or repeated ADP addition does not cause apparent uncoupling. The ADP/O ratio is maintained near its theoretical value and respiratory control is reduced from 5.4 to 1.6 only after the third ADP addition.

The spleen mitochondria just after isolation have rather low ADP/O and respiratory control values. The second addition of ADP causes the release of respiratory control, and 30- to 60-min ageing in an icebath leads to complete uncoupling (Table 2, Fig. 3b). Hence, liver cells resistant to alkylating agents differ from sensitive cells of the spleen by the higher stability of their mitochondrial membranes in extreme conditions.

Differences in functional stability of mitochondrial membranes could be seen more clearly by comparison of mitochondria from tumors sensitive and resistant to alkylating agents (Table 2, Fig. 4).

Freshly isolated mitochondria from all tumors under study do not differ from each other in terms of their ADP/O or respiratory control values. However, both values are lower than in liver mitochondria, probably due to some damage to tumor mitochondria during isolation.

Differences between the mitochondria of tumors sensitive and resistant to alkylating agents are seen during their ageing and after repeated ADP treatment.

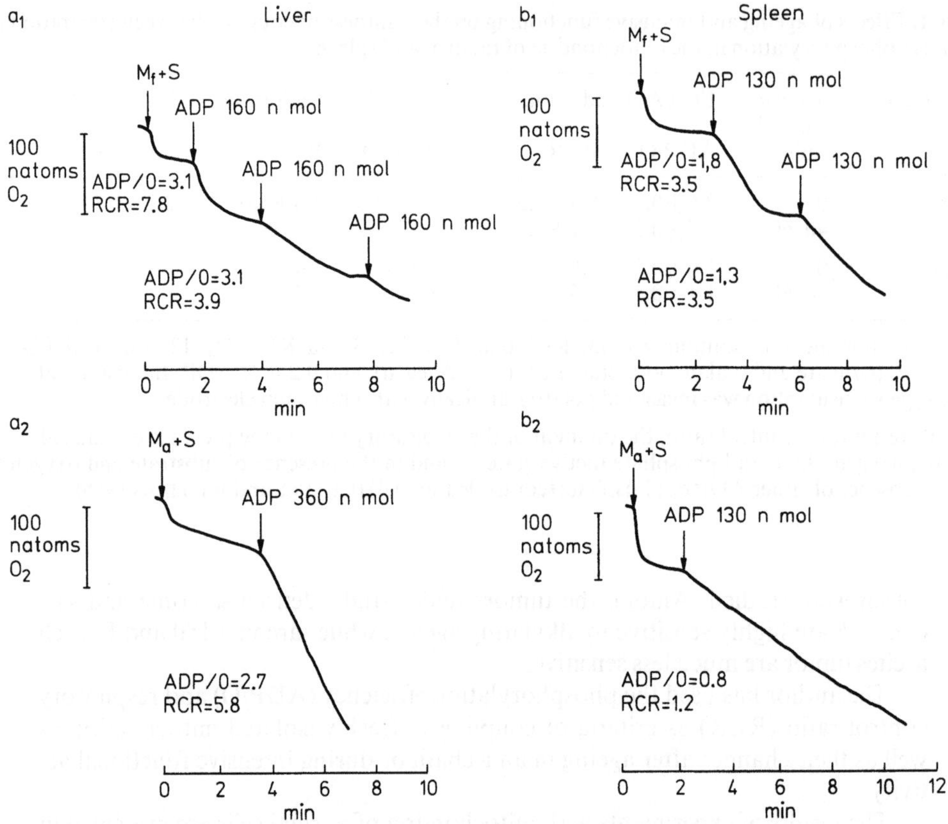

Fig. 3. Polarographic measurements of changes in the coupling of oxidative phosphorylation in isolated mitochondria from the rat liver and spleen after repeated ADP additions or after 60 min maintenance in an icebath. Added mitochondria (*M*) contain approximateley 1 mg protein. Respiratory substrates (*S*), pyruvate and malate (15 m*M* each) (BIRK 1967). M_f, freshly isolated mitochondria; M_a, aged mitochondria; *RCR*, respiratory control ratio

Mitochondria of sarcoma 45 and Jensen sarcoma are uncoupled almost completely after the second ADP addition, or after 30 min maintenance in an icebath (Table 2, Fig. 4a).

Mitochondria from resistant tumors, sarcoma 180 and Ehrlich ascites tumor, retain rather high ADP/O and respiratory control values even after the second ADP addition or againg in an icebath (Table 2, Fig. 4b).

Thus mitochondria of normal and tumor cells resistant to cytostatic action of alkylating agents retain high phosphorylation efficiency and respiratory control even when placed under conditions of intensive work or of cold stress. This could explain why, during the course of chemotherapy, resistant cells would keep the energy level sufficient to maintain their viability.

These conclusions have recently been confirmed by ROMANOVA et al. (1979), who compared mitochondria of normal tissues and tumors sensitive and resistant to alkylating agents in terms of their ultrastructure and tightness of coupling of

Table 2. Effects of ageing and intensive functioning on the tightness of coupling between respiration and oxidative phosphorylation in tumor mitochondria[a]

Mitochondria	Time in ice bath (min)	First ADP addition		Second ADP addition		Third ADP addition	
		ADP/O	RCR	ADP/O	RCR	ADP/O	RCR
Jensen sarcoma	0	2.0±0.3	3.6±1.0	1.5±1.0	2.4±0.5	0.7	–
	30–60	0.8±0.2	2.2±0.8	–	–	–	–
Sarcoma 45	0	1.9±0.5	2.2±1.0	1.2±0.3	1.9±1.0	0.9	–
	30–60	0.8±0.5	1.6±0.3	–	–	–	–
Sarcoma 180	0	2.2±0.3	3.7±1.0	2.4±0.4	3.2±1.0	1.9	–
	30–60	1.7±1.0	1.7±0.3	–	–	–	–
Ehrlich	0	2.4±0.1	2.5±1.0	1.8±0.1	1.9±0.5	1.7	–
	30–60	1.4±0.3	1.8±0.6	1.2±0.4	1.6±0.3	1.1	–

[a] The conditions of incubation are the same as in Table 1

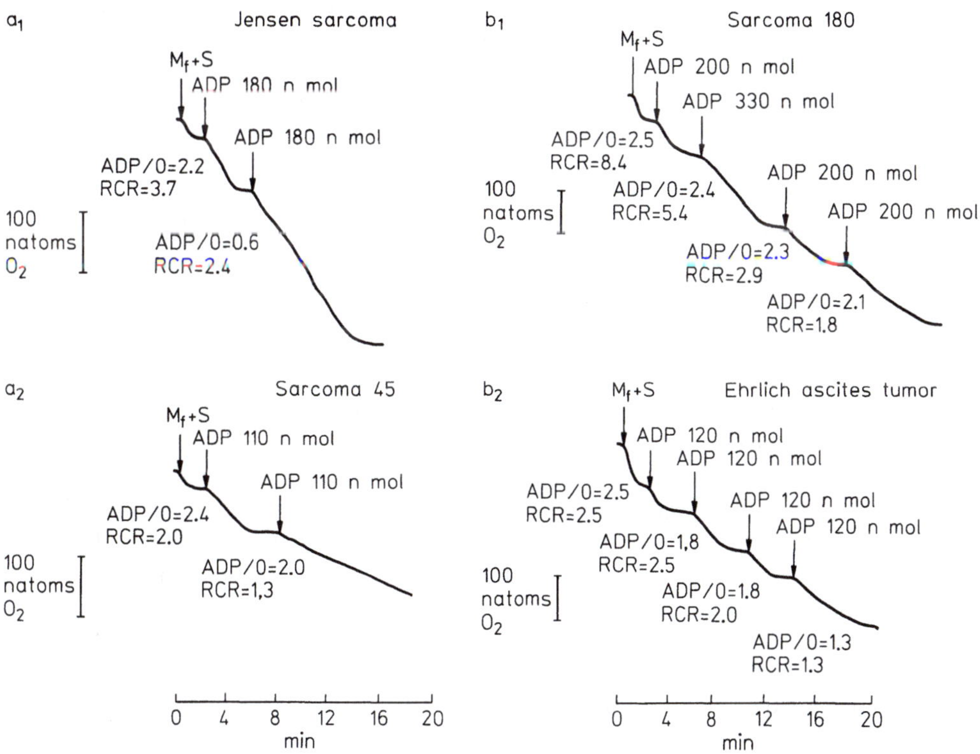

Fig. 4. Polarographic measurements of changes in the coupling of oxidative phosphorylation in the freshly isolated mitochondria (M_f) of tumors sensitive and resistant to alkylating agents. Added mitochondria contain approximately 1 mg protein. Respiratory substrates (*S*), pyruvate and malate (15 m*M* each); *RCR*, respiratory control ratio

Table 3. Parameters of coupling of respiration and phosphorylation in mitochondria of normal and tumor cells[a]

Mitochondria	No. of experiments	ADP/O	Respiratory control ratio	
			RCR_1	RCR_2
Rat liver	11	2.5±0.2	5.3±1.3	5.8±1.9
Rat thymus	7	2.6±0.3	2.1±0.7	1.9±0.3
Zajdela hepatoma	6	2.4±0.5	5.1±2.5	4.6±2.0
Adenocarcinoma 755	6	2.7±0.4	2.3±0.5	3.0±0.7
Jensen sarcoma	6	–	2.4±0.5	–
Sarcoma 45	10	–	2.0±0.5	–

[a] Mitochondria were incubated at 30 °C in medium containing 75 m*M* KCl; Tris-HCl buffer, pH 7.4; 125 m*M* KH_2PO_4; 1 m*M* EDTA; 1 m*M* $MgCl_2$; and 5 m*M* succinate as the respiratory substrate. Oxygen consumption was measured polarographically. RCR_1 and RCR_2 are the respiratory control ratios after the first and second ADP addition respectively

oxidative phosphorylation. Mitochondrial integrity or injury was assesed by studying their ultrastructure, ADP/O and respiratory control ratios as well as the basal ATPase level and enzyme response to DNP, Mg^{2+} and oligomycin.

Mitochondria from liver and thymus were isolated without special precautions by the method of SORDHAL and SCHWARTZ (1971). The tumor mitochondria, in view of their membrane fragility, were isolated in the presence of ethylenediaminetetraacetate (EDTA), mannitol and bovine serum albumin by the method of PEDERSEN et al. (1971).

It is known that thymus is highly sensitive to alkylating agents (GILMAN and PHILIPS 1946). The tumors under study are arranged in accordance to their sensitivity in the following order: sarcoma 45 = Jensen sarcoma > adenocarcinoma 755 > Zajdela hepatoma.

ROMANOVA et al. (1979) have shown that freshly isolated mitochondria of liver and thymus have fully intact ultrastructure with undamaged outer and inner membranes and cristae, as well as an electron-dense matrix.

Tightly coupled liver mitochondria have high ADP/O and respiratory control values, as shown in Table 3. The integrity of liver mitochondria is also suggested by the extremely low basal ATPase level. The enzyme is stimulated 20- to 40-fold by DNP and is Mg^{2+} independent and highly sensitive to oligomycin (Table 4).

Thymus mitochondria differ from those of liver by the loose coupling of oxidative phosphorylation. They exhibit a rather low respiratory control ratio and high basal ATPase activity which is stimulated to a greater extent by Mg^{2+} than by DNP and partly loses its oligomycin sensitivity (Tables 3 and 4).

In these experiments a surprising similarity between thymus and tumor mitochondria was found. These comparisons show that mitochondria of all tumors under study, except those of Zajdela hepatoma, can be distinguished by a rather loose coupling of phosphorylation which is expressed in low ADP/O and respiratory control values and some unusual properties of ATPase (Tables 3 and 4).

Table 4. ATPase activity in the mitochondria of rat thymus, liver and transplanted tumors [a]

Mitochondria	ATPase activity (nmol P_i/min mg protein)			
	Basal	With DNP	With Mg^{2+}	With Mg^{2+} + DNP
Rat liver ($n-10$)	5.2±1.0	233.0±9.0	8.0± 0.6	148.0± 6.0
Rath thymus ($n=3$)	43.2	125.4	222.0	260.0
Zajdela hepatoma ($n=10$)	28.4±2.4	122.0±36.0	79.0± 5.0	187.0±18.0
Adenocarcinoma 755 ($n=8$)	18.8±8.2	68.1±12.0	90.0±21.0	–
Jensen sarcoma ($n=5$)	14.7±4.0	52.7± 8.0	113.0±13.0	148.0±16.0
Sarcoma 45 ($n=20$)	15.4±1.6	31.1± 4.0	187.0±47.0	–

[a] Mitchondria were incubated for 10 min at 30 °C in the medium containing 75 m*M* KCl; 0.5 m*M* EDTA; 68 m*M* sucrose; 50 m*M* Tris-HCl buffer, pH 7.4; and, where shown, 5 m*M* $MgCl_2$ and 1–500 μ*M* DNP (Romanova et al. 1979). *n*, number of experiments

The basal ATPase level of tumor mitochondria is four to five times higher that of liver mitochondria. In mitochondria of Zajdela hepatoma the enzyme is activated by DNP much more than by Mg^{2+} and is sensitive to oligomycin. In adenocarcinoma 755 mitochondria both agents activate ATPase equally, but in mitochondria of sarcoma 45 and Jensen sarcoma ATPase is only slightly activated by DNP and much more by Mg^{2+}. It is insensitive to oligomycin in the presence of Mg^{2+} (Table 4).

These results are in general agreement with the data of some authors who have also reported unusual properties of tumor mitochondria (Feo and Garcea 1973; Kolarov et al. 1973; Pedersen and Morris 1974; Senior et al. 1975; Kaschnitz et al. 1976).

It has been shown that mitochondria of transplanted tumors showing intact ultrastructure and sufficiently high ADP/O and respiratory control ratios differ from mitochondria of homologous normal tissue by possessing unusually high basal ATPase levels. The enzyme is scarcely stimulated by DNP, but is Mg^{2+} dependent. The aim of these authors was to identify some correlation between characteristics of mitochondrial ATPase and growth rates of animal tumors.

In experiments of Romanova et al. (1979) some structural and functional features of tumor mitochondria were compared with tumor-cell sensitivity to the cytotoxic action of alkylating agents.

In the light of recent knowledge concerning the structure of the ATPase complex and mechanisms of uncoupler action one can suggest that in mitochondria of normal tissues and tumors sensitive to alkylating agents the interaction between the head (factor F_1) and the basepiece (factor F_0) of the ATPase complex is loosened or completely lost. As a result, free F_1 can function as a Mg^{2+} dependent ATPase insensitive to oligomycin.

In order to satisfy the energy needs of actively proliferating tumor cells, such a deficient oxidative phosphorylation system has to work at the limit of its capacity and, hence, is likely to be extremely sensitive to the variety of damaging agents.

Mitochondria of normal tissues and tumors resistant to alkylating agents have tightly coupled phosphorylating systems and usually only partially utilize their potential energy capacity for needs of growth and metabolism. Partial damage of ATPase complexes in mitochondria of these cells by alkylating agents does not lead to a significant impairment of the energy supply.

Thus, the experimental data suggest that the damage due to alkylating agents plays an essential role in the structural and functional changes of normal and tumor mitochondria in respect of their cytotoxic and antitumor effects. Cell sensitivity toward this class of antitumor drugs depends on the structure of the inner mitochondrial membrane and especially that of the ATPase complex. In general, there is a positive correlation between the tightness of the ATPase complex attachment to the inner membrane of mitochondria and resistance of normal and tumor cells to the cytotoxic action of alkylating agents.

References

Belousova AK (1965) Biochemical approaches to chemotherapy of tumors (in Russian). Medicine, Leningrad, p 395

Belousova AK (1977) The mechanisms of action of antitumor compounds. Cancer Inst Monogr 45:183–193

Belousova AK (1978) Molecular mechanisms of the acquirement of tumor drug resistance and some to overcome it (in Russian). Vopr Onkol 24:92–104

Belousova AK, Gerasimova GK (1980) Search for biochemical paramters of tumor cell sensitivity and resistance to antimetabolites. In: Mihich E, Eckhardt S (eds) Design of cancer chemotherapy. Experimental and clinical approaches. Antibiot Chemother 28:48–52

Belousova AK, Romanova IN (1971) The effects of alkylating agents on the structure and functions of mitochondrial membranes (in Russian). In: Blokhin NN (ed) Proceedings of the 7th annual conference of institute of experimental and clinical oncology. Institute of Experimental and Clinical Oncology, AMS USSR, pp 29–37

Belousova AK, Romanova IN, Kuzmina ZV (1964) The selectivity of alkylating agents action on the oxidative phosphorylation in tumor cells related to some features of cell structure (in Russian). In: 1st all-union biochemical congress, Leningrad, vol 1, pp 47–48

Belousova AK, Romanova IN, Kuzmina ZV, Zefirova LI (1966) On the mechanism of cytotoxic action of alkylating agents (in Russian). Biokhimia 31:13–20

Birk RV (1967) Study on the energetics of tumors with different sensitivity to alkylating agents (in Russian). Vopr Med Khim 13:307–313

Boyer PD (1975) Energy transformation and protein translocation by adenosine triphosphate. FEBS Lett 50:91–94

Brockman RW (1974) Mechanisms of resistance. In: Sartorelli AC, Johns DG (eds) Antineoplastic and immunosuppressive agents, 1st edn, part 1. Springer, Berlin Heidelberg New York, p 352–410

Carter SK, Slavik M (1977) Current investigational drugs of interest in the chemotherapy program of the national cancer institute. Cancer Inst Monogr 45:102–121

Chance B, Williams GR (1955) Respiratory enzymes in oxidative phosphorylation. III. The steady state. J Biol Chem 217:409–427

Feo F, Garcea R (1973) Acceptor-control ratio of mitochondria. Factors affecting it in Morris hepatoma 5123 and Yoshida hepatoma AG 130. Eur J Cancer 9:203–214

Gilman A, Philips FS (1946) The biological actions and therapeutic applications of the β-chloroethylamines and sulfides. Science 103:409–415

Glaser E, Norling B, Ernster L (1980) Reconstitution of mitochondrial oligomycin and dicyclohexylcarbodiimide sensitive ATPase. Eur J Biochem 225:225–235

Gomez-Puyou TM, Gavilani M, Delaisse JM, Gomez-Puyou A (1978) Conformational change of soluble mitochondrial ATPase as controlled by hyrodrophobic interaction within the enzyme. Biochem Biophys Res Commun 82:1028–1033

Green D (1974) The electrochemical model for energy coupling in mitochondria. Biochim Biophys Acta 346:27–78

Gudz TI, Yaguzhinsky LS, Skulatchev VP (1974) Alkylating compounds as inhibitors of ATP synthetase of mitochondria. Biochemistry (USSR) 40:72–76

Hanstein WG (1976) Uncoupling of oxidative phosphorylation. Biochim Biophys Acta 456:129–148

Kaschnitz RM, Hatefi RM, Morris HP (1976) Oxidative phosphorylation properties of mitochondria isolated from transplanted hepatoma. Biochim Biophys Acta 449:224–238

Klamerth DL (1973) Abnormal base-pairing under the influence of nitrogen mustards. FEBS Lett 24:35–37

Kolarov J, Kuzela S, Krempasky V (1973) Some properties of coupled mitochondria exhibiting uncoupler insensitive ATPase activity. Biochem Biophys Res Commun 55:1173–1179

Kozlov IA (1975) Oligomycin-sensitive ATPase (in Russian). Bioorg Chem 1:1545–1568

Kozlov IA, Milgrom IM (1980) The non-catalytic nucleotide-binding site of mitochondrial ATPase is localized on the α-subunits of factor F_1. Eur J Biochem 106:457–462

Lawley PD, Brookes P (1967) Interstrand cross-linking of DNA by difunctional alkylating agents. J Mol Biol 25:143–150

Loveless A (1966) Genetic and allied effects of alkylating agents. Butterworths, London, p 225

Mitchell P (1977) A commentary on alternative hypothesis of proton coupling in the membrane system catalysing oxidative phosphorylation. FEBS Lett 79:1–20

Mitskevitsh LG, Roset EG, Kukushkina GV, Gorbatsheva LB (1972) The study of the RNA polymerase activity in nuclei of Ehrlich ascites carcinoma in relation to the mechanism of action of *N*-alkyl-*N*-nitroseureas. Biochemistry (USSR) 37:711–714

Pedersen PL (1975) Adenosine triphosphatase from rat liver mitochondria: separate sites involved in ATP hydrolysis and in the reversible high affinity binding of ATP. Biochem Biophys Res Commun 64:610–616

Pedersen PL, Morris HP (1974) Uncoupler-stimulated adenosine triphosphatase activity deficiency in intact mitochondria from hepatoma and ascites tumor cells. J Biol Chem 249:3327–3334

Pedersen PL, Eska T, Morris HP, Catterall A (1971) Deficiency of uncoupler-stimulated adenosine triphosphatase activity in tightly coupled hepatoma mitochondria. Proc Natl Acad Sci USA 68:1079–1082

Racker E (1976) A new look at mechanisms in bioenergetics. Academic, New York, p 216

Recktenwald D, Hess B (1980) Classification of nucleotide-binding sites on mitochondria F_1-ATPase from yeast. Biochim Biophys Acta 592:377–384

Roberts JJ (1980) DNA repair mechanisms and cytotoxicity of antitumor alkylating agents and neutral platinum compounds. Antibiot Chemother 28:109–114

Romanova IN (1971) On the site of the uncoupling effects of alkylating agents in energy-transforming reactions (in Russian). Biokhimia 36:1119–1129

Romanova IN (1972) Effects of alkylating agents on ATPase activity of liver mitochondria. Biochemistry (USSR) 37:707–710

Romanova IN, Sofina ZP (1969) The effects of sarcolysine and of two stereoisomeres of asaphane on oxidative phosphorylation in mitochondria of liver and sarcoma 45 (in Russian). Vopr Med Khim 15:47–55

Romanova IN, Lebedeva MV, Filippova NA (1979) Characteristics of ATPase from tumor mitochondria. Biochemistry (USSR), v 43, N 12, p 2:1781–1789

Ross WC (1962) Biological alkylating agents. Fundamental chemistry and the design of compounds for selective toxicity. Academic, London, p 260
Ross WC, Ewig RA, Kohn KW (1978) Differences between melphalan and nitrogen mustard in the formation und removal of DNA cross-links. Cancer Res 38:1502–1506
Senior AE, McGowan EC, Hilf P (1975) A comparative study of inner membrane enzymes and transport system in mitochondria from R3230 AC mammary tumors and normal rat mammary glands. Cancer Res 35:2001–2007
Slater EC (1966) Oxidative phosphorylation. Compr Biochem 14:327–350
Sordhal LA, Schwartz A (1971) Tumor mitochondria. Methods Cancer Res 6:158–186
Spasskaja IG, Gratsheva NK, Belousova AK (1968) Some experimental data about the protective effect of cystaphos against lethal doses of sarcolysine and cyclophosphane. In: 1st all-union conference on the chemotherapy of malignant tumors (in Russian). Riga, pp 381–382
Tsagaloff A (1971) Structure and biosynthesis of the membrane adenosine triphosphatase of mitochondria. Curr Top Membr Transp 2:157–205
Verovsky VN, Gorbatsheva LB (1979) Use of models of the template RNA synthesis in the study of mechanisms of *N*-nitrosourea antitumor action (in Russian). Chimikopharmaceut J 10:24–29
Wilson DF, Fairs K (1974) A novel property of mitochondrial oxidative phosphorylation. Biochem Biophys Res Commun 56:635–640
Yaguzhinsky LS, Volkov AG, Boguslavsky LI (1976) Investigation of the mechanism of the action of a specific inhibitor of respiration and phosphorylation in the mitochondria – p-(*N*,*N*-DL-2-chloroethyl)aminophenyl acetic acid. Biochemistry (USSR) 41:983–986
Zubrod CG (1972) Chemical control of cancer. Proc Natl Acad Sci USA 69:1042–1045

CHAPTER 15

Mechanism of "Resistance" Towards Specific Drug Groups

T. A. CONNORS

The bifunctional alkylating agents were among the first chemicals to be used in scientific attempts at the chemotherapy of cancer. Although many other classes of anticancer agents such as the nitrosoureas and dialkyltriazenes also act by alkylation of cellular macromolecules, the bifunctional alkylating agents are distinct as a class because of their requirement for two alkylating arms for antitumour activity. Thus in Fig. 1 the difunctional agents are active in the Walker tu-

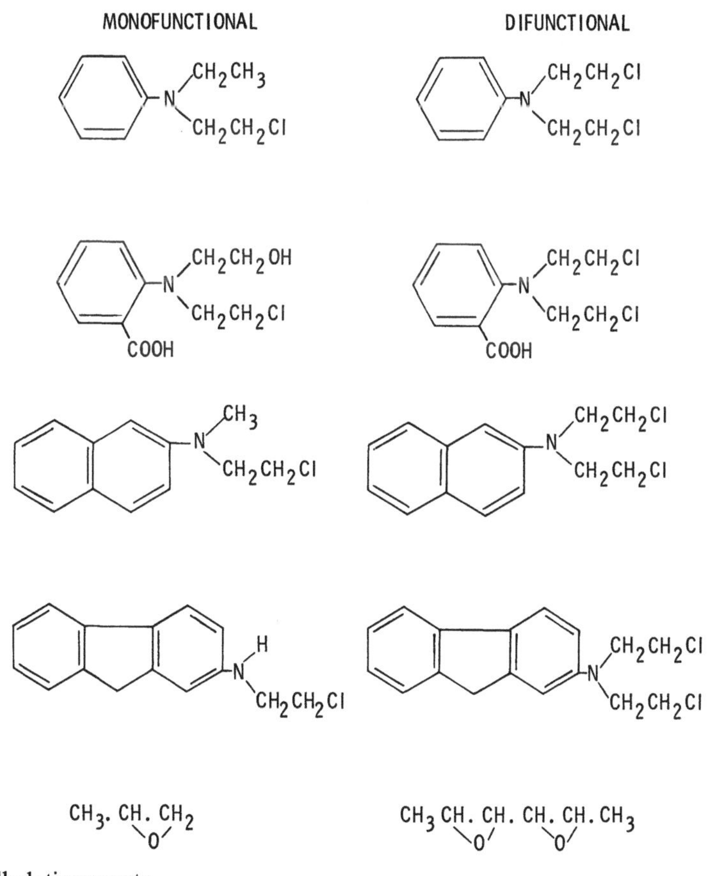

Fig. 1. Alkylating agents

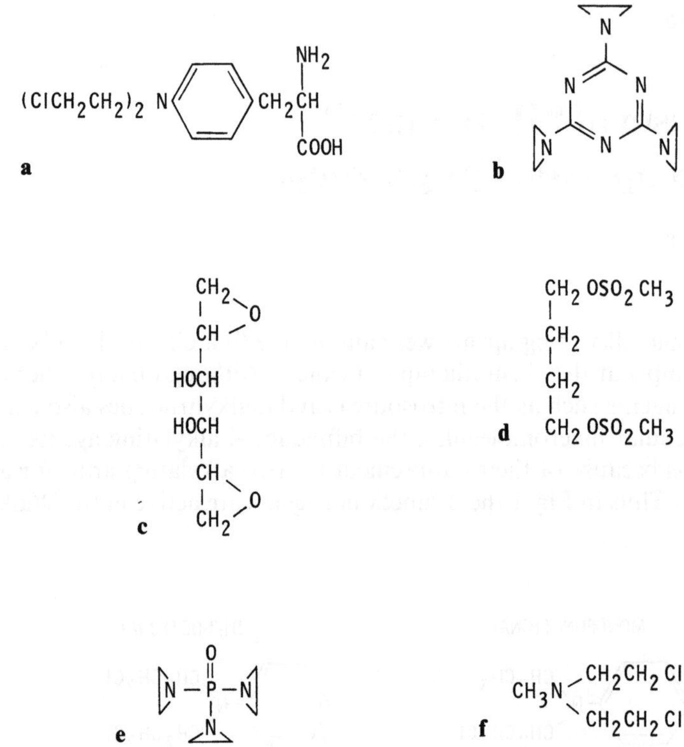

Fig. 2 a–f. Structures of different classes of bifunctional alkylating agents. **a** melphalan; **b** TEM; **c** dianhydrogalacticol; **d** myleran; **e** triethyleneiminophosphoramide; **f** HN2

mour inhibition test while the corresponding monofunctional analogues are not. The monofunctional derivatives may, however, be just as toxic, mutagenic and carcinogenic as the difunctional analogues and sometimes even more so.

A. Mechanisms of Alkylation

Four major classes of bifunctional alkylating agent have anticancer properties, the nitrogen mustards, e.g. melphalan (Fig. 2a), the aziridines, e. g. triethylenemelamine (TEM) (Fig. 2b), the epoxides, e.g. dianhydrogalacticol (Fig. 2c) and the sulphonoxyalkanes, e.g. myleran (Fig. 2d).

In most cases alkylation proceeds through a second order nucleophilic substitution (S_N2) as exemplified by the aziridines (ethyleneimines):

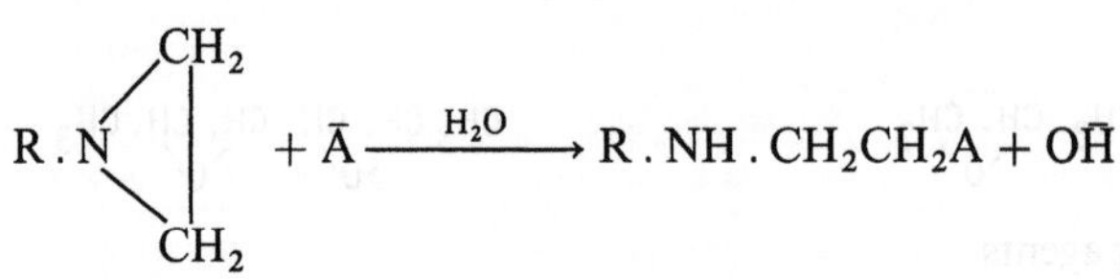

or the epoxides:

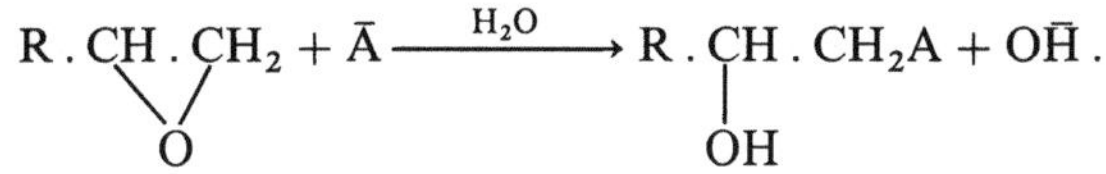

Since both classes of agent act by a bimolecular mechanism, their rate of reaction with nucleophilic centres will be dependent on the concentration of such centres. Both epoxides and ethyleneimines are more reactive under acidic conditions. Ethyleneimides such as triethyleneiminophosphoramide (Fig. 2e) are more reactive than ethyleneimines because the electron-withdrawing properties of the oxygen atom makes the methylene group of the ethyleneimine ring more susceptible to nucleophilic attack.

The aliphatic nitrogen mustards act similarly after formation of a cyclic immonium ion. The unimolecular conversion to the immonium ion is relatively fast and once formed it reacts by an S_N2 mechanism at a rate dependent on the concentration of nucleophilic centres:

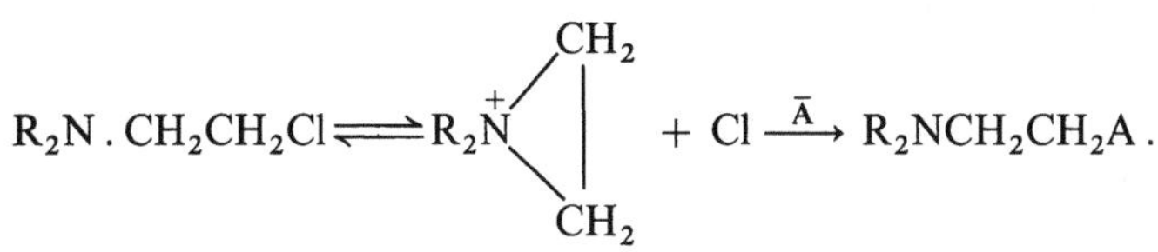

There is some question as to the mechanism of alkylation of the less basic aromatic nitrogen mustards and sulphur mustard. In these chemicals the lower basicity of the nitrogen or sulphur atom does not favour the formation of a stable cyclic immonium ion analogous to the aliphatic nitrogen mustards. They may also show first-order kinetics in that their rate of alkylation may be independent of the concentration of nucleophilic centres. This difference in mechanism can make them different from other alkylating agents in some of their biological properties. The toxicity of the aliphatic nitrogen mustard HN2 (Fig. 2f) in rats can be considerably reduced by prior administration of sodium thiosulphate, since by increasing the concentration of nucleophilic centres in the blood, it increases the rate of reaction of the nitrogen mustard so that less intact agent reaches sensitive tissues such as the bone marrow. There is no similar increase in the rate of reaction of aromatic nitrogen mustards in extracellular fluid and their toxicity cannot be reduced by thiosulphate (CONNORS et al. 1964a). Because most aromatic nitrogen mustards release equal amounts of chloride and hydrogen ions on hydrolysis, it has been suggested that they react through initial formation of a carbonium (or carbenium) ion formed by unimolecular loss of chloride ion (ROSS 1962):

$$R_2N.CH_2CH_2Cl \longrightarrow R_2NCH_2CH_2^+ \xrightarrow{\bar{A}} R_2NCH_2CH_2A.$$

It is not certain that aromatic nitrogen mustards act via carbonium ion formation (PRICE et al. 1969; BARDOS et al. 1969; EHRSSON et al. 1980) and some have been shown to lose chloride ion at a significantly faster rate than alkylating activity disappears, implying the formation of a relatively stable reactive intermediate (WILLIAMSON and WITTEN 1967). However, there is no doubt that for most aromatic nitrogen mustards there is no accumulation of a cyclic intermediate and the rate-determining step is first-order ionisation of the halogen atom.

B. Mechanisms of Cytotoxicity and Antitumour Action

Cells in cycle are usually much more sensitive to the toxic action of the alkylating agents than non-cycling cells and from a review of many different model systems using bacterial, plant and animal cells, in vivo and in vitro, it has been concluded that alkylation may itself be a relatively non-toxic event, unless cells are forced into division before repair of alkylation can take place (CONNORS 1975). It has also been proposed that although alkylating agents are relatively non-specific in the molecules they alkylate, some form of DNA alkylation is usually responsible for the characteristic toxicity induced by the difunctional alkylating agents. In the DNA molecule, phosphate groups may be esterified and the oxygen group of thymine and guanine alkylated as well as the exocyclic and ring nitrogen atoms of all the bases. Because the nucleophilic character of the various groups may be altered by hydrogen bonding or by association with nucleoprotein and because steric factors may be important, the actual alkylation that occurs under physiological conditions is dependent on many variables and may differ from cell to cell. Mutagenic and carcinogenic events may be initiated by a specific monofunctional alkylation of DNA (e.g. in the O^6-position of guanine) but it is likely that cross-linking reactions are a more acutely cytotoxic effect in dividing cells. A number of cross-linked DNA products, especially N^7-diguanyl products, have been identified following reaction of DNA with alkylating agents. If cross-linking were a highly toxic event it would satisfactorily explain why difunctional alkylating agents have antitumour activity whereas the analogous monofunctional agents do not. At least three types of cross-linking can occur, namely between protein and DNA, between the adjacent strands of DNA and between groups of the same strand. There is no convincing evidence that any one of these reactions is more cytotoxic than the others.

C. Selectivity of Antitumour Action of the Alkylating Agents

Many transplanted rodent tumors used in studying alkylating agents have a large proportion of cells in cycle and are sensitive to most alkylating agents provided they are difunctional. The also have a minimal degree of chemical reactivity under physiological conditions and are also not so reactive that they will alkylate or hydrolyse completely at the site of injection, which may be distant from the tumour. A large number of alkylating agents have these properties, and are therefore active against transplanted tumours such as the PC6 plasma-cell tumour growing in the mouse. Activity is simply measured by the therapeutic index (for example, the ratio of the LD_{50} as a measure of normal tissue toxicity and the ED_{90}, the dose that causes 90% regression of the tumour cell mass and usually cure of the animals). The majority of bifunctional agents will have a therapeutic index of about 20–50 against this tumour type (Table 1). A few agents, however, such as mel-

Table 1. Therapeutic indices of some alkylating agents on the PC6 plasma cell tumour

Melphalan	166
Cyclophosphamide	100
Aniline mustard	92
4-Mcthylcyclophosphamidc	54
Chlorambucil	44
Methylenedimethanesulphonate	30
Triethylenemelamine	20

phalan, cyclophosphamide and aniline mustard, have significantly larger therapeutic indices and may be thought of as having two components. The first component is a measure of the inherent "sensitivity" of the tumour to bifunctional alkylating agents compared with normal sensitive tissues such as bone marrow and is determined by such features as the growth fraction of the tumour, the cell-cycle time and the levels of various DNA repair enzymes. the second component is a characteristic feature of the drug which enables it to be more toxic to tumour cells than other alkylating agents and thus have a higher therapeutic index. These special features of particular alkylating agents will be considered in more detail later. For melphalan and HN2, increased selectivity is probably due to active transport mechanisms which result in more drug being concentrated in tumours with these carrier systems. For cyclophosphamide the selectivity is due to a complex pathway of metabolism which results in more cytotoxic metabolites forming in the tumor, and for aniline mustard, the presence of β-glucuronidase in the tumour which activates a relatively non-toxic metabolite to a highly toxic one.

D. Patterns of Resistance

It follows that for a group of alkylating agents different patterns of resistance might be shown by a tumour such as the PC6 plasma-cell tumour. For instance, if tumour cells acquired a mechanism for repairing or recovering from DNA cross-links one might see a partial or complete resistance to all bifunctional alkylating agents. On the other hand if the active transport mechanism for melphalan were lost then the "selective" component of the melphalan would disappear, its therapeutic index would fall to the level shown by most other alkylating agents and there would be no development of cross-resistance. Thus the development of a degree of resistance to one alkylating agent not associated with resistance to others cannot be taken as proof that the agents do not act by similar mechanisms (e.g. alkylation of DNA).

In a study of patterns of resistance among alkylating agents (SCHABEL et al. 1978) the response of cyclophosphamide (CPA), melphalan (L-phenylalanine mustard) and thiotriethylenephosphoramide (thio TEPA) was compared using the L1210 leukaemia sensitive to a range of alkylating agents and lines with acquired resistance to either cyclophosphamide or melphalan (Table 2). ThioTEPA killed 10^4 leukaemia cells at its optimal dose while melphalan and cyclophosphamide

Table 2. Log_{10} reduction in viable tumour cells by three alkylating agents against L1210 leukaemia and sublines resistant to L-PAM and cyclophosphamide (CPA). (SCHABEL et al. 1978)

	L1210	L1210/L-PAM	L1210/CPA
L-PAM	6	2	4
CPA	6	4	0
ThioTEPA	4	2	2

killed 10^6. Thus the "selective" component of the latter two chemicals might account for a killing of 10^2 cells while the response of the tumour due to its inherent sensitivity to bifunctional alkylating agents may be 10^4 cells as observed with thioTEPA. Melphalan kills only 10^2 cells of the $L1210_{PAM}$ tumour, indicating that resistance is due to the loss of the selective component of 10^2 cells plus a loss of general sensitivity of 10^2 cells. The loss of general sensitivity of 10^2 cells is confirmed by the finding of a reduced response (by 10^2 cells) to both cyclophosphamide and thioTEPA. Similarly resistance to cyclophosphamide is acquired both by a loss of the pathway of selectivity and a generally reduced tumour sensitivity since although the resistance to cyclophosphamide is greatest there is also a 10^2 reduction in response to melphalan and thioTEPA. The mulitfactorial acquisition of resistance has been demonstrated before, for example, by GOLDENBERG et al. (1970) and by HIRONO et al. (1962), who showed that acquisition of resistance to nitromin could be correlated with the combination of increased thiol content and reduced cell permeability. For other alkylating agents such as the nitrosoureas there is often no cross-resistance, suggesting that they act by a completely different mechanism.

E. Mechanisms of Resistance

The response of a tumour to an alkylating agent will clearly depend on the concentration of drug that reaches it, and this will be dependent on numerous factors such as the site of the tumour and its blood supply, as well as the pharmacokinetic properties of the drug. Even a high concentration of drug in the extracellular fluid of a tumour may not necessarily result in a high level of cytotoxicity since there are various factors which can greatly reduce the amount of drug that binds to the DNA target molecule. Some of these variables are shown in Fig. 3 using as an example a nitrogen mustard that requires metabolic activation before it can cause cytotoxicity. Resistance to alkylating agents could arise from an alteration in one or more of these variables. Initially the agent may enter the cell by passive diffusion or by active transport (Fig. 3, *R1*) and resistance could develop if the cell membrane became less permeable to drugs entering by passive diffusion or the cells lost the processes required for active transport (or perhaps "facilitated diffusion"). Some alkylating agents are not cytotoxic under physiological conditions but require intracellular metabolism, which converts them to reactive and toxic species (Fig. 3, *R2*). Resistance could clearly be acquired if the tumour cell lost this ac-

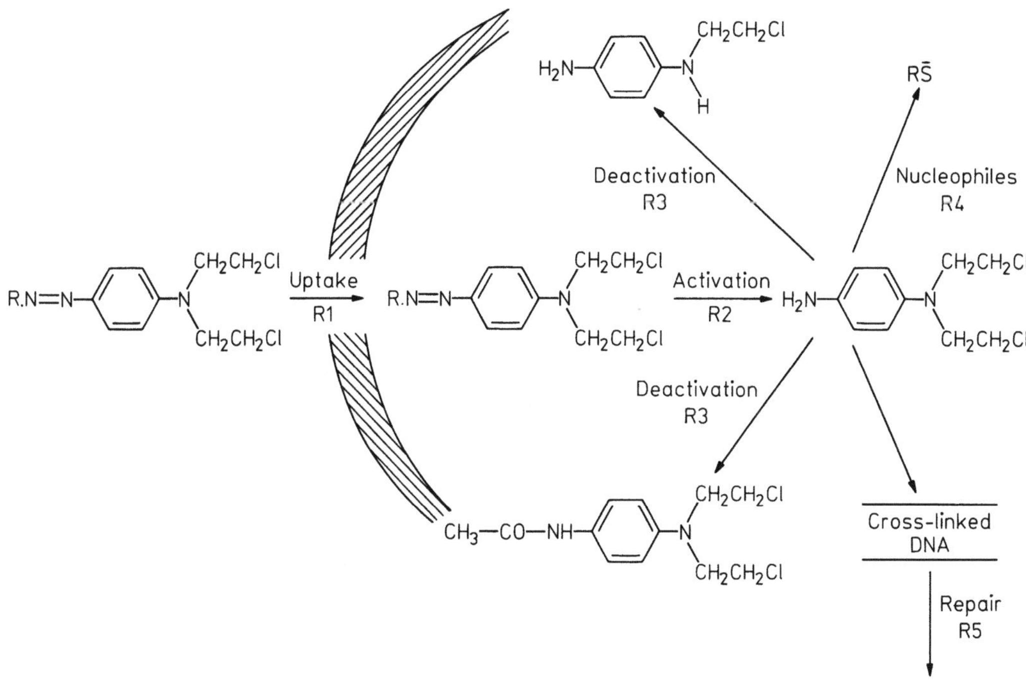

Fig. 3. Factors influencing the sensitivity of a malignant cell to alkylating agents

tivating mechanism. Conversely a metabolic pathway which detoxified a reactive alkylating agent would also lead to resistance since the amount of drug available for reaction with DNA would be reduced (Fig. 3, *R3*). The rate of reaction of most alkylating agents with a nucleophile is dependent on the concentration of that nucleophile and its "nucleophilic strength", which is usually expressed as a competition factor, comparing it with the nucleophilicity of hydroxyl ions. An increased concentration of any one of a number of cellular nucleophiles would reduce reaction with DNA and lead to resistance (Fig. 3, *R4*). A final mechanism could be the result of an increase of the different repair processes, which could repair alkylated DNA before irreversible toxicity occurred (Fig. 2, *R5*). These repair mechanisms are discussed elsewhere.

I. Resistance Through Decreased Cellular Uptake (Fig. 3, *R1*)

It has been shown that in L5178Y Lymphoblasts in vitro, HN2 is concentrated against a gradient as high as 35-fold and that this transport can be inhibited by low temperatures (4 °C) or partially by ouabain and 2,4-dinitrophenol. Since the monofunctional and the di-2-hydroxyethylamino analogues of HN2 could also prevent uptake of labelled HN 2 with the kinetics of competitive inhibition it was suggested that the mustard was incorporated into cells by an active transport mechanism (GOLDENBERG et al. 1970). L5178Y cells which slowly acquire resistance to HN2 after several exposures to the agent incorporate HN2 at a much slower rate, suggesting that the resistance is at least in part due to a reduced ac-

Choline HN2 Ethyleneimmonium Ion

Fig. 4. Comparison of the structure of choline with the enthyleneimmonium ion of HN2

tivity of the specific active transport mechanism (GOLDENBERG 1969). The specificity of the carrier system for HN2 was demonstrated by the finding that cyclophosphamide, chlorambucil and melphalan did not interfere with this active transport (GOLDENBERG et al. 1970). It appears that HN2 is taken into cells by the choline transport carrier (GOLDENBERG et al. 1971 a) and there is a close structural similarity between choline and the ethyleneimonium ion that HN2 quickly forms in body fluids (Fig. 4). Transport of HN2 by an active carrier-mediated process that is competitive with choline has also been demonstrated in human normal and leukaemic lymphoid cells (LYONS and GOLDENBERG 1972) and in Walker carcinosarcoma cells (GOLDENBERG and SINHA 1973).

In a study of L5178Y cells with acquired resistance to HN2 a two- to threefold resistance was shown to a variety of alkylating agents but an 18-fold resistance to HN2. As already discussed this implied that the resistance of the cells to HN2 had at least two components, a "specific" acquisition of resistance to HN2 by loss of the specific carrier mechanism and a more general mechanism causing a two- to three fold cross-resistance among other bifunctional alkylating agents. In fact the transport K_m for the resistant cells was higher than for sensitive cells, suggesting a decreased affinity between the transport carrier and the drug and the V_{max} was lower, indicating a decreased transport capacity (GOLDENBERG et al. 1970; GOLDENBERG 1975).

It is of interest that log phase L5178Y cells are more sensitive to HN2 than stationary phase cells because of the more efficient transport system of the former (GOLDENBERG et al. 1971 b). Thus specific resistance to HN2 might occur if a prior treatment reduced the ratio of cycling to resting cells. It is also of interest that 1,3 bis 2-chlorethylnitrosourea (BCNU) may interfere with HN2 transport mechanisms by a non-competitive mechanism, probably through irreversible alkylation or carbamoylation of reactive sites on the carrier protein. Thus pretreatment of cells with BCNU might conceivably lead to a partial resistance to HN2. However, the situation is complicated since the uptake of melphalan (which may also be transported by an active process) is inhibited by methyl-1-(2-chloroethyl)3-cyclohexyl-1-nitrosourea (CCNU) but stimulated by BCNU (MARTIN et al. 1981 to be published). Reduced uptake of HN2 as a mechanism of resistance has been demonstrated in a variety of systems. Repeated in vivo exposure of Lettre'-Ehrlich ascites cells to high doses of HN2 led to the formation of a number of resistant sublines, some of which were more than 50 times more resistant to HN2 that the parent line. The resistant cells took up only a quarter of the amount of labelled HN2 taken up by sensitive cells when measured 60 min after intraperitoneal injection of the drug. This reduced uptake of HN2 was reflected in a smaller amount of alkylation of DNA and less cross-linking (RUTMAN et al. 1968). However, since cross-linking and DNA alkylation were proportional to dose and since this was only reduced by 50% in cells which were more than 50 times more resistant to HN2, it was concluded that while the resistance could be partially explained by a reduced permeability to HN2 other factors were also important (CHUN et al. 1969). Similar results were obtained by WOLPERT and RUDDON (1969), who showed that Ehrlich ascites cells in vitro which were resistant to HN2 accumulated only half as much labelled drug as sensitive cells over a concentration range of 10^{-6}–$10^{-4}M$. This difference in uptake was apparent 5 min after incubation. Since this difference persisted for up to 24 h it was thought that not only was a reduction in active transport responsible for the resistance but also differences in the retention of the drug were important, suggesting a difference in binding sites for HN2. In other experiments HN2 has been shown to be taken up by L1210 cells by a temperature-dependent process, unlike myleran, which was accumulated equally well at 0 °C and 37 °C. In this case the uptake of HN2 was not inhibited by dinitrophenol (KESSEL et al. 1969). HN2 inhibits the incorporation of C^{14} orotic acid into the nucleic acid of sensitive hepatoma cells to a greater extent than resistant hepatoma cells. Such an effect was not seen when nuclei rather than intact cells were used and demonstrates the importance of the cell membrane in determining the cellular sensitivity to HN2 (MIURA and MORIYAMA 1961).

A series of ascites hepatoma cells derived from different chemically induced liver tumours and which show a graded response to HN2 and its *N*-oxide, nitromin, have been studied. Tumours most resistant were generally less permeable to HN2 (measured by an indirect method) although the most important factors determining resistance were reduced permeability combined with an increased free thiol content (HIRONO et al. 1962). The decreased permeability of these resistant cells to nitromin could be increased in vitro by administration of Tween 80, with a concomitant increase in drug sensitivity (YAMADA et al. 1963).

In L cells with a small degree of acquired resistance to sulphur mustard (and significantly smaller in cell volume from the line from which they were derived) there was 25% less labelled sulphur mustard taken up compared with the sensitive line and 50% less radioactivity associated with DNA. However, because of the rather small degree of resistance, the fluctuation of acid-soluble SH and cell volume associated with cell density and differences in cell cycle time it was not possible to define the mechanism(s) of resistance (REED and WALKER 1966). It is of interest that the cells with acquired resistance showed less tendency to form colonies and a greater tendency to migrate, a property also observed with cells treated with nitrogen mustard (LEVIS and COLUSSI 1963). This property was stable, being maintained without further exposure to alkylating agents. Differences in aggregatability of tumour cells have also been related to differences in permeability to HN2 and its *N*-oxide (HIRONO et al. 1962).

In other experiments using tumour cells and tumour-bearing animals, sometimes bilaterally transplanted with the sensitive and resistant tumours, there was no evidence of decreased permeability of resistant cells or decreased binding of label to DNA using a variety of alkylating agents including sulphur mustard, HN2, myleran, TEM, cyclophosphamide, sarcolysine and thioTEPA (Wheeler and Alexander 1964; Novikova 1961; Crathorn and Roberts 1965).

The cytotoxicity of melphalan to L1210 cells in vitro is reduced in growth media containing amino acids particularly leucine and glutamine (Vistica et al. 1976). Leucine can reduce the uptake of melphalan by certain cells (Vistica et al. 1978) and there is evidence that melphalan is actively transported by L1210 cells by a process partially dependent on sodium ions and mediated by two separate high-affinity leucine carriers (Vistica 1979). This active uptake can be reduced by removal of glucose from the growth medium or addition of carbonyl cyanide 3-chlorophenylhydrazone, an inhibitor of oxidative phosphorylation, or by low temperatures (Vistica and Rabinovitz 1979). One system is presumed to be system L since it exhibits no dependence on sodium and is sensitive to 2-aminobicyclo[2,2,1]heptane-2-carboxylic acid (BCH) and leucine while the other system is sodium dependent and insensitive to BCH and α-aminoisobutyric acid (Vistica 1980). Similar active transport processes for melphalan have been demonstrated in two other tumour lines, the LPCl plasmacytoma and L5178Y cells (Goldenberg et al. 1979). Evidence has also recently been obtained that melphalan is taken up by both a human breast cancer cell line and peripheral blood lymphocytes from normal humans by an active process involving two amino acid carriers (Begleiter et al. 1980). However, at equilibrium there was about four times as much melphalan in the breast cancer cells because the V_{max} values for both carrier systems were at least 50-fold greater in the tumour cells whereas the Michaelis constants were similar for both cell types.

It follows that resistance could arise by loss of these active transport systems similar to the acquisition of resistance by HN2. Melphalan would still be cytotoxic because it could still enter cells by passive diffusion but it would be markedly less potent and would have a small therapeutic index if the active transport process is more efficient in tumour cells as indicated above. The D isomer of melphalan, medphalan, is not as efficiently concentrated and is about 30 times less potent than melphalan (Elliot and Ling 1981; Vistica et al. 1979). In this connection it is of interest that peptichemio, a tripeptide containing an analogue of melphalan, was some 200–800 times more cytotoxic than melphalan, indicating that it might also be transported by an active process (Morasca and Erba 1980). Evidence that resistance to melphalan may arise from a loss or reduction of one or more active transport carriers has come from studies on L1210 and P388 leukaemia cells in vivo, in comparison with lines with acquired resistance to melphalan. The former tumours accumulated greater amounts of radioactivity following intraperitoneal injection of labelled melphalan than the latter (Brown et al. 1980). However, not all resistant cell lines show a reduced uptake of melphalan. A colchicine-resistant permeability mutant chinese hamster ovary (CHO) cell line was cross-resistant to melphalan because of reduced drug uptake. On the other hand, two CHO lines with acquired resistance to melphalan accumulated similar amounts of labelled drug but less penetrated the nucleus, suggesting that resistance in this case was associated with an alteration of the nuclear membrane (Elliot and Ling 1981). In experiments on a human melanoma cell line with acquired resistance to melphalan, both the parent and the resistant line reached a steady-state concentration of melphalan of three times the concentration in the medium after 2½ min. From a study of covalent binding of the drug and amount of cross-linking it was concluded that the toxicity of melphalan was a result of DNA cross-linking and that resistance arose because of decreased susceptibility of resistant cells to this form of DNA damage (PARSONS et al. 1981). ZWELLING et al. (1981) obtained similar results on L1210 cells with acquired resistance to melphalan. They concluded that DNA cross-linking was the important cytotoxic event since it correlated with the sensitivity of the tumour to bifunctional agents, but there was no good evidence to suggest that any one specific mechanism such as reduced uptake could account for the resistance observed.

Cyclophosphamide is taken up by L5178Y lymphoblasts and chick embryo liver cells by a carrier-mediated system consisting of two components, one which is active at low drug concentrations and is saturable and one which operates at high drug concentrations and is apparently non-saturable. Like the transport systems described for HN2 and melphalan it is temperature dependent. Other alkylating agents (melphalan, HN2 and phosphamide) do not compete with this transfer system, suggesting a very specific carrier, but the natural substrate was not identified (GOLDENBERG et al. 1974). However, since cyclophosphamide requires activation mainly by liver microsomes (CONNORS et al. 1974), loss of the specific carrier for cyclophosphamide could not be a mechanism for development of resistance unless the transport form of "activated" cyclophosphamide, 4-hydroxycyclophosphamide (JUMA et al. 1980; DOMEYER and SLADER 1980a), is also transported by the same mechanism. This is not likely since cyclophosphamide activated by liver microsomes and presumably containing the transport form did not compete with cyclophosphamide for active transport (GOLDENBERG et al. 1974).

Most bifunctional alkylating agents presumably enter cells by passive diffusion although the transport characteristics of most have not been investigated. As lipid water partition coefficient is an important factor for the effective entry of chemicals into cells one might predict that tumours might acquire resistance by acquiring a more lipophilic membrane so that alkylating agents with the appropriate partition coefficient for sensitive cells would not have the optimum value for resistant cells. A colchicine-resistant mutant which has an altered membrane permeability and which is cross-resistant to melphalan has already been mentioned.

It is also known that resistance to some drugs such as adriamycin may arise not only from an impaired facilitated diffusion (INABA and JOHNSON 1978) but also from an increased efflux of the drug from the cells (SKOVSGAARD 1978; KAYE and BODEN 1980). There is, however, no good evidence to show that resistance to alkylating agents may occur by this mechanism.

II. Resistance by Inhibition of the Activation of Prodrugs (Fig. 3 *R2*)

Table 3 shows that in general there is a correlation between the chemical reactivity of the bifunctional alkylating agents and their toxicity (BARDOS et al. 1969; ROSS 1962). Clearly if an alkylating agent has only poor reactivity the majority of it will be excreted unchanged before alkylation of important target molecules

Table 3. Relationship between alkylating activity and toxicity of a series of closely related alkylating agents. As the basicity of the nitrogen increases so does the alkylating activity, while the LD_{50} falls. (Data from BARDOS et al. 1969)

Compound	Alkylating activity ($K'_{80} \times 10^3$)	Toxicity (LD_{50} µmol/kg)
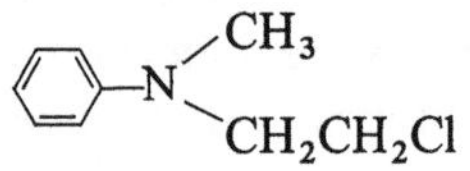	4.9	3,000
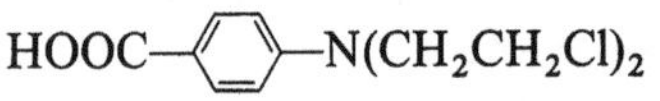	4.6	915
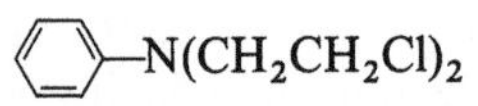	13.0	367
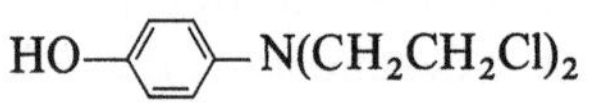	48.6	74
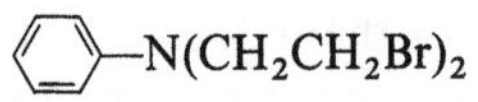	123.0	39

takes place and it will therefore not be highly cytotoxic. In fact there is probably an optimum level of activity for the best antitumour effect since some alkylating agents such as sulphur mustard may be so reactive that they do not reach the tumour but alkylate or hydrolyse close to the site of injection. This property of alkylating agents has been taken advantage of in the design of prodrugs which are themselves chemically unreactive but which can be converted by metabolism into reactive species. Selectivity would occur if the drug were activated only in the tumour cell and not in sensitive host tissues (CONNORS 1978, 1980). Resistance would occur if a tumour normally activating prodrugs lost this property. Thus the azo mustard (Fig. 3) was designed to be activated in malignant hepatocytes which had a reasonably high level of azo reductase and which convert the prodrug into the active *p*-aminophenyl mustard. The loss of the enzyme responsible for activating the azo mustard prodrug would lead to complete resistance to this nitrogen mustard but would not alter the response of the cells to other alkylating agents. For most prodrugs the development of resistance by loss of the activating enzyme has not been investigated, but it has been shown that this is the mechanism by which human tumours acquire resistance to aniline mustard. Aniline mustard (Fig. 5) can be considered to be a prodrug since it is rapidly converted in the liver to the *O*-glucuronide, which is a relatively non-toxic alkylating agent. In some tumours such as the mouse PC6 plasma cell tumour there is a high cytosolic concentration of *β*-glucuronidase which is functional at the physiological pH of the tumour (WHISSON and CONNORS 1965; CONNORS and WHISSON 1966; CONNORS et al. 1973) and converts aniline mustard *O*-glucuronide to the highly cytotoxic *para*-hydroxy aniline mustard. Attempts to obtain a line of the plasma cell tumour resistant to aniline mustard by loss of *β*-glucuronidase activity were unsuccessful, the tumour not changing in sensitivity despite a large number

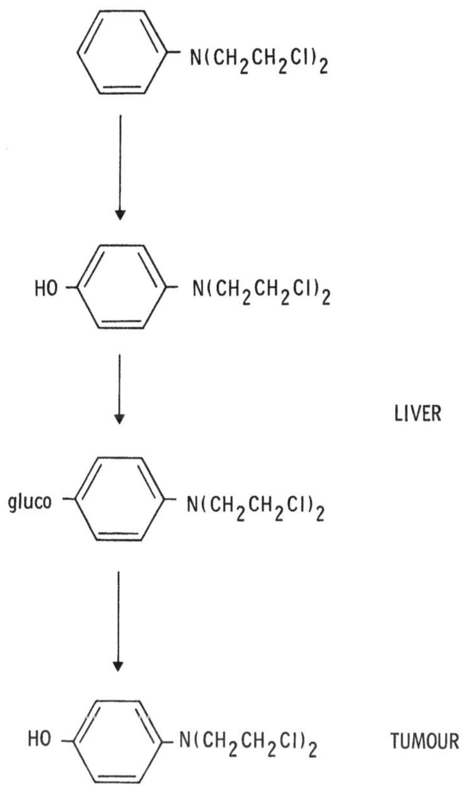

Fig. 5. Detoxification of aniline mustard in the liver by formation of *O*-glucuronide and activation in the region of tumours high in β-glucuronidase

of passages in the presence of aniline mustard. In a clinical study of aniline mustard on seventy-eight patients with advanced cancer a correlation was found between high β-glucuronidase activity of the tumours (measured histochemically) and response to aniline mustard. However, in two patients with high tumour enzyme levels and showing a good response to the drug, the tumour eventually regrew, had little or no glucuronidase activity and did not respond to aniline mustard (YOUNG et al. 1976).

Other alterations in the cellular environment besides loss of enzymes which activate prodrugs can also greatly alter the response of a tumour to alkylating agents. The rate coefficient for the acid-catalysed addition of water of TEM, for example, is extremely high [$K_2 = 2.98 \times 10^4$ (ROSS 1950)]. As a result a small increase in acidity will cause a large increase in chemical reactivity and cytotoxicity. Tumour cells have been reported to be more acid than normal cells (KAHLER and ROBERTSON 1943; EDEN et al. 1955; ASHBY 1966) although this difference has not been confirmed using more recent methods to measure intracellular pH (DICKSON and CALDERWOOD 1979). The cytotoxicity of TEM can be increased by treating tumour-bearing animals with glucose which by increasing the formation of lactic acid may further lower the tumour pH (CONNORS et al. 1964 b). Tumour cells with relatively low pH values and sensitive to ethyleneimines and epoxides because of

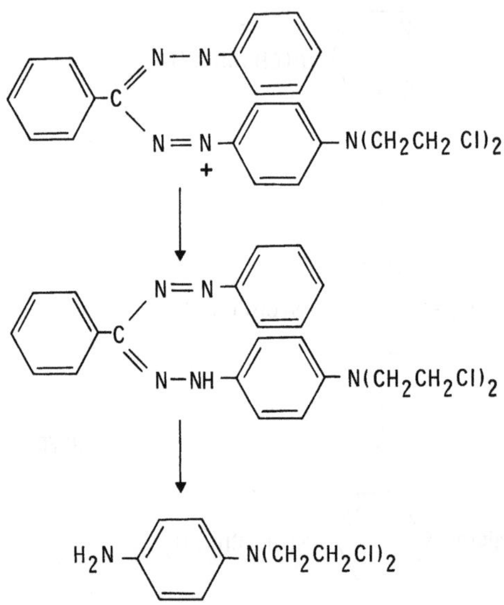

Fig. 6. Reduction of the chemically unreactive tetrazolium nitrogen mustard to a highly active metabolite

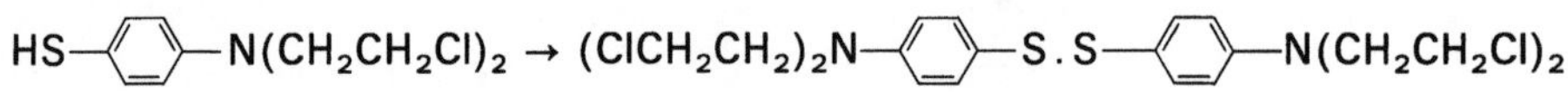

Fig. 7. Deactivation of a thiol mustard by formation of the disulphide

their acid catalysis properties might acquire resistance to these classes of agents if they had pH normal values. On the other hand nitrogen mustards are less active at low pH and there would be no cross-resistance by a mechanism relying on alterations of intracellular pH.

The redox potential of tumour cells will depend on their blood supply and hence on their level of oxygenation. Certain nitrofurans and nitroimidazoles can be selectively toxic against anoxic tumour cells due to their selective reduction in these cells to the corresponding amine with the formation of highly toxic intermediates (CHAPMAN et al. 1981). A cell could theoretically acquire resistance to agents activated by reduction by an increase in oxygen tension. Alkylating agents that might be more readily reduced by anoxic cells, and where resistance would be acquired by increased oxygen tension, would be the tetrazolium mustard (Fig. 6), which is chemically unreactive and a prodrug, releasing the highly toxic *p*-phenylenediamine mustard via the formazan on reduction (TSOU and SU 1963), mitomycin C, which is more toxic to cells under anoxic conditions (TEICHER et al. 1981), and the thiol mustard (Fig. 7), which would be converted to its less reactive disulphide in oxygenated cells. The *N*-oxide of nitrogen mustard might similarly rely on reduction for its activity and thus might be less effective in oxygenated cells. On the other hand ethyleneimine hydroquinones are less reactive than the corresponding quinone (Fig. 8) so that, in this case, an increase in oxygen tension would increase the chemical reactivity of the drug and its cytotoxicity (ROSS 1962).

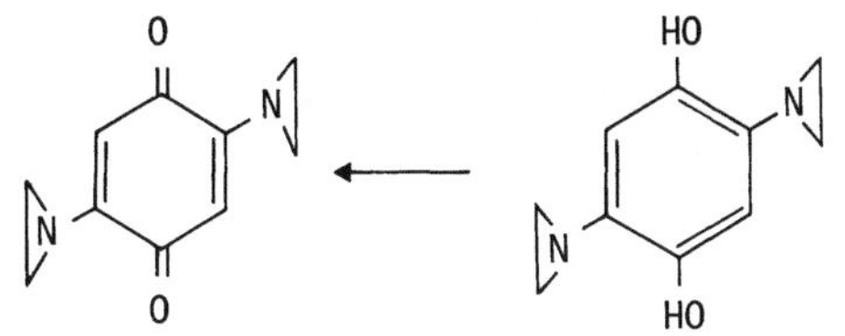

Fig. 8. Activation of an ethyleneimino hydroquinone by formation of the quinone

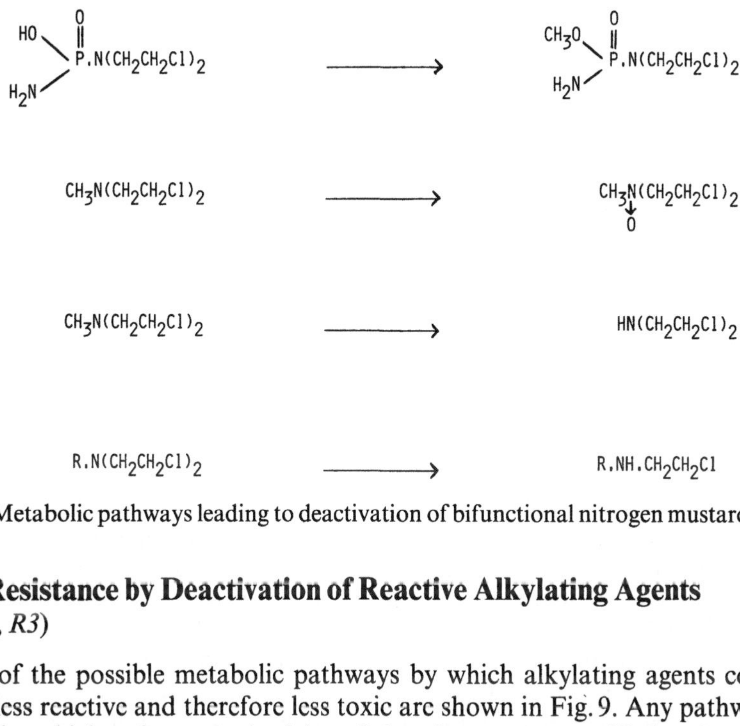

Fig. 9. Metabolic pathways leading to deactivation of bifunctional nitrogen mustard

III. Resistance by Deactivation of Reactive Alkylating Agents
(Fig. 3, *R3*)

Some of the possible metabolic pathways by which alkylating agents could be made less reactive and therefore less toxic are shown in Fig. 9. Any pathway, for example, which reduces the basicity of the nitrogen atom will therefore reduce chemical reactivity and cytotoxicity: thus phosphoramide mustard is very toxic to whole animals and to tumour cells in culture whereas its methyl ester is more than 100 times less toxic. If a cell acquired the ability to methylate phosphoramide mustard it would be much less sensitive to this agent than normal cells. A similar detoxification of nitrogen mustard would occur if it were converted to the *N*-oxide but there are no examples of either of these metabolic pathways occurring in rodents. Demethylation of nitrogen mustard would form norHN2, a much less toxic nitrogen mustard, but while this is a known metabolic pathway it occurs primarily in the liver and not in tumour cells. A mechanism which would lead to general cross-resistance amongst nitrogen mustards (but not to other types of alkylating agents) would be dechloroethylation since monofunctional nitrogen mustards as already discussed have little antitumour activity. Dechloroethylation has been observed with a number of nitrogen mustards and in some cases is quite considerable but this process once again occurs predominantly in the liver and there are no examples of tumours acquiring resistance by this mechanism.

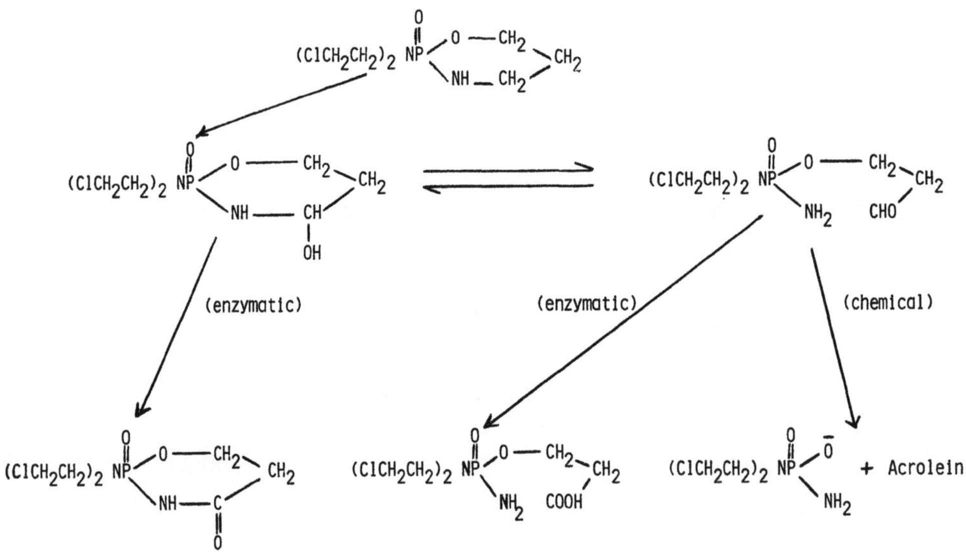

Fig. 10. Pathways of metabolism of cyclophosphamide

Cyclophosphamide is metabolised by the pathways shown in Fig. 10. Primary metabolism is in the liver to the 4-hydroxy derivative, which is in equilibrium with its ring-opened tautomer aldophosphamide. Either metabolite can undergo further metabolism to 4-ketocyclophosphamide in the case of 4-hydroxycyclophosphamide or to the propionic acid derivative in the case of aldophosphamide. Both compounds have poor alkylating ability, are relatively non-toxic and are excretory products in a number of species (COLVIN 1978). 4-Hydroxycyclophosphamide is probably the transport form of "active" cyclophosphamide (JUMA et al. 1980; DOMEYER and SLADEK 1980a). Cyclophosphamide is selective for some types of tumour because unlike other tissues sensitive to alkylating agents (bone marrow, for example) they do not have the ability to form stable non-toxic metabolites from 4-hydroxycyclophosphamide and aldophosphamide, and decomposition to acrolein and the highly toxic phosphoramide mustard occurs to a greater extent in these cells with a consequently higher toxicity. Detoxification of 4-hydroxycyclophosphamide/aldophosphamide is catalysed predominantly by NAD-linked aldehyde dehydrogenases (DOMEYER and SLADEK 1980b), and tumour cells could acquire resistance specifically to cyclophosphamide by an increase in this enzyme. Some preliminary data have been obtained which suggest that this occurs in the development of resistance of L1210 leukaemia cells to cyclophosphamide (P. Cox, personal communication).

IV. Resistance by Interaction with Non-essential Nucleophiles
(Fig. 3, *R4*)

Different cellular molecules will react at different rates with alkylating agents and their rate of reaction will depend both on their concentration and on their "nu-

Table 4. Competition factors for reaction with sulphur mustard in aqueous solution at 25 °C. (Ross 1962)

Substance	Competition factor	pH
Thiosulphate	2.7×10^4	8
Cysteine ethyl ester	1.3×10^3	7
Phosphate	75	8
Chloride	21	7
Acetate	10	7
Formate	3	7
Nitrate	0.2	7
Glucose	0	7

cleophilicity". The relative susceptibility of different molecules to alkylation can be measured in the form of competition factors (Ross 1962). In one example the competition factor measures the reactivity of a nucleophile relative to water. The competition factor of a chemical (F_a) is given by $F_a = K_a/K_o[H_2O]$ where K_a and K_o are the velocity constants for the second-order reaction with nucleophiles and water. The simplest way of measuring competition factors is to measure the extent of acid production of the alkylating agent in water under standard conditions in the presence and absence of the nucleophile since a nitrogen mustard, for example, will form acid when it hydrolyses but not when it alkylates an ionised nucleophile. The competition factors of a range of nucleophiles for sulphur mustard are shown in Table 4. Some nucleophiles can be seen to be a thousand times more reactive than other nucleophiles at physiological pH and hence a small change in the concentration of chemicals with high competition factors could greatly decrease alkylation of a target molecule if its nucleophilicity were not very high. The concept of competition factors is particularly important for agents that act by an SN_2 mechanism since their rate of reaction is dependent on the concentration of the nucleophile. For agents that react by an SN_1 mechanism nucleophilicity is not so important since rate of ionisation is the limiting step. Once the reactive species is formed it will alkylate or hydrolyse almost immediately so what will be important in this case are the nucleophiles in the area where the ionisation takes place.

Although nucleophiles such as chloride ion have been shown to reduce the alkylation of DNA in vitro (Ball and Connors 1967) and ascorbic acid has been suggested as a powerful "natural" protector of important molecules (Edgar 1974), thiols have been the only chemicals for which there is some direct evidence of involvement in the development of resistance. Hirono (1961) found that in three rat tumours with acquired resistance to nitromin the non-protein thiol values of the cells measured by amperometric titration were higher by 1.4- to 2.3-fold than the original sensitive cells from which they were derived. Ball et al. (1966), using a different technique for the measurement of soluble SH, also found that the Yoshida tumour with acquired resistance to melphalan had a level of free SH 1.6-fold higher than the sensitive tumour. The administration of thiols such as cysteine can increase the free SH content of tissues by up to 2.5-fold and can protect tissues including tumours from alkylating agent cytotoxicity (Calcutt et al. 1963; Connors et al. 1965; Connors 1966).

Many chemicals are metabolised in liver and other tissues to alkylating agents or related electrophilic reactants, and glutathione protects DNA and proteins from the potentially toxic effects of these intermediates. Thus paracetamol is metabolised by liver microsomes to a reactive intermediate but whether covalent binding and liver necrosis occurs is dependent on the level of glutathione. Overdoses of paracetamol are hepatotoxic since they deplete reserves of glutathione, but this toxicity may be prevented by giving cysteine, which restores the normal glutathione levels of liver (BUCKPITT et al. 1979). This reaction between electrophilic reactants and glutathione is catalysed by a variety of glutathione *S*-transferases (SMITH et al. 1977; NEMOTO et al. 1975). Tumours might thus acquire resistance to alkylating agents by increasing their levels of glutathione and the appropriate transferases. Resistance to electrophilic reactants may also be associated with an increase in γ-glutamyl transferase since it has been shown that resistance to the acute toxicity of aflatoxin B_1 (which forms a reactive epoxide) occurs in cells which have a high level of transferase enzyme (MANSON et al. 1981). The mechanism for this acquired resistance is not clear but the transferase enzyme is located on the plasma membrane with its active site externally located (DING et al., to be published). Its function could possibly be to transfer glutathione into cells as cysteinylglycine, whose competition factor is ten times higher than glutathione, and this might possibly be a substrate for transferase enzymes. However, in one resistant tumour where the level of γ-glutamyl transferase was measured there was no difference from the sensitive line from which it was derived (HARRAP et al. 1969).

It has also been shown that tumours which have different degrees of "natural" resistance to alkylating agents show a correlation between resistance and protein SH : soluble SH ratios. Thus tumours which did not respond to treatment with the alkylating agent merophan had low protein SH : soluble SH ratios and those which were very sensitive had high ratios. There was, however, no correlation between the total free SH and the sensitivity of the tumour so it was thought the ratio indicated that the role of the free SH was to protect important SH-containing macromolecules from alkylation (CALCUTT and CONNORS 1963).

Since thiols such as cysteine can protect most tissues against the toxicity of alkylating agents and since the glutathione *S*-transferase system has been demonstrated to protect animals against liver toxicity induced by alkylating agents and related compounds, it seems likely that tumours might acquire resistance by the development of such mechanisms. However, although small rises in free SH have been detected in a number of tumours and other tissues when resistance has developed, no such protective mechanism has been described.

F. Conclusions

Tumours can acquire resistance to alkylating agents by a number of different mechanisms. In many cases more than one mechanism is operating and the acquisition of resistance has often been described as multifactorial. As a result a tumour with acquired resistance to one alkylating agent may be completely cross-resistant to a wide spectrum of related agents as is the case with the Yoshida sarcoma (BALL et al. 1966) and the Walker tumour (SCHMID et al. 1980) or show a high resistance to the inducing agent and a smaller degree of resistance to related agents. In extreme cases a tumour with acquired resistance to one alkylating agent may show virtually no cross-resistance even to closely related agents (WAMPLER et al. 1978). However, this does not imply that the agents have a different site of action, merely that, for reasons discussed above, mechanisms are operating which can selectively prevent one alkylating agent from interacting with the DNA target site.

References

Ashby BS (1966) pH Studies in human malignant tumours. Lancet II:312–315

Ball CR, Connors TA (1967) Reduction of the toxicity of "radiomimetic" alkylating agents by thiol pretreatment VI. Biochem Pharmacol 16:509–519

Ball CR, Connors TA, Double JA, Ujhazy V, Whisson ME (1966) Comparison of nitrogen mustard-sensitive and -resistant Yoshida sarcomas. Int J Cancer 1:319–327

Bardos TJ, Chmielewicz ZF, Hebborn P (1969) Structure-activity relationships of alkylating agents in cancer chemotherapy. Ann NY Acad Sci 163:1006–1025

Begleiter A, Froese EK, Goldenberg GJ (1980) A comparison of melphalan transport in human breast cancer cells and lymphocytes in vitro. Cancer Lett 10:243–251

Brown RK, Duncan G, Hill DL (1980) Distribution and elimination of melphalan in rats and monkeys and distribution in tumours of mice bearing L1210 or P388 leukaemias sensitive and resistant to this agent. Cancer Treat Rep 64:643–648

Buckpitt, AR, Rollins DE, Mitchell JR (1979) Varying effects of sulfhydryl nucleophiles on acetaminophen oxidation and sulfhydryl adduct formation. Biochem Pharmacol 28:2941–2946

Calcutt G, Connors TA (1963) Tumour sulphydryl levels and sensitivity to the nitrogen mustard merophan. Biochem Pharmacol 12:839–845

Calcutt G, Connors TA, Elson LA, Ross WCJ (1963) Reduction of the toxicity of "radiomimetic" alkylating agents in rats by thiol pretreatment II. Biochem Pharmacol 12:833–837

Chapman JD, Franko AJ, Sharplin J (1981) A marker for hypoxic cells in tumours with potential clinical applicability. Br J Cancer 43:546–550

Chun EHL, Gonzales L, Lewis FS, Jones J, Rutman RJ (1969) Differences in the in vivo alkylation and cross-linking of nitrogen mustard sensitive and resistant lines of Lettre-Ehrlich ascites tumours. Cancer Res 29:1184–1194

Colvin M (1978) A review of the pharmacology and clinical use of cyclphosphamide. In: Pinedo HM (ed) Clinical pharmacology of anit-neoplastic drugs. Elsevier/North Holland, Amsterdam, pp 245–261

Connors TA (1966) Protection against the toxicity of alkylating agents by thiols. The mechanisms of protection and its relevance to cancer chemotherapy. Eur J Cancer 2:293–305

Connors TA (1975) Mechanism of action of 2-chloroethylamine derivatives, sulfur mustards, epoxides and aziridines. In: Sartorelli AC, Johns DG (eds) Antineoplastic and immunosuppressive agents. Springer, Berlin Heidelberg New York, pp 18–34 (Handbuch der experimentellen Pharmakologie, Vol 38/2)

Connors TA (1978) Antitumour drugs with latent activity. Biochimie 60:979–987

Connors TA (1980) Possible pro-drugs in cancer chemotherapy. Chem Ind (London) 447–450

Connors TA, Whisson ME (1966) Cure of mice bearing plasma cell tumours with aniline mustard. Nature 210:866–867

Connors TA, Jeney A, Jones M (1964a) Reduction of the toxicity of "radiomimetic" alkylating agents in rats by thiol pretreatment III. Biochem Parmacol 13:1545–1550

Connors TA, Mitchley BCV, Rosenoer VM, Ross WCJ (1964b) The effect of glucose pretreatment on the carcinostatic and toxic activities of some alkylating agents. Biochem Pharmacol 13:395–400

Connors TA, Jeney A, Whisson ME (1965) Reduction of the toxicity of radiomimetic alkylating agents in rats by thiol pretreatment V. Biochem Pharmacol 14:1681–1683
Connors TA, Farmer PB, Foster AB, Gilsenan AM, Jarman M, Tisdale MJ (1973) Metabolism of aniline mustard (*N,N*-di-(2-chloroethyl)aniline. Biochem Pharmacol 22:1971–1980
Connors TA, Cox PJ, Farmer PB, Foster AB, Jarman M (1974) Some studies of the active intermediates formed in the microsomal metabolism of cyclophosphamide and isophosphamide. Biochem Pharmacol 23:115–129
Crathorn AR, Roberts JJ (1965) reactions of cultured mammalian cells of varying radiosensitivity with the radiomimetic alkylating agent mustard gas. Prog Biochem Pharmacol 1:320–326
Dickson JA, Calderwood SK (1979) Effects of hyperglycaemic and hyperthermia on the pH, glycolysis and respiration of the Yoshida sarcoma in vivo. J Nat Cancer Inst 63:1371–1381
Ding JL, Smith GD, Peters TJ (to be published) Subcellular localisation and isolation of γ-glutamyl transferase from rat hepatoma cells. Biochem Biophys Acta
Domeyer BE, Sladek NE (1980a) Kinetics of cyclophosphamide biotransformation in vivo. Cancer Res 40:174–180
Domeyer BE, Sladek NE (1980b) Metablism of hydroxycyclophosphamide/aldophosphamide in vitro. Biochem Pharmacol 29:2903–2912
Eden M, Haines B, Kahler H (1955) The pH of rat tumour measured in vivo. JNCI 16:541–545
Edgar JA (1974) Ascorbic acid and biological alkylating agents. Nature 248:136–137
Ehrsson H, Eksborg S, Wallin I, Nilsson S (1980) Degradation of chlorambucil in aqueous solution. J Pharm Sci 69:1091–1094
Elliot EM, Ling V (1981) Selection and characterisation of Chinese hamster ovary cell mutants resistant to melphalan (L-phenylalanine mustard). Cancer Res 41:393–400
Goldenberg BE (1975) The role of drug transport in resistance to nitrogen mustard and other alkylating agents in L5178Y lymphoblasts. Cancer Res 35:1687–1692
Goldenberg GJ (1969) Properties of L5178Y lymphoblasts highly resistant to nitrogen mustard. Ann NY Acad Sci 163:936–953
Goldenberg GJ, Sinha BK (1973) Nitrogen mustard sensitivity and choline transport in Walker 256 carcinosarcoma cells in vitro. Cancer Res 33:2584–2587
Goldenberg GJ, Vanstone CL, Israels LG, Ilse D, Bimler I (1970) Evidence for a transport carrier of nitrogen mustard in nitrogen mustard-sensitive and -resistant L5178Y lymphoblasts. Cancer Res 30:2285–2291
Goldenberg GJ, Vanstone CL, Bimler I (1971a) Transport of nitrogen mustard on the transport carrier for choline in L5178Y lymphoblasts. Science 172:1148–1149
Goldenberg GJ, Lyons RM, Lepp JA, Vanstone CL (1971b) Sensitivity to nitrogen mustard as a function of transport activity and proliferative rate in L5178Y lymphoblasts. Cancer Res 31:1616–1619
Goldenberg GJ, Land HB, Cormack DV (1974) Mechanism of cyclophosphamide transport by L5178Y lymphoblasts in vitro. Cancer Res 34:3274–3282
Goldenberg GJ, Lam PH, Begleiter A (1979) Active carrier mediated transport of mephalan by two separate amino acid transport systems in LPC-1 plasmacytoma cells in vitro. J Biol Chem 254:1057–1064
Harrap KR, Jackson RC, Hill BT (1969) Some effects of chlorambucil on enzymes of gluthione metabolism in drug-sensitive and -resistant strains of the Yoshida ascites sarcoma. Biochem J 111:603–606
Hirono I (1961) Mechanism of natural and acquired resistance to methyl-bis-(β-chlorethyl) amine N-oxide in ascites tumours. Gann 52:39–48
Hirono I, Kachi H, Ohashi A (1962) Mechanism of natural and acquired resistance to methyl-bis(2-chloroethyl)-amine N-oxide in ascites tumours. Gan 53:73–80.
Inaba, M, Johnson RK (1978) Uptake and retention of adriamycin and daunorubicin by sensitive and anthracycline resistant sublines of P388 leukaemia, Biochem Pharmacol 27:2123–2130

Juma FD, Rogers HJ, Trounce JR (1980) The pharmacokinetics of cyclophosphamide, phosphamide mustard and nor nitrogen mustard studied by gas chromatography in patients receiving cyclophosphamide therapy. Br Clin Pharmacol 10:327–335

Kahler H, Robertson WB (1943) pH of normal liver and hepatic tumours. J Natl Cancer Inst 3:495–501

Kaye SB, Boden JA (1980) Cross-resistance between actinomycin-D, adriamycin and vincristine in a murine solid tumour in vivo. Biochem Pharmacol 29:1081–1084

Kessel D, Myers M, Wodinsky I (1969) Accumulation of two alkylating agents, nitrogen mustard and busulfan, by murine leukaemia cells in vitro. Biochem. Pharmacol 18:1229–1234

Levis AG, Colussi M (1963) Caratteristiche di cloni isolati doppo trattamento con una iprite azotata da un ceppo di cellue di cavia coltivate in vitro. Caryologia 16:353–369

Lyons RM, Goldenberg GJ (1972) Active transport of nitrogen mustard and choline by normal and leukaemic human lymphoid cells. Cancer Res 32:1679–1685

Manson MM, Legg RF, Watson JV, Green JA, Neal GE (1981) An examination of the relative resistances to aflatoxin B_1 and susceptibilities to γ-glutamyl *p*-phenylene diamine mustard of γ-glutamyl transferase negative and positive cells. Carcinogenesis 2:661–670

Martin AD, Beerring, Bosanquet AG, Gilby ED (to be published) The effect of alkylating agents and other drugs in the uptake of melphalan by murine L1210 leukaemia cells in vitro.

Miura Y, Moriyama A (1961) Studies on the metabolism of the rat ascites tumour with nitrogen mustard V. J Biochem (Tokyo) 50:362–366

Morasca L, Erba E (1980) In vitro cytotoxicity of peptichemio compared to melphalan and meta-DL sarcolysin. Eur J Cancer 16:1105–1109

Nemoto N, Gelboin HV, Habig WH, Ketley JN, Jakoby WB (1975) K region benzo(a)-pyrene-4,5-oxide in conugation by homogenous glutathione *S*-transferases. Nature 255:512

Novikova MA (1961) Distribution of sarcolysin-C^{14} in rats with sarcoma 45 and with a drug resistant variant of the ssme tumour. Vopr Onkol 7:48–56

Parsons PG, Carter FB, Morrison L, Mary SR (1981) Mechanism of melphalan resistance developed in vitro in human melanonia cells. Cancer Res 41:1525–1534

Price CC, Gaucher GM, Koneru P, Shibakawa R, Sowa JR, Yamaguchi M (1969) Mechanism of action of alkylating agents. Ann NY Acad Sci 163:593–600

Reed BD, Walker IG (1966) Resistance to sulfur mustard. A comparison of some properties of strain-L cells and a resistant subline. Cancer Res 26:1801–1805

Ross WCJ (1950) The reactions of certain epoxides in aqueous solutions. J Chem Soc:2257–2272

Ross WCJ (1962) Biological alkylating agents. Butterworths, London

Rutman RJ, Chun EHL, Lewis RS (1968) Permeability difference as a source of resistance to alkylating agents in Ehrlich tumor cells. Biochem Biophys Res Commun 32:650–657

Schabel FM, Trader WM, Laster WR, Wheeler GP, Witt MH (1978) Patterns of resistance and therapeutic synergism among alkylating agents. In: Schabel FM (ed) Antibiotics and chemotherapy, vol 23. Fundamentals in cancer chemotherapy. Karger, Basel, pp 200–214

Schmid FA, Otter GM, Stock CC (1980) Resistance patterns of Walker carcinosarcoma 256 and other rodent tumours to cyclophosphamide and L-phenylalanine mustard. Cancer Res 40:830–833

Skovsgaard T (1978) Carrier mediated transport of daunorubicin, adriamycin and rubidazone in Ehrlich ascites tumour cells. Biochem Pharmacol 27:1221–1227

Smith GJ, Ohl VS, Litwack G (1977) Ligandin the glutathione *S*-transferases and chemically induced hepatocarcinogenesis. A review. Cancer Res 37:8–14

Teicher BA, Lazo JS, Sartorelli AC (1981) Classifiction of antineoplastic agents by their selective toxicities toward oxygenated and hypoxic tumor cells. Cancer Res 41:73–81

Tsou KC, Su HCF (1963) Synthesis of possible cancer chemotherapeutic compounds based on enzyme approach. J Med Chem 6:693–696

Vistica DT (1979) Cytotoxicity as an indicator for transport mechanism. Biochim Biophys Acta 550:309–317
Vistica DT (1980) Cytotoxicity as an indicator for transport mechanism: evidence that murine bone marrow progenitor cells lack a high-affinity leucine carrier that transports melphalan in murine L1210 leukaemia cells. Blood 56:427–429
Vistica DT, Rabinovitz M (1979) Concentrative uptake of melphalan, a cancer chemotherapeutic agent which is transported by the leucine-preferring carrier system. Biochem Biophys Res Commun 86:929–932
Vistica DT, Toal JN, Rabinovitz M (1976) Amino acid conferred resistance to melphalan. I. Structure activity relationship in cultured murine L1210 leukaemia cells. Cancer Treat Rep 60:1363–1367
Vistica DT, Toal JN, Rabinovitz M (1978) Amino acid-conferred protection against melphalan. Biochem Pharmacol 27:2865–2870
Vistica DT, Rabon A, Rabinovitz M (1979) Cytotoxicities of the L and D isomers of phenylalanine mustards in L1210 cells. Biochem Pharmacol 28:3221–3225
Wampler GI, Regelson W, Bardos TJ (1978) Absence of cross resistance to alkylating agents in cyclophosphamide-resistant L1210 leukaemia. Eur J Cancer 14:977–982
Wheeler GP, Alexander JA (1964) Studies with mustards. In vivo fixation of C^{14} of labelled alkylating agents by bilterally grown sensitive and resistant tumors. Cancer Res 24:1331–1337
Whisson ME, Connors TA (1965) Cure of mice bearing advanced plasma cell tumours with aniline mustard. Nature 206:689–691
Williamson CE, Whitten B (1967) Reaction mechanism of some aromatic nitrogen mustards. Cancer Res 27:33–38
Wolpert MK, Ruddon RW (1969) A study on the mechanism of resistance to nitrogen mustard (HN2) in Ehrlich ascites tumor cells; comparison of uptake of HN2-^{14}C into sensitive and resistant cells. Cancer Res 29:873–879
Yamada T, Iwanami Y, Baba T (1963) The transport of ^{14}C-labelled nitrogen mustards N-oxide through cellulose membrane treated with Tween 80 in vitro. Gann 54:171–176
Young CW, Yagoda A, Bittar ES, Smith SW, Gribstald H, Whitmore W (1976) Therapeutic trial of aniline mustard in patients with advanced cancer. Cancer 38:1887–1895
Zwelling LA, Michaels S, Schwartz H, Dobson PP, Kohn KW (1981) DNA cross linking as an indicator of sensitivity and resistance of mouse L1210 leukemia to *cis*-diamminedichloroplatinum (II) and L-phenylalanine mustard. Cancer Res 41:640–649

CHAPTER 16

Nitrosoureas

K. D. TEW and P. S. SCHEIN

A. Pharmacology

Under physiological conditions the nitrosoureas decompose spontaneously (COLVIN et al. 1976; MONTGOMERY et al. 1975). The chemical half-lives of individual compounds in phosphate-buffered saline (pH 7.4) vary from 5 min to as long as 2 h. In the process of degradation, a number of alkylating moieties are formed of which an alkyldiazohydroxide precursor and the chloroethyl carbonium ion are considered the most important. Organic isocyanates are also generated that may carbamoylate intracellular proteins and nucleic acids. Thus, there are two chemical activities, alkylation and carbamoylation (WHEELER et al. 1974). Generally, amino, carboxyl, imidazole, sulphydryl and phosphate groups are preferential targets for alkylation. Carbamoylation occurs at nucleophilic sites in amino acids, such as the ε-amino group of lysine or guanidinium group of arginine. Alkylation is widely accepted as the principal mechanism of antitumor activity; however, studies have failed, with a wide range of nitrosoureas, to show a linear relationship between in vitro alkylating activity and the chloroethyl antitumor activity for the murine L1210 leukemia. Studies with water-soluble analogues have suggested a parabolic relationship with an optimal relative alkylating activity of 60% that of chlorozotocin. In addition, there was no correlation between carbamoylating activity and antitumor activity (WHEELER et al. 1974), granulocyte suppression (PANASCI et al. 1977), or lethal toxicity (HEAL et al. 1979b). Both chlorozotocin and streptozotocin contain carbon-2-sugar-substituted moieties in their R-groups and possess neglible carbamoylating activity but retain antitumor activity. Comprehensive studies on the breakdown products of chlorozotocin have demonstrated internal carbamoylation of the 1- or 3-hydroxyl groups of the glucose ring as well as dimer product formation (HAMMER et al. 1981). These internal reactions presumably explain the low carbamoylating potential of chlorozotocin and, by extrapolation, streptozotocin.

In addition to their spontaneous chemical dissociation, the nitrosoureas are now known to be metabolized by the liver microsomal mixed function oxidase system to more polar hydroxylated products which retain both the cyclohexyl ring structure and the cytotoxic nitrosoureido moiety (REED and MAY 1975). Current data indicate that the rate of metabolic hydroxylation of 1-(2-chloroethyl)-3-cyclohexyl-1-nitrosourea (CCNU) exceeds the rate of chemical dissociation (WALKER and HILTON 1976) and that, as a result, it is probable that hydroxylated metabolites are the immediate precursors of the therapeutic and toxic moieties. Metabolism of CCNU produces products in which the chemical properties of the parent compound are significantly modified. WHEELER et al. (1977) have shown that all of the hydroxylated derivatives of CCNU are more water soluble, have higher alkylating activities and in some cases have lower carbamoylating activities than CCNU.

B. Mechanisms of Drug Resistance

Acquired resistance to nitrosoureas must be mediated through an alteration in the genetic material of the cell, conferring phenotypic properties which permit cell survival during drug attack. During nitrosourea therapy in patients, such tumor cells that possess resistance will be selected, while those with "normal genotypes" will be killed. From this point, the tumor may be repopulated by clones of cells which are refractory to conventional drug treatment. Since multiple resistance develops in many cases, the rational, though still empirical, approach of combination drug regimens may remain ineffectual in eradicating the patient's tumor.

Both acquired and intrinsic resistance to antitumor nitrosoureas may be associated with any or all of the following:

1. Impaired uptake of the drug
2. Increased levels of drug-catabolizing enzymes
3. Enhanced repair of drug-damaged macromolecules (particularly DNA)
4. Differential sites of alkylation within chromatin.

Immunological and tumor-cell kinetic properties can also play determinant roles in mechanisms of resistance to drugs. In fact, it is likely that the overall expression of drug resistance will be a composite phenomenon, determined severally by the aforementioned properties.

Logically, the site of chromatin alkylation and the rate of repair of damage (if indeed repair does occur) would seem to be interdependent. Indeed, there are numerous reports of differential repair rates of alkylated DNA, dependent upon the location of the damage within the chromatin structural architecture (RAMANATHAN et al. 1976; BODELL 1977; AHLGREN et al. 1982).

Since nitrosoureas possess the same pharmacological properties as bifunctional alkylating agents, by necessity, mechanisms of resistance to nitrosoureas will be similar to (or may even overlap) mechanisms of alkylating agent resistance. In addition to the formation of alkylated monoadducts and cross-links, the capacity of most nitrosoureas to carbamoylate proteins cannot be overlooked when considering mechanisms of drug resistance.

At the cellular level there are two widely accepted resistance mechanisms which have been studied in mammalian cells: decreased drug uptake and increased repair of drug lesions. For example, in a study employing Ehrlich ascites cells it was found that uptake of nitrogen mustard into resistant cells was one-half that of the sensitive line, but resistance to the drug was 10- to 100-fold (WOLPERT and RUDDON 1969). Such quantitative differences suggested that factor(s) other than impaired uptake were involved in the expression of resistance.

Nitrogen mustard has an active mode of transport, involving at least two separate transport systems (LYONS and GOLDENBERG 1972). It is less easy to correlate nitrosourea resistance to an impaired uptake, since nitrosoureas have been shown to diffuse passively into cells in culture (BEGLEITER et al. 1977). These same authors demonstrated that both 1,3 bis 2-chlorethylnitrosourea (BCNU) and CCNU entered cells as intact molecules or as metabolites which were known to be cytotoxic. Since activation of nitrosoureas is spontaneous under physiological conditions, it is possible that differential uptake of drug metabolites could account for resistance. It has been suggested that the alkylating function of nitrosoureas is responsible for antitumor activity (COLVIN et al. 1976) and that the carbamoylation by isocyanates is of minor importance to cytotoxicity (PANASCI et al. 1979). Thus, a preferential uptake of isocyanates with reduced uptake of alkylating species may reduce the effectiveness of the drug and result in resistance. It remains unlikely that reduced drug uptake will provide a complete explanation for drug resistance. More recent studies have suggested that the rate and degree of repair of drug lesions may be more relevant. This phenomenon is closely linked to the site of drug interaction within the nucleus (for review see TEW 1981).

C. Significance of Molecular Considerations

Eukaryotic DNA is tightly complexed to proteins to form nucleoprotein fiber, chromatin. Electron microscopy has demonstrated a beaded appearance of chromatin composed of spheres (nucleosomes) containing some 140 base pairs of DNA complexed with histones. Between nucleosomes, a variable length of DNA (< 80 base pairs) is thought to be associated with histone H1 and various nonhistone proteins. Regions of chromatin that are actively transcribing RNA, euchromatin, have a more open structure than heterochromatin, the more condensed transcriptionally inactive material. Many lines of evidence point to structural and chemical differences between euchromatin and heterochromatin. Although both are organized into repeating structures, euchromatin differs from heterochromatin in both composition and DNA conformation.

It is axiomatic that nuclear-reactant drugs enact cell kill through modification of nuclear macromolecules, especially DNA. It is clear from the nucleosomal structural organization of chromatin that there is potential for differences in sites of drug interaction to exist between cells. Drug resistance and sensitivity may be explained by differences in the distribution of drug lesions within specific domains of chromatin, notwithstanding the possibility that one region may be more critical for cytotoxicity than another. This theory will be relevant both at the level of extended (euchromatin) versus condensed (heterochromatin) chromatin, and at the subnucleosome level.

Since nitrosoureas are known to interact extensively with cellular proteins both by alkylation and carbamoylation, there is a rationale for considering these modifications as potential cytotoxic events. There is evidence that protein modifications per se can modulate cytotoxicity and/or carcinogenicity (PITOT and HEIDELBERGER 1963). Alternatively, drug interactions with histone or nonhistone proteins could induce toxicity indirectly by (a) altering structural components of the cell nucleus, (b) inactivating functional proteins, which may be enzymes or receptors, (c) decreasing effectiveness of repair enzymes, (d) modifying the numerous interactions with DNA – thereby affecting both structure of function, and (e) inducing error-prone transcription and replication.

Recently, evidence has emerged to suggest that an intimate correlation between plasma membrane functions and the regulation of cell division exists (GERSTEN and BOSMAN 1975; EDELMAN 1976). Additionally, there is data to suggest that replicating chromatin is closely associated with the nuclear membrane (DIJKWEL et al. 1979). Since both types of membrane consist of molecular species which are susceptible to alkylation or carbamoylation, it is reasonable to suggest that they may play an important role in ultimate drug cytotoxicity. In fact, there is preliminary evidence that the alkylating agent Trenimon, at therapeutic concentrations, caused extensive alterations of the plasma membrane and that alkylation of this membrane may, per se, be sufficient for cytotoxicity (IHLENFELDT et al. 1981). The nuclear membrane and matrix contribute to the overall structural stabilization of the nucleus (see TEW 1982). Direct membrane protein alkylation or carbamoylation (WANG et al. 1983) may interfere with this stability, and direct alkylation of membrane-associated chromatin, plausibly replicative, may be of considerable importance to resultant drug cytotoxicity (TEW et al. 1983).

D. Monoadducts and Cross-Linking

In many cell lines, the increased cytotoxic potential of the haloethylnitrosoureas when compared with methylnitrosoureas has been attributed to the ability of the former to cross-link nuclear macromolecules (KOHN 1979). The methylnitrosoureas are capable of causing monoadducts which, unlike the chloroethyl, do not undergo conversion to cross-links. In V79 Chinese hamster cells, 1-methyl-1-nitrosourea (MNU) and streptozotocin required 40 times the drug concentration to produce toxicity equal to a wide range of haloethylnitrosoureas (ERICKSON et al. 1978a). Formation of either DNA-DNA or DNA-protein cross-links from an initial monoadduct alkylation is a time-dependent phenomenon. It is probable that the speed and efficiency of repair of these monoadducts will be predeterminate to the occurrence of cross-links. In other words, a more efficient removal and repair of alkylated nucleic acids or proteins would reduce the likelihood of cross-link formation with a presumed concomitant reduction in cytotoxicity. Thus, increased resistance to the haloethylnitrosoureas could be a consequence of either (a) enhanced repair of alkylated bases or amino acids or (b) reduced conversion of these monoadducts to cross-links. In addition, an enhanced ability to repair these cross-links may confer an increased drug tolerance. Indeed, it has been reported that a drug-resistant human colon xenograft (HT) grown in nude mice exhibited substantially less cross-linking than did a nitrosourea-sensitive line following methyl-CCNU (MeCCNU) treatment (THOMAS et al. 1978). Using the alkaline elution methodology, MeCCNU was found to produce DNA strand breaks and DNA cross-links in both resistant (HT) and sensitive (Be) cells in culture. The DNA cross-links were completely repaired in the resistant line by 48 h after drug removal, but in the sensitive BE line, little or no cross-link repair was observed during this interval (ERICKSON et al. 1978b). More recent studies have demonstrated that the HT cell line possessed the most competent Mer^+ repair function (monoadduct repair capacity) when compared with 14 human cell lines including BE (ERICKSON et al. 1980). Furthermore, in HT cells, the majority of the observed cross-links were DNA-protein, whereas in BE cells the cross-links were DNA interstrand (personal communication, L. C. Erickson). These findings have two major implications relating to drug resistance mechanisms: (a) the ability to repair monoadducts prior to their conversion to cross-links may confer phenotypic resistance to haloethylnitrosoureas and this is determined by an efficient Mer^+ repair capacity and (b) DNA-DNA cross-links are more cytotoxic than DNA-protein. Hence, occurrence of the latter in certain cells may result in the expression of drug resistance. By connotation, the possession of an efficient Mer^+ repair function should confer resistance not only to anticancer drugs such as nitrosoureas, but also to carcinogens and other methylating compounds such as the methylnitrosoureas.

Mechanistically, recent evidence has suggested that repair of O^6-methyl and O^6-ethyl guanine involves destruction rather than excision of these residues from DNA (ROBINS and CAIRNS 1979; KARRAN et al. 1979; RENARD and VERLY 1980). Since O^6-alkylation alters the bond conjugation in the guanine ring, this could be the recognition feature for an enzyme which acts on the ring regardless of the identity of the alkylating group. Thus, it has been suggested that O^6-methyl guanine and O^6-2-chloroethyl guanine (resultant monoadduct formed by chloroethylnitrosoureas) residues may be destroyed and repaired by the same enzyme (ERICKSON et al. 1980). Such a "chromatin factor" has been found in large quantities in rat liver (RENARD and VERLY 1980).

E. Interference with the DNA Repair Process

The importance of the carbamoylation potential of nitrosoureas to overall cytotoxicity is not altogether clear. Certainly there is much evidence that both chloroethylnitrosoureas (TEW et al. 1978b; SUDHAKAR et al. 1979b) and methylnitrosoureas (SUDHAKAR et al. 1979b; PINSKY et al. 1979) carbamoylate a large proportion of nuclear histone and nonhistone proteins. Because of the large numbers, adequate duplication, and high turnover rates of most of these proteins, it is plausible that the repair and/or replacement of these molecules will be achieved with minimal resultant cytotoxicity (TEW 1981). However, there are reports that 2-chloroethyl isocyanate, the carbamoylating moiety resulting from decomposition of BCNU, interferes with the ligase step of the excision process of X-ray damage repair (KANN et al. 1974; FORNACE et al. 1978). Inactivation of the enzyme system would presumably possess stoichiometry, relative to isocyanate pools and quantities of the repair ligase enzymes. These two parameters provide potential variables which might determine the expression of drug resistance, since a decreased potential to overcome the drug-induced ligase block would result in increased cytotoxicity.

It is not certain that the isocyanate inhibition of X-ray damage repair can be extrapolated to inhibition of drug damage repair. The effect of the nitrosoureas streptozotocin and 3-β-D-glucopyranosyl-1-methyl-1-nitrosourea (GMNU) on the repair of alkylating damage has been reported (HEAL et al. 1979b). The two drugs have comparable alkylating activity and produce similar numbers of single-strand breaks in L1210 cells in vitro. However, streptozotocin produces 3% carbamoylation of [^{14}C]lysine, as compared with 42% for GMNU. The rate of repair of L1210 DNA after exposure to GMNU was significantly slower than after streptozotocin, supporting the concept of carbamoylation-mediated interference with the repair process. The relevance of these data to cytotoxicity is equivocal, since either in vitro or in vivo the ID_{50} or LD_{50} values for streptozotocin are indistinguishable from those for GMNU (Heal et al. 1979a).

F. Subnucleosomal Nitrosourea Binding

The premise that the site of chromatin drug binding is important to eventual cytotoxicity has been mentioned previously. The relevance of such a theory relates to the potential of certain cells to repair drug damage in specific chromatin regions more efficiently than others. Preferential alkylation and/or repair of specific subnucleosomal regions of chromatin has been reported for a number of carcinogens (Bodell 1977; Cleaver 1977; Metzger et al. 1977; Ramanathan et al. 1976). The relative complexity of the eukaryotic repair system when compared with prokaryotes substantiates the concept that eukaryotic chromatin exerts a restraint upon the rate and possible efficiency of the repair process.

Our previous studies have shown preferential alkylation by MNU of HeLa-cell chromatin susceptible to the enzyme micrococcal nuclease (Sudhakar et al. 1979b), whereas both CCNU and chlorozotocin alkylated chromatin which was more accessible to DNase I (Tew et al. 1978b; Sudhakar et al. 1979b). It has been possible to correlate cytotoxicity with site of internucleosomal alkylation of chloroethylnitrosoureas. In vitro studies with murine bone marrow and L1210 cells demonstrated that chlorozotocin alkylation was 1.3 times higher in L1210 cells (Panasci et al. 1979) and in addition, the major proportion of this alkylation occurred in the DNA associated with the nucleosome core particle (Tew et al. 1978a). Conversely, alkylation of bone marrow DNA occurred preferentially between nucleosomes in the linker region. This site specificity may account for the observed quantitative differences in drug binding and may correlate with the low myelosuppressive activity of chlorozotocin in murine bone marrow. CCNU has an L1210: bone marrow DNA alkylation ratio of 0.6 and was found to alkylate DNA preferentially in the nucleosome core of bone marrow cells (Tew et al. 1978a). These findings were consistent with the known myelosuppressive properties of CCNU. Further validation of these findings was obtained by comparing the subnucleosome-binding sites of two nonmyelosuppressive nitrosoureas chlorozotocin and 1-(2-chloroethyl)-3-(β-D-glucopyranosyl)-1-nitrosourea (GANU) with two myelosuppressive nitrosoureas, CCNU and ACNU [*N'*-((4-amino-2-methyl-5-pyrimidinyl)-methyl)-*N*-(2-chloroethyl)-*N*-nitrosourea]. All four drugs were found to alkylate DNA associated with the core particle in L1210 cells, while in murine bone marrow, CCNU and ACNU alkylated DNA, but chlorozotocin and GANU alkylated linker DNA (Green et al. 1982). This relationship may be dependent upon the glucose carrier group which both chlorozotocin and GANU possess; however, their reduced cytotoxicity was not mediated by differential cellular uptake, since this process is passive for glucose-containing nitrosoureas (Begleiter et al. 1977). Such data are interpreted as meaning that drug lesions within regions of linker DNA are less deleterious to the cell. Preliminary data (AHLGREN et al. 1982) would suggest that these lesions are more easily repaired within bone marrow cells, findings which are consistent with similar studies using other carcinogens (BODELL 1977; CLEAVER 1977; METZGER et al. 1977; RAMANATHAN et al. 1976). Thus, this increased repair potential may account for the increased resistance of bone marrow to chlorozotocin and GANU.

Studies in other tissues with MNU and 1-ethyl-1-nitrosourea (ENU) have demonstrated a differential repair of O^6-alkylguanine in rat brain (these drugs are both neuro-oncogenic) when compared with other tissues (KLEIHUES and BUCHELER 1977). Repair of O^6-alkylguanine was complete in liver, lung and kidney after 7,28 and 84 days respectively. At 184 days approximately 25% of these drug lesions remained in brain tissue. By extrapolation, repair of drug damage would require approximately 1 year. The different components of the repair in rat brain may have been indicative of (a) the chromatin complex having different accessibility to repair enzymes or (b) an initial preferential subnucleosomal alkylation pattern; these factors are possibly interrelated.

G. Effects on Pyridine Nucleotides

It has been demonstrated that any compound with a basic $R\text{-}\overset{\overset{\textstyle NO}{|}}{N}\text{-}CH_3$ or $R\text{-}\overset{\overset{\textstyle NO}{|}}{N}\text{-}C_2H_5$ structure could reduce intracellular NAD and NADH concentrations in murine liver and L1210 leukemia (SCHEIN 1969). In fact, the acute reduction of NAD in the islets of Langerhans serves as an explanation for the diabetogenic properties of streptozotocin and has been shown to be prevented by concurrent administration of nicotinamide (SCHEIN et al. 1973a). The cytotoxic group of streptozotocin, MNU, is itself diabetogenic, although a 3.5-fold increase in the in vivo dose is required to achieve the same effect as with streptozotocin. The glucose (glucosamine) carrier facilitates a more efficient islet cell uptake of streptozotocin (ANDERSON et al. 1974) which explains the relative efficacy of this drug in pancreatic tumors. The addition of a halide moiety, as in chlorozotocin, eliminates both the reduction of pyridine nucleotides and the diabetogenic properties of the glucose nitrosourea.

A correlation between methylnitrosourea-induced reductions in NAD and stimulation of poly(ADP-ribose) polymerase activity has been established in HeLa cells (SMULSON et al. 1977). While the precise function of this enzyme has yet to be elucidated, its chromatin location (SUDHAKAR et al. 1979a) is suggestive of intranuclear regulation and there is evidence to suggest an involvement in the DNA repair process, especially repair of single-strand breaks (see SMULSON et al. 1979). This explanation is consistent with the propensity of methylnitrosoureas to induce single-strand breaks in chromatin, while chloroethylnitrosoureas do not. Resistance and/or sensitivity to methyl- versus chloroethylnitrosoureas may be a function of variations in cellular NAD or poly(ADP-ribose) polymerase concentrations.

H. Modulation of Drug Effect with Steroids and Other Transcriptional Modifiers

It has proved feasible to manipulate the cytotoxic properties of nuclear-reactant drugs, such as nitrosoureas, with chemicals which themselves modulate nuclear functions. Alterations of nuclear morphology and transcriptional activity following sodium butyrate (Nudel et al. 1977), dimethyl sulfoxide (Scher et al. 1978), prednisolone (Wilkinson et al. 1979), and hydrocortisone (Tew et al. 1980a, b, 1982) have, in some cases, modified the subsequent interaction of alkylating agents and nitrosoureas with nuclear macromolecules. For example, previous studies have shown that the corticosteroid prednisolone could potentiate the antitumor efficacy of chlorambucil in a resistant strain of a Yoshida sarcoma cell line (Harrap et al. 1977). Steroids have been shown to enact chromatin disaggregation in a number of cell lines (Whitfield et al. 1968; Wilkinson et al. 1979; Tew et al. 1980b). Alkylated nucleophilic sites in bases and amino acids have been identified, but their location within the nuclear structural and functional architecture has not been fully elucidated (Tew 1981, 1982). Similarly, steroid-mediated effects are preceded by initial binding of the steroid to a cytosol receptor, translocation to the nucleus, and eventual binding to nuclear receptors. The nature of these receptors has not been resolved, although there is evidence that both histones and nonhistones (Tsai and Hnilica 1971) are involved. The presence of common sites of drug and hormone binding within the nucleus lends credence to their increased efficacy in combination. Pretreatment of HeLa cells with physiological concentrations of hydrocortisone has been shown to modify the binding of chlorozotocin and CCNU to various chromatin fractions (Tew et al. 1980a, b). By exposing HeLa cells to micromolar concentrations of hydrocortisone for 22 h, transcriptional activity was stimulated approximately tenfold and chromatin disaggregation was identified by electron microscopy. Subsequent incubations with chlorozotocin or CCNU (0.6 m*M* for 2 h) demonstrated that, although cellular and nuclear drug uptake were unaffected, there was a greater proportion of drug binding in transcriptionally active chromatin fractions which were sensitive to DNase I and DNase II. The observation that "extended" chromatin regions are preferential drug targets has relevance to the manipulation of nuclear structure to enhance drug cytotoxicity and thereby overcome phenotypically expressed drug resistance. Our microscopic studies (Tew et al. 1980b) have detailed chromatin rearrangement which was consistent with an increased availability of disaggregated transcriptional chromatin for drug interaction. This resulted in a 1.5- to 2-fold increased alkylation and carbamoylation by both chlorozotocin and CCNU within that portion of the genome which was actively transcribing. As yet, there is no definitive evidence that drug lesions within transcriptional chromatin regions have greater cytotoxic potential; however, there is evidence of cytotoxic synergism (as measured by soft agar colony assays) when nitrosoureas and hormones are tested in combination against HeLa cells (Tew et al. 1982). These findings, together with those for prednisolone and chlorambucil, suggest that modulation of the properties of nuclear reactant drugs may be achieved with steroids, thereby sensitizing otherwise resistant cells. The precise scheduling of these combinations is critical to cytotoxic efficacy and may vary for specific steroids/drugs and, moreover, for particular tumor cell populations.

Similar studies using HeLa cells and sodium butyrate were designed to cause chromatin structural alterations via nuclear protein modifications and to result in an increase in transcriptional activity. Increased cellular uptake of chlorozotocin and CCNU in butyrate-treated cells demonstrated that butyrate had an effect upon the cell membrane. Whereas drug uptake into the cytoplasm of butyrate-treated cells was increased by a factor of 1.8, nuclear incorporation was 2.4 times greater than in control cells. This increase may have resulted from an effect on nuclear membrane permeability, or from an increase in the number of available binding sites within the chromatin structure. The latter explanation would be consistent with the corticosteroid effect, insofar as the stimulation of transcriptional activity by butyrate (Tew et al. 1978 b) would create more target sites for drug interaction. The effect of compounds such as butyrate on the cell-killing potential of drugs such as nitrosoureas is undetermined. However, there appears to be a rational basis for exploiting such combinations to eradicate tumor cell populations which are otherwise refractory to drug treatments.

J. Overcoming Resistance to Alkylating Agents with Nitrosoureas

In clinical situations it is usual to administer combinations of antitumor drugs in an empirical attempt to circumvent tumor cell resistance to one or more of the drugs. In such instances, nitrosoureas are assumed to act as bifunctional alkylating agents, with the underlying premise that cells resistant to alkylating agents will be cross-resistant to nitrosoureas. However, recent studies on the Walker 256 rat carcinoma cell line have provided data to suggest differential sensitivity to the two classes of drugs. An alkylating-agent-resistant cell line was established from the original sensitive line by Tisdale and Phillips (1976). By exposing an in vitro culture to increasing concentrations of chlorambucil they were able to select a stable cell line which exhibited resistance to chlorambucil (see Wilkinson et al. 1978). The tumor was found to be totally cross-resistant to nitrogen mustard, phenyl acetic mustard, melphalan, and cyclophosphamide. Using soft-agar colony assays, we have demonstrated that the resistant cell line does not possess cross-resistance to the chloroethylnitrosoureas, chlorozotocin, and CCNU (Tew and Wang 1982). Despite the ID_{50} value in Walkerresistant cells for chlorozotocin (5.0 μ*M*) being similar to that for CCNU (2.0 μ*M*), at higher concentrations CCNU was found to be more effective than chlorozotocin in eradicating resistant cells (Tew and Wang 1982). The increased efficacy of CCNU was also demonstrated as a function of exposure time. At 5.0 μ*M* total cell kill for CCNU was reached at 24 h. At this time, chlorozotocin had caused 85% cell death, with 100% lethality at 48 h. Thus, in addition to the ability of the haloethylnitrosoureas to overcome the acquired resistance to alkylating agents, there existed a differential in the sensitivity of Walker cells to CCNU and chlorozotocin. The precise mechanism of this differential drug effect is yet to be determined; however, the increased carbamoylation potential of CCNU [45% carbamoylated lysine versus 2% for chlorozotocin (see Panasci et al. 1979)] may prove to be significant. This concept is supported by survival studies in Walker-resistant cells when exposed to a nitrosocarbamate of 19-nortestosterone, LS 1727 (HARTLEY-ASP et al. 1981). This compound possessed properties of classical alkylating agents, with negligible carbamoylating potential. At concentrations as high as 50 μg/ml there was no effect on Walker-resistant cell survival, whereas the corresponding sensitive cell line was reduced to 40% survival in an in vitro colony assay procedure. Furthermore, there is evidence that the TLX5 lymphoma is sensitive to CCNU and cyclohexylisocyanate (the active carbamoylating moiety of CCNU) but resistant to alkylating agents of the nitrogen mustard type and only marginally sensitive to chlorozotocin (GIBSON and HICKMAN 1982). The specific mechanisms by which carbamoylation induces cytotoxicity in these cells is not defined, but presumably will relate to the inactivation of one or more crucial cellular proteins. This effect may be cytotoxic per se or may interfere indirectly with the storage, processing, or functioning of nucleic acids in the nucleus.

Since the uptake and metabolism of nitrosoureas are passive in cell culture, it is probable that this resistance to bifunctional alkylating agents and concomitant sensitivity of nitrosoureas will be determined at the level of the nucleus. Notwithstanding reports of alkylating-agent-induced cell death through plasma membrane interactions (GRUNICKE et al. 1978; IHLENFELDT et al. 1981), it is possible that no individual nuclear perturbation will be responsible for ultimate cell death. The determinants of drug resistance (or, conversely, sensitivity) may be a composite of nuclear protein, RNA, and DNA modifications, with resultant effects upon the cellular repair process. Only a greater understanding of the relative potential of nuclear chromatin domains to act as potential drug targets will lead to a knowledge of how these resistant cells have overcome drug-induced damage and, thereby, remain viable.

Information gained from Walker cells and certain other cell lines would indicate that nitrosoureas and alkylating agents have different cytotoxic properties which could be considered as effective additively in drug combinations at the clinical level. Such a possibility will have to be balanced with possible additive toxicity to the various dose-limiting normal tissues.

K. Clinical Therapeutic Activity

The initial phase I trial of BCNU, conducted in 1962, demonstrated clinical activity in lymphomas. Unfortunately, the problem of delayed and cumulative bone marrow toxicity was not appreciated in the initial animal toxicology studies, and the original schedule of frequent drug administration produced serious and lethal toxicity. In recognition of this inherent treatment-limiting toxicity, recently designed studies have employed intermittent schedules of treatment, to allow for full bone marrow recovery between each course. This represents an important limitation of this class of agents, which prevents the use of intensive courses and complicates the design of drug combinations. The most commonly employed dose schedules for the chloroethylnitrosoureas, when used as single agents in previously untreated patients, include the following: BCNU, 150–200 mg/m^2 intravenously ever 6–8 weeks; MeCCNU, 150–200 mg/m^2 orally every 6–8 weeks (WAS-

SERMAN et al. 1975). The intermittency of schedule can be presumed to allow resistant clones of cells to arise between the widely spaced treatments.

The chloroethylnitrosoureas have been demonstrated to possess a broad spectrum of activity against human malignancies. The major indications include gliomas, lymphoproliferative diseases, small-cell carcinomas of the lung, melanoma, and gastrointestinal cancer (WASSERMAN et al. 1975). The use of nitrosoureas for gliomas represents an attempt to exploit the lipid solubility of most members of this class of antitumor agent. The reported response rates for BCNU and CCNU are 45% and 37% respectively, whereas MeCCNU appears to be less active, 23%. The Brain Tumor Study Group has carried out an important controlled randomized trial of nitrosourea chemotherapy for patients with glioblastoma who had undergone a "definitive" surgical resection (WALKER and GEHAN 1976). Patients were randomized to receive one of four postoperative treatment options: (a) BCNU, 80 mg/m^2/day on three successive days every 6–8 weeks; (b) radiation therapy (5,000–6,000 rads over 6–8 weeks); (c) a combination of BCNU plus radiation therapy; and (d) best conventional care. An analysis of survival data for patients who received at least 5,000 rads of irradiation or two courses of BCNU revealed the following: the median survival for conventional care was 17 weeks; this was contrasted with a 25-week median for BCNU, 37.5 weeks for radiation therapy, and 40.5 weeks for the combination. All forms of active therapy, including BCNU alone, provided a statistically superior survival than conventional postoperative care. The difference between radiation therapy and the combined modality approach, however, is not significant. The survival at 18 months following radiation therapy was 9% versus 18% for BCNU plus irradiation, a marginal improvement, but achieved without appreciable additive toxicity (WALKER and GEHAN 1976).

The principal indication for nitrosourea therapy in lymphoproliferative disorders is Hodgkin's disease. Five independent clinical trials of BCNU chemotherapy, following relapse from previous therapy, have shown an overall objective response rate of 47%, with a range of 34%–55% (SELAWRY and HANSEN 1972; ANDERSON et al. 1976). Responses usually occur early, within 2 weeks, and with a median duration of 4 months. The Cancer and Acute Leukemia Group B (CALGB) has tested the activity of three chloroethylnitrosoureas in patients with advanced previously treated Hodgkin's disease. CCNU proved superior to both BCNU and MeCCNU (SELAWRY and HANSEN 1972).

The CALGB subsequently initiated a comparative trial of four regimens of combination chemotherapy for stage III B and IV disease, with substitutions of CCNU for the standard alkylating agent, nitrogen mustard, in two treatment arms; stage III A cases relapsing from radiation therapy were also included. The chemotherapy programs compared included: nitrogen mustard, vincristine, procarbazine, and prednisone (MOPP); nitrogen mustard, vinblastine, procarbazine, and prednisone (MVPP); CCNU, vincristine, procarbazine, and prednisone (CCNU–OPP); and CCNU, vinblastine, procarbazine, and prednisone (CCNU–VPP). The CCNU-containing combinations have produced complete remission rates that are either equivalent or superior to MOPP; these included patients without prior therapy as well as those with stage III A disease, relapsed after primary radiation therapy. In addition, the CCNU-containing programs have resulted in a significantly longer duration of complete remission. It is apparent that the chloroethylnitrosoureas have an established role in the treatment of advanced Hodgkin's disease.

Streptozotocin has also been demonstrated to have single-agent activity for advanced stage and heavily pretreated Hodgkin's disease. In phase II trials involving 16 patients, 44% achieved at least a partial response without evidence of myelosuppression. Of particular interest was the failure to demonstrate cross-resistance between this methyl nitrosourea and the chloroethylnitrosoureas. Of eight patients previously treated and whose disease proved refractory to BCNU and/or CCNU, three obtained a partial response and one achieved a complete response with streptozotocin (SCHEIN et al. 1974). In the one case where streptozotocin was used first, a subsequent response was obtained with CCNU.

The nitrosoureas have been actively employed in the treatment of advanced gastrointestinal cancer. They have demonstrated only modest activity as single agents, with response rates of 8%–18% in gastric cancer, 0%–9% in pancreatic cancer, and 9%–13% in advanced colorectal carcinoma (WASSERMAN et al. 1975). Nevertheless combinations of nitrosoureas with 5-fluorouracil have in some studies resulted in response rates better than those achieved with either drug used individually. KOVACH et al. (1974) have reported a 40% objective response with 5-fluorouracil (5-FU) plus BCNU in patients with advanced gastric cancer, with a significant improvement in survival at the 18-month period of follow-up. A trial of 5-FU plus MeCCNU conducted by the Eastern Cooperative Oncology Group has produced a similar response rate (DOUGLASS et al. 1976). Adriamycin, a drug with relatively high activity for gastric cancer, has now been successfully added to this regimen in studies conducted by the Gastrointestinal Tumor Study Group. A 33% response was recorded for patients with advanced pancreatic cancer treated with 5-FU plus BCNU, but without an apparent impact on survival (KOVACH et al. 1974). There had been great enthusiasm for the combination of 5-FU, MeCCNU, and vincristine for advanced colorectal cancer following the report of a 43% response rate in the initial controlled trial conducted at the Mayo Clinic (MOERTEL et al. 1975). While two other randomized trials have confirmed a somewhat increased activity of this regimen, compared with 5-FU (BAKER et al. 1976; FALKSON and FALKSON 1976), many large and well-designed studies have failed (ENGSTROM et al. 1978). As a consequence, the role of MeCCNU for colorectal cancer is undecided at present. The current controlled trials of 5-FU plus MeCCNU as adjuvant therapy for Dukes B2 and C colon cancer will hopefully produce a definitive answer within the next 2 years.

The chemotherapeutic agent most actively employed for the treatment of malignant islet cell tumors is streptozotocin, a naturally occurring methyl nitrosourea isolated from the fermentation cultures of *Streptomyces achromogenes*. A single dose of this compound in rodents, dogs, and monkeys is capable of producing a permanent diabetic state, an action mediated through the selective destruction of the pancreatic beta cell. Biochemically, the acute diabetogenic activity of streptozotocin has been related to the drug's ability to be taken up selectively into islets and depress the concentrations of the pyridine nucleotides, NAD and NADH (see Sect. C); this activity can be prevented in animals with pharmacological doses of nicotinamide (SCHEIN et al. 1973 a).

In a series of 12 patients with metastatic islet-cell carcinoma, treated with streptozotocin as a single agent, three patients achieved a complete clinical disappearance of tumor and hormone production. This included a patient with advanced malignant insulinoma who evidenced an objective response for 1 year after a single intravenous course at a daily dose of 500 mg/m^2 for five consecutive days (SCHEIN et al. 1973a). Two patients with "pancreatic cholera" and islet-cell carcinoma achieved a complete or near complete response to treatment with intra-arterial streptozotocin (KAHN et al. 1975). Before therapy they had stool volumes from 2 to 8 liters/day and required 200–300 mEq/day of supplemental potassium. After three to five doses of streptozotocin, 1.5 g/m^2 at weekly intervals, both stool volume and number and size of hepatic metastases decreased markedly. Partial remissions, averaging 4 months in duration, have been demonstrated in three additional patients with tumors that produced insulin, gastrin, or serotonin. These results are in general agreement with data compiled by the Cancer Therapy Evaluation Branch of the National Cancer Institute, which analyzed the records of 52 patients treated with streptozotocin (BRODER and CARTER 1973). In patients with functioning tumors, 60% were reported to have experienced a lessening in severity of hypoglycemia or hyperinsulinemia, and in 26% these hormonal variables returned to normal levels. Objectively, reduction of tumor mass had been reported in 48% of patients with functioning tumors; 17% were considered to have obtained a complete remission. Five of eight patients with islet-cell carcinoma without demonstrable hormone secretion also had a reduction in tumor size. The median duration of objective remission was approximately 1 year. The median survival of patients who had responded to streptozotocin was 4.5 years compared with 1.5 years for nonresponders. The latter figure is similar to the median survival recorded prior to the advent of specific chemotherapy. While streptozotocin is quite specific for the beta cell of the animal islet, it is of interest that this drug has proven an effective therapy for patients with non-beta-cell neoplasms. In addition to the cases with "pancreatic cholera" and serotonin secretion, there have been series of patients with pure gastrin-secreting (Zollinger-Ellison), non-beta-cell carcinomas which have responded similarly to treatment with streptozotocin (STADIE et al. 1976).

Despite the excellent antitumor activity of the chloroethylnitrosoureas in rodent systems, the full promise of this class of chemotherapeutic agents has not been realized in actual clinical use. While one could attribute this to differences in the high growth fraction and rapid cell proliferation of the L1210 leukemia and other rodent tumors, compared with the corresponding kinetic features of human malignancies, this argument is not sufficient. A clear example is the failure of MeCCNU to provide superior clinical therapeutic activity, despite its unique antitumor effect against the murine Lewis lung carcinoma, a tumor with growth kinetics quite similar to those found in solid tumors in man. As the biochemical mechanisms of resistance become better appreciated from laboratory and in vivo murine studies, it will be necessary to apply these concepts to the clinical setting. The development of prospective predictive tests for selecting patients for treatment is an obvious long-term goal.

The intermittent schedule of administration of nitrosoureas required because of the delayed nature of the bone-marrow toxicity offers a possible target for study. Certainly the current administration of a single dose every 6–8 weeks provides an optimal situation for the emergence of resistant clones of tumor cells. There are now attempts to design nitrosourea compounds with reduced myelosuppressive properties, as in the case of the two glucose analogues chlorozotocin and 1-(2-chloroethyl)-3-(β-D-glucopyranosyl)-1-nitrosourea (GANU), which may allow for more frequent administration.

There are several instances where chloroethyl- and methylnitrosoureas are used successfully in combination with no evidence of tumor cell cross-resistance. For example, in colon cancer the addition of streptozotocin to the basic combination of 5-FU, MeCCNU, and vincristine for advanced disease has resulted in a reported 20% increase in response rate (KEMENY et al. 1980). Similar combinations of the two classes of nitrosoureas are now being employed in the management of Hodgkin's disease, as in the case of the SCAB (streptozotocin, CCNU, adriamycin and bleomycin) regimen, which includes both streptozotocin and BCNU (KEMENY et al. 1980); a response and duration rate of response comparable to MOPP has recently been reported (DIGGS et al. 1981).

These observations confirm the potential for additive cytotoxic potential of chloroethyl- and methylnitrosoureas in combination. This is not unreasonable since the two classes of drug differ in their: (a) subnucleosomal binding sites (TEW et al. 1978 b; SUDHAKAR et al. 1979 b), (b) quantitative and qualitative nuclear protein alkylation and carbamoylation (TEW et al. 1978; SUDHAKAR et al. 1979 b; PINSKY et al. 1979), (c) capacity of chloroethylnitrosoureas only to form cross-links from monoadducts (KOHN 1979), (d) the selective effect of methylnitrosoureas on NAD concentrations and poly(ADP-ribose) polymerase activity (SCHEIN 1969; SUDHAKAR et al. 1979 a) and (e) their present clinical application.

L. Conclusions

In either the experimental or clinical treatment of tumor cells with nuclear reactant drugs, there is evidence that chloroethylnitrosoureas may be used in combination with methylnitrosoureas and/or bifunctional alkylating agents. Their respective mechanisms of cytotoxicity appear, in certain situations, to be complementary rather than duplicative, although the precise pharmacological mechanisms whereby these drugs induce cell death remains vague.

The nitrosoureas possess carbamoylating potential and, in the case of methylnitrosoures, interfere significantly with pyridine nucleotide biosynthesis: properties which distinguish these compounds from other classes of drugs. While carbamoylation has been shown to interfere with cellular repair mechanisms and reduced NAD concentrations are known to kill pancreatic cell populations, drug interactions with DNA are still believed to be the primary cause of cytotoxicity following exposure to nitrosoureas. In the final determination, the type of base lesion must be compared with the site of drug interaction within the chromatin architecture. The expression of drug resistance may prove to be a composite of the cell's efficiency in repairing certain regions of chromatin and to withstand other drug effects in "noncritical" chromatin targets. The potential for "directing" drug attack by concomitant treatment with steroid hormones or other transcriptional modifiers has proved effective in overcoming resistance to certain drugs. The scheduling of such combinations appears critical and may vary from one cell to another.

At present the phenomenon of drug resistance is a major obstacle in the successful application of chemotherapy. Understanding the molecular rationale for this process is prerequisite to overcoming the problem. The nitrosoureas provide an excellent probe through which a molecular explanation may be achieved and, in addition, provide an integral part of our present approaches to clinical combination chemotherapy.

References

Ahlgren JD, Green DC, Tew KD, Schein PS (1982) Repair of chloroethylnitrosourea DNA alkylation in L1210 leukemia and murine bone marrow. Cancer Res 42:2605–2608

Anderson T, Schein PS, McMenamin M, Cooney DA (1974) Streptozotocin diabetes: correlation with extent of depression and pancreatic islet nicotinamide adenine dinucleotide. J Clin Invest 54:672–677

Anderson T, DeVita VT, Young RC (1976) BCNU (NSC-409962) in the treatment of advanced Hodgkins disease: its role in remission induction and maintenance. Cancer Treat Rep 60:761–767

Baker LH, Vaitkevicius VK, Gehan E (1976) Randomized prospective trial comparing 5-fluorouracil (NSC 19893) to 5- fluorouracil and methyl-CCNU (NSC 95441) in advanced gastrointestinal cancer. Cancer Treat Rep 60:733–737

Begleiter A, Hing-Yat PL, Goldenberg GJ (1977) Mechanism of uptake of nitrosoureas by L5178Y lymphoblasts in vitro. Cancer Res 37:1022 1027

Bodell WJ (1977) Nonuniform distribution of DNA repair in chromatin after treatment with methyl methanesulfonate. Nucleic Acids Res 4:2619–2628

Broder LE, Carter SK (1973) Pancreatic islet cell carcinoma II results of therapy with streptozotocin in 52 patients. Am J Int Med 79:108–118

Cleaver JE (1977) Nucleosome structure controls rates of excision repair in DNA of human cells. Nature 270:451–453

Colvin M, Brundrett RB, Cowens JW, Jardine I, Ludlum DB (1976) A chemical basis for the antitumor activity of chloroethylnitrosoureas. Biochem Pharmacol 25:695–700

Diggs CH, Wiernik PH, Sutherland JC (1981) Treatment of advanced untreated Hodgkins disease with SCAB – an alternative to MOPP. Cancer 47:224–228

Dijkwel P, Mullenders L, Wanka F (1979) Analysis of the attachment of replicating DNA to a nuclear matrix in mammalian interphase nuclei. Nucleic Acids Res 6:219–230

Douglass HO, Lavin PT, Moertel CG (1976) Nitrosoureas: useful agents for the treatment of advanced gastrointestinal cancer. Cancer Treat Rep 60:769–780

Edelman G (1976) Some new views of the cell surface. J Biochem 79:1–12

Engstrom PF, MacIntyre J, Douglass H, Carbone P (1978) Combination chemotherapy of advanced bowel cancer. Proc Am Soc Clin Oncol 19:384

Erickson LC, Bradley MO, Kohn KW (1978a) Measurements of DNA damage in Chinese hamster cells treated with equitoxic and equimutagenic doses of nitrosoureas. Cancer Res 38:3379–3384

Erickson LC, Osieka R, Kohn KW (1978b) Differential repair of 1-(2-chloroethyl)-3-(4-methylcyclohexyl)-1-nitrosourea-induced DNA damage in two human colon tumor cell lines. Cancer Res 38:802–808

Erickson LC, Laurent G, Sharkey NA, Kohn KW (1980) DNA cross linking and monoadduct repair in nitrosourea-treated human tumor cells. Nature 288:727–729

Falkson G, Falkson HC (1976) Fluorouracil, methyl-CCNU and vincristine in cancer of the colon. Cancer 38:1468–1470

Fornace AJ, Kohn KW, Kann HE (1978) Inhibition of the ligase step of excision repair by 2-chloroethyl isocyanate, a decomposition product of 1,3-bis(2-chloroethyl)-1-nitrosourea. Cancer Res 38:1064–1069

Gersten D, Bosmann H (1975) Surface properties of plasma membrane following ionizing radiation exposure. Exp Cell Res 96:215–223

Gibson NW, Hickman JA (1982) The role of isocyanates in the toxicity of antitumor haloalkylnitrosoureas. Biochem Pharmacol 31:2795–2800

Green D, Tew KD, Hisamatsu T, Schein PS (1982) Correlation of nitrosourea murine bone marrow toxicity with DNA alkylation and chromatin binding sites. Biochem Pharmacol 31:1671–1679

Grunicke H, Gantner G, Holzweber F, Ihlenfeldt M, Puschendorf B (1978) New concepts on the interference of alkylating antitumor agents with the regulation of cell division. Adv Enzyme Regul 17:291–305

Hammer CF, Loranger RA, Schein PS (1981) The structures and decomposition products of chlorozotocin: new intramolecular carbamates of 2-amino-2-deoxyhexoses. J Organic Chem 46:1521–1531

Harrap KR, Riches PG, Gilby ED, Sellwood SM, Wilkinson R, Konyves I (1977) Studies on the toxicity and antitumor activity of prednimustine, a prednisolone ester of chlorambucil. Eur J Cancer 13:873–881

Hartley-Asp B, Wilkinson R, Venitt S, Harrap KR (1981) Studies on the mechanism of action of LS1727, a nitrosocarbamate of 19-nortestosterone. Acta Pharmacol Toxicol 48:129–138

Heal JM, Fox PA, Schein PS (1979a) A structure-activity study of seven new water soluble nitrosoureas. Biochem Pharmacol 28:1301–1306

Heal JM, Fox PA, Schein PS (1979b) Effect of carbamoylation on the repair of nitrosourea induced DNA alkylation damage in L1210 cells. Cancer Res 39:82–89

Ihlenfeldt M, Gantner G, Harrer M, Puschendorf B, Putzer H, Grunicke H (1981) Interaction of the alkylating antitumor agent 2,3 5-Tris(ethyleneimino)-benzoquinone with the plasma membrane of Ehrlich ascites tumor cells. Cancer Res 41:289–293

Kahn R, Levy A, Gardner J, Gorden P, Schein PS (1975) Successful treatment of "pancreatic cholera" by streptozotocin. N Engl J Med 292:941–945

Kann HE, Kohn KW, Lyles JM (1974) Inhibition of DNA repair by the 1,3-bis(2-chloroethyl)-1-nitrosourea breakdown product, 2-chloroethyl isocyanate. Cancer Res 34:398–402

Karran P, Lindahl T, Griffin B (1979) Adaptive response to alkylating agents involves alteration in situ of 0^6-methylguanine residues in DNA. Nature 280:76–77

Kemeny N, Yagoda A, Golbey R (1980) A prospective randomized study of methyl CCNU, 5-fluorouracil and vincristine (MOF) vs MOF plus streptozotocin (MOF-strep) in patients with metastatic colorectal carcinoma. Proc Am Assoc Cancer Res 21:417

Kleihues P, Bucheler J (1977) Long-term persistence of O^6 methylguanine in rat brain DNA. Nature 269:625–626

Kohn KW (1979) Drug-induced macromolecular damage of nuclear DNA. In: Busch H, Crookes S, Daskal Y (eds) Effects of drugs on the cell nucleus. Academic, New York, pp 208–240

Kovach JS, Moertel CG, Schutt AJ, Hahn RG, Reitemeier J (1974) A controlled study of combined 1,3-bis-(2-chloroethyl)-1-nitrosourea and 5-fluorouracil therapy for advanced gastric and pancreatic cancer. Cancer 33:563–567

Lyons RM, Goldenberg GJ (1972) Active transport of nitrogen mustard and choline by normal and leukemic human lymphoid cells. Cancer Res 32:1679–1685

Metzger G, Wilhelm FX, Wilhelm ML (1977) Non-random binding of a chemical carcinogen to DNA in chromatin. Biochem Biophys Res Commun 75:703–710

Moertel CG, Schutt AJ, Hahn RG, Reitemeier RJ (1975) Therapy of advanced colorectal cancer with a combination of 5-fluorouracil, methyl-1,3-cis(2-chloroethyl)-1-nitrosourea and vincristine. J Natl Cancer Inst 54:69–71

Montgomery JA, James R, McCaleb GS, Kirk MC, Johnston TP (1975) Decomposition of *N*-(2-chloroethyl)-*N*-nitrosoureas in aqueous media. J Med Chem 18:568–571

Nudel V, Salmon JE, Terada M, Bank A, Rifkind A, Marks PA (1977) Differential effects of chemical inducers on expression of β-globin genes in murine erythroleukemia cells. Proc Natl Acad Sci USA 74:1110–1104

Panasci LC, Green D, Nagourney R, Fox PA, Schein PS (1977) A structure-activity analysis of chemical and biological parameters of chloroethylnitrosoureas in mice. Cancer Res 37:2617–2618

Panasci LC, Green D, Schein PS (1979) Chlorozotocin mechanism of reduced bone marrow toxicity in mice. J Clin Invest 64:1103–1111

Pinsky S, Tew KD, Smulson ME Woolley PV (1979) Modification of L1210 chromatin-associated proteins by MNU and MNNG. Cancer Res 39:923–928

Pitot HC, Heidelberger C (1963) Metabolic regulatory circuits and carcinogenesis. Cancer Res 23:1694–1700

Ramanathan R, Rajalakshmi S, Sarma DSR, Farber E (1976) Nonrandom nature of in vivo methylation by dimethylnitrosamine and the subsequent removal of methylated products from rat liver chromatin DNA. Cancer Res 36:2073–2079

Reed DJ, May HE (1975) Alkylation and carbamoylation intermediates from the carcinostatic 1-(2-chloroethyl)-3-cyclohexyl-1-nitrosourea (CCNU) Life Sci 16:1263–1270

Renard A, Verly WG (1980) A chromatin factor in rat liver which destroys 0^6-ethylguanine in DNA. FEBS Lett 114:98–102

Robins P, Cairns J (1979) Quantitation of the adaptive response to alkylating agents. Nature 280:74–76

Schein PS (1969) 1-Methyl-1-nitrosourea and dialkylnitrosamide depression of nicotinamide adenine dinucleotide. Cancer Res 29:1226–1232

Schein PS, Cooney DA, McMenamin MG, Anderson T (1973a) Streptozotocin diabetes: further studies on the mechanism of depression of nicotinamide adenine dinucleotide concentrations in mouse pancreatic islets and liver. Biochem Pharmacol 22:2625–2631

Schein PS, Kahn R, Gorden P, Wells S, DeVita VT (1973b) Streptozotocin treatment of malignant insulomas and carcinoids: report of eight cases and review of the literature. Arch Intern Med 132:555–561

Schein PS, O'Connell MJ, Blom J, Hubbard S, Magrath IT, Bergevin Pa, Wiernik PH, Ziegler JL, DeVita VT (1974) Clinical antitumor activity and toxicity of streptozotocin (NSC 85998). cancer 34:993–1000

Scher W, Tsuei D, Sassa S, Price P, Gabelman N, Friend C (1978) Inhibition of dimethylsulfoxide-stimulated Friend cell erythrodifferentiation by hydrocortisone and other steroids. Proc Natl Acad Sci USA 75:3851–3855

Selawry OS, Hansen HH (1972) Superiority of CCNU over BCNU in treatment of advanced Hodgkin's disease. Proc Am Assoc Cancer Res 13:46

Smulson ME, Schein PS, Mullins DW, Sudhakar S (1977) A putative role for nicotinamide adenine dinucleotide-promoted nuclear protein modification in the antitumor activity of *N*-methyl-*N*-nitrosourea. Cancer Res 37:3006–3012

Smulson ME, Sudhakar S, Tew KD, Butt TR, Jump DB (1979) The influence of nitrosoureas on chromatin nucleosomal structure and function. In: Busch H, Brooke S, Daskal Y (eds) Effects of drugs on the cell nucleus. Academic, New York, pp 333–357

Stadie F, Stage G, Rehfeld JF, Efsen F, Fischerman K (1976) Treatment of Zollinger-Ellison syndrome with streptozotocin. N Engl J Med 294:1440–1442

Sudhakar S, Tew KD, Smulson ME (1979a) Effect of 1-methyl-nitrosourea on poly(adenosine diphosphate-ribose) polymerase activity at the nucleosomal level. Cancer Res 39:1405–1410

Sudhakar S, Tew KD, Schein PS, Woolley PV, Smulson ME (1979b) Nitrosourea interaction with chromatin and effect on poly(adenosine diphosphate ribose) polymerase activity. Cancer Res 39:1411–1417

Tew KD (1981) Chromatin and associated nuclear components as potential drug targets. In: Prestayko A, Crooke S, Baker L, Carter S, Schein P (eds) Nitrosoureas: current status and new developments. Academic, New York, pp 107–121

Tew KD (1982) The interaction of nuclear reactant drugs with structural macromolecules of the nucleus. In: Maul G (ed) The nuclear envelope and nuclear matrix. Alan R. Liss, Inc. New York, p 279–292

Tew KD, Wang AL (1982) Selective toxicity of haloethylnitrosoureas in a carcinoma cell lines resistant to bifunctional alkylating agents. Mol Pharmacol 21:729–738

Tew KD, Green D, Schein PS (1978a) Chlorozotocin binding to chromatin: a possible mechanism for reduced murine myelotoxicity. Proc Am Assoc Cancer Res 19:113
Tew KD, Sudhakar S, Schein PS, Smulson ME (1978b) Binding of chlorozotocin and CCNU to chromatin fractions of normal and sodium butyrate treated HeLa cells. Cancer Res 38:3371–3378
Tew KD, Pinsky S, Schein PS, Smulson ME, Woolley PV (1980a) Molecular aspects of nitrosamide carcinogenicity. In: Human cancer. Its characterization and treatment, vol 5. Excerpta Medica, Amsterdam, pp 387–395
Tew KD, Schein PS, Lindner DJ, Wang AL, Smulson ME (1980b) Influence of hydrocortisone on the binding of nitrosoureas to nuclear chromatin subfractions. Cancer Res 40:3697–3703
Tew KD, Wang AL, Lindner D, Schein PS (1982) Enhancement of nitrosourea cytoxicity in vitro using hydrocortisone. Biochem Pharmacol 31:1179–1180
Tew KD, Wang AL, Schein PS (1983) Putative mechanism for chloroethylnitrosourea cytotoxicity: interaction with the nuclear matrix and inhibition of matrix-DNA associations. Biochem Pharmacol 32:3509–3516
Thomas CB, Osieka R, Kohn KW (1978) DNA cross-linking by in vivo treatment with 1-(2-chloroethyl)-3-(4-methylcyclohexyl)-1-nitrosourea of sensitive and resistant human colon carcinoma xenografts in nude mice. Cancer Res 38:2448–2454
Tisdale MJ, Phillips BJ (1976) Alterations in adenosine 3′,5′-monophosphate-binding protein in Walker carcinoma cells sensitive or resistant to alkylating agents. Biochem Pharmacol 25:1831–1836
Tsai YH, Hnilica LS (1971) Interaction of histones with corticosteroids hormones. Biochim Biophys Acta 238:277–287
Walker MD, Gehan EA (1976) Clinical studies in malignant gliomas and their treatment with the nitrosoureas. Cancer Treat Rep 60:713–716
Walker MD, Hilton J (1976) Nitrosourea pharmacodynamics in relation to the central nervous system. Cancer Treat Rep 60:725–728
Wang AL, Schein PS, Tew KD (1983) Nitrosourea interactions with the nuclear envelope, nuclear matrix and associated chromatin. Oncology 40:367–371
Wasserman TH, Slavik M, Carter SK (1975) Clinical comparion of the nitrosoureas. Cancer 36:1258–1268
Wheeler GP, Bowden BJ, Grimsley J, Lloyd HH (1974) Interrelationships of some chemical, physicochemical and biological activities of several 1-(2-haloethyl)-1-nitrosoureas. Cancer Res 34:194–200
Wheeler GP, Johnston TP, Bowden BJ, McCaleb GS, Hill DL, Montgomery JA (1977) Comparison of the properties of metabolites of CCNU. Biochem Pharmacol 26:2331–2336
Whitfield JF, Perris AD, Youdale T (1968) Destruction of the nuclear morphology of thymic lymphocytes by the corticosteroid cortisol. Exp Cell Res 52:349–362
Wilkinson R, Gunnarsson PO, Plym-Forshell G, Renshaw J, Harrap KR (1978) The hydrolysis of prednimustine by enzymes from normal and tumour tissues. Excerpta Med Int Congr Ser 420:260–273
Wilkinson R, Birbeck M, Harrap KR (1979) Enhancement of the nuclear reactivity of alkylating agents by prednisolone. Cancer Res 39:4256–4262
Wolpert MK, Ruddon RW (1969) A study on the mechanism of resistance to nitrogen mustard in Ehrlich ascites tumor cells: comparison of uptake of HN_2-^{14}C into sensitive and resistant cells. Cancer Res 29:873–878

Section V: Antimetabolites

CHAPTER 17

Antipurines

D. M. TIDD

A. Introduction

The antipurines comprise a group of structural analogues of naturally occurring purine bases and nucleosides which exhibit cell growth inhibitory properties. A large number of purine and purine nucleoside analogues have been investigated for antitumour activity, but of these only a few have proved of sufficient interest as potentially useful clinical anticancer agents to warrant detailed studies of resistance. Such compounds include: 8-azaguanine (AzaG), 6-mercaptopurine (MP), 6-thioguanine (TG), 6-methylthioinosine (MMPR) and 9-β-D-arabinofuranosyladenine (AraA). The chemical structures of these drugs are presented in Fig. 1.

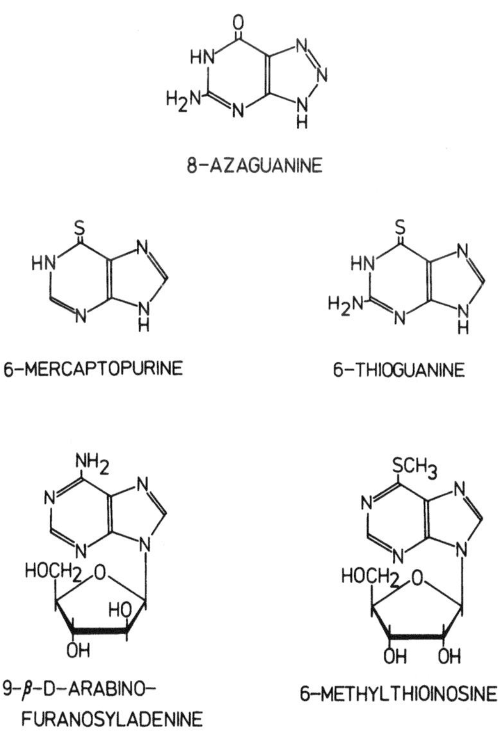

Fig. 1. Chemical structures of the major antineoplastic purine and purine nucleoside analogues

The 6-thiopurines, MP and TG, are the only antipurines to achieve widespread routine clinical use in cancer chemotherapy, and consequently they have received considerable attention in the laboratory.

Very few of the antipurines are active as such, most requiring "activation" within the target cells through their metabolism to nucleotide forms, which as enzyme inhibitors, or following incorporation into nucleic acids, are actually responsible for the biological effects of the drugs (BROCKMAN 1974; HENDERSON 1977). The few antipurines which appear to elicit their effects without this requirement for cellular metabolism include: 9-β-D-arabinofuranosyl-6-mercaptopurine, an inhibitor of cytidylate reductase (KIMBALL et al. 1964), psicofuranine and decoyinine, allosteric inhibitors of guanylate synthetase (MONTGOMERY 1974), puromycin and nucleocidin, inhibitors of protein synthesis (MONTGOMERY 1974), 9-β-D-xylofuranosyl-6-mercaptopurine (LEPAGE AND NAIK 1975) and certain growth inhibitory 9-alkylpurines (MONTGOMERY 1974). This section is concerned with resistance to the more widely studied antitumour purine and purine nucleoside analogues, all of which have an absolute requirement for cellular metabolism to pharmacologically active phosphorylated derivatives. In the course of and to the extent of their cellular metabolism, the antipurines behave as alternative substrates for enzymes of normal purine metabolism, a three-dimensional view of which is reproduced for reference in Fig. 2. One or more of these enzyme reactions may be responsible for conversion of an antipurine to its active form (HENDERSON 1977), namely:

1. Synthesis of a nucleoside monophosphate derivative
2. Phosphorylation of a nucleoside monophosphate to a diphosphate and/or triphosphate
3. Metabolism of the antipurine base part of the drug nucleotide molecule
4. Reduction of the ribose moiety to produce a 2′-deoxyribonucleotide
5. Incorporation of a nucleotide into nucleic acids.

There are several theoretical biochemical mechanisms which may conceivably endow resistance to the antipurines, and these are relevant to both acquired resistance and to natural or innate insensitivity (HENDERSON and BROCKMAN 1975). One or a combination of the following mechanisms may be responsible for antipurine resistance (HENDERSON 1977; EPPS et al. 1975; BROCKMAN 1974; ROY-BURMAN 1970):

1. Low or reduced permeability of the cell membrane to the antipurine or reduced access to its intracellular activation site
2. Low or decreased formation of the antipurine nucleoside monophosphate due to:
   a) Low or decreased activity of the nucleotide-forming enzyme
   b) Altered substrate specificity of the nucleotide-forming enzyme resulting in reduced catalysis of the antipurine reaction
   c) Low or reduced availability of the second substrate for the nucleotide-forming enzyme, e.g. 5-phosphoribosyl-pyrophosphate (PRPP)

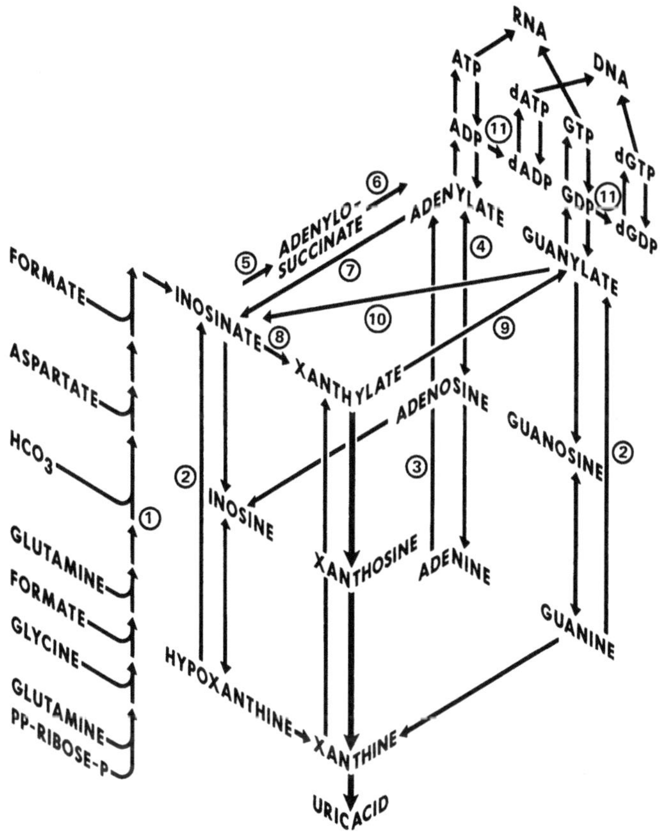

Fig. 2. Pathways of purine metabolism (*1*) purine biosynthesis de novo; (*2*) hypoxanthine-guanine phosphoribosyltransferase; (*3*) adenine phosphoribosyltransferase; (*4*) adenosine kinase; (*5*) adenylosuccinate synthetase; (*6*) adenylosuccinate lyase; (*7*) adenylate deaminase; (*8*) inosinate dehydrogenase; (*9*) guanylate synthetase; (*10*) guanylate reductase; (*11*) ribonucleotide reductase. (From HENDERSON 1977)

3. Low or decreased further metabolism of an antipurine nucleotide to its pharmacologically active form, or reduced incorporation into nucleic acids
4. High or increased capacity for catabolism of the antipurine to forms which are no longer precursors of pharmacologically active species by:
   a) Oxidation or reduction
   b) Deamination
   c) Methylation
   d) Cleavage of the purine ring
   e) Removal of the sugar moiety
5. High or increased capacity for conversion of antipurine nucleotides to inactive forms by:
   a) Dephosphorylation
   b) Metabolism of the antipurine base portion of the nucleotide molecule, e.g. by desulphuration or methylation

6. High or increased production of normal nucleotide metabolites capable of competing effectively with intermediate phosphorylated antipurine derivatives for enzymes involved in their further metabolism to pharmacologically active forms
7. Low or reduced effect at the drug target due to:
   a) High or increased effective concentration of a target enzyme
   b) Low or reduced affinity of activated drug for the target
   c) High or increased concentration of protecting metabolites
   d) Low or decreased relative importance of the target for cell survival, e.g. as a result of the existence or emergence of alternative metabolic pathways capable of bypassing the metabolic restriction imposed by the antipurine.

Specific examples of most of these possible types of resistance mechanisms have been observed in practice. In addition, it should be stressed that the antitumour purine and purine nucleoside analogues are cell cycle specific agents, that is, they are only effective against cells that are actively progressing around the mitotic cycle. Temporarily non-dividing or resting G_0 cells are resistant to the cytotoxic effects of these drugs. Several of the antipurines are also cell cycle phase specific, being only active against proliferating cells during a particular phase of the cell cycle, namely the DNA synthetic S-phase. These are agents that either specifically inhibit DNA synthesis or act through their incorporation into DNA. Consequently, the antipurines are most active against rapidly proliferating malignancies with high growth fractions and short cell generation times. Such cell kinetic considerations may account for two particular instances of innate antipurine resistance, rather than the direct biochemical mechanisms outlined above. Firstly, the general resistance of solid tumours to antipurines may result in large part from their low growth fraction, most cells existing in the resistant G_0 state in these malignancies (MONTGOMERY 1974; BROCKMAN 1974). Secondly, neoplasms with long cell-generation times are resistant to S-phase-specific antipurines since insufficient cells will enter the drug-sensitive DNA-synthetic phase during the time that the drug is available, whilst toxicity to normal stem cells in the marrow and gastrointestinal tract precludes attempts to overcome this difficulty by increasing the period of uninterrupted exposure. SKIPPER (1975) has suggested that neoplasms in which less than 50% of the cells initiate DNA replication in 24 h will not respond to S-phase-specific antipurines even though their capacity for drug activation is unimpaired. Resistance of this nature may be viewed in terms of the "target" concept of drug action; in cells outside S-phase the target concentration is nil and is obviously unimportant for cell survival (HENDERSON 1974).

HENDERSON and BROCKMAN (1975) have emphasized that resistance is a property of a particular tumour-host-drug system as a whole and not the tumour cell alone. Even low growth fraction solid tumours might be expected to respond to antipurines if continuous exposure were possible. Theoretically, in studying resistance no single element of the tumour-host-drug system should be isolated from the other two, although sometimes there may be overriding factors at one level which are responsible for the lack of drug effect (HENDERSON et al. 1975). This ideal is difficult to achieve and much of the biochemical work on antipurine resistance has considered only the tumour.

Resistance is a relative characteristic and varying degrees of unresponsiveness to antipurines have been observed. Most of the early work was concerned with resistant animal tumour and cell culture sublines generated under conditions of extremely high selection pressure. Resistant animal neoplasms were developed by direct intraperitoneal administration of high doses of the antipurine into ascitic tumours, with repetitive transplantation and treatment of surviving cells, whilst tissue culture permitted escalation of drug concentrations beyond the point where host toxicity would have become limiting in vivo. Such cell sublines were highly resistant, and often discrete mutations involving loss of activating enzymes were shown to be responsible for lack of drug sensitivity. Other more subtle biochemical changes of the types listed above may also have been present, but were obscured by the principal mutation, unless cross-resistance to other antipurines by the additional mechanisms was observed. Whilst these investigations were of undoubted importance in establishing clear-cut evidence for the mode of action of the drugs, they have proved of limited relevance to the problem of clinical resistance. Host toxicity, pharmacodynamic effects and inaccessibility of the neoplastic cells limit the selection pressure for cellular resistance applied in human cancer chemotherapy. Unresponsive cells may be only moderately resistant to antipurines in comparison with the animal tumour and cell culture models (HENDERSON et al. 1975; LEPAGE 1975a). In many cases human cellular resistance, either innate or acquired, may be due to the composite effect of various biochemical mechanisms acting in concert to reduce drug efficacy rather than being the result of a discrete mechanism or mutational event. Consequently, animal tumour sublines of low degrees of resistance to antipurines have been used as possible models for clinical resistance.

Resistance to the major antitumour antipurines, AzaG, MP, TG, MMPR, and AraA, is discussed in the first part of this section. The latter part describes other antipurine derivatives which have been synthesized and metabolic manipulations which have been investigated in attempts to overcome or circumvent resistance mechanisms. The antipurines may induce a number of cellular metabolic effects which are unrelated to the irreversible cytotoxic actions of the drugs responsible for their antineoplastic activity. At most these secondary effects might have reversible cytostatic or growth inhibitory consequences and, historically, investigations of resistance have often preceded elucidation of mechanisms of action and have enabled cytotoxic effects to be distinguished from superfluous biochemical perturbations. However, in this review, the metabolism and mechanisms of action of the major antipurines are described briefly prior to the discussion of their resistance mechanisms.

B. 8-Azaguanine

8-Azaguanine (AzaG) was the first antipurine to be synthesized and shown to have growth inhibitory activity. Although the drug did not prove to be an effective clinical antitumour agent, it has been widely studied and its properties have formed the basis for an understanding of antipurine action in general.

I. Metabolism and Mechanism of Action

The metabolism of guanine is compared with that of its analogue, 8-azaguanine, in Fig. 3. [For detailed discussions of the metabolism and mechanism of action of AzaG, see reviews by Parks and Agarwal (1975) and Grunberger and Grunberger (1979).] Briefly, AzaG is converted to its ribonucleoside 5′-monophosphate by IMP-GMP: pyrophosphate phosphoribosyltransferase (hypoxanthine-guanine phosphoribosyltransferase, HGPRT). This enzyme is also responsible for conversion of MP and TG to their respective ribonucleoside 5′-monophosphates. AzaG ribonucleoside 5′-monophosphate is phosphorylated further to the di- and tri-phosphates, and the drug is incorporated into RNA, but not DNA. Preferential incorporation of AzaG into mRNA and tRNA has been observed, whilst inhibition of maturation of preribosomal RNA has been reported for AzaG-treated cells (Rivest et al. 1982). AzaG may replace up to 5% of the guanine residues in RNA of bacteria, viruses and mammalian cells (Parks and Agarwal 1975; Grunberger and Grunberger 1979).

AzaG undergoes catabolic deamination by guanine deaminase to 8-azaxanthine, which is pharmacologically inactive; this derivative is the major urinary excretion product of the drug.

Growth inhibition by AzaG results from rapid inhibition of protein synthesis, which is apparently related to its incorporation into mRNA. It has been suggested that errors of translation might result from ionization of AzaG incorporated in RNA (AzaG $pK_a = 6.5$; cf. guanine $pK_a = 9.2$). Alternatively, the loss of steric hindrance between C-H at the purine 8-position and the sugar moiety, due to the substitution by nitrogen, might permit nucleic acid incorporated AzaG to adopt a *syn* conformation, thereby lowering the template activity of the RNA molecules. Guanine protects against the antitumour activity of AzaG but this almost

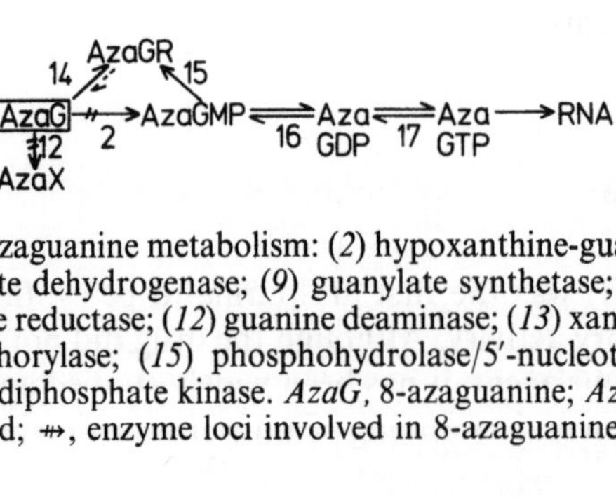

Fig. 3. Guanine and 8-azaguanine metabolism: (*2*) hypoxanthine-guanine phosphoribosyltransferase; (*8*) inosinate dehydrogenase; (*9*) guanylate synthetase; (*10*) guanylate reductase; (*11*) ribonucleotide reductase; (*12*) guanine deaminase; (*13*) xanthine oxidase; (*14*) purine nucleoside phosphorylase; (*15*) phosphohydrolase/5′-nucleotidase; (*16*) guanylate kinase; (*17*) nucleoside diphosphate kinase. *AzaG*, 8-azaguanine; *AzaX*, 8-azaxanthine; *X*, xanthine; *U/A*, uric acid; ⇸, enzyme loci involved in 8-azaguanine resistance

certainly results from competition for HGPRT and other enzymes involved en route to incorporation of AzaG into RNA.

II. Resistance

AzaG may elicit cytostatic rather than cytotoxic effects where growth is inhibited during exposure but readily resumes when the drug is withdrawn (PARKS and AGARWAL 1975). In such cases the cells are essentially resistant since effective cancer chemotherapy requires that a reduction in cellular proliferative ability be achieved. It was originally observed that the degree of innate or spontaneous insensitivity to AzaG in a series of mouse tumours correlated with their cellular levels of guanine deaminase and consequently their ability to deaminate AzaG to the inactive catabolite 8-azaxanthine (HIRSCHBERG et al. 1952). The toxicity of AzaG to skin was attributed to the low amount of guanine deaminase present in this tissue (GELLHORN 1953), whilst in clinical trials oral administration of AzaG was found to be inferior to the parenteral route, presumably due to deamination of the drug by intestinal mucosa and liver (PARKS and AGARWAL 1975). However, drug-induced tumour resistance to AzaG involving increased guanine deaminase activity has not been reported, and further investigations of AzaG's therapeutic spectrum against animal tumour models revealed no consistent relationship between innate insensitivity and deaminase activity (SCHACTER and LAW 1957; MANDEL 1959; KONDO and MARUYAMA 1955). It was apparent that whilst deamination might contribute to insensitivity it was not the sole mechanism of resistance. These early results have recently been reaffirmed by MEYERS and SHIN (1981), who showed that there was some correlation between sensitivity to AzaG and guanine deaminase levels in their cell lines. However, although they observed transient increases in enzyme activity during exposure to sublethal concentrations of AzaG, they were unable to demonstrate induction of elevated levels of guanine deaminase during development of resistance to the drug in cells which retained appreciable HGPRT activity.

The extent of acquired resistance to AzaG in animal tumours and bacteria has generally been shown to correlate with decreases in the capacity of cells to convert AzaG to its ribonucleotide, due to a deficiency at the level of the enzyme HGPRT (BROCKMAN et al. 1957, 1959a, b; BROCKMAN 1963; DAVIDSON et al. 1962). For example, LITTLEFIELD (1963), MORROW (1970) and ALBERTINI and DE MARS (1970) showed that reductions in the cellular concentrations of active HGPRT correlated with the degree of resistance to AzaG.

Where studied, the structural gene for HGPRT has been found to be located on the X chromosome of mammalian cells (CASKEY and KRUH 1979; CHASIN and URLAUB 1976; BRENNAND et al. 1982). As a consequence of this, male cells are hemizygous and female cells are functionally hemizygous for this locus, whilst female tissues are mosaics due to random X-chromosome inactivation. Many normal cell types and most, if not all, malignant cells are able to synthesize their total purine nucleotide requirements de novo, and therefore in such cases the presence of HGPRT is superfluous to requirements for individual cell survival. The foregoing considerations account for the common occurrence of considerable reductions in HGPRT activity with development of resistance to AzaG, MP and TG under conditions of high selection pressure. Mutation in the HGPRT structural gene in man is responsible for the Lesch-Nyhan syndrome, an inborn error of metabolism in male children characterized by severe neurological disease, developmental retardation, spasticity, accelerated rates of purine biosynthesis de novo and hyperuricaemia (LESCH and NYHAN 1964; SEEGMILLER et al. 1967; MCDONALD and KELLEY 1971; RUBIN et al. 1971; BAKAY and NYHAN 1972; CHANGAS and MILMAN 1977). Similarly, a mutant HGPRT was identified in cells of a hyperuricaemic patient where the affinity of the enzyme for PRPP was reduced ten fold without affecting binding of purine bases (BENKE et al. 1973). However, in this case the activity of the mutant enzyme was sufficient to prevent development of the Lesch-Nyhan syndrome. Extracts of cells from this patient appeared normal under the usual assay conditions for HGPRT where saturating concentrations of PRPP are used, and BENKE et al. (1973) pointed out that in studies of antipurine resistance, high apparent HGPRT activities measured in cell extracts by the standard assay do not necessarily preclude a defect at this enzyme locus. Purine overproduction by HGPRT-deficient cells does not result from increased capacities for purine nucleotide biosynthesis de novo. THOMPSON et al. (1978) showed that in the absence of exogenous hypoxanthine the rates of purine nucleotide biosynthesis de novo in normal and HGPRT-deficient cells were similar, whilst the enzyme-deficient cells excreted greater amounts of newly synthesized hypoxanthine which they were unable to reutilize. Reutilization of exogenous and newly synthesized hypoxanthine normally attenuates de novo synthesis through competition for available PRPP and feedback inhibition of the pathway by nucleotide metabolites of the purine base. The authors concluded that the purine "overproduction" could be better defined as resistance to inhibition normally produced by hypoxanthine.

The HGPRT locus has become the most extensively studied mammalian cell gene as a result of:

1. Its known location on the X chromosome
2. The high frequency of mutation resulting from the presence of a single active copy of the gene in mammalian cells
3. The facile selection for mutants with AzaG or TG
4. The ease of characterization of the gene product
5. The ability to isolate revertants using culture media containing hypoxanthine, aminopterin (or amethopterin) and thymidine (HAT media), where the antifolate drug inhibits de novo purine and thymidylate biosynthesis and thereby restricts survival to those cells which can utilize the preformed nucleic acid precursors (CASKEY and KRUH 1979).

Thus, much of the recent work on AzaG resistance (and to some extent TG resistance) has been undertaken from the point of view of mammalian somatic-cell genetics rather than cancer chemotherapy. In many cases, resistant-cell clones have been isolated under extreme selection pressure following treatment of cell populations with high concentrations of mutagens, and consequently the results of such studies may possibly have limited relevance to the problems of drug resistance in cancer treatment.

Cells selected for resistance to AzaG may be cross-resistant to TG and sensitive to cytotoxic effects of HAT media as a result of profound reductions in HGPRT activity (Fox et al. 1976; Fox and Hodgkiss 1981). However, stable AzaG-resistant clones have also frequently been isolated which (a) retain appreciable HGPRT activity or even wild-type levels of the enzyme, (b) grow well in HAT media and (c) remain sensitive to TG (van Diggelen et al. 1979; Meyers et al. 1980; Meyers and Shin 1981; Fox and Hodgkiss 1981). Whereas, in some cases, the degree of HGPRT deficiency has correlated with the concentration of AzaG used for selection, in others wild-type levels of the enzyme have been observed in clones isolated with high concentrations of the drug. In contrast to the situation with AzaG, resistance to high concentrations of TG is invariably accompanied by profound deficiencies in HGPRT, and therefore this antipurine is the preferred selective agent for mutations or deletions at the HGPRT locus (Sharp et al. 1973; van Diggelen et al. 1979; Meyers et al. 1980; Hodgkiss et al. 1980; Fox and Hodgkiss 1981). The anomalous observation of AzaG sensitivity in TG-resistant, HAT-sensitive clones appeared to reflect a supplementary cytostatic rather than cytotoxic action of the agent against cells at low density which occurred in the absence of AzaG nucleotide synthesis (Fox et al. 1976; Fox and Hodgkiss 1981). The differences between AzaG and TG undoubtedly reflect the very poor substrate activity of AzaG with HGPRT compared with the kinetics of the enzyme with TG which are similar to those of the natural substrates. HGPRT isolated from mouse sarcoma 180 cells exhibited the following K_m values: guanine, 5.4 μM; TG, 4.0 μM; AzaG, 300 μM (Ross et al. 1973). van Diggelen et al. (1979) reported a similar trend in apparent K_m values with purified mouse HGPRT, i.e. hypoxanthine, 0.7 μM; TG 0.9 μM; AzaG 300 μM; whilst AzaG showed no detectable reaction as substrate for the enzyme partly purified from mouse adenocarcinoma 755 cells (Hill 1970). Low activity of HGPRT with AzaG compared with hypoxanthine was reported for the rat enzyme (Berman et al. 1980) and K_m values recorded for HGPRTs of V79A and V79S Chinese hamster cell lines were respectively: hypoxanthine, 10 and 10 μM; TG, 3.0 and 12 μM; and AzaG, 100 and 100 μM (Fox and Hodgkiss 1981). AzaG was also shown to bind poorly to human HGPRT on the basis of the high value of the AzaG inhibition constant for the [^{14}C]hypoxanthine reaction compared with those of guanine, hypoxanthine, TG and MP (Krenitsky et al. 1969). Using human erythrocytic HGPRT, Kong and Parks (1974) demonstrated that the K_m values for substrates and analogues were dependent on the pH of measurement and that only the un-ionized forms of the purines were effective substrates for the enzyme. The poor apparent affinity of AzaG for HGPRT was explained by its high acidity (pK_a, 6.5) relative to guanine (pK_a, 9.2), TG (pK_a, 8.2) and MP (pK_a, 7.7), since at physiological pH much of the AzaG would be dissociated and therefore unable to bind to the enzyme. V_{max} values were relatively similar with the different substrates, including AzaG, at any selected pH. The poor substrate activity of AzaG with HGPRT accounted for the profound effects of exogenous purines in reducing cytotoxity of the drug compared with the situation with TG, and this has led workers in the field to recommend that dialyzed serum be used in selection experiments with AzaG (van Diggelen et al. 1979; Fox and Hodgkiss 1981). AzaG nucleotide formation in cell-free extracts of Chinese hamster cells was inhibited non-competitively by hypoxanthine, suggesting that the substrates occupied different binding sites on the HGPRT molecule whilst inhibition of inosinate formation from hypoxanthine by TG was largely competitive (FOX and HODGKISS 1981). The mouse tumour sarcoma 180 is naturally insensitive to AzaG and it has been suggested that this may be due to the low apparent affinity of its HGPRT for AzaG; as recorded above, the Michaelis constant for AzaG was approximately 60 times greater than the Michaelis constant for guanine in the reaction catalyzed by HGPRT from this neoplasm (AGARWAL et al. 1971; PARKS and AGARWAL 1975). Similarly, mouse P388 and L1210 cells are insensitive to the cytotoxic effects of AzaG, probably for the same reason (ANDERSON 1975). Thus conversion of AzaG to its nucleotide is an inefficient process at the outset and it would appear that stable adaptational changes in cell biochemistry may reduce net AzaG nucleotide formation to the extent that cells become resistant to high concentrations of the agent without there necessarily being very considerable reductions in HGPRT levels. Activity of the enzyme may be reduced to a degree at which sublethal concentrations of AzaG nucleotides accumulate whilst the TG-sensitive, HAT-resistant phenotype is retained. Decreased intracellular transport of AzaG (HARRIS and WHITMORE 1974) and excessive nucleotidase activity (BERMAN et al. 1980) have also been observed in AzaG-resistant cells containing high levels of HGPRT, and decreased availability of PRPP or increased dependence on purine nucleotide synthesis de novo has been invoked as a possible explanation for the occurrence of AzaG resistance without change in HGPRT activity (MEYERS and SHIN 1981). In contrast, the consistent association of the HGPRT-negative phenotype with resistance to high concentrations of TG is almost certainly related to the efficient substrate activity of this drug with the enzyme.

In addition to such adaptational changes, there have also been numerous examples where true mutations in the HGPRT structural gene have been selected by exposure to high concentrations of AzaG. AzaG-resistant cells carrying HGPRT structural gene mutations may survive and grow in HAT media if the mutant enzyme activity is sufficiently high (SHARP et al. 1973; FENWICK et al. 1977b; CASKEY and KRUH 1979; MEYERS et al. 1980; KRUH et al. 1981). This has caused some confusion in discriminating between resistance to AzaG arising through adaptation and resistance achieved by classical mutational events. The following characteristics exhibited by resistant clones have served to establish that the cells carry mutations in the HGPRT structural gene:

1. Long-term stability of the resistant phenotype in the absence of selective pressure and very low or immeasurable spontaneous reversion frequencies (GILLIN et al. 1972; FOX et al. 1976; FOX and RADACIC 1978)
2. The presence of residual HGPRT activity, AzaG resistance revertible by mutagens (missense point mutations); no detectable HGPRT activity or residual enzyme with altered subunit molecular weight, revertible by mutagens (frameshift or possibly nonsense point mutations); no detectable HGPRT activity or residual enzyme with reduced subunit molecular weight, irrevertible (deletion) (BAUDET et al. 1973; SHIN 1974; FOX et al. 1976; FENWICK et al. 1977b; FOX and RADACIC 1978; FOX and HODGKISS 1981)

3. Altered antigenic properties of residual HGPRT or of HGPRT in mutagen-induced revertants (SHIN 1974; FENWICK et al. 1977 a)
4. Altered kinetic constants of residual HGPRT (BAUDET et al. 1973; SHIN 1974; CHASIN and URLAUB 1976; FENWICK et al. 1977 b; CASKEY and KRUH 1979; MEYERS et al. 1980; FOX and HODGKISS 1981; SHARP et al. 1973)
5. Enhanced heat sensitivity of residual HGPRT or of the enzyme from revertant clones (SHARP et al. 1973; SHIN 1974; FOX et al. 1976; FOX and HODGKISS 1981; KRUH et al. 1981)
6. Different tryptic peptide analyses for wild-type and mutant HGPRT (KRUH et al. 1981)
7. The presence of protein cross-reacting with HGPRT antiserum (CRM^+) in HGPRT-negative cells, i.e. defective enzyme protein (BAUDET et al. 1973; FENWICK et al. 1977 b; CASKEY and KRUH 1979; KRUH et al. 1981)
8. Altered isoelectric points, electrophoretic mobility and subunit molecular weights of residual enzyme and immunologically cross-reactive protein from AzaG-resistant cells (FOX et al. 1976; CHASIN and URLAUB 1976; FENWICK et al. 1977 b; FOX and HODGKISS 1981; KRUH et al. 1981).

Mutant HGPRTs have been observed in AzaG-resistant lines where the affinities of the enzymes for PRPP were much reduced without there being any significant effects on binding of the drug or the normal purine substrates (FENWICK et al. 1977 b; CASKEY and KRUH 1979; FOX and HODGKISS 1981). However, one of the resistant lines isolated by FENWICK et al. (1977 b) contained HGPRT with reduced affinity for both PRPP and hypoxanthine. Cells of some of these clones were able to utilize exogenous hypoxanthine when purine ribonucleotide biosynthesis de novo was inhibited with aminopterin or azaserine. CHASIN and URLAUB (1976) described an AzaG-resistant Chinese hamster ovary cell line containing mutant HGPRT with a 20-fold higher K_m for PRPP than the wild-type enzyme, but concluded that the low specific activity of the enzyme rather than reduced substrate affinity was the primary cause of the mutant growth phenotype. Conversely, AzaG-resistant clones have been isolated where mutation in the HGPRT structural gene resulted in enzymes with considerably reduced activity towards AzaG without significant reduction in affinities for hypoxanthine and TG (SHARP et al. 1973; VAN DIGGELEN et al. 1979; MEYERS et al. 1980; MEYERS and SHIN 1981). The resistant lines grew in HAT media, which in some cases were used in conjunction with AzaG for their selection. Mutants of this phenotype are rare even in mutagenized populations and have never arisen spontaneously in cell populations exposed to the selection media alone (MEYERS et al. 1980). Residual HGPRT activities with reduced affinities for hypoxanthine have also been observed in AzaG-resistant clones although low V_{max} values or specific activities were probably the primary cause of drug resistance (SHIN 1974; KRUH et al. 1981). An AzaG-resistant clone derived from a mouse renal adenocarcinoma cell line contained neither HGPRT enzyme activity nor protein cross-reacting with HGPRT antiserum, whilst the HGPRT of revertants was indistinguishable from the normal mouse enzyme in terms of electrophoretic mobility and heat sensitivity (SHIN 1974). It was suggested that the resistant line might be a recessive regulatory mutant in which the synthesis of HGPRT was repressed by changes in control of expression of an unaltered structural gene. The idea of AzaG resistance arising through regulatory mutations receives some support from the observation that the frequency of occurrence of AzaG resistance was apparently independent of the ploidy level of cells (HARRIS 1971). Alternatively, this might equally well reflect the development of resistance through phenotypic adaptation rather than by genetic change. Dominant regulatory mutations would account for the suppression of HGPRT activity achieved when irradiated HGPRT-negative cells were fused with wild-type cells (KADOURI et al. 1978). Similarly, the re-expression of the suppressed HGPRT in hybrids between HGPRT-negative cells and HGPRT-positive cells of different species suggests that recessive regulatory mutations may possibly have been responsible for the variant phenotypes (see VAN ZEELAND et al. 1974). However, deliberate attempts to isolate hypothetical regulatory mutants have consistently failed (CHASIN and URLAUB 1976). HGPRT is a multimeric enzyme which probably exists as a tetramer in the native form, although this has been the subject of some controversy (JOHNSON et al. 1979). Hybrid enzyme molecules containing mutant and wild-type HGPRT subunits were detected in a hybrid clone formed from the fusion of mutant and wild-type cells (CHASIN and URLAUB 1976). Also, defective HGPRT subunits from an AzaG-resistant clone and a TG-resistant clone were able to combine in hybrid cells to yield an enzyme that was functional enough under intracellular conditions to impart a wild-type growth phenotype (CHASIN and URLAUB 1976). These results accounted for genetic complementation in hybrid cells derived from HGPRT-deficient clones, and cast doubt on the existence of *trans*-acting regulatory mutants of the HGPRT locus (SEKIGUCHI et al. 1974, 1975).

Whilst resistance to high concentrations of AzaG may occur through either mutational or adaptive changes, resistance to low concentrations of the drug appears to arise during chronic exposure by phenotypic evolution alone (TERZI 1974; VAN ZEELAND et al. 1974; FOX et al. 1976; FOX and RADACIC 1978, 1982). Chinese hamster cells gradually developed resistance to AzaG during long-term exposure to low concentrations of the agent, and at the same time there was a slow loss of ability to grow in HAT medium and a progressive reduction in, but never total loss of, HGPRT activity without change in kinetic constants or physical properties of the enzyme (FOX and RADACIC 1978, 1982). Drug treatment apparently induced increases in the proportion of resistant cells and of cells with unstable abnormal chromosome numbers (>22) in the cultures, although there was no direct correlation between the frequency of heteroploid cells and the level of AzaG resistance acquired (FOX and RADACIC 1982). In summary, resistant cell lines isolated under these conditions exhibited variable stability of phenotype in the absence of the drug, high "reversion" frequencies, variable chromosome numbers and karyotypic instability (TERZI 1974; VAN ZEELAND et al. 1974; FOX and RADACIC 1978, 1982). The frequency of occurrence of variants of this class was not increased by treatment with mutagens. FOX and RADACIC (1978) concluded that "many, though not all drug-resistant lines, which arise both in vitro and probably in vivo, during tumour chemotherapy are of non-mutational origin". They suggested that resistance to low concentrations of AzaG in Chinese hamster cells was "the result of gene dosage effects at autosomal loci controlling either catabolic enzymes of the purine synthetic pathway or a dominant suppressor of HGPRT activity" (FOX and RADACIC 1982).

C. 6-Mercaptopurine and 6-Thioguanine

6-Mercaptopurine (MP) and 6-thioguanine (TG) have been widely used as components of drug combinations in the clinical chemotherapy of acute leukaemia. MP is most effective against acute lymphoblastic leukaemia in children, whereas TG is superior to MP in the treatment of acute myelogenous leukaemia, particularly when administered in combination with arabinosylcytosine (GRINDEY 1979).

I. Metabolism and Mechanism of Action

The metabolism and mechanisms of action of MP and TG have been reviewed by PATERSON and TIDD (1975), LEPAGE (1977), HENDERSON (1977), CRABTREE (1978), ELION (1975) and GRINDEY (1979). The metabolism of hypoxanthine and guanine is compared with that of their analogues, MP and TG, in Fig. 4. As in the case of AzaG, MP and TG are converted to their ribonucleoside 5′-monophosphate derivatives by HGPRT. 6-Thioguanylate undergoes further phosphorylation to di- and triphosphates whereas higher levels of phosphorylation of 6-thioinosinate have not been observed. The mono-, di- and triphosphates of TG deoxyribonucleoside are formed following reduction of 6-thioguanosine diphosphate by ribonucleotide reductase. Incorporation of TG deoxyribonucleotide into DNA is responsible for the antileukaemic activity of TG, although it is not known how the nucleic acid-incorporated analogue exerts its cytotoxic effect. MP acts through further metabolism of 6-thioinosinate, via inosinate dehydrogenase and guanylate synthetase, to 6-thioguanylate, and its subsequent incorporation as TG deoxyribonucleotide into DNA. Consequently, in terms of their mechanism of action, MP and TG represent alternative ways of administering the same drug. Both agents induce delayed cytotoxic effects where cells exposed for approximately one cell generation time may continue to divide and undergo one or two further divisions after drug removal before the lethal effects of treatment are observed (TIDD and PATERSON 1974a, b). A cell cycle progression block in G2 phase characterized the delayed cytotoxic effects of TG in mouse lymphoma L5178Y (D. M. TIDD, unpublished observations) and mouse leukaemia L1210 cell cultures (WOTRING and ROTI ROTI 1980). The latter authors suggested that G2 arrest might result from inhibition of RNA transcription by TG incorporated in DNA of the cells or from inhibition of chromosomal segregation. LEE and SARTORELLI (1981a) reported that exposure to TG induced single-strand breaks in DNA of L1210 cells and therefore delayed cytotoxicity could conceivably be due to fragmentation of the chromosomes during a subsequent round of DNA replication. Specific inhibitors of DNA synthesis were shown to afford partial protection against the cytotoxicity of MP and TG (TIDD and PATERSON 1974a; NELSON et al. 1975a; LEE and SARTORELLI 1981a). TG and MP, after its conversion to TG nucleotide, are also incorporated into RNA. However, this does not appear to affect cell viability.

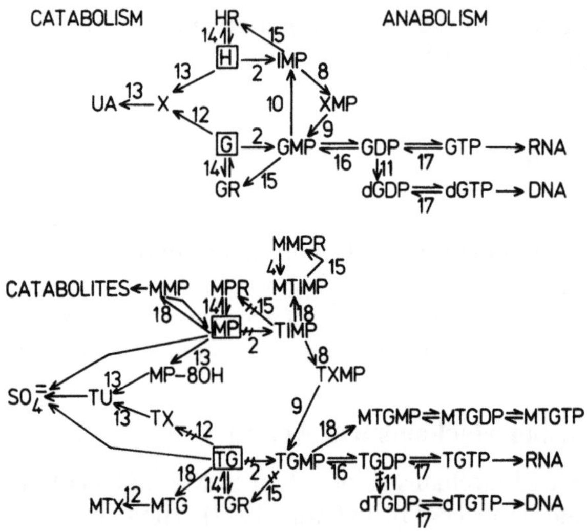

Fig. 4. Metabolism of hypoxanthine, guanine and their analogues 6-mercaptopurine and 6-thioguanine: (*2*) hypoxanthine-guanine phosphoribosyltransferase; (*4*) adenosine kinase; (*8*) inosinate dehydrogenase; (*9*) guanylate synthetase; (*10*) guanylate reductase; (*11*) ribonucleotide reductase; (*12*) guanine deaminase; (*13*) xanthine oxidase; (*14*) purine nucleoside phosphorylase; (*15*) phosphohydrolase/5′-nucleotidase; (*16*) guanylate kinase; (*17*) nucleoside diphosphate kinase; (*18*) methyltransferase; *MP*, 6-mercaptopurine; *TG*, 6-thioguanine; *MMPR*, 6-methylthioinosine; *TX*, 6-thioxanthine; *TU*, 6-thiouric acid; *MP-8OH*, 8-hydroxy-6-mercaptopurine; *M*, methyl substituent on 6-thiol; *TIMP*, 6-thioinosinate; *MTIMP*, 6-methylthioinosinate; →, enzyme loci involved in resistance

In addition to their incorporation into nucleic acids, several metabolic effects of MP and TG have been observed. These include:

1. Inhibition by 6-thioinosinate and 6-thioguanylate of PRPP amidotransferase, the first enzyme unique to the pathway of purine nucleotide biosynthesis de novo (path 1, Fig. 2). This has been described as pseudofeedback inhibition of the purine biosynthetic pathway by the analogue nucleotides.
2. Inhibition of inosinate dehydrogenase (enzyme 8, Fig. 2) by 6-thioinosinate and 6-thioguanylate.
3. Inhibition of adenylosuccinate synthetase (enzyme 5, Fig. 2) and adenylosuccinate lyase (enzyme 6, Fig. 2) by 6-thioinosinate.

A major difference between the thiopurines and their normal counterparts lies in the ability of the former to undergo S-methylation, catalysed by cellular methyltransferases (Fig. 4). Methylated TG nucleotides are pharmacologically inactive, but 6-methylthioinosinate, also a metabolite of MMPR, is a very potent inhibitor of PRPP amidotransferase, and in some cases this metabolite of MP may be responsible for a major part of the inhibition of purine synthesis observed in MP-treated cells. These enzyme inhibitions are not in themselves responsible for the antileukaemic activity of MP and TG, although inhibition of purine nucleotide biosynthesis de novo may represent a self-potentiating mechanism for the drugs:

1. By reducing the concentration of normal nucleotides competing for enzymes involved in drug metabolism along the pathway to incorporation into DNA
2. By enhancing further formation of drug nucleotides through the accumulation of PRPP normally consumed in the PRPP amidotransferase reaction.

Studies of drug resistance have led to an appreciation of the secondary role of inhibition of purine nucleotide synthesis de novo in the action of MP and TG. This pathway was shown to be inhibited to the same extent in sensitive and resistant lines of several animal tumours treated with MP and TG (LePage and Jones 1961 a; Hitchings and Elion 1967). It is noteworthy that MMPR, the most potent purine synthesis inhibitor, is itself without clinical antileukaemic activity, although it might be argued that this could conceivably result from pharmacokinetic effects to which MP and TG would not be subject.

MP undergoes catabolic oxidation catalysed by xanthine oxidase with formation of 6-thiouric acid, whilst TG may be deaminated by guanine deaminase to 6-thioxanthine which is then oxidized by xanthine oxidase to 6-thiouric acid. Both thiopurines are also metabolized to methylated derivatives, and, in addition, inorganic sulphate is a major oxidative breakdown product.

II. Resistance

Cellular resistance to MP and TG is almost invariably the result of effects at the level of their metabolism which lead to low incorporation of the drugs into DNA.

High capacities for cellular catabolism of MP and TG may contribute to both spontaneous and acquired resistance. Increased deamination of TG to 6-thioxanthine was observed in some TG-resistant tumour cell lines (Sartorelli et al. 1958; LePage 1977), whilst Higuchi (1974) suggested that rapid conversion of MP to 6-thiouric acid by xanthine oxidase was a possible mechanism of resistance in human leukaemia cells. Degradation of TG to the inactive metabolites 6-thioxanthine and 6-thiouric acid may also play a part protecting normal gastrointestinal mucosa and skin from drug toxicity (Moore and LePage 1958; Marchesi and Sartorelli 1963). Skin toxicity was reported in patients receiving β-2'-deoxythioguanosine, which is not degraded by guanine deaminase, whilst patients treated with TG did not develop this complication (LePage and Gottlieb 1973). Bone marrow, which has low guanine deaminase activity, accumulates higher concentrations of TG nucleotides than gastrointestinal mucosa, and is the normal proliferating tissue which is most susceptible to the toxic effects of TG (Sartorelli and LePage 1957; Marchesi and Sartorelli 1963). However, in contrast to AzaG, TG was found to be unreactive with guanine deaminase from mouse liver and some mouse tumours, and consequently the presence of high enzyme levels will not necessarily impart insensitivity to the thiopurine (Ellis and LePage 1963; Bieber and Sartorelli 1964; Ross et al. 1973). Variations in HGPRT activity were also associated with the differential sensitivities of normal tissues to TG (Marchesi and Sartorelli 1963).

The Mecca and 6C3HED lymphosarcomas are naturally insensitive to TG and little incorporation of the drug into DNA was observed, although it was readily metabolized to acid-soluble nucleotide(s) by the tumour cells, and was incorporated into RNA to a limited extent (LEPAGE et al. 1964; LEPAGE and JONES 1961 a, b). It was postulated that the Mecca lymphosarcoma may have a low capacity for reduction of 6-thioguanosine diphosphate to the deoxyribonucleoside diphosphate via ribonucleotide reductase (BROCKMAN 1974). However, the level of incorporation of TG into RNA of this neoplasm, though significant, was considerably lower than that observed in TG-responsive tumours (LEPAGE and JONES 1961 b). This could possibly mean that the tumour was also defective in converting TG nucleoside 5′-monophosphate to higher phosphorylated forms.

Acquired resistance to MP and TG is most frequently associated with decreased cellular accumulation of drug nucleoside 5′-monophosphate derivatives. This effect may result from one of three distinct types of biochemical mechanism, or a combination thereof, namely:

1. Reduction in HGPRT activity
2. Reduction in PRPP availability
3. Increase in catabolic activity towards drug nucleoside 5′-monophosphates.

Acquired resistance to MP and TG in bacteria and experimental tumour systems has most often involved reduction in or essentially total loss of HGPRT activity as the overriding mechanism, especially under conditions of high selection pressure (HUTCHISON 1963; BROCKMAN 1960;1963; STUTTS and BROCKMAN 1963; BROCKMAN and CHUMLEY 1965; DAVIDSON 1960; BROCKMAN et al. 1961; ELLIS and LEPAGE 1963). These observations provided the initial indication that formation of MP and TG nucleoside monophosphates was a prerequisite for drug activity; experimental tumours resistant to MP were cross-resistant to TG and vice versa where loss of HGPRT had occurred. However, LEPAGE and JONES (1961 a) described a TG-resistant tumour-cell line that was not cross-resistant to MP. It was apparent that in this example an alternative mechanism such as enhanced deamination of TG was responsible for resistance. VAN DIGGELEN et al. (1979) reported that they were unable to isolate mutants simultaneously resistant to both TG and HAT media, whereas others have described TG-resistant cell lines containing mutant HGPRT with enhanced heat lability that were TG resistant and HAT resistant at 33 °C, and TG resistant and HAT sensitive at 39 °C (FENWICK and CASKEY 1975; FRIEDRICH and COFFINO 1977). The temperature-sensitive enzyme from one of the clones was characterized and shown to have reduced affinity for PRPP (FRIEDRICH and COFFINO 1977). The ability to grow in HAT medium probably resulted from the elevation in cellular PRPP concentrations induced by antifolate treatment.

Mutations in the HGPRT structural genes of TG-resistant cells have been identified on the basis of the types of evidence discussed above in the section on AzaG resistance (FENWICK and CASKEY 1975; EPSTEIN et al. 1977; FRIEDRICH and COFFINO 1977; HODGKISS and FOX 1980; FOX and HODGKISS 1981). Reductions in the affinity of the enzyme for either PRPP or TG have frequently been observed in addition to mutations affecting its overall specific activity (CHASIN and URLAUB 1976; EPSTEIN et al. 1977; FRIEDRICH and COFFINO 1977; HODGKISS and FOX 1980; FOX and HODGKISS 1981). High concentrations of TG were effective in selecting irrevertible deletions within the HGPRT gene, presumably because complete resistance to this efficient substrate of the enzyme may only be achieved by total enzyme loss (HODGKISS et al. 1980). The same authors pointed out that the reported "reversion" of TG-resistant cell lines to growth ability in HAT media was an insufficient criterion by itself for reversion at the HGPRT locus, since this may be due to the acquisition of amethopterin resistance. Such "reversions" had been taken as evidence that the original forward mutations were not deletions. However, true reversions to TG sensitivity and growth in HAT media, with reappearance of antigenically altered HGPRT, are indicative of forward mutations in the structural gene, and imply that inactive proteins may have been produced by the original HGPRT-negative cells. BRENNAND et al. (1982) demonstrated that reversion of a TG-resistant, HGPRT structural gene mutant of a mouse neuroblastoma cell line to a HGPRT-positive phenotype occurred in one clone, not by a compensating mutation, but by a 50-fold amplification of the defective gene such that nearly normal cellular HGPRT activity was achieved with the variant protein. The reappearance of 45%–55% of wild-type HGPRT activity was observed in revertant clones from another TG-resistant mouse neuroblastoma cell line (SKAPER et al. 1977). The enzyme of the revertants was indistinguishable from wild-type HGPRT in terms of kinetic constants and physical properties, whilst the resistant cell line was negative for HGPRT and immunologically cross-reactive material. The authors suggested that these results could be interpreted in terms of a regulatory mutation or a structural gene mutation leading to an increased rate of degradation of HGPRT protein.

KIM et al. (1981) have explained the observations of SCHMID et al. (1976), who found that resistance of L1210 leukaemia in mice to combination chemotherapy with MMPR, MP, TG, methotrexate, 5-fluorouracil and cytosine arabinoside developed more rapidly when the agents were administered sequentially as single doses than when they were given simultaneously on a daily schedule for 6 days as fractions of the same total dosages. Resistance to the six-drug combination coincided with development of resistance to TG and MP through overgrowth of HGPRT-deficient mutant cells present in the original L1210 population at a level of one cell 10^4. Methotrexate alone was responsible for delaying the appearance of TG resistance on the simultaneous schedule as a consequence of its enhanced ability to kill HGPRT-deficient cells which are unable to circumvent the antifolate-induced blockade of purine nucleotide biosynthesis de novo through utilization of preformed hypoxanthine (KIM et al. 1981). An extended period of inhibition was apparently required to eliminate TG-resistant cells and consequently methotrexate administered as a single dose on the sequential schedule was unable to achieve the same result.

Resistance to low concentrations of TG appears to arise by phenotypic adaptation, as discussed in the section on AzaG resistance (TERZI 1974; FOX and RADACIC 1978).

MP- and TG-resistant cell sublines, particularly those generated under conditions of low selection pressure, may accumulate reduced intracellular concentrations of drug nucleotides, although their HGPRT activity, measured by the standard assay in cell-free extracts, is similar to that of the sensitive parent lines (ELLIS and LEPAGE 1963). Such observations were originally taken as evidence that alternative mechanisms other than effects at the HGPRT reaction were responsible for resistance. However, HGPRT activity assayed in cell-free extracts is usually greater, by up to three orders of magnitude, than that observed in intact cell suspensions (Higuchi 1974; Higuchi et al. 1976) and, consequently, Henderson et al. (1975) suggested that wherever technically feasible, it is preferable to base comparisons of different cell lines on measurements made using intact cells.

The intracellular concentration of PRPP varies widely among different cell types and is often considerably lower than its Michaelis constant for PRPP amidotransferase and phosphoribosyltransferases (Higuchi et al. 1976; Higuchi 1974; Fox and Kelley 1971; Henderson and Khoo 1965). The availability of PRPP is thus an important factor in the regulation of purine nucleotide synthesis by both the de novo route and through utilization of preformed bases (Thompson et al. 1978). It has been demonstrated that not only the level of HGPRT but also the concentration of PRPP may limit the cellular anabolism of MP and TG (Higuchi et al. 1976, 1977; Higuchi 1975). Inhibition of purine nucleotide biosynthesis de novo by MMPR or azaserine potentiates the cytotoxic action of MP and TG in large part by enhancing drug nucleotide formation through the accumulation of PRPP normally consumed by the pathway (Paterson and Moriwaki 1969; Scholar et al. 1972; Paterson and Wang 1970; Nelson and Parks 1972). In addition, pretreatment with adenosine has been shown to antagonize the cytotoxicity of TG and MP towards normal cells through selective depletion of PRPP pools (Jackson et al. 1980). Low rates of PRPP synthesis in the presence of high HGPRT levels may be responsible for the thiopurine insensitivity of some leukaemias (Higuchi et al. 1976, 1977; Higuchi 1975).

High or increased catabolism of 6-thioinosinate and 6-thioguanylate reduces the net rate of their cellular accumulation during and/or persistence after drug exposure and represents a major mechanism of innate insensitivity and resistance acquired under conditions of low selection pressure. An MP/TG-resistant subline of mouse sarcoma 180, S180/TG, achieved lower intracellular concentrations of TG nucleotides than the parent S180 line during exposure to TG. After treatment the concentration of acid-soluble drug metabolites decreased more rapidly in S180/TG than in S180 cells (Sartorelli et al. 1975; Wolpert et al. 1971; Lee et al. 1978). Both lines:

1. Were equally permeable to TG and MP which entered the cells by passive diffusion
2. Possessed equivalent guanine deaminase activity
3. Contained similar PRPP pools
4. Possessed similar levels of HGPRT activity.

It was concluded that an enhanced capacity for dephosphorylation of 6-thioinosinate and 6-thioguanylate was responsible for resistance in the S180/TG subline. Combination treatment with MMPR restored sensitivity to TG in the resistant line, not only by increasing PRPP availability, but, in addition, by inhibiting dephosphorylation of 6-thioguanylate, an effect that was ascribed to competition by 6-methylthioinosinate for the catabolic enzymes (Nelson and Parks 1972). The enhanced capacity for catabolism of 6-thioinosinate and 6-thioguanylate correlated with a large increase in the activity of particulate bound alkaline phosphohydrolase present in S180/TG cells, although when measured at physiological pH both lines appeared to possess roughly equivalent total phosphohydrolase activity (WOLPERT et al. 1971; LEE et al. 1978). It was suggested that in S180/TG cells the physiological nucleotides are protected from the enhanced catabolic activity since these exist primarily at the triphosphate level. In contrast, only the monophosphate of MP riboside is formed in MP-treated cells, and 6-thioguanylate is the predominant nucleotide in cells exposed to TG, as a consequence of its poor substrate activity with guanylate kinase (PATERSON 1959; CRABTREE et al. 1977). Nucleoside monophosphates, but not the triphosphates, were susceptible to hydrolysis catalysed by particulate bound alkaline phosphohydrolase prepared from S180/TG cells (LEE et al. 1978; SARTORELLI et al. 1975). However, labelling experiments indicated that inosine monophosphate was not extensively catabolized in cells of the S180/TG subline, an apparent discrepancy which has not been explained (LEE et al. 1978). On the basis of the foregoing it might be predicted that S180/TG cells would be cross-resistant to MMPR, since this drug is metabolized predominantly to its monophosphate derivative. A significant portion of the alkaline phosphohydrolase activity of S180/TG cells was shown to reside on the external surface of the cell membrane and it was suggested that specific targeting of drugs such as alkylators against thiopurine-resistant cells of this type might be achieved by administering them in the form of phosphorylated prodrugs where the active species would be released by the action of the phosphohydrolases (LEE et al. 1980). Although the high alkaline phosphohydrolase phenotype of S180/TG was stable when the line was passaged weekly in mice in ascites cell form, LEE and SARTORELLI (1981c) reported that a subline of this tumour which was transferred to culture and maintained in vitro for 3 years spontaneously lost the high levels of this enzyme activity without loss of resistance to the cytotoxic action of TG. The cultured cells were resistant by virtue of the fact that they synthesized less TG nucleoside 5′-monophosphate from TG than did the corresponding drug-sensitive S180 cells. In contrast, cultured S180/TG cells converted guanine to guanine nucleotides in much greater amounts than did S180 cells. The S180 and cultured S180/TG lines were similar in (a) their capacity to transport TG and guanine across the cell membrane, (b) their ability to synthesize and accumulate PRPP, (c) the levels and properties of HGPRT assayed in cell-free extracts and (d) their rates of hydrolysis of phosphate groups from newly synthesized TG nucleoside 5′-monophosphate. The authors concluded that either high particulate bound alkaline phosphohydrolase activity was not involved in the mechanism of resistance of S180/TG to TG in vivo, or that catabolism of TG nucleotide by alkaline phosphohydrolase was important for the expression of drug insensitivity, but that the cell line was a double variant in which more than one mechanism was involved in the expression of drug resistance. They suggested that the low rate of TG nucleotide synthesis in cultured S180/TG cells might reflect the existence of HGPRT either in a different state in situ compared with cell-free extracts, or in a cellular location from which TG was preferentially excluded in the resistant cells.

An MP-resistant subline of the Ehrlich ascites carcinoma (EAC), designated EAC-R1, was shown to be highly resistant to MP and cross-resistant to MP-ribonucleoside and TG (PATERSON 1960; HENDERSON et al. 1975). Intact cells formed very low amounts of the nucleotides of these drugs, but were similar to cells of the parent MP-sensitive EAC line in their ability to utilize hypoxanthine, guanine and adenine for nucleotide synthesis (PATERSON and HORI 1962). That resistance was an intact-cell phenomenon was evident from the demonstration that cell-free extracts of the EAC-R1 and EAC lines formed 6-thioinosinate from MP at similar rates in the presence of added PRPP (PATERSON 1962). Uptake of MP may have been impaired in the resistant line, although entry of purine and purine antimetabolite bases into mammalian cells has generally been found to occur by diffusion (HAKALA 1974; BIEBER and SARTORELLI 1964). It is conceivable that the thiopurines were taken up by EAC-R1 cells but failed to gain access to a cell compartment where nucleotide synthesis could occur. The EAC-R1 subline was later shown to be cross-resistant to MMPR as a result of enhanced nucleotide dephosphorylation, accelerated purine nucleotide biosynthesis de novo and partial loss of sensitivity of PRPP amidotransferase to inhibition by 6-methylthioinosinate (HENDERSON et al. 1975). Increased nucleotide dephosphorylation may have contributed to resistance to MP and TG, although in contrast to the low nucleotide synthesis with these agents the initial rate of 6-methylthioinosinate formation from MMPR was nearly normal in intact EAC-R1 cells. Cross resistance to MP was demonstrated in an EAC subline, EAC-R2, which was originally selected for resistance to MMPR (HENDERSON et al. 1975). The initial rate of nucleotide synthesis from MP in EAC-R2 cells was nearly as high as in sensitive EAC cells, and resistance was ascribed to reduced drug persistence caused by enhanced dephosphorylation of MP metabolites.

SCANNELL and HITCHINGS (1966) reported that an MP-resistant subline of the adenocarcinoma 755 tumour incorporated twice as much radiolabelled MP as TG deoxynucleotide into DNA as did the sensitive line. However, LEPAGE (1977) has pointed out that the level of incorporation obtained in both lines in this labelling experiment was below the threshold for lethality observed in treatment of adenocarcinoma 755 and other ascites tumours with TG. The mechanism of resistance in the adenocarcinoma 755 subline is not known. It is conceivable that resistance to MP and TG might arise through suppression of the cytotoxic effect of the DNA-incorporated analogue.

LEE and SARTORELLI (1981 b) reported significant metabolism of TG to its ribonucleoside by intact S180 and S180/TG cells in a reaction catalysed by intracellular purine nucleoside phosphorylase (enzyme 14, Fig. 4). Efflux of the product from the cells occurred via the nucleoside transport system and the nucleoside accumulated in the incubation media. The authors hypothesized that formation of TG ribonucleoside by purine nucleoside phosphorylase may be important to the expression of cell sensitivity to TG in that it decreases the availability of TG for direct conversion to the nucleotide level by HGPRT.

Clinical cellular resistance to MP is often associated with reduced accumulation of drug nucleotides (KESSEL and HALL 1969). The effects may not be as pronounced as those found in many resistant animal tumours and cell culture lines as a result of the lower selection pressure inherent in human cancer chemotherapy. It is likely that clinical resistance occurs predominantly by phenotypic adaptation rather than by mutational mechanisms (FOX and RADACIC 1978).

Loss of or substantial reduction in HGPRT activity as assayed in cell-free extracts does occur, but is not a common mechanism of thiopurine resistance in human leukaemia (DAVIDSON and WINTER 1964; ROSMAN et al. 1974; SARTORELLI et al. 1975; ROSMAN and WILLIAMS 1973; SMITH et al. 1971). Severe HGPRT deficiency accounted for approximately 12% of resistant cases of acute non-lymphocytic leukaemia, and moderate enzyme loss was responsible for an additional 23% (SARTORELLI et al. 1975). Decreased HGPRT activity was not found in any case of MP-resistant acute lymphocytic leukaemia. It has been postulated that the relatively lower frequency of HGPRT loss found in human leukaemic cells compared with transplantable animal tumours may be related to the obligatory utilization of preformed bases by the former to satisfy their purine requirements (SARTORELLI et al. 1975). A number of authors have reported little or no activity of the de novo pathway of purine biosynthesis in human bone marrow and leukaemic leucocytes (SCOTT 1962; SMELLIE et al. 1958; SCHOLAR and CALABRESI 1973). In contrast, SCOTT et al. (1966) reported that leucocytes from two cases of acute myelogenous leukaemia exhibited high rates of purine de novo synthesis which coincided with clinical resistance to MP. They suggested that increased purine biosynthetic reserves may be a mechanism of MP resistance in some human leukaemias. Enhanced purine nucleotide biosynthesis de novo may confer resistance to thiopurines through increased competition for available PRPP and elevated concentrations of normal purine nucleotides which would compete with drug nucleotides for further anabolism. Enhanced catabolism of drug nucleoside monophosphates to nucleosides which are lost from the cells may play an important part in resistance of human leukaemic cells to MP and TG, particularly in cases of acute lymphocytic leukaemia (ROSMAN et al. 1974; SARTORELLI et al. 1975). Development of resistance to these thiopurines in acute lymphocytic leukaemia was attributed at least in part to increases in the intracellular levels of particulate bound alkaline phosphohydrolases. Similarly, increases in activity of alkaline phosphohydrolases were observed in leukaemic cells from acute myelocytic and acute myelomonocytic leukaemia patients during development of resistance to 6-thiopurine therapy (SCHOLAR and CALABRESI 1979). TIDD and DEDHAR (1978) noted that intracellular 6-thioguanylate concentrations decreased to below the level of detection by a specific and sensitive fluorescence technique within minutes of removing the drug during in vitro incubations of human acute myelogenous leukaemia cell samples. However, the product of drug nucleotide catabolism was not identified. This contrasts with the results for mouse leukaemia cells, where thiopurine nucleotides may persist for several hours after drug exposure, and undoubtedly reflects a difference in sensitivity between the mouse and human cells. MARTIN et al. (1972) found no apparent relationship between MP resistance of human acute lymphocytic leukaemia cells and the ability of cell extracts to dephosphorylate 6-thioinosinate. However, they did demonstrate a correlation between insensitivity of the cells and the extent of dethiolation of 6-thioinosinate by cell extracts to produce the physiological nucleotide, inosinate. These data suggested that clinical resistance to MP might develop as a result of enhanced catabolism of 6-thioinosinate by:

1. Dethiolation to normal metabolites
2. Dephosphorylation to 6-thioinosine, or
3. A combination of both mechanisms.

In addition, low or reduced availability of PRPP may play a key role in clinical resistance to the thiopurine bases when normal levels of HGPRT activity are present (HIGUCHI 1975; HIGUCHI et al. 1976, 1977). The PRPP content of human leukaemic cells was shown to be far less than the amounts required for the observed formation of 6-thioinosinate from MP during in vitro incubations. Therefore it was apparent that PRPP synthesis occurred during the period of exposure to MP. The extent of thiosinosinate synthesis in vitro varied widely with cells from different patients but correlated with the phosphate-stimulated production of PRPP by such cells.

TG is usually administered orally in combination chemotherapy protocols for acute myelogenous leukaemia. BROX et al. (1981) measured plasma concentrations of TG in patients receiving standard oral dosages of the drug and demonstrated that absorption was erratic and that frequently only low peak plasma levels were attained which may have been insufficient to elicit antileukaemia effects. The ingestion of food at the time of drug administration tended to lower peak plasma levels and increased the time taken for their achievement. Such cases would probably have appeared to be resistant to TG had the drug been administered as a single agent. The authors quoted the findings of a recent large clinical trial of acute myelogenous leukaemia in which the addition of oral TG to a regimen of daunorubicin, cytosine arabinoside and prednisone failed to increase the remission rate (FINNISH LEUKAEMIA GROUP 1979). BROX et al. (1981) suggested that the intravenous formulation of TG may be superior to the same drug given orally, a possibility which is currently the subject of several phase-II clinical trials sponsored by the US National Cancer Institute.

DOOLEY and MADDOCKS (1982) suggested that delivery of thiopurines to the bone marrow (and other tissues) may occur predominantly via red blood cells in which the drugs are present as their nucleotide metabolites. Inefficiency in this process could conceivably be an additional factor in clinical resistance.

D. 6-Methylthioinosine

6-Methylthioinosine (MMPR) was first synthesized in an attempt to overcome mechanisms of resistance to MP. The rationale for its design is discussed in the later section on circumvention of resistance. MMPR is growth inhibitory to a number of experimental tumours but has not shown clinical activity when used alone. The sole clinical application of this agent has been its experimental use in combination with MP for treatment of acute granulocytic leukaemia (BODEY et al. 1968). However, MMPR has received considerable attention as a result of interest in its biochemical properties.

I. Metabolism and Mechanism of Action

The metabolism and mechanism of action of MMPR have been reviewed by PATERSON and TIDD (1975) and LEPAGE (1977). Unlike MP, which acts as a hypoxanthine antipurine, MMPR behaves as an analogue of adenosine. The explanation for this difference lies in the molecular configuration at the purine N-1 position. At physiological pH, MP and TG exist in solution predominantly in the form of their thioketo tautomers in which the N-1 nitrogen is protonated. In this respect their structures are completely analogous to those of hypoxanthine and guanine. In contrast, MMPR is locked in the thiol form by S-methylation and like adenosine the N-1 position carries no proton. MMPR is readily phosphorylated by adenosine kinase with formation of its monophosphate derivative, the principal drug metabolite. Di- and triphosphates of MMPR are produced but at considerably slower rates than the monophosphate and incorporation into nucleic acids has not been observed. 6-Methylthioinosinate is a potent inhibitor of purine nucleotide biosynthesis de novo through its interaction with PRPP amidotransferase, the first enzyme unique to the pathway. The antipurine nucleotide is thought to bind to the enzyme at the site of feedback inhibition by normal purine nucleotides, thereby inducing so-called pseudofeedback inhibition of purine synthesis. This effect appears to be the sole action of MMPR, and growth inhibition is completely reversed by 4-amino-imidazole-5-carboxamide and preformed purines. 6-Methylthioinosinate is also a metabolite of MP and in some MP-treated cells its concentration may be of the same order as that of 6-thioinosinate.

Like adenosine, MMPR ist not a substrate for purine nucleoside phosphorylase and consequently it is not degraded to 6-methylmercaptopurine, nor is it extensively catabolized by other routes.
The lack of clinical activity of MMPR may be related to two factors:

1. MMPR may inhibit growth reversibly to a considerable extent without affecting cell viability. Extremes of concentration or exposure duration may be required to produce cytolysis and hence a permanent antitumour response
2. Growth inhibition is reversed by preformed purines which may be readily available to human malignant cells.

There would appear to be little obvious justification for treating human leukaemias with inhibitors of purine nucleotide biosynthesis de novo when the cells have limited or no dependence on this pathway. However, it is possible that the malignant stem cells may have greater reliance on de novo synthesis than is implied by measurements on leukaemic cell populations as a whole.

II. Resistance

Resistance to MMPR may develop quite readily through reduction in or loss of adenosine kinase activity (Caldwell et al. 1967; Bennett et al. 1966a). A good correlation was found between the level of the enzyme and sensitivity to MMPR in a series of mouse tumours (Ho et al. 1968). However, no relationship was found between adenosine kinase levels and MMPR toxicity in normal tissues of mouse and man.

Cells of an MMPR-resistant subline of the Ehrlich ascites carcinoma (EAC-R2) were shown to have lost the capacity to phosphorylate MMPR and other adenosine analogues whilst the ability to phosphorylate adenosine itself was retained (Lomax and Henderson 1972). Adenosine kinase continued to be produced by the cells and resistance was ascribed to an alteration in the specificity of the enzyme such that MMPR was no longer accepted as a substrate. EAC-R2 cells also possessed an enhanced capacity for drug nucleotide dephosphorylation as evidenced by their cross-resistance to MP (HENDERSON et al. 1975). MP was metabolized at near normal initial rates by the EAC-R2 subline, but the intracellular half-life of drug nucleotide metabolites was much reduced. Another EAC subline designated EAC-R1 was originally selected for resistance to MP and only later shown to be cross-resistant to MMPR (HENDERSON et al. 1967, 1975). Resistance to MMPR was associated with multiple biochemical changes in the face of near normal initial rates of 6-methylthioinosinate formation. The cells were shown to have an enhanced capacity for dephosphorylation of the drug nucleotide and also synthesized purine nucleotides by the de novo route at an elevated rate. In addition, the latter process was less sensitive to inhibition by MMPR, apparently as a result of an alteration in PRPP amidotransferase which reduced the effectiveness of 6-methylthioinosinate as an inhibitor of this enzyme.

E. 9-β-D-Arabinofuranosyladenine

9-β-D-Arabinofuranosyladenine (AraA) was originally developed as an antiviral agent and was only later found to inhibit a number of experimental tumours in mice. The clinical usefulness of AraA both as an antitumour and antiviral agent has been limited by its suspectibility to deamination. However, the recent development of powerful deaminase inhibitors and protected derivatives of AraA has led to renewed interest in its clinical application. Methods of overcoming rapid catabolism of AraA are described in the section on circumvention of resistance.

I. Metabolism and Mechanism of Action

The metabolism and mechanism of action of AraA have been reviewed by CASS (1979). Figure 5 compares the metabolism of AraA and its normal counterpart 2′-deoxyadenosine. In most cells the drug is probably phosphorylated to its monophosphate derivative predominantly by deoxyadenosine-deoxyguanosine kinase, although adenosine kinase and deoxycytidine kinase may contribute to

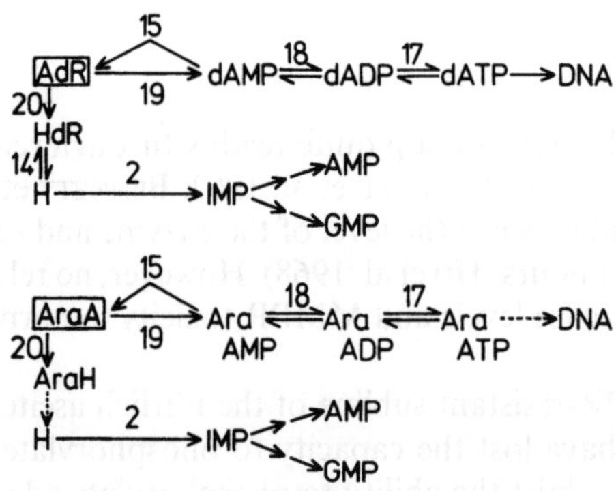

Fig. 5. 2′-Deoxyadenosine and 9-β-D-arabinofuranosyladenine metabolism: (*2*) hypoxanthine-guanine phosphoribosyltransferase; (*14*) purine nucleoside phosphorylase; (*15*) phosphohydrolase/5′-nucleotidase; (*17*) nucleoside diphosphate kinase; (*18*) adenylate kinase; (*19*) deoxyadenosine-deoxyguanosine kinase; (*20*) adenosine deaminase. *AraA*, 9-β-D-arabinofuranosyladenine. *AraH*, 9-β-D-arabinofuranosylhypoxanthine

this reaction. The monophosphate is readily phosphorylated further to AraA triphosphate, the major anabolite found in AraA-treated cells. Although initially the subject of some controversy, it is now clear that the drug is incorporated into internucleotide linkage in DNA at a very low level. Limited incorporation of AraA into RNA of ascites tumours has also been reported. AraA is rapidly deaminated by adenosine deaminase to give 9-β-D-arabinofuranosylhypoxanthine, a derivative which is devoid of antitumour activity. This catabolite is a major urinary excretion product of AraA in normal mice and man. AraA is not a substrate for purine nucleoside phosphorylase, although some cellular utilization of the purine moiety of the drug molecule in normal purine nucleotide synthesis is observed. This probably occurs via deamination of AraA and subsequent cleavage of 9-β-D-arabinofuranosylhypoxanthine.

AraA triphosphate is the pharmacologically active form of AraA, and inhibition of DNA synthesis by this metabolite is responsible for the cytotoxic activity of the nucleoside. Both ribonucleotide reductase and DNA polymerase are inhibited in AraA-treated cells. However, DNA polymerase is more sensitive to inhibition by AraA triphosphate and is almost certainly the predominant site of action of AraA.

II. Resistance

Excessive deamination of AraA to the inactive catabolite, 9-β-D-arabinofuranosylhypoxanthine, is a major mechanism of resistance to this antipurine. Spontaneous insensitivity to the drug in experimental neoplasms correlated with their cellular levels of adenosine deaminase (LePage 1970; 1975 b; Koshiura and LePage 1968). Tumours with low or moderate deaminase activity, such as carcinoma 1025, Ridgeway osteogenic sarcoma, 6C3HED lymphosarcoma, Ehrlich carcinoma and ascitic TA3 tumours were responsive to AraA, whereas mouse leukaemia L1210 and Sarcoma 180, with high levels of the enzyme, were resistant. Formation of AraA triphosphate with profound inhibition of DNA synthesis occurred initially in tumours containing high deaminase activity following injections of AraA. However, decay of intracellular drug nucleotide and recovery from inhibition of DNA synthesis was more rapid in such neoplasms than in those with low enzyme activity. The rate of recovery was directly related to the amount of deaminase present in the cells (LePage 1975b). The resistant tumours responded to AraA when the drug was administered in combination with an inhibitor of adenosine deaminase (LePage et al. 1976).

In addition to tumour resistance, the general lack of toxicity of AraA towards the host, particularly the absence of immunosuppressive effects, is explained by the general abundance of adenosine deaminase. In view of the rapid deamination of AraA by normal tissues the optimum mode of clinical therapy with the single agent has been by continuous i.v. infusions (LePage 1977; LePage and Khaliq 1979).

LePage (1975) has observed wide variations in the adenosine deaminase: AraA kinase ratio for human tumour cells and leukaemic leucocytes which might be expected to result in differences in suspectibility to AraA between individual human malignancies. However, he later reported that, in contrast to the results with mouse neoplasms, high cellular deaminase activities did not appear to be responsible for insensitivity to AraA in human tumours (LEPAGE and KHALIQ 1979). An inhibitor of adenosine deaminase did not affect the extent of inhibition of DNA synthesis by AraA in clinically unresponsive human malignant cells under conditions of in vitro incubation. Changes in DNA polymerases may be responsible for some cases of clinical resistance to AraA. This mechanism was observed in cells of an AraA-resistant line of the 6C3HED lymphosarcoma and in cells from a patient with chronic myelogenous leukaemia in blastic crisis, which did not respond to chemotherapy with AraA (LEPAGE 1978a).

Mutant cells of a Morris rat hepatoma which lacked adenosine kinase but not deoxyadenosine kinase activity were as sensitive to AraA in the presence of an adenosine deaminase inhibitor as were cells of the parent line (SUTTLE et al. 1981). Phosphorylation of AraA is thought to be mediated, for the most part, by deoxyadenosine-deoxyguanosine kinase, an enzyme which also phosphorylates cytidine. Whilst resistance to AraA involving loss of this enzyme is theoretically possible, such a mechanism has not been reported. Deoxyadenosine and deoxyguanosine are also substrates for deoxycytidine kinase and on the basis of their Michaelis constants it has been suggested that this enzyme might be the actual physiological kinase for the purine deoxyribonucleosides (HAKALA 1974). Human T-cell leukaemic lines in culture were shown to phosphorylate AraA mainly via deoxycytidine kinase (CARSON et al. 1980). Deoxycytidine protected cells against the growth inhibitory effects of AraA by inhibiting phosphorylation of the drug and thereby reducing the intracellular concentrations of AraA triphosphate. Human B-Lymphocytic cell lines were more resistant to the toxic effects of AraA in the presence of an adenosine deaminase inhibitor than were human malignant T-cell lines (CARSON et al. 1980). The differential sensitivity of the latter was ascribed to their greater capacity to accumulate AraA triphosphate as a result of their high AraA phosphorylating and low deoxyribonucleotide dephosphorylating activities. These observations suggested a possible application of AraA plus adenosine deaminase inhibitor combinations in treatment of T-cell leukaemias.

It would appear that deoxycytidine kinase activity is not consistently a significant factor in phosphorylation of AraA; cells resistant to arabinofuranosylcytosine through loss of this enzyme were not cross-resistant to AraA, although they were resistant to 9-β-D-arabinofuranosyl-2-fluoroadenine (BROCKMAN et al. 1979).

F. Adenine and Adenosine Antipurines

A large number of adenine and adenosine antipurines have been synthesized and some have shown growth inhibitory activity against experimental neoplasms.

I. Metabolism

Generally the adenine antipurines are converted to their nucleoside 5′-monophosphate derivatives by adenosine 5′-monophosphate (AMP): pyrophosphate phosphoribosyltransferase (adenine phosphoribosyltransferase, APRT), whereas the adenosine antipurines are substrates for adenosine kinase. The absence of a proton on the N-1 position of the purine ring is more critical for activity with adenosine kinase than is the nature of the group at the 6-position. Consequently several ribonucleosides bearing little direct resemblance to adenosine are phosphorylated by this enzyme. Catabolism of adenosine analogues is usually mediated by adenosine deaminase and as in the case of AraA the widespread occurrence of this enzyme has limited the usefulness of these agents (see reviews: BLOCH 1975; NICHOL 1975). Thus the cytotoxicity of O^6-methylinosine and 6-chloropurine ribonucleoside is destroyed through their conversion to inosine by adenosine deaminase. However, tubercidin is an adenosine analogue which is not extensively deaminated.

II. Resistance

Resistance to the adenine antipurines, 2-fluoroadenine and 2,6-diaminopurine, has often been associated with reduction in or loss of APRT activity (HENDERSON 1977; HAKALA 1973; BENNETT et al. 1966b; HENDERSON and BROCKMAN 1975). Resistant cells were generally cross-resistant to other adenine analogues but retained adenosine kinase activity and sensitivity to adenosine antipurines. Resistance of tumour cells in culture to 4-aminopyrazolo(3,4-*d*)pyrimidine was associated with increased degradation of the antipurine ribonucleotide (BENNETT et al. 1969).

Loss of or reduction in adenosine kinase activity has been found in cases of resistance to the adenosine analogues, 2-fluoroadenosine, formycin A, isopentenyladenosine, N^6-furfuryladenosine, tubercidin, toyocamycin and sangivamycin (BENNETT et al. 1966a; CALDWELL et al. 1967; HAKALA 1970; DIVEKAR et al. 1972; GUPTA and SIMINOVITCH (1978). The wild-type line and a deoxycytidine kinase-deficient mutant of Chinese hamster ovary cells were shown to convert 9-β-D-xylofuranosyladenine to its triphosphate and to be approximately equivalent in their sensitivity to the cytotoxic effects of this analogue, whereas an adenosine kinase-deficient line failed to phosphorylate the nucleoside and was highly resistant (HARRIS et al. 1981). Reduction in adenosine kinase activity was also associated with development of resistance to pyrazofurin, a result which provided direct evidence that the antipyrimidine is activated by this enzyme (SUTTLE et al. 1981). Mutants selected for resistance to both 2-fluoroadenine and 2-fluoroadenosine were deficient in both APRT and adenosine kinase (BENNETT et al. 1966b). In addition, catabolism of adenosine antipurines by adenosine deaminase may contribute to tumour resistance; this mechanism was shown to be responsible for insensitivity of experimental neoplasms to 9-β-D-xylofuranosyladenine (LEPAGE 1970).

G. Circumvention of Resistance

Efforts to circumvent resistance are equally relevant to both acquired resistance and natural or innate insensitivity, since their causes are the same at the molecular level (HENDERSON and BROCKMAN 1975). Success in overcoming acquired resistance may lead to effective chemotherapy of neoplasms which are naturally unresponsive to antipurines. Several types of manipulation have been investigated in attempts to overcome mechanisms of resistance to the antipurines. These include:

1. Use of derivatives of the antipurines capable of undergoing anabolism by alternative routes
2. Coadministration of a second agent which specifically potentiates the action of the antipurine
3. Use of derivatives of the antipurines which are not affected by degradative enzymes but which act as depot or slow release forms of the drugs
4. Coadministration of inhibitors of degradative enzymes
5. Molecular alteration of the antipurines to reduce substrate activity towards degradative enzymes, whilst the ability to undergo conversion to nucleotides with the activity of the parent drug nucleotides is retained
6. Use of phosphorylated "prodrug" derivatives of the antipurine nucleotides.

Specific examples of attempts to circumvent resistance mechanisms are described below.

I. Derivatives Metabolized by Alternative Routes

6-Thioinosine was synthesized on the basis that if it were phosphorylated directly by a kinase it might have potential for treatment of neoplasms that were resistant to MP through loss of HGPRT. However, it was found that 6-thioinosine was rapidly cleaved to MP by purine nucleoside phosphorylase, and many MP-resistant tumours were completely cross-resistant to the nucleoside (Paterson and Sutherland 1964; Brockman 1963). The activity of 6-thioinosine against MP-sensitive cells was interpreted in terms of its initial cleavage to MP and subsequent conversion of the latter to nucleotide by HGPRT. A similar situation was found with 6-thioguanosine (LePage and Junga 1963). 6-Thioinosine and 6-thioguanosine did have some activity in a few experimental neoplasms that were resistant to the bases as a result of HGPRT deficiency (Skipper et al. 1959; Brockman and Chumley 1965). It was suggested that in these cases direct phosphorylation of the antipurine nucleosides occurred to a limited extent, catalysed by low levels of inosine-guanosine kinase, an enzyme that has not been well characterized (Pierre and LePage 1968; Pierre et al. 1967). It is also possible that ribose-1-phosphate released through phosphorolysis of the nucleoside might be utilized for PRPP synthesis via its conversion to ribose-5-phosphate by phosphoribomutase (Fox and Kelley 1971). Increased intracellular pools of PRPP might stimulate thiopurine nucleotide synthesis from the free bases, produced by phosphorolysis, if, as is often the case, a low residual level of HGPRT were present in the resistant cells. Such a mechanism would be reflected in greater sensitivity of the cells to 6-thioinosine and 6-thioguanosine than to MP and TG. Resistance to the thiopurine nucleosides involving reduction in inosine-guanosine kinase activity has not been demonstrated.

β-2′-Deoxythioguanosine was designed to overcome at least three possible mechanisms of resistance to TG, namely: loss of HGPRT, increased guanine deaminase activity and impaired conversion of 6-thioguanylate to TG deoxyribonucleotides (LePage et al. 1964). The derivative was shown to be active against TG-resistant tumour lines and against the TG-insensitive Mecca lymphosarcoma, in which negligible incorporation of TG into DNA is observed. β-2′-Deoxythioguanosine was incorporated into the DNA of Mecca lymphosarcoma cells more rapidly than was TG, suggesting that the deoxynucleoside was phosphorylated directly, presumably by deoxyadenosine-deoxyguanosine kinase (LEPAGE and JUNGA 1967). Direct phosphorylation of β-2′-deoxythioguanosine by murine and human malignant cells has been reported, and some remissions were obtained with the deoxynucleoside in clinical treatment of leukaemias that were refractory to TG (NAKAI and LEPAGE 1972; PEERY and LEPAGE 1969; LEPAGE and GOTTLIEB 1973; OMURA 1975). However, β-2′-deoxythioguanosine is also rapidly cleaved to TG by purine nucleoside phosphorylase (LEPAGE 1968). In contrast to the foregoing, NELSON et al. (1975a, b) obtained a poor response with β-2′-deoxythioguanosine against the Mecca lymphosarcoma and also found that cell lines resistant to MP through loss of HGPRT activity were cross-resistant to both TG and its deoxyriboside. In no instance has resistance to β-2′-deoxythioguanosine been observed involving loss of deoxyadenosine-deoxyguanosine kinase activity.

α-2′-Deoxythioguanosine is not a substrate for purine nucleoside phosphorylase (LEPAGE 1968). This anomer of TG deoxyriboside is phosphorylated directly and incorporated into DNA of tumour cells as chain termini (PEERY and LEPAGE 1969; TAMAOKI and LEPAGE 1975). A preferential antitumour action is claimed for this derivative which is phosphorylated by responsive neoplastic cells but not by normal human bone marrow cells (LEPAGE 1968; PEERY and LEPAGE 1969). The latter characteristic in conjunction with the lack of cleavage to TG makes α-2′-deoxythioguanosine a comparatively non-toxic drug.

II. Potentiation by a Second Agent

In many cases, particularly in clinical chemotherapy, resistance to the antipurines may be operative only to the dosage limits imposed by normal tissue toxicity and might be overcome if higher concentrations of the agents could be safely maintained. One approach to this problem is to administer the antipurine in combination with another drug where either:

1. The second agent is able preferentially to protect vital normal tissues against toxicity and thereby permit higher doses of the first, and/or
2. Where the second drug potentiates the action of the first against malignant tissues but not against normal elements, such that the "synergistic" activity of the combination is greater than the sum of the effects of each agent alone.

As discussed above, treatment of mice bearing TG-resistant S180/TG cells with MMPR in combination with TG resulted in a TG-induced antitumour response (NELSON and PARKS 1972). MMPR may also potentiate the action of MP in treatment of human acute granulocytic leukaemia (BODEY et al. 1968).

Arabinofuranosylcytosine is a drug which like AraA inhibits DNA synthesis through the interaction of its triphosphate with DNA polymerase. The combination of arabinosylcytosine and MP was shown to be therapeutically synergistic against mouse leukaemia L1210, whilst toxicity to normal tissues appeared to be less than additive (BURCHENAL and DOLLINGER 1967). Marked therapeutic synergism was also reported for the combination of arabinosylcytosine and TG against mouse and human leukaemias when the two agents were administered simultaneously. With this schedule of drug administration toxicity to vital normal cells was less than additive (GEE et al. 1969; LEPAGE and WHITE 1973; SCHMIDT et al. 1970; SCHABEL 1975). Synergism, though to a lesser degree, was also observed when the combination was used in treatment of mice bearing arabinosylcytosine-resistant L1210 cells (SCHABEL 1975). The effects may be rationalized in terms of an arabinosylcytosine-induced reversible inhibition of DNA synthesis in normal bone marrow cells which protected these cells from TG toxicity by preventing incorporation of the thiopurine into their DNA (LEPAGE 1978b). This permitted higher doses of TG to be administered against the relatively TG-insensitive L1210 leukaemia (SCHABEL 1975). Apparently the arabinosylcytosine-sensitive L1210 leukaemia cells recovered from inhibition of DNA synthesis more rapidly than the normal bone marrow cells and at such time they were synchronized for entry into or continuation through the TG-sensitive phase of the cell cycle. Therefore, by protecting normal cells and increasing the doses of TG enhanced therapeutic responses were achieved against a comparatively insensitive leukaemia.

III. Protected Slow-Release Depot Derivatives

Azathioprine (6-[(1-methyl-4-nitro-5-imidazolyl)thio]purine, "Imuran", Fig. 6), an S-substituted 6-mercaptopurine, was originally synthesized as a depot form of MP, in which the sulphydryl is reversibly protected, in order to overcome resistance due to rapid host catabolism of MP through oxidation by xanthine oxidase and methylation with subsequent oxidation at the sulphur. However, the derivative was found to be metabolized readily in vivo (ELION and HITCHINGS 1975). Free MP is released from azathioprine in vivo or in vitro by non-enzymatic reactions with sulphydryl compounds such as glutathione, cysteine and certain proteins. The drug was active against a variety of experimental tumours but was not accepted as a substitute for MP in clinical cancer chemotherapy (ELION et al. 1961). On the other hand, azathioprine has superseded MP as an immunosuppressive agent for preventing graft rejection in organ transplantation (HITCHINGS and ELION 1969; ELION and HITCHINGS 1975).

The 5′-monophosphate of AraA has been shown to be superior to the parent nucleoside as a clinical cancer chemotherapeutic agent (LEPAGE et al. 1972, 1975; LEPAGE and KHALIQ 1979). The phosphorylated derivative is considerably more soluble than AraA, thus permitting the administration of large doses by i.v. injection and, in addition, the nucleotide is not susceptible to catabolic deamination by adenosine deaminase, the major mechanism of resistance to AraA. Following i.v. injection, AraA monophosphate is largely confined to the plasma space and

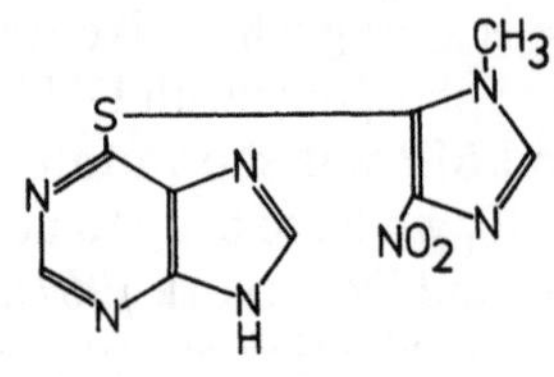

Fig. 6. Chemical structure of azathioprine

acts as a slow release form of AraA through its hydrolysis by phosphomonosterases. The levels of these hydrolytic enzymes in human kidney are low and consequently sustained plasma levels of AraA are achieved following a single injection of the nucleotide. Treatment with AraA monophosphate in this way effectively approximates i.v. infusions of AraA, the optimum mode on therapy with the nucleoside. AraA released from the monophosphate by extracellular hydrolysis is taken up by cells and rephosphorylated to the pharmacologically active triphosphate metabolite. In addition, AraA monophosphate may slowly enter cells as the intact nucleotide without prior dephosphorylation (COHEN and PLUNKETT 1975). Similarly, although arabinosyl-6-mercaptopurine is active as such and does not require phosphorylation by tumour cells for activity, it is claimed that administration of this drug as its 5′-monophosphate achieves the advantages of increased solubility, slower excretion and sustained release of the nucleoside (LEPAGE et al. 1972; LEPAGE and NAIK 1975).

IV. Coadministration of Inhibitors of Degradative Enzymes

One approach to the problem of overcoming resistance due to enhanced catabolism of the antipurines has been to administer the drugs in combination with specific inhibitors of the degradative enzymes.

Allopurinol, a xanthine oxidase inhibitor, was shown to prevent the oxidation of MP to 6-thiouric acid in vivo, and to increase the activity of MP against mouse tumours (ELION et al. 1963; ELION 1967, 1975). Much higher concentrations of 6-thioinosinate were found in tumour cells from mice treated with the combination of allopurinol and MP than in cells from animals treated with MP alone. It was suggested that more free MP was available for nucleotide formation when the antipurine was protected from oxidation. However, no significant changes in the pharmacokinetic parameters of MP in man were found when the drug was administered in combination with allopurinol (COFFEY et al. 1972).

Resistance to AraA and adenosine analogues involving high levels of adenosine deaminase activity may be overcome by the use of specific inhibitors of the enzyme in combination with the antipurine. Coformycin, 2′-deoxycoformycin and *erythro*-9-(2-hydroxy-3-nonyl)adenine (EHNA) are potent inhibitors of adenosine deaminase and have been shown to confer sensitivity to AraA and adenosine analogues on previously unresponsive neoplasms (PLUNKETT and COHEN 1975; LEPAGE et al. 1976; CASS and AU-YEUNG 1976; SCHABEL et al. 1976; JOHNS and ADAMSON 1976; ADAMSON et al. 1977; CASS 1979; PLUNKETT et al. 1980; HARRIS and PLUNKETT 1981; LEE et al. 1981). These effects were accompanied by increases in the intracellular concentrations of phosporylated antipurine derivatives (ROSE and BROCKMAN 1977; PLUNKETT et al. 1979; HARRIS and PLUNKETT 1981). The effectiveness of AraA monophosphate against L1210 cells in culture was also substantially enhanced in the presence of inhibitors of adenosine deaminase since AraA released by dephosphorylation of the nucleotide was susceptible to deamination by the high enzyme levels present in these cells (CASS et al. 1979). However, PLUNKETT et al. (1981) reported increased concentrations of deoxyadenosine triphosphate which exceeded the concentrations of AraA triphosphate in leukaemic cells of patients receiving therapy with combinations of

AraA and 2′-deoxycoformycin. This effect of the drug combination would tend to counteract inhibition of DNA synthesis by the AraA metabolite.

Inhibitors of phosphohydrolases have been sought in an effort to develop effective therapy for human leukaemia where elevated drug nucleotide catabolism may represent a major mechanism of antipurine resistance. SARTORELLI et al. (1975) have developed a series of α-(*N*)-heterocyclic carboxaldehyde thiosemicarbazones which possess the capacity to bind zinc ions. Since alkaline phosphohydrolases are zinc-requiring enzymes, one approach to the development of effective inhibitors of their activity is to screen zinc-ion-chelating compounds. The zinc-chelating potential of the α-(*N*)-heterocyclic carboxaldehyde thiosemicarbazones was shown to correlate with their biochemical effects on particulate bound alkaline phosphohydrolases isolated from S180/TG cells. In addition, tetramisole analogues have been investigated as inhibitors of these enzymes (LI et al. 1979).

V. Molecular Alteration to Prevent Catabolism but not Anabolism

The administration of an antipurine in combination with an inhibitor of its catabolism suffers from the practical disadvantages that the appropriate scheduling of two agents rather than one must be considered, as well as possible toxic effects of the second drug. For example, inhibitors of adenosine deaminase used to prevent rapid degradation of AraA may cause a variety of undesirable side effects (AVRAMIS and PLUNKETT 1982).

BENNETT et al. (1978) have adopted an approach to overcoming antipurine resistance which does not involve coadministration of a second agent to inhibit catabolic enzymes. They have introduced structural modifications into drug molecules which eliminate substrate activity with catabolic enzymes whilst the ability to undergo phosphorylation, usually by alternative enzymes, is retained. By this means the properties of insensitivity to catabolism and of utilizing alternative routes of anabolism are built into a single molecule. Finally, the derivatives are required to have the same ultimate mechanism of action and degree of activity as the original antipurine. Unfortunately, although the metabolic aims have been achieved in a number of examples, the molecular alterations introduced to manipulate metabolism have almost invariably resulted in agents with no antitumour activity or with different mechanisms of action from the parent drugs, metabolic resistance to which they were designed to circumvent.

As discussed above, 6-thioinosine was not significantly active against experimental tumours resistant to MP through loss of HGPRT activity. The nucleoside was readily cleaved to MP by purine nucleoside phosphorylase, and little direct conversion to the nucleotide occurred as a consequence of such phosphorolysis and the generally low activities of inosine-guanosine kinase. A carbocyclic analogue of 6-thioinosine was synthesized in order to replace the phosphorylase-susceptible glycosidic linkage with a stable C-N bond. However, this compound was found to be metabolically inert and pharamcologically inactive (BENNETT et al. 1968). MMPR, another structural derivative of 6-thioinosine, was synthesized in a further effort to bypass MP-resistance mechanisms (BENNETT et al. 1965). MMPR behaves as an adenosine analogue, is not cleaved by purine nucleoside phosphorylase and is rapidly phosphorylated by adenosine kinase. Although growth inhibitory towards some MP-resistant experimental neoplasms, the mechanism of action of MMPR was shown to be different from that of MP (BENNETT et al. 1978). Unlike MP, MMPR is not incorporated into DNA, and inhibition of purine nucleotide biosynthesis de novo appears to be its sole metabolic effect. It was apparent that MMPR represented a new drug rather than an improved form of 6-thioinosine. In addition, resistance to MMPR itself may develop with comparative ease, usually through loss of adenosine kinase activity (CALDWELL et al. 1967).

An HGPRT-deficient HEp No. 2 cell subline was shown to be highly resistant to 6-thioinosine and 8-azahypoxanthine, but not to 8-azainosine (BENNETT et al. 1973). The 8-aza nucleoside was only cleaved to a limited extent by purine nucleoside phosphorylase and nucleoside hydrolases, apparently because replacement of carbon by a nitrogen at the purine-8 position, adjacent to the glycosidic bond, altered the chemical equilibria for the reactions in favour of the nucleoside. Furthermore, 8-azainosine was phosphorylated directly by adenosine kinase although the analogue was not a good substrate for the enzyme. This effect was rationalized in terms of the increased acidity of the molecule compared with inosine. Substantial ionization of the azapurine N-1 proton occurs at physiological pH, and through loss of this proton a structural requirement for substrate activity with adenosine kinase is fulfilled. On the basis of these observations it was predicted that 8-aza-6-thioinosine would be phosphorylated by adenosine kinase and would not be cleaved appreciably by purine nucleoside phosphorylase (BENNETT et al. 1979). The azathiopurine nucleoside was shown to be metabolized as expected; however, its mechanism of action and that of a spontaneous rearrangement product were different from that of MP. The derivative was inferior to MP in terms of both its cytotoxicity in cell cultures and its antileukaemic activity in mice.

Resistance to adenosine and deoxyadenosine analogues involving high levels of adenosine deaminase may be overcome by the use of inhibitors of the enzyme in combination with the antipurine. An alternative approach has been to develop analogues which are not substrates for adenosine deaminase but which retain substrate activity with cellular phosphorylating enzymes and the inhibitory properties of the original drugs (BENNETT et al. 1978). Considerable effort has been directed towards the development of derivatives of AraA which inhibit DNA synthesis without being subject to degradative deamination. α-Arabinosyladenine and α-arabinosyl-8-azaadenine were investigated on the basis of observations that the α-anomers of adenosine and deoxyadenosine are not substrates for adenosine deaminase (CODDINGTON 1965). The α-arabinosyl analogues were phosphorylated by cells and were not susceptible to deamination. These agents exhibited some cytotoxic activity but were ineffective against the high deaminase, AraA-insensitive mouse leukaemia L1210 (BENNETT et al. 1978). Biochemical studies demonstrated that α-arabinosyladenine and α-arabinosyl-8-azaadenine had different mechanisms of action from AraA and were not true analogues of the latter. 9-β-(2′-Azido-2′-deoxy-D-arabinofuranosyl) adenine (arazide), a derivative of AraA, represented a somewhat improved form of the drug, being more water soluble and less susceptible to deamination. However, coadministration of an adenosine deaminase inhibitor was still required for maximal effects with this agent (LEE et al. 1981). Arazide in combination with 2′-deoxycoformycin was markedly superior to AraA plus the same inhibitor in chemotherapy experiments with mouse P388 leukaemia. A potent and longer-lasting inhibition of DNA synthesis appeared to constitute the biochemical basis for the greater efficacy of the former combination (LEE et al. 1981).

Fluorination of adenosine in the purine-2 position had previously been shown to produce a derivative which was phosphorylated by adenosine kinase, but which was not a substrate for adenosine deaminase (SHIGIURA et al. 1965; PARKS et al. 1975: SCHNEBLI et al. 1967; BAER et al. 1966). 2-Fluoroadenosine was found to be highly toxic and to have little or no selective antitumour activity. However, consideration of its metabolism led to the synthesis of 9-β-D-arabinofuranosyl-2-fluoroadenine (BENNETT et al. 1978). It was envisaged that this derivative would be phosphorylated by tumour cells, would not be deaminated, and might have similar antiproliferative activity to that of AraA. BROCKMAN et al. (1977) reported that the substitution of fluorine in the purine-2 position of AraA did indeed eliminate suspectibility to deamination without significantly affecting drug activity. In contrast to AraA, 9-β-D-arabinofuranosyl-2-fluoroadenine was phosphorylated by deoxycytidine kinase and not deoxyadenosine kinase (BROCKMAN et al. 1979, 1980). However, the derivative was converted to the triphosphate to about the same extent as AraA when the latter was administered in the presence of an inhibitor of adenosine deaminase, and like AraA the fluoro analogue elicited selective inhibition of DNA synthesis (BROCKMAN et al. 1977; PLUNKETT et al. 1980; AVRAMIS and PLUNKETT 1982). 9-β-D-Arabinofuranosyl-2-fluoroadenine was found to be active against the L 1210 leukaemia in mice, producing some 50-day survivors, whereas AraA, in the absence of adenosine deaminase inhibitors, had no significant activity against this experimental neoplasm. It would appear that the combination of properties required for circumvention of resistance were realized in the 2-fluoro analogue.

VI. Phosphorylated "Prodrug" Derivatives of Antipurine Nucleotides

It has not been possible to circumvent resistance mechanisms involving loss of drug-nucleotide-forming enzymes by administration of preformed antipurine nucleotides. Nucleoside monophosphates may slowly permeate cell membranes; however, it is generally found that high activities of cell-surface-bound phosphohydrolases lead to rapid dephosphorylation of the nucleotides, with the result that negligible uptake of the intact molecules occurs. A few examples have been reported where significant uptake of intact nucleotides was evident in cells with low surface phosphohydrolase activity (PLUNKETT and COHEN 1977; WAGAR et al. 1979). LEPAGE and NAIK (1975) demonstrated that xylofuranosyl 6-mercaptopurine 5′-monophosphate is not a substrate for phosphohydrolases and very little conversion to xylofuranosyl 6-mercaptopurine occurred in mice. However, the nucleotide was as effective or even more active than the nucleoside against certain mouse neoplasms, suggesting that the intact xylofuranosyl 6-mercaptopurine 5′-monophosphate molecule was taken up by the tumour cells.

Animal cells are resistant to 2′,3′-dideoxyadenosine, a DNA chain terminator in bacteria, apparently because they have limited ability to phosphorylate the nucleoside. However, mouse L cells were suspectible to the cytotoxic effects of the nucleotide 2′,3′-dideoxyadenosine 5′-monophosphate (COHEN and PLUNKETT 1975). This observation was tentatively interpreted in terms of cellular uptake of the intact phosphorylated compound. Loss of cell viability was delayed in 2′,3′-dideoxyadenosine 5′-monophosphate-treated cultures, possibly reflecting slow cellular penetration by the nucleotide.

COHEN and PLUNKETT (1975) demonstrated that AraA 5′-monophosphate was more lethal to L cells than AraA itself. They proved, using ^{32}P,^{3}H dual-labelled nucleotide, that intracellular transport of the intact molecule occurred, although at a considerably slower rate than uptake of the nucleoside. The greater efficacy of AraA 5′-monophosphate than AraA was ascribed to the lack of deamination and hence inactivation of the nucleotide and its relatively low susceptibility to dephosphorylation. In contrast to AraA-treated cells where viability decreased rapidly, cultures exposed to AraA 5′-monophosphate exhibited a delayed but subsequently sustained reduction in cell viability due to the slow rate of cellular uptake of the phosphorylated drug.

In contrast to the above, no appreciable differences have been observed between 6-thioinosinate, 6-thioguanylate or 6-methylthioinosinate and their parent nucleosides in terms of activity against both thiopurine-sensitive and resistant cells (HO 1971; MONTGOMERY et al. 1963; MONTGOMERY 1974). The apparent equivalence of the thiopurine nucleosides and their nucleotides is due presumably to extensive extracellular dephosphorylation of the latter. For example, the growth inhibitory action of 6-thioinosinate against MP-sensitive cells undoubtedly involves extracellular dephosphorylation to yield 6-thioinosine, uptake of 6-thioinosine, cleavage of 6-thioinosine to MP by purine nucleoside phosphorylase and intracellular conversion of MP to 6-thioinosinate by HGPRT.

A number of different types of derivatives of the antipurine nucleotides have been synthesized in attempts to develop "prodrugs" of the normal phosphorylated drug metabolites which would bypass resistance mechanisms involving loss of nucleotide-forming enzymes. Such prodrugs are required to possess the following properties:

1. Insusceptibility to extracellular degradation, e.g. by phosphohydrolases
2. The ability to penetrate tumour cells
3. Susceptibility to intracellular cleavage with release of the normal antipurine nucleotides.

It is generally accepted that intracellular transport of intact nucleotides is hindered by the negative charges on the phosphate groups. Therefore, in order to enhance cell uptake, the design of most prodrugs has involved reduction in the total charge on the antipurine nucleotide molecules through further esterification (or derivatization) of the phosphates. The resulting phosphodiesters are not subject to dephosphorylation by phosphohydrolases, whilst cleavage by phosphodiesterases may liberate the free antipurine nucleoside phosphates. In addition, acylation of the nucleoside moieties with carboxylic acids increases the lipophilicity of the molecules and may enhance permeation of cell membranes. The types of compound investigated as potential prodrugs of antipurine nucleotides include:

1. Simple alkyl esters of nucleoside monophosphates
2. Complex esters of nucleoside monophosphates
3. Dinucleoside monophosphates
4. Dinucleoside pyrophosphates
5. Nucleoside 3′,5′-cyclic monophosphates
6. Acylated nucleoside 3′,5′-cyclic monophosphates
7. Acylated dinucleoside monophosphates and pyrophosphates.

A series of simple alkylesters of 6-thioinosinic acid were prepared in an effort to overcome resistance to MP involving lack of HGPRT (MONTGOMERY et al. 1961). It was envisaged that reduction in the phosphate charge might facilitate cell uptake of the derivatives and that cytotoxic concentrations of 6-thioinosinate would be generated intracellularly through cleavage of the compounds by phosphodiesterases. However, MONTGOMERY et al. (1963) reported that none of the ester derivatives had more than minimal ability to inhibit an HGPRT-deficient human epidermoid cell subline, HEp No. 2/MP, in culture. In discussing this result they cited the work of ANDERSON and HEPPEL (1960), who found that simple esters of nucleoside 5′-phosphates were not substrates for a partially purified leukaemia-cell phosphodiesterase, and suggested that the presence of a nucleoside group on each side of the phosphodiester bond was a requisite for cleavage by this enzyme.

The 5-iodo-3-indolyl phosphodiester of MMPR was shown to inhibit growth of an adenosine kinase-deficient line of HEp No. 2 cells (TSOU et al. 1975). However, interpretation of this result was complicated by the inferred cytotoxicity of the indoxyl portion of the molecule which would be released by phosphodiesterase action.

MONTGOMERY et al. (1963) synthesized the 6-thioinosinyl ester of 6-thioinosine, bis(thioinosine)-5′,5‴-phosphate, and demonstrated that it was active against the MP-resistant HEp No. 2/MP cell line. In contrast, both 6-thioinosine and 6-thioinosinate were ineffective against the resistant cells. The dinucleoside phosphate was shown to be a good substrate for phosphodiesterase present in cell-free extracts of HEp No. 2 cells and for the enzyme in snake venom. It was concluded that the intact derivative may have penetrated HEp No. 2/MP cells and undergone intracellular hydrolysis to generate cytotoxic concentrations of 6-thioinosinate. However, bis(thioinosine)-5′,5‴-monophosphate was not developed further, presumably because it did not exhibit similar activity against MP-resistant experimental tumours. The MP dinucleoside phosphate inhibited proliferation of HGPRT-deficient mouse leukaemia L1210 cells in culture, but at much higher concentrations than those reported for HEp No. 2/MP cell cultures (TIDD et al. 1982a). It was shown that phosphodiesterases present in the serum components of tissue culture media degraded the derivative and hence at least partially limited its efficacy against thiopurine-resistant cells. Other antimetabolite dinucleoside phosphates were found to be no more effective than the parent drugs against sensitive and resistant neoplasms (see review by KUSMIEREK and SHUGAR 1979).

The dinucleoside pyrophosphate derivative, P^1,P^2-bis(thioinosine-5′) pyrophosphate, which carries two ionizable phosphate hydroxyl groups, was active against an HGPRT-deficient human bone marrow cell subline in culture (TIDD et al. 1982b). However, the pyrophosphate was approximately equivalent to 6-thioinosine in its effects on thiopurine-resistant L1210 and V79 Chinese hamster lung cells (TIDD et al. 1981, 1982b).

3′,5′-Cyclic phosphate derivatives of antipurine nucleosides have been investigated as prodrugs of the nucleoside 5′-monophosphates in which the charge on the phosphate is reduced by internal esterification (KUSMIEREK and SHUGAR 1979). The cyclic nucleotides require intracellular conversion to 5′-monophosphates by cyclic nucleotide phosphodiesterases in order to exert cytotoxic effects in cells resistant to the antipurines through loss of nucleotide-forming enzymes. MEYER et al. (1979), THOMAS and MONTGOMERY (1968) and KOONTZ and WICKS (1977) have reported that 6-thioinosine 3′,5′-cyclic phosphate was not significantly different from MP in terms of its effects on MP-sensitive and HGPRT-deficient cells, presumably as a consequence of extracellular breakdown of the derivative. In contrast, LEPAGE and HERSH (1972) demonstrated inhibition of an MP-resistant tumour line by relatively high doses of the cyclic nucleotide.

MMPR 3′,5′-cyclic monophosphate was shown to inhibit the growth of tumour lines resistant to MMPR through loss of MMPR kinase activity (LEPAGE and HERSH 1972; EPPS et al. 1975). The derivative was converted to MMPR 5′-monophosphate by tumour-cell cyclic phosphodiesterase and inhibition of purine nucleotide biosynthesis de novo was demonstrated in MMPR resistant cells treated with high concentrations of the antipurine cyclic nucleotide (EPPS et al. 1975).

AraA 3′,5′-cyclic monophosphate inhibited DNA synthesis in intact cells and was rapidly converted to AraA 5′-monophosphate by cell homogenates (HUGHES and KIMBALL 1972). However, the activity of AraA cyclic nucleotide was not greater than that of AraA 5′-monophosphate (PLUNKETT and COHEN 1975; COHEN and PLUNKETT 1975).

MEYER et al. (1979) demonstrated that although 6-thioinosine 3′,5′-cyclic monophosphate was not significantly more effective than MP against HGPRT-deficient lymphoma cells, the addition of a removable lipophilic group by acylation of the molecule gave compounds which were more active than the parent drug. They synthesized and tested a series of MP cyclic nucleotide derivatives in which the sugar was acylated at the 2′-hydroxyl by carboxylic acids of various chain lengths. A progressive increase in cytotoxicity of the compounds was observed as the number of carbon atoms in the carboxylic acid was increased. The maximum effect against the MP-resistant cell line was recorded with 2′-*O*-palmityl-6-thioinosine cyclic 3′,5′-phosphate. In terms of the concentrations giving 50% inhibition of growth (EC_{50} values) this derivative was approximately six times more effective than 6-thioinosine. Esterification of the sugar hydroxyls of bis(thioinosine)-5′,5‴-monophosphate with butyric acid afforded a lipophilic compound that was considerably more resistant to degradation by serum enzymes than the unesterified derivative, whilst at the same time exhibiting enhanced activity against thiopurine-resistant L1210 cells (TIDD et al. 1982a). Similarly, whilst P^1,P^2-bis(thioinosine-5′) pyrophosphate was ineffective against

HGPRT-deficient L1210 cells in culture, the butyrated derivative, P^1,P^2-bis (2′,3′-*O*-dibutyrylthioinosine-5′) pyrophosphate, and the hexanoylated derivative, P^1,P^2-bis(2′,3′-*O*-dihexanoylthioinosine-5′)pyrophosphate, showed appreciable activity against these cells (TIDD et al. 1982 b). Dinucleoside pyrophosphates may have some advantage in overcoming resistance due to increased alkaline phosphohydrolase activities since P^1,P^2-bis(thioinosine-5′) pyrophosphate was cleaved initially to 6-thioinosine 5′-diphosphate, which is not susceptible to hydrolysis by these enzymes.

H. Conclusion

Most cytotoxic anticancer agents that have become widely used in clinical chemotherapy are drugs that affect DNA preferentially through one of three mechanisms, namely:

1. Inhibition of DNA replication
2. Incorporation into newly synthesized DNA chains
3. Binding to, or chemical reaction with, preformed DNA molecules.

Many drugs with other loci of action and of proven activity in experimental animal systems have been tested clinically but have failed to become accepted. In the case of the antipurines the two analogues that have been used routinely in treatment of human disease are MP and TG. Both are incorporated into DNA. In addition, the 5′-monophosphate of the DNA synthesis inhibitor, AraA, appears to have clinical potential. Although effective against certain experimental animal tumours, AzaG and MMPR have not proved to be of use in human cancer chemotherapy. As discussed above, AzaG is an antipurine which exerts its cytotoxic effect through incorporation into RNA, and MMPR is an inhibitor of purine nucleotide biosynthesis de novo, an action that may affect many cellular processes including both RNA and DNA synthesis.

Resistance to the antipurines is most commonly associated with effects at the level of their metabolism where either excessive catabolism or low rates of anabolism lead to sublethal cellular concentrations of the pharmacologically active species. Diminished sensitivity of drug targets or increased production of protecting metabolites have rarely been observed with these agents. It may be concluded from consideration of the nature of the actions of the antipurines as cycle-specific agents that improved forms of greater efficacy against slow-growing tumours are unlikely to be developed. However, the antipurines may induce substantial responses against rapidly proliferating neoplasms with short cell generation times, and on the basis of an understanding of biochemical mechanisms of resistance it will be possible to develop better drugs for the treatment of these diseases. It seems likely that in the future antipurines will be administered routinely as phosphorylated derivatives with improved pharmacokinetic properties and/or as prodrugs of the active nucleotide metabolites specifically designed to overcome cellular resistance to the conventional purine and purine nucleoside antimetabolites. Administration as nucleotide prodrugs may also permit the use of purine nucleoside analogues which would not normally be phosphorylated by cells.

References

Adamson RH, Zaharevitz DW, Johns DG (1977) Enhancement of the antileukemic activity of 9-β-D-xylofuranosyladenine (xylo-A) and other adenosine analogs by 2′-deoxycoformycin (2′-DCF) and by *erythro*-9-(2-hydroxy-3-nonyl) adenine (EHNA). Proc Am Assoc Cancer Res 18:147

Agarwal KC, Chu S-H, Ross AF, Gorske AF, Parks RE Jr (1971) Antitumor action of 6-selenoguanine and 6-selenoguanosine. Pharmacologist 13:210

Albertini RJ, De Mars R (1970) Diploid azaguanine-resistant mutants of cultured human fibroblasts. Science 169:482–485

Anderson D (1975) Attempts to produce systems for isolating spontaenous and induced variants in various lymphoma cells using a variety of selective agents. Mutat Res. 33:407–416

Anderson EP, Heppel LA (1960) Purification and properties of a leukemic cell phosphodiesterase. Biochim Biophys Acta 43:79–89

Avramis VI, Plunkett W (1982) Metabolism and therapeutic efficacy of 9-β-D-arabinofuranosyl-2-fluoroadenine against murine leukemia P388. Cancer Res 42:2587–2591

Baer H-P, Drummond GI, Duncan EL (1966) Formation and deamination of adenosine by cardiac muscle enzymes. Mol Pharmacol 2:67–76

Bakay B, Nyhan WL (1972) Electrophoretic properties of hypoxanthine-guanine phosphoribosyltransferase in erythrocytes of subjects with Lesch-Nyhan syndrome. Biochem Genet 6:139–146

Baudet AL, Roufa DA, Caskey CT (1973) Mutations affecting the structure of hypoxanthine-guanine phosphoribosyl transferase in cultured Chinese hamster cells. Proc Natl Acad Sci USA 70:320–324

Benke PJ, Herrick N, Hebert A (1973) Hypoxanthine-guanine phosphoribosyltransferase variant associated with accelerated purine synthesis. J Clin Invest 52:2234–2240

Bennett LL Jr, Brockman RW, Schnebli HP, Chumley S, Dixon GJ, Schabel FM Jr, Dulmadge EA, Skipper HE, Montgomery JA, Thomas HJ (1965) Activity and mechanism of action of 6-methylthiopurine ribonucleoside in cancer cells resistant to 6-mercaptopurine. Nature 205:1276–1279

Bennett LL Jr, Schnebli HP, Vail MH, Allan PW, Montgomery JA (1966a) Purine ribonucleoside kinase activity and resistance to some analogs of adenosine. Mol Pharmacol 2:432–443

Bennett LL Jr, Vail MH, Chumley S, Montgomery JA (1966b) Activity of adenosine analogs against a cell culture line resistant to 2-fluoroadenine. Biochem Pharmacol 15:1719–1728

Bennett LL Jr, Allan PW, Hill DL (1968) Metabolic studies with carbocyclic analogs of purine nucleosides. Mol Pharmacol 4:208–217

Bennett LL Jr, Allen PW, Smithers D, Vail MH (1969) Resistance to 4-aminopyrazolo (3,4-*d*) pyrimidine. Biochem Pharmacol 18:725–740

Bennett LL Jr, Vail MH, Allan PW, Laster WR Jr (1973) Studies with 8-azainosine, a cytotoxic nucleoside with antitumor activity. Cancer Res 33:465–471

Bennett LL Jr, Montgomery JA, Brockman RW Shealy YF (1978) Design of analogs of purine nucleosides with specifically altered activities as substrates for nucleoside metabolizing enzymes. In: Weber G (ed) Advances in enzyme regulation, vol 16. Pergamon, Oxford p 255

Bennett LL Jr, Rose LM, Allan PW, Smithers D, Adamson DJ, Elliot RD, Montgomery JA (1979) Metabolism and metabolic effects of 8-aza-6-thioinosine and its rearrangement product, *N*-β-D-ribofuranosyl-[1, 2, 3] thiadiazolo [5, 4,-d)-pyrimidin-7-amine. Mol Pharmacol 16:981–996

Berman JJ, Tong C, Williams GM (1980) Differences between rat liver epithelial cells and fibroblast cells in sensitivity to 8-azaguanine. In Vitro 16:661–668

Bieber AL, Sartorelli AC (1964) The metabolism of thioguanine in purine analogue-resistant cells. Cancer Res 24:1210–1215

Bloch A (ed) (1975) Chemistry, biology and clinical uses of nucleoside analogs. Ann NY Acad Sci 255

Bodey GP, Brodovsky HS, Issassi AA, Samuels ML, Freireich EJ (1968) Studies of combination 6-mercaptopurine (NSC-755) and 6-methylmercaptopurine riboside (NSC-40774) in patients with acute leukemia and metastatic cancer. Cancer Chemother Rep. 52:315–320

Brennand J, Chinault AC, Konecki DS, Melton DW, Caskey CT (1982) Cloned cDNA sequences of the hypoxanthine/guanine phosphoribosyltransferase gene from a mouse neuroblastoma cell line found to have amplified genomic sequences. Proc Natl Acad Sci USA 79:1950–1954

Brockman RW (1960) A mechanism of resistance to 6-mercaptopurine: metabolism of hypoxanthine and 6-mercaptopurine by sensitive and resistant neoplasms. Cancer Res 20:643–653

Brockman RW (1963) Mechanisms of resistance to anticancer agents. In: Haddow A, Weinhouse S (eds) Advances in cancer research, vol. 7 Academic, New York p 129

Brockman RW (1974) Mechanism of resistance. In: Sartorelli AC, Johns DG (eds) Antineoplastic and immunosuppressive agents. Springer, Berlin Heidelberg New York (Handbook of experimental pharmacology, vol 38/1, p 352)

Brockman RW, Chumley S (1965) Inhibition of formylglycinamide ribonucleotide synthesis in neoplastic cells by purines and analogs. Biochim Biophys Acta 95:365–379

Brockman RW, Sparks MC, Simpson MS (1957) A comparison of the metabolism of purines and purine analogs by susceptible and drug-resistant bacterial and neoplastic cells. Biochim Biophys Acta 26:671–672

Brockman RW, Sparks MC, Hutchison DJ, Skipper HE (1959a) A mechanism of resistance to 8-azaguanine I. Microbiological studies on the metabolism of purines and 8-azapurines. Cancer Res 19:177–188

Brockman RW, Bennett LL Jr, Simpson MS, Wilson AR, Thomson JR, Skipper HE (1959 b) A mechanism of resistance to 8-azaguanine. II. Studies with experimental neoplasms. Cancer Res. 19:856–869

Brockman RW, Kelley GG, Stutts P, Copeland V (1961) Biochemical aspects of resistance to 6-mercaptopurine in human epidermoid carcinoma cells in culture. Nature 191:469–471

Brockman RW, Schabel FM Jr, Montgomery JA (1977) Biologic activity of 9-β-D-arabinofuranosyl-2-fluoroadenine, a metabolically stable analog of 9-β-D-arabinofuranosyladenine. Biochem Pharmacol 26:2193–2196

Brockman RW, Cheng Y-C, Schabel FM Jr, Montgomery JA (1979) Metabolism and chemotherapeutic effects of 9-β-D-arabinofuranosyl-2-fluoroadenine (F-AraA) and evidence for its activation by deoxycytidine kinase. Proc Am Assoc Cancer Res 20:37

Brockman RW, Cheng Y-C, Schabel FM Jr, Montgomery JA (1980) Metabolism and chemotherapeutic activity of 9-β-D-arabinofuranosyl-2-fluoradenine against murine leukemia L1210 and evidence for its phosphorylation by deoxycytidine kinase. Cancer Res 40:3610–3615

Brox LW, Birkett L, Belch A (1981) Clinical pharmacology of oral thioguanine in acute myelogenous leukemia. Cancer Chemother Pharmacol 6:35–38

Burchenal JH, Dollinger MR (1967) Cytosine arabinoside (NSC-63878) in combination with 6-mercaptopurine (NSC-755), methotrexate (NSC-740), or 5-fluorouracil (NSC-19893) in L1210 mouse leukaemia. Cancer Chemother Rep 51:435–438

Caldwell IC, Henderson JF, Paterson ARP (1967) Resistance to purine ribonucleoside analogues in an ascites tumor. Can J Biochem 45:735–744

Carson DA, Kaye J, Seegmiller JE (1980) Metabolism and toxicity of 9-β-D-arabinofuranosyladenine in human malignant T cells and B cells in tissue culture. In: Rapado A, Watts RWE, De Bruyn CHMM (eds) Purine metabolism in man. III. Biochemical, immunological and cancer research. Plenum, New York p 299

Caskey CT, Kruh GD (1979) The HPRT locus. Cell 16:1–9

Cass CE (1979) 9-β-D-Arabinofuranosyladenine (AraA). In: Hahn FE (ed) Mechanism of action of antieukaryotic and antiviral compounds. Springer, Berlin Heidelberg New York (Antibiotics, vol 5–2, p 85)

Cass CE, Au-Yeung TH (1976) Enhancement of 9-β-D-arabinofuranosyl-adenine cytotoxicity to mouse leukemia L1210 *in vitro* by 2′-deoxycoformycin. Cancer Res. 36:1486–1491

Cass CE, Tan TH, Selner M (1979) Antiproliferative effects of 9-β-D-arabinofuranosyladenine 5′-monophosphate and related compounds in combination with adenosine inhibitors against mouse leukemia L1210/C2 cells in culture. Cancer Res. 39:1563–1569

Changas GS, Milman G (1977) Hypoxanthine phosphoribosyltransferase: two dimensional gels from normal and Lesch-Nyhan hemolyzates. Science 196:1119–1120

Chasin LA, Urlaub G (1976) Mutant alleles for hypoxanthine phosphoribosyltransferase: codominant expression, complementation, and segregation in hybrid Chinese hamster cells. Somatic Cell Genet 2:453–467

Coddington A (1965) Some substrates and inhibitors of adenosine deaminase. Biochim Biophys Acta 99:442–451

Coffey JJ, White CA, Lesk AB, Rogers WI, Serpick AA (1972) Effect of allopurinol on the pharmacokinetics of 6-mercaptopurine (NSC 755) in cancer patients. Cancer Res 32:1283–1289

Cohen SS, Plunkett W (1975) The utilization of nucleotides by animal cells. Ann NY Acad Sci 255: 269

Crabtree GW (1978) Mechanisms of action of pyrimidine and purine analogs. In: Brodsky I, Kahn SB, Conroy JF (eds) Cancer chemotherapy III. 46th Hahnemann symposium. Grune & Stratton, New York, p 35

Crabtree GW, Nelson JA, Parks RE Jr (1977) Failure of 6-thio GMP to inhibit guanylate kinase in intact cells. Biochem Pharmacol 26:1577–1584

Davidson JD (1960) Studies on the mechanism of action of 6-mercaptopurine in sensitive and resistant L1210 leukemia in vitro. Cancer Res 20:225–232

Davidson JD, Winter TS (1964) Purine nucleoside pyrophosphorylases in 6-mercaptopurine sensitive and -resistant human leukemias. Cancer Res 24:261–267

Davidson JD, Bradley TR, Roosa RA, Law LW (1962) Purine nucleotide pyrophosphorylases in 8-azaguanine-sensitive and -resistant leukemias. J Natl Cancer Inst 29:789–800

Divekar AY, Fleysher MH, Slocum HK, Kenny LN, Hakala MT (1972) Changes in sarcoma 180 cells associated with drug-induced resistance to adenosine analogs. Cancer Res 32:2530–2537

Dooley T, Maddocks JL (1982) Assay of an active metabolite of 6-thioguanine, 6-thioguanosine 5′-monophosphate, in human red blood cells. J Chromatogr 229:121–127

Elion GB (1967) Biochemistry and pharmacology of purine analogues. Fed Proc 26:898–908

Elion GB (1975) Interaction of anticancer drugs with enzymes. In: Pharmacological basis of cancer chemotherapy. Williams & Wilkins, Baltimore, p 547

Elion GB, Hitchings GH (1975) Azathioprine: In: Sartorelli AC, Johns DG (eds) Antineoplastic and immunosuppressive agents. Springer, Berlin Heidelberg New York (Handbook of experimental pharmacology, vol 38/2, p 404)

Elion GB, Callahan S, Bieber S, Hitchings GH, Rundles RW (1961) A summary of investigations with 6-[(1-methyl-4-nitro-5-imidazolyl) thio] purine (B.W. 57-322). Cancer Chemother Rep 14:93–98

Elion GB, Callahan S, Nathan H, Bieber S, Rundles RW, Hitchings GH (1963) Potentiation by inhibition of drug degradation: 6-substituted purines and xanthine oxidase. Biochem Pharmacol 12:85–93

Ellis DB, LePage GA (1963) Biochemical studies of resistance to 6-thioguanine. Cancer Res 23:436–443

Epps D, Chang I-M, Sherwood E, Kimball AP (1975) Feedback inhibition by 6-methylthioinosine 3′,5′-cyclic monophosphate in tumor cells resistant to the nucleoside. Proc Soc Exp Biol Med 150:578–580

Epstein J, Leyva A, Kelley WN, Littlefield JW (1977) Mutagen-induced diploid human lymphoblast variants containing altered hypoxanthine guanine phosphoribosyl transferase. Somatic Cell Genet 3:135–148

Fenwick RG Jr, Caskey CT (1975) Mutant Chinese hamster cells with a thermosensitive hypoxanthine-guanine phosphoribosyltransferase. Cell 5:115–122

Fenwick RG Jr, Wasmuth JJ, Caskey CT (1977a) Mutations affecting the antigenic properties of hypoxanthine-guanine phosphoribosyltransferase in cultured Chinese hamster cells. Somatic Cell Genet 3:207–216

Fenwick RG Jr, Sawyer TH, Kruh GD, Astrin KH, Caskey CT (1977b) Forward and reverse mutations affecting the kinetics and apparent molecular weight of mammalian HGPRT. Cell 12:383–391

Finnish Leukaemia Group (1979) The effect of thioguanine on a combination of daunorubicine, cytarabine and prednisone in the treatment of acute leukaemia in adults. Scand J Haematol 23:124–128

Fox M, Hodgkiss RJ (1981) Mechanism of cytotoxic action of azaguanine and thioguanine in wild-type V79 cell lines and their relative efficiency in selection of structural gene mutants. Mutat Res 80:165–185

Fox IH, Kelley WN (1971) Phosphoribosylpyrophosphate in man: biochemical significance. Ann Intern Med 74:424–433

Fox M, Radacic M (1978) Adaptational origin of some purine analogue resistant phenotypes in cultured mammalian cells. Mutat Res 49–275–296

Fox M, Radacic M (1982) Variations in chromosome numbers and their possible relationship to the development of 8-azaguanine resistance in V79 Chinese hamster cells. Cell Biol Int Rep 6:39–48

Fox M, Boyle JM, Fox BW (1976) Biological and biochemical characterisation of purine analogue resistant clones of V79 Chinese hamster cells. Mutat Res 35:289–310

Friedrich U, Coffino P (1977) Hypoxanthine-guanine phosphoribosyl transferase with altered substrate affinity in mutant mouse lymphoma cells. Biochim Biophys Acta 483:70–78

Gee TS, Yu KP, Clarkson BD (1969) Treatment of adult acute leukemia with arabinosylcytosine and thioguanine. Cancer 23:1019–1032

Gellhorn A (1953) Laboratory and clinical studies on 8-azaguanosine. Cancer 6:1030–1033

Gillin FD, Roufa DJ, Beaudet AL, Caskey CT (1972) 8-Azaguanine resistance in mammalian cells I. Hypoxanthine-guanine phosphoribosyltransferase. Genetics 72:239–252

Grindey GB (1979) Clinical pharmacology of the 6-thiopurines. Cancer Treat Rev [Suppl] 6:19–25

Grunberger D, Grunberger G (1979) 8-Azaguanine. In: Hahn FE (ed) Mechanism of action of antieukaryotic and antiviral compounds. Springer, Berlin Heidelberg New York (Antibiotics, vol 5/2, p 110)

Gupta RS, Siminovitch L (1978) Genetic and biochemical studies with the adenosine analogs toyocamycin and tubercidin: mutation at the adenosine kinase locus in Chinese hamster cells. Somatic Cell Genet 4:715–735

Hakala MT (1970) Properties of sarcoma 180 (S-180) cells resistant to kinetin riboside (KR). Fed Proc. 29:884

Hakala MT (1973) Enzyme changes in resistant tissues. In: Mihich E (ed) Drug resistance and selectivity. Biochemical and cellular basis. Academic, New York, p 263

Hakala MT (1974) Transport of antineoplastic agents. In: Sartorelli AC, Johns DG (eds) Antineoplastic and immunosuppressive agents. Springer, Berlin Heidelberg New York (Handbook of experimental pharmacology, Vol 38/1, p 240)

Harris BA, Plunkett W (1981) Biochemical basis for the cytotoxicity of 9-β-D-xylofuranosyladenine in Chinese hamster ovary cells. Cancer Res 41:1039–1044

Harris BA, Saunders PP, Plunkett W (1981) Metabolism of 9-β-D-xylofuranosyladenine by the Chinese hamster ovary cell. Mol Pharmacol 20:200–205

Harris JF, Whitmore GF (1974) Chinese hamster cells exhibiting a temperature-dependent alteration in purine transport: J Cell Physiol 83:43–52

Harris M (1971) Mutation rates in cells at different ploidy levels. J Cell Physiol 78:177–184

Henderson JF (1974) Biochemical aspects of selective toxicity. In: Sartorelli AC, Johns DG (eds) Antineoplastic and immunosuppressive agents. Springer, Berlin Heidelberg New York (Handbook of experimental pharmacology, vol 38/1, p 341)

Henderson JF (1977) Analogs of purines and purine nucleosides: biological and biochemical effects. In: Quagliariello E, Palmieri F, Singer TP (eds) Horizons in biochemistry and biophysics, vol 4. Addison-Wesley, Reading, p 130

Henderson JF, Brockman RW (1975) Biochemical mechanisms of drug resistance in cancer chemotherapy. In: Pharmacological basis of cancer chemotherapy. Williams & Wilkins, Baltimore, p 629
Henderson JF, Khoo MKY (1965) Synthesis of 5-phosphoribosyl 1-pyrophosphate from glucose in Ehrlich ascites tumor cells in vitro. J Biol Chem 240:2349–2357
Henderson JF, Caldwell IC, Paterson ARP (1967) Decreased feedback inhibition in a 6-(methylmercapto)purine ribonucleoside-resistant tumor. Cancer Res 27:1773–1778
Henderson JF, Brox LW, Fraser JH, Lomax CA, McCoy EE, Snyder FF, Zombor G (1975) Models and methods for biochemical studies of resistance in man: In: Pharmacological basis of cancer chemotherapy. Williams & Wilkins, Baltimore, p 663
Higuchi T (1974) Phosphorylation of 6-mercaptopurine in human leukemic cells. Acta Haematol Jpn 37:282–288
Higuchi T (1975) Phosphorylation of 6-mercaptopurine in human leukemic cells and phosphoribosylpyrophosphate. Acta Haematol Jpn 38:248–258
Higuchi T, Nakamura T, Wakisaka G (1976) Metabolism of 6-mercaptopurine in human leukemic cells. Cancer Res 36:3779–3783
Higuchi T, Nakamura T, Uchino H, Wakisaka G (1977) Comparative study of 6-mercaptopurine metabolism in human leukemic leukocytes and L1210 cells. Antimicrob Agents Chemother 12:518-522
Hill DL (1970) Hypoxanthine phosphoribosyltransferase and guanine metabolism of adenocarcinoma 755 cells. Biochem Pharmacol 19:545–557
Hirschberg E, Kream J, Gellhorn A (1952) Enzymatic deamination of 8-azaguanine in normal and neoplastic tissues. Cancer Res 12:524–528
Hitchings GH, Elion GB (1967) Mechanisms of action of purine and pyrimidine analogs. In: Brodsky I, Kahn SB, Moyer JH (eds) Cancer chemotherapy. Grune & Stratton, New York, p 26
Hitchings GH, Elion GB (1969) The role of antimetabolites in immunosuppression and transplantation. Acc Chem Res 2:202–209
Ho DHW (1971) Metabolism of 6-methylthiopurine ribonucleoside 5′-phosphate. Biochem Pharmacol 20:3538–3539
Ho DHW, Luce JK, Frei E (1968) Distribution of purine ribonucleoside kinase and selective toxicity of 6-methylthiopurine ribonucleoside. Biochem Pharmacol 17:1025–1035
Hodgkiss RJ, Fox M (1980) Characteristics of revertants induced by EMS and UV light from a 6-thioguanine resistant HGPRT deficient V79 Chinese hamster cell line. Carcinogenesis 1:189–198
Hodgkiss RJ, Brennand J, Fox M (1980) Reversion of 6-thioguanine resistant Chinese hamster cell lines: agent specificity and evidence for the repair of promutagenic lesions. Carcinogenesis 1:175–187
Hughes RG Jr, Kimball AP (1972) Metabolic effects of cyclic 9-β-Arabinofuranosyladenine 3′,5′-monophosphate in L1210 cells. Cancer Res 32:1791–1794
Hutchison DJ (1963) Cross-resistance and collateral sensitivity studies in cancer chemotherapy. In: Haddow A, Weinhouse S (eds) Advances in cancer research, vol 7. Academic, New York, p 235
Jackson RC, Ross DA, Harkrader RJ, Epstein J (1980) Biochemical approaches to enhancement of antitumor drug selectivity: selective protection of cells from 6-thioguanine and 6-mercaptopurine by adenosine. Cancer Treat Rep 64:1347–1353
Johns DG; Adamson RH (1976) Enhancement of the biological activity of cordycepin (3′-deoxyadenosine) by the adenosine deaminase inhibitor 2′-deoxycoformycin. Biochem Pharmacol 25:1441–1444
Johnson GG, Eisenberg LR, Migeon BR (1979) Human and mouse hypoxanthine-guanine phosphoribosyltransferase: dimers and tetramers. Science 203:174–176
Kadouri A, Kunce JJ, Lark KG (1978) Evidence for dominant mutations reducing HGPRT activity. Nature 274:256–259
Kessel D, Hall TC (1969) Retention of 6-mercaptopurine derivatives by intact cells as an index of drug response in human and murine leukemias. Cancer Res 29:2116–2119
Kim K, Blechman WJ, Riddle VGH, Pardee AB (1981) Basis of observed resistance of L1210 leukemia in mice to methotrexate, 6-thioguanine, 6-methylmercaptopurine

riboside, 6-mercaptopurine, 5-fluorouracil, and 1-β-D-arabinofuranosylcytosine administered in different combinations. Cancer Res 41:4529–4534

Kimball AP, LePage GA, Bowman B (1964) The metabolism of 9-arabinosyl-6-mercaptopurine in normal and neoplastic tissues. Can J Biochem 42:1753–1768

Kondo T, Maruyama T (1955) The influence of 8-azaguanine on tumors and its enhancement. Gan 42:503-506

Kong CM, Parks RE Jr (1974) Human erythrocytic hypoxanthine-guanine phosphoribosyltransferase: effect of pH on the enzymatic reaction. Mol Pharmacol 10:648–656

Koontz JW, Wicks WD (1977) Comparison of the effects of 6-thio- and 6-methylthiopurine ribonucleoside cyclic monophosphates with their corresponding nucleosides on the growth of rat hepatoma cells. Cancer Res 37:651–657

Koshiura R, LePage GA (1968) Some inhibitors of deamination of 9-β-D-arabinofuranosyladenine and 9-β-D-xylofuranosyladenine by blood and neoplasms of experimental animals and humans. Cancer Res 28:1014–1020

Krenitsky TA, Papaioannou R, Elion GB (1969) Human hypoxanthine phosphoribosyltransferase 1. Purification, properties and specificity. J Biol Chem 244:1263–1270

Kruh GD, Fenwick RG Jr., Caskey CT (1981) Structural analysis of mutant and revertant forms of Chinese hamster hypoxanthine-guanine phosphoribosyltransferase. J Biol Chem 256:2878-2886

Kusmierek JT, Shugar D (1979) Nucleotides, nucleoside phosphate diesters and phosphonates as antiviral and antineoplastic agents – an overview. In: Chandra P (ed) Antiviral mechanisms in the control of neoplasia. Plenum, New York (NATO) advanced study institutes, ser A, vol 20, p 481)

Lee SH, Sartorelli AC (1981 a) The effects of inhibitors of DNA biosynthesis on the cytotoxicity of 6-thioguanine. Cancer Biochem Biophys 5:189–194

Lee SH, Sartorelli AC (1981 b) Conversion of 6-thioguanine to the nucleoside level by purine nucleoside phosphorylase of sarcoma 180 and sarcoma 180/TG ascites cells. Cancer Res 41:1086–1090

Lee SH, Sartorelli AC (1981 c) Biochemical mechanism of resistance of cultured sarcoma 180 cells to 6-thioguanine. Biochem Pharmacol 30:3109–3114

Lee MH, Huang Y-M, Sartorelli AC (1978) Alkaline phosphatase activities of 6-thiopurine-sensitive and -resistant sublines of sarcoma 180. Cancer Res 38:2413–2418

Lee SH, Shansky CW, Sartorelli AC (1980) Evidence for the external location of alkaline phosphatase activity on the surface of sarcoma 180 cells resistant to 6-thioguanine. Biochem Pharmacol 29:1859–1861

Lee SH, Thomas LK, Unger FM, Christian R, Sartorelli AC (1981) Comparative antineoplastic activity against P388 leukemia of 9-β-D-arabinofuranosyladenine (araA) and 9-β-(2'-azido-2'-deoxy-D-arabinofuranosyl)adenine (arazide). Int J Cancer 27:703–708

LePage GA (1968) The metabolism of α-2'-deoxythioguanosine in murine tumor cells. Can J Biochem 46:655–661

LePage GA (1970) Alterations in enzyme activity in tumors and the implications for chemotherapy. In: Weber G (ed) Advances in enzyme regulation, vol. 8. Pergamon, Oxford, p 323

LePage GA (1975 a) Introduction to resistance to cancer chemotherapy section. In: Pharmacological basis of cancer chemotherapy. Williams & Wilkins, Baltimore, p 627

LePage GA (1975 b) Purine arabinosides, xylosides and lyxosides. In: Sartorelli AC, Johns DG (eds) Antineoplastic and immunosuppressive agents. Springer, Berlin Heidelberg New York (Handbook of experimental pharmacology, vol 38/2, p 426)

LePage GA (1977) Purine antagonists. In: Becker FF (ed) Chemotherapy. Plenum, New York (Cancer: a comprehensive treatise, vol 5, p 309)

LePage GA (1978 a) Resistance to 9-β-D-arabinofuranosyladenine in murine tumor cells. Cancer Res 38:2314–2316

LePage GA (1978 b) some model systems in cancer chemotherapy. In: Scholefield PG (ed) Proceedings of the 10th Canadian Cancer Conference. University of Toronto Press, Toronto, p 171

LePage GA, Gottlieb JA (1973) Deoxythioguanosine and thioguanine. Clin Pharmacol Ther 14:966–969

LePage GA, Hersh EM (1972) Cyclic nucleotide analogs as carcinostatic agents. Biochem Biophys Res Commun 46:1918–1922
LePage GA, Jones M (1961 a) Purinethiols as feedback inhibitors of purine synthesis in ascites tumor cells. Cancer Res 21:642–649
LePage GA, Jones M (1961 b) Further studies on the mechanism of action of 6-thioguanine. Cancer Res 21:1590–1594
LePage GA, Junga IG (1963) Use of nucleosides in resistance to 6-thioguanine. Cancer Res 23:739–743
LePage GA, Junga IG (1967) The utilization of α-2′-deoxythioguanosine by murine tumor cells. Mol Pharmacol 3:37–43
LePage GA, Khaliq A (1979) Responses of patients to arabinosyladenine-5′-phosphate correlated with an in vitro test. In: Weber G (ed) Advances in enzyme regulation, vol. 17. Pergamon, Oxford p 437
LePage GA, Naik S (1975) Biochemical pharmacology of a new thiopurine nucleoside derivative. Ann NY Acad Sci 255:481
LePage GA, White SC (1973) Scheduling of arabinosylcytosine and 6-thioguanine therapy. Cancer Res 33:946–949
LePage GA, Junga IG, Bowman B (1964) Biochemical and carcinostatic effects of 2′-deoxythioguanosine. Cancer Res 24:835–840
LePage GA, Lin YT, Orth RE; Gottlieb JA (1972) 5′-Nucleotides as potential formulations for administering nucleoside analogs in man. Cancer Res 32:2441–2444
LePage GA, Naik SR, Kattakar SB, Khaliq A (1975) 9-β-D-Arabinofuranosyladenine-5′-phosphate metabolism and excretion in humans. Cancer Res 35:3036–3040
LePage GA, Worth LS, Kimball AP (1976) Enhancement of the antitumor activity of arabinofuranosyladenine by 2′-deoxycoformycin. Cancer Res 36:1481–1485
Lesch M, Nyhan WL (1964) A familial disorder of uric acid metabolism and central nervous system function. Am J Med 36:561–574
Li CL, Lee MH, Sartorelli AC (1979) Synthesis and biological evaluation of tetramisole analogues as inhibitors of alkaline phosphatase of the 6-thiopurine-resistant tumor Sarcoma 180/TG. J Med Chem 22:1030–1033
Littlefield JW (1963) The inosinic acid pyrophosphorylase activity of mouse fibroblasts partially resistant to 8-azaguanine. Proc Natl Acad Sci USA 50:568–576
Lomax CA, Henderson JF (1972) Phosphorylation of adenosine and deoxyadenosine in Ehrlich ascites carcinoma cells resistant to 6-(methylmercapto)purine ribonucleoside. Can J Biochem 50:423–427
Mandel HG (1959) The physiological disposition of some anticancer agents. Pharmacol Rev 11:743–838
Marchesi SL, Sartorelli AC (1963) The biochemical basis for the differential sensitivity of intestinal mucosa and bone marrow to 6-thioguanine. Cancer Res 23:1769–1773
Martin WR, Crichton IK, Yang RC, Evans AE (1972) The metabolism of thioinosinic acid by 6-mercaptopurine sensitive and resistant leukemic leukocytes. Proc Soc Exp Biol Med 140:423–428
McDonald JA, Kelley WN (1971) Lesch-Nyhan syndrome: altered kinetic properties of mutant enzyme. Science 171:689–691
Meyer RB Jr, Stone TE, Ullman B (1979) 2′-*O*-Acyl-6-thioinosine cyclic 3′,5′-phosphates as prodrugs of thioinosinic acid. J Med Chem 22:811–815
Meyers MB, Shin S (1981) Specific resistance to 8-azaguanine in cells with normal hypoxanthine phosphoribosyltransferase (HPRT) activity: the role of guanine deaminase. Cytogenet Cell Genet 30:118-128
Meyers MB, Van Diggelen OP, Van Diggelen M, Shin S (1980) Isolation of somatic cell mutants with specified alterations in hypoxanthine phosphoribosyltransferase. Somatic Cell Genet 6:299–306
Montgomery JA (1974) Rational design of purine nucleoside analogs. In: Sartorelli AC, Johns DG (eds) Antineoplastic and immunosuppressive agents. Springer, Berlin Heidelberg New York (Handbook of experimental pharmacology, vol 38/1, p 76)
Montgomery JA, Thomas HJ, Schaeffer HJ (1961) Synthesis of potential anticancer agents. XXVIII. Simple esters of 6-mercaptopurine ribonucleotide. J Org Chem 25:1929–1933

Montgomery JA, Dixon GJ, Dulmage EA, Thomas HJ, Brockman RW, Skipper HE (1963) Inhibition of 6-mercaptopurine-resistant cancer cells in culture by bis-(thioinosine)-5′,5‴-phosphate. Nature 199:769–772

Moore EC, LePage GA (1958) The metabolism of 6-thioguanine in normal and neoplastic tissues. Cancer Res 18:1075–1083

Morrow J (1970) Genetic analysis of azaguanine resistance in an established mouse cell line. Genetics 65:279–287

Nakai Y, LePage GA (1972) Characterization of the kinase(s) involved in the phosphorylation of α- and β-2′deoxythioguanosine. Cancer Res 32:2445–2451

Nelson JA, Parks RE Jr (1972) Biochemical mechanism for the synergism between 6-thioguanine and 6-(methylmercapto)purine ribonucleoside in sarcoma 180 cells. Cancer Res 32:2034–2041

Nelson JA, Carpenter JW, Rose LM, Adamson DJ (1975 a) Mechanism of action of 6-thioguanine, 6-mercaptopurine, and 8-azaguanine. Cancer Res 35:2872–2878

Nelson JA, Kuhns JN, Carpenter JW (1975 b) Lack of activity of β-2′-deoxythioguanosine against two tumors resistant to 6-thioguanine. Cancer Res 35:1372–1374

Nichol CA (1975) Antibiotics resembling adenosine: tubercidin, toyocamycin, sangivamycin, formycin, psicofuranine and decoyinine. In: Sartorelli AC, Johns DG (eds) Antineoplastic and immunosuppressive agents. Springer, Berlin Heidelberg New York (Handbook of experimental pharmacology, vol 38/2, p 434)

Omura GA (1975) Phase II trial of beta-deoxythioguanosine (β-TGdR, NSC 71261) in refractory adult acute leukemia. Proc Am Assoc Cancer Res 16:140

Parks RE Jr, Agarwal KC (1975) 8-Azaguanine. In: Sartorelli AC, Johns DG (eds) Antineoplastic and immunosuppressive agents. Springer, Berlin Heidelberg New York (Handbook of experimental pharmacology, vol 38/2, p 458)

Parks RE Jr, Crabtree GW, Kong CM, Agarwal RP, Agarwal KC, Scholar EM (1975) Incorporation of analog purine nucleosides into the formed elements of human blood: erythrocytes, platelets and lymphocytes. Ann NY Acad Sci 255:412

Paterson ARP (1959) The formation of 6-mercaptopurine riboside phosphate in acites tumor cells. Can J Biochem Physiol 37:1011–1023

Paterson ARP (1960) The development of resistance to 6-mercaptopurine in a subline of the Ehrlich ascites carcinoma. Can J Biochem Physiol 38:1117–1127

Paterson ARP (1962) Resistance to 6-mercaptopurine. II. The synthesis of thioinosinate in a 6-mercaptopurine-resistant subline of the Ehrlich ascites carcinoma. Can J Biochem Physiol 40:195–206

Paterson ARP, Hori A (1962) Resistance to 6-mercaptopurine. I. Biochemical differences between the Ehrlich ascites carcinoma and a 6-mercaptopurine-resistant subline. Can J Biochem Physiol 40:181–194

Paterson ARP, Moriwaki A (1969) Combination chemotherapy: synergistic inhibition of lymphoma L5178Y cells in culture and in vivo with 6-mercaptopurine and 6-(methylmercapto)purine ribonucleoside Cancer Res 29:681–686

Paterson ARP, Sutherland A (1964) Metabolism of 6-mercaptopurine ribonucleoside by Ehrlich ascites carcinoma cells. Can J. Biochem 42:1415–1423

Paterson ARP, Tidd DM (1975) 6-Thiopurines. In: Sartorelli AC, Johns DG (eds) Antineoplastic and immunosuppressive agents. Springer, Berlin Heidelberg New York (Handbook of experimental pharmacology, vol 38/2, p 384)

Paterson ARP, Wang MC (1970) Mechanism of the growth inhibition potentiation arising from combination of 6-mercaptopurine with 6-(methylmercapto)purine ribonucleoside. Cancer Res 30:2379–2386

Peery A, LePage GA (1969) Nucleotide formation from α- and β-2′-deoxythioguanosine in extracts of murine and human tissues. Cancer Res 29:617–623

Pierre KJ, LePage GA (1968) Formation of inosine-5′-monophosphate by a kinase in cell-free extracts of Ehrlich ascites cells in vitro. Proc Soc Exp Biol Med 127:432–440

Pierre KJ, Kimball AP, LePage GA (1967) The effect of structure on nucleoside kinase activity. Can J Biochem 45:1619–1632

Plunkett W, Cohen SS (1975) Two approaches that increase the activity of analogs of adenine nucleosides in animal cells. Cancer Res 35:1547–1554

Plunkett W, Cohen SS (1977) Penetration of mouse fibroblasts by 2′-deoxyadenosine 5′-phosphate and incorporation of the nucleotide into DNA. J Cell Physiol 91:261–270
Plunkett W, Alexander L, Chubb S, Loo TL (1979) Biochemical basis of the increased activity of 9-β-D-arabinofuranosyladenine in the presence of inhibitors of adenosine deaminase. Cancer Res 39:3655–3660
Plunkett W, Chubb S, Alexander L, Montgomery JA (1980) Comparison of the toxicity and metabolism of 9-β-D-arabinofuranosyl-2-fluoroadenine and 9-β-D-arabinofuranosyladenine in human lymphoblastoid cells. Cancer Res 40:2349–2355
Plunkett W, Benjamin R, Feun L, Keating M, Freireich EJ (1981) Cellular concentrations of dATP and araATP in peripheral blood leukemic cells and erythrocytes from patients treated with deoxycoformycin and arabinosyladenine. Proc Am Assoc Cancer Res 22:177
Rivest RS, Irwin D, Mandel HG (1982) Purine analogs revisited: interference in protein formation. Adv Enzyme Regul 20:351–373
Rose LM, Brockman RW (1977) Analysis by high pressure liquid chromatography of 9-β-D-arabinofuranosyladenine 5′-triphosphate (AraATP) levels in murine leukaemia cells. J Chromatogr 133:335–343
Rosman M, Williams HE (1973) Leukocyte purine phosphoribosyltransferases in human leukemias sensitive and resistant to 6-thiopurines. Cancer Res 33:1202–1209
Rosman M, Lee MH, Creasey WA, Sartorelli AC (1974) Mechanisms of resistance to 6-thiopurines in human leukemia. Cancer Res 34:1952–1956
Ross AF, Agarwal KC, Chu S-H, Parks RE Jr (1973) Studies on the biochemical actions of 6-selenoguanine and 6-selenoguanosine. Biochem Pharmacol 22:141–154
Roy-Burman P (1970) Analogues of nucleic acid components. Springer, Berlin Heidelberg New York (Recent results in cancer research, vol 25)
Rubin CS, Dancis J, Yip LC, Nowinski RC, Balis ME (1971) Purification of IMP: pyrophosphate phosphoribosyltransferases, catalytically incompetent enzymes in Lesch-Nyhan disease. Proc Natl Acad Sci USA 68:1461–1464
Sartorelli AC, LePage GA (1957) Modification of thioguanine toxicity in tumor-bearing mice with bone marrow transplants. Proc Am Assoc Cancer Res 2:246
Sartorelli AC, LePage GA, Moore EC (1958) Metabolic effects of 6-thioguanine. I. Studies on thioguanine-resistant and -sensitive Ehrlich ascites cells. Cancer Res 18:1232–1239
Sartorelli AC, Lee MH, Rosman M, Agrawal KC (1975) Mechanisms of resistance to 6-thiopurines by neoplastic cells. In: Pharmacological basis of cancer chemotherapy. Williams & Wilkins, Baltimore, P 643
Scannell JP, Hitchings GH (1966) Thioguanine in deoxyribonucleic acid from tumors of 6-mercaptopurine-treated mice. Proc Soc Exp Biol Med 122:627–629
Schabel FM Jr (1975) Synergism and antagonism among antitumor agents. In: Pharmacological basis of cancer chemotherapy. Williams & Wilkins, Baltimore, p 595
Schabel FM Jr, Trader MW, Laster WR Jr (1976) Increased therapeutic activity of 9-β-D-arabinofuranosyladenine against leukemia P388 and L1210 by an adenosine deaminase inhibitor. Proc Am Assoc Cancer Res 17:46
Schacter B, Law LW (1957) Azaguanine-deaminase activity of several lymphocytic leukemias of mice. J Natl Cancer Inst 18:77–81
Schmid FA, Hutchison DJ, Otter GM, Stock CC (1976) Development of resistance to combinations of six antimetabolites in mice with L1210 leukemia. Cancer Treat Rep 60:23–27
Schmidt LH, Montgomery JA, Laster WR Jr, Schabel FM Jr (1970) Combination therapy with arabinosylcytosine and thioguanine. Proc Am Assoc Cancer Res 11:70
Schnebli HP, Hill DL, Bennett LL Jr (1967) Purification and properties of adenosine kinase from human tumor cells of type H.Ep.No.2. J Biol Chem 242:1997–2004
Scholar EM, Calabresi P (1973) Identification of the enzymatic pathways of nucleotide metabolism in human lymphocytes and leukemia cells. Cancer Res 33:94–103
Scholar EM, Calabresi P (1979) Increased activity of alkaline phosphatase in leukemic cells from patients resistant to thiopurines. Biochem Pharmacol 28:445–446
Scholar EM, Brown PR, Parks RE Jr (1972) Synergistic effect of 6-mercaptopurine and 6-methylmercaptopurine ribonucleoside on the levels of adenine nucleotides of sarcoma 180 cells. Cancer Res 32:259–269

Scott JL (1962) Human leukocyte metabolism in vitro. I. Incorporation of adenine-8-C^{14} and formate-C^{14} into the nucleic acids of leukemic leukocytes. J Clin Invest 41:67–79

Scott JL, Marino JV, Gabor EP (1966) Human leukocyte metabolism in vitro. II. The effect of 6-mercaptopurine on formate-C^{14} incorporation into the nucleic acids of acute leukemic leukocytes. Blood 28:683–691

Seegmiller JE, Rosenbloom FM, Kelley WN (1967) Enzyme defect associated with a sex-linked human neurological disorder and excessive purine synthesis. Science 155:1682–1684

Sekiguchi T, Sekiguchi F, Tomii S (1974) Complementation in hybrid cells derived from mutagen-induced mouse clones deficient in hypoxanthine-guanine phosphoribosyltransferase activity. Exp Cell Res 88:410–414

Sekiguchi T, Sekiguchi F, Tomii S (1975) Genetic complementation in hybrid cells derived from mutagen-induced mouse clones deficient in HGPRT activity. Exp Cell Res 93:207–218

Sharp JD, Capecchi NE, Capecchi MR (1973) Altered enzymes in drug-resistant variants of mammalian tissue culture cells. Proc Natl Acad Sci USA 70:3145–3149

Shigiura HT, Boxer GE, Sampson SD, Meloni ML (1965) Metabolism of 2-fluoroadenosine by Ehrlich ascites cells. Arch Biochem Biophys 111:713–719

Shin S-I (1974) Nature of mutations conferring resistance to 8-azaguanine in mouse cell lines. J Cell Sci 14:235–251

Skaper SD, Spector EB, Seegmiller JE (1977) Reversion in expression of hypoxanthine-guanine phosphoribosyltransferase in 6-thioguanine resistant neuroblastoma: evidence for reduced enzyme levels associated with unaltered catalytic activity. J Cell Physiol 92:275–284

Skipper HE (1975) Closing remarks. In: Pharmacological basis of cancer chemotherapy. Williams & Wilkins, Baltimore, p 713

Skipper HE, Montgomery JA, Thomson JR, Schabel FM Jr (1959) Structure-activity relationships and cross-resistance observed on evaluation of a series of purine analogs against experimental neoplasms. Cancer Res 19:425–437

Smellie RMS, Thomson RY, Davidson JN (1958) The nucleic acid metabolism of animal cells in vitro. I. The incorporation of ^{14}C-formate. Biochim Biophys Acta 29:59–74

Smith JL, Omura GA, Krakoff IH, Balis ME (1971) IMP: and AMP: pyrophosphate phosphoribosyltransferase in leukemic and normal human leukocytes. Proc Soc Exp Biol Med 136:1299–1303

Stutts P, Brockman RW (1963) A biochemical basis for resistance of L1210 mouse leukemia to 6-thioguanine. Biochem Pharmacol 12:97–104

Suttle DP, Harkrader RJ, Jackson RC (1981) Pyrazofurin-resistant hepatoma cells deficient in adenosine kinase. Eur J Cancer 17:43–51

Tamaoki T, LePage GA (1975) Inhibition of DNA chain growth by α-2′-deoxythioguanosine. Cancer Res 35:1103–1105

Terzi M (1974) Chromosomal variation and the origin of drug-resistant mutants in mammalian cell lines. Proc Natl Acad Sci USA 71:5027–5031

Thomas HJ, Montgomery JA (1968) Deriatives and analogs of 6-mercaptopurine ribonucleotide. J Med Chem 11:44–48

Thompson LF, Willis RC, Stoop JW, Seegmiller JE (1978) Purine metabolism in cultured human fibroblasts derived from patients deficient in hypoxanthine phosphoribosyltransferase, purine nucleoside phosphorylase, or adenosine deaminase. Proc Natl Acad Sci USA 75:3722–3726

Tidd DM, Dedhar S (1978) Specific and sensitive combined high-performance liquid chromatographic-flow fluorometric assay for intracellular 6-thioguanine nucleotide metabolites of 6-mercaptopurine and 6-thioguanine. J Chromatogr 145:237–246

Tidd DM, Paterson ARP (1974 a) Distinction between inhibition of purine nucleotide synthesis and the delayed cytotoxic reaction of 6-mercaptopurine. Cancer Res 34:733–737

Tidd DM, Paterson ARP (1974 b) A biochemical mechanism for the delayed cytotoxic reaction of 6-mercaptopurine. Cancer Res 34:738–746

Tidd DM, Gibson I, Dean PDG (1981) Acylated dinucleoside phosphate derivatives as agents to overcome resistance to purine antimetabolites. Br J Cancer 43:733
Tidd DM, Johnston HP, Gibson I (1982a) Effects of bis(6-mercaptopurine-9-β-D-ribofuranoside)-5′, 5‴-phosphate and its butyryl derivative on mouse leukaemia L1210 and a 6-mercaptopurine-resistant subline in culture. Biochem Pharmacol 31:2903–2912
Tidd DM, Gibson I, Dean PDG (1982b) Partial circumvention of resistance to 6-mercaptopurine by acylated P^1, P^2-bis(6-mercaptopurine-9-β-D-ribofuranoside-5′) pyrophosphate derivatives. Cancer Res 42:3769–3775
Tsou KC, Ledis S, Bennett LL (1975) Synthesis of 5-iodo-3-indolyl phosphodiester of 6-methylthiopurine ribonucleoside (MeMPR) and its activity in an MeMPR-resistant tissue culture line. In: Pharmacological basis of cancer chemotherapy. Williams & Wilkins, Baltimore, p 239
Van Diggelen OP, Donahue TF, Shin S-I (1979) Basis for differential cellular sensitivity to 8-azaguanine and 6-thioguanine. J Cell Physiol 98:59–72
Van Zeeland AA, De Ruijter YCEM, Simons JWIM (1974) The role of 8-azaguanine in the selection from human diploid cells of mutants deficient in hypoxanthine-guanine-phosphoribosyl-transferase (HGPRT). Mutat Res 23:55–68
Wagar MA, Taber RL, Huberman JA (1979) Studies on the penetration of mammalian cells by deoxyribonucleoside-5′-phosphates. J Cell Physiol 101:251–259
Wolpert MK, Damle SP, Brown JE, Sznycer E, Agarwal KC, Sartorelli AC (1971) The role of phosphohydrolases in the mechanism of resistance of neoplastic cells to 6-thiopurines. Cancer Res 31:1620–1626
Wotring LL, Roti Roti JL (1980) Thioguanine-induced S and G_2 blocks and their significance to the mechanism of cytotoxicity. Cancer Res 40:1458–1462

CHAPTER 18

Ribofuranose-containing Analogues of Uridine and Cytidine

A. D. WELCH and N. K. AHMED

A. Introduction

The development of a stable state of insensitivity of mammalian neoplastic cells to cytotoxic analogues of pyrimidine-containing nucleosides results primarily from the selection by the compounds of spontaneously occurring enzyme-deficient mutant cells. These become the progenitors of new populations, the proliferation of which is but little affected by the otherwise cytotoxic agents. Occasionally, however, cells that are less sensitive to drugs may emerge as the result of metabolic alterations that are of epigenetic origin. With certain exceptions, analogues of pyrimidines or their nucleosides are anabolized, using the same pathways as those followed by the naturally occurring compounds they resemble, i.e., uracil (Ura), uridine (Urd), or cytidine (Cyd), with the utilization of which they may compete. In addition, after conversion to nucleotide forms, analogous to either uridine 5′-monophosphate (UMP) or cytidine 5′-monophosphate (CMP), these anabolites may interfere with either the biosynthesis or the metabolic functions of complexes containing either UMP or CMP, such as either the corresponding di- or triphosphates or complexes containing diphosphate linkages. Some of the analogues may interfere with the formation of either RNA or even DNA, into which some analogues may be incorporated to the potential detriment of the function of the macromolecules.

In this chapter, several analogues of Urd and Cyd (other than 5-fluorouridine, FUrd) will be reviewed, concerning which specific knowledge of drug resistance in neoplastic cells has been developed, together with the fundamental principles of their mechanisms of action and their main biological effects. Most of these compounds have been employed not only in cell culture and in the chemotherapy of experimental neoplasms, but also as antineoplastic agents in clinical cancer chemotherapy. Among other reviews that have some bearing on this subject are those of WELCH (1945, 1959), ŠKODA (1963, 1975), BROCKMAN (1963, 1974), ROY-BURMAN (1970), VESELÝ and ČIHÁK (1973), ČIHÁK and RADA (1976), RADA and DOSKOČIL (1980), and JONES (1980).

B. 6-Azauridine

6-Azauridine (6-azaUrd) is generally prepared from synthetic 6-azauracil (6-azaUra), i.e., 3,5-dioxo-2,3,4,5-tetrahydro-1,2,4-triazine (SEIBERT 1947; BARLOW and WELCH 1956; FALCO et al. 1956), by incubation of the pyrimidine analogue with cultures of strains of *Escherichia coli* (ŠKODA et al. 1957 a, b), although it also has been prepared synthetically, as well as with the aid of *Streptococcus faecalis* (HANDSCHUMACHER 1957, 1960). The molecule termed 6-azaUrd (Fig. 1) contains β-D-ribofuranose in the *anti*conformation, as is the case with uridine. A weak acid (pK_a ~6.7), 6-azaUrd is transported into mammalian cells, at least in part by a facilitated process that can be inhibited by *p*-nitrobenzyl-6-thioinosine (PATERSON et al. 1979); this process utilizes the uncharged 6-azaUrd molecule (BELT and WELCH 1983). 6-AzaUrd is anabolized in such cells (HANDSCHUMACHER and PASTERNAK 1958; PASTERNAK and HANDSCHUMACHER 1959; HABERMAN and ŠORM 1958), as well as by certain microorganisms (ŠKODA and ŠORM 1959), to the corresponding 5'-monophosphate (6-azaUMP), but appreciable amounts of either 5'-di- or 5'-triphosphate esters ordinarily cannot be formed by mammalian cells (HANDSCHUMACHER 1957, 1958, 1960). Certain bacterial species convert 6-azaUrd to 6-azaUra, but this does not appear to occur in mammalian cells; indeed, the parenteral administration of 6-azaUrd leads to a rapid and nearly quantitative urinary excretion of 6-azaUrd per se, e.g., ~75% within 4 h and ~95% within 8 h (WELCH et al. 1960; HANDSCHUMACHER et al. 1962a), although a very small amount of opening of the aglycone ring may occur.

The blood level of 6-azaUrd, after its appropriate intravenous administration to man, falls from a peak of over 0.6 m*M* to less than 0.2 m*M* within 1 h and to a barely measurable level within 4 h (HANDSCHUMACHER et al. 1962b). The phosphorylation of 6-azaUrd by high-energy phosphate, e.g., ATP (or dATP), is catalyzed by Urd-Cyd kinase (HANDSCHUMACHER 1960; SKÖLD 1960), and Urd competes with 6-azaUrd. The product, 6-azaUMP, is a competitive inhibitor of orotidine 5'-phosphate (OMP) decarboxylase; thus, it interferes with the last (a rate-limiting) step in the biosynthesis of pyrimidines de novo (HANDSCHUMACHER and PASTERNAK 1958; HABERMAN and ŠORM 1958, HANDSCHUMACHER 1960). Were it not for the very rapid dephosphorylation of OMP to the ribonucleoside (orotidine), 6-azaUMP would cause the intracellular accumulation of OMP; in addition, the actual precursor of OMP, i.e., orotic acid (OA; 6-carboxyuracil), also accumulates. OMP is formed by the reaction of OA with 5-phosphoribosyl-1-pyrophosphate (PRPP), catalyzed by OA phosphoribosyltransferase, which, in mammalian cells, appears to be closely associated with OMP decarboxylase, apparently within a single protein molecule (TRAUT and JONES 1977; JONES 1980). When 6-azaUrd is administered, OA is found in experimental tumors of mice (PASTERNAK and HANDSCHUMACHER 1959). Interference with the intracellular utilization of OA, a stronger acid than 6-azaUrd, leads to its entrance into tissue fluids and blood, from which it is very poorly transported into most mammalian cells and tissues, with the exception of the liver and kidneys [in the latter, as with 6-azaUrd, both glomerular filtration and tubular excretion occur (VOLLE et al. 1962)]. The liver excretes OA rapidly into the bile (HANDSCHUMACHER and COLERIDGE 1979), but this probably does not occur with 6-azaUrd, because intestinal microorganisms then would cleave 6-azaUra from it, the absorption of which would lead to toxic effects within the central nervous system (WELCH et al. 1960; CALABRESI et al. 1975). In general, mammalian cells do not appear to cleave either orotidine to OA (an apparent exception will be noted below) or 6-azaUrd to 6-azaUra; a small proportion of the aglycone-moiety of 6-azaUrd may be further degraded in some instances in mammalian systems, as well as by certain microor-

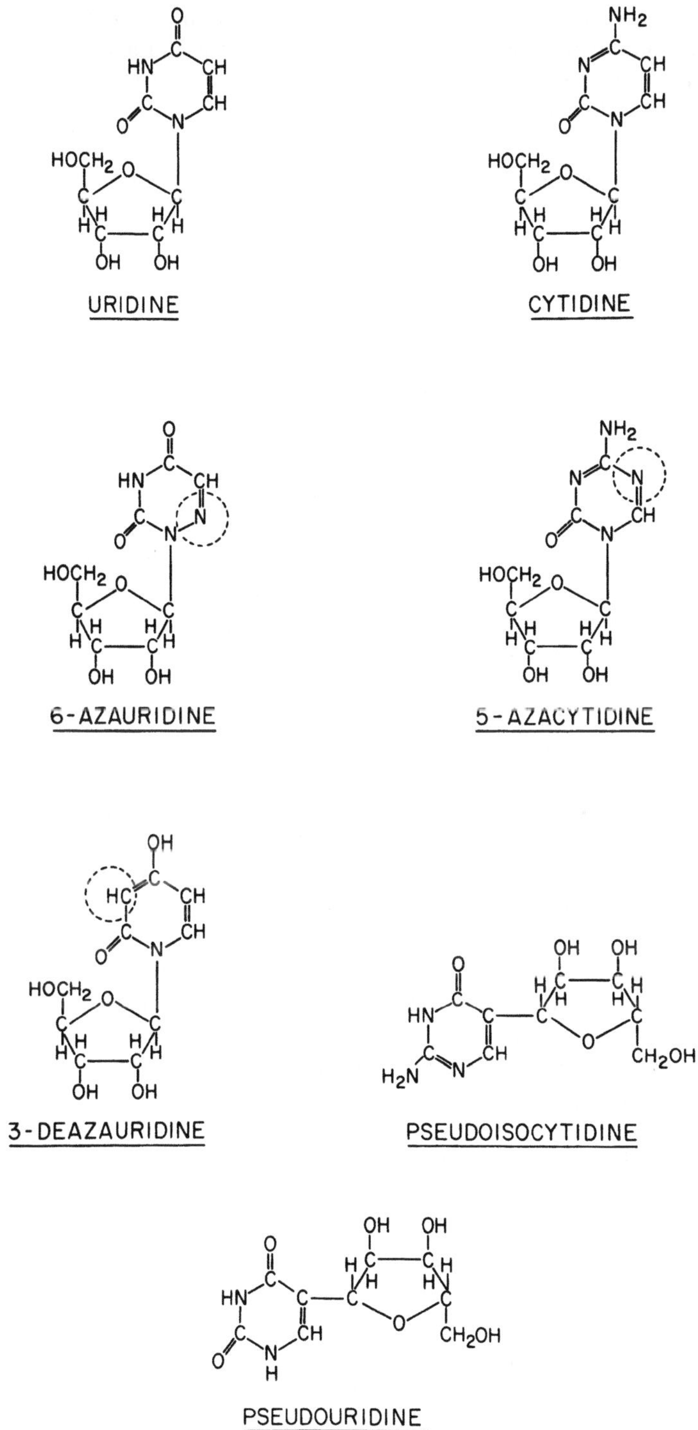

Fig. 1. Structural formulas of uridine, cytidine, and some of their analogues

ganisms (WELCH et al. 1960; WIESENFELD and CROKAERT 1969; LÍSMANE et al. 1977). In human urine, 6-azaUra rarely appears unless contact of 6-azaUrd with intestinal microorganisms has occurred (HANDSCHUMACHER et al. 1962b; CALABRESI et al. 1975). 5′-Polyphosphates of 6-azaUrd can be formed by *Trypanosoma equiperdum* (RUBIN et al. 1962). A claim (WELLS et al. 1963) that 6-azaUrd can enter the RNA of brain, when the drug has been injected into that tissue, has not yet been confirmed; furthermore, it has been shown (LISÝ et al. 1968; ŠKODA 1975) that synthetic codons containing 6-azaUMP in place of UMP are not functional. 6-AzaUrd (unlike 6-azaUra) is not significantly transported across the "blood-brain barrier" (CALABRESI et al. 1975); hence, circulating 6-azaUrd is not proffered to the brain cells, even if it were possible for the analogue to enter RNA.

A cell-line resistant to 6-azaUrd was selected by PASTERNAK et al. (1961) from murine lymphoblastic cells, L5178Y (L5178Y/6-azaUrd), grown in culture; with this cell-line, both 6-azaUrd and Urd were converted to their 5′-monophosphates at a very limited rate. The biochemical lesion in these resistant cells was related to an observed deficiency in the activity of Urd-Cyd kinase, while alterations in permeability were ruled out.

Inhibition of the proliferation of L5178Y/6-azaUrd cells in culture required a concentration of the analogue that was ~1,500-fold greater than that needed for the parent line, while the formation of nucleotides from Urd by the parental strain of cells was only 30-fold higher than that of resistant cells (PASTERNAK et al. 1961). The contribution of phosphorolytic cleavage of Urd and FUrd has been suggested by some studies, e.g., with a human cell-line resistant to 6-azaUrd (see below); however, recent studies with L5178Y/6-azaUrd cells by ULLMAN et al. (1979) have indicated that both Urd phosphorylase and Urd-Cyd kinase activities are deficient. Of interest also is the report of the selection of 6-azaUrd-resistant Ehrlich ascites cells in vivo that apparently did not exhibit changes in the activities of either Urd-Cyd kinase or Urd phosphorylase (BLAIR and HALL 1969); subsequent studies of mutants that overproduce the enzyme activities involved with the utilization of OA and OMP may bear on these observations. A cell line (A9), resistant to 6-azaUrd, was selected from a mouse cell line deficient in hypoxanthine-guanine phosphoribosyltransferase and adenine phosphoribosyltransferase activities; these cells were also resistant to otherwise cytotoxic levels of adenosine (HASHMI et al. 1975). The resistant cells were sensitive to FUrd, however, which suggests that part of the salvage pathway for pyrimidine biosynthesis might be intact. Conceivably, however, the sensitivity of these cells to FUrd could involve the cleavage of the latter to 5-fluorouracil (FUra), which, in turn, is converted by pyrimidine phosphoribosyltransferase, in the presence of PRPP, to 5-fluorouridine 5′-monophosphate (FUMP), from which can be formed the corresponding 2′-deoxyribonucleotide (FdUMP), an inhibitor of thymidylate synthetase activity.

In any case, L5178Y/6-azaUrd cells (in mice, cell cultures, cell suspensions, and extracts thereof) exhibited defective formation of 6-azaUMP from 6-azaUrd and of UMP from Urd (PASTERNAK et al. 1961).

A clone, AU-200-1, derived from a mouse lymphoma of T-cell origin (S49), was isolated by virtue of its resistance to 6-azaUrd (ULLMAN et al. 1979). Extracts of these cells lacked over 90% of the capacity of extracts of wild-type cells to phosphorylate either Urd or Cyd. This cell line, deficient in Urd-Cyd kinase activity, was also resistant to FUrd; hence, in this mutant line, FUMP apparently was not formed, presumably because FUra was not formed from FUrd by Urd phosphorylase. If mutational alterations had also involved a severe deficiency of orotate phosphoribosyltransferase activity, the enzyme that appears to react with FUra, the apparently compensatory increase in the biosynthesis de novo of UMP, which entailed a six-fold increase in the activity of OMP decarboxylase, as compared with that of the wild-type cells, presumably could not have occurred (see below).

Brief mention should be made of 6-azacytidine, studied by HANDSCHUMACHER et al. (1963). Although deaminated (about one-third) in mice to 6-azaUrd, it is also converted to the 5′-monophosphate (6-azaCMP); the latter is about one-tenth as active as 6-azaUMP as an inhibitor of OMP decarboxylase activity.

I. Another Mechanism for Resistance to 6-Azauridine

A mechanism for the development of cells with a relatively low level of resistance to certain pyrimidine nucleosides (particularly pertinent to 6-azaUrd) should now be described. The biochemical basis of this phenomenon has been reviewed recently by JONES (1980), who, together with her associates, has been especially involved in obtaining the now convincing evidence that, in the *six* steps of the enzymically catalyzed pathways to UMP de novo in those mammalian cells studied, only *three* enzyme proteins appear to be involved directly. The first of these proteins behaves as a single cytosolic protein possessing *three* enzymatic activities: (a) carbamoylphosphate synthetase, (b) L-aspartate transcarbamoylase, and (c) dihydroorotase. From the cytosol, the third product of this sequence, i.e., 5,6-dihydroorotate, passes to the outer surface of the inner membrane of the mitochondrion, where it is converted by dihydrorotate dehydrogenase to OA. The two final steps in the formation of UMP appear to be accomplished by a single cytosolic protein, with *two* enzymic capabilities: (a) orotate phosphoribosyltransferase (OA PRTase), which, together with PRPP, leads to the conversion of OA into its ribonucleotide (OMP), and (b) OMP decarboxylase, which specifically catalyzes the decarboxylation of OMP to form UMP; thus, OMP from (a) appears to be "channeled" directly to (b). The apparent K_m of OMP for the decarboxylase (depending on the source of the enzyme) is $\sim 3 \times 10^{-7} M$, while the relative velocity of the decarboxylation is about twice that of the phosphoribosylation of OA (JONES 1980). Accordingly, OMP would not tend to accumulate unless OMP decarboxylase activity were inhibited. Indeed, as previously mentioned, significant inhibition of the decarboxylase does not lead to a measurable accumulation of OMP, because of its very rapid dephosphorylation, with the consequent accumulation of the ribonucleoside of OA. This compound, orotidine, has been generally regarded as a "dead-end" compound, since evidence that it could be cleaved to OA had not been observed until the work of JANEWAY and CHA (1977), utilizing a homogenate of murine L5178Y cells, which, in the presence of phosphate, formed OA from orotidine. It may be, therefore, that the accumulation of OA, when OMP decarboxylase is inhibited, may not be entirely accounted for by product inhibition of the activity of OA PRTase.

In this de novo pathway, many inhibitors have been studied; among the most potent are *N*-[phosphonacetyl]-L-aspartate (PALA), which inhibits the non-rate-limiting reaction catalyzed by L-aspartate transcarbamoylase, while several compounds inhibit OMP decarboxylase, functioning either as feedback inhibitors (e.g., UTP, UDP, UDP glucose, CTP, dUDP, and dUTP), or as antagonists that inhibit the enzyme in a competitive manner. Among this latter group, of the many compounds now known, those of greatest current interest are 6-azaUMP (K_i $\sim 1 \times 10^{-7} M$; TRAUT and JONES 1977), pyrazofurin 5′-monophosphate (K_i $\sim 5 \times 10^{-8} M$; GUTOWSKI et al. 1975), and the ribonucleotide of oxipurinol (K_i $\sim 1 \times 10^{-8} M$; FYFE et al. 1973); oxipurinol is a metabolite of allopurinol.

In view of the primary objective of this chapter, attention must now be directed to the manner in which the information concerning the enzymic formation of OMP and UMP can provide a mechanism for low-level resistance to such an analogue of Urd as 6-azaUrd.

SUTTLE and STARK (1979) and LEVINSON et al. (1979) used mutant cells that overproduce a bifunctional protein with OA PRTase and OMP decarboxylase activities; these cells had significantly reduced sensitivities to both 6-azaUMP and pyrazofurin 5′-monophosphate. In the cells studied by SUTTLE and STARK, the level of OA PRTase activity (which, per se, is not inhibited significantly by these compounds) was increased by as much as 67-fold. The concentrations of both 6-azaUrd and pyrazofurin (the phosphorylation of the latter is not catalyzed by Urd-Cyd kinase, but rather by adenosine kinase) required for inhibition by 50% of the proliferation of such cells were increased by $\sim$20-fold, as compared with the wild-type cells (C13/SV28, a cloned line of Syrian hamster BHK 21 cells transformed by simian virus 40). LEVINSON et al. (1979) studied several stable variants, obtained by mutagenizing the cells of a murine lymphoma (S49); one of these mutants, AU-11, required a 10- to 12-fold increase in the concentration of 6-azaUrd required for 50% inhibition of proliferation to be exerted, as compared with that necessary for the inhibition of parent cells. The levels of Urd-Cyd kinase activity in these two cell lines were the same, although other mutant cells were obtained in which Urd-Cyd kinase activity was deficient (and the cells were then very resistant to both 6-azaUrd and FUrd). Although PINSKY and KROOTH (1967) had described the "induction" by 6-azaUrd of the two enzyme activities (OA-PRTase and OMP decarboxylase) in cultured human fibroblasts, presumably reflecting gene amplification, such an "induction" of OMP decarboxylase activity did not occur with the AU-11 cells, the mutational events in which had resulted from exposure of the parent cells to *N*-methyl,*N*′-nitro-*N*-nitrosoguanidine.

C. 5-Azacytidine

5-Azacytidine (5-azaCyd)(4-amino-1-β-D-ribofuranosyl-1,3,5-triazine-2-one) (Fig. 1) is an unusual synthetic analogue of cytidine in that it also occurs naturally in an actinomycete, *Streptoverticillium lakadanus* (HANKA et al. 1966). Most studies of 5-azaCyd have been carried out with the synthetic compound, as first prepared by PÍSKALA and ŠORM (1964), while early biological studies were described by ŠORM et al. (1964) and by EVANS and HANKA (1968), as reviewed recently by VESELÝ and ČIHÁK (1978) and by RADA and DOSKOČIL (1980).

5-AzaCyd enters mammalian cells by way of the nucleoside-transport mechanism (PATERSON et al. 1979) and is phosphorylated to the corresponding 5′-mono-, di-, and triphosphate levels; it is incorporated into the RNA of mouse liver (ČIHÁK et al. 1965), and also that of Ehrlich ascites tumor cells in vivo (JUROVČIK et al. 1965). 5-AzaCyd also is converted metabolically into the corresponding 2′-deoxy form (ČIHÁK et al. 1980) (presumably this occurs at the level of the 5′-diphosphate); thus, the analogue is also incorporated into DNA and causes chromosomal damage in L1210 cells (LI et al. 1970a, b). The initial phosphorylation of 5-azaCyd is generally attributed to catalysis by cytosolic Urd-Cyd kinase (e.g., LI et al. 1970a; LEE et al. 1974; LIACOURAS and ANDERSON 1975; DRAKE et al. 1977); however, a mutational change, with deletion of over 99% of the Urd-Cyd kinase activity of the parent cells, which imparted high resistance to 3-deazaUrd in human lymphoblastoid lines of RPMI-6410, resulted in relatively little diminution in the sensitivity of the mutants to either 5-azaCyd or 6-azaUrd (AHMED et al. 1980). 5-AzaCMP also depresses the biosynthesis of pyrimidines de novo by inhibiting OMP decarboxylase activity (VESELÝ et al. 1968a; ČIHÁK and BROUČEK 1972).

The effect of 5-azaCyd on protein synthesis in mammalian cells appears to be related to its incorporation into newly synthesized RNA and to changes in polyribosome patterns, especially the loss of heavy polyribosomes in regenerating rat liver (ČIHÁK et al. 1968; LEVITAN and WEBB 1969). Since the antileukemic effects of 5-azaCyd in mice with L1210 leukemia can be reversed by Cyd, but not by dCyd (VADLAMUDI et al. 1970), the predominant effect would appear to involve the synthesis of RNAs (and possibly other derivatives of Cyd). On the other hand, 5-azaCyd inhibits mitosis and it is most toxic to mammalian cells in culture when they are in S-phase (LI et al. 1970b). 5-AzaCyd is extensively deaminated in biological systems (CHABNER et al. 1973) and the products of the degradation of 5-azaUrd, a relatively unstable molecule, can be found (COLES et al. 1974). Indeed, in *Escherichia coli,* ŠKODA et al. had identified ribosyl biuret in 1962 as the main decomposition product of 5-azaUrd. In addition to 5-azaUrd, two products of the degradation of 5-azaCyd have been identified as *N*′-(formylamidino)-*N*′-β-D-ribofuranosylurea and 1-β-D-ribofuranosyl-3-guanylurea (BEISLER 1978). Similarly, a product of the degradation of 5-aza-2′-deoxyCyd has been identified as *N*-amidino-*N*′-deoxy-β-D-ribofuranosylurea (ČIHÁK et al. 1980).

The development of resistance of experimental tumor cells to 5-azaCyd has been investigated extensively, primarily in vivo, by VESELY et al. (1967, 1968a, b, 1970, 1971); resistance to 5-azaCyd of murine AKR leukemic cells was accompanied by a reduction in Urd-Cyd kinase activity in the third transplant period (VESELÝ et al. 1967). The decreased survival of the leukemic mice treated with 5-azaCyd was associated with an impaired uptake of 5-azaCyd into liver RNA. Urd-Cyd kinase activity decreased simultaneously with the development of resistance (VESELY et al. 1968b). The 5-azaCyd-resistant subline exhibited increased DNA-dependent RNA and DNA polymerase activities. The enhancement of these polymerase activities, however, did not appear to be related directly to the development of resistance; rather, it may have represented a compensatory response to impairment of salvage pathways for pyrimidine nucleosides (VESELÝ 1971). A partially purified form of Urd-Cyd kinase, isolated from the 5-azaCyd-resistant murine leukemic cells (VESELÝ et al. 1971), was considerably more stable toward heating and to the action of *p*-chloromercuribenzoate than was the enzyme derived from the parent line of cells; accordingly, possible conformational or structural changes in the enzyme of the resistant cells were suggested.

Cells selected for resistance to 5-azaCyd were also almost completely resistant to 5-aza-2′-deoxyCyd, a circumstance attributed to reduction in the activity of dCyd kinase (VESELÝ et al. 1970). It was unexpected to find, therefore, that the incorporation of [2-^{14}C]-dCyd into the DNA of both the resistant and the sensitive lines was comparable. It was concluded that, despite the reduction in dCyd kinase activity in the resistant line, sufficient activity remained to supply [2-^{14}C]-dCMP for its subsequent conversion to the triphosphate and incorporation into DNA.

A subline of L1210 leukemia that is resistant to 5-azaCyd (BEISLER et al. 1977) was also cross-resistant to 5,6-dihydro-5-azaCyd hydrochloride [initially described by VOYTEK et al. (1976) and BEISLER et al. (1976)]; this and other findings by VOYTEK et al. (1977), as well as the similar inhibitory effects of 5-azaCyd and 5,6-dihydro-5-azaCyd on the methylation and synthesis of 5 and 4S nuclear RNA of L1210 (GLAZER and HARTMAN 1979), suggested that the 5,6-dihydro-form may serve as a prodrug. Other interpretations must be considered, however, because (a) the kinetics of the responses of L1210 cells in culture to 5,6-dihydro-5-azaCyd are very different from those to 5-azaCyd (PRESANT et al. 1979), and (b) proliferation of HeLa cells, although inhibited completely by 5-azaCyd (10 μ*M*), was not inhibitied by the dihydro derivative (200 μ*M*), except in the presence of a Cyd deaminase inhibitor, which did *not* augment the cytotoxicity of 5-azaCyd (FUTTERMAN et al. 1978), while (c) studies of the metabolism and urinary elimination of [4-^{14}C]-5,6-dihydro-5-azaCyd led to the appearance of no 5-azaCyd, although ~30% of the dihydro derivative was excreted unchanged (MALSPEIS and DESOUZA 1981).

In a phase II study of 5-azaCyd in 177 patients with solid tumors (WEISS et al. 1977), insensitivity to the drug developed rapidly. Remissions were seen in patients whose tumors appeared to be resistant to FUra, arabinosylcytosine (araC), methotrexate, and alkylating agents; thus, there appeared to be no clinically demonstrable cross-resistance to these agents. Although 5-azaCyd appears to have only limited effects on solid tumors, investigation is continuing in this area.

5-AzaCyd inhibited the differentiation of a rat myeloblast line in culture (NG et al. 1976). Variants resistant to the cytotoxic effect of 5-azaCyd were obtained and the resistant cells were more susceptible than the parental line to the lethal actions of both 5-bromo-dUrd and adenosine, but not to those of either araC or 8-azaguanine. The resistant cells were capable of transporting Urd, thymidine, and 5-azaCyd, but their Urd-Cyd kinase activity was reduced to only from one-half to one-third that of the parental cells (NG et al. 1976). Two variants showed a two- to three-fold increase in the activity of OMP decarboxylase. This latter enzyme activity, derived from the resistant cells, in contrast to that of the parental cells, was completely insensitive to the inhibitory effect of a nucleotide generated from ATP and 5-azaCyd in cell extracts, in contrast to the inhibition of Urd-Cyd kinase activity by the 5′-triphosphates of Urd and Cyd: UTP and CTP, respectively (AN-

DERSON and BROCKMAN 1964), as well as by other metabolites (see JONES 1980) and by 6-azaUMP. These observations led to the suggestion that this type of resistance to 5-azaCyd may arise in myeloblasts from alterations in components of two target pathways: (a) the de novo pathway to UMP and (b) an undefined sequence leading to the synthesis of membrane components (NG et al. 1976). 3-DeazaUrd (see below) has been used to increase the phosphorylation of 5-azaCyd (GRANT and CADMAN 1980); presumably this occurs because the formation of 3-deazaUTP inhibits the formation of CTP from UTP and thus of compounds derived from CTP, which are antagonistic to the cytotoxic effects of 5-azaCyd.

D. Pseudoisocytidine

This atypical ribonucleoside, in which carbon-1 of the β-D-ribofuranose moiety is linked to carbon-5 of the aglycone, in a manner analogous to that in pseudouridine (Fig. 1), was synthesized by CHU et al. (1975) and studied extensively by BURCHENAL et al. (1976), as well as by CHOU et al. (1979) and ZEDECK (1979). The analogue is converted to the 5′-di- and 5′-triphosphate forms, since it appears in both DNA and RNA. Although highly effective in the chemotherapy of a variety of murine leukemias, pseudoisocytidine (ψisoCyd) proved to be too hepatotoxic in man for chemotherapeutic utility. Uptake of the analogue by perfused mouse livers can be prevented by an inhibitor of nucleoside transport, i.e., *p*-nitro-benzyl-6-thioinosine (PATERSON et al. 1980).

Lines of the murine mastocytoma, P815, were selected for resistance to ψisoCyd, and reductions in their levels of Urd-Cyd kinase activities were reported (CHOU et al. 1979; ZEDECK 1979). Despite these observations, however, the meaning of which is not yet clear, ψisoCyd did not compete significantly (at ~7 × the K_m for Urd) with the phosphorylation of Urd by ATP, as catalyzed by preparations of Urd-Cyd kinase obtained from L1210 cells (AHMED and BAKER 1980); in addition, the proliferation of cells of RPMI 6410/6-MP/3-deazaUrd, which were essentially devoid of Urd-Cyd kinase activity, was inhibited significantly by ψisoCyd (AHMED et al. 1980). As will be discussed below, a system other than Urd-Cyd kinase may be responsible for the initial phosphorylation of ψisoCyd. It has not yet been established, however, that the ψisoCyd-resistant variants of P815 have lost the postulated route for this phosphorylation.

E. 3-Deazauridine

3-Deazauridine (3-deazaUrd) (Fig. 1) and 3-deazaCyd are analogues of Urd and Cyd, respectively, in which the nitrogen in position-3 of the pyrimidine ring can be regarded as having been replaced by a carbon atom (with one associated hydrogen atom, because the oxygen in position-4 is predominantly in the enol form, unlike the corresponding oxygen of Urd). An initial report of the synthesis of 3-deazaUrd by ROBINS and CURRIE (1968) was followed by a more detailed study of the syntheses of 3-deazaUrd and 3-deazaCyd by CURRIE et al. (1970). The analogues were studied in neoplastic cells by WANG and BLOCH (1972), who demonstrated the conversion of 3-deazaUrd to the 5′-mono-, -di-, and -triphosphate forms, as also was done by BROCKMAN et al. (1975) and by CYSYK et al. (1978).

Other groups have studied the powerful inhibitory effect of 3-deazaUrd on the proliferation of mammalian cell lines in culture, as well as on the growth of a variety of transplantable murine neoplasms in vivo (ROBINS et al. 1969; BLOCH et al. 1973). 3-DeazaUrd also potentiates the cytotoxic action of araC on two lines of human neoplastic cells in culture: HeLa (carcinoma) and RPMI-6410 (lymphoblastoid cells of B-cell origin) (MILLS-YAMAMOTO et al. 1978).

The primary site of the cytotoxic action of 3-deazaUrd ($pK_a \sim 6.5$), functioning as 3-deazaUTP, appears to be CTP synthetase ($K_i \sim 5.3 \times 10^{-6} M$), which catalyzes the conversion of UTP to CTP (MCPARTLAND et al. 1974; BROCKMAN et al. 1975; MCPARTLAND and WEINFELD 1976); this inhibition results in a profound diminution in intracellular levels of cytosine-containing nucleotides. It is of particular importance, in view of the formation of the higher phosphate esters of 3-deazaUrd, that the latter did *not* lead to the appearance of 3-deazaUrd in the nucleic acids of Ehrlich ascites carcinoma cells in vivo (WANG and BLOCH 1972).

Although 3-deazaUrd is generally regarded as catabolically stable (WANG and BLOCH 1972), BENVENUTO et al. (1979) reported that 3-deazaUrd is cleaved by humans to some extent to 3-deazaUra (i.e., 2,4-dihydroxypyridine), which was found in the plasma but not in the urine of patients given the nucleoside by rapid infusion; the small amounts of the parent drug excreted in the urine suggested its elimination in the bile. Of potential importance for the treatment of cerebral leukemias was the accumulation of the triphosphate ester of 3-deazaUrd in the brain.

Selection of mammalian cells resistant to 3-deazaUrd was reported by MILLS-YAMAMOTO et al. (1978), using two lines of human lymphoblastoid cells, RPMI 6410 [one already resistant to 6-mercaptopurine (6-MP)]. These 3-deazaUrd-resistant cells were very low in Urd-Cyd kinase activity; thus, the initial phosphorylation of the Urd analogue by the mutant cells was markedly diminished and only minimal formation of cytotoxic 3-deazaUTP could occur.

In view of the selection by 3-deazaUrd of stably resistant cells, deficient in Urd-Cyd kinase activity, it was not anticipated that the proliferation of such cells (e.g., RPMI 6410/3-deazaUrd and RPMI 6410/6-MP/3-deazaUrd) would be inhibited by other cytotoxic nucleosides known to serve as substrates for Urd-Cyd kinase. Thus, the marked inhibition of the proliferation of such 3-deazaUrd-resistant mutant cells by 6-azaUrd was unexpected (A. R. P. Paterson, personal communication). As previously indicated, 6-azaUrd is an excellent substrate for Urd-Cyd kinase; hence, this observation led to collaborative studies being initiated (AHMED et al. 1980). After doubly cloning the two 3-deazaUrd-resistant lines, the levels of Urd-Cyd kinase activity were even further reduced; thus, in the resistant lines this enzyme activity was less than 1% of that found in the parent line (RPMI 6410/0), i.e., below levels that could be accurately quantified. It was confirmed, however, that the proliferation of these Urd-Cyd kinase-deficient cells was indeed markedly inhibited, not only by 6-azaUrd but also by 5-azaCyd. Proof that [5-^{3}H]-6-azaUrd was converted into 6-azaUMP was obtained with RPMI 6410/6-MP/3-deazaUrd, as was reported by AHMED et al. (1980). Either the miniscule amount of Urd-Cyd kinase activity (< 1% of that in the parent cells) in the 6410/6-MP/3-deazaUrd cells was responsible for the phosphorylation of 6-azaUrd by ATP or another mechanism for the formation of 6-azaUMP from 6-azaUrd appeared to exist (AHMED et al. 1980); to be excluded, however, are the nucleoside-phosphotransferases that utilize phenylphosphate, and certain other monophosphates, as donors, because these cells do not possess such enzyme activity (Ahmed and Green, unpublished observations). Nevertheless, the possibility of another nucleoside-phosphorylating system was suggested by (a) the ~1,000-fold reduction in the sensitivity of 6410/6-MP/3-deazaUrd to 3-deazaUrd, as compared with that of the parent strain of these cells (AHMED et al. 1980), (b) the findings with ψisoCyd in cultures of 6410/6-MP/3-deazaUrd, and (c) unpublished studies of the mutant in culture, the proliferation of which also was inhibited significantly by 5-hydroxyuridine and 5-aminouridine. The latter derivatives of Urd and Cyd have not interfered significantly (at 1.75 mM; ~7× the K_m for Urd) with the phosphorylation of Urd by ATP, as catalyzed by Urd-Cyd kinase activities of a human lymphoma and of murine L1210 cells (AHMED and WELCH, 1979; AHMED and BAKER 1980).

This human lymphoblastoid (B-cell) line (RPMI-6410) is not unique in that its proliferation is markedly inhibited by 6-azaUrd and 5-azaCyd, when selected for resistance to 3-deazaUrd; this has also been found with the human T-lymphoblastoid line of cells, CCRF-CEM. In this case, however, the mutant cells are *not* deficient in Urd-Cyd kinase activity (WELCH et al. 1982). Consequently, another type of mutation has been sought, although the Urd-Cyd kinase appears also to have been altered in the resistant cells. Thus, the affinity for Urd of the cytosolic kinase in the parent cells, CEM/O, is indicated by the K_m, 0.42 (±0.06) mM, while that of CEM/3-deazaUrd is 0.87 (±0.15) mM. Of even greater significance, however, is the surprising finding that the cytosolic Urd-Cyd kinase of the parent cells, CEM/O, has no detectable affinity for [5-^{3}H]-3-deazaUrd (in concentrations ranging from 1 μM to 60 mM), despite its ability to catalyze the phosphorylation of Urd, Cyd, and 6-azaUrd. DRAKE et al. (1977) had noted the very low affinity of 5-azaCyd for the Cyd kinase of their "wild strain" of CEM cells; thus, using an unpurified supernatant fraction of the homogenized cells, they reported a K_m of ~11 mM, as measured under rather difficult conditions with respect to solubility and instability of 5-azaCyd. With slightly purified Urd-Cyd kinase of our CEM/O cells, the affinity for the stable analogue of Urd, i.e., 3-deazaUrd, is so low that no K_m has been determinable; however, the K_m values for Urd, Cyd, and 6-azaUrd are reasonable, although higher than with most Urd-Cyd kinase preparations (Welch et al., unpublished observations).

The findings with 3-deazaUrd, highly cytotoxic for CEM/O cells proliferating in culture, indicate clearly that these neoplastic cells must possess another nucleoside-phosphorylating system, able to utilize 3-deazaUrd (based on the reasonable assumption that its 5′-monophosphate must be formed initially, as a precursor of 3-deazaUTP). As noted previously, this analogue of UTP markedly inhibits the activity of CTP synthetase, but does not modify the structure of either RNA or DNA (MCPARTLAND et al. 1974). The mutation that confers resistance to 3-deazaUrd does not alter significantly the sensitivity of the CTP synthetase to inhibition by synthetic 3-deazaUTP, as shown by studies of the effect of the latter on the enzymatic conversion of UTP into CTP by extracts of CEM/0 cells and of CEM/3-deazaUrd cells (Welch and Panahi, unpublished results). The formation of CTP was measured by high performance liquid chromatography (HPLC), using the system devised by MOYER and HANDSCHUMACHER (1978).

A significant source of nucleoside-phosphorylating activity has been found in both very crude homogenates and thrice-washed nuclei of CEM/0 cells, incubated at 37 °C in a nutrient medium containing 0.24 *M* sucrose; added ATP and Mg^{2+} are essential (AMP is ineffective). This nuclear enzyme catalyzes the phosphorylation of 3-deazaUrd, unlike the cytosolic enzyme of CEM/0 cells, while both enzymes lead to the formation of the phosphate esters of Urd and 6-azaUrd (Welch and Panahi, unpublished results).

It should be emphasized that the striking deficiency of the cytosolic Urd-Cyd kinase of CEM/0 cells, with respect to its lack of affinity for 3-deazaUrd, is *not* characteristic of the Urd-Cyd kinases of all other cells so far studied, e.g., human 6410/0 (AHMED et al. 1980), murine L1210 (AHMED and BAKER 1980), and murine Ehrlich ascites carcinoma (Welch and Panahi, unpublished results).[1] That the nuclear enzyme is not a "nascent" form of the cytosolic kinase is shown by the striking inability of the latter to utilize 3-deazaUrd, while retaining the ability to catalyze the phosphorylation of Urd, Cyd, and 6-azaUrd.[2]

Further studies will be done with the nuclei of other cells, especially CEM/3-deazaUrd, but also of 6410 and its drug-resistant mutants, with a view to disclosing the effects of these mutations on the activities of the nucleoside-phosphorylating enzyme of the various nuclei. Of particular interest will be investigations of 5,6-dihydro-5-azaCyd, in view of the observations of many workers (initially SKÖLD 1960) that neither 5,6-dihydroUrd nor 5,6-dihydroCyd is a substrate for the Urd-Cyd kinases investigated. Indeed, the very low affinity of even 5-azaCyd for the supernatant fraction of homogenized CEM/0 cells, observed by DRAKE et al. (1977), suggests the possibility that the high cytotoxicity of 5-azaCyd for proliferating CEM/0 cells may reflect a participation of the nucleoside-phosphorylating system of the nuclei. A similar suggestion may apply to 6410/MP/3-deazaUrd with respect to its sensitivity to 6-azaUrd and 5-azaCyd, as well as to ψisoCyd, 5-aminoUrd, and 5-hydroxyUrd, which exhibit significant cytotoxicity for various lines of proliferating cells (WELCH et al. 1982), but only weakly affect the phosphorylation of Urd, as catalyzed by the Urd-Cyd kinase of L1210 cells (AHMED and BAKER 1980).

It is of interest to note that the proliferation of 6410/6-MP/3-deazaUrd cells (shown to be free of mycoplasma) can still be inhibited markedly by FUrd. This phenomenon is attributed to the cleavage of FUrd by Urd phosphorylase to FUra, the toxicity of which for these cells is indistinguishable from that exhibited by FUrd, especially when the cloned cells used were derived from RPMI 6410/6-MP/3-deazaUrd, but selected further for resistance to 6-azaUrd (Welch et al., unpublished findings). Indeed, these triply drug-resistant cells phosphohydrolytically cleave FUrd to FUra (Belt and Germain, unpublished findings), while FUra, by reaction with PRPP, is converted to FUMP, as catalyzed by OAPRTase. Indeed,

---

1 We are grateful to Dr. T. W. Traut, University of North Carolina School of Medicine, Chapel Hill, NC, for supplying a partially purified fraction, containing Urd-Cyd kinase activity, derived from Ehrlich ascites carcinoma cells (PAYNE and TRAUT 1982)

2 Quantification of the enzymic phosphorylation of the acidic nucleosides, 6-azaUrd (pK_a ~6.7) and 3-deazaUrd (pK_a ~6.5), is outlined in an abstract (WELCH et al. 1983) and is fully described in a paper in press (WELCH et al. 1984)

using discs of DEAE-cellulose (DE-81) and [6-^{3}H]-FUra as a substrate (AHMED 1981), this PRPP-requiring enzyme activity has been shown to be present in these cells (Ahmed, unpublished results).

It is appropriate to suggest, however, that any attempt to obtain an additional mutant line, also insensitive to FUra, may not be feasible, because the necessary depletion of enzyme activity would appear to involve OAPRTase, which is believed to be identical with the enzyme that catalyzes the reaction between FUra and PRPP (JONES 1980).

F. Concluding Statement

We may conclude, therefore, by emphasizing that studies of the mechanisms of resistance of mammalian cells to cytotoxic analogues of pyrimidine-containing ribonucleosides have shown not only that highly drug-resistant mutant cells can be obtained (especially with 3-deazaUrd, 6-azaUrd, and 5-azaCyd) in which one type of mutational event has resulted in either the partial or the essentially complete deletion of Urd-Cyd kinase activity. Low levels of resistance to 6-azaUrd at times can be attributed to accumulation of an enzymically bifunctional protein; in addition, however, another mechanism of resistance may exist (see below). Thus, the proliferation of such cells as RPMI 6410/6-MP/3-deazaUrd (essentially devoid of cytosolic Urd-Cyd kinase activity: $<1\%$ of that of the parent cells), for which the sensitivity to 3-deazaUrd is reduced $\sim$1,000-fold, is markedly inhibited by 6-azaUrd (from which 6-azaUMP is formed) and by 5-azaCyd. In addition, less marked inhibition of proliferation by *certain* other cytotoxic nucleosides, such as 5,6-dihydro-5-azaCyd, ψisoCyd, 5-aminoUrd, and 5-hydroxyUrd, is retained. From such cells, stable mutants have been selected that also are additionally resistant to 6-azaUrd; these triply drug-resistant cells have afforded new tools for (a) exploring the mechanisms of transport of Urd, Cyd, and their analogues, separate from their intracellular phosphorylation (PATERSON et al. 1979; BELT and WELCH 1983), and (b) investigating potentially useful inhibitors of the residual multistep de novo pathway to UMP.

In addition to the findings with drug-resistant lines of the 6410(B) cells, recent studies with another type of human lymphoblast, CCRF-CEM (a T-cell), also selected for resistance to 3-deazaUrd (CEM/3-deazaUrd), have shown that cytosolic Urd-Cyd kinase activity is *not* deleted from this drug-resistant mutant. Drug resistance in these cells also is not attributable to an alteration in the sensitivity of CTP synthetase to 3-deazaUrd 5′-triphosphate; rather, it may be suggested that a hitherto unrecognized nucleoside-phosphorylating enzyme activity, found in the nuclei of CEM/0 cells, may be related to the resistance of such mutants as CEM/3-deazaUrd, with which further studies will be done. Conceivably, this nuclear enzyme activity could be related to one of those described by LENGER (1982), which are associated with the nuclear chromatin, as derived from a hepatoma (Morris 9121) grown in rats; although the phosphorylation of thymidine was studied primarily, phosphorylations of Urd and Cyd were noted in the presence of ATP and Mg^{2+}.

The clinical significance of studies of the mechanisms of resistance to antitumor drugs, in general, needs no emphasis. These investigations of resistance to cytotoxic ribonucleosides, however, have also yielded an important molecular pharmacological dividend. Thus, there has been disclosed another nucleoside-phosphorylating system, hitherto unrecognized, which occurs in the nuclei of certain human neoplastic cells and presumably also in their normal precursors. It is suggested that this nuclear enzymic activity may be mutationally altered and thus can be involved in the selection by certain cytotoxic ribonucleosides, such as 3-deazaUrd, 6-azaUrd, and 5-azaCyd, of mutant cells resistant to these and related chemotherapeutic agents.

Acknowledgements. The authors acknowledge their indebtedness for grants that contributed to the support of investigations in their laboratories: A.C.S.: NP-351; N.S.F.: PCM-8012099; N.C.I.: CA21677, and ALSAC.

References

Ahmed NK (1981) Determination of pyrimidine phosphoribosyltransferase and uridine kinase activities by an assay with DEAE-paper discs. J Biochem Biophys Meth 4:123–130

Ahmed NK, Baker DR (1980) Properties of uridine-cytidine kinase derived from L1210 leukemia cells. Cancer Res 40:3559–3563

Ahmed NK, Welch AD (1979) Some properties of uridine-cytidine kinase from a human malignant lymphoma. Cancer Res 39:3102–3106

Ahmed NK, Germain GS, Welch AD, Paterson ARP, Paran JH, Yang S (1980) Phosphorylation of nucleosides catalyzed by a mammalian enzyme other than uridine cytidine kinase. Biochem Biophys Res Commun 95:440–445

Anderson EP, Brockman RW (1964) Feedback inhibition of uridine kinase by cytidine triphosphate and uridine triphosphate. Biochim Biophys Acta 91:380–386

Barlow RB, Welch AD (1956) A synthesis of "6-azauracil" (1,2,4-triazine-3,5(2H,4H)-dione, an analog of uracil. J Am Chem Soc 78:1258–1259

Beisler JA (1978) Isolation, characterization, and properties of a labile hydrolysis product of the antitumor nucleoside, 5-azacytidine. J Med Chem 21:204–208

Beisler JA, Abbasi MM, Driscoll JS (1976) Dihydro-5-azacytidine hydrochloride, a biologically active and chemically stable analog of 5-azacytidine. Cancer Treat Rep 60:1671–1674

Beisler JA, Abbasi MM, Kelley JA, Driscoll JS (1977) Synthesis and antitumor activity of dihydro-5-azacytidine, a hydrolytically stable analogue of 5-azacytidine. J Med Chem 20:806–812

Belt JA, Welch AD (1983) Transport or uridine and 6-azauridine in human lymphoblastoid cells. Specificity for the uncharged 6-azauridine molecule. Mol Pharmacol 23:153–158

Benvenuto JA, Hall SW, Farquhar D, Stewart DJ, Benjamin RS, Loo TL (1979) Pharmacokinetics and disposition of 3-deazauridine in humans. Cancer Res 39:349–352

Blair DGR, Hall AD (1969) Specific activites of uridine phosphorylase and uridine kinase in Ehrlich ascites carcinoma cells and 6-azauracil and azauridine treated sublines in successive transplant generations. Br J Cancer 23:875–896

Bloch A, Dutschman G, Currie BL, Robins RK, Robins MJ (1973) Preparation and biological activity of various 3-deazapyrimidines and related nucleosides. J Med Chem 16:294–297

Brockman RW (1963) Mechanism of resistance to anticancer agents. Adv Cancer Res 7:129–234

Brockman RW (1974) Mechanisms of resistance. In: Sartorelli AC, Johns DG (eds) Antineoplastic and immunosuppressive agents. Springer, Berlin Heidelberg New York pp 352–440 (Handbook of experimental pharmacology, vol 38/1)

Brockman RW, Shaddix SC, Williams M, Nelson JA, Rose LM, Schabel FM (1975) The mechanism of action of 3-deazauridine in tumor cells sensitive and resistant to arabinosylcytosine. Ann NY acad Sci 255:501–521

Burchenal JH, Ciovacco K, Kalaher K, O'Toole T, Kiefner R, Dowling MD, Chu CK, Watanabe KA, Wempen I, Fox JJ (1976) Antileukemic effects of pseudoisocytidine, a new synthetic pyrimidine C-nucleoside. Cancer Res 36:1520–1523

Calabresi P, Doolittle CH, Heppner GH, McDonald CV (1975) Nucleoside analogs in the treatment of nonneoplastic diseases. Chemistry, biology and clinical uses of nucleoside analogs. Ann NY Acad Sci 255:190–201

Chabner BA, Drake JC, Johns DG (1973) Deamination of 5-azacytidine by a human leukemia cell cytidine deaminase. Biochem Pharmacol 22:2763–2765

Chou T-C, Burchenal JH, Fox JJ, Watanabe KA, Chu CK, Philips FS (1979) Metabolism and effects of 5-(β-D-ribofuranosyl)-isocytosine in P-815 cells. Cancer Res 39:720–728

Chu CK, Watanabe KA, Fox JJ (1975) Nucleosides XXCII: A facile synthesis of 5-(β-D-ribofuranosyl)-isocytosine. J Heterocycl Chem 12:817–818

Čihák A, Brouček J (1972) Dual effect of 5-azacytidine on the synthesis of liver RNA. Lack of the relationship between metabolic transformation of orotic acid in vitro and its incorporation in vivo. Biochem Pharmacol 21:2497–2507

Čihák A, Rada B (1976) Uridine kinase: properties, biological significance and chemotherapeutic aspects (a review). Neoplasma 23:233–257

Čihák A, Veselý J, Šorm F (1965) Incorporation of 5-azacytidine into liver ribonucleic acids of leukemic mice sensitive and resistant to 5-azacytidine. Biochim Biophys Acta 108:516–518

Čihák A, Veselý H, Šorm F (1968) Thymidine kinase and polyribosome distribution in regenerating rat liver following 5-azacytidine. Biochim Biophys Acta 166:277–279

Čihák A, Veselý J, Hynie S (1980) Transformation and metabolic effects of 5-aza-2′-deoxycytidine in mice. Biochem Pharmacol 29:2929–2932

Coles E, Thayer PS, Reinhold V, Gaudio L (1974) Pharmacokinetics of excretion of 5-azacytidine and its metabolites. Proc Am Assoc Cancer Res 15:286

Currie BL, Robins RK, Robins MJ (1970) Synthesis of 3-deazapyrimidine nucleosides related to uridine and cytidine and their derivatives. J Heterocycl Chem 7:323–329

Cysyk RL, Gormley PE, D'Anna ME, Adamson RH (1978) The disposition of 3-deazauridine in mice. Drug Metab Dispos 6:125–132

Drake JC, Stoller RG, Chabner BA (1977) Characteristics of the enzyme uridine-cytidine kinase isolated from a cultured human cell line. Biochem Pharmacol 26:64–66

Evans JS, Hanka LJ (1968) The in vivo activity of combinations of 5-azacytidine and cytidine on leukemia L1210. Experientia 24:922–923

Falco EA, Pappas E, Hitchings GH (1956) 1,2,4-triazine analogs of the natural pyrimidines. J Am Chem Soc 78:1938–1971

Fyfe JA, Miller RL, Krenitsky TA (1973) Kinetic properties and effects of some allopurinol metabolites on the enzyme and inhibition of orotidine 5′-phosphate decarboxylase. J Biol Chem 248:3801–3809

Glazer RI, Hartman KD (1979) The comparative effects of 5-azacytidine and dihydro-5-azacytidine on 4S and 5S nuclear RNA. Mol Pharmacol 17:250–255

Grant S, Cadman E (1980) Altered 5-azacytidine metabolism following 3-deazauridine treatment of L5178Y and human myeloblasts. Cancer Res 50:4000–4006

Gutowski GE, Sweeney MJ, DeLong DC, Hamill RL, Gerzon K, Dyke RW (1975) Biochemistry and biological effects of the pyrazofurine (pyrazomycins): initial clinical trial. Ann NY Acad Sci 255:544–551

Habermann V, Šorm F (1958) Mechanism of the cancerostatic action of 6-azauracil and its riboside. Coll Czech Chem Commun 23:2201–2206

Handschumacher RE (1957) Studies of bacterial resistance to 6-azauracil and its riboside. Biochim Biophys Acta 23:428–430

Handschumacher RE (1958) Inhibition of orotidylic acid decarboxylase, a primary site of carcinostasis by 6-azauracil. Biochim Biophys Acta 30:451–452

Handschumacher RE (1960) Orotidylic acid decarboxylase: inhibition studies with azauridine 5′-phosphate. J Biol Chem 235:2917–2919

Handschumacher RE, Coleridge J (1979) Hepatic and biliary transport of orotate and its metabolic consequences. Biochem Pharmacol 28:1977–1981

Handschumacher RE, Pasternak CA (1958) Inhibition of orotidylic acid decarboxylase, a primary site of carcinostasis by 6-azauracil. Biochim Biophys Acta 30:451–452

Handschumacher RE, Calabresi P, Welch AD, Bono VH Jr, Fallon JH, Frei E III (1962a) Summary of current information on 6-azauridine. Cancer Chemother Rep 21:1–18

Handschumacher RE, Creasey WA, Fink ME, Calabresi P, Welch AD (1962b) Pharmacological and clinical studies with triacetyl 6-azauridine. Cancer Chemother Rep 16:267–269

Handschumacher RE, Škoda J, Šorm F (1963) Metabolic and biochemical effects of 6-azacytidine in mice with Ehrlich ascites carcinoma. Coll Czech Chem Commun 28:2983–2990

Hanka LJ, Evans JS, Mason DJ, Dietz A (1966) Microbiological production of 5-azacytidine. I. Production and biological activity. Antimicrob Agents Chemother 616–624

Hashmi S, May SR, Krooth RS, Miller OJ (1975) Concurrent development of resistance to 6-azauridine and adenosine in a mouse cell line. J Cell Physiol 86:191–200

Janeway CM, Cha S (1977) Effects of 6-azauridine on nucleotides, orotic acid, and orotidine in L5178Y mouse lymphoma cells in vitro. Cancer Res 37:4382–4388

Jones ME (1980) Pyrimidine nucleotide biosynthesis in animals: Genes, enzymes, and regulation of UMP biosynthesis. Annu Rev Biochem 49:253–279

Jurovčik M, Raška K, Šormova Z, Šorm F (1965) Anabolic transformation of a novel antimetabolite, 5-azacytidine, and evidence for its incorporation into ribonucleic acid. Coll Czech Chem Commun 30:3370–3376

Lee T, Karon M, Momparler RL (1974) Kinetic studies on phosphorylation of 5-azacytidine with the purified uridine-cytidine kinase from calf thymus. Cancer Res 34:2484–2488

Lenger K (1982) Isolation of nucleoside phosphotransferases from chromatin of Morris hepatoma 9121. Int J Biochem 14:53–61

Levinson BB, Ullman B, Martin DW Jr (1979) Pyrimidine pathway variants of cultured mouse lymphoma cells with altered levels of both orotate phosphoribosyltransferase and orotidylate decarboxylase. J Biol Chem 254:4376–4401

Levitan IB, Webb TE (1969) Effects of 5-azacytidine on polyribosomes and on the control of tyrosine transaminase activity in rat liver. Biochim Biophys Acta 182:491–500

Li LH, Olin EJ, Buskirk HH, Reineke LM (1970a) Cytotoxicity and mode of action of 5-azacytidine on L1210 leukemia. Cancer Res 30:2760–2769

Li LH, Olin EJ, Fraser TJ, Bhuyan BK (1970b) Phase specificity of 5-azacytidine against mammalian cells in tissue culture. Cancer Res 30:2770–2775

Liacouras AS, Anderson EP (1975) Uridine-cytidine kinase. Purification from a murine neoplasm and characterization of the enzyme. Arch Biochem Biophys 168:66–73

Lísmane A, Muiznieks I, Vitols M, Čihak A, Škoda J (1977) Catabolic degradation of 6-azauracil and 6-azauridine by *Pseudomonas putida*. Coll Czech Chem Commun 42:2586–2593

Lisý V, Škoda J, Rychlík I, Smrt J, Holý A, Šorm F (1968) Changes in coding properties of poly- and oligonucleotides containing 6-azapyrimidine ribonucleosides. Coll Czech Chem Commun 33:4111–4119

Malspeis L, DeSouza JJV (1981) Metabolism and elimination of 5,6-dihydro-5-azacytidine. Proc Am Assoc Cancer Res 22:868

McPartland RP, Weinfeld H (1976) Cytidine 5′-triphosphate synthetase of calf liver. J Biol Chem 251:4372–4378

McPartland RP, Wang MC, Bloch A, Weinfeld H (1974) Cytidine 5′-triphosphate synthetase as a target for inhibition by the antitumor agent 3-deazauridine. Cancer 34:3107–3111

Mills-Yamamoto C, Lauzon GJ, Paterson ARP (1978) Toxicity of combinations of arabinosylcytosine and 3-deazauridine toward neoplastic cells in culture. Biochem Pharmacol 27:181–186

Moyer JD, Handschumacher RE (1978) Selective inhibition of pyrimidine synthesis and depletion of nucleotide pools by *N*-phosphonacetyl-L-aspartate. Cancer Res 39:3089–3094

Ng SK, Rogers J, Sanwal BO (1976) Alterations in differentiation and pyrimidine pathway enzymes in 5-azacytidine resistant variants of a myeloblast line. J Cell Physiol 90:361–374

Pasternak CA, Handschumacher RE (1959) The biochemical activity of 6-azauridine: interference with pyrimidine metabolism in transplantable mouse tumors. J Biol Chem 234:2992–2997

Pasternak CA, Fischer GA, Handschumacher RE (1961) Alteration in pyrimidine metabolism in L5178Y leukemia cells resistant to 6-azauridine. Cancer Res 21:110–117

Paterson ARP, Yang S, Lau EY, Cass CE (1979) Low specificity of the nucleoside transport mechanism of RPMI 6410 cells. Mol Pharmacol 16:900–908

Paterson ARP, Kolassa N, Chou T-C (1980) Inhibition of pseudoisocytidine uptake in isolated perfused livers of mice by nitrobenzylthioinosinate (NBMPR-P). Proc Am Assoc Cancer Res 21:1140

Payne RC, Traut TW (1982) Regulation of uridine kinase quaternary structure. Dissociation by the inhibitor CTP. J Biol Chem 257:12485–12488

Pinsky L, Krooth RS (1967) Studies on the control of pyrimidine biosynthesis in human diploid cell strains. II. Effects of 5-azaorotic acid, barbituric acid, and pyrimidine precursors on cellular phenotypes. Proc Natl Acad Sci 57:925–932

Pískala A, Šorm F (1964) Nucleic acid components and their analogues. LI. Synthesis of l-glycosyl derivatives of 5-azauracil and 5-azacytosine. Coll Czech Chem Commun 29:2060–2076

Presant CA, Valeriote F, Vietti TJ, Perez C (1979) Kinetics of dihydroazacytidine cytotoxicity differ from 5-azacytidine. Proc Am Assoc Cancer Res 20:113

Rada B, Doskočil J (1980) Azapyrimidine nucleosides. Pharmac Ther 9:171–217

Robins MJ, Currie BL (1968) The synthesis of 3-deazauridine [4-hydroxy-l-(β-D-ribofuranosyl)-2-pyridone]. Chem Commun 2:1547–1548

Robins MJ, Currie BL, Robinson RK, Bloch A (1969) The biological activity of 3-deazapyrimidine nucleosides. Proc Am Assoc Cancer Res 10:290

Roy-Burman P (1970) Analogues of nucleic acid components. Springer, Berlin Heidelberg New York, pp 1–113 (Recent results in cancer research, vol 25)

Rubin RJ, Jaffe JJ, Handschumacher RE (1962) Qualitative differences in the pyrimidine metabolism of *Trypanosoma equiperdum* and mammals, as characterized by 6-azauracil and 6-azauridine. Biochem Pharmacol 11:563–572

Seibert W (1947) Über den Mechanismus der Reaktion von Kishner-Wolff-Staudinger. Ber Dtsch Chem Ges 80:494–502

Škoda J (1963) Mechanism of action and application of azapyrimidines. In: Davidson JM, Cohn WE (eds) Progress in nucleic acid research and molecular biology, vol 2, Academic, New York, pp 197–210

Škoda J (1975) Azapyrimidine nucleosides. In: Sartorelli AC, Johns DG (eds) Antineoplastic and immunosuppressive agents. Springer, Berlin Heidelberg New York, pp 348–372 (Handbook of experimental phamacology, vol 38/2)

Škoda J, Šorm F (1959) The accumulation of orotic acid, uracil and hypoxanthine by *Escherichia coli* in the presence of 6-azauracil and the biosynthesis of 6-azauridylic acid. Coll Czech Chem Commun 24:1331–1337

Škoda J, Hess VF, Šorm F (1957a) The biosynthesis of 6-azauracil riboside by *Escherichia coli* growing in the presence of 6-azauracil. Experientia 13:150–151

Škoda J, Hess VF, Šorm F (1957b) Production of 6-azauracil riboside by *Escherichia coli* growing in the presence of 6-azauracil. Coll Czech Chem Commun 22:1330–1333

Škoda J, Kára J, Čihák A, Šorm F (1962) Formation of the ribonucleoside of 5-azauracil by *Escherichia coli* and isolation of ribosyl biuret as the main decomposition product of 5-azauridine. Coll Czech Chem Commun 27:1692–1693

Sköld O (1960) Uridine kinase from Ehrlich ascites tumor: purification and properties. J Biol Chem 235:3273–3279

Šorm F, Pískala A, Čihák A, Veselý J (1964) 5-Azacytidine, a new, highly effective cancerostatic. Experientia 20:202–203

Suttle DP, Stark GR (1979) Coordinate overproduction of orotate phosphoribosyltransferase and orotidine-5-phosphate decarboxylase in hamster cells resistant to pyrazofurin and 6-azauridine. J Biol Chem 254:4602–4607

Traut TW, Jones ME (1977) Inhibitors of orotate phosphoribosyltransferase and orotidine-5′-phosphate decarboxylase from mouse Ehrlich ascites cells: a procedure for analyzing the inhbition of a multienzyme complex. Biochem Pharmacol 26:2291–2296

Ullmann B, Levinson BB, Ullmann DH, Martin DW (1979) Isolation and characterization of cultured mouse T-lymphoma cells deficient in uridine-cytidine kinase. J Biol Chem 254:8736–8739

Vadlamudi S, Chaudry JN, Waravdekar JS, Kline I, Goldin A (1970) Effect of combination treatment with 5-azacytidine and cytidine on the life-span and spleen and bone marrow cells of leukemic (L1210) and nonleukemic mice. Cancer Res 30:362–369

Veselý J (1971) Resistance to pyrimidine analogs. In: Clark RL, Cumley RW, McCay JF, Copeland MM (eds). Oncology 1970, vol. 2, experimental cancer therapy. Yearbook Medical Publishers, Chicago, pp 265–274

Veselý J, Čihák A (1973) Resistance of mammalian tumor cells toward pyrimidine analogs (a review). Oncology 28:204–226

Veselý J, Čihák A (1978) 5-Azacytidine: mechanism of action and biological effects in mammalian cells. Pharmacol Ther A2:813–840

Veselý J, Čihák A, Šorm F (1967) Development of resistant to 5-azacytidine and simultaneous depression of pyrimidine metabolism in leukemic mice. Int J Cancer 2:639–646

Veselý J, Čihák A, Šorm F (1968 a) Biochemical mechanism of drug resistance. VII. Inhibition of orotic acid metabolism by 5-azacytidine in leukemic mice sensitive and resistant to 5-azacytidine. Biochem Pharmacol 17:519–524

Veselý J, Čihák A, Šorm F (1968 b) Characteristics of mouse leukemic cells resistant to 5-azacytidine and 5-aza-2′-deoxycytidine. Cancer Res 28:1995–2000

Veselý J, Čihák A, Šorm F (1970) Association of decreased uridine and deoxycytidine kinase with enhanced RNA and DNA polymerase in mouse leukemia cells resistant to 5-azacytidine. Cancer Res 30:2180–2186

Veselý J, Čihák A, Šorm F (1971) Enhanced stability of uridine kinase from mouse leukemic cells resistant to 5-azacytidine. Thermal inactivation and effect of *p*-chloro-mercuribenzoate. Eur J Biochem 22:551–556

Volle RL, Green RE, Peters L, Handschumacher RE, Welch AD (1962) Renal tubular excretion studies with pyrimidine derivatives and analogs. J Pharmacol Exp Ther 136:353–360

Voytek P, Beisler J, Wolpert-DeFilippes M, Driscoll J (1976) Initial studies on the cytotoxic action and metabolism of 5,6-dihydro-5-azacytidine. Pharmacologist 18:126

Voytek P, Beisler J, Abbasi MM, Wolpert-DeFilippes MK (1977) Comparative studies of the cytostatic action and metabolism of 5-azacytidine and 5,6-dihydro-5-azacytidine. Cancer Res 37:1956–1961

Wang MC, Bloch A (1972) Studies on the mode of action of 3-deazapyrimidines 1. Metabolism of 3-deazauridine and 3-deazacytidine in microbial and tumor cells. Biochem Pharmacol 21:1063–1073

Weiss AJ, Metter GE, Nealon TF, Keanan JP, Ramierz G, Swaiminathan A, Fletcher WS, Moss SE, Manthei RW (1977) Phase II study of 5-azacytidine in solid tumors. Cancer Treat Rep 61:55–58

Welch AD (1945) Interference with biological processes through the use of analogs of essential metabolites. Physiol Rev 25:687–715

Welch AD (1959) The problem of drug resistance in cancer chemotherapy. Cancer Res 19:359–371

Welch AD, Handschumacher RE, Finch SC, Jaffe JJ, Cardoso SS, Calabresi P (1960) A synopsis of recent investigations of 6-azauridine (NSC 32074). Cancer Chemother Rep 9:39–45

Welch AD, Germain GS, Ahmed NK (1982) Mechanisms of resistance of human lymphoblastoid cells to 3-deazauridine. Proc Am Assoc Cancer Res 23:4

Welch AD, Nemec J, Panahi J (1983) Quantitative determination of 3-deazauridine, 6-azauridine and their phosphate esters. FEBS Abstracts FR-247, p 293

Welch AD, Nemec J, Panahi J (1984) Quantitative determination of nucleosides and their phosphate esters. 1. The acidic nucleosides, 3-deazauridine and 6-azauridine. Int J Biochem (in press)
Wells W, Gaines D, Koenig H (1963) Studies of pyrimidine metabolism in the central nervous system. I. Metabolic effects and metabolism of 6-azauridine. J Neurochem 10:709–723
Wiesenfeld M, Crokaert R (1969) Effect of aza derivatives of uracil on *Saccharomyces cerevisiae*. III. Catabolic products of 6-azauracil. Bull Soc Chim Biol 51:951–960
Zedeck MS (1979) Incorporation of Ψ-isocytidine, a new antitumor C-nucleoside, into mammalian RNA and DNA. Biochem Pharmacol 28:1440–1443

CHAPTER 19

5-Halogenated Pyrimidines and Their Nucleosides

J. A. HOUGHTON and P. J. HOUGHTON

A. Introduction

The 5-halogenated pyrimidines and their nucleosides comprise a class of agents that have diverse biological effects upon eukaryotic cells. The thymidine (dThd) analogues 5-bromo-2′-deoxyuridine (BrdUrd) and 5-iodo-2′-deoxyuridine (IdUrd) are mutagenic (CHU et al. 1972; HUBERMAN and HEIDELBERGER 1972; STARK and LITTLEFIELD 1974), teratogenic (DI-PAOLO 1964; MURPHY 1965; PERCY 1975), and oncogenic (GOZ 1978). In addition, these agents have been shown to prevent, or reverse, cellular differentiation (HOLTZER et al. 1972; SILAGI and BRUCE 1970), sensitize cells to ionizing radiation (DJORDEVIC and Szybalski 1960; BERRY and ANDREWS 1962), and are cytotoxic at appropriate concentrations (JAFFE and PRUSOFF 1960; MATHIAS et al. 1959). Many of these effects are considered to be a consequence of incorporation of the analogue into DNA (PRUSOFF and GOZ 1974; GOZ 1978). In contrast, 5-fluorouracil (FUra), its ribonucleoside (FUrd), and 2′-deoxyribonucleoside (FdUrd) are not incorporated into the DNA of eukaryotic cells (HEIDELBERGER 1965, 1974).

Experimentally, 5-halogenated pyrimidines have shown cytotoxic activity against neoplastic cells in culture, and have been shown to prolong the lives of tumor-bearing animals, but only FUra and its derivatives appear to have clinical utility in the treatment of human malignancy. 5-Fluorouracil is at present one of the most effective agents for the palliative treatment of carcinomas of the breast, stomach, large bowel, pancreas, and ovary (CARTER 1972; 1974; MOERTEL and REITEMEIER 1969; YOUNG et al. 1974). This agent is curative therapy for noninvasive multiple basal-cell carcinomas (WILLIAMS and KLEIN 1970). Clinical responsiveness to FUra has been reviewed by HALL (1974). The majority of human cancers are naturally resistant (Table 1), and in patients who do respond to FUra therapy, the tumor response is often of short duration.

It is apparent that mechanisms conferring resistance to 5-halogenated pyrimidines are diverse. It is the purpose of this work to review factors that have been associated with both natural and acquired resistance to this class of antitumor agents, and to examine how a knowledge of these may be used in the design of therapy that may overcome such resistance.

B. Metabolism and Mechanism of Action

The biological activities of 5-halogenated pyrimidines and the mechanisms proposed by which they exert their effects upon prokaryotic and eukaryotic cells have

Table 1. Innate clinical resistance to 5-fluorouracil. (HALL 1974)

Tumor type	(%)
ALL	95
AML	95
CLL	100
Breast	75
Colon	75
Lung	90
Hodgkins lymphoma	95
Renal cell	95

ALL, acute lymphocytic leukemia; AML, acute myelocytic leukemia; CCL, chronic lymphocatic leukemia

been extensively reviewed by PRUSOFF and GOZ (1974), GOZ (1978), PRUSOFF et al. (1979), HEIDELBERGER and ANSFIELD (1963), HEIDELBERGER (1965, 1967, 1973, 1974), MANDEL (1969), and MANDEL et al. (1977). However, it is pertinent to the understanding of mechanisms of resistance to summarize briefly both the pathways utilized in the metabolism of these agents and the proposed mechanisms responsible for their cytotoxicity. The close chemical and structural similarities between dThd and IdUrd or BrdUrd allow utilization of these compounds as substrates for various enzymes concerned with the biosynthesis of DNA. These dThd analogues are incorporated into the DNA of mammalian cells and may prove cytotoxic as a consequence. The biochemical and physical effects that result from incorporation of halogenated uracils into nucleic acids have been reviewed by KIT (1962), SZYBALSKI (1962), BROCKMAN and ANDERSON (1963), ELION and HITCHINGS (1965), and PRUSOFF et al. (1965). In addition, 5-iodo-2′-deoxyuridine-5′-triphosphate (IdUTP) and 5-bromo-2′-deoxyuridine-5′-triphosphate (BrdUTP) act as allosteric effectors of enzymes in the de novo pathway for pyrimidine biosynthesis. PRUSOFF and CHANG (1969/1970) have shown that IdUTP was more inhibitory than thymidine-5′-triphosphate (dTTP) in exerting feedback inhibition on dThd kinase and also 2′-deoxycytidine-5′-monophosphate (dCMP) deaminase (PRUSOFF and CHANG 1968); BrdUTP and IdUTP are also better inhibitors of the enzyme ribonucleotide reductase than is dTTP (MEUTH and GREEN 1974). It is possible therefore that BrdUrd, IdUrd, and dThd may have a similar cytotoxic mechanism by depleting cells of 2′-deoxycytidine (dCyd) nucleotides (REICHARD et al. 1961; MORRIS and FISCHER 1960; BJURSELL and REICHARD 1973; ROLLER and COHEN 1976; REYNOLDS et al. 1979; FOX et al. 1979a).

5-Fluorouracil utilizes the same metabolic pathways as uracil (Ura) (Fig. 1) and may be cytotoxic to mammalian cells by one of at least two mechanisms. After intracellular conversion to 5-fluoro-2′-deoxyuridine-5′-monophosphate (FdUMP), this metabolite forms a tight binding quasi-irreversible complex with the enzyme thymidylate (dTMP) synthetase and N^5N^{10}-methylenetetrahydrofolate, the cofactor used in the conversion of 2′-deoxyuridine-5′-monophosphate (dUMP) to dTMP. This interaction and the consequences of inhibiting dTMP

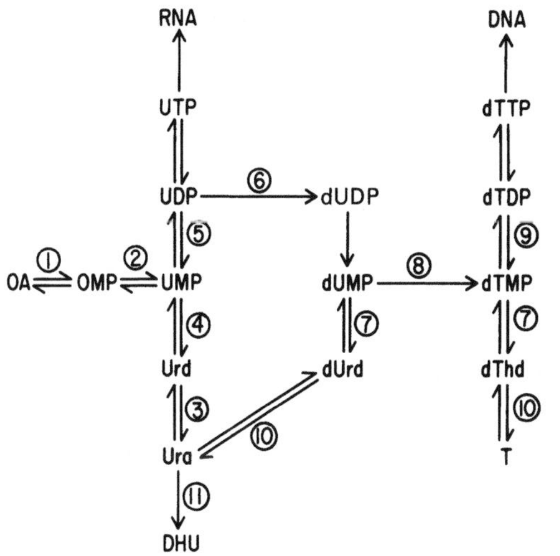

Fig. 1. *1*, orotate phosphoribosyltransferase; *2*, orotidine-5′-monophosphate decarboxylase; *3*, uridine phosphorylase; *4*, uridine kinase; *5*,, uridylate kinase; *6*, ribonucleotide reductase; *7*, thymidine kinase; *8*, thymidylate synthetase; *9*, thymidylate kinase; *10*, thymidine phosphorylase; *11*, dihydrouracil dehydrogenase

biosynthesis de novo have been reviewed by HEIDELBERGER (1965, 1974), DANENBERG (1977), and SANTI (1980). As shown in Fig. 1, FUra can be metabolized to FUTP and incorporated into RNA during transcription. The consequence of this is obscure, but after incorporation of analogue the post-transcriptional processing of rRNA is impaired (WILKINSON and PITOT 1973; WILKINSON et al. 1975; WILKINSON and CRUMLEY 1976; CARRICO and GLAZER 1979). LU et al. (1976) have suggested that the reduction in the content of 5-methyluridine, pseudouridine, and dihydrouridine, but not of 3-(3-amino-3-carboxypropyl) uridine in tRNA from the livers of mice treated with FUrd, was not simply due to analogue incorporation into tRNA; a direct action by some metabolite upon the activity of tRNA methyltransferase has been proposed (TSENG et al. 1978). The mechanism by which 5-fluoropyrimidines are cytotoxic may depend upon the characteristics of the cells studied and the experimental conditions employed (UMEDA and HEIDELBERGER 1968; EVANS et al. 1980; MAYBAUM et al. 1980).

C. Development and Stability

The development of resistance to FUra in tumor cells in vivo is relatively slow. In L1210 leukemia cells, complete resistance to FUra required 20 transplant generations, although only eight transplant generations in the presence of 1-(tetrahydrofuran-2yl)-5-fluorouracil (Ftorafur) (GARIBJANIAN et al. 1976). KASBEKAR and GREENBERG (1963) induced resistance in 16 transfers in the Gardner lymphosarcoma, although REICHARD et al. (1959) induced resistance to FUra comparatively rapidly within five passages, in both Ehrlich ascites carcinoma cells and L1210 leukemia in vivo. ROOSA et al. (1962) reported difficulty in deriving lines resistant to FUra and FUrd in vivo, while in P388 leukemia FOX and ANDERSON (1974) were unable to isolate clones of L5178Y cells in vitro resistant to IdUrd.

Resistance, based on genetic mutation where mutants arise spontaneously and are subsequently selected in the presence of a drug, is characterized by its stability (BROCKMAN 1974). FOX et al. (1969) demonstrated DNA-mediated transfer of IdUrd resistance in mammalian cells. Other data derived using mammalian cells in vitro, where resistant clones have been isolated using multiple-step techniques, or by single-step selection subsequent to mutagenesis, indicate a genetic basis for resistance to 5-halogenated pyrimidines (MULKINS and HEIDELBERGER 1980; PASZTOR et al. 1973; PASZTOR and HU 1972; CLIVE and VOYTEK 1977; CABOCHE 1974; ANDERSON and FOX 1974; WILKINSON et al. 1977; SLACK et al. 1976; MORSE and POTTER 1965; KIT et al. 1963). CABOCHE (1974) has estimated the rate of spontaneous mutation resulting in resistance to be less than 8.5×10^{-8}/cell per generation and that mutagenesis occurs during stepwise selection using BrdUrd. Consequently, where the selecting agent is also a mutagen, the frequency with which resistant clones are isolated may not be a measure of truly spontaneous mutation; this may account for the ten fold lower frequency reported for dThd compared with IdUrd (FOX and ANDERSON 1974).

Failure to maintain a resistant phenotype in the absence of selection pressure may indicate that resistance was due to epigenic factors, or alternatively to a high revertant frequency. HEIDELBERGER et al. (1960a) reported that a line of the Ehrlich ascites tumor reverted to FUra sensivitiy, and that another FUra-resistant line became more sensitive to this agent after 40 – 45 transplant generations in untreated mice. A line of L1210 leukemia, resistant to Ftorafur in vivo and cross-resistant to FUra, also regained sensitivity to the latter agent after only three serial transfers in the absence of selecting agent (GARIBJANIAN et al. 1976). Whether such instability of resistance is due to a small population of wild-type cells that originally were not eradicated by treatment complicates the interpretation of data derived from in vivo experiments. Two variant cell lines of C1300 mouse neuroblastoma resistant to FdUrd have been reported to be unstable in vitro. In one line characterized by elevated dTMP synthetase levels, resistance was lost exponentially in the absence of drug, with a 50% decline in activity during ten generations (BASKIN et al. 1975). Resistance in this line was reported subsequently to have stabilized (BASKIN et al. 1977). In the second line, dThd kinase deficient, resistance declined by 50% in 15 generations, representing a reversion rate of approximately 5×10^{-3}/cell per generation (BASKIN et al. 1977). This is far higher than that reported by SLACK et al. (1976) for spontaneous reversion to FdUrd sensitivity in DON cells (1×10^{-5}/cell per generation). The rate of spontaneous reversion in P388 cells resistant to IdUrd (1 to 9×10^{-7} cell/generation) was lower than the rate of forward mutation to resistance (FOX and ANDERSON 1974). CABOCHE (1974) reported a similar rate of spontaneous reversion to BrdUrd, but showed also that mutagenesis with ethyl methane sulfonate (EMS) could increase revertant rates. KAUFMAN and DAVIDSON (1979) observed a slight increase in sensitivity in an IdUrd-resistant melanoma line subcultured in the absence of drug. Recently, ADAIR and CARVER (1979) isolated clones of Chinese hamster ovary cells resistant to 5-trifluoromethyl-2′-deoxyuridine, trifluorothymidine (F_3dThd). The apparent spontaneous mutation rate, calculated from the

Luria-Delbrück fluctuation analysis (LURIA and DELBRÜCK 1943, was 1.5×10^{-6} cell per generation. Of interest is that none of these clones retained their resistance to F_3dThd when directly plated into drug-containing medium, indicating an unstable nonmutational expression of resistance, although F_3dThd has selected for stable dThd kinase-deficient mutants in a TK^{+-}heterozygote of L5178Y cells (BROWN and CLIVE 1977). FOX (1971) reported also that after selective doses of IdUrd (28 μM), no heritable resistance could be demonstrated in P388 mouse cells.

Data obtained using cells cloned in vitro show that resistance to 5-halogenated pyrimidines is a stable characteristic, indicative of a genetic basis. In contrast, resistance in tumors growing in laboratory animals shows greater variability, possibility a consequence of a heterogeneous tumor-cell population.

D. Transport

While resistance to amethopterin may be related to a decrease in a specific transport system (FISCHER 1962; KESSEL et al. 1965; SIROTNAK et al. 1968), the characterization of transport mutants resistant to halogenated pyrimidines and their nucleosides is less certain. In part this is due to the difficulty in dissociating membrane transport from intracellular metabolism to nucleotides, which are unable to exit freely from the cell. In Ehrlich cells in vitro, transport of FdUrd exceeded the rate of phosphorylation during the first 15 – 20 s (BOWEN et al. 1979). Rapid sampling and techniques that can separate transport from metabolism (PLAGEMANN and ERBE 1973; PLAGEMANN et al. 1978) are therefore necessary to characterize transport mutants. Thus early reports of transport variants must be considered with respect to these findings.

In a haploid frog-cell line, resistance to BrdUrd correlated with the absence of a specific dThd transport reaction (FREED and MEZGER-FREED 1973). These variants demonstrated between 40% and 100% of the dThd kinase activity of the wild-type cells, while the uptake of Urd and Cyd was decreased by approximately 50%. FOX and ANDERSON (1974) isolated two clones of P388 cells and one clone from the L5178Y murine lymhoma, resistant to dThd, that were considered to be "membrane mutants," since a reduction in incorporation of radiolabeled dThd was not associated with a change in dThd kinase activity. Similar mutants were not isolated using IdUrd. Variants of DON Chinese hamster fibroblasts resistant to dThd maintained high levels of dThd kinase and also incorporated radiolabeled dUrd (BRESLOW and GOLDSBY 1969). LYNCH et al. (1977) reported a line of HeLa cells resistant to BrdUrd and cross-resistant to FdUrd in which dThd kinase activity was comparable to that of parental cells. Rates of BrdUrd, FdUrd, and dThd uptake into resistant cells were considerably reduced, indicating an altered affinity of the transport systems for dThd and its analogues.

The dThd-transporter system appears tolerant to replacement of the 5-methyl group by Br, F, or H (LEUNG and VISSER 1976) or by I (PLAGEMANN and ERBE 1974). Thus from the available data, a deletion of dThd transport would be expected to confer resistance to other pyrimidine 2′-deoxynucleosides. In erythrocytes both dThd and Urd appeared to be transported by the same mechanism with equal facility (CASS and PATERSON 1972), and ATP-depleted Novikoff cells transported all nucleosides by the same system although with different efficiencies (PLAGEMANN et al. 1976; 1978). The reports of dThd-transport-deficient lines, which take up pyrimidine ribonucleosides (FREED and MEZGER-FREED 1973) or dUrd (BRESLOW and GOLDSBY 1969), may indicate a change in the structural requirements of the transporter.

The transport of pyrimidine bases is not resolved. JACQUEZ (1962) showed that Ura, Thy, and FUra entered Ehrlich cells by simple diffusion, the rate of uptake being directly proportional to the extracellular concentration. In Novikoff cells, however, the uptake of Ura was shown to be a saturable process in the absence of phosphoribosylation (PLAGEMANN and RITCHEY 1974). More recent reports indicate a K_m (zero time) of about 6.3 m*M* for Ura (PLAGEMANN et al. 1978). It has also been suggested that FUra and BrUra are actively transported by a pyrimidine transport system of the intestine (SCHANKER and JEFFREY 1961). Failure to transport halogenated pyrimidine bases, as distinct from failure to metabolize them further intracellularly, has not been reported to be responsible for acquired resistance in neoplastic cells.

Where transport has been adequately dissociated from the subsequent metabolism of halogenated nucleosides, rates of uptake have been demonstrated to be reduced in resistant cells. As these compounds appear to enter cells by a common nucleoside transporter, cross-resistance between these drugs would be anticipated.

E. Decreased Lethal Synthesis

I. Thymidine Kinase

In cell lines that acquire resistance to dThd analogues, including BrdUrd, IdUrd, F_3dThd, or the derivative of dUrd, FdUrd, there is often an associated decrease in the incorporation of radiolabeled dThd into both the nucleotide pool and DNA (SLACK et al. 1976; KIT et al. 1963; DUBBS and KIT 1964; WOLBERG 1970; FOX and ANDERSON 1974; ZIELKE 1979). Acquired resistance has most frequently been associated with a decrease in dThd kinase activity (KIT et al. 1963; UMEDA and HEIDELBERGER 1968; SCHIMMER et al. 1974; CABOCHE 1974; KIT et al. 1973; ROUFA et al. 1973).

MORRIS and FISCHER (1960) isolated a subline of the murine mast-cell tumor that was resistant to both FdUrd and dThd. KIT et al. (1963) demonstrated that a mouse fibroblast cell line chronically exposed to BrdUrd was dThd kinase deficient. By treatment of wild-type fibroblasts with 3–5 μg/ml or 30 μg/ml of BrdUrd, LITTLEFIELD (1965) obtained sublines that were partially or highly resistant to this analogue, and partially or essentially deficient in dThd kinase activity. Resistance to BrdUrd was associated with a decrease in dThd kinase activity to 2% of that observed in wild-type BHK 21/13 Syrian hamster kidney cells (CABOCHE 1974). Similarly, using chemical mutagens and a single-step selection procedure with FdUrd (10 μ*M*), MULKINS and HEIDELBERGER (1980) isolated L1210 and P388 mouse leukemic cells that were 4000- to 25000-fold more resistant to this agent than were the respective wild-type cells, and contained only 0.04% of the dThd kinase acitivity. KIT et al. (1972) demonstrated the presence of the mitochondrial form of dThd kinase in BrdUrd-resistant cell lines of mouse and human origin, despite the loss of high-speed supernatant (cytosol) enzyme from the mutant cells. The BrdUrd-resistant subline of Hela S3 cells showed normal levels of mitochondrial dThd kinase and preferentially incorporated radiolabeled dThd into superhelical mitochondrial DNA (BERK and CLAYTON 1973). Thymidine kinase from the mutant line was able to utilize ATP, UTP, GTP, and CTP as phosphate donors, in contrast to the mitochondrial enzyme in wild-type cells, which utilized only ATP. Residual dThd kinase activity in mouse L cells resistant to BrdUrd was found to be exclusively associated with mitochondria (KAUFMAN and DAVIDSON 1977a). SLACK et al. (1976) using autoradiographic techniques have demonstrated, however, that small numbers of grains are associated specifically with the nuclei of FdUrd-resistant Chinese hamster cells incubated with radiolabeled dThd.

Although many studies have related the development of resistance to dThd or dUrd analogues to changes in dThd kinase activity, there are several exceptions. In clones of a hamster melanoma cell line resistant to BrdUrd, analogue incorporation correlated with the ability of these cells to utilize exogenous dThd (KAUFMAN and DAVIDSON 1977a). There was no such relationship, however, between analogue incorporation and the activity in vitro of dThd kinase, and this could not be explained by a change in the substrate specificity of dThd kinase. Resistant cell lines were found to grow equally well in HAT medium (medium containing hypoxanthine, amethopterin, and thymidine) and in medium lacking aminopterin, indicating the ability of these cells to utilize preformed dThd. Similarly, MORSE and POTTER (1965) demonstrated that a line derived from the Novikoff hepatoma, resistant to high concentrations of dThd (1 m*M*), retained a very high level of dThd kinase. KAUFMAN and DAVIDSON (1979) have also shown in one cell line that resistance to IdUrd was not associated with a decrease in dThd kinase activity, although other studies have demonstrated decreased activity of this enzyme in P388 mouse leukemic cells resistant to IdUrd (FOX 1971; FOX and ANDERSON 1974; ANDERSON and FOX 1974).

II. Uridine Phosphorylase; Uridine Kinase

Reduction in the activities of enzymes involved in the conversion of FUra or FUrd to nucleotides has been shown to be responsible for resistance to these agents in a variety of experimental tumors. A reduced, but not complete, loss of the formation of nucleotides from FUra and decreased incorporation of FUra into RNA in FUra- and FUrd-resistant sublines of the P815 mast-cell neoplasm (BROCKMAN and LAW 1960) and in L1210 leukemia resistant to both 6MP and FUra (LAW 1962) has been reported. In N_1S_1/FdUrd cells, cross-resistant to FUra, WILKINSON and CRUMLEY (1977) found that, in addition to the loss of dThd kinase activity, the conversion of FUra to ribonucleotides was also greatly depressed, while levels of ribonucleotide reductase were identical in both sensitive and resistant lines. A FUra-resistant line, of the P388 murine leukemia was found, however, to contain a decreased level of uridine-5′-monophosphate (UMP) kinase (ARDALAN et al. 1980).

Almost complete, but not absolute, resistance to prolonged treatment with FUra in vivo was reported by the fifth passage in a line of the Ehrlich ascites tumor by REICHARD et al. (1959). Resistance was characterized by the absence of both uridine (Urd) and 2′-deoxyuridine (dUrd) phosphorylases, with some decrease in the activity of Urd kinase, while that of dUrd kinase was virtually unchanged. A FUra-resistant line of the L1210 ascites tumor was found also to have reduced activity of Urd kinase, and a smaller decrease in Urd phosphorylase, while the phosphorylase and kinase of dUrd remained at low levels. In a later report, four FUra-resistant lines of the Ehrlich ascites tumor were developed in vivo (REICHARD et al. 1962). In each line, the activity of Urd kinase (but not that of Urd or dUrd phosphorylase, dUrd kinase, or the enzymes involved in the conversion of orotic acid to UMP) gradually decreased, beginning at approximately the tenth passge. Concentrations of FUra nucleotides were lower in the resistant lines than in the parent tumor, although drug permeability was similar between the five lines. Cross-resistance of FUrd and FdUrd was obtained after 25 – 30 passages. In two lines, resistance to FUra was obtained, however, before Urd kinase activity was decreased, and at this time, one of these lines was cross-resistant to FdUrd but not to FUrd. KESSEL et al. (1971) demonstrated reduced activities of both Urd phosphorylase and Urd kinase in a FUra-resistant line of P388 leukemia, while in lines of the P815 ascitic mast-cell tumor resistant to FUra or FUrd, ANDERSON et al. (1962) reported a decrease in both the rate and extent of UMP synthesis; these lines demonstrated reduced activity of Urd kinase and reduced conversion of [^{14}C]FUra to nucleotides. GOLDBERG et al. (1966) found that L1210 cells incorporated more FUra into FUrd, phosphorylated intermediates, and RNA than did L1210 cells that were resistant to FUra due to a decrease in Urd phosphorylase activity.

KESSEL et al. (1971) selected P388 leukemia cells for resistance to FUrd, after prior exposure to a terephthalanilide (P388/38280); these cells were deficient in the activities of both Urd phosphorylase and Urd kinase. More recently, MULKINS and HEIDELBERGER (1980) treated L1210 and P388 cells with mutagens prior to the selection of cells for resistance to FUrd. The clones selected in 10^{-6} M FUrd were 100- to 200-fold more resistant to growth inhibition by this agent, and were found to contain only 3% – 20% of the Urd kinase activity of the wild-type cells.

III. Orotate Phosphoribosyltransferase; Orotidine-5′-Monophosphate Decarboxylase

KASBEKAR and GREENBERG (1963) selected a FUra-resistant line of the Gardner lymphosarcoma in vivo; with increasing resistance, orotic acid decarboxylating activity decreased, and no 5-fluorouridine-5′-monophosphate (FUMP) was formed from FUra in resistant cells, suggesting the absence of orotate phosphoribosyltransferase (OPRTase), while dTMP synthetase levels were unchanged.

A mutant of S49 cultured mouse T-lymhoma cells that contained 50% of the wild-type levels of both OPRTase and orotidine-5′-monophosphate (OMP) decarboxylase was obtained by initial exposure of the mutagen *N*-methyl-*N*′-nitro-*N*-nitrosoguanidine (MNNG), followed by selection for resistance to FUra (ULL-

MAN and KIRSCH 1979; LEVINSON et al. 1979). Using similar procedures, others have also demonstrated reduced levels of OPRTase in L1210 and P388 cells selected for resistance to FUra (MULKINS and HEIDELBERGER 1980). The 745A strain of erythroleukemic cells, after exposure to MNNG, and subsequently to 5-fluoroorotate (FO) and Urd, was found to require Urd for growth and was deficient in OPRTase, 5-fluoroorotate phosphoribosyltransferase (FOPRTase), and OMP decarboxylase in comparison to the parent line; other enzymes tested, namely carbamyl phosphate synthetase, aspartate transcarbamylase, dihydroorotase, dihydroorotic acid dehydrogenase, Urd phosphorylase, and Urd kinase, remained at similar levels in sensitive and resistant lines (KROOTH et al. 1979).

The predominant mechanism by which cells are resistant to 5-halogenated pyrimidines is therefore through a decreased ability to form phosphorylated derivatives. For nucleoside analogues, decreased activity of the respective kinase is a frequent observation; presumably such cells must subsequently depend upon synthesis of nucleotides de novo. In addition, resistance to 5-halogenated bases has been characterized by failure to form nucleotides, although this may occur at the level of the phosphorylase, the kinase, or, in certain instances, be due to the decreased activity of pyrimidine phosphoribosyltransferase.

F. Changes in Enzyme Characteristics

I. Altered (Mutated) Enzymes

There are several reports providing data supportive of biophysical changes in certain enzymes involved in the metabolism of 5-halogenated pyrimidines during the induction of resistance. SKÖLD (1963) observed changes in the physical properties of Urd kinase from Ehrlich ascites tumor lines resistant to FUra, including changes in the elution profile on diethylaminoethanol (DEAE) cellulose and decreased stability to heat inactivation. Such properties may be explained in part by a change in the ratio of isoenzymes from the adult form (type I) to the embryonic (type II) variant, found in normal tissues, observed during the induction of resistance to FUra (GREENBERG et al. 1977). It is of interest that isoenzyme II demonstrated a lower affinity for FUrd. HEIDELBERGER et al. (1960b) isolated a line of the Ehrlich ascites tumor resistant to 5-fluorinated pyrimidines. The structure of the active site of the enzyme dTMP synthetase was altered in such a way that it could discriminate between the natural substrate dUMP and the potent inhibitor FdUMP. Similar changes were not observed in other studies (HÄGGMARK 1962; ARDALAN et al. 1980). However, a variant of the C1300 mouse neuroblastoma resistant to FdUrd demonstrated 30% of the activity of dTMP synthetase that was not inhibited in the presence of 5 m*M* FdUrd in cultured cells. It was concluded that either the enzyme had a reduced affinity for FdUMP or that some portion of the enzyme was compartmentalized so as to be inaccessible to this inhibitor (BASKIN et al. 1977). WOLBERG (1964) also suggested that the failure of some human cancers to respond to treatment with fluorinated pyrimidines may be due to an insensitive dTMP synthetase. Data consistent with a structural gene mutation in a variant of the S49 mouse T-lymphoma mutagenized initially by MNNG and subsequently selected for growth in medium containing FUra have been reported (LEVINSON et al. 1979). Although no major changes in OPRTase or OMP decarboxylase were observed by K_m or K_i analysis, heat stability, or isoelectric point, there was a three- to four-fold increase in the apparent K_m of OPRTase for FUra. KAUFMAN and DAVIDSON (1979) reported that a line of Syrian hamster melanoma cells selected for resistance to high levels of IdUrd readily incorporated dThd and BrdUrd and possessed normal levels of dThd kinase. In contrast to the wild-type cell, this variant was unable to phosphorylate IdUrd beyond the monophosphate, suggesting that resistance in this line involved a change in the substrate specificity of dTMP kinase. CABOCHE (1974) also reported a slight but significant change in the substrate affinity of dThd kinase from a spontaneous revertant of BrdUrd-resistant Syrian hamster kidney cells.

II. Increased Enzyme Activities

In contrast to the association of resistance with a decreased lethal synthesis, increased levels of target enzymes have been reported. Thus the intracellular concentration of agent, or its active metabolite, may no longer be sufficient to inhibit the metabolic pathway and subsequently achieve cytotoxicity. Examples of this are illustrated by the increase in the level of dihydrofolate reductase during the development of resistance to methotrexate (MTX) (FISCHER 1971; MISRA et al. 1961), or the increase in activity of OMP decarboxylase during the development of resistance to 6-azauridine (LEVINSON et al. 1979). A clone of C1300 mouse neuroblastoma, 2000-fold resistant to FdUrd, demonstrated an eightfold elevation in the level of dTMP synthetase while maintaining normal levels of dThd kinase (BASKIN et al. 1975). Further studies showed that this increase in activity was not associated with a change in cytoplasmic inhibitors or activators, a decreased rate of degradation of the enzyme, or the synthesis of a new species with an increased V_{max} (BASKIN and ROSENBERG 1975). WILKINSON et al. (1977) found increased dTMP synthetase activity in a FdUrd-resistant variant of the Novikoff hepatoma, which also had decreased activity of dThd kinase (MORSE and POTTER 1965). This cell line, in addition, possessed slightly elevated activities of both dCMP deaminase and ribonucleotide reductase. The possibility that the increase in dTMP synthetase activity in these cells was either an adaptive response, which allowed biosynthesis of dTMP de novo to compensate for decreased dTMP formation via the salvage pathway, or was an essential part of the resistance to FdUrd, was not determined. HARDS et al. (1979) reported that two lines of Chinese hamster ovary cells, highly resistant to FUra, exhibited enhanced levels of ribonucleotide reductase. Of interest are reports that MTX and other folate antagonists may elevate the level of dTMP synthetase (ROBERTS and LOEHR 1971; MALEY and MALEY 1971; CHELLO et al. 1976). Under these conditions cells would be expected to be less sensitive to FdUrd cytotoxicity.

Several reports have indicated changes in enzyme characteristics in cells resistant to 5-halogenated pyrimidines. Most frequently the alteration is one that allows the enzyme to discriminate between its natural substrate and the analogue.

Table 2. Resistance to 5-halogenated pyrimidines and their nucleosides in experimental tumors

Tumor	Sensitivity	Selecting agent	Retention of sensitivity	Cross-resistance	Collateral sensitivity	References
Ehrlich	FUra, FdUrd, FUrd	FUra	FUrd	FdUrd (partial)		HEIDELBERGER et al. (1958a)
	FUra, FdUrd, FUrd	FUra		FUrd, FdUrd		HEIDELBERGER et al. (1960a)
	FUra, FdUrd, FUrd	FUra	FUrd	FdUrd		REICHARD et al. (1962)
		FUra		FUrd, FdUrd		
	FUra, FdUrd, F_3Thy, F_3dThd	FdUrd		F_3dThd, FUra (incomplete) F_3Thy (partial)		HEIDELBERGER and ANDERSON (1964)
L1210	FUra, FdUrd, FUrd, FO, FdCyd	FUra		FdUrd, FUrd (partial), FO (partial), FdCyd		HUTCHISON et al. (1962)
	FUra, FdUrd, FUrd, FO	6MP/FUra		FUrd, FdUrd, FO		LAW (1962)
	FUra, Ftorafur	FUra		Ftorafur		GARIBJANIAN et al. (1976)
		Ftorafur		FUra		
P815	FUra, FUrd, FO	FUra		FUrd, FO		BROCKMAN and LAW (1960)
		FUrd		FUra, FO		
P388	FUra, FdUrd, FUrd	FUra		FdUrd, FUrd (partial)		ROOSA et al. (1962)
		FUrd	FdUrd	FUra (incomplete)		
		FdUrd	FUra	FUrd (partial)		
	FUra, FdUrd, FUrd	NSC38280/FUrd		FUra, FdUrd		KESSEL et al. (1971)
		FUra		FdUrd	FUrd	
Novikoff	FUra, FdUrd	FdUrd		FUra		MORSE and POTTER (1965)
	FUra, FdUrd, FUrd	FdUrd		FUra		CORY et al. (1977)
	FUra, FUrd	FUra		FUrd		GREENBERG et al. (1977)
	FUra, FdUrd, FUrd, F_3dThd, IdUrd, DHFdUrd	FdUrd		FUra, FUrd, F_3dThd, IdUrd, DHFdUrd (partial)		UMEDA and HEIDELBERGER (1968)

Table 2. (continued)

Tumor	Sensitivity	Selecting agent	Retention of sensitivity	Cross-resistance	Collateral sensitivity	References
HeLa	FUra, FdUrd, BrdUrd	BrdUrd	FUra	FdUrd		LYNCH et al. (1977)
Syrian hamster melanoma	FdUrd, BrdUrd, IdUrd, CldUrd	CldUrd		BrdUrd, FdUrd (partial), IdUrd (partial)		KAUFMAN and DAVIDSON (1977b)
		IdUrd	FdUrd	BrdUrd (partial) CldUrd (partial)		
L5178Y	FUra, FdUrd, FUrd, IdUrd, F_3Thd, DHFdUrd	FdUrd	FUrd, DHFdUrd	IdUrd, F_3dThd	FUra	UMEDA and HEIDELBERGER (1968)
	FUra, FUrd, FUMP, FUMP-methylester, FUMP-decylester, FUMP-hexadecylester, FUMP-benzylester	MNNG/FUrd		FUMP, FUra (partial), FUMP-methylester, FUMP-decylester, FUMP-benzylester, FUMP-hexadecyl-ester (partial)		KANZAWA et al. (1979)

G. Cross-Resistance and Collateral Sensitivity

5-Halogenated pyrimidines and their nucleosides that have been used in the induction of resistance in a variety of neoplastic cell lines are shown in Table 2. From the references cited, the original sensitivity of the parent lines to these agents, together with the retention of sensitivity, cross-resistance, and collateral sensitivity after resistance development, if studied, have also been documented.

H. Tolerance

There are several reports describing cells that have developed resistance to the cytotoxic actions of dThd analogues, where the formation of the putative cytotoxic metabolite or incorporation of the analogue into nucleic acid has not changed. In some reports, cell lines became dependent upon the drug for continued proliferation (DAVIDSON and BICK 1973). KAUFMAN and DAVIDSON (1977 a) isolated clones of melanoma cells resistant to BrdUrd that demonstrated up to 72% substitution of dThd by BrdUrd in nuclear DNA. This suggested that exclusion of BrdUrd from the cells was not a primary mechanism of resistance. In further studies (KAUFMAN and DAVIDSON 1977 b), two cell lines, both requiring high concentrations of BrdUrd for optimal growth, could substitute 5-chloro-2′-deoxyuridine (CldUrd) but not other dThd analogues. 5-Bromo-2′-deoxyuridine-tolerant variants from B16 melanoma have also been described (PASZTOR et al. 1973). An interesting observation made by HENDERSON and STRAUSS (1975) was that cell lines derived either from individuals recovering from infectious mononucleosis, or from healthy adult donors, were, with one exception, unable to replicate for more than one division in the presence of BrdUrd. The analogue was incorporated into only one strand of DNA. In contrast, lymphoblastoid lines derived from Burkitt's lymphoma were capable of at least two rounds of DNA replication in the presence of BrdUrd and produced DNA with analogue substitution in both strands.

Although many of the effects on cells can be related to the incorporation of 5-halogenated pyrimidines into nuclear DNA (see review by GOZ 1978), it has been suggested that the cytotoxic effects of BrdUrd may be due to the inhibition of ribonucleotide reductase by BrdUTP and subsequent depletion of deoxycytidine nucleotides (MEUTH and GREEN 1974). Addition of dCyd to the growth medium reversed the toxic effects, but reduced the incorporation of BrdUrd into DNA. Such reversal was not observed in the presence of aminopterin (KAUFMAN and DAVIDSON 1978). MORSE and POTTER (1965) isolated a line of Novikoff hepatoma cells resistant to high levels of dThd, but possessing dThd kinase activity. An alteration in cytidine diphosphate (CDP) reductase, such as to render it less sensitive to feedback control by dTTP, was hypothesized.

For many 5-halogenated pyrimidines the lesion responsible for cytotoxicity is unclear. For cell tolerance to be more readily understood, it is apparent that the precise mechanism responsible for cytotoxicity must be elucidated.

J. Natural Resistance

The great majority of human cancers, with the exception of basal-cell carcinoma of the skin (WILLIAMS and KLEIN 1970), fail to respond to therapy with halogenated pyrimidine analogues at dose levels causing acceptable host toxicity (HALL 1974; CARTER 1974; MOERTEL 1978). Such tumors are naturally resistant. Although kinetics of cell proliferation and drug distribution must influence the efficacy of an agent, mounting evidence suggests that differential metabolism between normal and neoplastic tissues is a critical factor in determining the efficacy of 5-fluoropyrimidines.

I. Formation of Nucleotides

KESSEL et al. (1966) indicated the importance of nucleotide formation as a determinant of sensitivity to FUra in murine leukemias. The efficacy of FUra in extending the life span of tumor-bearing mice correlated with the capacity of each tumor line for nucleotide formation in vitro. Further, REYES and HALL (1969) demonstrated a significant correlation between the activity of OPRTase in murine leukemias and their sensitivity to FUra. Similar observations were made in bovine leukemias (KESSEL et al. 1973). Other reports have suggested that natural resistance may be due to factors other than nucleotide formation. In P388/38280, a murine leukemia selected for resistance to the terephthalanilide, 2-chloro-4′,4″-di-2-imidiazolin-2-yl, dihydrochloride (NSC-38280, BURCHENAL et al. 1962), conversion of FUra to nucleotides was significantly reduced compared with wild-type P388 cells, although both lines showed similar sensitivity to FUra (KESSEL et al. 1969). KESSEL and WODINSKY (1970) found an inverse correlation between the level of dThd kinase and the response of murine leukemias to FdUrd in vivo. Cell lines most capable of converting FdUrd to FdUMP, also, therefore, possessed an increased ability to salvage preformed dThd, thereby circumventing the blockade of dTMP biosynthesis de novo. Further reports by this group have shown tumor sensitivity to FUrd to be inversely correlated with the activity of Urd phosphorylase in P388 leukemia (KESSEL et al. 1971). Subsequently, it was suggested that a low activity of dThd kinase and a high level of OPRTase would be favorable for responsiveness to FUra (NAHAS et al. 1974). Activities of dTMP synthetase, dThd kinase, and OPRTase did not correlate with FUra responsiveness in patients with colon carcinoma, and comparison of the tumor/normal tissue ratios of OPRTase did not allow identification of patients responsive to FUra therapy. It is worthy of note that 5-fluorocytosine (FCyt), an agent that is not metabolized by mammalian cells, is inactive as an anticancer agent in several experimental tumors (HEIDELBERGER et al. 1958b; LAW 1958), while its 2′-deoxynucleoside, FdCyd, which is converted to nucleotides, is active (BURCHENAL et al. 1959).

II. Formation of 5-Fluoro-2′-Deoxyuridylate

Conversion to the nucleotide level may prove, therefore, only an initial, although essential, step in a complex series of interactions that ultimately result in cell death. Both the level and duration of inhibition of dTMP synthetase may also prove to be critical factors in the determination of responsiveness. ARDALAN et al. (1978) reported the peak concentration of FdUMP and the kinetics of its clearance to correlate with the responsiveness of two murine colon tumors. Similarly, KLUBES et al. (1978) concluded that the failure of the Walker 256 carcinosarcoma to respond to FUra was due to rapid elimination of FdUMP and not to an inability to form this metabolite. HOUGHTON and HOUGHTON (1980a) examined the metabolism of FUra, FUrd and FdUrd in four lines of human colon adenocarcinoma maintained in immune-deprived mice. In these studies, the agent producing the greatest concentration and maintenance of free FdUMP within a sensitive line was also the most effective at inhibiting tumor growth. Concentrations of FdUMP were equally as high, however, within the insensitive tumors, suggesting that failure to synthesize the putative active metabolite was not the final determinant of sensitivity. RUSTUM et al. (1979) also related FUra sensitivity in L1210 and L1210/Fura leukemias to peak levels and retention of FdUMP. Unbound FdUMP has also been determined in vivo after FUra administration by others (MYERS et al. 1975; CHADWICK and ROGERS 1972; CHADWICK and CHANG 1976; MURINSON et al. 1979). In vitro, however, free FdUMP has been detected only after inhibition of dTMP synthetase activity (MORAN et al. 1979b), or only if present in excess of dTMP synthetase (LASKIN et al. 1979), or after heat dissociation of the ternary complex (WASHTIEN and SANTI 1979). Differences observed between in vitro and in vivo data may be caused by artifacts from tissue sampling in vivo, leading to dissociation of the complex, or, alternatively, conditions in vivo may not prove ideal for formation of the ternary complex, particularly in solid tumors.

III. Accumulation of 2′-Deoxyuridylate

The duration of inhibition of dTMP synthetase may depend upon the maintenance of a critical level of FdUMP. Several studies have shown, however, that concentrations of unbound FdUMP remain relatively high for prolonged periods of time after FUra administration (ARDALAN et al. 1978; MYERS et al. 1975; HOUGHTON and HOUGHTON 1980a). Accumulation of dUMP after inhibition of dTMP synthetase has been shown (MYERS et al. 1975; EVANS et al. 1980; JACKSON 1978). Although dUMP does not displace FdUMP, or alter the rate of dissociation of FdUMP, from the ternary complex (DANENBERG and DANENBERG 1978), it may protect newly synthesized or regenerated enzyme from inactivation by competing with FdUMP. The accumulation of dUMP, particularly in cells of normal limiting tissues, may prove important in determining the selectivity of fluorinated pyrimidines. MYERS et al. (1975) showed that recovery of dTMP biosynthesis appeared to correlate with both the maximum accumulation of dUMP and a decline in the concentration of free FdUMP. ARDALAN et al. (1978) and KLUBES et al. (1978) related the recovery of dTMP biosynthesis de novo (using incorporation of [6-^{3}H]dUrd into DNA) to a decrease in levels of free FdUMP. However, with [6-^{3}H]dUrd incorporation studies, compensation for isotope dilution by dUMP pool expansion may be inadequate, as JACKSON (1978) has demonstrated a greater expansion of the dUrd pool in FdUrd-treated N_1S_1 cells in vitro.

IV. Concentration of N^5N^{10}-Methylenetetrahydrofolate

It has generally been considered that inhibition of dTMP synthetase by FdUMP is essentially irreversible in vivo. However, the original kinetic studies using extracts from Ehrlich ascites tumor demonstrated classical competitive inhibition (HARTMAN and HEIDELBERGER 1961). REYES and HEIDELBERGER (1965) demonstrated also that enzyme which had been inhibited by incubation with FdUMP and cofactor regained full activity after dialysis for 16 h. Accordingly, the rate of enzyme reactivation, and factors that may influence this, should be considered as determinants of the chemotherapeutic effectiveness of 5-fluoropyrimidines. Dissociation of the dTMP synthetase-FdUMP-N^5N^{10}-methylenetetrahydrofolate complex in the presence of either dUMP or FdUMP is quite rapid ($t\frac{1}{2}=36$ min) at 37 °C (DANENBERG and DANENBERG 1978). SANTI et al. (1974) also showed that this dissociation was a temperature-dependent first-order process and concluded that the enzyme itself catalyzes the breakdown to regenerate FdUMP and free dTMP synthetase. The rate was independent of FdUMP or dUMP (DANENBERG and DANENBERG 1978), but was a function of N^5N^{10}-methylenetetrahydrofolate concentration. Hence, at the low concentrations of cofactor reported in neoplastic cells (3 – 6 µ*M* in L1210 cells in vitro) (MORAN et al. 1976; JACKSON and HARRAP 1973), recovery of enzyme activity may be quite rapid. Low N^5N^{10}-methylenetetrahydrofolate concentrations can therefore determine both the level of enzyme inhibition by 5-fluoropyrimidines and the stability of that inhibition. ULLMAN et al. (1978) have shown a definitive relationship between the sensitivity to FdUrd in L1210 cells in vitro and the availability of reduced folates. Of interest was that concentrations of folinic acid (5-formyltetrahydrolate), optimal for cell proliferation, were suboptimal for FdUrd cytotoxicity, and for formation of the ternary complex. Data from studies using human colorectal adenocarcinomas growing in immune-deprived mice also support the role of reduced folate cofactors as determinants of tumor sensitivity to 5-fluoropyrimidines (HOUGHTON et al. 1981). Addition of N^5N^{10}-methylenetetrahydrofolate was required to achieve maximum ternary complex formation in nonresponsive tumor lines, but not in sensitive tumors, where sufficient endogenous cofactor was available. The data suggested that, in nonresponsive tumors in situ, levels of cofactor were inadequate to allow complete inactivation of dTMP synthetase, even in the presence of excess FdUMP. Using a direct assay of enzyme activity (see Fig. 2, HxVRC$_5$), incubation with FdUMP produced only 50% inhibition, while addition of cofactor decreased activity by 95%. In responsive lines (e.g., HxHC$_1$), incubation either with or without N^5N^{10}-methylenetetrahydrofolate resulted in almost complete inhibition of enzyme activity in the presence of FdUMP.

V. Enzyme Activities

In view of the finding that FdUrd resistance was associated with an increase in the activity of dTMP synthetase (BASKIN et al. 1974), the activity of this enzyme may be a determinant of tumor sensitivity. HALL et al. (1968) found no correlation between the activities of Urd kinase, dThd kinase, and dTMP synthetase in various tumor cells, and their sensitivities to FUra. HOUGHTON et al. (1981) also could not relate the activity of dTMP synthetase to 5-fluoropyrimidine sensitivity in human colorectal tumor xenografts.

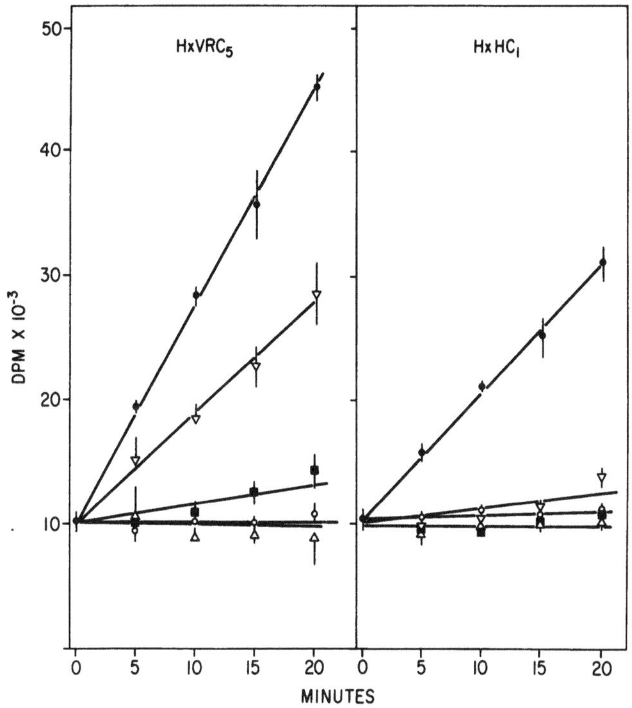

Fig. 2. Activity of dTMP synthetase in cytosols preincubated with excess FdUMP with or without added N^5N^{10}-methylenetetrahydrofolate. Preincubation: ●, cytosol+buffer; ○, cytosol+buffer; △, cytosol+FdUMP; ▽, cytosol+FdUMP; ■, cytosol+FdUMP+N^5N^{10}-methylenetetrahydrofolate. Postincubation: [5^3H]dUMP was added to each reaction mixture, and either excess N^5N^{10}-methylenetetrahydrofolate (●, ▽, ■) or buffer (○, △). Results show the mean ±SD for triplicate determinations from representative experiments using cytosols from $HxVRC_5$ and $HxHC_1$ tumors. (HOUGHTON et al. 1981)

VI. Catabolism

Few data are available to indicate whether sensitivity is determined by the rate of catabolism of halogenated pyrimidines by tumor cells, although high catabolism/anabolism ratios would, presumably, favor insensitivity (CANO et al. 1980). The behavior of the activity of opposing pathways of dThd utilization with respect to growth rate has been studied in a series of rat hepatomas (FERDINANDUS et al. 1971). With increasing growth rate the ratio of anabolism to catabolism increased by some five orders of magnitude, although whether this correlated with an increased sensitivity to dThd analogues was not reported. Fox et al. (1979a) correlated the sensitivity of cultured leukemic lymphocytes to dThd with reduced activity of the catabolic enzyme dThd phosphorylase and sustained elevation of the dTTP pool. QUEENER et al. (1971) also showed that the activity of dihydrouracil (DHU) dehydrogenase, considered to be the rate-limiting enzyme in the catabolic pathway of Ura and thymine (Thy), decreased in parallel with the increase in the growth rate of hepatomas. Studies using Ehrlich ascites cells failed to demonstrate catabolism of FUra in either parent or resistant lines (CHAUDHURI et al. 1958; MUKHERJEE and HEIDELBERGER 1960), but found degradation in normal tissues. In this system catabolism may not relate to tumor sensitivity, but may correlate with drug selectivity. 5-Fluorouridine and FdUrd were degraded by Ehrlich cells (BIRNIE et al. 1963). The 5-substituted dThd analogues are rapidly degraded in man (CALABRESI et al. 1961) and are better substrates for dThd phosphorylase than is dThd (NAKAYAMA et al. 1980). Further studies on the role of drug catabolism in tumors as a determinant of sensitivity to halogenated pyrimidines are required before its importance in the effectiveness of these agents can be understood.

The mechanisms responsible for intrinsic resistance of tumor cells to 5-halogenated pyrimidines and their nucleosides are diverse and are not necessarily similar to those reported for cell lines where acquired resistance has been studied. For 5-fluoropyrimidines, cells acquiring resistance may form lower levels of nucleotide due to decreased anabolism or increased catabolism. Alternatively, it is now established that the inhibitory complex formed between thymidylate synthetase, FdUMP, and 5,10-methylenetetrahydrofolate is unstable at low cofactor concentrations. Such conditions in vivo may favor rapid dissociation of the complex. Hence, accumulation of dUMP would reduce FdUMP reassociation and lead to continued synthesis of dTMP de novo.

K. Overcoming Resistance

I. Metabolic Modulation

1. Naturally Occurring Pyrimidine Metabolites

Attempts have been made to increase the selectivity of pyrimidine antimetabolites, notably 5-fluoropyrimidines, by combining these agents with naturally occurring pyrimidine bases and nucleosides. BURCHENAL et al. (1960) reported that various pyrimidine derivatives, including dThd, markedly potentiated the antileukemic effects of small doses of FUra or FdUrd in vivo. Of importance was the finding that the therapeutic ratio was not enhanced in these combinations. More recently, MARTIN and STOLFI (1977) reported that dThd treatment potentiated the growth inhibition in $CD8F_1$ mammary carcinoma treated with low doses of FUra. Pretreatment with dThd was also reported to increase the therapeutic efficacy of FUra in mice bearing colon 26 tumors, and it was postulated that this effect was due to increased incorporation of analogue into RNA (MARTIN et al. 1978; SPIEGEL-MAN et al. 1980). Thymidine also potentiated FUra cytotoxicity in AKR leukemia (SANTELLI and VALERIOTE 1978). However, in studies where the efficacy of dThd-FUra combinations were compared with the optimal schedule of FUra alone, therapeutic synergism was demonstrated for lymphocytic leukemia P388, but not for AKR leukemia, colon tumors 26 or 38 (TRADER et al. 1979), or hepatoma 3924A (HOPKINS et al. 1980). It is of interest that administration of dThd before FUra increased toxicity of this antimetabolite in mice (MARTIN et al. 1978; SPIEGELMAN et al. 1980; TRADER et al. 1979), in rats (HOPKINS et at. 1980; DANHAUSER and RUSTUM 1979), and in humans (KIRKWOOD et al. 1980; VOGEL et al. 1979; WOODCOCK et al. 1980). The major interaction between FUra and dThd appears to be at the level of degradation; they can compete with FUra for the rate-limiting enzyme in the catabolic pathway, DHU dehydrogenase, located primarily in the liver (QUEENER et al. 1971; MUKHERJEE and HEIDELBERGER 1960). Combination of dThd with FUra increased the half-life of FUra in the serum and plasma of patients (KIRKWOOD et al. 1980; WOODCOCK et al. 1980), increased concentrations of Thy, and markedly reduced the formation of $^{14}CO_2$ from [2-^{14}C]FUra (WOODCOCK et al. 1980). Whether dThd given at high dose levels inhibits ribonucleotide reductase after conversion to dTTP and leads to increased substitution of FUra in RNA remains speculative. Hydroxyurea, an inhibitor of ribonucleotide reductase, was reported not to increase the incorporation of FUra into RNA (NAYAK et al. 1978). However, in man, combination of dThd with FUra resulted in the rapid appearance of FdUrd in plasma (WOODCOCK et al. 1980) and may cause a greater inhibition of dTMP synthetase (WOLBERG 1979).

Enhancement of FUra cytotoxicity in experimental tumors has been demonstrated in vivo for Thy (SANTELLI and VALERIOTE 1980), Ura (SANTELLI and VALERIOTE 1980; IKENAKA et al. 1979); Cyd (SPIEGELMAN et al. 1980; SANTELLI and VALERIOTE 1980; OSSWALD and YOUSSEF 1979), Urd (SPIEGELMAN et al. 1980; SANTELLI and VALERIOTE 1980), dCyd (SANTELLI and VALERIOTE 1980), and dUrd (SANTELLI and VALERIOTE 1980; JATO and WINDHEUSER 1973; JATO et al. 1975). The cytotoxicity of FdUrd was also potentiated by pyrimidine nucleosides and bases, but host toxicity was similarly increased (BURCHENAL et al. 1960; IKENAKA et al. 1979; JATO et al. 1975). Data at this time suggest that, while pyrimidine nucleosides and bases do modify the potency of 5-fluoropyrimidines, these combinations generally do not appear to increase drug selectivity or increase therapeutic index.

2. Purines and Purine Analogues

The availability of ribose-1-phosphate and 2′-deoxyribose-1-phosphate are reported to be limiting in the conversion of FUra to FUrd (GOTTO et al. 1969; LASKIN et al. 1979) or to FdUrd (LASKIN et al. 1979), respectively. Thus nucleosides such as inosine (Ino), adenosine (Ado), or guanosine (Guo), which may be converted to the base by purine nucleoside phosphorylase with the release of ribose-1-phosphate, enhanced the conversion of FUra to nucleotides (CORY et al. 1977; GOTTO et al. 1969; KESSEL and HALL 1969; LASKIN et al. 1979) and have potentiated FUra cytotoxicity both in vivo (SANTELLI and VALERIOTE 1980; OSSWALD and YOUSSEF 1979) and in cell culture (CORY et al. 1977; LASKIN et al. 1979). Inosine did not increase the therapeutic index of FUra in mice bearing murine leukemias (KESSEL and HALL 1969), while Ino and 2′-deoxyinosine (dIno) protected cells from FUra cytotoxicity in vitro (ULLMAN and KIRSCH 1979). Purine deoxynucleosides have been shown to increase the cytotoxicity of FUra or FdUrd in vivo (SANTELLI and VALERIOTE 1980; BURCHENAL et al. 1960).

An area in pyrimidine metabolism that may offer potential, for increasing the selectivity of FUra is in its conversion to FUMP. Conversion of FUra by OPRTase may be inhibited by depleting the concentration of cosubstrate, 5-phosphoribosyl-1-pyrophosphate (PRPP), or by accumulation of orotic acid, which competes favorably with FUra for the enzyme. In cells utilizing Urd phosphorylase and Urd kinase in the conversion of FUra to FUMP, nucleotide formation should not be reduced. Thus, hypoxanthine (Hx) reduced the cytotoxicity of

FUra in L5178Y leukemia (Yoshida et al. 1978a), S49, L1210, and Novikoff cells in culture (Ullman and Kirsch 1979), an effect attributed to the depletion of PRPP. Hypoxanthine also reduced the toxicity of FUra in mice (Houghton and Houghton 1980b). Allopurinol, an inhibitor of xanthine oxidase, antagonized the cytotoxicity of FUra in murine leukemias and sarcoma 180 cells, but not in Walker 256 or HeLa cells in culture (Schwartz and Handschumacher 1979). Allopurinol also reduced the toxicity of FUra in humans (Fox et al. 1979b, c; Howell et al. 1980) and in rodents at both high (Schwartz et al. 1980) and low (Houghton and Houghton 1980b) dose levels. Allopurinol and FUra in combination increased the growth inhibition in murine colon tumor 38 by 100% (Schwartz and Dunigan 1980); but did not antagonize FUra cytotoxicity in sarcoma 180 in vivo (Sartorelli and Creasey 1967), although antagonism in vitro was reported (Schwartz and Handschumacher 1979).

Given simultaneously with potentially lethal dose levels of FUra, low doses of Hx and allopurinol (HPP) gave superior protection from FUra toxicity than did FUra combined with only one of these purines (Houghton and Houghton 1980b). This combination is of interest as it reduces host toxicity and could potentiate the metabolism of FUra in tumors via the Urd phosphorylase-Urd kinase pathway by indirectly increasing the availability of ribose-1-phosphate. Indeed, in two human tumors growing in mice, the total concentration of FUra anabolites, but particularly the nucleoside FUrd, was increased (Houghton and Houghton 1980b). Whether such combinations increase the therapeutic index of FUra remains to be proven. As discussed, cytotoxicity may be determined by factors other than nucleotide formation.

3. Methotrexate

Extensive studies by Kessel and his colleagues established a relationship between nucleotide formation and the sensitivity of various murine leukemic cells to FUra or FUrd (Kessel et al. 1966, 1973). Thus, increasing nucleotide formation in such cells may increase the antitumor effectiveness of these agents. Cadman et al. (1979) found elevated concentrations of FUra nucleotides and increased cytotoxicity in L1210 cells in vitro when MTX administration preceded that of FUra. Increased nucleotide formation correlated with an elevated concentration of PRPP, which could be utilized in the formation of FUMP by OPRTase. Others have demonstrated an MTX-induced increase in levels of PRPP and have suggested that this was due to decreased utilization of the substrate in purine biosynthesis de novo rather than an increase in the activity of PRPP synthetase (Buesa-Perez et al. 1980).

In experimental tumor systems both in vivo and in vitro, combinations of FUra or FdUrd with MTX have produced antitumor effects that were additive or synergistic (Kline et al. 1966; Bertino et al. 1977; Cadman et al. 1979; Benz et al. 1980; Jackson and Weber 1976; Brown and Ward 1978) or less than additive or antagonistic (Bertino et al. 1977; Tattersall et al. 1973; Jackson and Weber 1976; Ullman et al. 1978; Bowen et al. 1978; Brown and Ward 1978; Moran et al. 1979a; Benz et al. 1980) and also dose dependent (Tattersall et al. 1973).

Schedule dependency of the antitumor effects of MTX and FUra were found for the treatment of sarcoma 180 (BERTINO et al. 1977) and murine mammary tumors (HEPPNER and CALABRESI 1977; BROWN and WARD 1978) in vivo. Pretreatment of tumor-bearing mice with MTX either 1 h (HEPPNER and CALABRESI 1977), 2 h (BERTINO et al. 1977), or 6 – 12 h (BROWN and WARD 1978) before FUra was therapeutically superior to simultaneous administration, whereas the reverse schedule was found to be antagonistic. It has been proposed that inhibition of dihydrofolate reductase by MTX may allow accumulation of dihydrofolate polyglutamates, which may form inhibitory complexes with FdUMP and dTMP synthetase (FERNANDES and BERTINO 1980). These complexes, however, are less stable than that formed with N^5N^{10}-methylenetetrahydrofolate (LOCKSHIN and DANENBERG 1979; SANTI et al. 1974; SANTI 1980). The proposed mechanism for synergism is of considerable interest as this may provide a means by which resistance due to low levels of N^5N^{10}-methylenetetrahydrofolate may be circumvented. However, ULLMAN et al. (1978) demonstrated that MTX antagonized FdUrd cytotoxicity, an effect reversible by folinic acid, in L1210 cells in culture; they deduced that MTX depleted cells of intracellular tetrahydrofolate to levels insufficient for optimal formation of ternary complex between FdUMP, N^5N^{10}-methylenetetrahydrofolate, and dTMP synthetase. Schedules in which MTX is administered before FUra, based on the rationales discussed, are now under clinical evaluation with MTX being administered 1 h (PITMAN et al. 1980; GEWIRTZ and CADMAN 1981), 4 h (SOLAN et al. 1980), or 24 h (E. Cadman, personal communication) before FUra.

4. Inhibitors of Pyrimidine Biosynthesis de Novo

It has been suggested that depletion of endogenous Ura nucleotide pools by inhibitors of pyrimidine biosynthesis de novo may enhance the activity of pyrimidine analogues. Pyrazofurin, an inhibitor of OMP decarboxylase after conversion to its monophosphate, has been shown to enhance FdUrd cytotoxicity in vitro (CADMAN et al. 1978). In contrast, pyrazofurin reduced both host toxicity and the antitumor activity of FUra in P388 and L1210 tumors, while the combination was more effective than FUra alone in colon tumor 38 in vivo (JOHNSON et al. 1980). Inhibition of OMP decarboxylase probably results in the accumulation of orotic acid, which prevents the conversion of FUra to nucleotides by OPRTase in normal tissues and leukemias, while colon tumor 38 may utilize the Urd phosphorylase-Urd kinase pathway in the formation of FUMP. The combination of PALA, a transition-state inhibitor of aspartate transcarbamylase with FUra, was more effetive than FUra alone against several experimental solid tumors, but not against murine leukemias (JOHNSON et al. 1980). Agents that decrease UTP pools have been shown to increase the formation of nucleotides from FUrd in vitro due to decreased feedback control of UTP on Urd kinase (HOLSTEGE et al. 1978). 5-Fluoro-2'-deoxyuridine has also been shown to sensitize L5178Y cells to acute cell death by cytosine arabinoside (CHU et al. 1976).

II. Congener Synthesis

1. Metabolic Activation

A knowledge of factors involved in the acquisition of resistance, or in natural resistance, is a prerequisite for the development of new agents that may prove more effective in the treatment of disease refractory to halogenated pyrimidines and their nucleosides. Thus, a logical goal has been to synthesize halogenated pyrimidine analogues that do not require conversion to nucleotides by kinases. KHWAJA and HEIDELBERGER (1967) reported that DHFdUrd was active against FdUrd-resistant lines of Novikoff hepatoma and L5178BF cells and was not a substrate for either dThd or Urd kinases; further studies (KENT and HEIDELBERGER 1970) suggested that the activity could be explained by nonenzymic cleavage to FUra. Nucleotides, due to their formal charge, do not readily enter cells, however. YOSHIDA et al. (1978b) showed that FUMP had a higher therapeutic efficacy against mice bearing L1210 leukemia than either FUrd or FUra. Administration of the putative active metabolite, FdUMP, was found to be less effective than its nucleoside in inhibiting the incorporation of [^{14}C]-formate into DNA-Thy (HEIDELBERGER 1965). Neutral derivatives of FdUMP capable of diffusion across cell membranes have been reported. The 5′-phosphorodiamidate of FdUMP was shown to be active against L1210 leukemia in vivo (DANENBERG and WOODMAN 1977). Antitumor activity and inhibition of dTMP synthetase appeared to correlate with the rate of non-enzymic hydrolysis (PHELPS et al. 1980). The 5′-nitrate of FdUrd, a possible neutral isostere of FdUMP, has shown greater therapeutic activity than FdUrd against mice bearing L1210 leukemia (CHWANG and AVERY 1980), and the phosphonate analogue of FdUMP inhibited dTMP synthetase from bacterial and phage sources and was cytotoxic to HEp-2 cells in culture (MONTGOMERY et al. 1979). MILLER et al. (1976) observed that resistance to FdUrd in mouse glioma 26 was characterized by a decrease in dThd kinase activity and an increase in the activity of 5′-nucleotide phosphodiesterase. 5′-Fluoro-2′-deoxyuridine 5′(5-iodo-4-indolyl)phosphate (TSOU et al. 1970), which was cleaved to FdUMP by the phosphodiesterase, was shown to be active in both parent and FdUrd-resistant lines.

2. Decreased Phosphorolytic Cleavage

Analogues of dThd with 5-substituents at least the size of a methyl group are good substrates for dThd phosphorylase (NAKAYAMA et al. 1980). FdUrd is also rapidly degraded to FUra, and this may limit its therapeutic effectiveness (BIRNIE et al. 1963). Pyrimidinediones substituted with small, hydrophobic groups at either C-5 or C-6, or both, inhibited cleavage of FdUrd by both mammalian dThd and Urd-dUrd phosphorylases (WOODMAN et al. 1980). 6-Aminothymine, the best inhibitor of dThd phosphorylase, was shown to increase incorporation of dThd into DNA of mouse tissues three- or fourfold, but that of IdUrd was at best only doubled (MATTHES et al. 1974). 6-Aminothymine also inhibited catabolism of pyrimidine bases and increased both incorporation of [6-^{3}H]FUra into tissue RNA and host toxicity. NIEDZWICKI et al. (1980) have reported that pyrimidine acyclonucleosides inhibit uridine phosphorylase in vitro. At present it is unknown whether inhibition of the catabolism of 5-halogenated pyrimidines by using specific phosphorylase inhibitors or competitive nucleosides and bases would result in greater drug selectivity. That such manipulations result in increased toxicity of FUra in both man and experimental animals is well established (KIRKWOOD et al. 1980; TRADER et al. 1979). There is, however, evidence to suggest that the toxicity of 5-fluoropyrimidines may be related to analogue incorporation into RNA, while tumor cytotoxicity may be due to inhibition of dTMP synthetase (HEIDELBERGER 1965; HOUGHTON et al. 1979). Accordingly, inhibition of the degradation of FdUrd to FUra may prove to have therapeutic significance.

3. Latentiation

Ftorafur, a clinically active agent in human gastrointestinal cancer (MOERTEL 1978), is hydrolyzed to FUra in vivo (COHEN 1975). Ftorafur was less toxic than FUra at equimolar doses in man, although its superior efficacy has yet to be proven (BLOKHINA et al. 1972; GARIBJANIAN et al. 1976). OKADA et al. (1974) reported extensive studies where FUra was conjugated with unsaturated fatty acids or with ethylene hydrocarbons. 1-Acetyl-FUra and 1-benzoyl-FUra have shown activity superior to that of FUra; 1-hexylcarbamoyl-FUra (IIGO et al. 1978) has been reported to be therapeutically more effective than 1(2-tetrahydro-furanyl)-FUra or FUra in experimental systems. Interestingly 1-hexylcarbamoyl-FUra and FUra have different distribution patterns after oral administration to mice (IIGO et al. 1979). This new agent is being evaluated clinically (TAGUCHI 1980a). The analogue 1,3-bis(tetrahydro-2-furanyl)-5-fluoro-2,4-pyrimidinedione, a slow-release prodrug of FUra has shown considerable activity in several animal tumor systems (TAGUCHI 1980b). KANZAWA et al. (1979) have reported that the hexadecylester of FUMP was active against a subline of L5178Y mouse leukemia cells resistant to FUrd. 5′-Deoxy-FUrd has also shown greater therapeutic efficacy against rodent tumors than FUra (ARMSTRONG and DIASIO 1980).

4. Increased Uptake

Orotic acid and FO are highly ionized at physiological pH, and hence penetrate most cells poorly (BOSCH et al. 1958). BONO et al. (1964) synthesized the methyl ester of FO, an un-ionized species, but this analogue was degraded by serum esterases and was spontaneously unstable.

There have been many attempts to increase the selectivity of FUra and hence overcome intrinsic or acquired resistance. These approaches have generally utilized pyrimidine or purine nucleosides and bases in order to modulate the metabolism of FUra. It is clear, however, that these techniques increase the potency of FUra but do not appear to increase its selectivity. An alternative approach has been to modulate FUra metabolism selectively by manipulating PRPP concentrations. Thus, decreasing PRPP levels in normal tissues only, or selectively increasing levels in tumor tissue, may lead to greater selectivity of FUra (or other cytotoxic agents that utilize PRPP in their metabolism). At present there is little convincing evidence either in laboratory animals or in man that selectivity of FUra is currently being increased by these procedures.

L. Conclusions

5-Halogenated pyrimidines have proven valuable tools in understanding the development of resistance in tumor cells. For thymidine analogues (BrdUrd, IdUrd), cytotoxicity appears to be a consequence of incorporation into DNA. Acquired resistance is associated, usually, with the exclusion of the analogue from DNA, most frequently due to deletion of thymidine kinase. However, there are examples in which cells become tolerant to analogue incorporation; this may be understood only after the consequence of analogue substitution into DNA has been elucidated. Mutants that show changes in transport and changes at the level of thymidylate kinase serve as examples of the diversity of mechanisms responsible for acquired resistance. It is apparent that the more complex the metabolism of the agent, the more loci may be involved in the resistance mechanism. This is demonstrated for FUra, in which enzyme deletions, elevations, or mutations have been implicated in the development of resistance. Acquired resistance appears to be a stable phenomenon indicating a genetic basis.

In contrast, intrinsic resistance implies a situation in which tumor and normal tissues have similar sensitivity to the agent used. Of the halogenated pyrimidines, only the 5-fluoro derivatives have demonstrated reasonable selectivity in vivo, although only a small proportion of human cancers respond to systemic therapy with these agents. The underlying mechanisms governing intrinsic resistance are, as yet, little understood, but may not be related to those determined for acquired resistance in animal models.

In examining acquired resistance it is apparent that the mechanisms involved are diverse and may depend upon the cell characteristics and the experimental conditions employed. For applying such information to the design of chemotherapy in human malignancies it becomes critical to know by which mechanism(s) particular types of cancer acquire resistance. With the development of more successful techniques for the culture of human malignant cells, it would appear possible to determine loci of resistance common to a high proportion of cell lines of a particular cancer type. Such an approach may aid in the development of chemotherapy programs, specific to certain cancer types, designed to prevent or circumvent acquired resistance.

Acknowledgements. This work was supported by grants CH-172 and CH-156 from the American Cancer Society, by grant CA-21677 from the National Cancer Institute, and by ALSAC.

References

Adair GM, Carver JH (1979) Unstable, non-mutational expression of resistance to the thymidine analogue, trifluorothymidine in CHO cells. Mutat Res 60:207–213

Anderson D, Fox M (1974) The induction of thymidine- and IUDR-resistant variants in P388 mouse lymphoma cells by x-rays, UV and mono- and bi-functional alkylating agents. Mutat Res 25:107–122

Anderson EP, Ciardi JE, Brockman RW, Law LW (1962) Uridine kinase activity in fluorouridine-resistant tumor cells. Fed Proc 21:384

Ardalan B, Buscaglia MD, Schein PS (1978) Tumor 5-fluorodeoxyuridylate concentration as a determinant of 5-fluorouracil response. Biochem Pharmacol 27:2009–2013

Ardalan B, Cooney DA, Jayaram HN, Carrico CK, Glazer RI, Macdonald J, Schein PS (1980) Mechanisms of sensitivity and resistance of murine tumors to 5-fluorouracil. Cancer Res 40:1431–1437

Armstrong RD, Diasio RB (1980) Metabolism and biological activity of 5′-deoxy-5-fluorouridine, a novel fluoropyrimidine. Cancer Res 40:3333–3338

Baskin F, Rosenberg RN (1975) A comparison of thymidylate synthetase activities from 5-fluorodeoxyuridine sensitive and resistant variants of mouse neuroblastoma. J Neurochem 24:233–238

Baskin F, Carlin SC, Kraus P, Friedkin M, Rosenberg RN (1975) Experimental chemotherapy of neuroblastoma. II. Increased thymidylate synthetase activity in a 5-fluorodeoxyuridine-resistant variant of mouse neuroblastoma. Mol Pharmacol 11:105–117

Baskin F, Davis R, Rosenberg RN (1977) Altered thymidine kinase or thymidylate synthetase activities in 5-fluorodeoxyuridine resistant variants of mouse neuroblastoma. J Neurochem 29:1031–1037

Benz C, Schoenberg M, Choti M, Cadman E (1980) Schedule-dependent cytotoxicity of methotrexate and 5-fluorouracil in human colon and breast tumor cell lines. J Clin Invest 66:1162–1165

Berk AJ, Clayton DA (1973) A genetically distinct thymidine kinase in mammalian mitochondria. Exclusive labeling of mitochondrial deoxyribonucleic acid. J Biol Chem 248:2722–2729

Berry RJ, Andrews JR (1962) Modification of radiation effect on mammalian tumor cells by pharmacological agents. Nature 196:185–186

Bertino JR, Sawicki WL, Lindquist CA, Gupta VS (1977) Schedule-dependent antitumor effects of methotrexate and 5-fluorouracil. Cancer Res 37:327–328

Birnie GD, Kroeger H, Heidelberger C (1963) Studies on fluorinated pyrimidines. XVIII. The degradation of 5-fluoro-2′-deoxyuridine and related compounds by nucleoside phosphorylasc. Biochcmistry 2:566–572

Bjursell G, Reichard P (1973) Effects of thymidine on deoxynucleoside triphosphate pools and deoxyribonucleic acid synthesis in Chinese hamster ovary cells. J Biol Chem 248:3904–3909

Blokhina NG, Vozny EK, Garin AM (1972) Results of treatment of malignant tumors with ftorafur. Cancer 30:390–392

Bono VH Jr, Cheng CC, Frei E, Kelly MG (1964) Methyl-5-fluoroorotate: synthesis and comparison with 5-fluoroorotic acid with respect to biological activity and cell entry. Cancer Res 24:513–517

Bosch L, Harbers E, Heidelberger C (1958) Studies in fluorinated pyrimidines. V. Effects on nucleic acid metabolism in vitro. Cancer Res 18:335–343

Bowen D, White JC, Goldman ID (1978) A basis for fluoropyrimidine-induced antagonism to methotrexate in Ehrlich ascites tumor cells in vitro. Cancer Res 38:219–222

Bowen D, Diasio RB, Goldman ID (1979) Distinguishing between membrane transport and intracellular metabolism of fluorodeoxyuridine in Ehrlich ascites tumor cells by application of kinetic and high performance liquid chromographic techniques. J Biol Chem 254:5333–5339

Breslow RE, Goldsby RA (1969) Isolation and characterization of thymidine transport mutants of Chinese hamster cells. Exp Cell Res 55:339–346

Brockman RW (1974) Mechanisms of resistance. In: Sartorelli AC, Johns DG (eds) Antineoplastic and immunosuppressive agents Springer, Berlin Heidelberg New York (Handbook of experimental pharmacology, vol 38/1, pp 352–410)

Brockman RW, Anderson EP (1963) Biochemistry of cancer (metabolic aspects). Annu Rev Biochem 32:463–512

Brockman RW, Law LW (1960) Metabolism of pyrimidines and 5-fluoropyrimidines by sensitive and resistant neoplasms. Proc Am Assoc Cancer Res 3:98

Brown I, Ward HWC (1978) Therapeutic consequences of antitumour drug interactions: methotrexate and 5-fluorouracil in the chemotherapy of C_3H mice with transplanted mammary adenocarcinoma. Cancer Lett 5:291–297

Brown MMM, Clive D (1977) The utilization of trifluorothymidine as a selective agent for $TK^{-/-}$ mutants in L5178Y mouse lymphoma cells. Mutat Res 53:116

Buesa-Perez JM, Leyva A, Pinedo HM (1980) Effect of methotrexate on 5-phosphoribosyl 1-pyrophosphate levels in L1210 leukemia cells in vitro. Cancer Res 40:139–144
Burchenal JH, Holmberg EAD, Fox JJ, Hemphill SC, Reppert JA (1959) The effects of 5-fluorodeoxycytidine, 5-fluorodeoxyuridine and related compounds on transplanted mouse leukemias. Cancer Res 19:494–500
Burchenal JH, Oettgen HF, Reppert JA, Coley V (1960) Studies on the synergism of fluorinated pyrimidines and certain pyrimidine and purine derivatives against transplanted mouse leukemia. Cancer Chem Rep 6:1–5
Burchenal JH, Lyman MS, Purple JR, Coley V, Smith S, Bucholz E (1962) Therapeutic, combination, and resistance studies on certain imidazolin phthalanilide derivatives in mouse leukemia. Cancer Chem Rep 19:19–29
Caboche M (1974) Comparison of the frequencies of spontaneous and chemically-induced 5-bromodeoxyuridine-resistance mutations in wild-type and revertant BHK-21/13 cells. Genetics 77:309–322
Cadman EC, Dix DE, Handschumacher RE (1978) Clinical, biological, and biochemical effects of pyrazofurin. Cancer Res 38:682–688
Cadman E, Heimer R, Davis L (1979) Enhanced 5-fluorouracil nucleotide formation after methotrexate administration: explanation for drug synergism. Science 205:1135–1137
Calabresi P, Cardoso SS, Finch SC, Kligerman MM, Von Essen CF, Chu MY, Welch AD (1961) Initial clinical studies with 5-iodo-2′-deoxyuridine. Cancer Res 21:550–559
Cano JP, Aubert C, Rigault JP, Seitz JF, Carcassone Y (1980) Pharmacokinetic studies of 5-fluorouracil (5FU) in cancer patients: relation with clinical response and implication of measurement of 5,6-dihydro-5-fluorouracil (FUH_2). Proc Am Assoc Cancer Res 21:152
Carrico CK, Glazer RI (1979) Augmentation by thymidine of the incorporation and distribution of 5-fluorouracil in ribosomal RNA. Biochem Biophys Res Commun 87:664–670
Carter SK (1972) Single and combination nonhormonal chemotherapy in breast cancer. Cancer 30:1543–1555
Carter SK (1974) Integration of chemotherapy into combined modality treatment of solid tumors. II. Large bowel carcinoma. Cancer Treat Rev 1:111–129
Cass CE, Paterson ARP (1972) Mediated transport of nucleosides in human erythrocytes. J Biol Chem 247:3314–3320
Chadwick M, Chang C (1976) Comparative physiologic dispositions of 5-fluoro-2′-deoxyuridine and 5-fluorouracil in mice bearing L1210 lymphocytic leukemia. Cancer Treat Rep 60:845–855
Chadwick M, Rogers WI (1972) The physiological disposition of 5-fluorouracil in mice bearing solid L1210 lymphocytic leukemia. Cancer Res 32:1045–1056
Chaudhuri NK, Mukherjee KL, Heidelberger C (1958) Studies on fluorinated pyrimidines VII–the degradative pathway. Biochem Pharmacol 1:328–341
Chello PL, McQueen CA, DeAngelis LM, Bertino JR (1976) Elevation of dihydrofolate reductase, thymidylate synthetase and thymidine kinase in cultured mammalian cells after exposure to folate antagonists. Cancer Res 36:2442–2449
Chu MY, Hoovis ML, Fischer GA (1976) Effects of 5-fluorodeoxyuridine on cell viability and uptake of deoxycytidine and [^{3}H]cytosine arabinoside in L5178Y cells. Biochem Pharmacol 25:355–357
Chu EHY, Sun NC, Chang CC (1972) Induction of auxotrophic mutations by treatment of Chinese hamster cells with 5-bromodeoxyuridine and black light. Proc Natl Acad Sci USA 69:3459–3463
Chwang TL, Avery TL (1980) Synthesis and preliminary biological evaluation of a new antitumor agent, 5′-*O*-nitro-5-fluoro-2′-deoxyuridine (5′-ONO_2FdUrd). Proc Am Assoc Cancer Res 21:298
Clive D, Voytek P (1977) Evidence for chemically-induced structural gene mutations at the thymidine kinase locus in cultured L5178Y mouse lymphoma cells. Mutat Res 44:269–278
Cohen AM (1975) The disposition of ftorafur in rats after intravenous administration. Drug Metab Dispos 3:303–308

Cory JG, Crumley J, Wilkinson DS (1977) Evidence for role of purine nucleoside phosphorylase in sensitivity of Novikoff hepatoma cells to 5-fluorouracil. Adv Enzyme Regul 15:153–166

Danenberg PV (1977) Thymidylate synthetase – a target enzyme in cancer chemotherapy. Biochim Biophys Acta 473:73–92

Danenberg PV, Danenberg KD (1978) Effect of 5,10-methylenetetrahydrofolate on the dissociation of 5-fluoro-2′-deoxyuridylate from thymidylate synthetase: evidence for an ordered mechanism. Biochemistry 17:4018–4024

Danenberg PV, Woodman PW (1977) Fed Proc 36:282 (abstr)

Danhauser LL, Rustum YM (1979) A method for continuous drug infusion in unrestrained rats: its application in evaluating the toxicity of 5-fluorouracil/thymidine combinations. J Lab Clin Med 93:1047–1053

Davidson RL, Bick MD (1973) Bromodeoxyuridine dependence–a new mutation in mammalian cells. Proc Natl Acad Sci USA 70:138–142

DiPaolo JA (1964) Polydactylism in the offspring of mice injected with 5-bromodeoxyuridine. Science 145:501–503

Djordevic B, Szybalski W (1960) Genetics of human cell lines III. Incorporation of 5-bromo- and 5-iododeoxyuridine into the deoxyribonucleic acid of human cells and its effect on radiation sensitivity. J Exp Med 112:509–531

Dubbs DR, Kit S (1964) Effect of halogenated pyrimidines and thymidine on growth of L-cells and a subline lacking thymidine kinase. Exp Cell Res 33:19–28

Elion GB, Hitchings GH (1965) Metabolic basis for the actions of analogs of purines and pyrimidines. Adv Chemother 2:91–177

Evans M, Laskin JD, Hakala MT (1980) Assessment of growth-limiting events by 5-fluorouracil in mouse cells and in human cells. Cancer Res 4113–4122

Ferdinandus JA, Morris HP, Weber G (1971) Behavior of opposing pathways of thymidine utilization in differentiating, regenerating, and neoplastic liver. Cancer Res 31:550–556

Fernandes DJ, Bertino JR (1980) 5-Fluorouracil-methotrexate synergy; enhancement of 5-fluorodeoxyuridylate binding to thymidylate synthetase by dihydropteroylpolyglutamates. Proc Natl Acad Sci USA 77:5663–5667

Fischer GA (1962) Defective transport of amethopterin (methotrexate) as a mechanism of resistance to the antimetabolite in L5178Y leukemic cells. Biochem Pharmacol 11:1233–1234

Fischer GA (1971) increased levels of folic acid reductase as a mechanism of resistance to amethopterin in leukemic cells. Biochem Pharmacol 7:75–77

Fox M (1971) Spontaneous and x-ray-induced genotypic and phenotypic resistance to 5-iodo-2′-deoxyuridine in lymphoma cells in vitro. Mutat Res 13:403–419

Fox M, Anderson D (1974) Characteristics of spontaneous and induced thymidine and 5-iodo-2-deoxyuridine resistant clones of mouse lymphoma cells. Mutat Res 25:89–105

Fox M, Fox BW, Ayad SR (1969) Evidence of genetic expression of integrated DNA in lymphoma cells. Nature 222:1086–1087

Fox RM, Tripp EH, Piddington SK, Dudman NP, Tattersall MHN (1979a) Thymidine sensitivity of cultured leukaemic lymphocytes. Lancet 2:391–393

Fox RM, Woods RL, Tattersall MHN, Brodie GM (1979b) Allopurinol modulation of high-dose-fluorouracil toxicity. Lancet 1:677

Fox RM, Woods RL, Tattersall MHN, Brodie GW (1979c) Allopurinol modulation of high-dose fluorouracil toxicity. Cancer Treat Rev[Suppl] 6:143–147

Freed JJ, Mezger-Freed L (1973) Origin of thymidine kinase deficient (TK^-) haploid frog cells via an intermediate thymidine transport deficient (TT^-) phenotype. J Cell Physiol 82:199–212

Garibjanian BT, Johnson RK, Kline I, Vadlamudi S, Gang M, Venditti JM, Goldin A (1976) Comparison of 5-fluorouracil and ftorafur. II. Therapeutic response and development of resistance in murine tumors. Cancer Treat Rep 60:1347–1361

Gewirtz AM, Cadman E (1981) Preliminary report on the efficacy of sequential methotrexate and 5-fluorouracil in advanced breast cancer. Cancer 47:2552–2555

Goldberg AR, Machledt JH Jr, Pardee AB (1966) On the action of fluorouracil on leukemia cells. Cancer Res 26:1611–1615

Gotto AM, Belkhode ML, Touster O (1969) Stimulatory effects of inosine and deoxyinosine on the incorporation of uracil-2-^{14}C, 5-fluorouracil-2-^{14}C, and 5-bromouracil-2-^{14}C into nucleic acids by Ehrlich ascites tumor cells in vitro. Cancer Res 29:807–811

Goz B (1978) The effects of incorporation of 5-halogenated deoxyuridines into the DNA of eukaryotic cells. Pharmacol Rev 29:249–272

Greenberg N, Schumm DE, Webb TE (1977) Uridine kinase activities and pyrimidine nucleoside phosphorylation in fluoropyrimidine-sensitive and -resistant cell lines of the Novikoff hepatoma. Biochem J 164:379–387

Häggmark A (1962) Studies on resistance against 5-fluorouracil II. Thymidylate synthetase from drug-resistant tumor lines. Cancer Res 22:568–572

Hall TC (1974) Clinical resistance to antipyrimidine anticancer drugs. Biochem Pharmacol [Suppl] 2:119–127

Hall TC, Kessel D, Godsill A, Roberts D (1968) Uridine phosphorylation, an overlooked pathway?; 5-fluorouridine, a neglected drug? Proc Am Assoc Cancer Res 9:27

Hards RG, Dick JE, Wright JA (1979) Altered levels of ribonucleotide reductase activity in drug-resistant mammalian cell lines. Proc XI Int Congr Biochem (Toronto) 11:317

Hartman KU, Heidelberger C (1961) Studies on fluorinated pyrimidines XIII. Inhibition of thymidylate synthetase. J Biol Chem 236:3006–3013

Heidelberger C (1965) Fluorinated pyrimidines. Proc Nucl Acid Res Mol Biol 4:1–50

Heidelberger C (1967) Cancer chemotherapy with purine and pyrimidine analogues. Annu Rev Pharmacol 7:101–124

Heidelberger C (1973) Pyrimidine and pyrimidine nucleoside antimetabolites. In: Frei E III, Holland JF (eds) Cancer medicine. Lea & Febiger, Philadelphia, pp 768–791

Heidelberger C (1974) Fluorinated pyrimidines and their nucleosides. In: Sartorelli AC, Johns DG (eds) Antineoplastic and immunosuppressive agents. Springer, Berlin Heidelberg New York (Handbook of experimental pharmacology, vol 38/2, pp 193–231)

Heidelberger C, Anderson SW (1964) Fluorinated pyrimidines XXI. The tumor-inhibitory activity of 5-trifluoromethyl-2′-deoxyuridine. Cancer Res 24:1979–1985

Heidelberger C, Ansfield FJ (1963) Experimental and clinical use of fluorinated pyrimidines in cancer chemotherapy. Cancer Res 23:1226–1243

Heidelberger C, Griesbach L, Cruz O, Schnitzer RJ, Grunberg E (1958 a) Fluorinated pyrimidines. VI. Effects of 5-fluorouridine and 5-fluoro-2′-deoxyuridine on transplanted tumors. Proc Soc Exp Biol Med 97:470–475

Heidelberger C, Griesbach L, Montag BJ, Mooren D, Cruz O, Schnitzer RJ, Grunberg E (1958 b) Studies on fluorinated pyrimidines. II. Effect on transplanted tumors. Cancer Res 18:305–317

Heidelberger C, Ghobar A, Baker RK, Mukherjee KL (1960 a) Studies on fluorinated pyrimidines. X. In vivo studies on tumor resistance. Cancer Res 20:897–902

Heidelberger C, Kaldor G, Mukherjee KL, Danneberg PB (1960 b) Studies on fluorinated pyrimidines. XI. In vitro studies on tumor resistance. Cancer Res 20:905–909

Henderson EE, Strauss B (1975) Differences in the incorporation of bromodeoxyuridine by human lymphoblastoid cell lines. Cell 5:381–387

Heppner GH, Calabresi P (1977) Effect of sequence of administration of methotrexate, leucovorin, and 5-fluorouracil on mammary tumor growth and survival in syngeneic C3H mice. Cancer Res 37:4580–4583

Holstege A, Herrmann B, Keppler DOR (1978) Increased formation of nucleotide derivatives of 5-fluorouridine in hepatoma cells treated with inhibitors of pyrimidine synthesis and *d*-galactosamine. Febs Lett 95:361–365

Holtzer H, Weintraub H, Mayne R, Mochan B (1972) The cell cycle, cell lineages and cell differentiation. Curr Top Dev Biol 7:229–256

Hopkins HA, Fager RS, Looney WB (1980) Effectiveness of 5-fluorouracil (5-FU) with or without prior thymidine on therapeutically responsive and resistant solid tumors. Proc Am Assoc Cancer Res 21:282

Houghton JA, Houghton PJ (1980a) On the mechanism of cytotoxicity of fluorinated pyrimidines in four human colon adenocarcinoma xenografts maintained in immune-deprived mice. Cancer 45:1159–1167

Houghton JA, Houghton PJ (1980b) 5-Fluorouracil in combination with hypoxanthine and allopurinol: toxicity and metabolism in xenografts of human colonic carcinomas in mice. Biochem Pharmacol 29:2077–2080

Houghton JA, Houghton PJ, Wooten RS (1979) Mechanism of induction of gastrointestinal toxicity in the mouse by 5-fluorouracil, 5-fluorouridine, and 5-fluoro-2′-deoxyuridine. Cancer Res 39:2406–2413

Houghton JA, Maroda SJ Jr, Phillips JO, Houghton PJ (1981) Biochemical determinants of responsiveness to 5-fluorouracil and its derivatives in xenografts of human colorectal adenocarcinomas in mice. Cancer Res 41:144–149

Howell SB, Wung W, Tamerius R (1980) Modulation of 5-fluorouracil (FU) toxicity by allopurinol (HPP) in man. Proc Am Assoc Res 21:336

Huberman E, Heidelberger C (1972) The mutagenicity to mammalian cells of pyrimidine nucleoside analogs. Mutat Res 14:130–132

Hutchison DJ, Robinson DL, Martin D, Ittensohn OL, Dillenberg J (1962) Effects of selected cancer chemotherapeutic drugs in the survival times of mice with L-1210 leukemia: relative responses of antimetabolite resistant strains. Cancer Res 22/2:57–72

Iigo M, Hoshi A, Nakamura A, Kuretani K (1978) Antitumor activity of 1-hexylcarbamoyl-5-fluorouracil in Lewis lung carcinoma and B16 melanoma. J Pharmacobiodyn 1:49–54

Iigo M, Nakamura A, Kuretani K, Hoshi A (1979) Distribution of 1-hexylcarbamoyl-5-fluorouracil and 5-fluorouracil by oral administration in mice. J Pharmacobiodyn 2:5–11

Ikenaka K, Shirasaka T, Kitano S, Fujii S (1979) Effect of uracil on metabolism of 5-fluorouracil in vitro. Gan 70:353–359

Jackson RC (1978) The regulation of thymidylate biosynthesis in Novikoff hepatoma cells and the effects of amethopterin, 5-fluorodeoxyuridine, and 3-deazauridine. J Biol Chem 253:7440–7446

Jackson RC, Harrap KR (1973) Studies with a mathematical model of folate metabolism. Arch Biochem Biophys 158:827–841

Jackson RC, Weber G (1976) Enzyme pattern directed chemotherapy. The effects of combinations of methotrexate, 5-fluorodeoxyuridine and thymidine on rat hepatoma cells in vitro. Biochem Pharmacol 25:2613–2618

Jacquez JA (1962) Permeability of Ehrlich cells to uracil, thymine and fluorouracil. Proc Soc Exp Biol Med 109:132–135

Jaffe JJ, Prusoff WH (1960) The effect of 5-iododeoxyuridine upon the growth of some transplantable rodent tumors. Cancer Res 20:1383–1388

Jato JG, Windheuser JJ (1973) 5-Fluorouracil and derivatives in cancer chemotherapy. III. In vivo enhancement of antitumor activity of 5-fluorouracil (FU) and 5-fluoro-2′-deoxyuridine (FUDR). J Pharm Sci 62:1975–1978

Jato JG, Lake LM, Grunden EE, Johnson BM (1975) Effect of deoxyuridine coadministration on toxicity and antitumor activity of fluorouracil and floxuridine. J Pharm Sci 64:943–946

Johnson RK, Clement JJ, Howard WS (1980) Treatment of murine tumors with 5-fluorouracil in combination with de novo pyrimidine synthesis inhibitors PALA or pyrazofurin. Proc Am Assoc Cancer Res 21:292

Kanzawa F, Hoshi A, Kuretani K (1979) Antitumor activity of alkylesters of 1-β-D-ribofuranosyl-5-fluorouracil-5′-phosphate against murine lymphoma L5178Y resistant to 1-β-D-ribofuranosyl-5-fluorouracil. Bull Cancer (Paris) 66:497–501

Kasbekar DK, Greenberg DM (1963) Studies on tumor resistance to 5-fluorouracil. Cancer Res 23:818–824

Kaufman ER, Davidson RL (1977a) Novel phenotypes arising from selection of hamster melanoma cells for resistance to BUdR. Exp Cell Res 107:15–24

Kaufmann ER, Davidson RL (1977b) Effects of thymidine analogs on Syrian hamster melanoma cells: phenotypes arising from selection for analog resistance. Somatic Cell Genet 3:649–661

Kaufmann ER, Davidson RL (1978) Biological and biochemical effects of bromodeoxyuridine and deoxycytidine on Syrian hamster melanoma cells. Somatic Cell Genet 4:587–601

Kaufman ER, Davidson RL (1979) Altered thymidylate kinase substrate specificity in mammalian cells selected for resistance to iododeoxyuridine. Exp Cell Res 123:355–363

Kent RJ, Heidelberger C (1970) Fluorinated pyrimidines – XXXV. The metabolism of 2′,3′-dehydro-5-fluoro-2′-deoxyuridine in Ehrlich ascites cells. Biochem Pharmacol 19:1095–1104

Kessel D, Hall TC (1969) Influence of ribose donors on the action of 5-fluorouracil. Cancer Res 29:1749–1754

Kessel D, Wodinsky I (1970) Thymidine kinase as a determinant of the response to 5-fluoro-2′-deoxyuridine in transplantable murine leukemias. Mol Pharmacol 6:251–254

Kessel D, Hall TC, Roberts D, Wodinsky I (1965) Uptake as a determinant of methotrexate response in mouse leukemias. Science 150:752–754

Kessel D, Hall TC, Wodinsky I (1966) Nucleotide formation as a determinant of 5-fluorouracil response in mouse leukemias. Science 154:911–913

Kessel D, Hall TC, Reyes P (1969) Metabolism of uracil and 5-fluorouracil in P388 murine leukemia cells. Mol Pharmacol 5:481–486

Kessel D, Bruns R, Hall TC (1971) Determinants of responsiveness to 5-fluorouridine in transplantable murine leukemias. Mol Pharmacol 7:117–121

Kessel D, Dodd DC, Hall TC (1973) Some determinants of drug responsiveness in bovine leukemia cells. Biochem Pharmacol 22:1161–1164

Khwaja TA, Heidelberger C (1967) Fluorinated pyrimidines XXIX. Syntheses of 2′,3′-dehydro-5-fluoro-2′-deoxyuridine and 2′,3′-dideoxy-5-fluorouridine. J Med Chem 10:1066–1070

Kirkwood JM, Ensminger W, Rosowsky A, Papathanasopoulos N, Frei E (1980) Comparison of pharmacokinetics of 5-fluorouracil and 5-fluorouracil with concurrent thymidine infusions in a phase-I trial. Cancer Res. 40:107–113

Kit S (1962) Physiochemical studies on the deoxyribonucleic acids of mouse tissues. In: The molecular basis of neoplasia. 15th Symposium on Fundamental Cancer Research, MD Anderson Hospital and Tumor Institute, Houston, Texas, 1961. University of Texas Press, Austin, pp 133–146

Kit S, Dubbs DR, Piekarski LJ, Hsu TC (1963) Deletion of thymidine kinase activity from L cells resistant to bromodeoxyuridine. Exp Cell Res 31:297–312

Kit S, Kaplan LA, Leung W-C, Trkula D (1972) Mitochondrial thymidine kinase of bromodeoxyuridine-resistant, kinase-deficient HeLa (BU25) cells. Biochem Biophys Res Commun 49:1561–1567

Kit S, Leung W-C, Trkula D (1973) Distinctive properties of mitochondrial thymidine (dT) kinase from bromodeoxyuridine (dBu)-resistant mouse lines. Biochem Biophys Res Commun 54:455–461

Kline I, Venditti JM, Mead JAR, Tyrer DD, Goldin A (1966) The antileukemic effectiveness of 5-fluorouracil and methotrexate in the combination chemotherapy of advanced leukemia L1210 in mice. Cancer Res 26:848–852

Klubes P, Connelly K, Cerna I, Mandel HG (1978) Effects of 5-fluorouracil on 5-fluorodeoxyuridine 5′-monophosphate and 2-deoxyuridine 5′-monophosphate pools, and DNA synthesis in solid mouse L1210 and rat Walker 256 tumors. Cancer Res 38:2325–2331

Krooth RS, Hsiao W-L, Potvin BW (1979) Resistance to 5-fluoroorotic acid and pyrimidine auxotrophy: a new bidirectional selective system for mammalian cells. Somatic Cell Genet 5:551–569

Laskin JD, Evans RM, Slocum HK, Burke D, Hakala MT (1979) Basis for natural variation in sensitivity to 5-fluorouracil in mouse and human cells in culture. Cancer Res 39:383–390

Law L (1958) The effect of fluorinated pyrimidines on neoplasms of the blood and blood-forming organs. Proc Am Assoc Cancer Res 2:318

Law LW (1962) Studies of inhibitory effects of terephthalanilide derivatives against several variants of leukemia L1210. Cancer Chem Rep 19:13–18

Leung KK, Visser DW (1976) Characteristics of deoxythymidine transport and deoxythymidine kinase in 3T3 cells. Biochem Med 16:127–137

Levinson BB, Ullman B, Martin DW (1979) Pyrimidine pathway variants of cultured mouse lymphoma cells with altered levels of both orotate phosphoribosyltransferase and orotidylate decarboxylase. J Biol Chem 254:4396–4401

Littlefield JW (1965) Studies on thymidine kinase in cultured mouse fibroblasts. Biochim Biophys Acta 95:14–22

Lockshin A, Danenberg PV (1979) Thymidylate synthetase and 2′-deoxyuridylate form a tight complex in the presence of pteroyltriglutamate. J Biol Chem 254:12285–12288

Lu LW, Chiang GH, Tseng W-C, Randerath K (1976) Effects of 5-fluorouridine on modified nucleosides in mouse liver tansfer RNA. Biochem Biophys Res Commun 73:1075–1082

Luria SE, Delbrück M (1943) Mutations of bacteria from virus sensitivity to virus resistance. Genetics 28:491–511

Lynch TP, Cass CE, Paterson ARP (1977) Defective transport of thymidine by cultured cells resistant to 5-bromodeoxyuridine. J Supramol Struct 6:363–374

Maley F, Maley GF (1971) The apparent induction of thymidylate synthetase by amethopterin. Ann NY Acad Sci 186:168–171

Mandel HG (1969) The incorporation of 5-fluorouracil into RNA and its molecular consequences. Prog Mol Subcell Biol 1:82–135

Mandel HG, Klubes P, Fernandes DJ (1977) Understanding the actions of carcinostatic drugs to improve chemotherapy: 5fluorouracil. Adv Enzyme Regul 16:79–93

Martin DS, Stolfi RL (1977) Thymidine (TdR) enhancement of antitumor activity of 5-fluorouracil (FU) against advanced murine ($CD8F_1$) breast carcinoma. Proc Am Assoc Cancer Res 18:126

Martin DS, Nayak R, Sawyer RC, Stolfi RL, Young CW, Woodcock T, Spiegelman S (1978) Enhancement of 5-fluorouracil chemotherapy with emphasis on the use of excess thymidine. Cancer Bull 30:219–224

Mathias AP, Fischer GA and Prusoff WH (1959) Inhibition of the growth of mouse leukemia cells in culture by 5-iododeoxyuridine. Biochim Biophys Acta 36:560–561

Matthes E, Bärwolff D, Langen P (1974) Inhibition by 6-aminothymine of the degradation of nucleosides (5-iododeoxyuridine, thymidine) and pyrimidine bases (6-iodouracil, uracil and 5-fluorouracil) in vivo. Acta Biol Med Germ 32:483–502

Maybaum J, Ullman B, Mandel HG, Day JL, Sadee W (1980) Regulation of RNA- and DNA-directed actions of 5-fluoropyrimidines in mouse T-lymphoma (S-49) cells. Cancer Res 40:4209–4215

Meuth M, Green G (1974) Induction of a deoxycytidineless state in cultured mammalian cells by bromodeoxyuridine. Cell 2:109–112

Miller EE, Ledis SL, Lo KW, Tsou KC (1976) 5′-Nucleotide phosphodiesterase activity of fluorodeoxyuridine-resistant mouse glioma. J Pharm Sci 65:384–387

Misra DK, Humphreys SR, Friedkin M, Goldin A, Crawford EJ (1961) Increased dihydrofolate reductase activity as a possible basis of drug resistance in leukemia. Nature 189:39–42

Moertel CG (1978) Current concepts in cancer: chemotherapy of gastrointestinal cancer. N Engl J Med 299:1049–1052

Moertel CG, Reitemeier RJ (1969) Advanced gastrointestinal cancer. Clinical management and chemotherapy. Hoeber, New York

Montgomery JA, Thomas HJ, Kisliuk RL, Gaumont Y (1979) Phosphonate analogue of 2′-deoxy-5-fluorouridylic acid. J Med Chem 22:109–111

Moran RG, Werkheiser WC, Zakrzewski SF (1976) Folate metabolism in mammalian cells in culture 1. Partial characterization of the folate derivatives present in L1210 mouse leukemia cells. J Biol Chem 254:3569–3575

Moran RG, Mulkins M, Heidelberger C (1979a) Role of thymidylate synthetase activity in development of methotrexate cytotoxicity. Proc Natl Acad Sci USA 76:5924–5928

Moran RG, Spears CP, Heidelberger C (1979b) Biochemical determinants of tumor sensitivity to 5-fluorouracil: ultrasensitive methods for the determination of 5-fluoro-2'-deoxyuridylate, 2'-deoxyuridylate and thymidylate synthetase. Proc Natl Acad Sci USA 76:1456–1460

Morris NR, Fischer GA (1960) Studies concerning inhibition of the synthesis of deoxycytidine by phosphorylated derivatives of thymidine. Biochim Biophys Acta 42:183–184

Morse PA, Potter VR (1965) Pyrimidine metabolism in tissue culture cells derived from rat hepatomas I. Suspension cell cultures derived from the Novikoff hepatoma. Cancer Res 25:499–508

Mukherjee KL, Heidelberger C (1960) Studies on fluorinated pyrimidines IX. The degradation of 5-fluorouracil-6-C^{14}. J Biol Chem 235:433–437

Mulkins M, Heidelberger C (1980) Isolation and characterization of mutant leukemic cell lines resistant to fluorinated pyrimidines. Proc. Am Assoc Cancer Res 21:285

Murinson DS, Anderson T, Schwartz HS, Myers CE, Chabner BA (1979) Competitive binding radioassay for 5-fluorodeoxyuridine 5'-monophosphate in tissues. Cancer Res 39:2471–2475

Murphy ML (1965) Dose-response relationships in growth inhibitory drugs in the rat: time of treatment as a teratologic determinant. In: Wilson JG, Warkany J (eds) Teratology. Principles and techniques. University of Chicago Press, Chicago, pp 161–184

Myers CE, Young RC, Chabner BA (1975) Biochemical determinants of 5-fluorouracil response in vivo. The role of deoxyuridylate pool expansion. J Clin Invest 56:1231–1238

Nahas A, Savlov ED, Hall TC (1974) Phosphoribosyl transferase in colon tumor and normal mucosa as an aid in adjuvant chemotherapy with 5-fluorouracil (NSC-19893). Cancer Chem Rep 58:909–912

Nakayama C, Wataya Y, Meyer RB, Santi DV (1980) Thymidine phosphorylase. Substrate specificity for 5-substituted 2'-deoxyuridines. J Med Chem 23:962–964

Nayak R, Martin D, Stolfi R, Furth J, Spiegeleman S (1978) Pyrimidine nucleosides enhance the anti-cancer activity of FU and augment its incorporation into nulcear RNA. Proc Am Assoc Cancer Res 19:63

Niedzwicki SH, Chu SH, el Kouni MH, Cha S (1980) Acyclopyrimidine nucleosides, a new class of specific inhibitors of uridine phosphorylase. Pharmacologist 22:241

Okada T, Nakayama M, Mitsui R (1974) A new approach to the development of anti-cancer agents-5-FU derivatives. Hiroshima J Med Sci 23:51–76

Osswald H, Youssef M (1979) Potentiation of the chemotherapeutic action of 5-fluorouracil by combination with cytidine or guanosine on HRS sarcoma. J Cancer Res Clin Oncol 93:241–244

Pasztor LM, Hu F (1972) Anamelanotic variant of B16 malignant melanoma. Cancer Res 32:1769–1774

Pasztor LM, Hu F, McNulty WP (1973) 5-bromodeoxyuridine-tolerant melanoma cells in vitro and in vivo. Yale J Biol Med 46:397–410

Percy DH (1975) Teratogenic effects of the pyrimidine analogues 5-iodo-deoxyuridine and cytosine arabinoside in late fetal mice and rats. Teratology 11:103–117

Phelps ME, Woodman PW, Danenberg PV (1980) Synthesis and biological activity of 5-fluoro-2'-deoxyuridine 5'-phosphorodiamidates. J Med Chem 23:1229–1232

Pitman SW, Kowal CD, Papac RJ, Bertino JR (1980) Sequential methotrexate-5-fluorouracil: a highly active drug combination in advanced squamous cell carcinoma of the head and neck. Proc Am Assoc Cancer Res 21:473

Plagemann PGW, Erbe J (1973) Nucleotide pools of Novikoff rat hepatoma cells growing in suspension culture. IV. Nucleoside transport in cells depleted of nucleotides by treatment with KCN. J Cell Physiol 81:101–111

Plagemann PGW, Erbe J (1974) The deoxyribonucleoside transport systems of cultured Novikoff rat hepatoma cells. J Cell Physiol 83:337–343

Plagemann PGW, Richey DP (1974) Transport of nucleosides, nucleic acid bases, choline and glucose by animal cells in culture. Biochim Biophys Acta 344:263–305

Plagemann PGW, Marz R, Erbe J (1976) Transport and counter-transport of thymidine in ATP depleted and thymidine kinase-deficient Novikoff rat hepatoma and mouse L cells: evidence for a high-K_m-facilitated diffusion system with wide nucleoside specificity. J Cell Physiol 89:1–18

Plagemann PGW, Marz R, Wohlhueter RM (1978) Uridine transport in Novikoff rat hepatoma cells and other cell lines and its relationship to uridine phosphorylation and phosphorolysis. J Cell Physiol 97:49–72

Prusoff WH, Chang PK (1968) 5-Iodo-2′-deoxyuridine 5′-triphosphate, an allosteric inhibitor of deoxycytidylate deaminase. J Biol Chem 243:223–230

Prusoff WH, Chang PK (1969/1970) Regulation of thymidine kinase activity by 5-iodo-2′-deoxyuridine 5′-triphosphate and deoxythymidine 5′-triphosphate. Chem Biol Interact 1:285–299

Prusoff WH, Goz B (1974) Halogenated pyrimidine deoxyribonucleosides. In: Sartorelli AC, Johns DG (eds) Antineoplastic and immunosuppressive agents. Springer, Berlin Heidelberg New York (Handbook of experimental pharmacology, vol 38/2, pp 272–347)

Prusoff WH, Bakhle YS, Sekely L (1965) Cellular and antiviral effects of halogenated deoxyribonucleosides. Ann NY Acad Sci 130:135–150

Prusoff WH, Chen MS, Fischer PH, Lins TS, Shiau GT, Schinazi RF, Walker J (1979) Antiviral iodinated pyrimidine deoxyribonucleosides: 5-iodo-2′-deoxyuridine; 5-iodo-2′-deoxycytidine; 5-iodo-5′-amino-2′,5′-dideoxyuridine. Pharmacol Ther 7:1–34

Queener SF, Morris HP, Weber G (1971) Dihydrouracil dehydrogenase activity in normal, differentiating, and regenerating liver and in hepatomas. Cancer Res 31:1004–1009

Reichard P, Sköld O, Klein G (1959) Possible enzymic mechanism for the development of resistance against fluorouracil in ascites tumours. Nature 183:939–941

Reichard P, Canellakis ZN, Canellakis ES (1961) Studies on a possible regulatory mechanism for the biosynthesis of deoxyribonucleic acid. J Biol Chem 236:2514–2519

Reichard P, Sköld O, Klein G, Révész L, Magnusson P-H (1962) Studies on resistance against 5-fluouracil I. Enzymes of the uracil pathway during development of resistance. Cancer Res 22:235–243

Reyes P, Hall TC (1969) Synthesis of 5-fluorouridine 5′-phosphate by a pyrimidine phosphoribosyltransferase of mammalian origin – II. Correlation between tumor levels of the enzyme and the 5-fluorouracil-promoted increase in survial of tumor bearing mice. Biochem Pharmacol 18:2587–2590

Reyes P, Heidelberger C (1965) Fluorinated pyrimidines. XXVI. Mammalian thymidylate synthetase: its mechanism of action and inhibition by fluorinated nucleotides. Mol Pharmacol 1:14–30

Reynolds EC, Harris AW, Finch LR (1979) Deoxyribonucleoside triphosphate pools and differential thymidine sensitivities of cultures of mouse lymphoma and myeloma cells. Biochim Biophys Acta 561:110–123

Roberts D, Loehr EV (1971) Elevation of thymidylate synthetase activity in CCRF-CEM cells. Cancer Res 31:1181–1187

Roller B, Cohen GH (1976) Deoxyribonucleoside triphosphate pools in synchronized human cells infected with herpes simplex virus types 1 and 2. J Virol 18:58–64

Roosa RA, Bradley TR, Law LW, Herzenberg LA (1962) Characterization of resistance to amethopterin, 8-azaguanine and several fluorinated pyrimidines in the murine lymphocytic neoplasm, P388. J Cell Comp Physiol 60:109–126

Roufa DJ, Sadow BN, Caskey CT (1973) Derivation of TK^- clones from revertant TK^+ mammalian cells. Genetics 75:515–530

Rustum YM, Danhauser L, Wang G (1979) Selectivity of action of 5-FU: Biochemical basis. Bull Cancer (Paris) 66:44–47

Santelli G, Valeriote F (1978) In vivo enhancement of 5-fluorouracil cytotoxicity to AKR leukemia cells by thymidine in mice. J Natl Cancer Inst 61:843–847

Santelli G, Valeriote F (1980) In vivo potentiation of 5-fluorouracil cytotoxicity against AKR leukemia by purines, pyrimidines, and their nucleosides and deoxynucleosides. J Natl Cancer Inst 64:69–72

Santi DV (1980) Perspectives on the design and biochemical pharmacology of inhibitors of thymidylate synthetase. J Med Chem 23:103–111
Santi DV, McHenry CS, Sommer H (1974) Mechanism of interaction of thymidylate synthetase with 5-fluorodeoxyuridylate. Biochemistry 13:471–481
Sartorelli AC, Creasey WA (1967) The antineoplastic and biochemical effects of some 5-fluoropyrimidines. Cancer Res 27:2201–2206
Schanker LS, Jeffrey JJ (1961) Active transport of foreign pyrimidines across the intestinal epithelium. Nature 190:727–728
Schimmer BP, Stevenson LF, Hofstede CT, Cheung NH, Marks A (1974) Glial tumor cells deficient in thymidine kinase: isolation and characterization. Exp Cell Res 86:425–428
Schwartz PM, Dunigan JM (1980) Allopurinol (HPP) modification of 5-fluorouracil (FUra) bone marrow toxicity and enhanced therapeutic index in the treatment of colon tumor # 38. Proc Am Assoc Cancer Res 21:276
Schwartz PM, Handschumacher RE (1979) Selective antagonism of 5-fluorouracil cytotoxicity by 4-hydroxypyrazolopyrimidine (allopurinol) in vitro. Cancer Res 39:3095–3101
Schwartz PM, Dunigan JM, Marsh JC, Handschumacher RE (1980) Allopurinol modification of the toxicity and antitumor activity of 5-fluorouracil. Cancer Res 40:1885–1889
Silagi S, Bruce SA (1970) Suppression of malignancy and differentiation in melanotic melanoma cells. Proc Natl Acad Sci USA 66:72–78
Sirotnak FM, Kurita S, Hutchison DJ (1968) On the nature of a transport alteration determining resistance to amethopterin in L1210 leukemia. Cancer Res 28:75–80
Sköld O (1963) Studies on resistance against 5-fluorouracil IV. Evidence for an altered uridine kinase in resistant cells. Biochim Biophys Acta 76:160–162
Slack C, Morgan RHM, Carritt B, Goldfarb PSG, Hooper ML (1976) Isolation and characterisation of Chinese hamster cells resistant to 5-fluoro-deoxyuridine. Exp Cell Res 98:1–14
Solan A, Vogl SE, Kaplan BH, Lanham R, Berenzwieg M (1980) 5-fluorouracil (FU) and methotrexate (MTX) in combination for colo-rectal cancer: Unacceptable toxicity when intermediate dose MTX precedes FU by 4 hours. Proc Am Assoc Cancer Res 21:335
Spiegelman S, Sawyer R, Nayak R, Ritzi E, Stolfi R, Martin D (1980) Improving the antitumor activity of 5-fluorouracil by increasing its incorporation into RNA via metabolic modulation. Proc Natl Acad Sci USA 77:4966–4970
Stark RM, Littlefield JW (1974) Mutagenic effect of BUdR in diploid human fibroblasts. Mutat Res 22:281–286
Szybalski W (1962) Properties and applications of halogenated deoxyribonucleic acids. In: The molecular basis of neoplasia. Uniersity of Texas Press, Austin, pp 147–171
Taguchi T (1980a) Review of a new antimetabolic agent 1-hexacarbamoyl-5-fluorouracil (HCFU). Recent Results Cancer Res 70:125–132
Taguchi T (1980b) Review of a new antimetabolic agent, 1,3,-bis(tetrahydro-2-furanyl)-5-fluoro-2,4-pyrimidinedione (FD-1). Recent Results Cancer Res 133–145
Tattersall MHN, Jackson RC, Connors TA, Harrap KR (1973) Combination chemotherapy: the interaction of methotrexate and 5-fluorouracil. Eur J Cancer 9:733–739
Trader MW, Schabel FM, Laster WR; Witt MH, Corbett TH (1979) Comparative therapeutic activity of 5-fluorouracil (FU) alone or thymidine (TdR) followed by FU against leukemia P388, spontaneous AKR leukemia, and colon carcinomas 26 and 38. Proc Am Assoc Cancer Res 20:95
Tseng W-C, Medina D, Randerath K (1978) Specific inhibition of transfer RNA methylation and modification in tissues of mice treated with 5-fluorouracil. Cancer Res 38:1250–1257
Tsou KC, Aoyagi S, Miller EE (1970) Synthesis of 5-iodo-4-indolyl-phosphodiesters of 5-fluorodeoxyuridine as possible chromogenic cancer chemotherapeutic agents. J Med Chem 13:765–768
Ullman B, Kirsch J (1979) Metabolism of 5-fluorouracil in cultured cells. Protection from 5-fluorouracil cytotoxicity by purines. Mol Pharmacol 15:537–366
Ullman B, Lee M, Martin DW, Santi DV (1978) Cytotoxicity of 5-fluoro-2′deoxyuridine: requirement for reduced folate cofactors and antagonism by methotrexate. Proc Natl Acad Sci USA 75:980–983

Umeda M, Heidelberger C (1968) Comparative studies of fluorinated pyrimidines with various cell lines. Cancer Res 28:2529–2538

Vogel SJ, Presant CA, Ratkin GA, Klahr C (1979) Phase-I study of thymidine plus 5-fluorouracil infusions in advanced colorectal carcinoma. Cancer Treat Rep 63:1–5

Washtien WL, Santi DV (1979) Assay of intracellular free and macromolecular-bound metabolites of 5-fluorodeoxyuridine and 5-fluorouracil. Cancer Res 39:3397–3404

Wilkinson DS, Crumley J (1976) The mechanism of 5-fluorouridine toxicity in Novikoff hepatoma cells. Cancer Res 36:4032–4038

Wilkinson DS, Crumley J (1977) Metabolism of 5-fluorouracil in sensitive and resistant Novikoff hepatoma cells. J Biol Chem 252:1051–1056

Wilkinson DS, Pitot HC (1973) Inhibition of ribosomal ribonucleic acid maturation in Novikoff hepatoma cells by 5-fluorouracil and 5-fluorouridine. J Biol Chem 248:63–68

Wilkinson DS, Tlsty TD, Hanas RJ (1975) The inhibition of ribosomal RNA synthesis and maturation in Novikoff hepatoma cells by 5-fluorouridine. Cancer Res 35:3014–3020

Wilkinson DS, Solomonson LP, Cory JG (1977) Increased thymidylate synthetase activity in 5-fluorodeoxyuridine-resistant Novikoff hepatoma cells. Proc Soc Exp Biol Med 154:368–371

Williams AC, Klein E (1970) Experiences with local chemotherapy and immunotherapy in premalignant and malignant skin lesions. Cancer 25:450–462

Wolberg WH (1964) Studies on the mechanism of human tumor resistance to the fluorinated pyrimidines. Cancer Res 24:1437–1447

Wolberg WH (1970) Development of resistance of Novikoff hepatoma to 5-fluoro-2′-deoxyuridine. Int J Cancer 6:261–269

Wolberg WH (1979) Enhancement by thymidine of 5-fluorouracil's inhibition of thymidylate synthetase in human tumors. Cancer Treat Rep 63:1817–1820

Woodcock TM, Martin DS, Damin LAM, Kemeny NE, Young CW (1980) Combination clinical trials with thymidine and fluorouracil: a phase-I and clinical pharmacologic evaluation. Cancer 45:1135–1143

Woodman PW, Sarrif AM, Heidelberger C (1980) Inhibition of nucleoside phosphorylase cleavage of 5-fluoro-2′-deoxyuridine by 2,4-pyrimidinedione derivatives. Biochem Pharmacol 29:1059–1063

Yoshida M, Hoshi A, Kuretani K (1978a) Prevention of antitumor effect of 5-fluorouracil by hypoxanthine. Biochem Pharmacol 27:2979–2982

Yoshida M, Kuretani K, Hoshi A (1978b) Bode of action of 5-fluorouridine 5′-phosphate in vivo and in vitro. Chem Pharm Bull 26:429–434

Young RC, Hubbard SP, DeVita VT (1974) The chemotherapy of ovarian carcinoma. Cancer Treat Rev 1:99–110

Zielke HR (1979) Isolation of thymidine-resistant cells from a thymidine-sensitive acute lymphoblastic leukemia cell line. Cancer Res 39:3373–3376.

CHAPTER 20

Resistance to Amino Acid Analogs

J. R. UREN

A. Definitions

Three types of resistance will be discussed in this chapter: natural resistance, acquired resistance, and cross-resistance. Natural resistance is the inherent difference in sensitivity of cell types to the lethal actions of various agents. Acquired resistance is the decrease in sensitivity of a cell population to an agent following repeated exposure to that agent. Cross-resistance is the concomitant decrease in sensitivity to two or more agents when cells are repeatedly exposed to only one of these agents. Acquired resistance will be primarily discussed, with only limited consideration of the other topics.

For the purpose of this review, amino acid analogs are compounds which resemble amino acids in structure and antagonize some aspect of amino acid metabolism. The first part of this definition is easy to identify, but many compounds have not been sufficiently characterized to be certain of the second. For example, the classical antifolate compounds like methotrexate could be considered glutamic acid analogs from the structural viewpoint like many of the other alpha-amino-substituted amino acids described in Table 1. Only the extensive body of experimental evidence which documents its site of action as a true folic acid antagonist prevents such a characterization. Recently, however, SCANLON and WAXMAN (1980) demonstrated that methotrexate will alter the transport of methionine into cells independent of its antifolate activity. Possibly under some experimental conditions these compounds are also functioning as amino acid analogs. The polypeptide and protein antitumor agents are also not included as amino acid analogs although structurally they are substituted amino acids.

B. Natural Resistance

Any compound which demonstrates antitumor activity in animals shows some degree of differential natural cellular resistance by virtue of the fact that a positive antitumor response means that the cytotoxic effects of the agent are directed at the tumor cells to a greater extent than normal host tissues. The reasons for these differential responses are complex, relating to the individual growth rates and overall metabolism of each cell type. It is beyond the scope of this chapter to review what is known about the 103 amino acid analogs compiled in Tables 1 and 2. The purpose of these tables is to illustrate the types of chemical alterations of amino acid structure which seem to show antitumor activity. The compounds with exceptional activity have been further evaluated with respect to acquired resistance and will be discussed in greater detail in the following section. The orga-

Table 1. Alpha-amino-substituted amino acids with in vivo antitumor activity

Substituent	Structure	Tumor test system	Reference
		Phenylalanine Analogs	
Carbobenzoxy	$PhCH_2OCO-$	Ehrlich carcinoma/mice	SCHLESINGER et al. (1971)
		Hepatoma AH60C/rats	FUKUSHIMA and TOYOSHIMA (1975)
(Vinyl ester)	$CH_2{=}CH-$	Ehrlich carcinoma/mice	LOEFFLER et al. (1977)
		Walker 256/rats	LOEFFLER et al. (1977)
(1,2-Dibromo-ethyl ester)	$CH_2BrCHBr-$	Ehrlich carcinoma/mice	LOEFFLER et al. (1977)
		Walker 256/rats	LOEFFLER et al. (1977)
Iodoacetyl	ICH_2CO-	Sarcoma 37/mice	FRIEDMAN and RUTENBERG (1950)
Methyl	CH_3-	Novikoff hepatoma/rats	MARTEL and BERLINGUET (1959)
		Leukemia SR 61/mice	FUKUSHIMA and TOYOSHIMA (1975)
		Ehrlich carcinoma/mice	FUKUSHIMA and TOYOSHIMA (1975)
Hydroxyethyl	$HOCH_2CH_2-$	Leukemia SR 61/mice	FUKUSHIMA and TOYOSHIMA (1975)
		Ehrlich carcinoma/mice	FUKUSHIMA and TOYOSHIMA (1975)
Isopentyl	$(CH_3)_2CHCH_2$-$-CH_2-$	Leukemia SR 61/mice	FUKUSHIMA and TOYOSHIMA (1975)
		Ehrlich carcinoma/mice	FUKUSHIMA and TOYOSHIMA (1975)
Carboxypropyl	$HOOC(CH_2)_3-$	Ehrlich carcinoma/mice	FUKUSHIMA and TOYOSHIMA (1975)
Propionyl	CH_3CH_2CO-	Leukemia SR 61/mice	FUKUSHIMA and TOYOSHIMA (1975)
		Ehrlich carcinoma/mice	FUKUSHIMA and TOYOSHIMA (1975)
Lauryl	$CH_3(CH_2)_{10}CO-$	Leukemia SR 61/mice	FUKUSHIMA and TOYOSHIMA (1975)
9-Fluorenylacetyl	$9\text{-}C_{13}H_9CH_2CO-$	Leukemia SR 61/mice	FUKUSHIMA and TOYOSHIMA (1975)
		Ehrlich carcinoma/mice	FUKUSHIMA and TOYOSHIMA (1975)
		Hepatoma AH60C/rats	FUKUSHIMA and TOYOSHIMA (1975)
2-Naphthalene-sulfonyl	$2\text{-}C_{10}H_7SO_2-$	Ehrlich carcinoma/mice	FUKUSHIMA and TOYOSHIMA (1975)
2-Nitrophenyl-sulfenyl	NO_2PhS-	Sarcoma 45/rats	LAUKAITIS and PAULIUKONIS (1976)
		Leucine Analogs	
Iodoacetyl	ICH_2CO-	Sarcoma 37/mice	FRIEDMAN and RUTENBERG (1950)
2-Furanylmethyl	$2\text{-}C_4H_3OCH_2-$	Leukemia SR 61/mice	FUKUSHIMA and TOYOSHIMA (1975)
		Ehrlich carcinoma/mice	FUKUSHIMA and TOYOSHIMA (1975)
Propionyl	CH_3CH_2CO-	Leukemia SR 61/mice	FUKUSHIMA and TOYOSHIMA (1975)
		Tryptophan Analogs	
Iodoacetyl	ICH_2CO-	Sarcoma 37/mice	FRIEDMAN and RUTENBERG (1950)
Carbobenzoxy	$PhCH_2OCO-$	Leukemia SR 61/mice	FUKUSHIMA and TOYOSHIMA (1975)
2-Naphthalene-sulfonyl	$2\text{-}C_{10}H_7SO_2-$	Leukemia SR 61/mice	FUKUSHIMA and TOYOSHIMA (1975)
		Ehrlich carcinoma/mice	FUKUSHIMA and TOYOSHIMA (1975)
		Hepatoma AH60C/rats	FUKUSHIMA and TOYOSHIMA (1975)
		Isoleucine Analogs	
Ethylcarbamino-methyl	$EtOCONHCH_2-$	Ehrlich carcinoma/mice	FUKUSHIMA and TOYOSHIMA (1975)
Pentadecanyl	$CH_3(CH_2)_{13}CO-$	Hepatoma AH60C/rats	FUKUSHIMA and TOYOSHIMA (1975)
		Aspargine Analogs	
Carbobenzoxy	$PhCH_2OCO-$	Ehrlich carcinoma/mice	SCHLESINGER et al. (1971)
		Mammary carcinoma/mice	SCHLESINGER et al. (1971)
		Lymphosarcoma/mice	SCHLESINGER et al. (1971)
		Serine Analogs	
Dichloroacetyl	Cl_2CHCO-	Sarcoma 37/mice	LEVI et al. (1960)
		Walker 256/rats	BLONDAL et al. (1961)

Table 1 (continued)

Substituent	Structure	Tumor test system	Reference
		Methionine Analogs	
Dichloroacetyl	Cl_2CHCO-	Ehrlich carcinoma/mice	ABE et al. (1960)
Chloroacetyl	$ClCH_2CO-$	Ehrlich carcinoma/mice	ABE et al. (1960)
2-Naphthylamino-methyl	$2\text{-}C_{10}H_7NHCH_2-$	Leukemia SR 61/mice	FUKUSHIMA and TOYOSHIMA (1975)
2-Furanylmethyl	$2\text{-}C_4H_3OCH_2-$	Leukemia SR 61/mice	FUKUSHIMA and TOYOSHIMA (1975)
		Ehrlich carcinoma	FUKUSHIMA and TOYOSHIMA (1975)
		Threonine Analogs	
2-Naphthylamino-methyl	$2\text{-}C_{10}H_7NHCH_2-$	Hepatoma AH60C/rats	FUKUSHIMA and TOYOSHIMA (1975)
		Valine Analogs	
Propionyl	CH_3CH_2CO-	Leukemia SR 61/mice	FUKUSHIMA and TOYOSHIMA (1975)
		Ehrlich carcinoma/mice	FUKUSHIMA and TOYOSHIMA (1975)
		Alanine Analogs	
Bischloroethyl	$(ClCH_2CH_2)_2-$	Ehrlich carcinoma/mice	SCHMID et al. (1965)
		Numerous/mice and rats	WHITE (1960a)
		Glycine Analogs	
Bischloroethyl	$(ClCH_2CH_2)_2-$	Ehrlich carcinoma/mice	SCHMID et al. (1965)
		Numerous/mice and rats	WHITE (1960a)
Carbobenzoxy-	$PhCH_2OCO-$	Ehrlich carcinoma/mice	LOEFFLER et al. (1977)
(1,2-Dibromo-ethyl ester)	$CH_2BrCHBr-$	Walker 256/rats	LOEFFLER et al. (1977)
Diazoacetyl	N_2CHCO-	Lewis lung metastasis/mice	GIRALDI et al. (1979)
(amide)	NH_2-		
Phenylacetyl	$PhCH_2CO-$	Ehrlich carcinoma/mice	LICHTENSTEIN et al. (1977)
(phenyl)	$Ph-$		
		Norvaline Analogs	
Hydroxylamino	$HO-$	Ehrlich carcinoma/mice	WILSON et al. (1959)
		Aspartic Acid Analogs	
Carbobenzoxy	$PhCH_2OCO-$	Lymphosarcoma/mice	SCHLESINGER et al. (1971)
(*β*-Benzyl ester)	$PhCH_2-$	Ehrlich carcinoma/mice	LICHTENSTEIN et al. (1977)
Phosphonacetyl	$H_2O_3PCH_2CO-$	Lewis lung/mice	JOHNSON et al. (1978)
		B16 melanoma/mice	JOHNSON et al. (1978)
		Glioma 26/mice	JOHNSON et al. (1978)
		Leukemia P388/mice	JOHNSON et al. (1976)
Phenylacetyl	$PhCH_2CO-$	Ehrlich carcinoma/mice	LICHTENSTEIN et al. (1977)
(*β*-Benzyl ester)	$PhCH_2-$		
		Arginine Analogs	
Acetyl	CH_3CO-	Leukemia SR 61/mice	FUKUSHIMA and TOYOSHIMA (1975)
		Homocysteine Thiolactone Analogs	
Arachidonyl	$CH_3(CH_2)_{18}CO-$	Adenocarcinoma/mice	MCCULLY and CLOPATH (1977)
		Tyrosine Analogs	
Carbobenzoxy	$PhCH_2OCO-$	Ehrlich carcinoma/mice	LICHTENSTEIN et al. (1977)
(*O*-Benzyl)	$PhCH_2-$	Ehrlich carcinoma/mice	LICHTENSTEIN et al. (1977)
Phenylacetyl	$PhCH_2CO-$	Ehrlich carcinoma/mice	LICHTENSTEIN et al. (1977)
(*O*-Benzyl)	$PhCH_2-$	Ehrlich carcinoma/mice	LICHTENSTEIN et al. (1977)
Phenylpropionyl	$PhCH_2CH_2CO-$	Ehrlich carcinoma/mice	LICHTENSTEIN et al. (1977)
(*O*-Benzyl)	$PhCH_2-$	Ehrlich carcinoma/mice	LICHTENSTEIN et al. (1977)

Table 2. Side-chain-substituted amino acids with in vivo antitumor activity

Substituent	Structure	Tumor test system	Reference
		Phenylalanine Analogs	
4′-Fluoro	F–	Taper tumor/mice	MACLEAN AND HUBER (1971)
4′-Bis(chloro-ethyl)amino	$(ClCH_2CH_2)_2N$–	Numerous/mice and rats	WHITE (1960b)
2′-Bis(chloro-ethyl)amino	$(ClCH_2CH_2)_2N$–	Leukemia L1210/mice	TYRER et al. (1969)
2′-Methyl-5′-bis-(chloroethyl)-amino	2′-CH_3-5′-$(ClCH_2CH_2)_2N$–	Sarcoma 180/mice	ZENG and YUNFENG (1979)
3′,4′-Dihydroxy (methylester) L and D isomer	3′,4′-HO–	Melanoma B16/mice	WICK (1977)
		Neuroblastoma/mice	WICK (1978)
		Leukemia L1210–P388/mice	WICK (1979)
α-Methyl	CH_3-	Leukemia L1210/mice	WICK 1979)
3′-4′-dihydroxy (methylester)	3′,4′-HO–	Leukemia P388/mice	WICK (1979)
3′-4′-Dihydroxy	3′-4′-HO–	Melanoma B16/mice	FUJITA et al. (1980)
5′-cysteinyl	$COOHCHNH_2$-CH_2S–	Leukemia L1210/mice	FUJITA et al. (1980)
		Glycine Analogs	
2,2-Tetra-methylene	$-(CH_2)_4-$	Novikoff hepatoma/rats	MARTEL and BERLINQUET (1959)
		Walker carcinoma/rats	CONNOR et al. (1960)
N-Hydroxy	HO–	Ehrlich carcinoma/mice	WILSON et al. (1959)
2,2-Tetramethylene	$-(CH_2)_4-$		
2,2-Pentamethylene	$-(CH_2)_5-$	Novikoff hepatoma/rats	MARTEL and BERLINQUET (1959)
N-Ethyl-2,2--pentamethylene	CH_3CH_2– $-(CH_2)_5-$	Novikoff hepatoma/rats	MARTEL and BERLINQUET (1959)
N-Methyl-2,2--pentamethylene	CH_3– $-(CH_2)_5-$	Novikoff hepatoma/rats	MARTEL and BERLINQUET (1959)
2-Allyl	CH_2=CH–	Novikoff hepatoma/rats	MARTEL and BERLINQUET (1959)
3′-Chloro-4′,5′--dihydro-5′--isoxazole	CCl — CH_2 ‖ | N–O–CH–	Leukemia L1210/mice	MARTIN et al. (1974)
		Leukemia P388/mice	HOUCHENS et al. (1978)
		Ovarian tumor/mice	HOUCHENS et al. (1978)
3′-Chloro-4′-hydroxy-4′-5′--dihydro-5′--isoxazole	CCl — CHOH ‖ | N–O–CH–	Leukemia L1210/mice	MARTIN et al. (1974)
2-*N*-Bis(chloro-ethyl)amino-phenylethyl	$(ClCH_2CH_2)_2N$– –Ph–CH_2CH_2–	Walker carcinoma/rats	STOCK (1958)
		Melanoma S91/mice	LUCK (1957)
4′-Formyl-3′--hydroxyphenyl	4′-OCH 3′-HO– Ph–	Carcinoma IMC/mice	UMEZAWA (1978)
		Gardner lymphosarcoma/mice	UMEZAWA (1978)
		Homocysteine Analogs	
S-Ethyl	CH_3CH_2–	UCLA fibrosarcoma/rats	LEVY et al. (1953)
		Jensen sarcoma/rats	LEVY et al. (1953)
		Leucine Analogs	
5,5,5-Trifluoro	5,5,5 F–	AKR leukemia/mice	RENNERT and ANKER (1964)
		Leukemia L4946/mice	RENNERT and ANKER (1964)

Table 2 (continued)

Substituent	Structure	Tumor test system	Reference
		Alanine Analogs	
β-3′-Thienyl	CH–C– ‖ ╲ CH–S–CH	Jensen sarcoma/rats	BRISTOW and WISSLER (1961)
		Walker carcinoma/rats	BRISTOW and WISSLER (1961)
		Lymphosarcoma/rats	HRUBAN and WISSLER (1960)
β-2′-Thienyl	CH–CH ‖ ╲ CH–S–C–	Sarcoma T241/mice	JACQUEZ et al. (1953)
		Ehrlich carcinoma/mice	WILSON et al. (1959)
α-Methyl	CH_3–	Novikoff hepatoma/rats	MARTEL and BERLINQUET (1959)
3-(N-Hydroxy- -N-nitroso)	HON(NO)–	Fibrosarcoma/hamster	MURTHY et al. (1966)
		Leukemia P388–L1210/mice	JAYARAM et al. (1979)
β-Seleno	Se–	Lymphosarcoma/rats	WEISBERGER and SUHRLAND (1956)
		Cysteine Analogs	
3,3-Dimethyl	3,3 CH_3–	Sarcoma 180/mice	LITTMANN et al. (1964)
		Melanoma S91/mice	HOURANI and DEMOPOULOS (1969)
S-Ethylcarbamoyl	CH_3CH_2NHCO–	Ehrlich carcinoma/mice	NEMETH et al. (1978)
		Sarcoma 37/mice	NEMETH et al. (1978)
S-Chloroethyl- carbamoyl	$ClCH_2CH_2$- -NHCO–	Ehrlich carcinoma/mice	NEMETH et al. (1978)
		Sarcoma 37/mice	NEMETH et al. (1978)
S-Trityl	$(Ph)_3C$–	Leukemia L1210/mice	ZEE-CHENG and CHENG (1972)
S-Carbamoyl	NH_2CO–	Adenocarcinoma/mice	SKINNER et al. (1958)
N-CBZ-S-benzyl	N $PhCH_2OCO$– S $PhCH_2$–	Ehrlich carcinoma/mice	SCHLESINGER et al. (1971)
1-N-Bis(chloro- ethyl)hydrazide	$(ClCH_2CH_2)_2$- NNH–	Myeloma P8/rats	GOLOVINSKY et al. (1977)
		Walker carcinoma/rats	GOLOVINSKY et al. (1977)
		Pliss lymphosarcoma/rats	GOLOVINSKY et al. (1977)
		Yoshida sarcoma/rats	GOLOVINSKY et al. (1977)
		Jensen sarcoma/rats	GOLOVINSKY et al. (1977)
		Sarcoma 180/mice	GOLOVINSKY et al. (1977)
S-2-Hydroxy- pentenal	CH_3CHOH- $(CH_2CHO)CH$–	Ehrlich carcinoma/mice	TILLIAN et al. (1976)
S-Crotonal	$CH_3(CH_2$- -CHO)CH–	Ehrlich carcinoma/mice	TILLIAN et al. (1976)
		Aspartic Acid Analogs	
D isomer		Lymphosarcoma/mice	MIURA et al. (1970)
N-Carbamoyl α (lactam)	–NHCO–	Lymphosarcoma/mice	MIURA et al. (1970)
β-Hyrazide	NH_2NH–	Sarcoma 180/mice	MICKELSON and FLIPPIN (1956)
β-Hydroxamate	HONH–	Lymphosarcoma/mice	MIURA et al. (1970)
		Leukemia L1210/mice	MIURA et al. (1970)
		Sarcoma 180/mice	MIURA et al. (1970)
		Yoshida sarcoma/mice	MIURA et al. (1970)
		Leukemia SN36/mice	MIURA et al. (1970)
β-Methylamide	CH_3NH–	Sarcoma 180/mice	UREN et al. (1977)
		Leukemia L1210/mice	UREN et al. (1977)
		Adenocarcinoma/mice	UREN et al. (1977)
		Tryptophan Analogs	
5′-Bis(chloro- ethyl)amino	$(ClCH_2CH_2)_2N$–	Plasma cell YPCl/mice	FISHBEIN et al. (1964)
		Mast cell P815/mice	FISHBEIN et al. (1964)
		Ehrlich carcinoma/mice	SCHMID et al. (1965)

Table 2 (continued)

Substituent	Structure	Tumor test system	Reference
		Norleucine Analogs	
6-Diazo-5-oxo	6 N_2–5 O=	Numerous/mice and rats	DUVALL (1960b)
6-Hydroxy	HO–	Novikoff hepatoma/rats	MARTEL and BERLINQUET (1959)
6-Methylthio	CH_3S–	Novikoff hepatoma/rats	MARTEL and BERLINQUET (1959)
		Serine Analogs	
O-Diazoacetyl	N_2CH_2CO–	Numerous/mice and rats	DUVALL (1960a)
O-Carbazyl	H_2NNHCO–	Adenocarcinoma/mice	SKINNER et al. (1958)
O-Bis(2-chloro-propyl)-carbamyl	$(CH_3CHClCH_2)_2$–NCO–	Plasma tumor/mice	FALKSON and FALKSON (1965)
		Ehrlich carcinoma/mice	FALKSON and FALKSON (1965)
		Dunning leukemia/mice	FALKSON and FALKSON (1965)
O-Bis(chloro-ethyl)carbamyl	$(ClCH_2CH_2)_2$-NCO–	Walker carcinoma/rats	STOCK (1958)
β-Phenyl	Ph–	Sarcoma 45/rats	STREUKAS et al. (1977)
		Norvaline Analogs	
5-Methylthio	CH_3S–	Novikoff hepatoma/rats	MARTEL and BERLINQUET (1959)
5-Bis(chloroethyl)-aminophenyl	$(ClCH_2CH_2)_2$-NPh–	Walker carcinoma/rats	STOCK (1958)
		Melanoma S91/mice	LUCK (1957)
5-Diazo-4-oxo	5-N_2– 4-O=	Leukemia L1210/mice	CONNEY et al. (1976)
5-Chloro-4-oxo	5-Cl– 4-O=	Leukemia L1210/mice	CONNEY et al. (1976)
		Glutamic Acid Analogs	
D isomer		Lymphosarcoma/mice	MIURA et al. (1970)
γ-4′-Hydroxy-anilide	HOPhNH–	Melanoma B16/mice	VOGEL et al. (1977)
		Lysine Analogs	
ε-*N*-Bis-chloroethyl	$(ClCH_2CH_2)_2$–	Sarcoma 45/rats	SPASSKAYA and LARIONOV (1966)
		Jenson sarcoma/rats	SPASSKAYA and LARIONOV (1966)
		Carcinoma RGl/rats	SPASSKAYA and LARIONOV (1966)
		Sarcoma 180, 298, 37/mice	SPASSKAYA and LARIONOV (1966)
		Ehrlich carcinoma/mice	SPASSKAYA and LARIONOV (1966)
		Melanoma S91/mice	SPASSKAYA and LARIONOV (1966)
ε-*N*-Benzoyl	PhCO–	Carcinoma/mice	LARIONOV (1965)
		Tyrosine Analogs	
3-Fluoro	F–	Jensen sarcoma/rats	MAY and LITZKA (1939)
3-Nitro	NO_2–	Taper tumor/mice	MACLEAN et al. (1971)
		Citrulline Analogs	
N^2,N^8-Bis-(*n*-butyloxy-carbonylamino-methyl)–	C_4H_9OCO-$NHCH_2$–	Hepatoma/rats	FUJITA et al. (1977)

nization of these tables is for structural comparisons only. Compounds which can be considered to be a structural analog of one amino acid can in fact antagonize the metabolism of another. For example, 4-bis-(chloroethyl)-amino-phenylalanine is antagonized by leucine, *O*-diazoacetyl-serine antagonizes glutamine, and gamma glutamyl-4-hydroxyanilide antagonizes tyrosine metabolism (see below).

C. Acquired and Cross-Resistance

I. Glutamine Antagonists

1. Biochemistry

The following compounds in Table 2 have been shown to antagonize glutamine metabolism in either prokaryotic or eukaryotic cells: 5-diazo-4-oxo-norleucine (DON), *O*-diazoacetylserine (azaserine), 3-chloro-4,5-dihydro-5-isoxazole-glycine (acivicin), 3-chloro-4-hydroxy-4,5-dihydro-5-isoxazoleglycine, *O*-carbazyl-serine, and *S*-carbamyl-cysteine. Also, the *N*-acetyl (duazomycin) and peptide derivatives (azotomycin and alazopeptin) of DON have demonstrated antitumor activity (LIVINGSTON et al. 1970). In mammalian cells glutamine is involved in the biosynthesis of purines and pyrimidines as described in Figs. 1 and 2. In addition, glutamine functions as an amino donor in the synthesis of NAD from deamido-NAD, glucosamine-6-phosphate from fructose-6-phosphate, and asparagine from aspartic acid.

Among these multiple possible sites of inhibition the FGAR to FGAM reaction (Fig. 1) seems to be the most sensitive to the best studied compounds, DON and azaserine (LEVENBERG et al. 1957). This inhibition has been shown to be irreversible and a valylcysteine azaserine complex has been isolated from the chicken liver enzyme (MIZOBUCHI and BUCHANAN 1968). FGAR accumulates in the cells at low DON levels, but this accumulation is abolished by higher levels of the drug, suggesting an inhibition of the earlier steps leading to FGAR synthe-

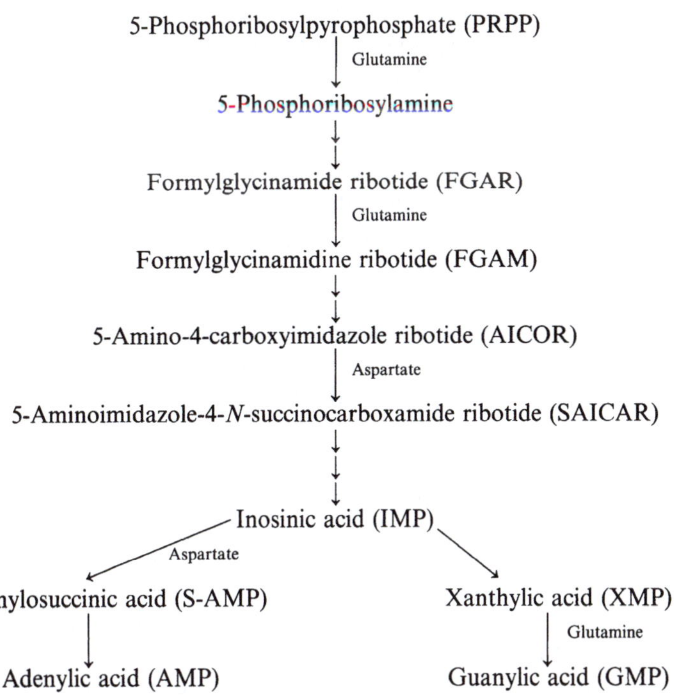

Fig. 1. Glutamine and aspartate requiring reactions of the purine biosynthetic pathway

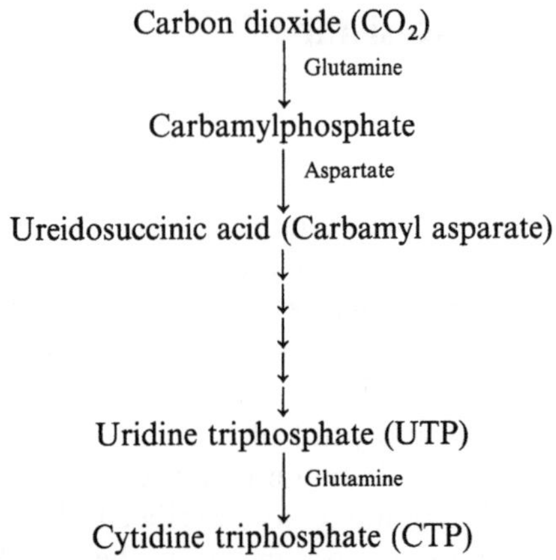

Fig. 2. Glutamine and aspartate requiring reactions of the pyrimidine biosynthetic pathway

sis (ANDERSON and BROCKMAN 1963). Likewise, low concentrations of DON effective at inhibiting purine biosynthesis actually stimulate pyrimidine biosynthesis from labeled orotic acid, possibly by increasing the availability of glutamine for cytidine triphosphate (CTP) synthetase (MOORE and HURLBERT 1961). At higher concentrations of DON these investigators found that both purine and cytidine formation was inhibited, yet cells were able to maintain 60% of RNA turnover, suggesting extensive salvage utilization of preformed nucleotides. With azaserine at high concentrations sites of inhibition independent of glutamine metabolism also seem to exist. Cells undergo morphological changes in the nucleolus characteristic of DNA-binding agents (SIMARD and BERNARD 1966), bacteria are mutagenized (HEMMERLY and DEMEREC 1955), and lysogenic bacteriophages are induced (GOTS et al. 1955). Radiation-resistant mutants of *Escherichia coli* were cross-resistant to azaserine (GREENBERG et al. 1961). These DNA-altering properties have not been found with DON (SZYBALSKI 1958; WOODY et al. 1961). It is reasonable to assume that these alternative sites for inhibition become much more important as cells express resistance mechanisms for the most sensitive sites.

2. Resistance

Azaserine resistance has been developed in three transplantable murine tumors by passage of the tumor through mice treated with azaserine. A plasma-cell tumor (70429), an ascites carcinoma TA3, and a leukemia L1210 resistant to azaserine have been developed by these techniques (POTTER and LAW 1957; SARTORELLI and LEPAGE 1958; JACQUEZ and HUTCHISON 1958). Resistance was developed in as few as six generations after transplantation in the treated animals and maximally expressed by 13 generations (SARTORELLI and LEPAGE 1958). In four of five different sublines obtained after a single generation in treated animals, the resistance was shown to be stable and heritable by the fact that it would not revert back to the sensitive state after further transplantation in animals not treated with azaserine (POTTER and LAW 1957). The resistance was also shown to be incomplete in that some measure of sensitivity to the drug was observed in the most resistant lines with all of these examples. In every case as well, cross-resistance to DON has been shown. The plasma-cell tumor and the carcinoma were also shown to be cross-resistant to *N*-methylformamide (a compound also shown to inhibit de novo purine biosynthesis; BARCLAY and GARFINKEL 1957) but not 6-mercaptopurine (POTTER and LAW 1958; SARTORELLI and LEPAGE 1958).

Earlier mechanistic studies suggested that the plasma cell tumor was resistant by virtue of its lower uptake of azaserine at concentrations below 10μg/ml. Likewise the naturally resistant lymphosarcoma 6C3HED took up less drug at all concentrations than the sensitive plasma cell lines (PINE 1958). But more detailed studies of the transport of azaserine in the plasma tumor showed no difference between the sensitive and resistant lines (ANDERSON and JACQUEZ 1961). Similarly, drug transport does not appear to be the mechanism for L1210 resistance (JACQUEZ and HUTCHISON 1958) and carcinoma TA3 resistance (SARTORELLI and LEPAGE 1957). In this carcinoma, resistance was related to a greater rate of recovery from inhibition by azaserine, suggesting a more rapid resynthesis of inhibited enzymes. In addition, these cells could utilize preformed purines by their salvage pathways to a greater extent than the sensitive cells (SARTORELLI and LEPAGE 1958).

Recently, studies on the newer glutamine antagonist acivicin (3-chloro-4,5-dihydro-5-isoxazoleglycine) have been described by JAYARAM et al. (1980). Using a resistant P388 leukemia they found that the V_{max} for transport of the resistant line was ten fold lower than the sensitive parent cell line, while the K_m was unchanged. Drug metabolism was minimal in both lines. Presumably as a consequence of this enhanced uptake of drug in the sensitive line, a therapeutic dose inhibited fructose-6-phosphate aminotransferase, PRPP aminotransferase (Fig. 1), and L-glutaminase only in the sensitive line while asparagine synthetase and carbamylphosphate synthetase (Fig. 2) were equally inhibited in both lines.

II. Aspartic Acid Antagonists

1. Biochemistry

N-Phosphonacetyl aspartate (PALA) and 3-(*N*-hydroxy-*N*-nitroso)-alanine (alanosine) are two analogs from Tables 1 and 2, respectively, which antagonize aspartic acid metabolism. PALA interferes with pyrimidine biosynthesis by preventing the conversion of carbamylphosphate to carbamylaspartate (Fig. 2). The compound functions as a transition-state analog and is competitive with respect to carbamylphosphate, with a K_i of about 1 n*M* (COLLINS and STARK 1971). The toxicity and antitumor activity can be reversed by uridine and carbamylaspartate, demonstrating the selectivity of the drug for only this reaction (JOHNSON 1977). The mechanism of growth inhibition by alanosine is more complex since the drug only weakly inhibits the enzymes of aspartic acid metabolism (JAYARAM and COONEY 1979). Interestingly, however, a metabolite of alanosine was shown to be a potent inhibitor of adenylosuccinate synthetase (HURLBERT et al. 1977). This metabolite was shown to be synthesized by SAICAR synthetase by the conjugation of alanosine to AICOR (see Fig. 1). The conjugate demonstrated a K_i of 0.2 μ*M* compared with 57 m*M* for unaltered alanosine toward adenylosuccinate synthetase (TYAGI and CONNEY 1980). Adenine but not hypoxanthine would reverse the inhibition of DNA synthesis the drug, demonstrating the significance of this site of inhibition (TYAGI and COONEY 1980). A similar antibiotic, hadacidin, (*N*-formyl-*N*-hydroxyglycine) also inhibits adenylosuccinate synthesis and is competitive with aspartate (CLARK and RUDOLPH 1976). Likewise, the toxicity of this compound is reversed by adenine but not hypoxanthine (PATTERSON 1976), but this analog demonstrates much less in vivo antitumor activity than alanosine (WHITE 1962).

2. Resistance

PALA resistance has been selected for by subculturing simian virus 40 transformed Syrian hamster cell lines and human breast cancer cell lines in the presence of various levels of the drug (KEMPE et al. 1976; COWAN and LIPPMAN 1980). In every case overproduction of aspartic transcarbamylase to as much as 100-fold has been the mechanism of resistance. With the hamster system this has been shown to be a spontaneous stocastic process with a frequency of $2–5 \times 10^{-5}$. The activities of carbamylphosphate sythetase and dihydroorotase which copurify with aspartic transcarbamylase also increased in parallel (KEMPE et al. 1976). To a large degree the level of natural resistance of various cell types to PALA also correlates with the level of aspartic transcarbamylase in the cell (JOHNSON et al. 1978; JAYARAM et al. 1979).

When mice bearing the PALA-sensitive Lewis lung carcinoma were repeatedly treated with subcurative doses of PALA, drug-resistant variants were isolated (KENSLER et al. 1980). Three of the four variants had marked increases in aspartic transcarbamylase while the fourth had normal levels of this enzyme. In an attempt to identify the nature of this resistance, it was demonstrated that the resistant lines had normal levels of salvage pathway enzymes, normal aspartic transcarbamylase enzyme kinetics, normal recovery time courses following the administration of a single dose of PALA, and normal uptake of labeled PALA in vitro. The only factor which might explain this resistance was a higher ratio of carbamylphosphate synthetase to aspartic transcarbamylase in the complex than was found with the sensitive line. It was suggested that an augmented pool of carbamylphosphate might competitively displace PALA from the enzyme and allow pyrimidine biosynthesis to continue. Support for this proposal was suggested by the therapeutic synergism between acivicin, a carbamylphosphate synthetase inhibitor (see previous section), and PALA (KENSLER et al. 1980).

Alanosine resistance was obtained in mice bearing the leukemias P388 and L1210 by repeated subcurative treatment of the animals with the drug (TYAGI et al. 1980). Biochemical studies demonstrated that the P388-resistant line had a lower specific activity for SAICAR synthetase, the enzyme which conjugates the inactive alanosine to AICOR forming the active inhibitor (Fig. 1), accounting for the lower level of the active anabolite in the resistant cells. In contrast, the L1210-resistant line had a normal specific activity for this enzyme. Both resistant lines, however, had much higher levels of the enzymes of the purine salvage pathways but unaltered levels of the alanosyl-AICOR degradative enzyme, adenylosuccinate lyase. Apparently the ability of the cells to salvage adenine from the blood imparts resistance.

III. Tyrosine Antagonists

1. Biochemistry

The following compounds from Table 2 have been shown to interfere with tyrosine metabolism: L- and D-3-4-dihydroxy-phenylalanine methylester (DOPA methylester), alpha methyl-3-4-dihydroxy-phenylalanine methylester (alpha-methyl-DOPA-methylester), 3-4-dihydroxy-5-cysteinyl-phenylalanine (5-cysteinyl DOPA), and gamma glutamyl-4-hydroxy-benzylamide (GHB). Tyrosine metabolism not only includes protein synthesis but also melanin formation (pigment production) and epinephrine formation (adrenal hormone synthesis). It is the involvement of these tyrosine analogs in melanin formation that has been exploited therapeutically, mostly toward melanoma tumors, and the involvement of these analogs in epinephrine synthesis that has produced host toxicity. Biochemical analysis has suggested that the tyrosine analogs are by themselves nontoxic, but in melanotic cells they undergo futher metabolism by tyrosinase to quinone derivatives which are highly toxic (WICK 1980). DNA synthesis has been shown to be most sensitive to these agents; and DNA polymerase, while not sensitive to the DOPA analogs alone, was very sensitive to the agents after their incubation with tyrosinase (WICK 1979). The activity of these agents toward cells other than melanomas suggests that other enzymes such as myeloperoxidases are capable of activating the agents to quinones (WICK 1980). Like alanosine, these compounds appear to require anabolism to their active agents, that is "lethal synthesis".

2. Resistance

Acquired resistance to these agents has not been selected, but a spontaneous amelanotic line of melanoma S91 was much less sensitive to the growth inhibitory properties of the DOPA analogs than the parent melanotic line (WICK et al. 1977). In addition, both leukemia L1210 and melanoma B16 are sensitive to the cytotoxic effect of a quinone derived from GHB by tyrosinase oxidation, but only the B16 melanoma was inhibited by GHB alone (VOGEL et al. 1977). These studies again point to the importance of tyrosinase in the selectivity of these agents.

IV. Asparagine Antagonists

1. Biochemistry

The following compounds from Table 2 have been shown to interfere with asparagine metabolism: 5-diazo-4-oxo-norvaline (DONV), 5-chloro-4-oxo-norvaline (CONV), beta-aspartyl hydrazide, beta-aspartyl hydroxamate, and beta-aspartyl methylamide. All of the above compounds will inhibit asparagine synthetase, with CONV being the most potent, producing irreversible inhibition (JAYARAM et al. 1976; UREN et al. 1977). In cell culture, however, asparagine could only reverse the cytotoxicity of the last three compounds, demonstrating their selectivity for asparagine metabolism (UREN et al. 1977; SUMMERS and HANDSCHUMACHER 1971). The most potent of these selective inhibitors, beta-aspartyl methylamide, inhibited asparagine synthetase, competitive with glutamine, with a K_i of 0.2 m*M* (UREN et al. 1977). Since asparagine reversed the toxicity of these compounds they should be investigated under conditions of asparagine depletion such as is produced by L-asparaginase therapy. Beta-aspartyl methylamide, unlike the other two compounds, was relatively resistant to cleavage by *E. coli* and *Erwinia* asparaginases (UREN et al. 1977). This compound, however, was a good reversible inhibitor of asparaginase ($K_i = 0.03$ m*M*), unlike DONV, which demonstrated irreversible inhibition with this enzyme (UREN et al. 1977; JACKSON and HANDSCHUMACHER 1970).

2. Resistance

Acquired resistance to these agents has not been investigated. Most of the therapeutic interest with these compounds has been for use with tumors which have become resistant to, or are naturally resistant to, L-asparaginase. Asparaginase resistance is due to the ability of cells to derepress their asparagine synthetase levels in response to asparaginase-induced plasma asparagine depletion. Asparaginase-sensitive cells cannot derepress their asparagine synthetase and succumb to the lack of this amino acid. Initial resistant mutants have regained their ability to derepress this enzyme and long-term selection results in constitutive expression of this enzyme (UREN et al. 1974). This mutation was shown to be a random event with a frequency of 9×10^{-7}/cell per generation (SUMMERS and HANDSCHUMACHER 1973). Asparaginase therapy is also restricted by cross-feeding of malignant cells within tissues of high asparagine biosynthetic capacity such as the liver (FULKERSON 1972). Because the basis of these limitations to asparaginase therapy is the asparagine biosynthetic ability of either the tumor or the host, combination therapy with some of the above asparagine synthetase inhibitors has been investigated. The ability of asparaginase either to degrade or to be inhibited by the above analogs has restricted such combined therapies, but beta-aspartyl methylamide has shown some therapeutic activity with asparaginase-resistant tumors (UREN et al. 1974). In addition, therapeutic synergism between asparaginase and CONV has been reported by BURCHENAL et al. (1971) but not confirmed by COONEY et al. (1976). A new potent asparagine synthetase inhibitor, *O*-homoserine adenylate ($K_i = 0.2$ μ*M* which is an analog of a proposed transitory intermediate beta-aspartyl adenylate, has been described (JAYARAM and COONEY 1979). This compound is neither a substrate nor an inhibitor of asparaginase, but unfortunately it is either not transported into cells or is too rapidly degraded by cells to demonstrate cytotoxicity. Possible analogs of this structure will yield the desired compound.

V. General Amino Acid Antagonists

1. Biochemistry

4-Bis-(chloroethyl)amino-phenylalanine (melphalan) and probably most of the other amino acid alkylating agents found in Tables 1 and 2 enter cells via an amino acid carrier transport process. With plasmacytoma LPC1 and leukemias L1210 and L5178Y, melphalan transport has been shown to utilize the L or leucine preferred carrier with some activity for the ASC (alanine, serine, cysteine) system (BEGLEITER et al. 1979; GOLDENBERG et al. 1979; VISTICA and RABINOVITZ

1979). Among the naturally occurring amino acids at physiological concentrations, leucine and glutamine were the most effective at reducing melphalan toxicity toward murine bone marrow precursor cells (CFU-C), but little difference between the pattern of L1210 leukemia and CFU-C protection by these amino acids was observed (VISTICA et al. 1979a). In vivo leucine administration would prevent the long-term survival of mice bearing L1210 leukemia produced by melphalan therapy (VISTICA et al. 1979b). Similarly, glutamine depletion in vitro by glutaminase would promote melphalan uptake and cytotoxicity, and combined treatment in L1210-bearing mice demonstrated an increased therapeutic response (VISTICA et al. 1978). Once inside cells, the toxicity of melphalan probably does not relate to its amino acid character but rather to its ability to cross-link DNA (see Chap. 15).

2. Resistance

Melphalan-resistant leukemia L1210 cells were obtained by repeated passage in mice receiving subcurative therapy. Marked resistance was obtained by the 10th –15th serial passage. This cell line showed incomplete resistance to melphalam, partial cross-resistance to cyclophosphamide, complete cross-resistance to *cis*-diaminodichloro-platinum (II), and undiminished sensitivity to *N,N*-bis(1-chloroethyl)-*N*-nitrosourea (BCNU) (SCHABEL et al. 1978). Transport studies revealed both a lower velocity of melphalan uptake and a lower final accumulation of drug at equilibrium for the resistant compared with the sensitive cells. In the presence of a specific inhibitor of the L transport system this transport difference was not observed. Therefore, it was concluded that the transport difference was due to a mutation in the L transport system (REDWOOD and COLVIN 1980). Certainly, transport changes are not the only possible mechanisms of resistance to these agents. In fact, L5178Y cells selected for resistance to nitrogen mustard (HN2) are cross-resistant to melphalan; yet these compounds do not share the same transport system (GOLDENBERG 1975). For other mechanisms of resistance to these agents see Chap. 15.

D. Summary

Amino acid analogs, like all other classes of antitumor chemotherapeutic agents, illustrate multiple sites of drug resistance. Decreased drug transport has been demonstrated following continued melphalan and acivicin therapy. Inhibition sites have been circumvented by increased levels of the enzymes in the salvage pathway for purines following continued azaserine and alanosine therapy, and higher levels of asparagine synthetase have been observed following asparaginase therapy. Changes in target enzymes are also observed. Enhanced levels (up to 100-fold) of aspartate transcarbamylase following continued PALA therapy have been documented and a rapid resynthesis of the inhibited enzyme has been proposed to overcome azaserine resistance. In one case, resistance was related to a higher level of the preceding enzyme in the metabolic pathway which was proposed to accumulate a product which would compete with the drug for binding to its target enzyme. Finally, decreases in the rate of synthesis of the active form of the drug have been observed following continued therapy with alanosine, and a similar mechanism may account for natural resistance to the various DOPA analogs.

References

Abe M, Chibata I, Horobawn H, Koneda Y, Mizano D (1960) Antitumor effect of amino acid analogs. Yakugaka Zasshi 80:1309

Anderson E, Brockman R (1963) Biochemical effects of duazomycin A in the mouse plasma cell neoplasm 70429. Biochem Pharmacol 12:1335–1354

Anderson E, Jacquez J (1962) Azaserine resistance in a plasma-cell neoplasm without change in active transport of the inhibitor. Cancer Res 22:27-37

Barclay R, Garfinkel E (1957) The influence of *N*-methylformamide on formate-C14 incorporation. II. In nucleic acids of tumor-bearing rats. Cancer Res 17:345–348

Begleiter A, Lam H-Y, Grover J, Froese E, Goldenberg G (1979) Evidence for active transport of melphalan by two amino acid carriers in L5178Y lymphoblasts in vitro. Cancer Res 39:353–359

Blondal H, Levi I, Latour J, Fraser W (1961) Observations on the antitumor effect of *N*-dichloroacetyl-DL-serine (FT-9045). Radiology 76:945–960

Bristow E, Wissler R (1961) Acute effects of beta-3-thienylalanine on neoplastic growth in the male albino rat. Lab Invest 10:31–38

Burchenal J, Clarkson B, Dowling M, Gee T, Haghbin M, Tan C (1970) Experimental and clinical studies of L-asparaginase in combination therapy. In: Bernard J, Boiron M, Jacquillat C, Weil M, Levy D (eds) La L-asparaginase. Centre National de la Recherche Scientifique, Paris, pp 243–248

Clark A, Rudolph F (1976) Regulation of purine metabolism. Adenylosuccinate synthetase from Novikoff ascities tumor cells. Biochim Biophys Acta 437:87–90

Collins K, Stark G (1971) Asparate transcarbamylase. Interaction with the transition state analogue *N*-(phosphonacetyl)-L-asparate. J Biol Chem 246:6599–6605

Connor T, Elson L, Haddow A, Ross W (1960) The pharmacology and tumor growth inhibitory activity of *l*-aminocyclopentane-*l*-carboxylic acid and related compounds. Biochem Pharmacol 5:108–129

Cooney D, Jayaram H, Milman H, Homan E, Pittillo R, Geran R, Rayan J, Rosenbluth R (1976) DON, CONV and DONV-III. Pharmacologic and toxicologic studies. Biochem Pharmacol 25:1859–1870

Cowan K, Lippman M (1980) Human breast cancer cells resistant to PALA (*N*-phosphonoacetyl-L-aspartate) Proc Am Assoc Cancer Res 21:41

Duvall L (1960a) Azaserine. Cancer Chemother Rep 7:65–86

Duvall L (1960b) 6-Diazo-5-oxo-L-norleucine. Cancer Chemother Rep 7:86–98

Falkson G, Falkson H (1965) DL-Serine-bis-(2-chloropropyl)carbamate ester (CD-3210; NSC-37023) for treatment of cancer patients–preliminary results. Cancer Chemother Rep 49:31–46

Fishbein W, Carbone O, Owens A, Kelly M, Rall D, Tarr N (1964) Preliminary studies with 5-bis-(2-chloroethyl)amino-DL-tryptophan (NSC-62403) in animals and man. Cancer Chemother Reps 42:19–24

Friedman O, Rutenburg A (1950) Possible usefulness of substituded amino acids for tumor growth inhibition. Proc Soc Exp Biol Med 74:764–766

Fujita H, Sakurai T, Ichimura H, Sato H, Toyoshima S (1977) A new antineoplastic amino acid derivative, A-924. Cancer Treat Rep 61:1577–1578

Fujita K, Ito S, Inoue S, Yamamoto Y, Takeuchi J, Shamoto M, Nagatsu T (1980) Selective toxicity of 5-*S*-cysteinylDOPA, a melanin precursor, to tumor cells in vitro and in vivo. Cancer Res 40:2543–2546

Fukushima K, Toyoshima S (1975) Antitumor activity of amino acid derivatives in the primary screening. Gan 66:29–36

Fulkerson J (1972) Evaluation and therapy of leukemia cell sanctuaries. MD thesis, Yale University

Giraldi T, Guarino A, Nisi C, Baldini L (1979) Selective antimetastatic effects of *N*-diazoacetylglycine derivatives in mice. Eur J Cancer 15:603–607

Goldenberg G (1975) The role of drug transport in resistance to nitrogen mustard and other alkylating agents in L5178Y lymphoblasts. Cancer Res 35:1687–1692

Goldenberg G, Lam H, Begleiter A (1979) Active carrier-mediated transport of melphalan by two separate amino acid transport sysems in LPC-1 plasmacytoma cells in vitro. J Biol Chem 254:1057–1064

Golovinsky E, Alexiev B, Spassov A, Stoev S, Emanuilov E, Angelov I, Maneva L, Stoychev T (1977) A new substance effective against transplantable tumors in vivo: L-cystine-bis-(*N,N*-chloroethyl)-hydrazide. Neoplasma 24:401–404

Gots J, Bird T, Mudd S (1955) L-Azaserine as an inducing agent for the development of phage in the lysogenic *Escherichia coli*, K-12. Biochim biophys acta 17:449–450

Greenberg J, Mandell J, Woody P (1961) A preliminary report: Resistance and cross-resistance of *Escherichia coli* mutants to radiomimetic agents. Cancer Chemother Rep 11:51-56

Hemmerly J, Demerec M (1955) Tests of chemicals for mutagenicity. Cancer Res [Suppl 3]:69–75

Houchens D, Ovejera A, Johnson R, Bogden A, Neil G (1978) Therapy of mouse tumors and human tumor xenografts by the antitumor antibiotic AT-125 (NSC-163501). Proc Am Assoc Cancer Res 19:40

Hourani B, Demopoulos H (1969) Inhibition of S91 mouse melanoma metastases and growth by D-penicillamine. Lab Invest 21:434–438

Hruban Z, Wissler R (1960) Effect of beta-3-thienylalanine and deoxypyridoxine on the growth of the Murphy-Sturm lymphosarcoma. Cancer Res 20:1530–1537

Hurlbert R, Zimmerman C, Carrington D (1977) Inhibition of adenylosuccinate synthetase by a metabolite of alanosine. Proc Am Assoc Cancer Res 18:234

Jackson R, Handschumacher R (1970) *Escherichia coli* L-asparaginase. Catalytic activity and subunit nature. Biochemistry 9:3585–3590

Jacquez J, Hutchison D (1959) Resistance in L1210 ascites without change in concentrative uptake of *O*-diazoacetyl-L-serine or 6-diazo-5-oxo-L-norleucine. Cancer Res 19:397–401

Jacquez J, Stock C, Barclay R (1953) Effect of beta-2-thienyl-DL-alanine on the growth of sarcoma T241 in C57 black mice. Cancer 6:828–836

Jayaram H, Cooney D (1979) Analogs of L-aspartic acid in chemotherapy for cancer. Cancer Treat Rep 63:1095–1108

Jayaram H, Cooney D, Milman H, Homan E, Rosenbluth R (1976) DON, CONV and DONV-I. Inhibition of L-asparagine synthetase in vitro. Biochem Pharmacol 25:1571–1582

Jayaram H, Cooney D, Vistica D, Kariya S, Johnson R (1979) Mechanisms of sensitivity or resistance of murine tumors to *N*-(phosphonacetyl)-L-aspartate (PALA). Cancer Treat Rep 63:1291–1302

Jayaram H, Cooney D, Swiniarski J, Johnson R (1980) Studies on the mechanism of resistance to L-[α*S*,5*S*]-alpha-amino-3-chloro-4,5-dihydro-5-isoxazoleacetic acid (acivicin). Proc Am Assoc Cancer Res 21:22

Johnson R (1977) Reversal of toxicity and antitumor activity of *N*-(phosphonacetyl(-L-aspartate by uridine or carbamyl-DL-aspartate in vivo. Biochem Pharmacol 26:81–84

Johnson R, Inouye T, Goldin A, Stark G (1976) Antitumor activity of *N*-(phosphonacetyl)-L-aspartic acid, a transition-state inhibitor of aspartate transcarbamylase. Cancer Res 36:2720–2725

Johnson R, Swyryd E, Stark G (1978) Effects of *N*-(phosphonacetyl)-L-aspartate on murine tumors and normal tissues in vivo and in vitro and the relationship of sensitivity to rate of proliferation and level of aspartate transcarbamylase. Cancer Res 38:371–378

Kempe T, Swyryd E, Bruist M, Stark G (1976) Stable mutants of mammalian cells that overproduce the first three enzymes of pyrimidine nucleotide biosynthesis. Cell 9:541–550

Kensler T, Mutter G, Hankerson J, Reck L, Harley C, Han N, Ardalan B, Cysyk R, Johnson R, Jayaram H, Cooney D (1981) Studies on the mechanism of resistance of variants of the Lewis lung carcinoma to *N*-(phosphonacetyl)-L-aspartic acid. Cancer Res 41:894–904

Larionov L (1965) Cancer chemotherapy. Pergamon, London, pp 238–239

Laukaitis V, Pauliukonis A (1976) Antineoplastic activity of *N*-*o*-nitrophenyl sulfenyl amino acid derivatives (in Russian) Liet. TSR Mokslu Akad Darb Ser C 115–118

Levenberg B, Melnick I, Buchanan J (1957) Biosynthesis of the purines. XV. The effect of aza-L-serine and 6-diazo-5-oxo-L-norleucine on inosinic acid biosynthesis de novo. J Biol Chem 225:163–176

Levi I, Blondal H, Lozinski E (1960) Serine derivative with antitumor activity. Science 131:666

Levy H, Montanez G, Murphy E, Dunn M (1953) Effect of ethionine on tumor growth and liver amino acids in rats. Cancer Res 13:507–512

Lichtenstein N, Grossowicz N, Schlesinger M (1977) Antitumor activity of aromatic acyl derivatives of amino acids. Isr J Med Sci 13:316–320

Littman M, Taguchi T, Shimizu Y (1964) Growth retarding effect of oral L-penicillamine on sarcoma 180. Nature 203:726–728

Livingston R, Venditti J, Cooney D, Carter S (1970) Glutamine antagonists in chemotherapy. Adv Pharmacol Chemother 8:57–120

Loeffler L, Sajadi Z, Hall I (1977) Antineoplastic agents. 2. Structure-activity studies on *N*-protected vinyl, 1,2-dibromoethyl, and cyanomethyl esters of several amino acids. J Med Chem 20:1584–1587

Luck J (1957) The action of the phenylalanine mustards and of several homologs on mouse melanoma. Cancer Res 17:1071–1076

MacLean S, Huber R (1971) The effects of DL-*p*-fluorophenylalanine and L-3-nitrotyrosine on the growth and biochemistry of the Taper liver tumor. Cancer Res 31:1669–1672

Martel F, Berlinguet L (1959) Impairment of tumor growth by unnatural amino acids. Can J Biochem Physiol 37:433–439

Martin D, Hanka L, Neil G (1974) A new antitumor agent, (alpha *S*,4*S*,5R)-alpha-amino-4-chloro-4hydroxy-4,5-dihydro-5-isoxazoleacetic acid (NSC-176324): Preliminary evaluation against L1210 mouse leukemia in vivo. Cancer Chemother Rep 58:935–9037

May H, Litzka G (1939) Über die Hemmung des Tumorwachstums durch Fluorotyrosin. Z Krebsforsch 48:376–383

McCully K, Clopath O (1977) Homocysteine compounds which influence the growth of a malignant neoplasm. Chemotherapy 23:44–49

Mickelson M, Flippin R (1956) The use of an amino acid analogue in the therapy of mouse sarcoma 180. Arch biochem Biophys 64:246–248

Miura M, Hirano M, Kakizawa K, Morita A, Uetani T, Yamada K (1970) Antitumor activity of L-beta-aspartohydroxamic acid in vivo. Screening data of 21 L-asparagine related compounds. Prog Antimicrobial Anticancer Chemother 2:170–174

Mizobuchi K, Buchanan J (1968) Biosynthesis of purines. XXX. Isolation and characterization of formylglycinamide ribonucleotide amidotransferase-glutamyl complex. J Biol Chem 243:4853–4862

Moore E, Hurlbert R (1961) Biosynthesis of RNA cytosine and RNA purines: Differential inhibition by diazo-oxo-norleucine. Cancer Res. 21:257–261

Murthy Y, Thiemann J, Coronelli C, Sensi P (1966) Alanosine, a new antiviral and antitumor agent isolated from a *Streptomyces*. Nature 211:1198–1199

Nemeth L, Somfai-Relle S, Kellner B, Sugar J, Bognar R, Farkas J, Balint J, Palyi I, Toth K, Szentirmay Z, Somosy Z, Pokorny E (1978) Study of the antitumoral activity of *S*-carbamoyl-L-cysteine derivatives in animal experiments. Arzneim Forsch 28:1119–1123

Patterson D (1976) Biochemical genetics of Chinese Hamster cell mutants with deviant purine metabolism III. Isolation and characterization of a mutant unable to convert IMP to AMP. Somatic Cell Genet 2:41–53

Pine E (1958) Concentrative uptake of azaserine by neoplastic plasma cells and lymphocytes. J Natl Cancer Inst 21:973–984

Potter M, Law L (1957) Studies of a plasma-cell neoplasm of the mouse. I. Characterization of neoplasm 70429, including its sensitivity to various antimetabolites with the rapid development of resistance to azaserine, DON, and *N*-methyl-formamide. J Natl Cancer Inst 18:413–441

Redwood W, Colvin M (1980) Transport of melphalan by sensitive and resistant L1210 cells. Cancer Res 40:1144–1149

Rennert O, Anker H (1964) Effect of 5,5,5-trifluoroleucine on a number of mouse leukemias. Nature 203:1256–1257

Sartorelli A, LePage G (1958) The development and biochemical characterization of resistance to azaserine in a TA3 ascites carcinoma. Cancer Res 18:457–463

Scanlon K, Waxman S (1980) Inhibition of methionine transport by methotrexate (MTX) in mouse leukemia L1210 cells. Proc Am Assoc Cancer Res 21:284

Schabel F, Trader M, Laster W, Wheeler G, Witt M (1978) Patterns of resistance and therapeutic synergism among alkylating agents. Fundamentals in Cancer Chemotherapy Antibiotics Chemother 23:200–215

Schlesinger M, Grossowicz N, Lichtenstein N (1971) Inhibition of murine tumors by carbobenzoxy derivatives of amino acids. Isr J Med Sci 7:547–552

Schmid F, Stern B, Schmid M, Tarnowski G (1965) Effect of alanine, glycine, phenylalanine, and tryptophan mustards on Ehrlich ascites carcinoma and Ridgway osteogenic sarcoma. Cancer Chemother Rep 49:1–7

Simard R, Bernhard W (1966) The phenomenon of nucleolar segregation: Specific action of certain antimetabolites. Int J Cancer 1:463–479

Skinner C, McKenna G, McCord T, Shive W (1958) Antitumor activity of some amino acid analogs. I. *S*-carbamylcysteine and *O*-carbazylserine. Tex Rep Biol Med 16:493–499

Spasskaya I, Larionov L (1966) Antitumor activity of epsilon-*N*,*N*-bis-(chloroethyl)-L-lysine (lysepsin). Vopr Onkol 129:66–70

Stock J (1958) Amino acid and peptide derivatives with potential antitumor properties. In: Woklenholme, O. Conner (eds) Amino acids and peptides with antimetabolic activity. Little Brown, Boston, pp 89–103

Streukas I, Dirvianskite N, Kersulis A (1977) Synthesis and antitumor activity of some aromatic amino acids and their *N*-arylidine derivatives (in Russian). Izuch Prot-Prot Mut Ves 14–24

Summers W, Handschumacher R (1971) L5178Y asparagine-dependent cells and independent clonal sublines: Toxicity of 5-diazo-4-oxo-L-norvaline. Biochem Pharmocol 20:2213–2220

Summers W, Handschumacher R (1973) The rate of mutation of L5178Y asparaginase-dependent mouse leukemia cells to asparagine-independence and its biological consequences. Cancer Res 33:1775–1779

Syzbalski W (1958) Special microbiological systems. II. Observations on chemical mutagenesis in microorganisms. Ann NY Acad Sci 76:475–489

Tillian H, Schauenstein E, Ertl A, Esterbauer H (1976) Therapeutic effects of cysteine adducts of alpha, beta-unsaturated aldehydes on Ehrlich ascities tumor of mice. Eur J Cancer 12:989–993

Tyagi A, Cooney D (1980) Identification of the antimetabolite of Lalanosine, L-alanosyl-5-amino-4-imidazolecarboxylic acid ribonucleotide, in tumors and assessment of its inhibition of adenylosucccinate synthetase. Cancer Res 40:4390–4397

Tyagi A, Conney D, Jayaram H, Swiniarski J, Johnson R (1980) Studies on the mechanism of resistance of selected murine tumors to L-alanosine. Biochem Pharmacol 30:915–924

Tyrer D, Kline I, Gang M, Goldin A, Venditti J (1969) Effectiveness of antileukemic agents in mice inoculated with a leukemia L1210 variant resistant to 5-¼3,3-bis(2-chloroethyl)-1-triazeno imidazole-4-carboxamide (NSC-82196). Cancer Chemother Rep 53:229–241

Umezawa H (1978) Advances in bioactive microbial secondary metabolites useful in the treatment of cancer. In: Umezawa H (ed) Advances in cancer chemotherapy. Jpn Sci Soc Press, Tokyo, p 27

Uren J, Summers W, Handschumacher R (1974) Enzymatic and nutritional evidence for two-stage expression of the asparagine synthetase locus in L5178Y murine leukemia mutants. Cancer Res 34:2940–2945
Uren J, Chang P, Handschumacher R (1977) Effects of asparagine synthetase inhibitors on asparaginase resistant tumors. Biochem Pharmacol 26:1405–1410
Vistica D, Rabinovitz M (1979) Concentrative uptake of melphalan, a cancer chemotherapeutic agent which is transported by the leucine-preferring carrier system. Biochem Biophys Res Commun 86:929–932
Vistica D, Rabon A, Rabinovitz M (1978) Enhancement of melphalan therapy with glutaminase: asparaginase. Res Commun Chem Pathol Pharmacol 22:83–92
Vistica D, Rabon A, Rabinovitz M (1979 a) Amino acid conferred protection against mephalan: Comparison of amino acids which reduce melphalan toxicity to murine bone marrow precusor cells (CFU-C) and murine L1210 leukemia cells. Res Commun Chem Pathol Pharmacol 23:171–183
Vistica D, Rabon A, Rabinovitz M (1979 b) Effect of L-alpha-amino-gamma-guanidinobutyric acid an melphalan therapy of the L1210 murine leukemia. Cancer Lett 6:345–350
Vogel F, Kemper L, Jeffs P, Cass M, Graham D (1977) Gamma-L-glutaminyl-4-hydroxybenzene, a inducer of cryptobiosis in *Agaricus bisporus* and a source of specific metabolic inhibitors for melanogenic cells. Cancer Res 37:1133–1136
Weisberger A, Suhrland L (1956) Studies on analogs of L-cysteine and L-cystine. II. The effect on selenium cystine on Murphy lymphosarcoma tumor cells in the rat. Blood 11:11–18
White F (1960 a) The nitrogen mustards of glycine and DL-alanine. Cancer Chemother Rep 7:99–103
White F (1960 b) Sarcolyse and related compounds. Cancer Chemother Rep 6:61–93
White F (1962) Hadacidin. Cancer Chemother Rep 23:81–85
Wick M (1977) L-DOPA methyl ester as a new antitumor agent. Nature 269:512–513
Wick M (1978) L-DOPA methyl ester: prolongation of survival of neuroblastoma-bearing mice after treatment. Science 199:775–776
Wick M (1979) Levodopa and dopamine analogs. DNA polymerase inhibitor and antitumor agents in human and murine melanoma. Clin Res 27:246a
Wick M (1979) Levodopa and dopamine analogs: melanin precusors as antitumor agents in experimental human and murine leukemia. Cancer Treat Rep 63:991–997
Wick M (1980) An experimental approach to the chemotherapy of melanoma. J Invest Dermatol 74:63–65
Wick M, Byers L, Frei III E (1977) L-DOPA: Selective toxicity for melanoma cells in vitro. Science 197:468–469
Wilson J, Irvin J, Suggs J, Liu K (1959) Inhibition of growth and protein biosynthesis in Ehrlich ascites carcinoma by alpha-hydroxylamino acids and alpha-oximino acids. Cancer Res 19:272–276
Woody P, Mandell J, Greenberg J (1961) Resistance and cross-resistance of *Escherichica coli* mutants to anticancer agents. Radiat Res 15:290–297
Zee-Cheng K, Cheng C (1972) Structural modification of *S*-trityl-L-cysteine. Preparation of some *S*-(substitued trityl)-L-cysteines and dipeptides of *S*-trityl-L-cysteine. J Med Chem 15:13–16
Zeng Y, Yunfeng R (1979) Synthesis of 2-methyl-5-bis(chloroethyl)-aminophenylalanine and 2-bis(chloroethyl)-aminomethyl-5-nitrophenylalanine (in Chinese). Acta Pharmacol Sinica 14:676–680

CHAPTER 21

Alkaloids

W. T. Beck

A. Introduction

Despite the historic roles of colchicine (and certain of its derivatives) and, subsequently, of the *Vinca* alkaloids, not only as probes that have expanded our fundamental knowledge of cell biology, but also as important therapeutic agents, there is comparatively little knowledge of the mechanisms by which tumor cells express resistance to these drugs. Moreover, of the information available, there appears to be no uniform agreement about these mechanisms of insensitivity. It is fortunate, however, that much knowledge of the transport, cellular pharmacology, and cytotoxic lesions of the alkaloids has been accumulated during the past 5–6 years, since many of these investigations bear on the studies of resistance to be described. Accordingly, those studies of the cellular pharmacology of the alkaloids will be discussed in this chapter as a prelude to a consideration of the cellular bases for resistance to these agents.

Alkaloids, which comprise a variety of important classes of drugs that have wide experimental and therapeutic application, may, in general, be defined as being (usually) structurally complex organic bases that are formed in plants and have pharmacological activity (Finar 1975). The *Vinca* alkaloids represent a class of natural or semisynthetic drugs derived the periwinkle plant, *Vinca rosea L.*, while colchicine and its important derivatives are found in the autumn crocus plants (*Colchicum autumnale*). Since the basic chemistry of these and other plant products has been outlined by Creasey (1975) in an earlier review in this series, this subject will not be discussed here.

The focus of this chapter will be on the *Colchicum* and *Vinca* compounds whose structures are shown in Fig. 1. These alkaloids have been instrumental in expanding our understanding of some fundamental processes in cell biology, ranging from cell division, to the secretion of proteins, to the underlying mechanisms in blastogenic transformation of lymphocytes. Moreover, the *Vinca* compounds are important antineoplastic agents, used now in combination with other drugs; indeed, vincristine is one of the mainstays in the induction of remissions in pediatric acute lymphoblastic leukemia, while vinblastine is used widely against a variety of pediatric and adult lymphomas and sarcomas. Although the clinical use of colchicine is limited to the treatment of gout and some inflammatory conditions, primarily because of its toxicity, it is still an important experimental tool, and because of certain similarities to the *Vinca* compounds it will be considered here. Newer drugs, such as maytansine, the epipodophyllotoxins, oncodazole, and the like, which are often considered with the former compounds, will not be

Vinca Colchicum

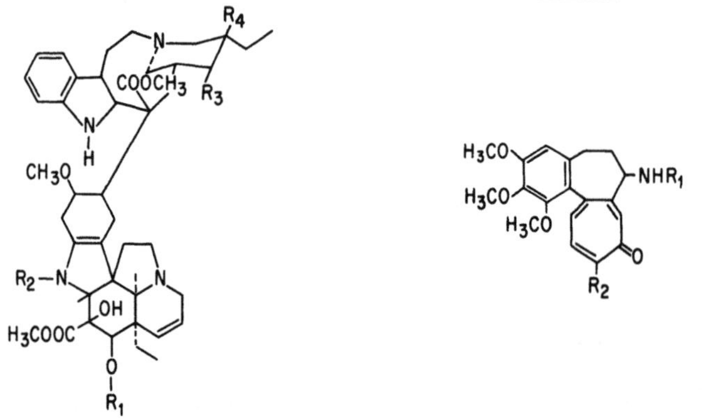

Name	R_1	R_2	R_3	R_4
Vincristine	CH_3CO	CHO	H	OH
Vinblastine	CH_3CO	CH_3	H	OH
Vindesine	NH_2	CH_3	H	OH

Name	R_1	R_2
Colchicine	$COCH_3$	OCH_3
Colcemid	CH_3	OCH_3

Fig. 1. Chemical structures of the major *Vinca* and *Colchicum* alkaloids to be discussed in this chapter

discussed in any detail here because there is at this time too little information concerning their cellular pharmacology and virtually no knowledge about cellular resistance to these agents.

The experimental and therapeutic uses of the alkaloids have been based on a generally accepted antimitotic action of these drugs, presumably mediated through their specific binding to subunit proteins of microtubules, tubulins. Indeed, early studies of actions of the *Vinca* and *Colchicum* alkaloids focused on their antimitotic effects, presumably as a consequence of their demonstrable binding to tubulin. The traditional biochemical lesions in DNA synthesis, produced by most of the effective anticancer drugs, were not seen with the *Vinca* compounds, and this may have discouraged subsequent exploration of those biochemical disruptions that might be a consequence of binding to tubulin. Recently, however, a number of studies of the cellular pharmacology and biochemistry of these alkaloids have examined mechanisms of (a) their accumulation by cells (including transport and binding), (b) their effects on membrane transport and other cell-surface phenomena, and (c) their cytotoxic manifestations that suggest other actions of these compounds. These areas will be discussed in this chapter, before considering resistance, because an understanding of alterations pertinent to resistance and critical evaluations of available data can best be achieved through an understanding of these aspects of the cellular pharmacology and biochemistry of the alkaloids.

Compared with other anticancer drugs, such as the major nucleoside antimetabolites and methotrexate, whose biochemical actions and mechanisms of resistance have been studied in detail, there is relatively little known about resistance to the *Vinca* alkaloids. This paucity of knowledge may be attributable, at least in part, to some early work in which assumptions were made on the basis of cross-resistance studies; additionally, the commercial unavailability of radiolabeled compounds until the mid-1970s has doubtless been a major deterrent to progress.

Finally, because this chapter must reflect the nature of this monograph, the subject matter has been restricted to studies carried out with mammalian cells, while work on alkaloid resistance with such other cell types as yeasts has been omitted. Similarly, some recent pharmacokinetic studies in man and other animals has been regarded, of necessity, as beyond the scope of this chapter. Additionally, because there is a considerable body of literature in some of the areas covered, it was necessary to be even more selective and to discuss only those papers deemed to be representative or particularly illuminating in the context of the chapter; any omissions are regretted. For discussions of the properties and regulation of microtubules, their assembly, and their tubulin subunits, the reader is referred to reviews by OLMSTED and BORISY (1973), SNYDER and MCINTOSH (1976), KIRSCHNER (1978), RAFF (1979), and TIMASHEFF and GRISHAM (1980); thorough considerations of the interactions of the alkaloid drugs with microtubular proteins are presented in reviews by WILSON and BRYAN (1974) and WILSON (1975a, 1975b). Moreover, three recent symposia (SOIFER 1975; BORGERS and DEBRABANDER 1975; DEBRABANDER and DEMAY 1980) and a book (ROBERTS and HYAMS 1979) on microtubule biology and pharmacology have also been published.

B. Cellular Pharmacology and Biochemistry of the *Vinca* and *Colchicum* Alkaloids

I. Mechanisms of Alkaloid Accumulation by Cells

There have been comparatively few studies of the mechanism(s) by which cells accumulate the *Colchicum* and *Vinca* alkaloids, and the results, summarized in Table 1, reveal that accumulation may occur by a variety of processes, ranging from passive diffusion to possibly a carrier-mediated transport, with contributions by some type of drug-binding within or on the cells. Indeed, only a few investigations have attempted to distinguish between cellular transport and binding, as will be discussed; accordingly, unless otherwise indicated, "accumulation" will be the general term used to describe alkaloid "uptake" by cells.

The accumulation of colchicine by cultured cells appears to be attributable primarily to passive diffusion of the drug across the cell membrane with subsequent binding to cellular components (TAYLOR 1965; BORISY and TAYLOR 1967; LING and THOMPSON 1974; MINOR and ROSCOE 1975). Although the uptake of colchicine is apparently limited by the rate of drug-binding to the tubulin subunits of microtubules, rather than by passage across the cell membrane (TAYLOR 1965), its rate of uptake can be enhanced by the nonionic detergent, Tween 80, a mem-

Table 1. Mechanisms of alkaloid accumulation by tumor cells and platelets

Drug studied	Cell type/line	Mechanisms of accumulation	Reference
[^{3}H]Colchicine	KB	Passive diffusion/binding	Taylor (1965)
	CHO	Passive diffusion	Ling and Thompson (1974); See et al. (1974)
	Various mouse and Syrian hamster lines	Binding	Minor and Roscoe (1975)
[^{3}H]Vinblastine	Ehrlich carcinoma	Binding to alkali-labile material	Creasey and Markiw (1966); Creasey (1968)
	Sarcoma 180	Ninefold drug concentration	Swerdlow and Creasey (1975)
	Rat platelets	Reversible, high-affinity binding	Secret et al. (1972)
	Rat lymphoma cells	Reversible binding	Gout et al. (1978)
	CCRF-CEM	Binding initially (temperature-dependent, energy-independent)	Beck (1981)
[^{3}H]Vincristine	L1210	Carrier-mediated	Bleyer et al. (1975)
	CCRF-CEM	Carrier-mediated	Bender and Nichols (1978)
	P388	Energy-independent, temperature-sensitive, nonsaturable process	Bender and Kornreich (1981)

brane-active agent (LING and THOMPSON 1974); this latter observation indicates that drug diffusion across the plasma membrane also has some effect on the rate of cellular drug-uptake. The free intracellular concentration of colchicine, calculated by TAYLOR (1965), by subtracting the "bound" from the total accumulated, was determined to be roughly equivalent to the extracellular concentration of the drug; increased binding in proportion to the intracellular levels of free drug supported the notion of passive penetration.

Kinetic analyses of [^{3}H]colchicine accumulation also support the conclusion that the uptake of this drug occurs by a passive process. For example, it was shown by SEE et al. (1974) that a double-reciprocal plot of velocity versus substrate concentration extrapolated back to zero, indicating that there was no saturation of the uptake over the concentration range studied (up to $\sim 5 \times 10^{-6}$ *M*). Although TAYLOR (1965) reported saturation kinetics at an external concentration of colchicine of 5×10^{-7}*M*, this was ascribed to binding rather than to transport, and was achieved over a period of hours, not minutes. It has been demonstrated that >90% of the accumulated colchicine is bound to a cytoplasmic protein(s) (BORISY and TAYLOR 1967; LING and THOMPSON 1974); indeed, some studies have not even attempted to ascertain the mechanism of passage of colchicine across the membrane, and have considered the accumulation of colchicine as synonymous with drug-binding (MINOR and ROSCOE 1975; KRALOVIC and VOELZ 1977).

While cells appear to accumulate colchicine by passive diffusion and subsequent binding, the literature for the cellular accumulation of *Vinca* compounds presents, in some cases, a more complex situation. The earliest studies of the accumulation of vinblastine came from the laboratories of CREASEY and of BEER. It was noted that [^{3}H]vinblastine was accumulated rapidly by Ehrlich ascites cells, reaching an equilibrium cell/medium ratio of 4 in 10 min (CREASEY and MARKIW 1966); similar observations were subsequently reported for Sarcoma 180 cells (SWERDLOW and CREASEY 1975). Moreover, by 60 min, roughly 10%–20% of the radioactivity was bound to an alkali-labile cellular component (CREASEY 1968).

This accumulation of vinblastine may represent, in part, some types of binding within or on the cells; for example, it was shown that after an injection of [^{3}H]vinblastine to rats, of the radioactivity found in the blood, ~60% of this was associated with platelets (~75% if the labeled compound was incubated in vitro with platelet-rich plasma) (HEBDEN et al. 1970). Subsequent analysis showed that the accumulation of [^{3}H]vinblastine by platelets was a temperature-sensitive, reversible binding (SECRET et al. 1972). Indeed, this binding can be demonstrated by the following exercise: the intracellular volume of 10^9 platelets can be calculated to be $\sim 14.1 \times 10^{-9}$ liters, using the formula $V = 0.523\ D^3$ [where V is the intracellular volume and D is the average diameter of a platelet [~3 μm]. Taking the data from Fig. 5 of SECRET et al. (1972), it can be determined that at an extracellular concentration of vinblastine of 1 μg/ml, 0.27 μg of the drug was associated with 10^9 platelets, a nearly 2000-fold accumulation of vinblastine after 2 h; such a high "cell"/medium ratio probably indicates that the drug is bound extensively by the platelets. These studies of BEER and his collaborators were extended to a comparison of the binding of [^{3}H]vinblastine and [^{3}H]vincristine by platelets, rat lymphoma cells, and murine L5178Y cells (GOUT et al. 1978). Differences in rates of accumulation of the two compounds were observed, and it was speculated that this might be due to differences in rates of transport of the two compounds, although this was not studied.

The accumulation of [^{3}H]vincristine by murine P388 cells has been studied recently by BENDER and KORNREICH (1981). These investigators found that the initial accumulation of this alkaloid was (a) sensitive to changes in temperature and pH, (b) independent of cellular energy metabolism, (c) nonsaturable, and (d) unaffected by the presence of either vinblastine or colchicine. Accordingly, the accumulation of [^{3}H]vincristine by these cells is consistent with a passive, rather than facilitated, diffusion mechanism. The accumulation of [^{3}H]vinblastine has been studied in cultured human leukemic lymphoblasts (CCRF-CEM) (BECK 1981). The initial uptake of this drug by these cells was also temperature sensitive and independent of cellular energy metabolism. The cell/medium ratios over a fourfold $\log_{10}$ range of external vinblastine-concentration for initial (10-min) net accumulation were between 5 and 28; even at zero time and 4 °C, the cell/medium ratios were considerably greater than 1.0. Moreover, the concentration of drug able to efflux from the cells far exceeded that which was present in the medium originally, indicating that it must have come from a large pool of vinblastine that was bound either in or on the cell. These results permit the suggestion that a significant component of the vinblastine accumulated by these cells represents bound material. Additionally, the achievement of high cell/medium ratios in energy-depleted cells lends further support to the suggestion that drug accumulation is attributable largely to binding, and also argues against these ratios being attained by an active transport process; however, it was not possible from these studies to determine whether some of the drug accumulation was a reflection of facilitated diffusion.

Likewise, the mode of accumulation of [^{3}H]vincristine by Ehrlich ascites cells could not be readily assessed in a study by SKOVSGAARD (1978a). It was shown that the cell/medium ratio for [^{3}H]vincristine at equilibrium (1–2 h) was ~10.0, and that the initial accumulation could be increased somewhat (~17%) by preincubation of the cells with inhibitors of cellular metabolism (azide and iodoacetate), the latter observation permitting the suggestion that these compounds inhibited a drug-efflux mechanism in these cells.

In contrast to the work cited above, other studies using murine and cultured human leukemia cells permitted the conclusions that the accumulation of [^{3}H]vincristine occurred by a carrier-mediated, energy-dependent mechanism. For example, it was shown by BLEYER et al. (1975) that the uptake of [^{3}H]vincristine was (a) highly temperature dependent (the temperature coefficient between 27 °C and 37 °C [Q_{10}] = 6.3), (b) exhibited typical Michaelis-Menton kinetics, (c) could be inhibited by fluoride, *p*-chloro-mercuribenzoate, ouabain, and vinblastine, and (d) led to cell/medium ratios of 5.2–18.7. Based on these results, the authors concluded that the uptake of [^{3}H]vincristine by these murine cells involved active transport. Similar conclusions were reached by BENDER and NICHOLS (1978) for the accumulation of this drug by cultured leukemic lymphoblasts (CCRF-CEM); cell/medium distribution ratios 45 and 16.1 were found for cells incubated in 0.1 and 1.0 μM [^{3}H]vincristine respectively.

That drug-binding is also important, however, was shown by the studies of BLEYER et al. (1975), in that 36%–41% of the [^{3}H]vincristine initially accumulated was bound and unable to exit from the cell during reincubation of the preloaded cells in drug-free medium; likewise, in the study by BENDER and NICHOLS (1978), roughly 20%–30% of the total cell-associated drug was bound within 60 min. Additionally, the amount of drug bound to the cell was shown to be an important determinant of cellular sensitivity to vincristine (BENDER and KORNREICH 1980), as this measurement correlated best with the increase in life span produced by vincristine when administered to mice bearing leukemias of differing degrees of resistance to this agent.

To summarize this section, then, tumor cells may accumulate the alkaloids by passive diffusion, or possibly by a carrier-mediated process. It appears that the apparent differences in the way cells accumulate colchicine, vinblastine, and vincristine may reside, in part, in the different cell lines and drugs used; however, it is likely that there are metabolic and other factors involved, since the accumulation of the alkaloids could be blocked by metabolic inhibitors in some studies (BLEYER et al. 1975; BENDER and NICHOLS 1978), but not in others (SKOVSGAARD 1978a; BENDER and KORNREICH 1981; BECK 1981). In addition, the binding of the drugs to the cells is extensive, and may interfere with the determination of free (osmotically active) intracellular drug levels. Colchicine is nearly completely bound to tubulin (BORISY and TAYLOR, 1967), but binding of the *Vinca* compounds may involve a displaceable (loose) component of 20%–40% or more (BLEYER et al. 1975; BENDER and NICHOLS 1978; BECK 1981), although the nondisplaceable fraction is probably the most important determinant of cytotoxicity (BENDER and KORNREICH 1980). Clearly, more studies are needed in this area to resolve these apparent discrepancies.

II. Effects of Alkaloids on Cellular Functions

While the predominant biological effects of the alkaloids on mitosis have been well studied, the biochemical perturbations have been somewhat more difficult to categorize. The actions of these drugs on the synthesis of DNA, RNA, and protein have been reviewed by CREASEY (1975); it has not been made clear, however, whether these were primary effects of these drugs or secondary actions subsequent to binding to microtubule subunits. Much recent work with alkaloids has focused on their effects on cellular function and activity. The presumption has been that the binding of these drugs to microtubule subunits prevents the further assembly of additional microtubules and causes the disassembly of these subcellular structures; as a consequence, various cellular processes would be perturbed. This concept will be examined in this section, and, while the results tend to support such a notion, there are clearly other factors involved in the actions of these alkaloids on various cellular functions.

1. Membrane Transport

There have been several studies demonstrating an effect of the alkaloids on the membrane transport of nucleosides, amino acids, and other drugs in tumor cells. For example, MIZEL and WILSON (1972) showed that colchicine can inhibit the uptake of thymidine, uridine, adenosine, and guanosine by HeLa cells, with inhibition constants $\sim 5 \times 10^{-5}$ M. This effect was apparently specific for nucleosides, since neither the uptake of 2-deoxyglucose, a nonmetabolizable sugar, nor the uptake of α-aminoisobutyric acid, a nonmetabolizable amino acid, was affected. This action of colchicine was apparently unrelated to its effect on microtubules, however, since it was shown that (a) colchicine inhibited the uptake of thymidine at 0 °C, a temperature at which binding of the alkaloid to microtubules is considerably reduced, and (b) lumicolchicine, the light-inactivated product of colchicine that neither binds to microtubule protein nor has antimitotic activity, also inhibited nucleoside transport. It is of interest that, while MIZEL and WILSON (1972) could demonstrate no effect of colchicine on the rates of phosphorylation of thymidine or uridine, CLINE (1967) and PLAGEMANN (1970) showed that vincristine and vinblastine, respectively, inhibited the incorporation of uridine into RNA. Thus, vincristine at $0.7–70 \times 10^{-6}$ M inhibited the incorporation of uridine by leukemic lymphoblasts in the former study, while vinblastine was shown to inhibit uridine incorporation into acid-soluble nucleotides of Novikoff rat hepatoma cells in the latter study, but only at very high concentrations ($2–6 \times 10^{-4}$ M). The interpretation of these observations is unclear.

While MIZEL and WILSON (1972) indicated that colchicine had no effect on the membrane transport of α-aminoisobutyric acid, work from GOLDMAN's laboratory (FYFE et al. 1975; GOLDMAN et al. 1977) showed that, in Ehrlich ascites cells, both colchicine and vincristine inhibited the active transport of this compound when compared with controls. The authors suggested the possibility that the alkaloids either inhibited cellular energy metabolism (glucose could, in part, prevent the alkaloid-produced decreased uptake of the amino acid) or interfered with the coupling of energy utilization to transport processes; a role for microtubules in transport, at least of amino acids, was proposed.

Additional studies demonstrated that these alkaloids affected the membrane transport of drugs. For example, vincristine increased the net accumulation of methotrexate by various murine and human tumor cells (FYFE and GOLDMAN 1973; ZAGER et al. 1973; GOLDMAN et al. 1976; WARREN et al. 1977; CHELLO et al. 1979a). This effect was attributed to an interference with the unidirectional efflux of methotrexate by the alkaloid, possibly through an inhibition of cellular energy metabolism by some mechanism(s) other than that of vincristine on microtubules (FYFE and GOLDMAN 1973). The potential therapeutic significance of these findings, however, was tempered by results of a study (BENDER et al. 1978) demonstrating no therapeutic benefit of the combination when administered to mice bearing the L1210 tumor. In that study, the methotrexate was given after the alkaloid, with an interval ranging from 0 to 2 h. It was subsequently shown by CHELLO et al. (1979a, b), however, that when vincristine was given ≧24 h *after* methotrexate to mice bearing the L1210 leukemia, therapeutic synergism, with long-term survivors in some combinations, could be achieved. While the mechanism of this effect has not been established, it is known that the delayed administration of the alkaloid had no effect on the very low levels of methotrexate remaining in the tumor cells. Thus, the results permitted the suggestion that the therapeutic synergism was probably *not* related to the interaction of the drugs shown in vitro.

Another alkaloid-drug interaction of interest was described by CARLSEN et al. (1976). It was shown that vinblastine stimulated the rate of uptake of colchicine by both sensitive- and colchicine-resistant Chinese hamster ovary (CHO) cells in a concentration-related manner. This effect was apparently independent of the action of the alkaloid on microtubules, however, because it also stimulated the uptake of puromycin, while daunorubicin and actinomycin D also enhanced the uptake of colchicine. Unlike the stimulation by vincristine of the uptake of methotrexate, as described above, which was thought to be due in part to an inhibition of cellular energy metabolism, CARLSEN et al. (1976) noted that vinblastine had no effect on cellular levels of ATP; it was concluded, therefore, that the stimulated uptake of colchicine was not a consequence of impaired cellular energy metabolism. Additionally, it was shown that this effect of vinblastine was not attributable to nonspecific "leakiness" of the cell membrane, because neither the transport of 2-deoxyglucose nor the mechanism of colchicine uptake was altered by the vinblastine. The authors proposed that the interaction of these agents with membranes resulted in increased "membrane-fluidity," which could permit enhanced drug passage.

2. Other Membrane-Related Actions

The most studied of these effects of the alkaloids have been concerned with the apparent microtubule regulation of various membrane functions, such as lectin-binding to lymphocytes, phagocytosis, and protein secretion; the first two phenomena, at least, appear to be associated with the lateral mobility of proteins in the plane of the membrane. It has been proposed (EDELMAN et al. 1973; BERLIN et al. 1979) that by binding to its receptor a ligand such as concanavalin A stimulates the anchoring of this receptor complex and other membrane proteins to microtubules; accordingly, interference with microtubule function by agents such as colchicine would free these bound receptors from their microtubular constraints, and allow their rearrangement on the cell surface into discrete polar accumulations known as "caps". These proposals were based largely on the evidence of the effects of the alkaloids on these processes. The various studies (reviewed by SCHREINER and UNANUE 1976) made the assumption that these drugs have highly specific actions on and bind almost exclusively to cellular microtubules, causing their disruption. AUBIN et al. (1975, 1980), using colchicine- and Colcemid-resistant mutants of CHO cells, provided strong support for the involvement of microtubules on this lectin-mediated membrane-receptor rearrangement. The validity of the interpretations of the studies of AUBIN et al., however, rests on the mechanism of drug resistance in these cells, a subject that will receive further attention in a subsequent section (Sect. C. II).

The microtubule–cell-membrane relationship may also have significance for another area: is tubulin an important constituent of cell membranes? This has been subject of much debate and controversy, and has been reviewed recently (BERLIN et al. 1979; WEATHERBEE 1981), with the conclusion that its role in membranes is still unclear and requires further study. Recent reports, however, have demonstrated that tubulin appears to be a significant component of the *external* surface membrane of leukemic lymphoblasts (BACHVAROFF et al. 1980; RUBIN et al. 1982). These results raise such questions as: (a) are the membranebound tubulins of leukemic lymphoblasts different from those of other cells or of cytoplasm? (if so, this may explain the exquisite sensitivity of such cells to *Vinca* alkaloids); (b) are altered *membrane* tubulins important in the expression of resistance of *Vinca* alkaloids and similar compounds? and (c) is glycosylation involved in the regulation of polymerization (or other functions) of membrane-bound or cytoplasmic tubulin? If glycosylation is so involved, it could help to explain why tubulin has not been found in the past to be a major constituent of membranes.

3. Cytotoxic Lesions

In order to understand the primary alterations in tumor cells that could permit the expression of resistance to the actions of the alkaloids, it would be helpful to examine the cytotoxic lesion(s) produced by these agents. In this regard, most opinion favors the explanation that the cytotoxicity of these alkaloids reflects their binding to tubulin, thereby blocking cells in metaphase. Indeed, there is much evidence to support this view, with several studies showing good correlations between drug-binding to microtubules and either metaphase arrest (reviewed by WILSON 1975a, b) or therapeutic activity in tumor-bearing mice (OWELLEN et al. 1977); another study demonstrated a relation between metaphase arrest and cytotoxicity, as measured by cloning assays (TUCKER et al. 1977). Moreover, recent investigations with alkaloid-insensitive lines that were resistant because of diminished ability of the drugs to bind to tubulin (LING et al. 1979; CABRAL et al. 1980) also tend to support this concept of cytotoxicity due to mitotic arrest.

It is not immediately clear, however, why this apparently reversible binding of the alkaloids to tubulin, with subsequent mitotic arrest, should be lethal to the cell [although it is possible that this may result in precipitation of microtubular proteins (WILSON et al. 1970) or even in unbalanced growth]. Indeed, the results of several studies have indicated that the cytotoxicity of the *Vinca* alkaloids may be attributable to actions other than those producing metaphase arrest. For example, STRYCKMANS et al. (1973) demonstrated that vincristine, when administered to a patient with acute lymphoblastic leukemia, caused radioactively prelabeled blasts to disappear from the blood and marrow. Since $\sim$95% of the cells were in G_1, the results supported the concept that the alkaloid had cytolytic actions in interphase cells; i.e., the drug effect could not be attributed to effects on processes concerned with mitosis. Likewise, ROSNER et al. (1975) showed that cultured human lymphoid cells were more sensitive to the toxic actions of vincristine when in the plateau phase of the culture, rather than in the log phase. Since the former (more sensitive) cells were presumably dividing at a much slower rate than the latter cells, the authors reasoned that a mechanism other than mitotic arrest was responsible for the cytotoxicity of the alkaloid, and that the drug has more than one site of action. Finally, MADOC-JONES and MAURO (1968) presented clear evidence that, when added to synchronized cultures of HeLa cells, vincristine and vinblastine produced their greatest cytotoxic effects (as measured by cloning assays) on cells in either the S-phase or in the late G_1- and S-phases of the cell cycle, respectively. This interphase action of these compounds has a number of implications: (a) the presumed alkaloid-binding to tubulin appears to be important in phases of the cell cycle other than mitosis; (b) DNA synthesis may be influenced significantly by the subcellular microtubular architecture, which can be disrupted by antimicrotubule agents; and (c) these alkaloids may prove to have important cytotoxic actions that are independent of their binding to tubulins.

Regarding these latter two points, work from CANELLAKIS' laboratory (CHEN et al. 1976) has demonstrated that vinblastine and colchicine inhibit the activity of ornithine decarboxylase (ODCase), the rate-limiting enzyme in the biosynthesis of polyamines. While these results promoted the hypothesis that the enzyme required an intact cytoskeleton for the expression of its activity, it is possible to view the data in the light of the late-G_1/S-phase cytotoxicity described in the study by MADOC-JONES and MAURO. Thus, ODCase is believed to be an enzyme that is necessary for cellular replication, the activity of which reaches a maximum in mid-G_1-(HEBY et al. 1976) or in the late G_1, early S-phase (FRIEDMAN et al. 1972; FULLER et al. 1977). Since the alkaloids inhibit this enzyme, possibly in these phases of the cell cycle, the expected consequences for cell replication would be those demonstrated by MADOC-JONES and MAURO, namely, their greatest cytotoxic effects would be exerted on interphase cells.

Finally, it is possible that the alkaloid inhibition of ODCase activity has little to do diretly with the binding of these drugs to tubulin, but is more likely a consequence of their inhibition of protein synthesis. Thus, studies in this laboratory have revealed that the effects of the alkaloids on the activity of ODCase are closely related to their effects on general protein synthesis (Beck, unpublished results). Additionally, recent work from this laboratory (BECK 1980a) has demonstrated that *Vinca* alkaloids cause a profound (reversible) elevation in the levels of oxidized glutathione (GSSG) in monolayer cultures of H-35 rat hepatoma cells. It was also shown in that study that protein synthesis was inhibited by vinblastine and that this was reciprocally related to the levels of GSSG in the cell. Consequently, it was proposed that GSSG, which is known to inhibit the synthesis of proteins, could be responsible for this action of the alkaloids; these observations may have implications for the cytotoxic action(s) of these agents. Clearly, these findings do not preclude a role for the binding of the alkaloids to tubulin, but they do permit the suggestion that the cytotoxicity of these drugs may not be caused directly by such interactions.

C. Manifestations of Resistance to the Alkaloids

I. Resistance and Cross-Resistance Characteristics of Alkaloid-Insensitive Cells

Several studies in cell culture and in vivo have explored the resistant features of alkaloid-insensitive cells; conversely, a number of tumor cell-lines selected for resistance to other agents have been shown to be cross-resistant to the alkaloids. Most of these findings are listed in Table 2, and can be summarized as follows: (a) in general, alkaloid-insensitive cells are cross-resistant to other "natural products," such as other alkaloids, anthracyclines, various antibiotics, and epipodophyllotoxins (semisynthetic derivatives of a natural product; (b) moreover, cells selected for resistance to such natural products are generally cross-resistant to the alkaloids; (c) the degree of cross-resistance is roughly related to the degree of resistance (but see below); and (d) alkaloid-resistant or cross-resistant cells retain their sensitivity to the antimetabolites, alkylating agents, and other classes of drugs studied. In some cases, alkaloid-resistant cells have been shown to exhibit collateral sensitivity to selected agents. As detailed below and in Sect. C.II.1.a, these broad resistance and cross-resistance features have been termed the "pleiotropic phenotype" by LING (1975) and his co-workers (BECH-HANSEN et al. 1976) in an attempt to describe a common basis for the insensitivity of the cells to such a wide range of compounds having such disparate structures and mechanisms of action.

Clinical resistance to *Vinca* alkaloids, that is, the lack of therapeutic response, either initially, or at some point after producing a tumor response to a course of therapy, is complex and attributable to many factors, as described below. It is of considerable interest, however, that while cross-resistance between the alkaloids and other natural products has been amply demonstrated experimentally, this phenomenon is not readily seen clinically. The reason(s) for this is not clear, but it may be related to both the heterogeneity and degree of resistance of the cells. For example, the experimental cells often represent cloned, homogeneous populations, rather than the heterogenous mixtures of drug-resistant and -sensitive cells which presumably occur clinically; more importantly, cells selected for drug-insensitivity in vitro or in animals are often many times more resistant to the drug than are the sensitive cells [e.g., $>1,000$ to $>100,000$ times (BIEDLER et al. 1975)]. Such high levels of resistance may be related to the homogeneity of the experimental cell population; however, such is probably not the case in the clinical situation, in which a slight (two- to four-fold) increase in the degree of drug resistance, as compared with that of sensitive cells, can probably lead to clinical manifestations of drug insensitivity.

The consequences of this difference in resistance for the cross-resistance properties of cells are illustrated in the following example (Table 3): it is seen that cells selected for lower resistance to vincristine (CEM/VCR_5) are considerably less resistant to daunorubicin and to the epipodophyllotoxin, VM-26, whereas cells that are highly resistant to the alkaloid (CEM/VCR_{100}) are more clearly cross-resistant to the other two agents. These results show that cross-resistance of cells to the other drugs is related to the degree of alkaloid resistance of these cells. Similar cross-resistance data have been reported for cells selected for resistance either to actinomycin D (BIEDLER and RIEHM 1970) or to colchicine (LING and THOMPSON 1974). Results such as these permit the suggestion that the "pleiotropic phenotype" may not be the first expression of resistance of a cell to these compounds, but, rather, initial resistance may be due to a more specific lesion.

The results given in Table 3 also allow an explanation for the discrepancy between experimental cross-resistance and its apparent lack of expression clinically: namely, cross-resistance (pleiotropy) may only become a problem when the cells are highly resistant to the particular agent, and it may be expressed only at a low level, if at all, in cells demonstrating lower levels of resistance. Indeed, clinical studies demonstrating a lack of apparent cross-resistance tend to support this assessment, but such results must be interpreted with caution. For example, it was

Table 2. Pattern of alkaloid resistance and cross-resistance

Alkaloid class	Resistance/cross-resistance	Drugs	Reference
Vinca alkaloids	*Primary resistance* in vivo or in vitro has been associated with cross-resistance to:	Daunorubicin	KESSEL et al. (1968)
		Adriamycin, other *Vinca* alkaloids	DANØ (1972)
		AD-32	WILKOFF and DULMADGE (1978)
		Actinomycin-D	BIEDLER et al. (1975)
		Maytansine	WOLPERT-DEFILLIPES et al. (1975)
		Colchicine, VM-26, VP-16-213	V. CONTER and W. T. BECK (unpublished)
	Cross-resistance to the *Vinca* alkaloids has been associated with *primary* resistance to:	Adriamycin	JOHNSON et al. (1978)
		Daunorubicin	BIEDLER and RIEHM (1970)
		Actinomycin-D	BIEDLER et al. (1975); KAYE and BODEN (1980)
		Colchicine	LING and THOMPSON (1974); LING (1975); BECH-HANSEN et al. (1976) MINOR and ROSCOE (1975)
Colchicum alkaloids	*Primary resistance* has been associated with cross-resistance to:	*Vinca* alkaloids, puromycin, emetine; anthracyclines	LING and THOMPSON (1974); BECH-HANSEN et al. (1976); MINOR and ROSCOE (1975)
	Cross-resistance to the *Colchicum* alkaloids has been associated with *primary* resistance to:	Actinomycin-D	BIEDLER and RIEHM (1970)
		Maytansine	ALDRICH (1979)
		Vincristine, vinblastine	V. CONTER and W. T. BECK (unpublished)

Table 3. Resistance and cross-resistance properties of vincristine-insensitive CCRF-CEM cells[a]

Cell line	Degree of resistance or cross-resistance to:		
	Vincristine	Daunorubicin	VM-26
CCRF-CEM[b]	1 (0.043 ± 0.027)[c]	1 (2.59 ± 0.63)	1 (11.1 ± 5.5)
CEM/VCR_5[d]	57[e]	3	5
CEM/VCR_{100}	653	19	32

[a] V. CONTER and W. T. BECK (unpublished)
[b] Human leukemic lymphoblast line established by FOLEY et al. (1965); culture conditions were as described by BECK et al. (1979)
[c] The concentrations of drugs ($M \times 10^{-8}$) that inhibit cell growth by 50% in 48 h (IC_{50}). Means ± S. D. of four to eight separate experiments
[d] Vincristine-resistant sublines were established as described (BECK et al. 1979) for vinblastine-resistant cells
[e] Degree of resistance or cross-resistance was obtained by dividing the IC_{50} value for the resistant line by the IC_{50} value of the sensitive CCRF-CEM cells

shown by WARREN et al. (1978) that vinblastine as a single agent could induce remissions in patients with advanced (stages III and IV) Hodgkin's disease who had either failed induction or had only a brief initial response to MOPP (a combination of nitrogen mustard, vincristine, prednisone, and procarbazine). The response rate of 62% with vinblastine was comparable to the rates of *initial* remission achieved with this drug. While it would seem that vinblastine was effective against disease apparently resistant to a combination that included vincristine, the actual situation, however, is too complex to assume that the tumor cells may have been originally resistant, in part even to vincristine; the amount of vincristine administered in combination was probably below the maximum tolerated dosage, whereas vinblastine, as a single agent, was given in corresponding higher doses. Indeed, since the response rate to vinblastine in these "induction failures" was the same as that for other patients treated initially with this drug, it seems clear that the bases for clinical resistance are much too difficult to elucidate.

Likewise, it was shown by MATHÉ et al. (1978 a, b) that vindesine was capable of inducing remissions in patients with acute lymphoblastic leukemia in whom prior therapy with vincristine, prednisone, and asparaginase (and in some cases, other drugs such as cyclophosphamide, 6-mercaptopurine, and methotrexate) had proven to be ineffective. Again, as with the study by WARREN et al. (1978), it is not clear from the results of MATHÉ et al. that the leukemic cells were initially insensitive to vincristine; a greater amount of vindesine was generally given as a single agent when compared with the usual doses of vincristine that were administered in combination with other drugs.

Recently, RIVERA et al. (1980) showed that a combination of VM-26 and cytosine arabinoside (araC) induced remissions (nine complete and one partial) in 10 of 33 leukemic patients, despite the fact that three of the patients had never achieved an initial remission, while seven had relapsed during therapy for the maintenance of remissions. The authors proposed that the effect of the combination was attributable to the epipodophyllotoxin, and suggested that cross-resistance between VM-26 and the other drugs to which the patients had been exposed, which had included vincristine and daunorubicin, as well as araC, did not occur. However, prior exposure to these drugs does not guarantee subsequent insensitivity, especially since therapy with the drugs in seven of the patients was discontinued before any appearance of clinical resistance. Indeed, although these authors proposed that the newly induced remissions were most likely due to the VM-26 and not to the araC, it could be argued as well that, since seven to ten patients had received the nucleoside (araC) previously, and six of these patients had gone into remission after being treated with a combination of drugs, including araC, the patients were still potentially responsive to the nucleoside. Thus, again, the appearance of or lack of clinical resistance or cross-resistance is difficult to assess.

It should be clear from these few examples that while cross-resistance between alkaloids and other natural products has been well documented experimentally, this is most difficult to demonstrate clinically; indeed, the converse has been indicated in patients: i.e., there appears to be little, if any, cross-resistance among these drug classes. The most likely explanations for this discrepancy reside in the following: (a) neoplastic cells within patients do not represent a relatively homogeneous resistant population; (b) at low levels of resistance, cross-resistance to other drugs is manifest to a lesser degree than is seen with cells expressing higher degrees of resistance; and (c) clinical insensitivity may be a reflection of the limitations imposed by drug toxicity to the patient. Thus, various demonstrations of clinical resistance, cross-resistance, or their lack must be evaluated with much caution; likewise, experimental demonstrations of cross-resistance, at least among "natural products," seem to be related clearly to degrees of resistance of the neoplastic cells that may not be attainable under clinical conditions.

II. Pharmacological Bases of Alkaloid Resistance

Traditionally, it has been accepted that alkaloid-resistant cells are less permeable to these drugs than are the sensitive cells, although this conclusion was based on cross-resistance studies, using uptake of other drugs and cytotoxicity as criteria (KESSEL et al. 1968; BIEDLER and RIEHM 1970; LING and THOMPSON 1974). In contrast, other investigations with colchicine- and anthracycline-resistant murine cells, which are cross-resistant to the *Vinca* alkaloids (Table 2), have offered the explanation that the basis of resistance to such natural compounds is decreased retention of drug (MINOR and ROSCOE 1975; DANØ 1973; SKOVSGAARD 1978b; INABA and JOHNSON 1977, 1978). Further, it has been proposed that this phenomenon may be mediated by a ubiquitous "active efflux pump," which is apparently capable of exporting such structurally disparate molecules as anthracyclines and *Vinca* alkaloids from resistant cells (DANØ 1973; SKOVSGAARD 1978a, b; INABA et al. 1979, 1981a; INABA and SAKURAI 1979). On close analysis, however, the

Table 4. Pharmacological bases of alkaloid resistance

Drug studied	Resistant cell line	Pharmacological alteration compared with sensitive cells	References
[^{3}H]Colchicine	CH^R5, others	Decreased permeability, possibly due to active permeability barrier	LING and THOMPSON (1974); SEE et al. (1974); CARLSEN et al. (1976)
	Various mouse and hamster lines	Diminished uptake, diminished retention, possibly due to altered binding component	ROSCOE and MINOR (1975)
	$3T3^r$ (maytansine)	Decreased drug uptake, possibly due to altered surface-binding	ALDRICH (1979)
[^{3}H]Vincristine	P388/VCR	Diminished drug uptake, diminished retention	BLEYER et al. (1975)
	EHR/VCR, EHR/DNR	Decreased drug uptake and retention, possibly due to "efflux pump"	SKOVSGAARD (1978 a)
	P388/ADR	Decreased uptake, enhanced efflux	INABA and SAKURAI (1979)
	P388/VCR	Decreased uptake, enhanced efflux	INABA et al. (1981 a)
[^{3}H]Vinblastine	Ehrlich ascites (vinblastine)	Decreased drug uptake	CREASEY (1968)
	CEM/VLB_{100}	Decreased drug uptake; decreased retention, possibly due to altered binding component	BECK (1981); BECK et al. (1983)

"pump" data are less clear and are subject to other interpretations, as will be discussed below. The various pharmacological alterations observed in alkaloid-resistant cells are summarized in Table 4.

1. Decreased Uptake of Drug

a) Colchicine

The major studies of the uptake of [^{3}H]colchicine by mammalian cells selected for resistance to this compound have been done by LING and his collaborators. Thus, LING and THOMPSON (1974) selected a series of cloned sublines of CHO cells for varying degrees of resistance to colchicine. They demonstrated that the resistant lines incorporated less [^{3}H]colchicine than did the sensitive parent line; moreover, in this and subsequent papers (SEE et al. 1974; CARLSEN et al. 1976), it was shown that colchicine uptake curves could be extrapolated back through the origin, as could the double-reciprocal plots for the uptake of this drug. The results indicated that the uptake of colchicine by these CHO cells could not be saturated, and this is consistent with the notion that the drug enters the cells by passive diffusion. Furthermore, an inverse relationship was found between the degree of resistance and the amount of drug accumulated. In exploring other possibilities to account for this decreased uptake of labeled drug by the resistant cells, these workers showed clearly that this was not due to decreased drug-binding to some cytoplasmic proteins, because [^{3}H]colchicine was bound equally well by cytoplasmic extracts of the sensitive parent line and by all resistant sublines. Additionally, it was shown that the colchicine-resistant sublines were cross-resistant not only to the colchicine analog, Colcemid, but also to such structurally unrelated compounds as vinblastine and actinomycin-D. Accordingly, these authors argued that cross-resistance to agents of such dissimilar molecular structure offered strong evidence that the basis of resistance was altered membrane permeability. Moreover, while the resistant lines showed no preferential cross-resistance to Colcemid, vinblastine, or actinomycin D, [^{3}H]colchicine that was bound to cytoplasmic extracts could be displaced only by Colcemid, which competes with colchicine for this binding. Again, this was taken as evidence that the cell lines were resistant by virtue of their diminished ability to allow passage of these molecules across the membrane, rather than by altered cytoplasmic drug-binding. Finally, these workers demonstrated that treatment of the parent line and two resistant mutant lines with noncytotoxic concentrations of the nonionic detergent, Tween 80, potentiated the cytotoxicity of colchicine in these cell lines, indicating that the detergent increased the permeability of the cells to colchicine.

In another thorough study, MINOR and ROSCOE (1975) performed experiments similar to those of LING and THOMPSON, and came to similar conclusions. Working primarily with mouse (3T6) and Syrian hamster (B_1) cell lines, these investigators selected independently cloned sublines with different degrees of resistance to colchicine. Generalized cross-resistance to puromycin, vinblastine, and actinomycin D was observed in these cells, and the authors indicated that such a phenomenon was difficult to explain in terms of anything *but* a permeability barrier. Additionally, these authors found, as did LING and THOMPSON, that the cytoplasmic extracts of cells with differing colchicine sensitivities bound [^{3}H]colchicine equally, but the rates of "binding" to whole cells (uptake) varied with the degree of drug insensitivity. Thus, it seems clear that a major basis of resistance to colchicine resides in diminished membrane permeability.

In characterizing the resistance to colchicine, LING and his collaborators (BECH-HANSEN et al. 1976) extended their earlier observations of cross-resistance to other "natural" compounds (puromycin, daunorubicin, emetine, ethidium bromide, cytochalasin B, vinblastine, etc.) and demonstrated that the degree of response of these compounds correlated with the degree of resistance to colchicine. Moreover, it was observed that the resistant lines demonstrated collateral sensitivity to classes of membrane-active agents (local anesthetics, steroids, some Triton X compounds). Such cross-resistant and collaterally sensitive behavior of the cells was termed the "pleiotropic phenotype," and these workers suggested that it was the result of the same mutation or mutations that conferred colchicine resistance on these cells. In this regard, BIEDLER and co-workers (BIEDLER and RIEHM 1970; BIEDLER et al. 1975) showed that resistance to actinomycin D was associated with cross-resistance to a series of "natural products," including anthracyclines, *Vinca* alkaloids, puromycin, and demecolcine (Colcemid); interestingly, these cells also appeared to exhibit a low degree of collateral sensitivity to hydrocortisone. Furthermore, BIEDLER et al. (1975) demonstrated that cross-resistance was generally correlated with the molecular weight of the compound: the higher the molecular weight, the greater the degree of cross-resistance. Thus, the parallels between the resistance, cross-resistance, and collateral sensitivity properties of cells selected for resistance to actinomycin-D are strikingly similar to those selected for resistance to colchicine. Such results add much support to the concept of the pleiotropic phenotype put forward by BECH-HANSEN et al. (1976), who proposed a model for resistance involving altered modulation of membrane fluidity, perhaps by some membrane component(s), in states of reduced permeability; PETERSON et al. (1974) also suggested that the membrane components are altered in actinomycin D resistance. This theory and its support will be examined critically in the subsection on biochemical lesions in alkaloid resistance (Sect. C.III).

b) *Vinca* Alkaloids

As indicated earlier, there have been but few studies of the uptake of [^{3}H]*Vinca* alkaloids by tumor cells, and fewer yet have attempted to characterize this phenomenon in cells selected for resistance to these drugs. Early work was based largely on assessments of cross-resistance and cytotoxicity, and on the accumulation of other compounds, such as [^{3}H]actinomycin-D and daunorubicin, because radiolabeled *Vinca* alkaloids were not then readily available. These studies promoted the ideas that resistance to the *Vinca* alkaloids was expressed as either (a) decreased uptake or (b) decreased retention of the drug. For example, as described above for [^{3}H]colchicine uptake by colchicine-resistant CHO cells, it was shown (PETERSON et al. 1974; BIEDLER et al. 1975) that the uptake of [^{3}H]actinomycin-D is inversely related to the degree of resistance of the various sublines. Moreover, these investigators found that the transport of actinomycin D did not require energy (PETERSON et al. 1974), and BOWEN and GOLDMAN (1975) demonstrated that actinomycin D enters Ehrlich ascites cells by a passive process. Such results permitted the conclusion that a common cellular attribute, such as nonspecific reduced permeability to these drugs, could account for the resistance. Conversely, it was proposed by KESSEL and his collaborators that decreased drug retention plays a role in the resistance of murine cells to daunorubicin (KESSEL et al. 1968) and to actinomycin D (KESSEL and WODINSKY 1968). Since cross-resistance had been demonstrated between these compounds and *Vinca* alkaloids, and because alkaloid-resistant lines also demonstrated decreased retention of the antibiotics, these investigators proposed that such compounds share a common mode of resistance, namely, the altered permeability barriers possibly related to diminished retention of the drugs.

While probably the first mention of the incorporation of a radiolabeled *Vinca* alkaloid by vinblastine-*resistant* murine cells was described as a minor part of a review by CREASEY (1968), the data presented did not fully support the interpretation given them, namely that the uptake of [^{3}H]vinblastine by vinblastine-resistant Ehrlich ascites cells in vitro and subsequent conversion to bound, alkali-labile material was slower than in the sensitive cells; unfortunately, these differences are not readily apparent from the figure presented.

The data presented by BLEYER et al. (1975), in a thorough study of the uptake and binding of [^{3}H]vincristine by murine leukemia cells (detailed in Sect. B.I), are more readily interpreted. While the experiment with vincristine-resistant P388 cells was not the primary focus of the paper, the data show clearly that these cells accumulated considerably less ($\sim$25%) [^{3} H]vincristine than did the sensitive parent line during a period of 60 min. Furthermore, SKOVSGAARD (1978 a) examined the pharmacological mechanism of cross-resistance between vincristine and daunorubicin in Ehrlich ascites cells and showed clearly that the 2-h uptake of [^{3}H]vincristine by both vincristine-resistant and daunorubicin-resistant cells was less than one-sixth that observed with the sensitive line. In our studies of resistance to *Vinca* alkaloids in cultured human leukemic lymphoblasts (CCRF-CEM), we have found that the net accumulation of [^{3}H]vinblastine is decreased in cells selected for resistance to this compund, when compared with the sensitive parent line (BECK 1979, 1981; BECK et al. 1983); thus, it would appear that diminished uptake may be a major mechanism of resistance to *Vinca* alkaloids, as was seen for colchicine.

2. Diminished Retention of Drug

Some data show that the decreased net accumulation of alkaloids by the resistant cells, described above, may be due to an altered retention of these agents. For example, SKOVSGAARD (1978 a), INABA and SKURAI (1979), and INABA et al. (1981 a) have presented data suggesting that *enhanced extrusion* of [^{3}H]vincristine via an "efflux pump" is the basis for diminished accumulation of this drug by vincristine-resistant Ehrlich ascites cells, when compared with the drug-sensitive parental line. Additionally, data from this laboratory for the diminished accumulation of [^{3}H]vinblastine by vinblastine-resistant leukemic cells (BECK 1979, 1981) may be interpreted to support the concept of an efflux pump. Because an efflux pump provides an important conceptual framework to describe a basis of resistance of

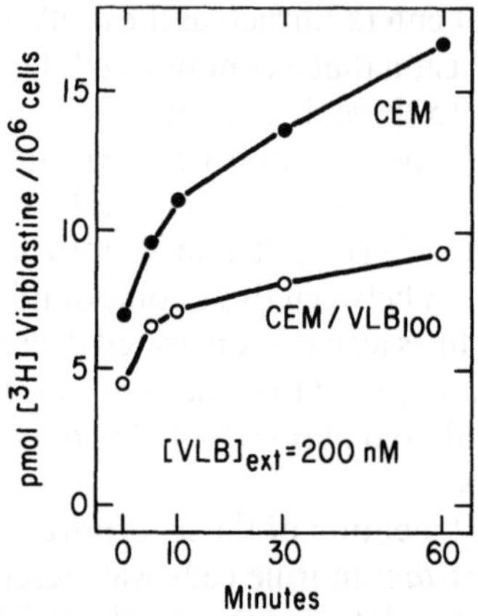

Fig. 2. Accumulation of [^{3}H]vinblastine by vinblastine-sensitive (●) and -resistant (o) cultured human leukemic lymphoblasts. Culture conditions, history, and selection of resistant cells are described in BECK et al. (1979). Cells were incubated in buffer containing 200 n*M* [^{3}H]vinblastine. At the times indicated, aliquots were removed to tubes containing silicone oil and were centrifuged at ~12,000 × g for 1 min. The medium and oil were aspirated, and the cell pellet was dissolved in sodium dodecylsulfate and then counted for radioactivity. Shown is a representative experiment. Each *point* is the mean of triplicate aliquots; the standard deviations were usually ≦15% of the mean values

tumor cells not only to *Vinca* alkaloids, but also to other natural products as well (the pleiotropic phenotype), it would be profitable to discuss here the key arguments in its favor and to determine if the data actually support such an hypothesis, at least for alkaloids.

Most of the work promoting the concept of an active efflux pump for natural products has been done in only a few laboratories, and has been developed through studies of the accumulation of the anthracyclines (DANØ 1973; SKOVSGAARD 1978 a, 1978 b; INABA and JOHNSON 1978; INABA et al. 1979) and more recently, vincristine (SKOVSGAARD 1978 a; INABA and SAKURAI 1979; INABA et al. 1981 a) in murine cells selected for resistance and cross-resistance to these agents. The most compelling argument, based on earlier studies of the transport of antifolates (HAKALA 1965; GOLDMAN 1969), is that resistant cells, which normally incorporate less drug than do the sensitive parent cells, can be made to incorporate more drug when depleted of sources of energy. One interpretation of these results is that an active efflux pump has been poisoned, and that the net accumulation under these conditions is due solely to unidirectional drug influx.

An experiment from this laboratory, which demonstrates the accumulation of [^{3}H]vinblastine, will suffice as an example of this poisoning of an apparent efflux pump; in this regard, it reflects accurately the findings of others (DANØ 1973; INABA and JOHNSON 1978; SKOVSGAARD 1978a, 1978b; INABA and SAKURAI 1979; INABA et al. 1981 a) concerning the accumulation of anthracyclines and vincristine by murine cells resistant to these agents. This experiment involved a subline of CCRF-CEM cells (designated as CEM) that was selected for resistance to vinblastine (CEM/VLB_{100}) (BECK et al. 1979). This work is detailed else-

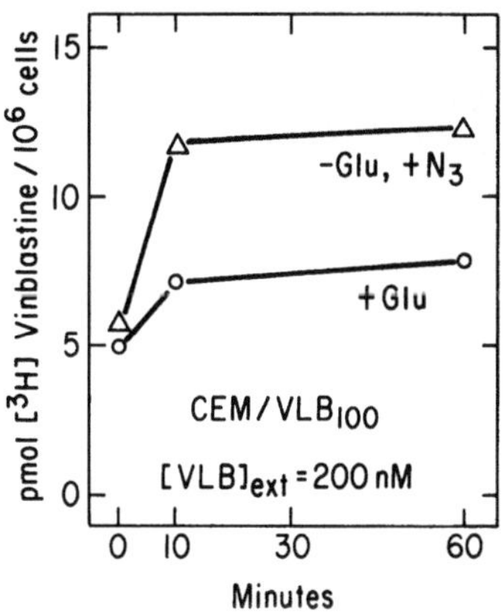

Fig. 3. Effect of depletion of cellular energy stores on the accumulation of [^{3}H]vinblastine by vinblastine-resistant CEM/VLB$_{100}$ cells. Normal buffer contained 10 m*M* glucose (+Glu); "depletion"-buffer contained 10 m*M* sodium azide, but no glucose (-Glu, +N$_3$). See legend to Fig. 2 for further details

where (Beck et al. 1983). When incubated in 200 n*M* [^{3}H]vinblastine, the resistant cells incorporated about half the amount of drug accumulated by the sensitive cells (see Fig. 2). When the drug-insensitive cells were depleted of cellular energy stores by removing glucose and adding azide to the medium, however, both the initial rate and total amount of [^{3}H]vinblastine accumulated were increased (Fig. 3); indeed, the net 10-min accumulation of drug by these energy-depleted resistant cells was essentially the same as that of the metabolically intact sensitive cells.

As a corollary of these observations demonstrating enhanced drug accumulation by metabolically deprived resistant cells, it has been shown for a number of natural products, including [^{3}H]vincristine, that upon the readdition of an energy source such as glucose, a rapid and pronounced loss of drug from the cells occurs (e.g., Skovsgaard 1978a, 1978b; Inaba et al. 1979, 1981a; Inaba and Sakurai 1979). We have made such observations also, employing [^{3}H]vinblastine-preloaded, energy-depleted CEM/VLB$_{100}$ cells, as illustrated by Fig. 4. Results of this type have been used to give further support to the concept of an active efflux pump, the hypothesis being that restoration of a source of metabolic energy activated the pump, causing a rapid extrusion of drug *against a concentration gradient,* even in the presence of a metabolic inhibitor.

The questions to be resolved, then, are these: Do the data fit the hypothesis that resistance to these classes of drugs is attributable to their decreased retention, mediated in part by an active efflux pump? Is it "active"? Is it a pump? Is this a universal phenomenon for all or most resistant lines, and all or most natural products, i.e., do the data support the concept of a pleiotropic phenotype? It should be recalled that others have proposed that resistance and cross-resistance to such naturally occurring drug molecules are reflections of a diminished cellular permeability (see Table 4). Moreover, See et al. (1974) suggested that the basis for colchicine resistance (and *Vinca* alkaloid cross-resistance) in CHO cells resided in an active (energy-requiring) permeability *barrier*. Upon close analysis, however,

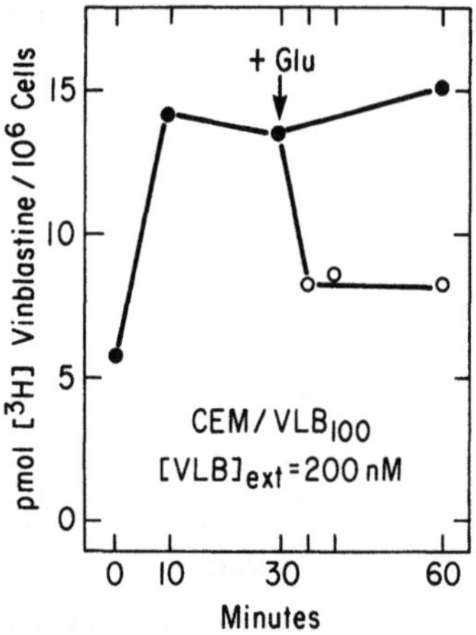

Fig 4. Effect of glucose on the levels of [^{3}H]vinblastine in preloaded, metabolically deprived CEM/VLB$_{100}$ cells. Cells incubated in "depletion" buffer (containing 10 m*M* azide, but not glucose) were preloaded with [^{3}H]vinblastine. After 30 min, glucose was added to some flasks to a final concentration of 10 m*M*. Aliquots were taken at the time points indicated and processed for the determination of [^{3}H] as described in the legend to Fig. 2. A representative experiment is shown

it seems that the data can be given yet another interpretation: that the *binding* of drug by resistant cells differs from drug-binding by sensitive cells, and what has been construed as a "pump" (or even a permeability barrier) may reflect primarily a change in drug-binding. Thus, it is appropriate at this time to examine the data with respect to: (*a*) intracellular concentration and binding of drug and (*b*) the metabolic status of the cell.

a) Intracellular Concentration and Binding of Drug

The problem of cellular drug-binding and its interference with the accurate determination of intracellular free drug concentrations has been discussed earlier (Sect. B. I) and in a recent report from this laboratory (BECK et al. 1983). It is critical to be able to assess the levels of intracellular free drug, because this is the form of the drug that is capable of traversing cell membranes, and is, consequently, available for export. In most studies of the transport of natural products, little attention has been given to the intracellular concentration of drug, either total accumulated or free. When examined, accurate measurements of intracellular concentrations of free drug have proved difficult to obtain, largely because of extensive binding of these large heterocyclic molecules either within or on the cell. For example, BOWEN and GOLDMAN (1975) showed that the high cell/medium ratios and the cellular accumulation of actinomycin D are attributable primarily to loose binding of this agent. Likewise, SKOVSGAARD (1977, 1978b, c) has shown very high cell/medium ratios for anthracyclines, which also implies extensive drug-binding by the cells. However, attempts to measure the concentrations of free intracellular drug (SKOVSGAARD 1977) by comparing the amount of anthracycline bound to homogenates with that amount of drug in the extracellular medium were not convincing: although it was concluded that cellular *free* drug/medium ratios were less than one, the likely redistribution of drug during homogenization of the cells imposes difficulties in the interpretation of such results.

Other studies by SKOVSGAARD (1978b) indicated that resistance to daunorubicin may be related to a decreased retention of drug; specifically, the resistant cells accumulated less daunorubicin than the sensitive cells because of an apparent enhanced efflux of drug. In another study comparing mechanisms of resistance and cross-resistance of vincristine and daunorubicin, similar results were obtained with a vincristine-insensitive line of Ehrlich ascites cells (SKOVSGAARD 1978a). Additionally, INABA and SAKURAI (1979) and INABA et al. (1981a) showed that the uptake of [^{3}H]vincristine by adriamycin-resistant and vincristine-resistant lines of P388 cells was diminished, as compared with that of the sensitive parental lines, and proposed a similar efflux mechanism for this compound.

Diminished drug retention by *Vinca* alkaloid-insensitive cells can be demonstrated by loading cells with drug, and then incubating them in drug-free-medium. Such cells will release drug until a plateau is reached; the drug remaining associated with the cells presumably represents bound material (GOLDMAN 1973; SIROTNAK et al. 1979). The amount of drug retained by resistant cells is considerably less than that retained by the sensitive line, often ranging from 10% to 25% of the total amount of drug accumulated (BECK 1979, 1981; BECK et al. 1983). Moreover, the evidence for the existence of an efflux pump has been obtained from the types of experiments shown in Figs. 3 and 4: the cellular accumulation of drug is enhanced in metabolically deprived resistant cells, and when an energy source is supplied there is an immediate and rapid loss of label from these cells.

By definition, an "active" efflux pump would be able to cause drug extrusion from preloaded cells *against* a concentration gradient, and this argument has been promoted by SKOVSGAARD (1978a, b) as a basis for resistance to vincristine and daunorubicin. It is not clear, however, that this exodus occurs against a gradient. As has been recognized for compounds that are extensively bound, the intracellular concentration of free drug is difficult to measure directly. Indeed, it would appear that the intracellular drug must exist in equilibrium with the bound material as:

$$F_x\text{-bound}_{cell} \rightleftharpoons F_x\text{-free}_{cell} \rightleftharpoons F_x\text{-medium},$$

where the fraction (F_x) designated as "bound" is very large, and that termed "free" is very small. At equilibrium, because of the binding, the cell/medium ratio will be very large, especially at lower concentrations of drug in the medium. If the binding is governed by the law of mass action, resuspension of the cells in drug-free medium will shift the equilibrium to the right, and loosely bound drug will be removed to the extracellular compartment. The glucose-induced drug extrusion appears to promote a similar shift of equilibrium to the right, causing the loosely bound drug to be removed to the extracellular medium, even in the presence of extracellular drug. The concentration of *total* intracellular drug is so much greater than that in the medium, however, that the extruded drug must be escaping from the cell *down its concentration gradient*. If, in fact, this is the case, then

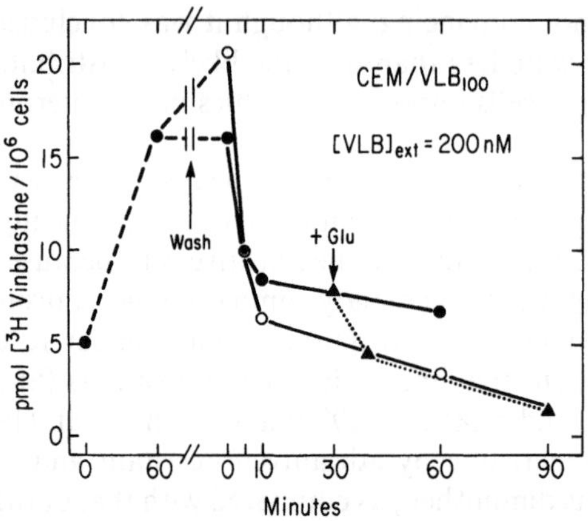

Fig. 5. Release of [^{3}H]vinblastine from CEM/VLB$_{100}$ cells. See text for experimental details and legend to Fig. 2 for details of the processing of samples. Symbols: ●, cells incubated or resuspended in buffer containing sodium azide (10 m*M*), but no glucose (−Glu, +N_3); ○, cells resuspended in (−Glu, +N_3) to which glucose was added at the time indicated to a final concentration of 10 m*M*; ▲ cells resuspended in (−Glu, +N_3) to which glucose was added at the time indicated to a final concentration of 10 m*M*

by definition the glucose-mediated drug extrusion cannot be an active process. Moreover, if the *concentration* of drug lost from the cells after the addition of glucose is calculated, it is evident that this value far exceeds the drug level that was present in the medium. Thus, it can be determined from Fig. 4 that glucose caused the extrusion of ~9.3 μ*M* [^{3}H]vinblastine into a medium containing 0.2 μ*M* drug. Likewise, it can be calculated from the data of SKOVSGAARD that glucose caused the extrusion of ~5 μ*M* [^{3}H]vincristine into medium containing 1 μ*M* vincristine and ~300 μ*M* daunorubicin into medium containing 5 μ*M* daunorubicin (SKOVSGAARD 1978a, Charts 2 and 3, respectively). Similar determinations can be made from the results of others (INABA and JOHNSON 1978; INABA et al. 1979).

Thus, it can be concluded from this exercise that: (a) natural compounds such as the *Vinca* alkaloids, anthracyclines, and other antibiotics are bound extensively to the cells, and much of this binding is in a readily exchangeable form; (b) the free intracellular drug-concentrations of such compounds cannot be determined readily; but (c) the amount of drug extruded from metabolically deprived, preloaded cells upon readdition of energy sources is far in excess of the concentration of drug in the medium; permitting the suggestion that (d) drug exodus is most likely *not* an active process.

Indeed, to illustrate this last point, the following experiment was done (BECK et al. 1983): metabolically depleted CEM/VLB$_{100}$ cells were preloaded with [^{3}H]vinblastine for 60 min, collected, washed, and resuspended in drug-free medium (a) without glucose, but containing azide (−Glu, +N_3); (b) with glucose (+Glu); and (c) without glucose initially, for 30 min, after which glucose was added (−, +Glu). The results, shown in Fig. 5, reveal the following: (a) preloaded cells rapidly lost most of the accumulated drug within 10 min when resuspended in drug-free medium, whether or not glucose was present (60% and 48%, respectively); (b) the rate of loss was slower thereafter, with the cells in (−Glu, +N_3) retaining about twice as much drug as those reincubated in +Glu; and (c) addition of glucose to cells in (−Glu, +N_3) led to a further loss of [^{3}H]vinblastine to a level and rate seen with the +Glu cells. These results demonstrate that [^{3}H]vinblastine is lost from resistant cells down its concentration gradient by a *passive* process; glucose has but little effect on this initial rate of loss, but it does seem to be able to enhance the subsequent drug loss to some extent. The data permit the suggestion that loosely bound drug is readily lost from the resistant cells by a passive process, and that glucose may cause the release of a more tightly bound fraction of [^{3}H]vinblastine.

With regard to the example shown above in Fig. 5, it is worth noting that similar results were obtained by MINOR and ROSCOE (1975) for the release of [^{3}H]colchicine from monolayer cultures of mammalian lines having varying degrees of sensitivity to this drug. Thus, when incubated in drug-free medium, two resistant lines lost the drug at a rate that was more than three times as fast as that from a relatively more sensitive line, and the investigators attributed this to an extra drug-binding pool, possibly on the cell surface within a glycocalyx (the glycoprotein and polysaccharide cover that surrounds many cells), which fills and empties rapidly.

Finally, in contrast, PETERSON et al. (1974) found that the rate and amount of release of [^{3}H]actinomycin D was greater from drug-*sensitive* Chinese hamster cells than from an actinomycin D-resistant line. It is likely, however, that these results reflect the initial loading concentration of the drug, the amount released from the cells being directly related, in part, to the amount accumulated. Thus, PETERSON et al. loaded both sensitive and resistant cells in 2 μg [^{3}H]actinomycin D/ml; they had shown, however, that while there was ready uptake of drug by the sensitive line when incubated in this concentration of actinomycin D, the resistant line incorporated essentially no drug, even when incubated in a ten-fold higher concentration. Accordingly, these results of PETERSON et al. with [^{3}H]actinomycin D must be evaluated with caution.

b) Metabolic Status of the Cell

The examples presented in the preceeding section indicate that cellular metabolism plays some role in the ability of resistant cells to retain the drug. Indeed, it has been shown for a number of "natural product" drugs that depletion of energy stores of drug-resistant cells permits enhanced drug accumulation; the presumed repletion of energy levels by the addition of glucose either prevents further accumulation or causes an extrusion of the accumulated drug. Furthermore, these glucose-like effects have been shown by SEE et al. (1974) in KCN-treated CHO cells to be mediated in part by such other sugars as ribose and xylose, which could be metabolized to produce energy via the pentose-phosphate pathway, but not by sugars such as fucose or 2-deoxyglucose. We have made similar observations with our leukemic cells: while mannose, a metabolizable sugar, mimicked the glucose effects, nonmetabolizable sugars, such as galactose, 2-deoxyglucose, and fucose, had no effect on cellular drug levels (BECK et al., unpublished). Such results strengthen the suggestion that cellular metabolism plays a role in the accumulation or binding (retention) of drug by both resistant and sensitive cells.

Thus, certain sugars, rather than activating a drug pump, may alter the accumulation of alkaloids through an energy-requiring binding mechanism. There appear to be precedents for such a concept. For example, COSTLOW and HAMPLE (1980) have shown that the specific binding of prolactin by rat mammary carcinoma cells is *enhanced* in the presence of such inhibitors of cellular metabolism as azide, cyanide, arsenate, and 2,4-dinitrophenol. This observation may indicate that energy is required to keep receptor proteins in an "off" state; removal of the source of energy may alter the structure of the receptor in some manner. Additionally, FRY et al. (1980) have presented data showing that 2,4-dinitrophenol and other inhibitors of cellular metabolism increase the non-exchangeable ("bound") fraction of methotrexate in Ehrlich ascites cells, and have suggested that such inhibitors interact directly with the methotrexate carrier in the membrane. Accordingly, such results may be relevant to the effects of cellular metabolic status in the accumulation of *Vinca* alkaloids and other drugs, as described above. Clearly, more studies, using membrane transport vesicles, cellular homogenates, membranes, and other subcellular fractions, are needed in this area to resolve these present uncertainties.

3. Role of Calcium

Some very recent work by TSURUO et al. (1981 a) and INABA et al. (1981 b) has provided fresh insights into a possible mechanism behind the diminished retention of alkaloids and anthracyclines by murine cells selected for resistance to vincristine. These investigators have shown that both verapamil, a coronary vasodilator, and reserpine, an antihypertensive agent, can overcome the resistance of murine leukemia cells to vincristine. It was proposed that the increased cytotoxicity of vincristine, vinblastine, or adriamycin toward the alkaloid- or anthracycline-resistant cells, respectively, is related in some way to perturbations (decreases) in cellular levels of calcium caused by verapamil or reserpine. Conversely, it was shown by SCHREK and STEFANI (1976) that the cytotoxicity of vincristine, colchicine (and X-rays) toward leukemic lymphocytes could be impaired by the calcium ionophore, A23187; accordingly, it was suggested that calcium was involved in the cytotoxicity of the alkaloids. Similarly, TSURUO et al. (1981 b) demonstrated that the cytotoxicity of vinblastine toward KB cells in culture could be reversed by the inorganic dye, ruthenium red. In this study, the dye, which has affinity for mucopolysaccharides, also inhibited Ca^{++}-ATPase in these cells, again implying a relationship between the metabolism of calcium and the action of the alkaloid. It should be noted, however, that at the concentration of ruthenium red that completely reversed the cytotoxicity of vinblastine, the Ca^{++}-ATPase was only inhibited about 12%. Thus, it appears that the relationship between cellular calcium and the cytotoxicity of and cellular resistance to alkaloids remains to be clarified; nevertheless, these interesting studies provide a starting point for further investigations of a possible role for calcium in the phenomenon of alkaloid resistance or cytotoxicity.

III. Biochemical Alterations Associated with Alkaloid Resistance

1. Membrane Alterations

There have been several studies exploring the biochemical lesions that may account for alkaloid resistance in mammalian cells. Most of these investigations documenting biochemical changes in alkaloid resistant or cross-resistant cell lines are summarized in Table 5. Some of the earliest work in this area was done by BOSMANN and KESSEL, using the various cell lines listed in the table, which were selected for resistance or cross-resistance to *Vinca* alkaloids. Because it had appeared that the plasma membrane is the site of the resistance lesion(s), as described in an earlier section, these investigators studied the membrane glycoproteins of the resistant cells and found them to be generally increased in amount when compared with the sensitive lines (BOSMANN 1971). Specifically, it was demonstrated that the levels of the glycoprotein synthetic enzymes (glycoprotein : glycosyl transferases) were generally increased and those of the glycoprotein degradative enzymes (glycosidases) were generally decreased in the drug-resistant lines, as compared with the drug-sensitive controls (BOSMANN 1971; KESSEL and BOSMANN 1970; BOSMANN and KESSEL 1970). The net effect of these alterations in enzyme activites would be one to increase generally the amounts of membrane glycoproteins; as will be discussed presently, however, such increases appear to be restricted to one or more discrete surface proteins. Finally, with respect to these early studies, it is notable that an L1210 subline selected for resistance to araC was also shown to have decreased glycosidase levels when compared with sensitive controls (BOSMANN and KESSEL 1970). Because resistance to this drug is generally attributed to either a decrease of the activity of the cytoplasmic enzyme, deoxycytidine kinase (MEYERS and KREIS 1978), or an increase in the activity of cytidine deaminase (STEUART and BURKE 1971), and because surface glycoproteins of similar resistant cells do not seem to differ from those found on araC-sensitive cells (BECK et al. 1979), the meaning of this early observation remains obscure.

As can be seen in Table 5, there have been several studies examining the surface glycoproteins of alkaloid-resistant or cross-resistant cells. The general observation, regardless of the cell line or selection agent, has been that resistant cells have on their surfaces a high molecular weight glycoprotein when they are compared with the drug-sensitive parent lines (JULIANO et al. 1976; JULIANO and LING 1976; PETERSON and BIEDLER 1978; BECK et al. 1979). The molecular weights of the resistance-associated glycoproteins have been reported to be 150,000 (PETERSON and BIEDLER 1978), 165,000 (JULIANO and LING 1976; JULIANO et al. 1976), and between 170,000 and 190,000 (BECK et al. 1979). While the weights, determined on sodium dodecylsulfate-polyacrylamide gels (SDS-PAGE), suggest that these may be different proteins, the range may reflect either differences in the degree of glycosylation of similar peptides or merely differences in calibrating the various gel systems. The glycoprotein(s) has been identified primarily by surface labeling, using the method of GAHMBERG and HAKOMORI (1973) or of STECK and DAWSON (1974), which consists of oxidation of the sugars with galactose oxidase (with or without neuraminidase) and subsequent reduction with [^{3}H]borohydride (NaB^3H_4). It is of interest that this glycoprotein could not be identified by the

Table 5. Biochemical changes associated with alkaloid-resistant or cross-resistant mammalian cell lines

Cell line	Origin	Selected for resistance to	Change(s) relative to drug-sensitive parent line	Detected by	References
P388/VCR P388/38280 L1210/CA	Murine leukemias	VCR Phthalanalide Cytosine arabinoside	↓Glycosidases	Enzyme assay	BOSMANN and KESSEL (1970)
L5178Y/D	Murine leukemia	Actinomycin D	↑Glycoprotein : glycosyl transferases	Enzyme assay	KESSEL and BOSMANN (1970)
DC-3F/ADX	Chinese hamster lung	Actinomycin D	↑Glycoprotein : glycosyl transferases; ↓glycosidases	Enzyme assay	BOSMANN (1971)
			↑Glycoprotein content of membranes	SDS-PAGE	
CH^RC4 CH^RC5 Others SV-40 transformed	Chinese hamster ovary Syrian hamster	Colchicine (varying degrees) Actinomycin D	165,000-dalton surface glycoprotein (↑ with ↑ resistance)	SDS-PAGE; surface-labeling (GO/NaB^3H_4); metabolic labeling ([^{14}C]$gluNH_2$)	JULIANO et al. (1976); JULIANO and LING (1976)
DC-3F/ADX	Chinese hamster lung	Actinomycin D	150,000-dalton surface glycoprotein	SDS-PAGE; surface-labeling (GO/NaB^3H_4); metabolic labeling ([^{3}H]-leu;[^{3}H]$gluNH_2$)	PETERSON and BIEDLER (1978)
DC-3F/DMXX DC-3F/VCRd	Chinese hamster lung	Daunorubicin Vincristine	↑150,000-dalton surface glycoprotein; concomitant ↓100,000-dalton surface glycoprotein	SDS-PAGE; surface labeling (GO/NaB^3H_4)	PETERSON and BIEDLER (1980)

GO, galactose oxidase; NaB^3H_4, sodium [^{3}H]borohydride; [^{14}C]$gluNH_2$, [^{14}C]glucosamine; [^{3}H]leu, [^{3}H]leucine; IEF, isoelectric focusing

Table 5. (continued)

Cell line	Origin	Selected for resistance to	Change(s) relative to drug-sensitive parent line	Detected by	References
CEM/VLB$_{100}$	Human leukemic lymphoblast	Vinblastine	↑ ~ 180,000-dalton surface glycoprotein; ↑ with ↑ resistance; concomitant ↓ ~ 90,000-dalton glycoprotein	SDS-PAGE; surface labeling (GO/NaB^3H_4)	Beck et al. (1979)
DC-3F/ADX	Chinese hamster	Actinomycin D	Incomplete set of gangliosides; hematosides (G_{M3}) only	Thin-layer chromatography; radioautography	Peterson et al. (1979)
CH^{R}C4 CH^{R}C5	Chinese hamster	Colchicine	↑ Phosphorylation of 165,000- and 200,000-dalton membrane proteins	SDS-PAGE; ^{32}P-labeling	Carlsen et al. (1977)
Cmd 4 Grs 2	Chinese hamster ovary	Colcemid Griseofulvin	Altered β-tubulin	Two-dimensional electrophoresis (IEF/SDS-PAGE)	Cabral et al. (1980)
DC-3F/VCRd-5	Chinese hamster fibroblast	Vincristine	Cytoplasmic, protein, 19,000-dalton; pI, 5.7	Two-dimensional electrophoresis (IEF/SDS-PAGE)	Meyers and Biedler (1981)
MAZ/VCR	Mouse tumor line	Vincristine			
DC-3F/VCRd-5	Chinese hamster fibroblast	Vincristine	Homogeneously staining region of chromosome	Giemsa-banding	Biedler et al. (1980)

surface-labeling method using ^{125}I and lactoperoxidase (JULIANO et al. 1976), suggesting that the glycoconjugate, at least on CHO cells, has no tyrosine or histidine residues available for iodination. The glycoprotein has also been identified by metabolic labeling with [^{3}H]- or [^{14}C]glucosamine (JULIANO et al. 1976; PETERSON and BIEDLER 1978; BECK et al. 1979).

The high molecular weight glycoprotein is apparently resistance-associated. Thus, it was shown that, in general, there was a correlation between the amount of this material (represented by increased peak height, peak size, or peak labeling) and the degree of resistance of either CHO cells to colchicine (JULIANO and LING 1976) or of CCRF-CEM cells to vinblastine (BECK et al. 1979). Moreover, concomitant with the resistance-associated increase in the high-molecular-weight species, there are decreases, compared with the sensitive parent lines, in the amounts of a glycoprotein(s) of ~90,000–100,000 (BECK et al. 1979; PETERSON and BIEDLER 1980). Whether these apparently reciprocal changes are related to each other has yet to be established.

An example of the resistance-associated surface alterations is shown in Fig. 6, which is a fluorogram of gels comparing a vinblastine-resistant subline (CEM/VLB_{100}) with the drug-sensitive parent (CEM). These cells were labeled on the surface with $NaB^{3}H_4$ after treatment with galactose oxidase (Fig. 6a) or galactose oxidase and neuraminidase (Fig. 6b). While the labeling profile is somewhat more complex after removal of the terminal sialic acids (Fig. 6b), the basic features remain: (a) band *1*, the high molecular weight, resistance-associated glycoprotein, is probably a series of proteins, as seen more clearly in Fig 6b, at least one of which appears to be unique to the CEM/VLB_{100} cells; (b) the broad band *2* is also probably a series of glycoproteins that are diminished in amount on the membranes of the resistant cells, as compared with those of the sensitive line. It is tempting to speculate not only that the decrease in band(s) *2* is related to the increase in band(s) *1*, when cells become resistant, but also that these changes possibly represent permeability-associated restricted "domains," similar to those proposed by JULIANO and LING (1976). (c) The broad bands designated *C* are common to both sensitive and resistant lines and are due to treatment with neuraminidase, while (d) the bands designated *NE* (and those below them) are nonenzymatically labeled and have been observed by others (ANDERSSON et al. 1977); neither the bands designated *C* nor those termed *NE* appear to be resistance associated.

Other discrete membrane and cytoplasmic differences between sensitive and alkaloid-resistant cells have been described, as indicated in Table 5. Of special interest is the observation that the synthesis of gangliosides is blocked at the level of hematosides (G_{M3}) in actinomycin D-resistant Chinese hamster cells as compared with those of the sensitive parent line (PETERSON et al. 1979). This observation permits the suggestion that membranes from drug-resistant cells may contain (areas of or domains of) less complex lipids than those found in the sensitive cells, and this may in some way contribute to the diminished drug permeability of these cells; it may, however, be a reflection of the altered glycoproteins seen on these cells. Moreover, these results may be related both to the findings of KITANO et al. (1972) and NICOLIN et al. (1972) that drug-resistant cells are more immunogenic (antigenic) than the sensitive parent lines, as well as to the prior results of

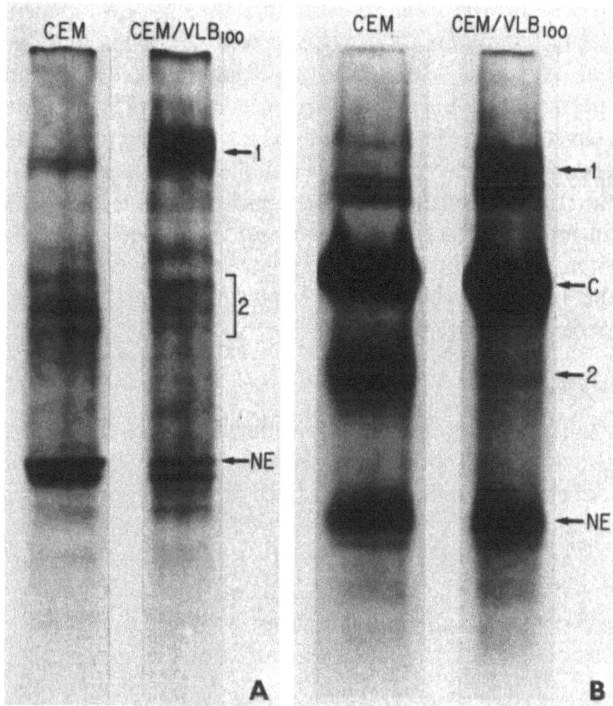

Fig. 6 a, b. Cell-surface glycoproteins of vinblastine-sensitive (CEM) and -resistant (CEM/VLB_{100}) human leukemic lymphoblasts. Cells were labeled on the surface with [^{3}H]borohydride after treatment with either galactose oxidase (**a**) or galactose oxidase and neuraminidase (**b**), as described by BECK et al. (1979). See text for details. *1*, Resistance-associated glycoproteins, ~180,000 daltons; *2*, region of ~90,000 daltons, prominent in neuraminidase-treated sensitive cells whose loss may be resistance related; *C*, prominant large bands (~130,000 daltons) appearing after treatment with neuraminidase; *NE*, nonenzymatically labeled bands

BIEDLER et al. (1975) that these drug-resistant cells are no longer capable of inducing tumors in animals.

Another important biochemical difference between drug-sensitive and -resistant cells was demonstrated by CARLSEN et al. (1977). These investigators found that the phosphorylation of two high molecular weight (165000 and 200000) membrane proteins was increased in colchicine-resistant cells when compared with the sensitive parent line. The suggestion was made that the resistance-associated glycoprotein acted in some way to promote a permeability barrier; furthermore, it was proposed that this protein had to be phosphorylated in order to restrict drug permeability. In support of this concept, these workers demonstrated that the phosphorylation of two high molecular weight (165000 and 200000) by sensitive and resistant cells (SEE et al. 1977), produced a rapid depletion of cellular ATP levels (CARLSEN et al. 1977); moreover, addition of glucose was shown to increase KCN-depleted cellular ATP content, and rotenone, another metabolic inhibitor, could also do the same, presumably through an independent mechanism. In all cases tested, depletion of cellular ATP levels led to an increase in the rate of uptake of colchicine, although it was found that the resistant cells could maintain the "permeability-barrier" at lower levels of ATP than could the sensitive cells. (One caveat is in order: rotenone, which was used to decrease ATP levels in the cell, has been shown by Brinkley et al. (1974) to have antimitotic properties; thus, it is not clear whether the depletion of cellular ATP by this compound is a direct or an indirect effect, the latter being a consequence of binding to tubulin; if the latter, this might have consequences for the uptake/binding of colchicine, and the proposed relationship between permeability and ATP levels would therefore be less apparent.)

2. Cytoplasmic Alterations

Three recent studies have presented data indicating that alkaloid-resistant cells contain altered cytoplasmic proteins when compared with the sensitive parent lines. Using independently selected CHO lines expressing resistance to Colcemid and to griseofulvin, Cabral et al. (1980) showed by two-dimensional electrophoresis that these mutants possessed an altered β-tubulin that was more basic than that obtained from cells of the wild type. This protein, which was present in addition to the wild-type β-tubulin in the mutants, was apparently a new gene product, rather than a post-translational modification of the normal protein, because it could be produced in vitro from mutant-cell mRNA, using a reticulocyte cell-free translation system. Further proof that this protein was an altered β-tubulin came from experiments with Triton X-100 extractions, peptide maps, and clonogenic assays; these latter experiments provided support for the concept that the cells were indeed tubulin mutants and not permeability mutants, in that they were resistant (in clonogenic assays) only to antimitotic drugs (colchicine, Colcemid griseofulvin, and vinblastine), but not to puromycin or ethidium bromide. Conversely, a colchicine-resistant permeability mutant was, as expected, demonstrably cross-resistant to these latter two drugs. The resistance of these CHO β-tubulin mutants was of a low degree (~two- to five-fold). In this regard, Ling et al. (1979) also selected mutants of CHO cells possessing low degrees of resistance to Colcemid. These investigators demonstrated that the most likely reason for the drug resistance of their mutants was impaired binding of Colcemid to tubulin. Indeed, detergent-enhanced drug permeability did not alter the relative resistance of these cells to Colcemid, and, although α- and β-tubulins purified from the mutant cells appeared the same as those purified from the wild-type line on one-dimensional SDS-PAGE, the Colcemid-binding capacity of the tubulin purified from the mutant lines was reduced, compared with the sensitive cells. Thus, it is possible that Ling et al. (1979) had selected cells having an altered β-tubulin, as was shown by Cabral et al. (1980).

In a recent report, Meyers and Biedler (1981) have presented data to indicate that the cells of a vincristine-resistant subline of Chinese hamster fibroblasts have a 19000-dalton cytoplasmic protein (*pI*, 5.7) that is not readily detected in the drug-sensitive parent, a sensitive revertant, an actinomycin D-resistant subline, or two antifolate-resistant lines. This cytoplasmic protein, which was also seen in a vincristine-resistant mouse tumor line designated MAZ/VCR, was detected by two-dimensional electrophoresis; its function at this time remains obscure. These authors speculated that the protein was probably associated with resistance to vincristine, but most likely not with the mechanisms of gene amplification or the formation of homogenously staining regions (HSRs) on chromosomes per se.

Related to this latter study, another preliminary report has been presented recently from the same laboratory (BIEDLER et al. 1980) indicating that these vincristine-resistant Chinese hamster fibroblasts also posses a marker chromosome identified by an HSR, which is considerably reduced in length in a less-resistant revertant subline. While it had been shown previously (BIEDLER and SPENGLER 1976) that HSRs were common to methotrexate-resistant cells, those of the vincristine-resistant cells appear to be quite distinct, and are associated with other chromosomes; their function at this time is obscure. It would be of considerable interest to determine whether these HSRs contain gene sequences that code for one or more specific glycoprotein: glycosyltransferases, tubulins, or the alkaloid-resistant glycoproteins.

3. Relationship Between Biochemical Changes and Alkaloid Resistance

While these various biochemical changes have been shown to be associated with resistance to certain alkaloids, an actual causal relationship has yet to be established. Thus, while it has been demonstrated that the amount of the high-molecular-weight surface membrane glycoprotein appears to be related to the degree of resistance of the cells (JULIANO and LING 1976; BECK et al. 1979), it has yet to be shown that its presence is required for the expression of resistance. Although CARLSEN et al. (1977) showed that the phosphorylation of membrane proteins, including the resistance-associated glycoproteins, apparently was required for the maintenance of an "active permeability barrier" by colchicine-resistant CHO cells, these results did not demonstrate that such changes do in fact mediate drug permeability.

We have attempted to address this question of the role of these surface glycoproteins in mediating drug resistance. Our results (BECK 1980b; BECK and CIRTAIN 1982) indicate that neither the apparent removal of the surface glycoproteins by proteolytic digestion with pronase, nor the prevention of their synthesis with tunicamycin, a specific inhibitor of *N*-acetyl-glucosaminyl-lipid synthesis (STRUCK and LENNARZ 1977), had much effect on the expression of resistance by the vinblastine-resistant CEM cells. Thus, pronase- or tunicamycin-treated CEM/VLB_{100} cells, which were shown by gel electrophoresis to be devoid of surface carbohydrate in the region of the resistance-associated glycoprotein, accumulated [^{3}H]vinblastine to the same extent as the untreated controls; moreover, exodus of [^{3}H]vinblastine from preloaded cells was qualitatively the same for both the treated and the control cells, although the treated cells appeared to retain about twice as much drug as did the controls after 60 min. The meaning of these results is not yet clear, because these treatments did not appear to be able to enhance the sensitivity of these resistant cells toward vinblastine in growth experiments, despite the apparent lack of resistance-associated glycoproteins on the cells. Other experiments with [^{14}C]glucosamine and [^{3}H]leucine revealed that treatment with tunicamycin did not affect the overall distribution of proteins in these cells. These data permit the suggestion that the carbohydrate moiety of the cell-surface resistance-associated glycoprotein does not mediate resistance per se. Clearly, more experiments must be done before definitive conclusions can be drawn; indeed, nothing is yet known about the role(s) of the noncarbohydrate component of the resistance-associated glycoprotein or its location in the plane of the membrane (e.g., is it a transmembrane protein?).

Discerning the relationship of the surface glycoprotein(s) to alkaloid resistance and cross-resistance will probably require more direct approaches, such as the following: (a) purification of the glycoprotein [which has been accomplished by RIORDAN and LING (1979), using affinity methods] and insertion of the holo- or asialo-glycoprotein into (i) membranes of sensitive whole cells, or (ii) membrane vesicles and subsequent fusion of these vesicles with sensitive cells; (b) hybridization of alkaloid-resistant auxotrophs with drug-sensitive cells that grow in a medium that supports only the growth of the sensitive cells; and (c) the use of recombinant DNA technique to isolate, clone in bacteria, and insert the gene(s) coding for the resistance-associated protein(s) or glycoprotein(s) into the drug-sensitive wild-type cells. Studies along these lines should provide direct evidence for the requirement of this membrane glycoprotein in conferring alkaloid resistance upon cells.

IV. Genetics of Alkaloid Resistance

Drug-resistant cells are frequently used for the study of mammalian cell genetics (SIMINOVITCH 1976), because they possess phenotypic markers that distinguish them from the drug-sensitive, parental lines. Moreover, insights into the expression of drug resistance can be obtained from "classic" hybridization experiments in which drug-sensitive cells are fused with drug-resistant mutants, and the hybrids are tested for drug responsiveness. Under these conditions, full resistance of the hybrids indicates that resistance to the drug of interest is a dominant characteristic; an intermediate level of resistance of the hybrid compared with the resistant mutant line demonstrates a codominant expression with the wild-type sensitive features, while full sensitivity of the hybrid indicates that the characteristics of resistance are expressed as recessive features. In this regard, it has been found (Table 6) that the mode of expression of alkaloid resistance in mammalian cells is either dominant or codominant (HARRIS 1973, 1974; LING 1975; CABRAL et al. 1980). It is of interest that this apparently applies to permeability mutants (LING 1975), as well as to β-tubulin mutants (CABRAL et al. 1980). It might be informative to determine whether the gene(s) coding for these different expressions of resistance are on the same or different alleles.

An interesting study by HARRIS (1974) attempted to determine whether the expression of drug resistance was genetic, reflecting an alteration or mutation in the gene(s) or chromosome(s) coding for the particular feature, or if resistance had an epigenetic basis, reflecting a change in gene *expression*, rather than in the information stored in the gene. HARRIS measured the frequency of appearance of vinblastine (dominant or codominant)- and araC(recessive)-resistant cells after mutagenizing diploid or tetraploid cells. It was argued that if resistance were due to genetic changes, the frequency of dominant mutations would be greater in tetraploid cells, when compared with diploid cells (because of the greater number

Table 6. Genetics of alkaloid resistance in mammalian cells

Cell line	Origin	Selected for resistance to	Observation	Detected by	References
V79	Chinese hamster	Vinblastine	VLB resistance is dominant or codominant	Cell hybridization	HARRIS (1973)
V79 (diploid) 991 (tetaploid)	Chinese hamster	Vinblastine araC	Frequency of selection of resistant colonies expressing dominant or recessive markers is independent of ploidy; suggests that resistance is epigenetic (altered gene expression)	Mutagenesis and cloning	HARRIS (1974)
EHR 2 EHR 2/VCR+ EHR 2/VLB+ EHR 2/DNR+ EHR 2/ADR+	Ehrlich ascites carcinoma	 Vincristine Vinblastine Daunorubicin Adriamycin	Sensitive and VCR-resistant line was near-tetraploid, but ADR-, DNR-, and VLB-resistant lines were near haploid; indicates VCR-resistant cells came from different clone, although sharing common mechanisms of resistance	Conventional Giemsa staining; Giemsa banding	HASHOLT and DANØ (1974)
E29 CH^RC4	Chinese hamster	Growth medium auxotroph Colchicine	Colchicine-resistant pleiotropic phenotype (permeability mutant) is (incompletely) dominant	Cell hybridization	LING (1975)
Cmd 4 Grs 2	Chinese hamster ovary	Colcemid Griseofulvin	β-Tubulin mutation is expressed codominantly with wild-type β-tubulin	Cell hybridization; clonogenic assay	CABRAL et al. (1980)

VLB, vinblastine; VCR, vincristine; ADR, adriamycin; DNR, daunorubicin of alleles), and, conversely, that recessive mutations would be seen with *less* frequency in tetraploid cells, as compared with diploid cells, because at least two or more genes would have to undergo simultaneous mutation, or one gene mutation would have to be accompanied by the loss of the remaining wild-type allele(s). HARRIS showed, however, that there was no difference in the frequency of expression of either dominant or recessive traits in the mutagenized cells, regardless of their ploidy. Thus, it was inferred from these data that resistance to either vinblastine, or to araC, may have an epigenetic basis, such as an alteration in gene expression, rather than an actual mutation in the gene(s) coding for the products ultimately responsible for the resistance phenotype.

The conclusions of HARRIS would appear to be supported by the results of BOSMANN and KESSEL, discussed in the previous section (Sect. C.III.1, Table 5), which demonstrated that, in drug-resistant cells, the anabolic glycoprotein: glycosyl transferases were in general increased in activity, and the catabolic glycosidase activities were decreased. These observations may be related to a gene-dosage effect, as described in a series of exceptional studies of SCHIMKE and colleagues (ALT et al. 1978; SCHIMKE et al. 1978). These investigators demonstrated that the overproduction of the enzyme dihydrofolate reductase by methotrexate-resistant murine tumor cells is attributable to the amplification of the gene coding for this protein; the amplified genes coding for dihydrofolate reductase in the resistant lines produce the same gene product as do the unamplified gene(s) in the sensitive cells. Technically, this does not represent a genetic mutation, in the strict sense of an alteration in the code leading to the production of an altered protein, but neither does it represent an epigenetic mutation conferred by altered gene expression, as defined by HARRIS (1974). LING and THOMPSON (1974) argued that their independently selected colchicine-resistant lines were true mutations because (a) the frequency of resistant colonies could be increased by mutagen treatment and (b) the resistant phenotype was stable when cells were grown in the absence of colchicine.

The amplified genes demonstrated in the methotrexate-resistant cells appear to be localized to HSRs on one or more chromosomes (BIEDLER and SPENGLER 1976). Recently, in a preliminary report (BIEDLER et al. 1980), it was demonstrated by a trypsin-Giemsa method that similar HSRs were present on chromosomes of Chinese hamster cells selected for resistance to vincristine, but that these were in different chromosomal locations than those HSRs of methotrexate-resistant cells. Whether these HSRs of vincristine-resistant cells code for proteins related to the pleiotropic phenotype remains to be investigated.

Finally, it was demonstrated by HASHOLT and DANØ (1974) that although vincristine-resistant cells, which were near-tetraploid, shared a common mechanism of resistance with vinblastine- and anthracycline-resistant cells, they must have come from different clones than did the other resistant lines, because the latter cells were all near-diploid.

D. Summary and Future Considerations

Several subjects pertinent to the mechanisms of resistance to certain cytotoxic alkaloids have been discussed in this chapter. For example, it has been shown that the *Colchicum* and *Vinca* alkaloids may be accumulated by cells differently, the former most likely by passive diffusion, and the latter possibly by some type of carrier-mediated process(es), although extensive binding of these drugs within or on the cells tends to obscure actual mechanism of accumulation. Future studies should investigate the role of this binding and attempt to define precisely the mode of accumulation of *Vinca* alkaloids by tumor cells.

Regarding expressions of resistance to alkaloids and cross-resistance to other "natural products," such phenomena are commonly observed in cell culture and in experimental murine systems, but these observations, especially concerning cross-resistance, are considerably more difficult to document clinically. It was speculated in this discussion that one basis for this discrepancy might reside in the usually extensive resistance and relative homogeneity of the experimental tumor lines as opposed to the situation that doubtless exists clinically, with cells of probably much lower degrees of resistance and considerable heterogeneity. Future efforts to examine drug-resistant cells in patients either for the purposes of detecting their presence or designing more effective chemotherapeutic regimens, will have to account for these factors, especially those related to the heterogeneity of tumor cell populations.

It has been shown in this chapter that the pharmacological bases of alkaloid resistance appear to be attributable either to diminished uptake or to decreased retention of the drugs; furthermore, the diminished retention may be the result either of some type of "pump" mechanism, which is capable of exporting drugs of disparate structure from the cell, or of altered binding, perhaps expressed as a larger fraction of "nonspecific" or loose-binding of drug by the resistant cells. Future studies of the accumulation of alkaloids by drug-resistant and -sensitive cells alike might employ isolated cell membranes, cytoplasmic fractions, or membrane transport vesicles, as well as, perhaps, immobilized or derivatized alkaloids, in order to resolve the mechanism(s) by which alkaloid-resistant cells display a diminished net accumulation of the drugs.

Finally, it has been shown in this chapter that a common feature of alkaloid resistance is the appearance of a surface glycoprotein of high molecular weight (ranging from ~150000 to ~180000, depending on the cell line), the amount of which is related to the degree of resistance. Although it has been proposed that this glycoprotein regulates membrane permeability (CARLSEN et al. 1977), its precise role in alkaloid resistance remains to be determined (BECK 1980b; BECK and CIRTAIN 1982). Further experiments with inhibitors of glycoprotein synthesis, hybrid cells, and sensitive cells into which either the purified resistance-associated glycoprotein or the genome for this protein has been inserted should establish the role of this glycoprotein in alkaloid resistance.

Answers to some of the questions raised in this review may expand our knowledge in such areas as drug action, resistance mechanisms, and somatic cell genetics, and might lead to improved ability to design courses of chemotherapeutic regimens, based on an awareness of the presence of specific subpopulations of drug-resistant cells.

Acknowledgments. I am indebted to Dr. Arnold D. Welch for his encouragement and support of my participation in this endeavor. The original studies reported here were done with the expert assistance of Margaret Cirtain, Janet Lefko, and Lee Tanzer, and were supported in part by Cancer Center (CORE) Grant CA-21765, by Program Grant CA-23099 from the NCI, and by ALSAC. I am grateful to Dolores Anderson and the Word Processing Center for excellent secretarial efforts.

References

Aldrich CD (1979) Pleiotropic phenotype of cultured murine cells resistant to maytansine, vincristine, colchicine, and adriamycin. J Natl Cancer Inst 63:751–757

Alt FW, Kellums RE, Bertino JR, Schimke RT (1978) Selective multiplication of dihydrofolate reductase genes in methotrexate-resistant variants of cultured murine cells. J Biol Chem 253:1357–1370

Andersson LC, Gahmberg CG, Nilsson K, Wigzell H (1977) Surface glycoprotein patterns of normal and malignant human lymphoid cells. I. T cells, T blasts and leukemic T cell lines. Int J Cancer 20:702–707

Aubin JE, Carlsen SA, Ling V (1975) Colchicine permeation is required for inhibition of concanavalin A capping in Chinese hamster ovary cells. Proc Natl Acad Sci USA 72:4516–4520

Aubin JE, Tolson N, Ling V (1980) The redistribution of fluoresceinated concanavalin A in Chinese hamster ovary cells and their colcemid-resistant mutants. Exp Cell Res 126:75–85

Bachvaroff RJ, Miller F, Rapaport FT (1980) Appearance of cytoskeletal components on the surface of leukemia cells and of lymphocytes transformed by mitogens and Epstein-Barr virus. Proc Natl Acad Sci USA 77:4979–4983

Bech-Hansen NT, Till JE, Ling V (1976) Pleiotropic phenotype of colchicine-resistant CHO cells: cross-resistance and collateral sensitivity. J Cell Physiol 88:23–32

Beck WT (1980a) Increase by vinblastine of oxidized glutathione in cultured mammalian cells. Biochem Pharmacol 29:2333–2337

Beck WT (1980b) Cell-surface glycoproteins (GP) and vinblastine (VLB) transport and toxicity in VLB-resistant leukemic cells. Proc Am Assoc Cancer Res 21:24

Beck WT (1981) Accumulation of vinblastine (VB) by sensitive and VB-resistant CCRF-CEM cells. Proc Am Assoc Cancer Res 22:204

Beck WT, Cirtain MC (1982) Continued expression of *Vinca* alkaloid-resistance by CCRF-CEM cells after treatment with tunicamycin or pronase. Cancer Res 42:184–189

Beck WT, Mueller TJ, Tanzer LR (1979) Altered surface membrane glycoproteins in *Vinca* alkaloid-resistant human leukemic lymphoblasts. Cancer Res 39:2070–2076

Beck WT, Cirtain MC, Lefco JL (1983) Energy-dependent reduced drug binding as a mechanism of *Vinca* alkaloid resistance in human leukemic lymphoblasts. Mol Pharmacol 24:485–492

Bender RA, Kornreich WD (1980) Cellular determinants of vincristine (VCR) sensitivity in murine leukemia cells. Proc Am Assoc Cancer Res 21:264

Bender RA, Kornreich WD (1981) Cellular entry of vincristine (VCR) in murine leukemia cells. Proc Am Assoc Cancer Res 22:227

Bender R, Nichols A (1978) Membrane transport of vincristine (VCR) in human lymphoblasts. Proc Am Assoc Cancer Res 19:35

Bender RA, Nichols AP, Norton L, Simon RM (1978) Lack of therapeutic synergism between vincristine and methotrexate in L1210 murine leukemia in vivo. Cancer Treat Rep 62:997–1003

Berlin RD, Caron JM, Oliver JM (1979) Microtubules and the structure and function of cell surfaces. In: Roberts K, Hyams JS (eds) Microtubules. Academic, London pp 443–485

Biedler JL, Riehm H (1970) Cellular resistance to actinomycin D in Chinese hamster cells in vitro: cross-resistance, radioautographic, and cytogenetic studies. Cancer Res 30:1174–1184

Biedler JL, Spengler BA (1976) Metaphase chromosome anomaly: association with drug resistance and cell-specific products. Science: 191:185–187

Biedler JL, Riehm H, Peterson RHF, Spengler BA (1975) Membrane-mediated drug resistance and phenotypic reversion to normal growth behavior of Chinese hamster cells. J Natl Cancer Inst 55:671–680

Biedler JL, Meyers MB, Peterson RHF, Spengler BA (1980) Marker chromosome with a homogeneously staining region (HSR) in vincristine-resistant cells. Proc Am Assoc Cancer Res 21:292

Bleyer WA, Frisby SA, Oliverio VT (1975) Uptake and binding of vincristine by murine leukemia cells. Biochem Pharmacol 24:633–639

Borgers M, DeBrabander M (1975) (eds) Microtubules and microtubule inhibitors. North-Holland, Amsterdam

Borisy GG, Taylor EW (1967) The mechanism of action of colchicine. Binding of colchicine-^{3}H to cellular protein. J Cell Biol 34:525–533

Bosmann HB (1971) Mechanism of cellular drug resistance. Nature 233:566–569

Bosmann HB, Kessel D (1970) Altered glycosidase levels in drug-resistant mouse leukemias. Mol Pharmacol 6:345–349

Bowen D, Goldman ID (1975) The relationship among transport, intracellular binding, and inhibition of RNA synthesis by actinomycin D in Ehrlich ascites tumor cells in vitro. Cancer Res 35:3054–3060

Brinkley BR, Barham SS; Barranco SC, Fuller GM (1974) Rotenone inhibition of spindle microtubule assembly in mammalian cells. Exp Cell Res 85:41–46

Cabral F, Sobel ME, Gottesman MM (1980) CHO mutants resistant to colchicine, colcemid or griseofulvin have an altered β-tubulin. Cell 20:29–36

Carlsen SA, Till JE, Ling V (1976) Modulation of membrane drug permeability in Chinese hamster ovary cells. Biochim Biophys Acta 455:900–912

Carlsen SA, Till JE, Ling V (1977) Modulation of drug permeability in chinese hamster ovary cells. Possible role for phosphorylation of surface glycoproteins. Biochim Biophys Acta 467:238–258

Chello PL, Sirotnak FM, Dorick DM (1979 a) Different effects of vincristine on methotrexate uptake by L1210 cells and mouse intestinal epithelia in vitro and in vivo. Cancer Res 39:2106–2112

Chello PL, Sirotnak FM, Dorick DM, Moccio DM (1979 b) Schedule-dependent synergism of methotrexate and vincristine against murine L1210 leukemia. Cancer Treat Rep 63:1889–1894

Chen K, Heller J, Canellakis ES (1976) Studies on the regulation of ornithine decarboxylase activity by the microtubules: the effect of colchicine and vinblastine. Biochem Biophys Res Commun 68:401–409

Cline MJ (1967) Prediction of in vivo cytotoxicity of chemotherapeutic agents by their effect on malignant leukocytes in vitro. Blood 30:176–188

Costlow M, Hample A (1980) Metabolic inhibitors increase prolactin binding to cultured mammary tumor cells. Biochem Biophys Res Commun 92:213–220

Creasey WA (1968) Modifications in biochemical pathways produced by the *Vinca* alkaloids. Cancer Chemother Rep 52:501–507

Creasey WA (1975) *Vinca* alkaloids and colchicine. In: Sartorelli AC and Johns DG (eds) Antineoplastic and immunosuppressive agents. II. Springer, Berlin Heidelberg New York (Handbook of experimental pharmacology, vol XXXVIII/2, pp 670–694)

Creasey WA, Markiw ME (1966) Uptake of vinblastine (VLB) by Ehrlich ascites carcinoma cells. Fed Proc 25:733

Danø K (1972) Cross resistance between *Vinca* alkaloids and anthracyclines in Ehrlich ascites tumor in vivo. Cancer Chemother Rep 56:701–708

Danø K (1973) Active outward transport of daunomycin in resistant Ehrlich ascites tumor cells. Biochim Biophys Acta 323:466–483

DeBrabander M, DeMey J (1980) (eds) Microtubules and microtubule inhibitors 1980. North-Holland, Amsterdam

Edelman GM, Yahara I, Wang JL (1973) Receptor mobility and receptor-cytoplasmic interactions in lymphocytes. Proc Natl Acad Sci USA 70:1442–1446

Finar IL (1975) Organic chemistry, vol II 5th edn. Longman, London, p 696

Foley GE, Lazarus H, Farber S, Uzman BG, Boone BA, McCarthy RE (1965) Continuous culture of human lymphoblasts from peripheral blood of a child with acute leukemia. Cancer 18:522–529

Friedman SJ, Bellantone RA, Canellakis ES (1972) Ornithine decarboxylase activity in synchronously growing Don C cells. Biochim Biophys Acta 261:188–193

Fry DW, White JC, Goldman ID (1980) Effects of 2,4-dinitrophenol and other metabolic inhibitors on the bidirectional carrier fluxes, net transport, and intracellular binding of methotrexate in Ehrlich ascites tumor cells. Cancer Res 40:3669–3673

Fuller DJM, Gerner EW, Russell DH (1977) Polyamine biosynthesis and accumulation during the G_1 to S phase transition. J Cell Physiol 93:81–88

Fyfe MJ, Goldman ID (1973) Characteristics of the vincristine-induced augmentation of methotrexate uptake in Ehrlich ascites tumor cells. J Biol Chem 248:5067–5073

Fyfe MJ, Loftfield S, Goldman ID (1975) A reduction in energy-dependent amino acid transport by microtubular inhibitors in Ehrlich ascites tumor cells. J Cell Physiol 86:201–212

Gahmberg CA, Hakomori S (1973) External labeling of cell surface galactose and galactosamine in glycolipid and glycoprotein of human erythrocytes. J Biol Chem 248:4311–4317

Goldman ID (1969) Transport energetics of the folic acid analogue, methotrexate, in L1210 cells: enhanced accumulation by metabolic inhibitors. J Biol Chem 244:3779–3785

Goldman ID (1973) Uptake of drugs and resistance. In: Mihich E (ed) Drug resistance and selectivity. Biochemical and cellular basis. Academic, London pp 299–358

Goldman ID, Gupta V, White JC, Loftfield S (1976) Exchangeable intracellular methotrexate levels in the presence and absence of vincristine at extracellular drug concentrations relevant to those achieved in high-dose methotrexate-folinic acid "rescue" protocols. Cancer Res 36:276–279

Goldman ID, Fyfe MJ, Bowen D, Loftfield S, Schafer JA (1977) The effect of microtubular inhibitors on transport of α-aminoisobutyric acid. Inhibition of uphill transport without changes in transmembrane gradients of Na^+, K^+, or H^+. Biochim Biophys Acta 467:185–191

Gout PW, Wijcik LL, Beer CT (1978) Differences between vinblastine and vincristine in distribution in the blood of rats and binding by platelets and malignant cells. Eur J Cancer 14:1167–1178

Hakala MT (1965) On the nature of permeability of sarcoma-180 cells to amethopterin in vitro. Biochim Biophys Acta 102:210–225

Harris M (1973) Phenotypic expression of drug resistance in hybrid cells. J Natl Cancer Inst 50:423–429

Harris M (1974) Comparative frequency of dominant and recessive markers for drug resistance in Chinese hamster cells. J Natl Cancer Inst 52:1811–1816

Hasholt L, Danø K (1974) Cytogenetic investigations on an Ehrlich ascites tumor, and four sublines resistant to daunomycin, adriamycin, vincristine and vinblastine. Hereditas 77:303–310

Hebden HF, Hadfield JR, Beer CT (1970) The binding of vinblastine by platelets in the rat. Cancer Res 30:1417–1424

Heby O, Gray JW, Lindl PA, Marton LJ, Wilson CB (1976) Changes in L-ornithine decarboxylase activity during the cell cycle. Biochem Biophys Res Commun 71:99–105

Inaba M, Johnson RK (1977) Decreased retention of actinomycin D as the basis for cross-resistance in anthracycline-resistant sublines of P388 leukemia. Cancer Res 37:4629–4634

Inaba M, Johnson RK (1978) Uptake and retention of adriamycin and daunorubicin by sensitive and anthracycline-resistant sublines of P388 leukemia. Biochem Pharmacol 27:2123–2130

Inaba M, Sakurai Y (1979) Enhanced efflux of actinomycin D, vincristine, and vinblastine in adriamycin-resistant subline of P388 leukemia. Cancer Lett 8:111–115

Inaba M, Kobayashi H, Sakurai Y, Johnson RK (1979) Active efflux of daunorubicin and adriamycin in sensitive and resistant sublines of P388 leukemia. Cancer Res 39:2200–2203

Inaba M, Fujikura R, Sakurai Y (1981a) Active efflux common to vincristine and daunorubicin in vincristine-resistant P388 leukemia. Biochem Pharmacol 30:1863–1865

Inaba M, Fujikura R, Tsukagoshi S, Sakurai Y (1981b) Restored in vitro sensitivity of adriamycin- and vincristine-resistant P388 with reserpine. Biochem Pharmacol 30:2191–2194

Johnson RK, Chitnis MP, Embrey WM, Gregory EB (1978) In vivo characteristics of resistance and cross-resistance of an adriamycin-resistant subline of P388 leukemia. Cancer Treat Rep 62:1535–1547

Juliano RL, Ling V (1976) A surface glycoprotein modulating drug permeability in Chinese hamster ovary cell mutants. Biochim Biophys Acta 455:152–162

Juliano R, Ling V, Graves J (1976) Drug-resistant mutants of Chinese ovary cells possess an altered cell surface carbohydrate component. J Supramol Struct 4:521–526

Kaye SB, Boden JA (1980) Cross-resistance between actinomycin-D, adriamycin and vincristine in a murine solid tumor in vivo. Biochem Pharmacol 29:1081–1084

Kessel D, Bosmann HB (1970) On the caracteristics of actinomycin D resistance in L5178Y cells. Cancer Res 30:2695–2701

Kessel D, Wodinsky I (1968) Uptake in vivo and in vitro of actinomycin D by mouse leukemias as factors in survival. Biochem Pharmacol 17:161–164

Kessel D, Botterill V, Wodinsky I (1968) Uptake and retention of daunomycin by mouse leukemic cells as factors in drug response. Cancer Res 28:938–941

Kirschner MW (1978) Microtubule assembly and nucleation. Int Rev Cytol 54:1–71

Kitano M, Mihich E, Pressman D (1972) Antigenic differences between leukemia L1210 and a subline resistant to methylglyoxalbis (guanylhydrazone). Cancer Res 32:181–186

Kralovic RC, Voelz H (1977) Vinblastine-enhanced colchicine binding to tubulin in mouse fibroblasts. Exp Cell Res 106:205–210

Ling V (1975) Drug resistance and membrane alteration in mutants of mammalian cells. Can J Genet Cytol 17:503–515

Ling V, Thompson LH (1974) Reduced permeability in CHO cells as a mechanism of resistance to colchicine. J Cell Physiol 83:103–116

Ling V, Aubin JE, Chase A, Sarangi F (1979) Mutants of Chinese hamster ovary (CHO) cells with altered colcemid-binding affinity. Cell 18:423–430

Madoc-Jones H, Mauro F (1968) Interphase action of vinblastine and vincristine: differences in their lethal action through the mitotic cycle of cultured mammalian cells. J Cell Physiol 72:185–196

Mathé G, Misset JL, DeVassal F, Gouveia J, Hayat M, Machover D, Belpomme D, Pico JL, Schwarzenberg L, Ribaud P, Musset M, Jasmin Cl, DeLuca L (1978a) Phase II clinical trial with vindesine for remission induction in acute leukemia, blastic crisis of chronic myeloid leukemia, lymphosarcoma, and Hodgkin's disease: absence of cross-resistance with vincristine. Cancer Treat Rep 62:805–809

Mathé G, Misset JL, DeVassal F, Hayat M, Gouveia J, Machover D, Belpomme D, Schwarzenberg L, Ribaud P, Pico JL, Musset M, Jasmin C, DeLuca L (1978b) Traitment de leucémies et hématosarcomes par la vindésine. Résultats d'un essai phase II en termes d'induction de rémission. Nouv Presse Méd 7:525–528

Meyers MB, Biedler JL (1981) Increased synthesis of a low molecular weight protein in vincristine-resistant cells. Biochem Biophys Res Comm 99:228–235

Meyers MB, Kreis W (1978) Comparison of enzymatic activities of two deoxycytidine kinases purified from cells sensitive (P815) or resistant (P815/ara-C) to 1-β-D-arabinofuranosylcytosine. Cancer Res 38:1105–1112

Minor PD, Roscoe DH (1975) Colchicine resistance in mammalian cell lines. J Cell Sci 17:381–396
Mizel SB, Wilson L (1972) Nucleoside transport in mammalian cells. Inhibition by colchicine. Biochemistry 11:2573–2578
Nicolin A, Vadlamudi S, Goldin A (1972) Antigenicity of L1210 leukemic sublines induced by drugs. Cancer Res 32:653–657
Olmsted JB, Borisy GG (1973) Microtubules. Ann Rev Biochem 42:507–540
Owellen RJ, Donigan DW, Hartke CA, Hains FO (1977) Correlation of biologic data with physico-chemical properties among the *Vinca* alkaloids and their congeners. Biochem Pharmacol 26:1213–1219
Peterson RHF, Biedler JL (1978) Plasma membrane glycoproteins from Chinese hamster cells sensitive and resistant to actinomycin D. J Supramol Struct 9:289–298
Peterson RHF, Biedler JL (1980) Comparison of plasma membrane glycopeptides and gangliosides of Chinese hamster cells sensitive and resistant to actinomycin D (AD), daunorubicin (DM) and vincristine (VCR). Proc Am Assoc Cancer Res 21:292
Peterson RHF, O'Neil JA, Biedler JL (1974) Some biochemical properties of Chinese hamster cells sensitive and resistant to actinomycin D. J Cell Biol 63:773–779
Peterson RHF, Beutler WJ, Biedler JL (1979) Ganglioside composition of malignant and actinomycin D-resistant nonmalignant Chinese hamster cells. Biochem Pharmacol 28:579–582
Plagemann PGW (1970) Vinblastine sulfate: metaphase arrest, inhibition of RNA synthesis, and cytotoxicity in Novikoff rat heptoma cells. J Natl Cancer Inst 45:589–595
Raff EC (1979) The control of microtubule assembly in vivo. Int Rev Cytol 59:1–98
Riordan JR, Ling V (1979) Purification of P-glycoprotein from plasma membrane vesicles of Chinese hamster ovary cell mutants with reduced colchicine permeability. J Biol Chem 254:12701–12705
Rivera G, Aur RJ, Dahl GV, Pratt CB, Wood A, Avery TL (1980) Combined VM-26 and cytosine arabinoside in treatment of refractory childhood lymphocytic leukemia. Cancer 45:1284–1288
Roberts K, Hyams JS (1979) Microtubules. Academic, London
Rosner F, Hirshaut Y, Grünwald HW, Dietrich M (1975) In vitro combination chemotherapy demonstrating potentiation of vincristine cytotoxicity by prednisone. Cancer Res 35:700–705
Rubin RW, Quillen M, Corcoran J, Ganapathi R, Krishan A (1982) Tubulin as a major cell surface protein in human lymphoid cells of leukemic origin. Cancer Res 42:1384–1389
Schimke RT, Kaufmann RJ, Alt FW, Kellems RF (1978) Gene amplification and drug resistance in cultured murine cells. Science 202:1051–1055
Schreiner GR, Unanue ER (1976) Membrane and cytoplasmic changes in B lymphocytes induced by ligand-surface immunoglobulin interaction. Adv Immunol 24:37–165
Schrek R, Stefani StS (1976) Inhibition by ionophore A23187 of the cytotoxicity of vincristine, colchicine and x-rays to leukemic lymphocytes. Oncology 33:132–135
Secret CJ, Hadfield JR, Beer CT (1972) Studies on the binding of [^{3}H]-vinblastine by rat blood platelets in vitro. Biochem Pharmacol 21:1609–1624
See YP, Carlsen SA, Till JE, Ling V (1974) Increased drug permeability in Chinese hamster ovary cells in the presence of cyanide. Biochim Biophys Acta 373:242–252
Siminovitch L (1976) On the nature of hereditable variation in cultured somatic cells. Cell 7:1–11
Sirotnak FM, Chello PL, Brockman RW (1979) Potential for exploitation of transport systems in anticancer drug design. In: DeVita VT, Busch H (eds) Methods in Cancer Research. Cancer drug development. Vol. XVI/part A. Academic, New York pp 382–447
Skovsgaard T (1977) Transport and binding of daunorubin, adriamycin, and rubidazone in Ehrlich ascites tumor cells. Biochem Pharmacol 26:215–222
Skovsgaard T (1978a) Mechanism of cross-resistance between vincristine and daunorubicin in Ehrlich ascites tumor cells. Cancer Res 38:4722–4727
Skovsgaard T (1978b) Mechanisms of resistance to daunorubicin in Ehrlich ascites tumor cells. Cancer Res 38:1785–1791

Skovsgaard T (1978c) Carrier-mediated transport of daunorubicin, adriamycin, and rubidazone in Ehrlich ascites tumor cells. Biochem Pharmacol 27:1221–1227
Snyder JA, McIntosh JR (1976) Biochemistry and physiology of microtubules. Ann Rev Biochem 45:699–720
Soifer D (1975) (ed) The biology of cytoplasmic microtubules. Ann NY Acad Sci 253:1–848
Steck TL, Dawson G (1974) Topographical distribution of complex carbohydrates in the erythrocyte membrane. J Biol Chem 249:2135–2142
Steuart CD, Burke PJ (1971) Cytidine deaminase and the development of resistance to arabinosyl cytosine. Nature New Biol 233:109–110
Struck DK, Lennarz WJ (1977) Evidence for the participation of saccharide-lipids in the synthesis of the oligosaccharide chain of ovalbumin. J Biol Chem 252:1007–1013
Stryckmans PA, Lurie PM, Manaster J, Vamecq G (1973) Mode of action of chemotherapy in vivo on human acute leukemia. II. Vincristine. Eur J Cancer 9:613–620
Swerdlow B, Creasey WA (1975) Binding of vinblastine in vitro to ribosomes of Sarcoma 180 cells. Biochem Pharmacol 24:1243–1245
Taylor EW (1965) The mechanism of colchicine inhibition of mitosis. I. Kinetics of inhibition and the binding of H^3-colchicine. J Cell Biol 25:145–160
Timasheff SN, Grisham LM (1980) In vitro assembly of cytoplasmic microtubules. Ann Rev Biochem 49:565–591
Tsuruo T, Iida H, Tsukagoshi S, Sakurai Y (1981a) Overcoming of vincristine resistance in P388 leukemia in vivo and in vitro through enhanced cytotoxicity of vincristine and vinblastine by verapamil. Cancer Res 41:1967–1972
Tsuruo T, Iida H, Tsukagoshi S, Sakurai Y (1981b) Prevention of vinblastine-induced cytotoxicity by ruthenium red. Biochem Pharmacol 30:213–216
Tucker RW, Owellen RJ, Harris SB (1977) Correlation of cytotoxicity and mitotic spindle dissolution by vinblastine in mammalian cells. Cancer Res 37:4346–4351
Warren RD, Nichols AP, Bender RA (1977) The effect of vincristine on methotrexate uptake and inhibition of DNA synthesis by human lymphoblastoid cells. Cancer Res 37:2993–2997
Warren RD, Bender RA, Norton L, Young RC (1978) The treatment of combination chemotherapy-resistant Hodgkin disease with single-agent vinblastine. Am J Hematol 4:47–55
Weatherbee JA (1981) Membranes and cell movement: Interactions of membranes with the proteins of the cytoskeleton. Int Rev Cytol [Suppl] 12:113–176
Wilkoff LJ, Dulmadge EA (1978) Resistance and cross-resistance of cultured leukemia P388 cells to vincristine, adriamycin, adriamycin analogs, and actinomycin D. J Natl Cancer Inst 61: 1521–1524
Wilson L (1975a) Microtubules as drug receptors: pharmacological properties of microtubule protein. Ann NY Acad Sci 253:213–231
Wilson L (1975b) Action of drugs on microtubules. Life Sci 17:303–310
Wilson L, Bryan J (1974) Biochemical and pharmacological properties of microtubules. Adv Cell Molec Biol 3:21–72
Wilson L, Bryan J, Ruby A, Mazia D (1970) Precipitation of proteins by vinblastine and calcium ions. Proc Natl Acad Sci USA 66:807–814
Wolpert-DeFillipes MK, Adamson RH, Cysyk RL, Johns DG (1975) Initial studies on the cytotoxic action of maytansine, a novel ansa macrolide. Biochem Pharmacol 24:751–754
Zager RF, Frisby SA, Oliverio VT (1973) The effects of antibiotics and cancer chemotherapeutic agents on the cellular transport and antitumor activity of methotrexate in L1210 murine leukemia. Cancer Res 33:1670–1676

Note Added in Proof. This review was completed in January, 1981, with some revisions in September, 1981. For more current discussion of the biochemistry and pharmacology of the alkaloid-resistant phenotype, see Beck, Cancer Treat

Rep 67:875–882 (1983); and Beck, Adv Enz Reg 22:207–227 (1984). Recent work on the genetics of alkaloid-resistance has been reviewed by Ling et al., Cancer Treat Rep 67:869–874 (1983); and for an update on recent advances in the circumvention of alkaloid resistance, see Tsuruo, Cancer Treat Rep 67:889–894 (1983), and Skovsgaard et al., Cancer Treat Reviews (1984, in press).

Section VI: Antifolates

CHAPTER 22

Folate Antagonists

J. R. BERTINO

A. Introduction

Drug resistance of bacterial, protozoan, and neoplastic disease of man continues to be a difficult and challenging problem. In the current era of combination chemotherapy, understanding the mechanisms of natural and acquired resistance at the cellular level becomes even more important, since it is usually not possible to challenge the patient with a single agent in maximally tolerated doses to establish without question that the patient has a drug-resistant tumor.

Mammalian cell lines both intrinsically resistant to methotrexate (MTX) and with acquired resistance to this drug have been particularly useful in the study of resistance. Cytogenetic as well as biochemical changes have been described in these cell lines, propagated in vitro. In this chapter, mechanisms of intrinsic, as well as acquired, resistance to MTX will be reviewed, both as described in experimental models and in patients with malignancy.

B. Intrinsic or Natural Resistance to Methotrexate and Other Folate Antagonists

In order to understand why cells are sensitive, or naturally or intrinsically resistant to MTX, the mechanism of action of this drug must first be described. It should also be appreciated that resistance to MTX may be a relative term, and this is determined when sensitivities of tumor and normal cell populations are compared.

MTX is an effective inhibitor of DNA synthesis both in normal and neoplastic cells (Fig. 1). All mammalian cells require folate coenzymes for the synthesis of amino acids (serine, methionine) and nucleic acids (purines, thymidylate). Since thymidylate synthesis occurs rapidly during S-phase of the cell cycle, cells in this DNA synthetic phase are particularly vulnerable to the action of MTX; cells in G_0- or in plateau phase growth will not be affected by this S-phase inhibitor (HRYNIUK et al. 1969; JOHNSON et al. 1978). In addition, for reasons that are not clear, inhibition of DNA synthesis by MTX of those cells in the plateau phase that are in the S-phase is less compared with logarithmically growing cells in the S-phase (HRYNIUK et al. 1969). These considerations presumably explain the relative resistance of normal stem-cell populations (marrow, gastrointestinal tract) to short (24 h or less) intensive exposure even to very high concentrations of this drug (10^{-4} *M*) and the relative sensitivity of these same populations to low or moderate drug concentrations (10^{-7} *M*) when exposure times exceed 48 h (KOIZUMI et al. 1980;

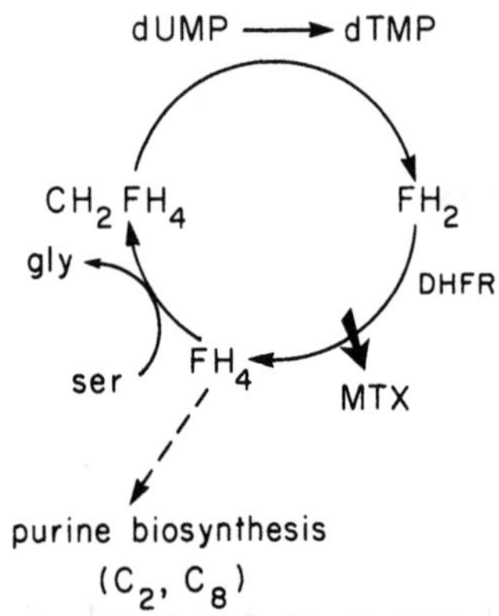

Fig. 1. Inhibition of DNA synthesis by methotrexate (MTX). *FH_2*, dihydrofolate; *DHFR*, dihydrofolate reductase; *FH_4*, tetrahydrofolate; *ser*, serine; *gly*, glycine; CH_2FH_4, N^5,N^{10}methylenetetrahydrofolate; *dUMP*, deoxyuridylate; *dTMP*, thymidylate

HRYNIUK and BERTINO 1969). In the latter case, presumably stem cells in G_0 are recruited and many of them are "in cycle."

Conditions which have already stressed normal stem-cell populations (infection, previous X-ray or drug therapy) will result in an increased sensitivity of these organs (marrow, gastrointestinal tract) to MTX (HARDING and MACLENNON 1977). Thus one form of intrinsic tumor resistance to MTX might actually be the inability of the physician to use adequate doses of the drug, because of the increased sensitivity of normal stem-cell populations.

It also follows that a major cause of apparent insensitivity of a tumor-cell population to MTX may be kinetic and not biochemical (Table 1). Tumors that are bulky and possess necrotic centers may have many stem cells "out of cycle", and thus relatively resistant to pulse doses of MTX. In general, cells with rapid growth rates and in logarithmic growth appear to be more sensitive to MTX treatment, e.g., treatment of acute lymphocytic leukemia (ALL) in remission. While it may be possible to treat patients with large tumor masses with MTX administered continuously or with repeated dosing (e.g., squamous-cell carcinoma of the head and neck, osteosarcoma, diffuse histiocytic lymphoma), these circumstances are ideal for development of acquired drug resistance (see below). The effectiveness of high-dose, very short exposures to MTX (requiring leucovorin rescue) in osteogenic sarcoma, either metastatic (JAFFE et al. 1974) or as initial treatment prior to surgery, is surprising in view of the relatively slow growth rate of this tumor and the large masses of tumor cells present. During recent years a possible explanation for the sensitivity of this tumor has emerged. It is now recognized that almost all cells form polyglutamates of not only folates but also MTX (BAUGH et al. 1973; NAIR and BAUGH 1973; WHITEHEAD et al. 1975; GALIVAN 1980). The addition of glutamates in γ-linkage to MTX is a mechanism whereby "free drug" in the cytoplasm [i.e., not bound to dihydrofolate reductase (DHFR)] may be retained in cells for a long period of time (GEWIRTZ et al. 1980; SCHILSKY et al. 1980; BALINSKA et al. 1981). Cells capable of efficiently forming MTX-polyglutamates

Table 1. Possible causes of intrinsic resistance to MTX

1.	Kinetic: cells in G_0- or plateau phase
2.	Low capacity for MTX polyglutamate formation
3.	Poor transport of MTX
4.	High dihydrofolate reductase levels
5.	Rapid synthesis of DHFR
6.	Inadequate NADPH levels to facilitate MTX binding to DHFR
7.	High intracellular folate levels
8.	Utilization of salvage pathways (thymidine, hypoxanthine)

may therefore be more sensitive to the action of this drug, since as new DHFR is synthesized this "free MTX" will inactivate the enzyme and the cell prevented from replicating DNA, even if the cell is triggered into cycle hours or days later. It is already clear that cells of the same tumor type (breast cancer cells) may have different capacities with regard to synthesis of MTX polyglutamates (CHABNER et al. 1982). It should also be noted that polyglutamation of MTX, apparently carried out by the same enzyme (folylpolyglutamate synthetase) that adds glutamates to folate coenzymes (MCGUIRE and BERTINO 1982) is not an inactivation process; the MTX polyglutamate forms are at least as tightly bound to DHFR as MTX (JACOBS et al. 1975).

Cells may also be intrinsically resistant to MTX because of poor transport of the drug. Evidence from several laboratories has shown that in most cells studied MTX is actively transported by a carrier mechanism that is the physiological carrier system for the reduced folates, 5-formyl-tetrahydrofolate and 5-methyl-tetrahydrofolate (GOLDMAN et al. 1968; NAHAS et al. 1972; HUENNEKENS et al. 1978; WARREN et al. 1978). Since both DHFR-binding and MTX-polyglutamate formation are "trapping" mechanisms for MTX, these events may influence what is regarded as "transport." However, it is also clear that even when initial rates are measured, before substantial polyglutamation can occur, cells vary in their ability to transport this drug (GOLDMAN et al. 1968). Relative resistance of the Walker carcinosarcoma, a rat tumor, to MTX has been ascribed to poor transport of MTX. In contrast, this tumor is highly sensitive to Baker's antifol, triazinate (TZT), as a consequence of the ability of this drug to accumulate rapidly in these cells (SKEEL et al. 1973). Relative resistance of several human tumors has also been thought to be due to this mechanism, but in light of recent data on polyglutamate formation as a trapping mechanism, this conclusion must be reexamined, since lack of polyglutamate formation would lead to rapid efflux of MTX and apparent "poor transport." MTX transport will be competitively inhibited by reduced folates and vice versa. Thus another mechanism of MTX action, in addition to inhibiting DHFR, is to prevent reduced folate uptake into cells. Furthermore, since MTX and reduced folates also compete for the active site of polyglutamate synthetase, MTX may also inhibit polyglutamate formation of the folate coenzymes, leading to increased efflux of folate monoglutamates and intensifying the relative folate deficiency already present by virtue of decreased influx and trapping of folate coenzymes as dihydrofolate.

Cells capable of synthesizing DHFR at a rapid rate (presumably with rapid turnover of the enzyme, since the steady-state level of enzyme activity does not vary appreciably in human neoplastic cells) are also more likely to be naturally resistant to this drug. Since MTX (and its polyglutamates) can protect DHFR from degradation processes in cells, the turnover rate of DHFR may be indirectly estimated by the rise in total DHFR that occurs after MTX treatment (BERTINO 1963; BERTINO et al. 1977). Most of this enzyme is bound to MTX, and this increase in enzyme concentration may only be detected by freeing the bound MTX from the enzyme, or assay at a high pH in the presence of salt, conditions favoring decreased binding of MTX to the enzyme (BERTINO et al. 1965). This increase in the level of DHFR may allow cells to survive MTX treatment since once efflux of drug occurs from the cell, a small amount of MTX dissociating from this high level of enzyme (four to ten times increase) may allow resumption of tetrahydrofolate biosynthesis, especially in the presence of elevated levels of dihydrofolate (BERTINO et al. 1977). This is possible because thymidylate synthetase rather than DHFR is the rate-limiting enzyme in thymidylate biosynthesis. In addition, insufficient NADPH may be present in cells at these DHFR levels to result in tight binding of MTX to DHFR, thus allowing NADH rather than NADPH to be used as the cofactor (see below).

MTX binding is maximal only in the presence of NADPH; thus intracellular DHFR without associated NADPH would not necessarily be stoichiometrically inhibited by MTX, as has been assumed in the past. In view of the polymorphism of DHFR, in part based upon the presence or absence of NADPH or folates (NIETHAMMER and JACKSON 1975), the finding that NADH can substitute for NADPH, without enhancing binding of MTX, may be significant (KAMEN and BERTINO 1978). Thus with NADH as a cofactor, even in the presence of MTX in excess of stoichiometric amounts with regard to DHFR, tetrahydrofolate synthesis would occur under conditions in which there would otherwise be no detectable enzyme activity if NADPH were the sole cofactor (KAMEN and BERTINO 1978). This enzyme polymorphism and use of an alternate pyridine nucleotide could in part explain the need for MTX to accumulate in the cell above the apparent DHFR concentration to be optimally effective, as previously reported (SIROTNAK and DONSBACH 1974; WHITE et al. 1975).

In several lines of human melanoma cells propagated in vitro, KUFE et al. (1980) concluded that natural resistance to MTX was due to high levels of DHFR found in these tumors. The mechanism of this relatively high level of enzyme has not been further characterized.

C. Acquired Resistance to Folate Antagonists

Acquired resistance to MTX develops when a tumor-cell population is initially decimated after exposure to this drug, but a few cells survive, presumably pre-existent mutants, that eventually give rise to a population of cells that requires more MTX to produce the equivalent amount of cell kill seen in the parent tumor. Resistance to MTX may be induced rapidly in malignant cells propagated in culture by the use of mutagens (FLINTOFF et al. 1976a), or by exposing cells to low concentrations of the drug, and growing the surviving cells in gradually increasing concentrations of the folate analog (FISCHER 1961; DOLNICK et al. 1979). The former technique has been used to produce a CHO subline resistant to MTX by virtue of an altered DHFR that binds MTX less well than the wild-type cell. However, even without the use of a mutagen, a subline of 3T6 cells has also been developed that is highly resistant to MTX and is characterized by an elevated DHFR (ca. 30-fold) and also by a markedly altered DHFR that binds MTX (I_{50}) only at concentrations 100 times the wild-type enzyme (HABER et al. 1981). Methotrexate may itself be a mild mutagen (GENTHER et al. 1977). In general, however, exposure of cells to stepwise increments of MTX leads to cell populations with either increased levels of DHFR, or the inability to transport MTX well (NIETHAMMER and JACKSON 1975). Treatment of mice with transplanted tumors with MTX also resulted in gradual elevations of DHFR in the tumor cells as resistance developed (MISRA et al. 1961; SCHRECKER et al. 1971). Cell lines have been developed utilizing the stepwise exposure techniques that have several hundred fold elevations of DHFR compared with the parent line (HAKALA et al. 1961; DOLNICK et al. 1979; BOSTOCK et al. 1979; CHANG and LITTLEFIELD 1976). With continued selection pressure, some lines developed an additional probable mutation, e.g., we isolated a subline of the L1210 leukemia characterized by a 35-fold elevation of DHFR and a decreased ability to transport the drug. The increase in DHFR occurred first, followed by the transport alteration (LINDQUIST 1979). FLINTOFF et al. (1980) also described a line with an elevated DHFR level, as well as DHFR with a decreased affinity for MTX. This line was intitially selected after mutagenesis and was found to have an altered DHFR (GUPTA et al. 1977). By subsequently subculturing the line in stepwise increased levels of MTX the altered DHFR was amplified as well.

I. Gene Amplification and Elevation of Dihydrofolate Reductase

In recent years, gene amplification has been shown to be the mechanism for the development of drug resistance associated with increase in DHFR levels (ALT et al. 1978). Several mammalian cell lines, resistant to MTX by virtue of an elevation of DHFR, have been described, and in every case examined there has been a corresponding increase in the level of DHFR mRNA and copies of the DHFR gene (ALT et al. 1978; DOLNICK et al. 1979; MELERA et al. 1980). It is still not clear as to what the molecular mechanism of gene amplification is, although various models have been proposed (SCHIMKE et al. 1979). A powerful tool for the study of cell populations with different levels of DHFR, and population dynamics, has been the use of fluoroscein-labeled MTX, with analysis by the fluorescence-activated cell sorter (KAUFMAN et al. 1978). This compound, a tight-binding inhibitor of DHFR, may be used to quantitate the amount of DHFR per cell. When MTX-resistant sarcoma-180 cells were analyzed with a 200-fold increase in DHFR, it was found that this subline was composed of a heterogeneous population with a wide distribution of DHFR levels and DHFR gene copies (KAUFMAN et al. 1979). After continued culture in the absence of MTX for 400 generations, a new stable state was reached, characterized by reversion to partial sensitivity to MTX. These cells were relatively homogeneous as regards DHFR content, and contained a seven fold increase in DHFR over the wild type. This, and other cell lines that are also unstably resistant, are characterized by DHFR gene location in double minute chromosomes, which increase in number as resistance increases and decrease proportionally as the population reverts to sensitivity to MTX (KAUFMAN et al. 1979). In stably resistant cells, most or all of the DHFR genes appear to be located in homogeneously staining regions (BIEDLER and SPANGLER 1976; BIEDLER et al. 1980). Further, with continued culture in MTX unstably resistant cells became stably resistant; this event was associated with loss of double minute chromosomes and presumed integration of this genetic material into homogeneous staining regions (HSRs) of chromosomes. Facilitation of gene amplification (i.e., an increased number of surviving cells with amplified DHFR genes) exposed to MTX by substances like TPA (12-*O*-tetradecanoylphorbal-13-acetate), a tumor promoter, and other growth regulatory substances, e.g., insulin, has been reported (VARSHAVSKY 1981).

1. Organization of the Dihydrofolate Reductase Gene

The mouse DHFR gene contains five intervening sequences, similar to the picture seen for other genes of higher eukaryotes (NUNBERG et al. 1980). The DHFR gene is very large, and is approximately 30 kilo base paris (kbp) in length, some 70 times larger than the coding portion required as present in the mature mRNAs for DHFR (DOLNICK and BERTINO 1981). The restriction map of nonamplified and amplified cell lines is similar; in addition DNA from normal mouse tissues was shown to have a similar restriction pattern (NUNBERG et al. 1980). These data indicate that no substantial gene reorganization occurred during the amplification process. The size of the amplified unit has been estimated to be as low as 135 kbp (HAMLIN 1982) and as large as 800 kbp, from crude estimates of the size of the HSRs of some cell lines (NUNBERG et al. 1978; DOLNICK 1979). Even if the lower amplified unit estimate is correct, it is clear that additional genetic information is amplified; what this is, and whether it varies from cell to cell, is not yet clear. Although in the MTX-resistant Lactobacillus *casei* strain, thymidylate synthetase is also amplified as well as DHFR, no example of a coamplified folate enzyme has been described. We recently developed a highly resistant subline of the human leukemia line K^{562} (BERTINO et al. 1982). Analysis of other folate-coenzyme-mediated enzymes showed no substantial elevation of folate enzymes, except for dihydrofolate reductase. Preliminary data indicate that this K^{562} line, resistant to MTX, has amplified DHFR genes, as determined qualitatively by restriction analysis (BERTINO et al. 1982). Differences in the restriction patterns between the human and mouse have been observed, as well as between hamster lines and mouse lines with amplified DHFR genes (DOLNICK and BERTINO 1982). It will be of interest to determine of these differences result from sequence divergence of the structural or the intervening sequence portions of the DHFR gene. The hamster DHFR gene may be much smaller than the mouse gene as a consequence of the loss of large amounts of intervening sequence (SCHONER and LITTLEFIELD 1981).

The availability of human amplified lines should allow a determination of the DNA sequence and thus the amino acid sequence of the human enzyme. It will be of great interest to determine whether heterogeneity exists in the enzyme sequence between tumor and normal cells. If such differ-

Table 2. Examples of enzyme or receptor elevation in response to drug treatment

Drug	Enzyme or receptor increased	Gene amplification
MTX	Dihydrofolate reductase	Yes
PALA	Aspartate transcarbamylase	Yes
Cd^{++}	Metallothionein	Yes
FuDR	Thymidylate synthetase	ND
Asparaginase	Asparagine synthetase	ND
Hydroxyurea	Ribonucleotide reductase	ND
Pyrazofurin	Orotidylate decarboxylase	ND
Methylornithine	Ornithine decarboxylase	ND

PALA, (*N*-phosphonoacetyl)-L-aspartate); CAD, the first three enzymes of de novo uridine-5-monophosphate synthesis; FuDR, 5-fluorodeoxyuridine; ND, not determined

ences exist, then BAKER's concept of designing tumor-specific drugs may be correct (1964).

2. Gene Amplification and Resistance to Other Drugs

The finding of gene amplification as a mechanism of resistance to MTX has led to the examination of other lines resistant to other drugs, characterized by an elevation in the target enzyme. Table 2 is a list of resistant sublines to drugs that have been shown to be associated with elevations of target enzymes or receptors. In PALA (*N*-(phosphonoacetyl)-L-aspartate) resistance, WAHL et al. (1979) have demonstrated elevation of the gene copies coding a multifunctional protein which catalyzes the first three reactions of de novo UMP biosynthesis. In addition, resistance to heavy metals, e.g., Cd^{++}, may be associated with an increase in the binding protein (metallothionein) associated with an increase in gene copies (BEACH and PALMITER 1981). It will be of interest to ascertain whether resistance to hydroxyurea (associated with an increase in the subunit that binds this drug), FuDR, associated in some circumstances with an elevation in thymidylate synthetase (PRIEST et al. 1980) and asparaginase, associated with elevated levels of asparagine synthetase may also be due to gene amplification.

II. Impaired Transport as a Mechanism of Resistance to Methotrexate

Decreased transport of MTX, characterized by a decreased K_t or a decreased V_{max} for transport, is also a common mechanism of resistance to MTX (FISCHER 1961 b; HAKALA 1965; HUENNEKENS et al. 1978; SIROTNAK et al. 1968). In some lines, virtual absence of transport is observed; in fact when care is taken to use MTX free of impurities, one resistant L1210 cell line essentially excludes MTX (KAMEN et al. 1980). This degree of transport alteration can be tolerated in vitro, since folic acid, a substance that enters cells by an alternate, albeit less efficient, transport system, can satisfy the cells' folate requirements. These cells do not exclude certain other nonclassical folate antagonists, characterized by the absence of the glutamate in MTX, and therefore are still sensitive to these agents [e.g., pyrimethamine, daraprim, JB-11 (Fig. 2)]. Differential protection of normal tissues, but not these transport mutants, may be possible by the use of a combination of a

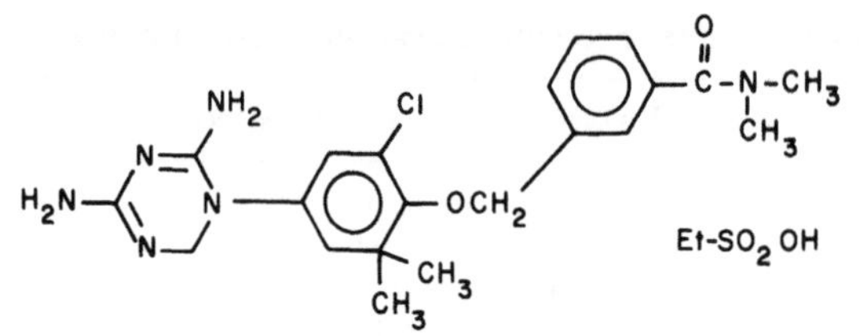

TZT, BAKER'S ANTIFOL, NSC 139105

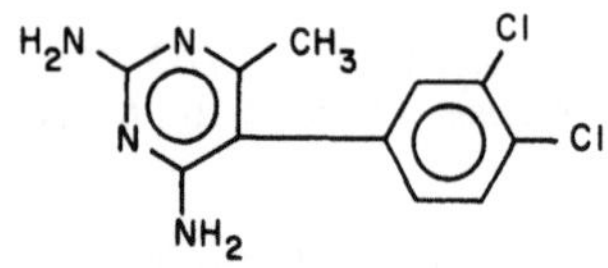

DDMP

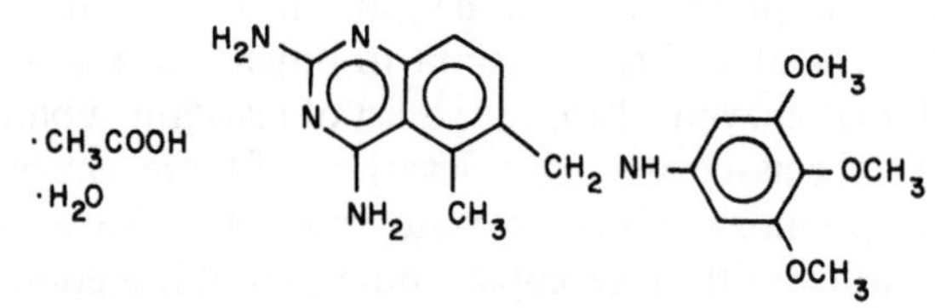

JB-II, NSC 249008

Fig. 2. Structure of three "nonclassical" folate antagonists: TZT, DDMP, and JB-11 (NSC 249008, "trimetrexate")

nonclassical antifolate with leucovorin. These normal cells, capable of transporting leucovorin, will be protected from the antifolate; the MTX-resistant cells will not, since the leucovorin cannot cross the membrane (HILL et al. 1977).

III. Altered Dihydrofolate Reductase as a Mechanism of Methotrexate Resistance

Several examples of cell lines resistant of MTX by virtue of an alteration in DHFR have been reported. This alteration, presumably in the gene coding for DHFR, leads to expression of an enzyme with a decreased affinity to MTX (BLUMENTHAL and GREENBERG 1970; ALBRECHT et al. 1972; JACKSON and NIETHAMMER 1977; FLINTOFF and ESSANI 1980; GOLDIE et al. 1980; HABER et al. 1981). The decrease in affinity to MTX observed has ranged from four fold to approximately 100,000-fold. The enzyme from 3T6 cells exhibiting this alteration has recently been purified and characterized by HABER et al. (1981). Of interest was the finding that the alteration in binding observed varied considerably between the 2,4-diamino antifolates studied. For example, JB-11 showed the greatest increase in I_{50}

(3,000-fold), while trimethoprim showed the least change (four fold). It will be of great interest to determine whether a single cell can synthesize both a normal and an altered enzyme, and to determine the amino acid sequence(s) of the altered enzyme that is responsible for the altered binding. These data also encourage the hope that inhibitors of DHFR may be found that have a *greater* affinity for the altered enzyme compared with the wild-type enzyme, which presumably is similar to normal-cell DHFR. If so, selective therapy with such an antifolate may be possible if the tumor-cell population is resistant to MTX by virtue of this mechanism.

D. Collateral Sensitivity Between Methotrexate-Resistant Cells and Other Agents

Collateral sensitivity, defined as the simultaneous sensitization of a cell population to one drug on acquiring resistance to another, has only been reported to occur for a few mammalian cell lines (see Chap. 24). A striking example of collateral sensitivity of MTX of adriamycin-resistant Chinese hamster ovary (CHO) cells was reported by HERMAN et al. (1979). Of interest is that the parent cells were highly sensitive to adriamycin, but strongly resistant to MTX. The authors suggested that the collateral MTX sensitivity of adriamycin-resistant CHO cells was due to reduced DHFR activity and increased net MTX uptake. HILL et al. (1976) also noted that MTX-resistant cells were sensitive to adriamycin (1976).

Another example of collateral sensitivity to dichloro-MTX of tumors resistant to an alkylating agent, methylene dimethane sulfonate, was reported by FOX and PILLINGER (1976). The mechanism of this increased sensitivity to the halogenated MTX derivatives has not been elucidated as yet.

The opposite phenomenon, i.e., concurrent development of resistance to MTX along with resistance developing to another agent of a different class, has also been recently described by this laboratory (unpublished observations). Thus lines selected for resistance to cytosine arabinoside were also found to be markedly resistant to MTX. Impaired transport and an elevated DHFR have been ruled out as possible mechanisms for this phenomenon.

E. Overcoming Resistance to Folate Antagonists

In this section, various strategies of overcoming resistance to MTX will be discussed, as well as the specific design of drugs to selectively kill cells that have acquired resistance.

I. Agents Promoting Methotrexate Transport into Resistant Cells or Tumors

If either intrinsic resistance or acquired resistance to MTX is present as a result of limited uptake of MTX into tumor cells, two general approaches are possible to overcome this resistance. Encapsulation of MTX into liposomes (KOSLOSKI et al. 1978) or modifying its structure so that it will be transported by a different mechanism are both approaches that have proved successful in experimental systems. MTX encapsulated in small cationic liposomes, when tested against mice bearing the Ridgway osteosarcoma, has increased activity, both in terms of tumor growth inhibition and toxicity to normal tissues (KAYE et al. 1981). These authors concluded that liposome entrapment acted as a slow release system, rather than a means of selective delivery to tumors. TODD et al. (1980) suggested that high doses of MTX delivered by liposomes could be potentially useful in overcoming drug transport resistance. A very clever extension of this type of approach for selective delivery of MTX was the use of "temperature-sensitive" liposomes containing MTX (WEINSTEIN et al. 1980). By heating (to 42 °C), selective tumor delivery was achieved in the extremity bearing the tumor, and an extra cell kill using this method (over animals not heated) was estimated to be 4- to 16-fold.

The carrier transport system present in most mammalian cells studied requires a 2–4,diamino pteridine structure (or a reduced 2-amino-4-hydroxy pteridine ring) as well as a terminal glutamate with both the α- and γ-carboxyl free (KESSEL 1969; HUENNEKENS et al. 1978). Modification of the MTX molecule by attaching substituents to the α- and/or γ-carboxyl has led to compounds that are taken up by cells by mechanisms other than the reduced-folate/MTX transport system. Thus serum albumin coupled to MTX is apparently taken up by tumor cells by an endocytic process (JACOBS et al. 1971). Furthermore, transport-resistant MTX cells are still sensitive to this compound (CHU and HOWELL 1981). Similarly, MTX coupled to poly(L-lysines) of various sizes exceeds the uptake of free drug in both drug-sensitive and MTX-transport-resistant CHO lines (RYSER and SHEN 1978, 1980). Since in both cases the conjugate is a less effective inhibitor of DHFR, the potent antitumor effects of these compounds indicate that free MTX is released intracellularly.

Cells resistant to MTX by virtue of impaired transport may also be attacked by modification of MTX to obtain more lipophilic derivatives, e.g., esterification of either or both of the glutamate carboxyls. Thus the dibutyl ester or the monobutyl ester of MTX is effective against MTX-transport-resistant cells (CURT et al. 1976; ROSOWSKY et al. 1980). Since reduced folate transport is impaired in these MTX-resistant cells, the opportunity for selective rescue with leucovorin also exists, i.e., normal tissues will be rescued by concurrent leucovorin while the MTX-transport-resistant cells will not be, when a lipophilic MTX derivative is used (CURT et al. 1976). These drugs also have the potential of improved penetration across pharmacological barriers, e.g., blood-brain barrier and blood-testis barrier (ABELSON et al. 1980).

These considerations also apply to folate antagonists of the "nonclassical" type (reviewed in BERTINO 1979) (Fig. 2). These drugs are taken up by cells via non-folate transport systems, and MTX-transport-resistant cells retain sensitivity to these agents (KAMEN 1981). Furthermore, the concept of selective rescue also applies to these drugs, as well as different pharmacological distribution compared with MTX (HILL et al. 1977). By appropriate structure activity modifications, it is possible to obtain compounds of this type that closely approximate the "stoichiometric" bonding of MTX to DHFR (SKEEL et al. 1973; BERTINO et al. 1979).

II. Effects of Dihydrofolate Reductase or Thymidylate Synthetase Inhibitors on Methotrexate-Resistant Cells

When MTX resistance occurs as a result of an increased level of DHFR, resistance may be partly overcome by use of drugs that accumulate intracellularly to higher levels than MTX, whose intracellular concentration is limited by the active transport process. Use of very high doses of MTX, requiring leucovorin rescue, will partially overcome this resistance since MTX will also leak into the cells by passive diffusion, but relatively high extracellular concentrations of drug are required to achieve small increments in the intracellular levels (BENDER 1975; BERTINO 1977).

A more selective strategy would be to design inhibitors that are converted by the increased levels of DHFR in resistant cells to reduced forms that are inhibitory to other folate enzymes. This approach was first suggested by FRIEDKIN (1967), and several compounds were screened as substrates for DHFR (as the reduced form) and as inhibitors of thymidylate synthetase. Homofolate and dihydrohomofolate satisfied these requirements and were found to be more inhibitory to MTX-high DHFR-resistant cells compared with sensitive lines (MISHRA et al. 1974). However, recent data indicate that tetrahydrohomofolate and 5-methyl tetrahydrohomofolate were also effective versus MTX-resistant cells, and thus the mechanism for the activity of this class of compounds against high-DHFR MTX-resistant cells may not be a consequence of the original lethal synthesis concept. Nevertheless, this approach is an attractive one, in view of the potential selectivity that may be produced.

Another approach to selectively killing MTX-resistant cells with elevated DHFR (or resistant to MTX by other mechanisms as well) was recently described (URLAUB et al. 1981). By using high-specific-activity tritiated deoxyuridine, MTX-resistant cells were selectively killed. Normal cells were protected by the use of hypoxanthine and thymidine, which in the presence of MTX allowed normal cells to survive in the absence of thymidylate synthesis.

III. Methotrexate-Resistant Cells with an Altered Dihydrofolate Reductase as a Target for Inhibitors

Although an alteration in the gene leading to production of DHFR with a decrease in affinity to MTX is a relatively uncommon mechanism of resistance to this drug, this event has the potential for therapeutic exploitation. MTX-resistant cell lines have been discussed with alterations in DHFR that result in as much as a 1,000-fold decrease in binding of MTX (HABER et al. 1981). As a result of this type of mutation a qualitatively different target enzyme than the parent line (and presumably from the normal tissue DHFR) is present in cells of the resistant line.

F. Clinical Studies

In the clinic tumors may be somewhat arbitrarily divided into those intrinsically highly sensitive to MTX (cure possible and complete remissions common), those moderately sensitive to MTX ($>30\%$ response rate), and those relatively insensitive to the drug ($<30\%$ response rate) (Table 3).

Table 3. Intrinsic sensitivity and resistance of human tumors to methotrexate

Tumors highly sensitive to MTX	*Tumors relatively insensitive to MTX*
Choriocarinoma	Acute nonlymphatic leukemia
Acute lymphatic leukemia	Chronic lymphocytic leukemia
Burkitt's lymphoma	Myeloma
Tumors moderately sensitive to MTX	Gastrointestinal cancer
Diffuse histiocytic lymphoma	Prostate cancer
Head and neck cancer	Lung cancer (non-oat cell)
Breast cancer	Neuroblastoma
Osteogenic sarcoma	Renal carcinoma
Bladder cancer	Melanoma

Since MTX is an S-phase-specific, cycle-active drug, it is perhaps surprising that even advanced solid tumors, with many cells in G_1, respond to this drug, even despite inherent insensitivity of cells not in cycle.

The reasons for the relative insensitivity of many human tumors to MTX have not been completely elucidated. The relative ease of studying leukemia cells from patients with an intrinsically sensitive disease (acute lymphocytic leukemia, ALL) and relatively resistant disease (acute nonlymphocytic leukemia, ANLL) has provided some information as to why the latter type of leukemia is more intrinsically resistant to MTX. In these patients, natural resistance appears to be due to a combination of a relatively long generation time, a rapid turnover of DHFR, "induction" of DHFR due to stabilization by MTX (and its polyglutamates), and poor transport (lack of retention, perhaps due to relatively low polyglutamate formation (BERTINO et al. 1977).

Acquired resistance may be best studied in patients with ALL, who are almost always initially sensitive to MTX. The study of development of resistance is made more difficult by the use of drug combinations, which are employed not only to obtain additive cell kill, but also to prevent drug resistance. Since 50% of children with this disease are apparently cured; the strategy is effective in some, but not all, patients.

A valuable screening test used in this laboratory to detect biochemical resistance in cells from patients with ALL in relapse has been the measurement of DNA synthesis (HRYNIUK and BERTINO 1969; SKEEL and BERTINO 1973). Tritiated deoxyuridine incorporation into DNA is measured in the absence and presence of various concentrations of MTX, usually after a 1-h incubation with this drug. While of no value under those conditions for detecting natural resistance [there was no difference in acute myeloblastic leukemia (AML) versus ALL cells in degree of inhibition by MTX before treatment (HRYNIUK and BERTINO 1969)], this test is useful in detecting acquired resistance to MTX, and thus for selecting patients for further study. In 12 patients with ALL treated with MTX, and who were considered clinically resistant to the drug, seven had a change in sensitivity to MTX as measured by this test (>90% inhibition of DNA synthesis at 2×10^{-6} *M* MTX).

When these patients were further studied, two had evidence for an altered DHFR possibly causing the resistance (SKEEL and BERTINO 1973). In another patient, high levels of DHFR may have been responsible for MTX resistance (Hryniuk and Bertino 1969). The availability of sensitive methods to measure gene copy numbers, MTX transport, and altered DHFR and improved culture techniques for leukemic cells should enable a reassessment of acquired drug resistance to be made in these patients.

Acknowledgment. Some of the work referred to in this chapter was supported by USPHS grant CA-08010 and the American Cancer Society (Research Professorship).

References

Abelson HT, Beardsley GP, Ensminger WD, Modest EJ, Rosowsky A (1980) Pharmacologic studies of methotrexate dibutyl and gamma-monobutyl esters in the rhesus monkey. Proc Am Assoc Cancer Res 21:265

Albrecht AM, Biedler JL, Hutchison DJ (1972) Two different species of dihydrofolate reductase in mammalian cells differentially resistant to amethopterin and methasquin. Cancer Res 32:1539–1546

Alt F, Kellems RE, Bertino JR, Schimke RT (1978) Multiplication of dihydrofolate reductase genes in methotrexate-resistant variants of cultured murine cells. J Biol Chem 253:1357–1370

Balinska M, Galivan J, Coward JK (1981) Efflux of MTX and its polyglutamate derivatives from hepatic cells in vitro. Cancer Res 41:2751–2756

Baker BR (1964) Factors in the design of active-site directed irreversible inhibitors. J Pharmaceutical Sci 53:347–364

Baugh CM, Krumdieck CL, Nair MG (1973) Polygammaglutamyl metabolites of methotrexate. Biochem Biophys Res Commun 52:27–34

Beach LR, Palmiter RD (1981) Amplification of the metallothionein-I gene in cadmium resistant mouse cells. Proc Natl Acad Sci 78:2110–2114

Bender RA (1975) Anti-folate resistance in leukemia: treatment with "high-dose" methotrexate and citrovorum factor. Cancer Treat Rev 2:215–224

Bertino JR (1963) The mechanism of action of the folate antagonists in man. Cancer Res 23:1286–1306

Bertino JR (1979) Toward improved selectivity in cancer chemotherapy: the Richard and Hinda Rosenthal Foundation Award Lecture. Cancer Res 39:203–304

Bertino JR (1977) "Rescue" techniques in cancer chemotherapy: use of leucovorin and other rescue agents after methotrexate treatment. Sem Oncology 4:203–216

Bertino JR, Skeel RT (1975) On natural and acquired resistance to folate antagonists in man. In: Pharmacological basis of cancer chemotherapy. Williams and Wilkins, Baltimore, pp 681–689

Bertino JR, Cashmore A, Fink M, Calabresi P, Lefkowitz E (1965) The "induction" of leukocyte and erythrocyte dihydrofolate reductase by methotrexate I. Clinical and pharmacologic studies. Clin Pharmacol Therap 6:673–770

Bertino JR, Sawicki WL, Cashmore AR, Cadman EC, Skeel RT (1977) Natural resistance to methotrexate in human acute nonlymphocytic leukemia. Cancer Treat Rep 61:667–673

Bertino JR, Sawicki WL, Moroson BA, Cashmore AR, Elslager EF (1979) 2,4-Diamino-5-methyl-6[3,4,5-trimethoxy anilino)methyl] quinazoline (TmQ), a potent non-classical folate antagonist. Biochem Pharmacol 28:1983–1987

Bertino JR, Dolnick BJ, Berenson RJ, Scheer DI, Kamen BA (1981) Cellular mechanisms of resistance to methotrexate. In: Sartorelli AC, Lazo TR, Bertino JR (eds) Molecular action and targets for cancer chemotherapeutic agents. Academic, New York, pp 385–397

Bertino JR, Srimatkandada S, Engel D, Medina WD, Scheer DI, Moroson BA, Dube S (1982) Gene amplification in a methotrexate-resistant human leukemia line, K-562. Cold Spring Harbor Symp Quartl Biol 23–27

Biedler JL, Spengler BA (1976) Metaphase chromosome anomaly: association with drug resistance and cell-specific products. Science 191:185–187

Biedler JL, Melera PN, Spengler BA (1980) Specifically altered metaphase chromosomes in antifolate-resistant Chinese hamster cells that overproduce dihydrofolate reductase. Cancer Genet Cytogenet 2:47–60
Blumenthal G, Greenberg DM (1970) Evidence for two molecular species of dihydrofolate reductase in amethopterin resistant and sensitive cells of the mouse leukemia L4946. Oncology 24:223–229
Bostock CJ, Clark EH, Harding NGL, Mounts PM, Tyler-Smith C, Heyningen M, Walker PMP (1979) The development of resistance to methotrexate in a mouse melanoma cell line. Chromosoma 74:153–177
Chabner BA, Schilsky R, Jolivet J (to be published) The synthesis, binding, and retention of methotrexate polyglutamates by human breast cancer cells. In: Bertino JR, Chabner BA, Goldman ID (eds) Folyl and anti-folylpolyglutamates.
Chang SE, Littlefield JW (1976) Elevated dihydrofolate reductase messenger RNA levels in methotrexate-resistant BHK cells. Cell 7:391–396
Chu BC, Fan CC, Howell SB (1981) Activity of free and carrier-bound methotrexate against transport-deficient and high dihydrofolate dehydrogenase-containing methotrexate-resistant L1210 cells. JNCK 66:121–124
Curt GA, Tobias JS, Kramer RA, Rosowsky A, Parker LM, Tattersall MH (1976) Inhibition of nucleic acid synthesis by the di-*N*-butyl ester of methotrexate. Biochem Pharmacol 25:1943–1946
Dolnick BJ, Bertino JR (1981) Multiple messenger RNAs for dihydrofolate reductase. Arch Biochem Biophys 210:691–697
Dolnick BJ, Bertino JR (1982) Gene amplification in human tumor systems. In: Owens AH, Coffey OS, Baylin SB (eds) Tumor cell heterogeneity. Academic, New York, pp 169–179
Dolnick BJ, Berenson RJ, Bertino JR, Kaufman RJ, Nunberg JH, Schimke RT (1979) Correlation of dihydrofolate reductase elevation with gene amplification in a homogenously staining chromosomal region of L5178Y cells. J Cell Biol 83:394–402
Fischer GA (1961) Increased levels of folic acid reductase as a mechanism of resistance to amethopterin in leukemic cells. Biochem Pharmacol 7:75–80
Fischer GA (1961) Defective transport of amethopterin (methotrexate) as a mechanism of resistance to the antimetabolite in L5178Y leukemia cells. Biochem Pharmacol 11:1233–1234
Flintoff WF, Essani K (1980) Methotrexate-resistant Chinese hamster ovary cells contain a dihydrofolate reductase with an altered affinity for methotrexate. Biochemistry 19:4321–4327
Flintoff WF, Spindler SM, Siminovitch L (1976a) Genetic characterization of methotrexate-resistant Chinese hamster ovary cells. In Vitro 12:749–757
Flintoff WF, Davidson SV, Sininovitch L (1976) Isolation and partial characterization of three methotrexate resistant phenotypes from Chinese hamster ovary cells. Somatic Cell Genet 2:245–261
Fox BW, Pillinger DJ (1976) Collateral sensitivity studies between halogenated methotrexates and an alkylating agent. Br J Cancer 34:322
Friedkin M (1967) Enzyme studies with new analogues of folic acid and homofolic acid. J Biol Chem 242:1466–1476
Galivan J (1980) Evidence for the cytotoxic activity of polyglutamate derivatives of methotrexate. Mol Pharmacol 17:105–110
Genther CS, Schoeny RS, Loper JC, Smith CC (1977) Mutagenic studies of folic acid antagonists. Antimicrob Agents Chemother 12:84–92
Gewirtz DA, White JC, Randolph JK, Goldman ID (1980) Transport binding and polyglutamylation of methotrexate in freshly isolated rat hepatocytes. Cancer Res 40:573–578
Goldie JH, Krystal G, Hartley D, Gudauskes G, Dedhar S (1980) A methotrexate-insensitive variant of folate reductase present in two lines of methotrexate-resistant L5178Y cells. Eur J Cancer 16:1539–1546
Goldman ID, Lichenstein NS, Oliverio VT (1968) Carrier-mediated transport of the folic acid analogue methotrexate in the L1210 leukemia cell. J Biol Chem 243:5007–5017

Gupta RS, Flintoff WF, Siminovitch L (1977) Purification and properties of dihydrofolate reductase from methotrexate-sensitive and methotrexate-resistant Chinese hamster ovary cells. Can J Biochem 55:445–452

Haber DA, Beverley SM, Kiely ML, Schimke RT (1981) Properties of an altered dihydrofolate reductase encoded by amplified genes in cultured mouse fibroblasts. J Biol Chem 256:9501–9510

Hakala MT (1965) On the role of drug penetration in amethopterin resistance of Sarcoma-180 cells in vitro. Biochim Biophys Acta 102:198–209

Hakala MT, Zakrewski SF, Nichol CA (1961) Relation of folic acid reductase to amethopterin resistance in cultured mammalian cells. J Biol Chem 236:952–958

Hamlin J (1982) Studies on the mechanism of dihydrofolate reductase gene amplification in Chinese hamster ovary cells. In: Schinke R (ed) Gene amplification. Cold Spring Harbor Laboratory

Hamrell MR, Sedwick D, Lazlo J (1980) Interrelationship of drug transport and target enzyme levels as determinants of methotrexate resistance. Proc Am Assoc Cancer Res 21:3

Harding B, MacLennan IC (1977) Myelotoxicity of methotrexate in animals with pyogenic infection. Br J Haematol 37(4):515–520

Harding NG, Martelli MF, Huennekens FM (1970) Amethopterin-induced changes in the multiple forms of dihydrofolate reductase from L1210 cells. Arch Biochem Biophys 137:295–296

Hermann TS, Cress AE, Gerner EW (1979) Collateral sensitivity to methotrexate in cells resistant to Adriamycin. Cancer Res 39:1937–1942

Hill TT, Price LA, Goldie JH (1976) The value of Adriamycin in overcoming resistance to methotrexate in tissue culture. Eur J Cancer 12:541–549

Hill BT, Price LA, Harrison SI, Goldie JH (1977) The difference between "selective folinic acid protection" and "folinic acid rescue" in 5178Y cell culture. Eur J Cancer 13:861–871

Hryniuk WM, Bertino JR (1969) Treatment of leukemia with large doses of methotrexate and folinic acid: Clinical-biochemical correlates. J Clin Invest 48:2140–2155

Hryniuk WM, Fischer GA, Bertino JR (1969) S-Phase cells of rapidly growing and resting populations. Differences in response to methotrexate. Mol Pharmacol 5:557–564

Huennekens FM, Vitols KS, Henderson GB (1978) Transport of folate compounds in bacterial and mammalian cells. Adv Enzymol 47:313–344

Jackson RC, Niethammer D (1977) Acquired methotrexate resistance in lymphoblasts resulting from altered kinetic properties of dihydrofolate reductase. Eur J Cancer 13:567–575

Jacobs SA, d'Urso-Scott M, Bertino JR (1971) Some biochemical and pharmacologic properties of amethopterin-albumin. Ann NY Acad Sci 186:284–286

Jacobs SA, Adamson RH, Chabner BA, Derr CJ, Johns DG (1975) Stoichiometric inhibition of mammalian dihydrofolate reductase by the γ-glutamyl metabolite of methotrexate, 4-amino-4-deoxy-N^{10}-methyl-pteroylglutamyl-γ-glutamate. Biochem Biophys Res Comm 63:692–798

Jaffe N, Frei III Em, Traggis D, Cassady J, Watts H, Filler RM (1974) High-dose methotrexate with citrovorum factor in osteogenic sarcoma. N Eng J Med 291:994–997

Johnson LF, Fuhrman CL, Abelson HT (1978) Resistance of resting 3T6 mouse fibroblasts to methotrexate cytotoxicity. Cancer Res 38:2408–2412

Kamen BA, Bertino JR (1978) Non-stoichiometric inhibition of dihydrofolic acid reductase (DHFR) by methotrexate in the presence of NADH. Blood 82:287

Kamen BA, Cashmore ArR, Dreyer RN, Moroson BA, Hseih P, Bertino JR (1980) Effect of [^{3}H]methotrexate impurities on apparent transport of methotrexate by a sensitive and resistant L1210 line. J Biol Chem 255:3254–3257

Kamen BA, Eibl B, Cashmore AR, Whyte WL, Moroson BA, Bertino JR (1981) Efficacy and transport of a new lipid soluble antifol, 2,4-diamino-5-methyl-6-[(3,4,5-trimethoxyanilino)methyl]quinazoline (TMQ JB-11) in methotrexate resistant cells. Proc Am Assoc Cancer Res 22:26

Kaufman RJ, Bertino JR, Schimke RS (1978) Quantitation of dihydrofolate reductase in individual parental and methotrexate-resistant murine cells. Use of a fluorescence-activated cell sorter. J Biol Chem 253:5852–5860
Kaufman RJ, Brown RC, Schimke RT (1979) Amplified dihydrofolate reductase genes in unstable methotrexate-resistant cells are associated with double minute chromosomes. Proc Natl Acad Sci 76:5669–5673
Kaye SB, Boden JA, Ryman BE (1981) The effect of liposome entrapment of actinomycin D and methotrexate on the in vivo treatment of sensitive and resistant solid murine tumors. Eur J Cancer 17:279–289
Kessel D (1969) A comparison of 4-amino-4-deoxy-N^{10}-methylpteroic acid and methotrexate transport by mouse leukemia cells. Mol Pharmacol 5:21–25
Koizumi S, Yamagami M, Ueno Y, Mirua M, Taniguchi N (1980) Resistance of human bone marrow CFU_c to high-dose methotrexate cytotoxicity. Exp Hematol 8:635–640
Kosloski MJ, Rosen R, Milholland RJ, Papahadjopoulos D (1978) Effect of lipid vesicle (liposome) encapsulation of methotrexate on its chemotherapeutic efficacy in solid rodent tumors. Cancer Res 38:2848–2853
Kufe DW, Wick MM, Abelson HT (1980) Natural resistance to methotrexate in human melanomas. J Invest Dermatol 75:357–359
Lindquist CA (1979) Characterization of a new murine leukemia line, L1210RR, and comparative studies of human dihydrofolate reductase enzymes. Ph. D. Thesis, Yale University School of Medicine
McGuire JJ, Bertino JR (1981) Enzymatic synthesis and function of folyl polyglutamates. Mol Cell Biochem 38:19–48
Melera PW, Lewis JA, Biedler JL, Hession C (1980) Antifolate-resistant Chinese hamster cells. Evidence for dihydrofolate reductase gene amplification among independently derived sublines overproducing different dihydrofolate reductases. J Biol Chem 255:7024–7028
Mishra LC, Parmar AS, Mead JA (1974) Regeneration of tetrahydrohomofolate in cells. Possible basis for antitumor activity of homofolate. Biochem Pharmacol 23:1827–1834
Misra DK, Humphreys SP, Friedkin M, Goldin A, Crawford EJ (1961) Increased dihydrofolate reductase activity as a possible basis of drug resistance in leukemia. Nature 189:39
Nahas A, Nixon PF, Bertino JR (1972) Uptake and metabolism of N^5-formyltetrahydrofolate by L1210 leukemia cells. Cancer Res 32:1416–1421
Nair MG, Baugh CM (1973) Synthesis and biological evaluation of poly-γ-glutamyl derivatives of methotrexate. Biochem 12:3923–3927
Niethammer D, Jackson RC (1975) Changes of molecular properties associated with the development of resistance against methotrexate inhuman lymphoblastoid cells. Eur J Cancer 11:845–854
Nunberg JH, Kaufman RJ, Schimke RT, Urlaub G, Crasin LA (1978) Amplified dihydrofolate reductase genes are localized to a homogeneously staining region of a single chromosome in a methotrexate-resistant Chinese hamster ovary cell line. Proc Natl Acad Sci 75:5553–5556
Nunberg JH, Kaufman RJ, Chang ACY, Cohen SN, Schimke RT (1980) Structure and genomic organization of the mouse dihydrofolate reductase gene. Cell 19:355–364
Priest DG, Ledford BE, Doig MT (1980) Increased thymidylate synthetase in 5-fluorodeoyuridine-resistant cultured hepatoma cells. Biochem Pharmacol 29:1549–1553
Rosowsky A, Lazarus H, Yuan GC, Beltz WR, Mangini L, Abelson HT, Modest EJ, Frei E (1980) Effects of methotrexate esters and other lipophilic antifolates on methotrexate-resistant human leukemic lymphoblasts. Biochem Pharmacol 29:648–652
Ryser HJ, Shen WC (1980) Conjugation of methotrexate to poly(1-lysine) as a potential way to overcome drug resistance. Cancer 45:1207–1211
Schilsky RL, Bailey BD, Chabner BA (1980) Methotrexate polyglutamate synthesis by cultured human breast cancer cells. Proc Natl Acad Sci USA 77:2919–2922
Schimke RT, Kaufman RJ, Nunberg JH, Dana SL (1979) Studies on the amplification of dihydrofolate reductase genes in methotrexate-resistant cultured mouse cells. Cold Spring Harbor Symp Quart Biol 43:1297

Schoner RG, Littlefield JW (1981) The organization of the dihydrofolate reductase gene of baby hamster kidney fibroblasts. Nucleic Acids Res 9:6601–6614

Schrecker AW, Mead JAR, Greenberg NH, Goldin A (1971) Dihydrofolate reductase activity of leukemia L1210 during development of methotrexate resistance. Biochem Pharmacol 20:716–718

Sirotnak FM, Donsbach RC (1974) The intracellular concentration dependence of antifolate inhibition of DNA synthesis in L1210 leukemia cells. Cancer Res 34:3332

Sirotnak FM, Furita S, Hutchison DJ (1968) On the nature of a transport alteration determining resistance of amethopterin in the L1210 leukemia. Cancer Res 28:75–80

Skeel RT, Bertino JR, Resistance to chemotherapeutic agents. Clinical aspects. Proc. 5th int. congr. pharmacol., San Francisco, 1972, vol 3. Karger, Basel, pp 376–392

Skeel RT, Sawicki WL, Cashmore AR, Bertino JR (1973) The basis for the disparate sensitivity of L1210 leukemia and Walker 256 carcinoma to a new triazine folate antagonist. Cancer Res 33:2972–2976

Todd JA, Levine AM, Tokes ZA (1980) Liposome-encapsulated methotrexate interactions with human chronic lymphocytic leukemia cells. JNCI 64:715–719

Urlaub G, Landzberg M, Chasin LA (1981) Selective killing of methotrexate-resistant cells carrying amplified dihydrofolate reductase genes. Cancer Res 41:1594–1601

Varshavsky A (1981) Phorbol ester dramatically increases incidence of methotrexate-resistant mouse cells: possible mechanisms and relevance of tumor promotion. Cell 25:561–572

Wahl GM, Padgett RA, Stark GR (1979) Gene amplification causes overproduction of the first three enzymes of UMP synthesis in *N*-(phosporoacetyl)-L-aspartate-resistant hamster cells. J Biol Chem 254:8679–8689

Warren RD, Nichols AP, Bender RA (1978) Membrane transport of methotrexate in human lymphoblastoid cells. Cancer Res 39:668–671

Weinstein JN, Magin RL, Cysyk RL, Zaharko DS (1980) Treatment of solid L1210 murine tumors with local hyperthermia and temperature-sensitive liposomes containing methotrexate. Cancer Res 40:1388–1395

White JC, Loftfield S, Goldman JD (1975) The mechanism of action of methotrexate: Free intracellular methotrexate is required for maximal suppression of ^{14}C-formate incorporation into nucleic acids and proteins. Mol Pharmacol 11:287–297

Whitehead VM, Perrault MM, Stelcner S (1975) Tissue-specific synthesis of methotrexate polyglutamates in the rat. Cancer Res 35:2985–2990

CHAPTER 23

Steroids

M. M. Ip

A. Introduction

I. Structure

The steroids are a group of compounds containing a four-ring structure termed the cyclopentanoperhydrophenanthrene nucleus (Fig. 1). As shown in Fig. 1b, the nucleus itself is composed of 17 carbon atoms; however, the synthesis of the steroid hormones involves the addition of one, two, or four additional carbon atoms to form the C18 estranes, C19 androstanes, and C21 pregnanes, respectively (Fig. 2). The C18 steroids include estradiol, estrone, and estriol. Estradiol is synthesized mainly in the ovary, with transformation to estrone and estriol taking place in the liver. Some synthesis also occurs in the adrenal as well as in the testis. Testosterone and dihydrotestosterone are examples of the C19 steroids. The major synthesis of testosterone occurs in the testis; however, androgen production has also been shown to occur in the adrenal and the ovary. The C21 steroids are produced mainly in the adrenal gland and include progesterone (also synthesized by the ovary), the glucocorticoids such as cortisol, and the mineralocorticoids such as aldosterone.

a

b

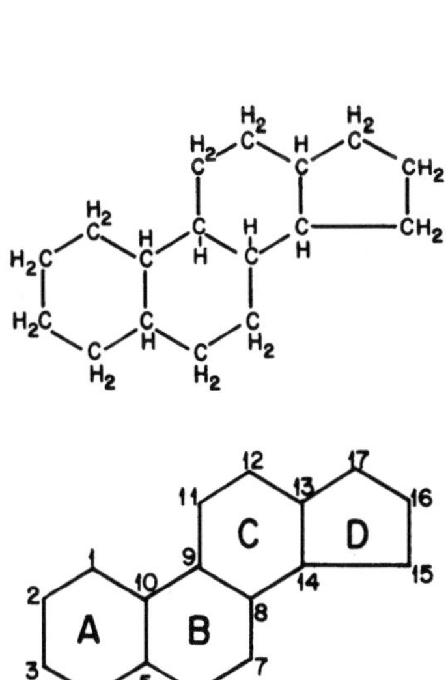

Fig. 1 a, b. The cyclopentanoperhydrophenanthrene nucleus of steroids: **a** structure **b** formula showing numbering system

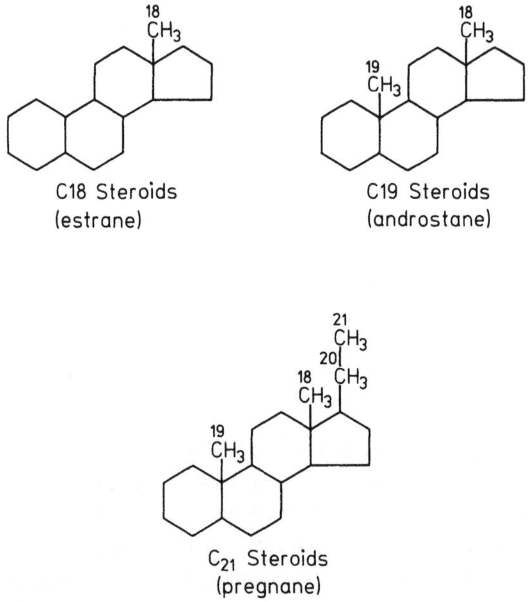

Fig. 2. Parent compounds of the various steroid hormone classes

II. Mechanism of Action of Steroid Hormones

The mode of action of all the steroid hormones is thought to be similar. Conventionally, the steroid enters the cell by passive diffusion and binds to a cytosol receptor. The steroid-receptor complex is then activated in a heat-dependent step and is translocated to the nucleus, where it binds to chromatin. As a result of this binding, RNA transcription is initiated, protein is synthesized, and a physiological effect is elicited (Fig. 3).

The actual details of this mechanism are somewhat more complicated. For example, although there appears to be good evidence in many tissues that steroids enter cells by passive diffusion, other data indicate the process may involve a facilitated or active transport system. Evidence suggestive of passive diffusion includes the fact that in several systems, including hepatoma (PLAGEMANN and ERBE 1976), thymocytes (MAYER et al. 1976), and the hepatoma tissue culture (HTC) cell line (SAMUELS and TOMKINS 1970), the amount of steroid accumulated in the cells is proportional to the external concentration. PLAGEMANN and ERBE (1976) also demonstrated that steroid uptake in hepatoma was not saturable, energy dependent, steroid specific, or affected by alterations of the cell surface with phospholipase or neuraminidase, all of which favor the theory that the process is passive. In contrast to these observations, however, HARRISON and co-workers (1974, 1975, 1977) have presented data suggesting that in the glucocorticoid responsive AtT-20/D-1 pituitary cell line, uptake of glucocorticoid involves a mechanism of specific, temperature-dependent transport through the cell membrane. In this cell line, treatments that perturbed the plasma membrane (e.g., treatment with neur-

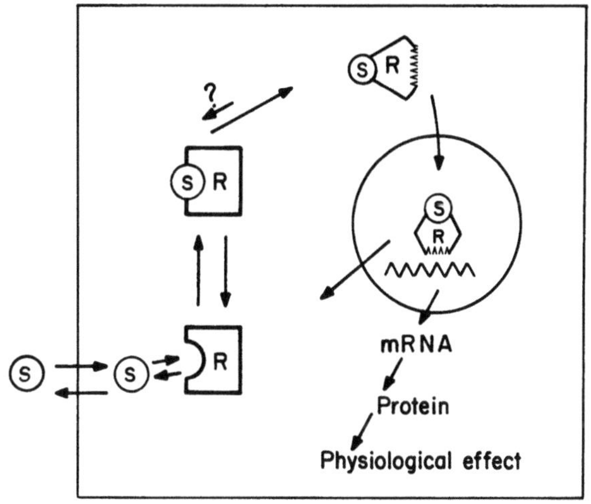

Fig. 3. Conventional mode of action of steroid hormones

aminidase, phospholipase A2, pronase, dimethylsulfoxide, or ethanol) decreased steroid uptake by the intact cell, yet had no effect on cell viability or on binding to the cytosol glucocorticoid receptor. RAO and co-workers (1976, 1977) have also described what they feel to be a carrier-mediated transport process in isolated rat liver cells, and concluded that the process contributed 88% to the total uptake of corticosterone within the physiological serum concentration range. Transport of corticosterone or cortisol was decreased by treatment of the cells with phospholipase, sulfhydryl reagents, or metabolic inhibitors (cortisol only). One criticism of these studies is that interpretation is complicated by the presence of receptors or other steroid-binding proteins within the cells; however, in more recent experiments (ALLÉRA et al. 1980) these workers have demonstrated the interaction of corticosterone with highly purified liver plasma membrane vesicles. Since membrane vesicles contain no steroid receptors or other cytoplasmic-binding proteins, this suggests that corticosterone is binding specifically to the plasma membrane at sites which may be involved in steroid transport into the cell. Similar observations have been made by KISLING and co-workers (1979), who reported in addition that binding of glucocorticoids to plasma membranes of rat liver was suppressed by pronase and phospholipase, but not by DNAse and RNAse. Taken together, these studies would seem to suggest that, in some cell types at least, both a diffusion and carrier-mediated process may be involved in steroid entry into the cell. However, in view of the sometimes conflicting data, it is not possible to make any definitive statement on the generality of either process for all cell types and for all steroids.

Once in the cell, the steroid binds with high affinity to a specific cytosol receptor. This steroid receptor complex must first be activated before it can be translocated to the nucleus or bind to chromatin. The process has recently been reviewed by HIGGINS and co-workers (1979) and by SIMONS (1979). Briefly, the complex can be activated by increasing the temperature or the ionic strength, by partial purification (e.g., by ammonium sulfate or gel filtration), or by dilution. The latter observations suggest that activation occurs by dissociation of a low-molecular-weight inhibitor, and in fact LITWACK and co-workers (CAKE et al. 1978; DI SORBO et al. 1980 b) have suggested that for the liver glucocorticoid receptor this inhibitor might be pyridoxal phosphate. While the actual mechanism of activation has not been detailed, it is clear that there is a change in the conformation of the steroid-receptor complex. Activated receptor complexes have an increased number of positive charges, contributed by lysine and arginine (CAKE et al. 1978; DI SORBO et al. 1980 a), and exhibit an increased affinity for various polyanions including DNA, phosphocellulose, hydroxylapatite, diethylaminoethyl (DEAE)-Sephadex, and DEAE cellulose. Most importantly, once activated, the complex can move into the nucleus, where it binds to some as yet undefined site and can initiate a chain of reactions, resulting in a physiological effect.

Little is really known about where the steroid-receptor complex binds in nuclei. Although most workers have assumed that binding is to chromatin, recent evidence also points to binding in the nuclear matrix as well (BARRACK and COFFEY 1980). All steroid receptors bind to some extent to DNA directly (reviewed by HIGGINS et al. 1979 but see also THRALL and SPELSBERG 1980), but this binding exhibits no saturability and is inhibited at an ionic strength greater than 0.10 *M* (MILGROM et al. 1976; SPELSBERG et al. 1977). In addition, steroid-receptor complex does not distinguish between DNA isolated from a variety of eukaryotes, prokaryotes, or bacteriophages, or when denatured DNA is used (MILGROM et al. 1976). These observations suggest that while DNA could be the physiological acceptor, other factors are responsible for the specificity of the binding, or alternatively that some other factor is the true acceptor.

Steroid-receptor complexes have also been shown to bind to chromatin. SPELSBERG et al. (1977), for example, have shown that in chick oviduct, acceptor activity was associated with two acidic proteins of mol. wt. 12,000 and 17,000, respectively. In contrast, PUCA et al. (1975) isolated a basic protein from calf uterine nuclei of mol. wt. 70,000, which bound estrogen receptor. MAINWARING et al. (1976) found a similar protein in androgen-sensitive tissues.Other investigators have probed for nuclear acceptor sites by treatment with nucleases. BAXTER and co-workers (1972) showed that treatment of HTC cell nuclei with DNAse I resulted in loss of 35% of nuclear DNA with loss of 90% of the capacity to bind steroid-receptor complexes. It was also demonstrated that while glucocorticoid binding to HTC cells and uterus was destroyed by DNAse I, that of estrogen binding to uterus was not (HIGGINS et al. 1973), so apparently it is not possible to generalize. Of more interest are those studies in which steroid-receptor complex has been bound to chromatin prior to limited nuclease digestion, so that some estimation could be made of its location. In these experiments, while some workers have only looked at solubilization of steroid-receptor complexes by various nucleases (BAXTER et al. 1972; CIDLOWSKI and MUNCK 1980), others have tried to determine whether the released receptor is associated with transcriptionally active chromatin. LEVY-WILSON and BAXTER (1976), for example, treated chromatin from cultured pituitary (GC) cells with DNAse II and looked at glucocorticoid binding in the unsheared chromatin fraction (pellet) and in the fraction released into the supernate. Their data showed that most of the glucocorticoid binding was associated with the pellet while most of the nascent RNA was in the supernate, and they concluded that the receptor was associated with template-inactive chromatin. SOCHER et al. (1976) also concluded that the majority of acceptor sites for the progesterone receptor in chick oviduct were associated with fractions low in template activity, based on experiments in which chromatin was sheared mechanically, the fractions separated on sucrose gradients and analyzed for progesterone binding, nascent RNA, and RNA polymerase activity. In contrast to these results, others have concluded that receptors are associated with template-active regions.

GOTTESFELD and BUTLER (1977) had earlier demonstrated that the 2 m*M* $MgCl_2$-soluble mononucleosomal fraction resulting after DNAse II treatment of nuclei was enriched in nascent RNA and sedimented at 14S rather than the usual 11S. The Mg^{++}-soluble fraction was shown to be rich in globin-coding regions in chick reticulocytes (HENDRICK et al. 1977) as well as in nascent RNA (GOTTESFELD and BUTLER 1977), suggesting that it is template active. When hen oviduct chromatin was digested with DNAse II and fractionated with $MgCl_2$, HEMMINKI (1976, 1977) found that the concentration of estrogen receptors was 4.5 times higher in $MgCl_2$-soluble chromatin (sedimenting at 14S) than in $MgCl_2$-insoluble chromatin (sedimenting at 11S). In immature chicks, this ratio was only 1.8, suggesting that the estrogen receptor was associated with template-active chromatin. In confirmation of this, ALBERGA et al. (1979) found an apparent enrichment of both the estrogen receptor and the vitellogenin gene in the Mg^{++}-soluble fraction of stimulated chick liver chromatin; in nonstimulated animals there was neither detectable receptor nor enrichment of the vitellogenin gene in this fraction. MASSOL et al. (1978) also found estrogen-binding sites in a 13–14S fraction from a micrococcal nuclease digest of oviduct nuclei; no such sites were found in kidney. More recently, SCOTT and FRANKEL (1980) have shown that digestion of chromatin from MCF-7 cells with micrococcal nuclease resulted in cofractionation of chromatin enriched in bound estrogen receptor and in transcribed sequences, as measured by a cDNA probe to cytoplasmic poly (A)-RNA sequences. This fraction was also depleted in globin sequences, which is presumably a nontranscribed gene in these cells.

It is important to note that in most of these studies receptor binding is found in all the chromatin fractions and the significance of this is not known at this time. What is significant, however, is the relative enrichment of receptor (relative to DNA) in fractions enriched in template-active areas, and the fact that this enrichment is not present in nonstimulated tissue or in nontarget tissue. As to the actual binding site, the factors that direct or specify this binding, and how RNA transcription is initiated, we must await further research.

B. Possible Mechanisms of Steroid Resistance

From the preceding discussion, it can be seen that natural resistance to steroids could arise at a number of different loci, with a defect at any step of the pathway resulting in failure of the cell to display the hormone response. Experiments on murine cell lines in culture (the S49 lymphoma and the WEHI-7 thymoma) suggested that the most common defect observed in steroid-resistant mutants was the absence of a receptor (or a defect in the steroid-binding site of the receptor since it was impossible to distinguish between the two) (Yamamoto et al. 1976; Pfahl et al. 1978; Gehring 1978; Sibley and Yamamoto 1979). Such a result may have been favored by the selection conditions, however, or be specific to the mouse, since it appears that in certain human cancers the absence of a receptor accounts for only a small proportion of the steroid-resistant states. In breast cancer, for example, recent studies, using better techniques for measurement, have demonstrated that 70%–85% of breast cancers contain the estrogen receptor (McGuire et al. 1975; Hawkins et al. 1980); yet the response rate in patients who are positive for the estrogen receptor is at best only 55%–60%. This suggests that only 15%–30% of breast cancers are resistant by virtue of having no receptor; a much larger majority have some other defect. Similar results have been reported in patients with various types of leukemia; virtually all of them have the glucocorticoid receptor (Konior-Yarbro et al. 1977; Konior et al. 1977b; Homo et al. 1978, 1980; Crabtree et al. 1978; Schmidt and Thompson 1978, 1979; Bell et al. 1979; Stevens et al. 1979; Ho et al. 1980; Bloomfield et al. 1980). Both examples are discussed in detail later in this chapter (Sects. E, F).

In addition to lack of receptor, steroid resistance could also arise at other loci. No defect has, as yet, been reported at the site of steroid transport into the cell. However, an example of resistance at the activation step was recently described by Schmidt and co-workers (1980). These workers identified a glucocorticoid-resistant mutant in a subclone (4R4) of CEM-C7, a cloned human leukemic T-cell line sensitive to the cytolytic action of glucocorticoids. Based on DEAE-cellulose chromatography, it was demonstrated that the receptors of the 4R4 clone were not able to form stable activated complexes with glucocorticoids. This is the first reported example of resistance at the activation step and it will be of interest to determine whether such a defect occurs in the cells of leukemia patients.

A lack of translocation of the steroid-receptor complex has frequently been observed, most notably in human breast cancers (Garola and McGuire 1977; Thorsen 1979; Fazekas and MacFarlane 1980; Hähnel et al. 1980; Romic-Stojkovic and Gamulin 1980) and in a series of S49 mouse lymphoma mutants (Yamamoto et al. 1976; Gehring 1978; Sibley and Yamamoto 1979). In such cases, there is no accumulation of the steroid-receptor complex in the nucleus; this could result from specific defects at the activation step, failure of the steroid-receptor complex to move across the nuclear membrane, or failure of the complex to bind in the nucleus. The latter could result from a defect in the receptor itself or at the nuclear acceptor site.

In many steroid-resistant cells, cytosol receptor is present and is translocated; however, the cell remains unresponsive to the cytolytic/growth stimulatory effect of the steroid [for example, the nt^i (increased nuclear transfer) S49 lymphoma mutants (Sect. C), the glucocorticoid-resistant line of the P1798 lymphosarcoma (Sect. D), human leukemias (Sect. E), and certain breast cancers (Sect. F)]. Paradoxically, in a few cases, certain parameters of steroid sensitivity remain unimpaired. Many types of human leukemia, for example, even though clinically insensitive to glucocorticoid, are sensitive in vitro, as measured by an inhibition of incorporation of nucleoside precursors into macromolecules (Sect. E). The growth of the MTW-9B rat mammary tumor is independent of estrogen, yet progesterone receptor levels in the tumor are very sensitive to circulating estrogen concentrations (IP et al. 1979). Approximately 27% of breast cancer patients whose tumors contain both the estrogen receptor and the progesterone receptor (presumably a gene product of estrogen) do not respond to endocrine therapy (Sect. F). It is somewhat more difficult to explain resistance in these cases; however, certain possibilities can be suggested, including the following:

1. In normal target tissue, such as the mammary gland, a protein or other factor is present that blocks or masks the specific gene site determining the growth response. When the estrogen receptor complex enters the nucleus, it binds to this protein (or elsewhere) and modifies it (e.g., by phosphorylation or acetylation) in such a way that the region of the DNA normally blocked is opened up and can be expressed. If we assume that there is a separate repressor protein for each estrogen-dependent function, it is reasonable to suggest that in some mammary tumors the specific repressor protein that blocks the gene site responsible for growth is lost or altered. In this case, estrogen would no longer exert any effect and growth would be "constitutive." In such a model, estrogen regulation of progesterone receptor synthesis would be possible if the repressor protein for the progesterone receptor region of the genome were still present. The model could also be applied to the cytolytic effects of glucocorticoids if it were assumed that in a normal lymphoid cell glucocorticoids induced a specific protein that resulted in cell lysis. In a malignant cell, the repressor protein for this induced protein could be altered such that the glucocorticoid receptor complex was no longer bound; hence the repression is not relieved and the protein could not be synthesized.
2. In normal target tissue the steroid-receptor complex binds to DNA directly (with specificity ensured by nearby proteins), opening up the DNA and allowing transcription to occur. It is possible that in a resistant cell a new protein is synthesized that blocks the site of interaction of the steroid-receptor complex with the region of the DNA that encodes for the growth response. This new protein would not block the region of DNA coding for synthesis of the progesterone receptor. The suggestion that a new protein might be made in an autonomous tumor is not entirely without foundation. KIM and DEPOWSKI (1975) have demonstrated, for example, that in the progression of the estrogen-dependent mammary tumor MTW-9A to the estrogen-independent MTW-9B, two extra chromosomes are added. Again, this model could also be applied to the lytic effects of glucocorticoids by assuming that the new protein blocked the interaction of the glucocorticoid receptor complex with the region of the DNA coding for the "lysis" protein.
3. Subtle alterations in the receptor are possible which interfere in some aspects of steroid action but not others.
4. The receptor or nuclear acceptor sites are not altered but some factor at the transcriptional or translational level is, the end result being the failure of one of the steroid responses.

All of the above explanations could apply to tumors in which the cytosol receptor complex was formed and was translocated into the nucleus and yet *none* of the steroid-induced responses were observed. A whole variety of other nuclear alterations are also possible.

The discussion so far assumes that resistance arises from some sort of defect in the cell. It is also possible that in certain receptor positive tumors resistance is only apparent because of tumor heterogeneity. In this situation, receptor-containing cells might still be sensitive to steroid; however, receptor-negative cells will not be. If objective response is defined as >50% tumor regression, it might appear that there was no clinical response even though all the sensitive cells disappeared. In such a situation, combined chemotherapy and hormonal therapy would probably be more appropriate as described later in Sect. F.

The remainder of this chapter is devoted to a detailed examination of a few specific steroid-resistant systems, with the goal of further developing some of the points outlined in this section.

C. S49 Lymphoma and WEHI-7 Thymoma Murine Cell Lines

The S49 cell line, an established line of glucocorticoid-responsive mouse lymphoma cells that has retained several properties of normal immature mouse T-lymphocytes (HORIBATA and HARRIS 1970), has proved extremely useful in the study of glucocorticoid resistance, and through these studies much has been learned of the mechanism of glucocorticoid action (reviewed by YAMAMOTO et al. 1976; GEHRING 1978; SIBLEY and YAMAMOTO 1979). These cells normally have a cloning efficiency of close to 100% when plated in soft agar with mouse fibroblasts as feeder cells; however, if the synthetic glucocorticoid, dexamethasone, is present in high concentrations, cloning efficiency approaches zero. Those colonies that do form are permanently steroid resistant. Using this selection technique, four types of mutant cell lines have been identified (Table 1). The vast majority of these are receptor negative (r^-) (YAMAMOTO et al. 1976; PFAHL et al. 1978; GEHRING 1978; SIBLEY and YAMAMOTO 1979). This category includes cells with no binding activity as well as cells with greatly decreased binding. However, until the critical experiments are carried out using specific antibodies, cells with no receptor protein cannot be distinguished from cells that contain receptor but have a lesion at the steroid-binding site.

Another category of mutants, the nuclear transfer negative (nt^-), includes those cell lines that have cytoplasmic receptor, but there is a defect in the ability of the receptors to translocate to and bind in the nucleus. From cell-free incubation studies in which nuclei and cytoplasm from wild-type (*wt*) and nt^- cells were mixed in various combinations, it was established that the defect was in the cytoplasm (GEHRING and TOMKINS 1974), most probably in the receptor itself (SIBLEY and YAMAMOTO 1979) since complementation studies ruled out the presence of a modulator of the nuclear interaction (GEHRING 1978; PFAHL et al. 1978). A third category of mutants is characterized by an increased binding to nuclei (nt^i), and in all nt^i mutants so far examined the cytoplasmic receptor is smaller, exhibiting a molecular weight of only 50,000, compared with 90,000 for the wild-type receptor (SIBLEY and YAMAMOTO 1979). A greater proportion of the nt^i receptor-steroid complexes bind to nuclei than in the wild-type cells and in addition it has been

Table 1. Characteristics of glucocorticoid-resistant S49 cell lines

Type	Defect	Comments
r^-	Receptor-negative	Majoritiy of mutants fall into this category. Cannot distinguish mutants that lack receptor from mutants whose receptor protein is present but deficient in steroid binding
nt^-	Nuclear-transfer-negative	Probably due to defect in cytoplasmic receptor; molecular weight is same, but sedimentation constant is slightly altered
nt^i	Increased nuclear transfer	Increased binding to nuclei. Molecular weight of cytoplasmic receptor is 50,000, compared with 90,000 for wild type
d^-	Deathless phenotype	Rare. Receptor is normal according to both physical and binding criteria. Defect is probably after nuclear-binding step

shown that the nt^i receptor complex binds more avidly to DNA-cellulose than does that from the parent steroid-sensitive cells (YAMAMOTO et al. 1974, 1976; SIBLEY and YAMAMOTO 1979). The final category of mutants, the so-called deathless phenotype (d^-), is rare. By both physical and binding criteria, the cytoplasmic receptor and its binding to nuclei appear to be equivalent to the wild type (SIBLEY and YAMAMOTO 1979), so the defect probably occurs after the nuclear-binding step. This particular group of mutants bears further examination since knowledge of the mechanism of their insensitivity to steroid could further our understanding of steroid action, especially at the point where it is least understood. In all these studies it is interesting to note that no mutant clone was isolated that was resistant to dexamethasone by virtue of its having a defect at the step of steroid transport. This could indicate that there is no active or facilitated process of steroid entry into this cell; on the other hand, the selection process, involving growth at high concentrations of dexamethasone, certainly did not favor selecting such a mutant.

In an interesting series of papers, BOURGEOIS and her co-workers (BOURGEOIS and NEWBY 1977; PFAHL et al. 1978; BOURGEOIS et al. 1978) have suggested that the S49 lymphoma cell line is functionally haploid (r^+/r^-) for a gene coding for the glucocorticoid receptor. The glucocorticoid-sensitive mouse thymoma line, WEHI-7, in contrast, appears to be diploid (r^+/r^+). Evidence for this is based on the following observations. First, there are twice as many receptors in the WEHI-7 cell line as in the S49 line, although the affinity for dexamethasone is similar. Second, while the frequency of spontaneous glucocorticoid-resistant mutants is high in the S49 cell line [3.5×10^{-6}/cell per generation (SIBLEY and YAMAMOTO 1979)], it is much lower for the WEHI-7 cell line [$<3 \times 10^{-9}$ (BOURGEOIS and NEWBY 1977)]. Furthermore, by growth of the WEHI-7 cell line in low concentrations of dexamethasone, it is possible to select mutants that are similar to the S49, i.e., that are less sensitive to glucocorticoid and that have one-half the receptor content of the parent WEHI-7 cell line. In addition, these variants, like the S49, give rise to fully resistant variants with a frequency of 2×10^{-6} (BOURGEOIS and NEWBY 1977; BOURGEOIS et al. 1978). These findings have led BOURGEOIS and

Table 2. Receptor content of parental lines and hybrids (Bourgeois and Newby 1979)

Cell line	Selective marker	Receptor alleles	No. of r^+ alleles/cell	Receptor sites/cell	$K_d \times 10^8$
W7TB	BrdUrd	r^+/r^+	2	28,000 ± 300 [a]	1.4 ± 0.2 [a]
W7TG	TG	r^+/r^+	2	30,100 ± 1,100	1.3 ± 0.1
MS1	BrdUrd	r^+/r^-	1	14,700 ± 1,100	1.5 ± 0.4
EO24	TG	r^+/r^-	1	13,200 ± 200	1.2 ± 0.2
AN6	BrdUrd	r^-/r^-	0	< 100	
SL3	TG	r^-/r^-	0	< 100	
W7TB × W7TG		$r^+/r^+ \times r^+/r^+$	4	57,500 ± 3,900 [b]	1.4 ± 0.2 [b]
W7TB × EO24		$r^+/r^+ \times r^+/r^-$	3	44,600 [c]	1.7 [c]
W7TG × MS1		$r^+/r^+ \times r^+/r^-$	3	41,000 [c]	1.8 [c]
W7TB × SL3		$r^+/r^+ \times r^-/r^-$	2	33,700 ± 1,700	1.5 ± 0.4
MS1 × EO24		$r^+/r^- \times r^+/r^-$	2	33,200 ± 1,500	1.7 ± 0.2
W7TG × AN6		$r^+/r^+ \times r^-/r^-$	2	30,700 [c]	1.2 [c]
MS1 × SL3		$r^+/r^- \times r^-/r^-$	1	12,700 ± 1,500 [d]	1.5 ± 0.3 [d]

[a] Mean ± SE
[b] Mean ± SE for two independent hybrid clones
[c] Single determinations
[d] Mean ± SE for four independent hybrid clones

her co-workers (1978) to suggest that in diploid lymphoma cell lines the development of resistance to high concentrations of glucocorticoid occurs in two steps:

$$r^+/r^+ \rightarrow r^+/r^- \rightarrow r^-/r^-$$

Each step occurs at a frequency of 10^{-6} and results in inactivation of one of the alleles of a gene coding for the receptor. It was also established that the receptor gene is autosomal and sensitivity is dominant over resistance (Bourgeois and Newby 1977; Pfahl et al. 1978; Gehring 1978).

Bourgeois and co-workers (1978) originally suggested that the reduced amount of receptor in the r^+/r^- phenotype leads to decreased sensitivity to steroid, and more recent studies have borne out this prediction. In an elegant series of experiments (Bourgeois and Newby 1979), various murine thymoma cell lines that are either homozygous (r^+/r^+ or r^-/r^-) or heterozygous (r^+/r^-) for the glucocorticoid structural gene were fused, producing hybrid clones that contained from one to four copies of the r^+ allele. In each of these hybrids and in the parent cell lines the number of glucocorticoid receptor sites was proportional to the number of r^+ alleles per cell (Table 2). Furthermore, by growth of each hybrid in various concentrations of dexamethasone, it was evident that sensitivity to dexamethasone, as measured by the cytolytic response, was determined by the number of receptors per cell (Fig. 4b). Thus the tetraploid line containing only one r^+ allele per cell (1 r^+/4n) was most resistant, and the tetraploid line with 4r^+ alleles (4r^+/4n) was most sensitive. For some reason that still has not been clarified, the parent diploid cell lines (2r^+/2n) were more sensitive than the tetra-

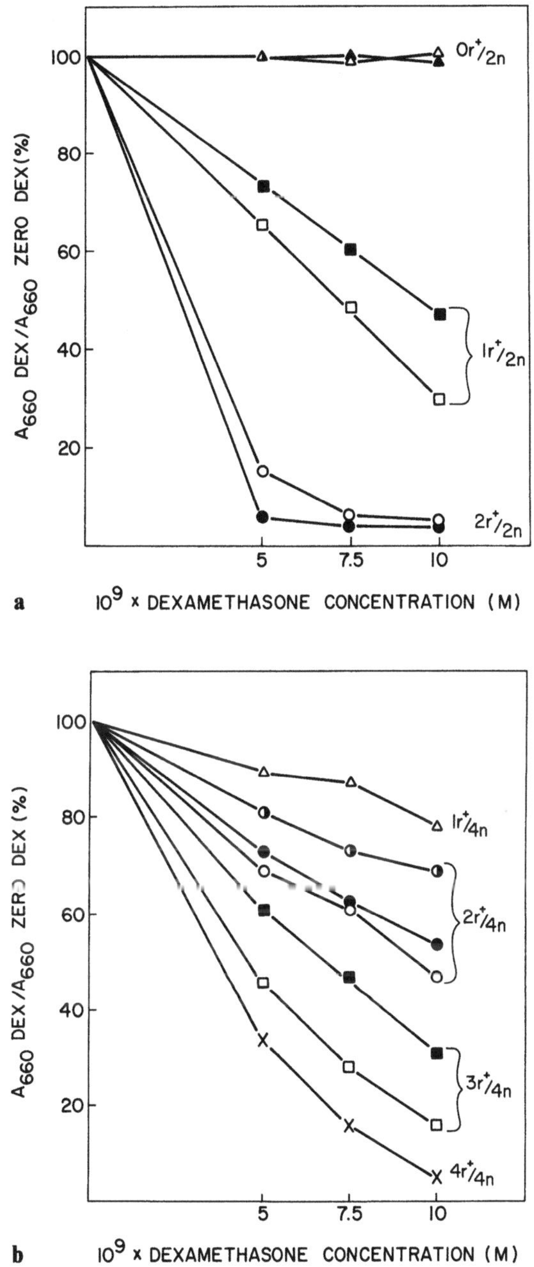

Fig. 4 a, b. Sensitivity to dexamethasone of parental and hybrid cell lines. The cellular material present in cultures after eight doublings was monitored by turbidity at 660 nm. The results obtained for the cultures with dexamethasone are expressed as percentages of the A_{660} reached in the control without steroid. **a** Parental lines: ●, W7TB; ○, W7TG; □, E024; ■, MS1; ▲, AN6; △, SL3. **b** Hybrid lines: X, W7TB × W7TG; □, W7TB × E024; ■, W7TG × MS1; ○, W7TG × AN6; ●, MS1 × E024; ◑, W7TB × SL3; △, MS1 × SL3. The number of r^+ alleles in each diploid (2n) or tetraploid (4n) line is indicated. (Bourgeois and Newby 1979)

ploid line ($4r^+/4n$) (compare Fig. 4a with Fig. 4b). These studies suggest that there is a relatively tight correlation between receptor concentration and steroid sensitivity and that in the absence of other factors limiting sensitivity steroid responsiveness is a function of receptor concentration.

D. The P1798 Mouse Lymphosarcoma

The P1798 mouse lymphosarcoma was originally described by LAMPKIN and POTTER (1958). The tumor arose as a large thymic mass in a BALB/c male mouse that had been implanted with a diethylstilbesterol pellet, and was extremely sensitive to cortisone, which caused an almost complete regression of tumor mass. Sensitivity to cortisone was maintained for several transplant generations (LAMPKIN and POTTER 1958; LAMPKIN-HIBBARD 1966) and is still being maintained today in several laboratories. It was also possible to develop a subline of the P1798 lymphosarcoma resistant to cortisone since it had been observed that after cortisone had caused an almost complete regression the tumor always regrew, although survival of the mouse was prolonged by cortisone treatment. The resistant subline was produced in one generation by repeated treatment with cortisone each time the tumor regrew. By the fourth and fifth such treatments the effect of cortisone was markedly reduced, and with the sixth treatment the tumor continued to grow in the presence of cortisone (LAMPKIN and POTTER 1958). This resistant subline has remained stable on repeated transplants.

In the ensuing years, numerous studies have been carried out in an attempt to assess biochemical differences between the cortisol-sensitive and -resistant lines of the P1798 lymphosarcoma and to determine the basis for the resistance. Early studies showed that the lack of sensitivity of the resistant tumor to the lytic effect of cortisol in vivo is correlated with a lack of in vitro sensitivity as well. Thus, cortisol administered in vivo or incubated in vitro with cell suspensions resulted in an early inhibition of glucose uptake, followed at later time periods by an inhibition of thymidine, uridine, and leucine uptake into DNA, RNA, and protein, respectively, in the cortisol-sensitive tumor. Inhibition in the resistant tumor was either absent or greatly reduced (RAINA and ROSEN 1969; ROSEN et al. 1970a, b, 1972; STEVENS et al. 1974).

A great deal of work has been carried out to try and determine the mechanism for the cortisol resistance of the P1798R subline, but comparison of results from one laboratory to another is complicated by the apparent divergence of the tumor which has resulted from repeated passages in different laboratories. Such changes are due to different transplantation techniques, including age of the tumor at the time of passage, routine passage in male or female mice, plus the inherent instability of the tumor itself. In any case, even if it is subsequently found that there are several sublines of the cortisol-resistant P1798 lymphosarcoma, the work done to date has been extremely useful in elucidating some of the possible modes of steroid resistance that occur in the in vivo situation.

The earliest studies were done with the original tumors of LAMPKIN (LAMPKIN and POTTER 1958; LAMPKIN-HIBBARD 1966). These showed that there were no differences in the uptake or metabolism of cortisol between the two lines (CHANG et al. 1964; HOLLANDER and CHIU 1966a); however, there were fewer specific glu-

Table 3. Comparison of the nuclear glucocorticoid receptors from the cortisol-sensitive and -resistant lines of the P1798 murine lymphosarcoma (STEVENS and STEVENS 1979)

	P1798S	P1798R
Sedimentation constant	3.70 ± 0.02	3.30 ± 0.03
Stokes radius (Å)	57.4 ± 0.7	29.1 ± 0.3
Molecular weight	90,000	40,000
Molecules/nucleus	$12{,}943 \pm 562$	$6{,}135 \pm 427$
Dissociation constant (n*M*)	10 ± 1	11 ± 2

cocorticoid receptors in the cytosol of resistant tumors compared with the sensitive tumors (HOLLANDER and CHIU 1966b; KIRKPATRICK et al. 1971, 1972; KAISER et al. 1974), suggesting that at least part of the resistance might be due to decreased receptor numbers. More recent transplants of the glucocorticoid-resistant line in our laboratory have, however, been shown to contain similar numbers of receptor molecules to the sensitive line (McPARTLAND et al. 1977). In addition to changes in receptor numbers, it has also been shown that the receptor isolated from the P1798R subline has altered properties. KAISER et al. (1974), for example, showed that the sedimentation constant of the receptor extracted with 0.15 *M* KCl from the crude nuclear pellet of a P1798R cell suspension sedimented at 3.7S on a sucrose gradient, in contrast to 4.1S for the receptor from the sensitive tumor. The corresponding values for the cytosol receptor (in 0.02 *M* Tris; no KCl) were 7.4S and 7.1S for resistant and sensitive, respectively. In spite of these changes in sedimentation constant, the binding affinity for both receptors was similar in the sensitive and resistant sublines of the tumor. A difference in sedimentation constants of the nuclear receptors from sensitive and resistant tumors was also reported by STEVENS and STEVENS (1979) (Table 3). Furthermore, analysis of the receptors by agarose gel filtration showed that the molecular weight of the sensitive receptor was 90,000, compared with 40,000 for the receptor from the resistant cells. Careful studies showed that the smaller size of the receptor from the P1798R tumor was not due to cleavage, nor the larger size of the P1798S receptor due to aggregation. The cytosol receptor from each cell type was similar in size to the corresponding nuclear receptor. These results are markedly similar to what has been described in the S49 cell line (see Sect. C). In that case the molecular weight of the receptor from the glucocorticoid-sensitive wild-type cell line was 90,000 and that from the nt^i (increased nuclear transfer) mutant, 50,000.

So far it has not been established whether the smaller receptor is responsible for the glucocorticoid resistance and if so, what the mechanism of action would be. In the case of the nt^i S49 mutant the result is actually an increased binding of steroid-receptor complex to nuclei (YAMAMOTO et al. 1974, 1976; SIBLEY and YAMAMOTO 1979). STEVENS and co-workers (1978) also concluded that interactions of [^{3}H]triamcinolone acetonide (TA) with nuclei from the resistant tumor were stronger than that observed with the sensitive tumor, based on experiments which showed that low concentrations of monovalent (KCl), divalent (Ca^{++} or Mg^{++}), or polyvalent (spermidine) cations extracted more [^{3}H]TA from P1798S than P1798R nuclei. These results are in contrast with those reported by McPARTLAND et al. (1977), who found that steroid-nuclear interactions were actually weaker in the resistant tumor and attributed resistance to this factor. The basis for the discrepancy between the results of STEVENS et al. (1978) and MCPARTLAND et al. (1977) is not readily apparent. However, the fact that the tumors used by each group have been maintained in the respective laboratories for several transplant generations offers one possible explanation. It is of interest that in both P1798R sublines the total number of steroid-receptor complexes associated with the nucleus was lower than that seen with the corresponding sensitive sublines.

Other workers have concluded that other factors may be, in part, responsible for the glucocorticoid resistance of the P1798R lymphosarcoma. TURNELL and co-workers (1973), for example, examined free fatty acid (FFA) pools in tumors of mice treated with cortisol and showed that pool size increased in the sensitive tumor and decreased in the resistant one. Further studies showed that the neutral fat content of the resistant tumor was one-half that of the sensitive, and, coupled with the fact that incubation of cells with FFA mimicked some of the nuclear effects of cortisol, they suggested that cytolysis results from an accumulation of FFA and resistance results from an enhanced capacity for FFA oxidation (TURNELL and BURTON 1974, 1975).

In this laboratory, MILHOLLAND and co-workers (1979) have shown that phosphorylation of three proteins that co-elute with the high mobility group (HMG) nuclear proteins is markedly reduced in the P1798S tumor after cortisol treatment in vivo; no effect of cortisol was noted in the P1798R tumor. The phosphorylation of another co-eluting protein, of molecular weight 90,000, was enhanced 75% by cortisol in the sensitive tumor, but again, cortisol was without effect in the resistant tumor. More recent studies (MILHOLLAND and IP, unpublished) have shown that the striking decrease in phosphorylation of the three proteins is associated with tumor regression rather than with cortisol treatment per se. When mice bearing the P1798S tumor were treated with cytosine arabinoside (araC) or mice bearing the P1798R tumor with 5-fluorouracil, in amounts calculated to give the same amount of tumor regression as seen with cortisol treatment of mice bearing the sensitive tumor, phosphorylation in both tumors was decreased to the extent seen with cortisol initially. Only the enhanced phosphorylation of the 90K protein appears to be specific for cortisol and for the sensitive tumor. The relevance of this protein to the mechanism of action of cortisol is still unknown. It is of interest that YOUNG and co-workers (NICHOLSON et al. 1979; VORIS et al. 1979) reported the synthesis of a new protein in P1798R tumors, but again the relevance of this is unknown at this time.

Many other differences have also been reported. Thus, NICHOLSON and YOUNG (1978, 1979) also found that nuclear fragility was increased 3 h after cortisol treatment of mice bearing the P1798S lymphosarcoma and 6 h after similar treatment of the P1798R tumor, and concluded that resistance to glucocorticoids developed by selection of cells with hardier membranes. BEHRENS and co-workers (1974, 1976) found differences in cell membrane properties of both the sensitive and resistant lines of the P1798 lymphosarcoma and concluded that sensitivity may be related to structural differences at the cell surface. These investigators determined the number of anionic sites on the cell membrane by fixing cell pellets with Alcian Blue 8GX and examining by electron microscopy (BEHRENS et al.

1974). This study showed definite histological differences between the sensitive and resistant tumors: dye complexes were present on cell surfaces of the P1798S tumors but were absent from the P1798R tumors. Some heterogeneity was noted in that a small number of the P1798S cells lacked cell coat, and a very small number of the P1798R cells had it. Further study showed that the negative charges on the P1798S cells were lost 6–8 h after glucocorticoid treatment; P1798R cells had no or few negative charges on the surface before or after steroid treatment (BEHRENS and HOLLANDER 1976). Both tumors were shown to contain sialoglycopeptides on the cell membrane, but these were different in the sensitive and resistant tumors. Interestingly, the glycopeptides of *both* tumors changed after cortisol treatment, but the differences between the sublines persisted. These investigators concluded that specific cell surface sialoglycoproteins are probably involved in mediating glucocorticoid sensitivity, perhaps by influencing cell-cell interactions (BEHRENS and HOLLANDER 1976). The data also suggest a reason why MCPARTLAND et al. (1977) only noted effects of concanavalin A on the sensitive tumor. As an aside, two other points are of interest in the work reported by BEHRENS and co-workers, in addition to the main data. The first, and perhaps most interesting point, is that a biochemical response to glucocorticoids was noted in the glucocorticoid-"resistant" tumor, specifically a change in cell surface glycoprotein. This suggests that in the P1798 lymphosarcoma as well as in leukemic cells (Sect. E) and in the MTW-9B mammary tumor (Sect. F) there might be a dissociation between the growth/lytic effects of steroid hormones and certain biochemical parameters. This should make the P1798 lymphosarcoma an important model to pursue. The second point of interest in the above experiments is the fact that both sublines of the tumor appeared to be heterogeneous since anionic sites were lacking on some cells from the sensitive tumor and were present on some cells from the resistant tumor. KAISER et al. (1974) had also concluded that the resistant tumor was heterogeneous, based on experiments in which cortisol administration to mice bearing the P1798R lymphosarcoma resulted in a decreased number of glucocorticoid receptors in the P1798R tumor compared with P1798S (30% of P1798S levels 73 h after cortisol). This reduction was attributed to the fact that the sensitive cells present in the P1798R tumor were killed by cortisol, and the remaining cells, all resistant, contained lower numbers of glucocorticoid receptors.

Recent data from the laboratory of THOMPSON and co-workers (DAVIS et al. 1980; THOMPSON et al. 1980), while intriguing, are difficult to fit into any of the above data, perhaps because the P1798 lymphosarcoma variant that they obtained from Litton Bionetics is unrelated to the other variants. THOMPSON and co-workers found that as the P1798 lymphosarcoma (the original cortisol sensitivity of the subline they used was unknown to them), implanted subcutaneously, grew larger, it abruptly lost its sensitivity to cortisol. Specifically, tumors with a radius^2 of >100 mm^2 were resistant to a single 100-mg/kg injection of cortisol, while tumors <100 mm^2 were sensitive. It was of interest that cells grown in the ascitic fluid were always sensitive to cortisol even though the cell suspension used for inoculation was prepared from large (cortisol-resistant) subcutaneous tumors. These results are in contrast to the original data of LAMPKIN (1958, 1966), who demonstrated that both large and small subcutaneous tumors of the P1798S subline were sensitive to cortisol, and that ascites cells were either sensitive or resistant to cortisol depending on the subline used for inoculation. In our own laboratory, the P1798S subline remains sensitive to cortisol up to the point at which the animal is ready to die as a result of the tumor burden. In our hands, for example, tumors as large as 32 mm in average tumor diameter ($r^2 \approx 256\ mm^2$) will regress by 50% 24 h after a single s.c. injection of 50 mg/kg hydrocortisone acetate (MILHOLLAND et al. 1979; IP et al., unpublished). THOMPSON and co-workers (1980) also showed that cortisol inhibited the DNA synthetic index and [^{3}H] thymidine incorporation in tumors with a radius^2 of less than 90 mm^2, but had no effect on tumors larger than this. These data, while different from those reported by other laboratories, are extremely interesting because they imply an entirely different mechanism for the development of resistance. In this P1798 variant, resistance develops in a size-dependent manner, rather than by a gradual increase in the proportion of resistant cells, and is reversible (by inoculation into the ascitic fluid). This suggests that in this case resistance does not result from any stable change in the genotype, but rather that this variant of the P1798 lymphosarcoma undergoes some epigenetic alteration in the phenotype, which leads to glucocorticoid resistance.

E. Human Leukemia

Although glucocorticoids either alone or in combination have been used for 30 years in the treatment of human leukemias and lymphomas (PEARSON and ELIEL 1950; FESSAS et al. 1954; RANNEY and GELLHORN 1957; GRANVILLE et al. 1958; SHANBROM and MILLER 1962; ROATH et al. 1964; HENDERSON 1973; CLINE 1974; CARTER 1978; DEBUSSCHER and STRYCKMANS 1978), the detailed mechanism of the lytic effect has still not been elucidated. What is clear, however, is that if the steroid is acting directly it must initially bind to its cytoplasmic receptor. In the absence of receptor, by implication, the cell is resistant to the steroid. Based on this assumption and also on the detailed work done with the S49 mouse lymphoma, in which it could be shown that 80%–90% of the glucocorticoid-resistant mutant clones were insensitive by virtue of having substantially decreased or altered binding activity (YAMAMOTO et al. 1976; PFAHL et al. 1978; GEHRING 1978; SIBLEY and YAMAMOTO 1979), it seemed logical to examine human leukemic cells for the glucocorticoid receptor. As used for treatment of the leukemias, the glucocorticoids are relatively toxic, and it was reasoned that a better selection of potential candidates for glucocorticoid therapy could be made based on a quantitation of the glucocorticoid receptor in the cells from each patient.

Initial results, in which the cytoplasmic glucocorticoid receptor was measured, were encouraging. Thus, LIPPMAN et al. (1973) and GAILANI et al. (1973) found significant glucocorticoid-binding activity in cells from 22/22 and 3/3, respectively, untreated patients with acute lymphoblastic leukemia (ALL), a disease in which the majority of patients show an objective response to glucocorticoids (HENDERSON 1973). Receptor levels were approximately tenfold higher than that found in peripheral blood lymphocytes from normal volunteers (LIPPMAN et al. 1973). Of interest was the fact that in relapsed patients previously treated with glucocorticoids six were now resistant to such therapy and their cells had no glucocorticoid-binding activity; six other patients continued to be sensitive and their cells contained the same amount of receptor as was found in untreated ALL patients (LIPPMAN et al. 1973). LIPPMAN et al. (1973) also showed that in these same patients the presence of the glucocorticoid receptor correlated with the ability of dexamethasone to inhibit [^{3}H]thymidine incorporation into the cells in vitro. Conversely, the absence of receptor was associated with lack of in vitro responsiveness. Using a similar cytosol assay, glucocorticoid receptors were also detected in a small number of patients with acute myelogenous leukemia (AML); specifically GAILANI et al. (1973) showed that the receptor was present in 2/6 of such patients and LIPPMAN et al. (1975) in 3/16. In the latter case, the presence of the receptor was positively correlated with dexamethasone inhibition of thymidine incorporation into myeloblasts in vitro, and its absence with lack of any effect. TERENIUS and co-workers (1976) demonstrated by the cytosol assay that the glucocorticoid receptor was present in 17/27 patients with chronic lymphatic leukemia (CLL), and in 4/6 patients with the receptor there was a clinical response to glucocorticoid therapy. GAILANI et al. (1973) found no receptors present in eight CLL patients, nor in two patients with chronic myelocytic leukemia (CML).

As mentioned above, these results were encouraging because they appeared to correlate the presence of the glucocorticoid receptor with sensitivity to glucocorticoid therapy, since ALL and CLL are relatively sensitive and AML and CML are not. The whole matter has become much more complicated, however, since it was demonstrated that by use of a whole cell assay receptors could be detected in all leukemic cells examined (KONIOR-YARBRO et al. 1977; KONIOR et al. 1977b; HOMO et al. 1978, 1980; CRABTREE et al. 1978; SCHMIDT and THOMPSON 1978; BELL et al. 1979; STEVENS et al. 1979; THOMPSON 1979; HO et al. 1980; BLOOMFIELD et al. 1980). The biological significance of these receptors is not yet known and in fact there is considerable controversy concerning the relationship of receptor levels with in vivo and in vitro sensitivity to glucocorticoids.

KONIOR and her co-workers in LIPPMAN's laboratory found that there is a good correlation between the number of glucocorticoid receptors in childhood ALL and complete remission duration (KONIOR-YARBRO 1977; KONIOR et al. 1977a; LIPPMAN 1979). Patients with ALL can be subdivided into two major categories, those with T-cell ALL (and a poorer prognosis) and those with null-cell ALL (the majority of patients). The latter category can be further subdivided based on the ability of the cells to stimulate allogeneic donors in mixed lymphocyte culture (MLC). When cells from each type were analyzed for glucocorticoid receptor, it was found that receptor levels were highest in null cells that stimulated in MLC (MLC+) and lowest in T cells (Table 4). Null cells that did not stimulate in MLC were intermediate (KONIOR-YARBRO et al. 1977). Interestingly, there appeared to be a correlation between receptor levels and prognosis of the patient, independent of whether the leukemia was of the T-cell or null-cell type. Thus KONIOR and co-workers (KONIOR et al. 1977a; LIPPMAN 1979) showed that in patients with T-cell ALL whose receptor levels were less than 2,500 sites/cell the median complete remission duration (CRD) was 7.6 months. In T-cell patients with receptor levels of 2501–6000 the CRD was 18.5 months, not significantly different from the 22.7 months observed in null-cell patients with receptors in the

Table 4. Glucocorticoid receptor levels in subpopulations of childhood acute lymphocytic leukemia (KONIOR-YARBRO et al. 1977)

ALL category	No. of patients	Glucocorticoid receptor (sites/cells)		
		Range	Median	Mean
Null cell (MLC+)	18	4,096–21,869	7,571	10,117
Null cell (MLC−)	9	2,936–16,469	4,484	6,729
T cell	18	0– 5,887	2,173	2,538

same range. The longest CRD (>26 months) was seen in patients with null-cell ALL who had glucocorticoid receptor levels in excess of 6000 sites/cell. Both null groups were equivalent in age and initial white blood cell count. These results are of great significance since they suggest that glucocorticoid receptor levels can be used as a separate prognostic indicator, independent of cell type or age or white blood cell count. It is important that they be confirmed in larger groups of patients and in other laboratories, however, since there already appears to be some controversy (HOMO et al. 1980).

HOMO and his colleagues (1980), for example, have reported that they found no difference in glucocorticoid receptor levels in male patients with null-cell or T-cell ALL. In this work, six patients with each disease were studied, and mean values of 10,128 and 10,365 sites/cell were found, respectively. Unfortunately the more appropriate median values and ranges were not reported and the null-cell patients were not further subdivided. HOMO et al. (1980) also found that receptor levels were twice as high in null cells from male patients as from females; such a difference was not found by KONIOR-YARBRO et al. (1977) and if anything the values from female patients were slightly higher. Of most importance in the work of HOMO et al. (1980) was the absence of any correlation between glucocorticoid receptor levels and in vivo and in vitro sensitivity to glucocorticoids. Eleven of their patients were treated with prednisolone (40 mg × ^{2}) for 2–4 days before starting combined chemotherapy. Only six of these responded by showing a decrease in both white blood cell levels and levels of circulating blast cells, and there was no relationship between receptor levels and response. In addition, in vitro sensitivity to glucocorticoids, as measured by inhibition of uridine or thymidine incorporation, was not dependent on glucocorticoid receptor levels, but for thymidine, at least, the effect was more related to the presence or absence of cells in the S-phase. They also showed that the sex differences in glucocorticoid receptor levels were not associated with sex differences in steroid sensitivity.

In agreement with this work are the studies of CRABTREE et al. (1978), which also demonstrated a lack of correlation between glucocorticoid receptor levels and steroid sensitivity. These workers showed that receptors were present in a whole range of hematological cancers, including the glucocorticoid-sensitive cancers such as ALL, CLL, and lymphoma; and the glucocorticoid-insensitive cancers such as AML, CML, acute myelomonocytic leukemia, and erythroleukemia. Moreover, as can be seen from Table 5, all cells were sensitive to glucocorticoids in vitro, independent of nuclear receptor concentration. It is also of interest that cells from 15 patients with acute non-lymphoblastic leukemia (ANLL), a set of

Table 5. Glucocorticoid receptors and sensitivity in normal lymphocytes and isolated leukemic and lymphoma cells (CRABTREE et al. 1978)

Cells	No. of subjects	Dexamethasone binding		Mean % decrease[c]				
		R_0[a] (sites/cell)	CNT[b]	Glucose uptake	Incorporation of			Viable cell count
					Leucine	Uridine	Thymidine	
Normal human peripheral lymphocytes	10	3,284 (840–6,720)[d]	4/4[e]	22 (15–30)	29 (20–36)			32 (19–49)
Peripheral lymphoblasts from patients with ALL[f]	6	4,600 (900–7,071)	5/5	58 (40–87)	55 (44–62)	69 (64–74)	41 (4–74)	47 (0–98)
Peripheral lymphocytes from patients with CLL	12	2,119 (400–4,620)	9/10	47 (0–80)	35 (12–60)	44 (20–70)		61 (18–95)
Lymph node and peripheral blood cells from lymphomas[g]	6	1,710 (477–2,690)	4/5	35 (14–53)	29 (17–53)	46 (18–74)	47 (40–53)	64 (38–79)
Blasts from patients with ANLL[h]	15	4,811 (1,920–13,230)	13/15	25 (−33–77)	16 (−62–54)	25 (−48–70)	3 (−64–70)	22 (−92–93)
Peripheral blasts from patients with CML in blast crisis	4	5,047 (2,610–6,300)	3/3	66 (0–51)	50 (−50–68)	42 (18–70)	53 (25–68)	40 (0–82)
Peripheral blood cells from patients with leukemic reticuloendotheliosis	2	4,940 (4,490–5,340)	2/2	20	41 (41–42)	36 (22–50)	42	34 (18–50)
Peripheral myelocytes from a patient with CML	1	2,607	1/1		38	22		0

[a] R_0, mean number of nuclear binding sites per cell

[b] CNT, cytoplasmic-to-nuclear translocation, scored positive if cells that had been incubated with 10 n*M* dexamethasone at 3 °C showed an increase in the ratio of nuclear to cytoplasmic binding when warmed to 37 °C

[c] The mean percentage decrease in glucose uptake was measured with a 30-s pulse of D[^{14}C]glucose after 4-h incubation with 1 μ*M* dexamethasone. The mean percentage decrease in isotope incorporation was measured after 24 h incubation with 100 n*M* dexamethasone. The mean percentage decrease in the viable cell count, based on final viable cell number in parallel control cultures without dexamethasone, was measured after 96–144 h incubation with 400 n*M* dexamethasone and was calculated as $100(C-E)/C$, where C and E are the control and experimental viable cell counts, respectively

[d] Numbers in parentheses indicate the range

[e] Number of positives/number tested

[f] This group included one patient with T-cell ALL (900 sites/cell) and two patients with null-cell ALL (5,020 and 2,511 sites/cell). Four of the patients were adults

[g] This group included three patients with poorly differentiated diffuse lymphoma, one patient with poorly differentiated nodular lymphoma, and one patient with well-differentiated diffuse lymphoma. The remaining patient had mycosis fungoides with large numbers of malignant cells in the peripheral blood

[h] This group included 11 patients with acute myelocytic leukemia, one patient with acute undifferentiated leukemia, one patient with erythroleukemia, and two patients with acute myelomonocytic leukemia

clinically less responsive leukemias, actually contained somewhat higher receptor levels than did the other groups. In vitro sensitivity to dexamethasone was demonstrated in these ANLL cells, but, as can be seen from Table 5, the effect was not as great as that observed with the other cell types, and in some cases a stimulation rather than an inhibition of precursor incorporation was observed (this was also noted by Homo et al. 1980). This variability suggests that it is probably not wise to lump all the ANLL patients into one group, but rather, since a portion of these patients might be clinically sensitive to glucocorticoid, a way should be devised to identify them, perhaps by running a battery of in vitro sensitivity tests.

From the results reported so far, it can be concluded that, based on the whole-cell receptor assay: (a) glucocorticoid receptors are present in most leukemia cells; (b) glucocorticoid receptor levels in various types of leukemias do not correlate with in vitro sensitivity to dexamethasone as measured by inhibition of uridine, thymidine, or leucine uptake, or to in vivo single agent glucocorticoid therapy [an exception to this is malignant lymphoma in which median glucocorticoid receptor levels were shown to be higher in patients that subsequently responded to single agent glucocorticoid therapy (Bloomfield et al. 1980)]; (c) glucocorticoid receptor levels correlate with an increase in median complete remission duration in acute lymphoblastic leukemia patients treated with a combined chemotherapy regimen that included glucocorticoids.

Many theories can be advanced for the lack of correlation between glucocorticoid receptor levels and in vitro and/or in vivo sensitivity to glucocorticoid. The most simplistic is that we are looking at a variety of diseases and it is simply not relevant to compare the absolute glucocorticoid receptor level in one type of leukemia with another, including the various subsets of ALL. This would be unlike the mouse lymphoma model systems where the actual receptor concentration does appear to be important (Bourgeois and Newby 1979). From the work reported above, it can be seen that the *presence* of the receptor is biologically significant, since in almost every case in vitro sensitivity to dexamethasone, measured in at least one test, was observed. What is striking, however, is the lack of association of in vitro sensitivity with an in vivo clinical response, suggesting that the process of cell lysis by glucocorticoids is dissociated from the biochemical effects of glucocorticoids on precursor incorporation into macromolecules. A precedent for this does exist in human and experimental mammary cancer. Thus, as described in Sect. F, in the MTW-9B rat mammary tumor there appears to be a dissociation between the effects of estrogen on progesterone receptor synthesis and on growth (Ip et al. 1979, 1981) and in human breast cancer approximately 27% of patients in which both the estrogen and progesterone receptors are present do not respond to endocrine manipulation (see Table 6).

Probably the most important finding to come out of these studies so far is the apparent relationship between glucocorticoid receptor levels in ALL and the clinical response to combination chemotherapy. While we know that the glucocorticoid receptor is required for a glucocorticoid-mediated response, its presence alone is not sufficient to guarantee that a response will be elicited. What the data suggest, however, is that the glucocorticoid receptor may act as a biological marker for factors such as the state of differentiation or the growth rate that determine the response to chemotherapy.

The reason for the discrepancy between the cytosol and whole-cell assays is yet to be resolved. It is well known that the glucocorticoid receptor is very susceptible to degradation, and as a result of homogenization and the consequent release of degradative enzymes much or all of the receptor could easily be lost. More work needs to be done to see if the cytosol receptor can be stabilized with reagents such as molybdate, and if so to compare results obtained in the modified cytosol assay with results obtained in the whole-cell assay. Still, the fact that the cytosol assay appears to correlate with clinical sensitivity and the whole-cell assay does not, is intriguing, and, as noted by THOMPSON (1979) in his report on the International Union against Cancer Workshop on Steroid Receptors in Leukemia, the receptors measured in the cytosol assay could represent a significant subset that are in some way relevant to the biological response.

F. Breast Cancer

I. Estrogen Receptors

Approximately 30% of human breast cancers will respond to some form of endocrine treatment, including ovariectomy, adrenalectomy, hypophysectomy, antiestrogens, androgens, progestins, or pharmacological doses of estrogens. JENSEN et al. (1967) was the first to suggest that measurement of estrogen receptor (ER) levels in breast tumors might improve the selection of patients for endocrine therapy. It was reasoned that since normal breast tissue contained the estrogen receptor and was dependent on estrogen for growth the presence of an estrogen receptor in a breast tumor might predict that the tumor was also dependent on estrogen for growth. This theory was tested by several investigators who presented their data at an International Workshop sponsored by the Breast Cancer Task Force in 1974. In brief, it was shown that 55%–60% of patients whose tumors contained the estrogen receptor responded to some form of endocrine manipulation, although 8% of patients whose tumors lacked the estrogen receptor also responded (MCGUIRE et al. 1975). [See HAWKINS et al. (1980) for a review of the relationship between individual hormonal therapies and the presence or absence of the estrogen receptor.] Earlier studies found the estrogen receptor present in about 50% of all tumors examined (MCGUIRE et al. 1975); however, with improvements in techniques, recent data have shown that 70%–85% of all tumors contain the estrogen receptor (MCGUIRE et al. 1975; HAWKINS et al. 1980).

II. Estrogen and Progesterone Receptors

Although the above results suggested that Jensen's hypothesis was essentially correct, it was obvious that in 40%–45% of ER+ tumors the estrogen receptor was not functional for one reason or another, and as a result it was thought desirable to improve the predictability of the estrogen receptor assay. Based on several animal studies in which estrogen modulation of progesterone receptor (PgR) levels had been demonstrated (SHERMAN et al. 1970; RAO and WIEST 1971; TOFT and O'MALLEY 1972), HORWITZ and co-workers (HORWITZ et al. 1975) proposed that the simultaneous presence in breast tumors of the progesterone receptor with the estrogen receptor might suggest that the estrogen receptor was functional. Sub-

Table 6. Estrogen and progesterone receptors and response to hormonal therapy in 334 breast cancer patients

Reference	ER+ PgR+	ER+ PgR−	ER− PgR+	ER− PgR−
LECLERCQ and HEUSON (1977)	1/3	1/3	0/1	–
KING et al. (1978)	8/9	1/7	1/2	1/ 5
MCGUIRE (1978)	13/16	7/17	–	0/11
SKINNER et al. (1978)	4/7	0/3	–	5/17
YOUNG et al. (1978)	13/18	1/7	1/1	1/ 3
ALLEGRA et al. (1979c)	11/14	8/14	0/4	0/12
BLOOM et al. (1980)	23/30	3/14	1/1	0/10
NOMURA et al. (1980)	20/30	12/37	1/4	4/34
Total	93/127	33/102	4/13	11/92
Percentage	73.2	32.4	30.8	12.0

Table 7. Estrogen and progesterone receptors and response to hormonal therapy in 334 breast cancer patients[a]

Reference	ER+	ER−	PgR+	PgR−
LECLERCQ and HEUSON (1977)	2/6	0/1	1/4	1/3
KING et al. (1978)	9/16	2/7	9/11	2/12
MCGUIRE (1978)	20/33	0/11	13/16	7/28
SKINNER et al. (1978)	4/10	5/17	4/7	5/20
YOUNG et al. (1978)	14/25	2/4	14/19	2/10
ALLEGRA et al. (1979c)	19/28	0/16	11/18	8/26
BLOOM et al. (1980)	26/44	1/11	24/31	3/24
NOMURA et al. (1980)	32/67	5/38	21/34	16/71
Totals	126/229	15/105	97/140	44/194
Percentage	55.0	14.3	69.3	22.7

[a] This table is derived from the values in Table 6

sequently, such a relation was shown in the 7,12-dimethylbenz(a)anthracene (DMBA)-induced rat mammary tumor (ASSELIN et al. 1977; TSAI and KATZENELLENBOGEN 1978) and in the MCF-7 human breast cancer cell line (HORWITZ and MCGUIRE 1978). Moreover, estrogen and progesterone receptors have now been measured simultaneously by a number of investigators in human breast tumors and the results correlated with response to endocrine therapy. Some of these studies, on a total of 334 patients, are combined in Tables 6 and 7. From Table 6, it can be seen that patients with both receptors have a 73% chance of responding to endocrine therapy, compared with a 55% chance in these same patients if only the estrogen receptor is considered (Table 7). Interestingly, progesterone receptor alone appeared to predict response as well as both receptors together (Table 7).

While of substantial value, these results also demonstrate that the theory of HORWITZ et al. (1975) is not completely correct. Thus 32% of patients who had the estrogen receptor but in whom the progesterone receptor was absent responded, whereas 27% of patients who had both receptors did not respond. A portion of these results could be ascribed to technical difficulties in the proges-

Table 8. The effect of ovariectomy and estradiol treatment on tumor weight and progesterone receptors in the MTW-9B rat transplantable mammary tumor (IP et al. 1979)

Treatment	Progesterone receptor (fmol/mg protein)	Tumor weight (g)
Sham-ovariectomized	269.0±22	7.21±0.65
Ovaricctomizcd	53.8±10.0	7.74±0.95
Ovariectomized + estradiol benzoate (25 μg/kg)	329.0±50	6.13±0.88

Table 9. The effect of estradiol and tamoxifen on progesterone receptors in the MTW-9B mammary tumor from ovariectomized rats (IP et al. 1981)

Treatment	Progesterone receptor (fmol/mg protein)	Tumor weight (g)
Ovariectomy	11.1± 4.8	2.65±0.60
Ovariectomy + estradiol benzoate (25 μg/kg)	422.0±72	2.29±0.57
Ovariectomy + tamoxifen (0.5 mg/kg)	79.5± 6.6	2.88±0.65
Ovariectomy + estradiol benzoate (25 μg/kg)+tamoxifcn (0.5 mg/kg)	185.0±16	2.83±0.48

terone receptor assay; however, it is most probable that for many breast tumors the situation is much more complex than originally envisioned. For example, although the progesterone receptor appears to be an estrogen gene product, it has not clearly been established that there is an association between the effects of estrogen on growth and progesterone receptor synthesis, and in fact there is some evidence against this, at least in animal model systems. The MTW-9B transplantable mammary tumor, in Wistar/Furth rats, is estrogen independent as evidenced by its equal growth rate in syngeneic males and females and also by the lack of effect of ovariectomy or hypophysectomy on its growth rate (KIM and DEPOWSKI 1975). However, as can be seen from Tables 8 and 9, progesterone receptor levels are very much dependent on the estrogen status of the host (IP et al. 1979, 1981). Moreover, the induction of the progesterone receptor by estrogen in ovariectomized rats is blocked, at least partially, by tamoxifen, even though tamoxifen has no effect on tumor growth. Possible reasons for this discrepancy have been discussed previously (IP et al. 1979, 1981, and see Sect. B). In spite of this clear limitation, the measurement of the progesterone receptor in breast tumors remains clinically useful. Indeed, based on experiments with the Dunning rat prostate adenocarcinoma in rats, in which the inducibility of the progesterone receptor by estrogen was able to predict successfully an antitumor effect of tamoxifen (IP et al. 1980), the concept might also be extended to prostate cancer. In the latter case, since the progesterone receptor might not normally be present the biopsy would probably have to be done after a short (2- to 3-day) course of estrogen therapy.

III. Estrogen Resistance

As with other cancers which are thought to be endocrine dependent, there are many sites at which resistance can occur. As noted earlier, the estrogen receptor is absent in 15%–30% of breast tumors (McGuire et al. 1975; Hawkins et al. 1980). Furthermore, it appears that not only is the presence of the estrogen receptor required for a response to hormonal therapy, but the actual amount of receptor determines the response, just as was noted with acute lymphatic leukemia in Lippman's laboratory (Konior-Yarbro et al. 1977) and in the WEHI-7-murine thymoma system by Bourgeois and Newby (1979). Specifically, Jensen (1975) reported that patients whose tumor estrogen receptor level was greater than 750 fmol/g tumor had a better chance of responding. In another series of patients, McGuire et al. (1978) reported that the response to hormonal therapy was 6%, 46%, and 81% in patients whose estrogen receptor levels were <3, 3–100, and 101–1,000 fmol/mg protein, respectively. Allegra et al. (1980) have recently reported similar findings. Although these results could be due to an effect of receptor number per se, it is more likely that the increased number of receptor sites reflects the proportion of hormone-sensitive cells in the tumor and therefore the increased likelihood of a response. Qualitative as well as quantitative differences in the estrogen receptor might also lead to resistance. Wittliff et al. (1978), for example, have suggested that the presence of an 8S receptor in a low-salt sucrose gradient frequently is associated with a clinical response, whereas the presence of only a 4–5S component usually is not. Surprisingly, there appeared to be no relationship between the dissociation constant of the estrogen receptor and the clinical response (Allegra et al. 1980).

Certain breast tumors in which a cytosol estrogen receptor has been demonstrated fail to translocate the steroid-receptor complex into the nucleus (Garola and McGuire 1977; Thorsen 1979; Fazekas and MacFarlane 1980; Hähnel et al. 1980; Romic-Stojkovic and Gamulin 1980), accounting for estrogen resistance in another group of patients. Interestingly, some patients whose tumors lacked a cytoplasmic estrogen receptor had a nuclear estrogen receptor (Panko and MacLeod 1978; Geier et al. 1979; Thorsen 1979; Hähnel et al. 1980; Romic-Stojkovic 1980). In some of these cases, cytoplasmic progesterone receptor was present (Thorsen 1979; Hähnel et al. 1980; Romic-Stojkovic 1980), suggesting that the nuclear estrogen receptor could be functional in the absence of the cytoplasmic estrogen receptor. These findings might account for the 8%–10% response rate in patients who lack the cytoplasmic estrogen receptor and suggest that measurements of nuclear estrogen receptor as well as the cytoplasmic progesterone receptor could be of value in predicting patient response. Several investigators have also demonstrated the presence of unoccupied estrogen receptors in the nuclei of human breast tumors (Garola and McGuire 1977; Kiang 1977; Panko and MacLeod 1978; Geier et al. 1979; Thorsen 1979; Hähnel et al. 1980; Romic-Stojkovic 1980). Based on a similar finding in the MCF-7 cell line Zava and McGuire (1977, but see also Edwards et al. 1980b) postulated that perhaps the free nuclear receptor could stimulate growth in the absence of estrogen and that, as a result, such a tumor would be insensitive to endocrine ablative procedures. Such a concept is of great interest even though the data do not fit the classical theory of steroid action, at least as it is known for normal target tissues. The results should be considered with a certain degree of caution, however, since artifacts could easily be generated depending on the particular assay used. In general, unoccupied receptors are measured by incubation with [^{3}H]estradiol at 4 °C; total (occupied + nonoccupied) receptors are measured in a similar assay, but at an elevated temperature so that exchange of bound with tritiated ligand can occur. In some human breast tumors exchange can occur at 4 °C (LAING et al. 1977), and we have found the same to be true in the MTW-9B rat mammary tumor (IP et al., unpublished). Breast tumors from different patients could behave differently, and even a small degree of exchange at 4 °C could make it appear that unoccupied nuclear receptors were present. Other potential factors that could interfere in the assay include contamination of nuclear preparations with unoccupied cytoplasmic receptors [as recently reported by EDWARDS et al. (1980b) in the MCF-7 cell line] or stripping endogenously bound steroid by high concentrations of salt which are used in some assays to extract the nuclear receptor prior to assay.

Still other possibilities exist for the estrogen resistance of certain breast tumors. These include the distinct possibility that since receptor measurements are generally only carried out on the primary tumor receptor levels in the metastases may be different although such is rarely the case (McGUIRE 1980). It is also possible that prior hormonal therapy or chemotherapy may have altered receptor levels from what was previously measured (either due to an effect on receptor levels per se, or by selective killing of one population of cells). While the effect of chemotherapeutic drugs on estrogen receptor levels is still controversial (DI CARLO et al. 1978; MÜLLER et al. 1980) the effect of certain steroid hormones such as androgens (RUH et al. 1975; ROCHEFORT et al. 1976; SCHMIDT et al. 1976), progestins (HSUEH et al. 1976; BHAKOO and KATZENELLENBOGEN 1977; DI CARLO et al. 1980b), and antiestrogens (JORDAN and DOWSE 1976; KATZENELLENBOGEN 1978), commonly used in breast cancer treatment, are well known. Another possible site of resistance in breast tumors is in the nucleus, involving either the interaction of the steroid receptor complex with chromatin or possibly a post-transcriptional block. No specific information is available on either possibility, but there are most certainly breast tumors that fall into either one of these broad categories (the MTW-9B mammary is probably one such tumor) and research directed at the mechanism of resistance of such tumors will go a long way toward helping us understand steroid action in normal tissue as well as to provide more appropriate therapy to breast cancer patients.

IV. Estrogen Receptor and Prognosis

In addition to predicting the response to hormonal therapy, measurement of estrogen receptor levels appears to provide an important clue to the prognosis of the patient, independent of other prognostic factors such as lymph node status, tumor size, age, or menopausal status (WALT et al. 1976; KNIGHT et al. 1977; MAYNARD et al. 1978; RICH et al. 1978; ALLEGRA et al. 1979a; BISHOP et al. 1979; HÄHNEL et al. 1979; CHEIX et al. 1980; HAWKINS et al. 1980). Patients whose tumors contain the estrogen receptor tend to have a longer disease-free interval, and in some studies an increased survival was noted. The best explanation for these findings is that, in general, ER-containing tumors are more differentiated (Maynard et al. 1978; Martin et al. 1979; Fisher et al. 1980; Parl and Wagner 1980; Silfverswärd et al. 1980) and have a lower growth rate (Meyer et al. 1978; Silvestrini et al. 1979; Meyer and Lee 1980).

More recently, the concept that the estrogen receptor can serve as a separate prognostic indicator has been disputed (Hilf et al. 1980; Meyer and Lee 1980). Meyer and Lee (1980) concluded that the estrogen receptor was not an independent prognostic variable, but rather its significance as a prognostic indicator resulted only from its inverse correlation with the SPF, or fraction of tumor cells in S-phase. This conclusion was based on a small number of patients, all of whom had relapsed, and many of whom had received prior therapy. Estrogen receptor measurements were made on the relapsed tumor. It would be of interest in future studies to compare SPF (or labeling index, LI) and estrogen receptor as prognostic indicators in patients in whom both measurements were made on the primary tumor. The results of Silvestrini and co-workers (1979) are of interest in this regard. These investigators found that the frequency distribution of LI as a function of ER content was different in pre- and postmenopausal patients. In ER+ cancers, a higher frequency of low LI values was found in the postmenopausal patients compared with the premenopausal patients. However, in ER− cancers, the results were more striking: premenopausal patients had a higher frequency of high LI values, whereas in postmenopausal patients low LI values predominated. Average LI values were lowest in ER+ postmenopausal patients (2.64) and highest in ER− premenopausal patients (9.49). It is the group of patients in between (ER− postmenopausal: LI, 4.26; ER+ premenopausal: LI, 5.19) in whom it would be of most interest to compare SPF and ER as prognostic indicators. Hilf et al. (1980) reported that when he examined the time to recurrence in 111 women who had received no therapy after mastectomy, there was no difference in women whose primary tumors were ER+ or ER−; no LI measurements were reported in this study. He noted that earlier studies were complicated by several factors, the most important of which was that either the majority of patients had received no postoperative therapy or that no statement was made regarding any adjuvant therapy.

V. Estrogen Receptor and Response to Chemotherapy

Based on the observation that the LI index was in general inversely correlated with the estrogen receptor (but note exceptions above), it was suggested that patients whose tumors were ER− might be more responsive to cytotoxic chemotherapy. Although some studies appeared to bear out this prediction (Jonat and Maas 1978; Lippman et al. 1978), others found just the opposite result (Kiang et al. 1978), and in many studies no differences were observed between ER+ and ER− patients. Twelve of these studies, involving a total of 488 ER+ and 420 ER− patients, are summarized in Table 10. The general impression gained from this table is that there is no real difference in response to cytotoxic chemotherapy in patients whose tumors are ER+ or ER−, even though statistical analysis suggests that the ER+ group had a somewhat better response. Based on very significant differences in how the studies were performed, however, it is difficult to

Table 10. Estrogen receptor and response to cytotoxic chemotherapy in 908 breast cancer patients

References	ER+	ER−
JONAT and MAAS (1978)	6/14	20/28
KIANG et al. (1978)	24/28	13/36
LIPPMAN et al. (1978)	3/25	34/45
SAMAL et al. (1978)	24/37	35/69
WEBSTER et al. (1978)	12/20	17/45
MARSLAND et al. (1979)	17/19	7/15
NOMURA et al. (1979)	6/14	3/22
ROSNER and NEMOTO (1979)	5/15	9/19
BONADONNA et al. (1980)		
Advanced cancer	24/46	16/30
Operable cancer	148/179	36/46
HAWKINS et al. (1980)	8/19	6/13
HILF et al. (1980)	17/35	21/35
RUBENS et al. (1980)	21/37	11/17
Totals	315/488	288/420
Percentage	64.5[a]	54.3[a]

[a] By chi-square analysis, applying the Yates correction, these values are significantly different ($P<.01$)

compare one study with another and statistical analysis is probably not really valid. Some of the factors complicating a comparison arise from the fact that most studies were retrospective, and include the following: the proportion of ER+ to ER− in the tumors of patients selected for study was usually not that found in the general population, suggesting that ER+ patients were more frequently given hormonal therapy and/or that patients whose tumor growth rate was high (more often ER−) were more frequently selected for chemotherapy; patient selection was biased in some instances based on the ability to biopsy for estrogen receptor assay (e.g., sometimes patients with osseous metastases were underrepresented); in many studies, patients had received some sort of prior therapy and in some studies it is not clear what this therapy actually was or indeed if there had been any prior therapy; a relationship of ER levels to adjuvant therapy was made in some studies and to cytotoxic chemotherapy of advanced cancer patients in others, with ER measurements frequently only being available on the primary tumor; the proportion of pre- to postmenopausal patients was not always clear; different drug regimens were used by different investigators, even within their own series. Unless it is possible to control these variables and to measure ER immediately prior to therapy, it will be very difficult to reach any general conclusion on the effect of ER status to chemotherapeutic response. However, it will be of interest to determine whether there is such a relationship in certain patient populations.

VI. Current and Future Directions in Research

Future research into the hormone dependence of breast cancer must proceed along several different lines, one of the most important being a continued investigation into the various mechanisms of resistance, in the hope that by this understanding we can predict with greater accuracy those patients that will respond to hormonal therapy. At the same time, other avenues must also be pursued. For example, many studies indicate the presence of receptors for other hormones including androgen (Wagner et al. 1973; Persijn et al. 1975; Maas et al. 1975; Allegra et al. 1979 b, c; Teulings et al. 1980), glucocorticoids (Fazekas and MacFarlane 1977; Allegra et al. 1979 b, c; Teulings et al. 1980), progesterone (see Table 6), and prolactin (Holdaway and Friesen 1977; Morgan et al. 1977; Partridge and Hähnel 1979; Di Carlo et al. 1980 a), and it is possible that growth could be dependent on or inhibited by some of these other hormones. Much more work needs to be done in this field, since many of the endocrine therapies employed involve one or more of these hormones. Teulings et al. (1980), for example, have shown that responsiveness to progestin therapy is strongly associated with the presence of the androgen receptor, and Allegra et al. (1979 c) found that there was a trend for the androgen receptor to predict response to the standard endocrine therapies [of 19 patients whose tumors contained the androgen receptor, 14 responded, compared with 11 of 35 patients whose tumors were androgen receptor netative ($P=0.10$)]. The presence of the androgen receptor with the estrogen receptor did not further increase the predictive power of the latter. Allegra et al. (1979 c) also noted that there was a trend for the glucocorticoid receptor to predict response, and although the numbers are still small, the data suggest that the presence of both the estrogen and glucocorticoid receptors increases the predictability over that seen with the estrogen receptor alone. Obviously, more information is badly needed in this area. It is also of interest to learn whether changes in receptor levels resulting from various hormonal manipulations have any therapeutic implications.

Future research should also include a search for estrogen-induced proteins in breast cancer such as has been described in the uterus (reviewed by Katzenellenbogen et al. 1980) and in the MCF-7 cell line (Westley and Rochefort 1979; Edwards et al. 1980 a) in the hope that, in conjunction with the progesterone receptor, they may be better able to predict the functionality of the estrogen receptor.

The degree of heterogeneity of breast tumors is now well recognized and future clinical protocols will have to take this into consideration. Using a fluorescent steroid histochemical technique, Lee (1979) has recently been able to determine the proportion of ER+/ER− cells in a series of 52 primary and metastatic breast tumors. While it is uncertain whether this technique could be applied on a routine basis, future research needs to be done with either this technique or a histoimmunofluorescent technique using the monoclonal antibodies currently being prepared in Jensen's laboratory, and correlating the results with cytosol estrogen receptor assays and with the response to endocrine therapy. It will also be of interest to determine the response to combined hormonal and chemotherapy or to estrogen-linked cytotoxic drugs (Leclercq and Heuson 1980) in patients in tumors that have varying proportions of ER+ and ER− cells.

G. Conclusions

From the preceding discussion, it can be seen that measurement of steroid receptors can provide valuable information both in terms of patient treatment and probably also in terms of prognosis, although, as noted earlier, there is some conflict on this point. With breast cancer in particular, significant strides have been made at improving the quality of life through the ability to select a more appropriate therapy, even though survival has not markedly increased in the last several years. With the more frequent use of adjuvant chemotherapy, however, including, where appropriate, hormonal therapy, this goal too will probably be attainable. Despite this substantial progress, at least one major problem remains unsolved: why certain tissues containing substantial levels of steroid receptor fail to respond to endocrine treatment. This has been observed both in breast cancer and in many types of leukemia, and research in the next few years will have to be directed at a resolution of this problem.

Acknowledgments. The author would like to thank Richard Milholland and Fred Rosen for critically reviewing this manuscript.

References

Alberga A, Tran A, Baulieu EE (1979) Distribution of estradiol receptor and vitellogenin gene in chick liver chromatin fractions. Nucleic Acids Res 7:2031–2044

Allegra JC, Lippman ME, Simon R, Thompson EB, Barlock A, Green L, Huff KK, Do HMT, Aitken S, Warren R (1979a) Association between steroid hormone receptor status and disease-free interval in breast cancer. Cancer Treat Rep 63:1271–1277

Allegra JC, Lippman ME, Thompson EB, Simon R, Barlock A, Green L, Huff KK, Do HMT, Aitken S (1979b) Distribution, frequency and quantitative analysis of estrogen, progesterone, androgen, and glucocorticoid receptors in human breast cancer. Cancer Res 39:1447–1454

Allegra JC, Lippman ME, Thompson EB, Simon R, Barlock A, Green L, Huff KK, Do HMT, Aitken SC, Warren R (1979c) Relationship between the progesterone, androgen and glucocorticoid receptor response rate to endocrine therapy in metastatic breast cancer. Cancer Res 39:1973–1979

Allegra JC, Lippman ME, Thompson EB, Simon R, Barlock A, Green L, Huff KK, Do HMT, Aitken S, Warren R (1980) Estrogen receptor status: an important variable in predicting response to endocrine therapy in metastatic breast cancer. Eur J Cancer 16:323–331

Alléra A, Rao GS, Breuer H (1980) Specific interactions of corticosteroids with components of the cell membrane which are involved in the translocation of the hormone into the intravesicular space of purified rat liver plasma membrane vesicles. J Steroid Biochem 12:259–266

Asselin J, Kelly PA, Caron MG, Labrie F (1977) Control of hormone receptor levels and growth of 7,12-dimethylbenz[a]anthracene-induced mammary tumors by estrogens, progesterone and prolactin. Endocrinology 101:666–671

Barrack ER, Coffey DS (1980) The specific binding of estrogens and androgens to the nuclear matrix of sex hormone responsive tissues. J Biol Chem 255:7265–7275

Baxter JD, Rousseau GG, Benson MC, Garcea RL, Ito J, Tomkins GM (1972) Role of DNA and specific cytoplasmic receptors in glucocorticoid action. Proc Natl Acad Sci 69:1892–1896

Behrens UJ, Hollander VP (1976) Cell membrane sialoglycopeptides of corticoid-sensitive and -resistant lymphosarcoma P1798. Cancer Res 36:172–180

Behrens UJ, Mashburn LT, Stevens J, Hollander VP, Lampen N (1974) Differences in cell surface characteristics between glucocorticoid-sensitive and resistant mouse lymphomas. Cancer Res 34:2926–2932

Bell PA, Sloman JC, Whittaker JA (1979) Glucorticoid receptors in myeloid leukemia. Cancer Treat Rep 63:1197

Bhakoo HS, Katzenellenbogen BS (1977) Progesterone modulation of estrogen-stimulated uterine biosynthetic events and estrogen receptor levels. Mol Cell Endocrinol 8:121–134

Bishop HM, Elston CW, Blamey RW, Haybittle JL, Nicholson RI, Griffiths K (1979) Relationship of estrogen receptor status to survival in breast cancer. Lancet 2:283–284

Bloom ND, Tobin EH, Schreibman B, Degenshein GA (1980) The role of progesterone in the management of advanced breast cancer. Cancer 45:2992–2997

Bloomfield CD, Peterson BA, Zaleskas J, Frizzera G, Smith KA, Hildebrandt L, Gajl-Peczalska J, Munck A (1980) In vitro studies for predicting glucocorticoid therapy in adults with malignant lymphoma. Lancet 1:952–955

Bonadonna G, Valagussa P, Tancini G, DiFronzo G (1980) Estrogen receptor status and response to chemotherapy in early and advanced breast cancer. Cancer Chemother Pharmacol 4:37–41

Bourgeois S, Newby RF (1977) Diploid and haploid states of the glucocorticoid receptor gene of mouse lymphoid cell lines. Cell 11:423–430

Bourgeois S, Newby RF (1979) Correlation between glucocorticoid receptor and cytolytic response of murine lymphoid cell lines. Cancer Res 39:4749–4751

Bourgeois S, Newby RF, Huet M (1978) Glucocorticoid resistance in murine lymphoma and thymoma lines. Cancer Res 38:4279–4284

Cake MH, DiSorbo DM, Litwack G (1978) Effect of pyridoxal phosphate on the DNA binding site of activated hepatic glucocorticoid receptor. J Biol Chem 253:4886–4891

Carter SK (1978) Acute lymphocytic leukemia. In: Staquet MJ (ed) Randomized trials in cancer: a critical review by sites. Raven, New York, pp 1–24

Chang E, Mittelman A, Rosen F (1964) The metabolism in vitro of [4-^{14C}] cortisone by lymphosarcoma P1798. Biochim Biophys Acta 90:600–605

Cheix F, Biron A, Bailly C, Mayer M, Pommatau E, Saez S (1980) Cancer du sein operable: valeur prognostique du nombres des recepteurs d'estradiol. Nouv Presse Med 9:933–935

Cidlowski JA, Munck A (1980) Differential solubilization of nuclear glucocorticoid receptors by DNAse I and DNAse II. Biochim Biophys Acta 630:375–385

Cline MJ (1974) Adrenal steroids in leukemia and lymphoma. Cancer Chemotherapy Rep 58 (part 1):521–525

Crabtree GR, Smith KA, Munck A (1978) Glucocorticoid receptors and sensitivity of isolated human leukemia and lymphoma cells. Cancer Res 38:4268–4272

Davis JM, Chan AK, Thompson EA (1980) Nonmutational alteration in glucocorticoid sensitivity of lymphosarcoma P1798. J Natl Cancer Inst 64:55–62

Debusscher L, Stryckmans PA (1978) Nonlymphocytic acute leukemia. In: Staquet MJ (ed), Randomized trials in cancer: a critical review by sites. Raven, New York, p 25–54

DiCarlo F, Reboani C, Conti G, Genazzani E (1978) Changes in the concentration of uterine cytoplasmic oestrogen receptors induced by doxorubicin and methotrexate. J Endocrinol 79:201–208

DiCarlo R, Muccioli G, Conti G, Reboani C, DiCarlo F (1980a) Estrogen and prolactin receptor concentrations in human breast tumors. In: Genazzani E, DiCarlo F, Mainwaring WIP (eds) Pharmacological modulation of steroid action, Raven, New York, pp 261–266

DiCarlo F, Reboani C, Conti G, Portaleone P, Viano I, Genazzani E (1980b) Changes in estrogen receptor levels induced by pharmacological agents. In: Genazzani E, DiCarlo F, Mainwaring WIP (eds) Pharmacological modulation of steroid action. Raven, New York, pp 61–74

DiSorbo DM, Phelps DS, Litwack G (1980a) Chemical probes of amino acid residues affect the active sites of the glucocorticoid receptor. Endocrinology 106:922–929

DiSorbo DM, Phelps DS, Ohl VS, Litwack G (1980b) Pyridoxine deficiency influences the behavior of the glucocorticoid receptor complex. J Biol Chem 255:3866–3870

Edwards DP, Adams DJ, Savage N, McGuire WL (1980a) Estrogen induced synthesis of specific proteins in human breast cancer cells. Biochim Biophys Acta 93:804–812

Edwards DP, Martin PM, Horwitz KB, Chamness GC, McGuire WL (1980b) Subcellular compartmentalization of estrogen receptors in human breast cancer cells. Exp Cell Res 127:197–213

Fazekas AG, MacFarlane JK (1977) Macromolecular binding of glucocorticoids in human mammary carcinoma. Cancer Res 37:640–645
Fazekas AG, MacFarlane JK (1980) Studies on cytosol and nuclear binding of estradiol in human breast cancer. J Steroid Biochem 13:613–622
Fessas P, Wintrobe MM, Thompson RB, Cartwright GE (1954) Treatment of acute leukemia with cortisone and corticotropin. Arch Int Med 94:384–401
Fisher ER, Redmond CK, Liu H, Rockette H, Fisher B (1980) Correlation of estrogen receptor and pathologic characteristics of invasive breast cancer. Cancer 45:349–353
Gailani S, Minowada J, Silvernail P, Nussbaum A, Kaiser N, Rosen F, Shimaoka K (1973) Specific glucocorticoid binding in human hemopoietic cell lines and neoplastic tissue. Cancer Res 33:2653–2657
Garola RE, McGuire WL (1977) An improved assay for nuclear estrogen receptor in experimental and human breast cancer. Cancer Res 37:3333–3337
Gehring U (1978) Genetic analysis of glucocorticoid action in neoplastic lymphoid cells. Adv Eng Regul 17:343–361
Gehring U, Tomkins GM (1974) A new mechanism for steroid unresponsiveness: loss of nuclear binding activity of a steroid hormone receptor. Cell 3:301–306
Geier A, Ginzburg R, Stauber M, Lunenfeld B (1979) Unoccupied binding sites for oestradiol in nuclei from human breast carcinomatous tissue. J Endocrinol 80:281–288
Gottesfeld JM, Butler PJG (1977) Structure of transcriptionally active chromatin subunits. Nucleic Acids Res 4:3155–3173
Granville NB, Rubio F Jr, Unugur A, Schulman E, Dameshek W (1958) Treatment of acute leukemia in adult with massive doses of prednisone and prednisolone. New Engl J Med 259:207–213
Hähnel R, Woodings T, Vivian AB (1979) Prognostic value of estrogen receptors in primary breast cancer. Cancer 44:671–675
Hähnel R, Partridge RK, Gavet L, Twaddle E, Ratajczak T (1980) Nuclear and cytoplasmic estrogen receptors and progesterone receptors in breast cancer. Eur J Cancer 16:1027–1033
Harrison RW, Fairfield S, Orth DN (1974) Evidence for glucocorticoid transport through the target cell membrane. Biochem Biophys Res Comm 61:1262–1267
Harrison RW, Fairfield S, Orth DN (1975) Evidence for glucocorticoid transport into AtT-20/D-1 cells. Biochemistry 14:1304–1307
Harrison RW, Fairfield S, Orth DN (1977) The effect of cell membrane alteration on glucocorticoid uptake by the AtT-20/D-1 target cell. Biochim Biophys Acta 466:357–365
Hawkins RA, Roberts MM, Forrest APM (1980) Oestrogen receptors and breast cancer: current status. Br J Surg 67:153–169
Hemminki K (1976) Distribution of estrogen receptors in subfractions of hen oviduct chromatin. Nucleic Acids Res 3:1499–1506
Hemminki K (1977) Differential distribution of oestrogen receptors in subfractions of oviduct chromatin. Acta Endocrinol 84:215–224
Henderson ES (1973) Acute lymphoblastic leukemia. In: Holland JF, Frei E (eds) Cancer medicine. Lea and Febiger, Philadelphia, pp 1173–1199
Hendrick D, Tolstoshev P, Randlett D (1977) Enrichment for the globin coding region in a chromatin fraction from chick reticulocytes by endonuclease digestion. Gene 2:147–158
Higgins SJ, Rousseau GG, Baxter JD, Tomkins GM (1973) Nature of nuclear acceptor sites for glucocorticoid-and estrogen-receptor complexes. J Biol Chem 248:5873–5879
Higgins SJ, Baxter JD, Rousseau GG (1979) Nuclear binding of glucocorticoid receptors. In: Baxter JD, Rousseau GG (eds) Glucocorticoid hormone action, Springer, Berlin Heidelberg New York, pp 135–160
Hilf R, Feldstein ML, Gibson SL, Savlov ED (1980) The relative importance of estrogen receptor analysis as a prognostic factor for recurrence or response to chemotherapy in women with breast cancer. Cancer 45:1993–2000
Holdaway IM, Friesen HG (1977) Hormone binding by human mammary carcinoma. Cancer Res 37:1946–1952

Hollander N, Chiu Y-W (1966a) Relation between cortisol metabolism and its lympholytic effect in P1978 lymphosarcoma. Endocrinology 79:168–174
Hollander N, Chiu Y-W (1966b) In vitro binding of cortisol -1,2-^{3}H by a substance in the supernatant fraction of P1798 mouse lymphosarcoma. Biochem Biophys Res Comm 25:291–297
Horwitz KB, McGuire WL (1978) Estrogen control of progesterone receptor in human breast cancer. Correlation with nuclear processing of estrogen receptor. J Biol Chem 253:2223–2228
Horwitz KB, McGuire WL, Pearson OH, Segaloff A (1975) Predicting response to endocrine therapy in human breast cancer: a hypothesis. Science 189:726–727
Ho AD, Hunstein W, Schmid W (1980) Determination of glucocorticoid receptors in human leukemias. Klin Wochenschr 58:43–45
Homo F, Duval D, Meyer P, Belas F, Debre P, Binet J-L (1978) Chronic lymphatic leukemia: cellular effects of glucocorticoid in vitro. Br J Haemat 38:491–499
Homo F, Duval D, Harousseau JL, Marie JP, Zittoun R (1980) Heterogeneity of the in vitro response to glucocorticoids in acute leukemia. Cancer Res 40:2601–2608
Horibata K, Harris AW (1970) Mouse myelomas and lymphomas in culture. Exp Cell Res 60:61–77
Hsueh AWJ, Peck EJ, Clark JH (1976) Control of uterine estrogen receptor levels by progesterone. Endocrinology 98:438–444
Ip MM, Milholland RJ, Rosen F, Kim U (1979) Mammary cancer: selective action of the estrogen receptor complex. Science 203:361–363
Ip MM, Milholland RJ, Rosen F (1980) Functionality of estrogen receptor and tamoxifen treatment of R3327 Dunning rat prostate adenocarcinoma. Cancer Res 40:2188–2193
Ip MM, Milholland RJ, Rosen F, Kim U (1981) Dichotomous effects of tamoxifen on a transplantable rat mammary tumor. Cancer Res 41:984–988
Jensen EV (1975) Estrogen receptors in hormone-dependent breast cancers. Cancer Res 35:3362–3364
Jensen EV, DeSombre ER, Jungblut PW (1967) Estrogen receptors in hormone responsive tissues and tumors. In: Wissler RW, Dao TL, Wood SJ Jr (eds) Endogenous factors influencing host-tumor balance. University of Chicago Press, Chicago, pp 15–30
Jonat W, Maass H (1978) Some comments on the necessity of receptor determination in human breast cancer. Cancer Res 38:4305–4306
Jordan VC, Dowse LJ (1976) Tamoxifen as an antitumor agent: effect on oestrogen binding. J Endocrinol 68:297–303
Kaiser N, Milholland RJ, Rosen F (1974) Glucocorticoid receptors and mechanism of resistance in the cortisol-sensitive and -resistant lines of lymphosarcoma P1798. Cancer Res 34:621–626
Katzenellenbogen BS (1978) Basic mechanisms of antiestrogen action. In: McGuire WL (ed) Hormones, receptors and breast cancer. Raven, New York, pp 135–157
Katzenellenbogen BS, Bhakoo HS, Hayes JR, Schmidt WN (1980) Uterine estrogen-induced protein: an index of uterine sensitivity to hormones. In: Beato M (ed) Steroid induced proteins, Elsevier, North Holland Biomedical, Amsterdam, pp 267–281
Kiang DT (1977) Nuclear oestrogen receptor and breast cancer. Lancet 2:714–715
Kiang DT, Frenning DH, Goldman AI, Ascensao VF, Kennedy BJ (1978) Estrogen receptors and response to chemotherapy and hormonal therapy in advanced breast cancer. N Engl J Med 299:1330–1334
Kim U, Depowski MJ (1975) Progression from hormone dependence to autonomy in mammary tumors as an in vivo manifestation of sequential clonal selection. Cancer Res 35:2068–2077
King RJB, Redgrave S, Rubens RD, Millis R, Hayward JA (1978) Cited by WL McGuire in: Steroid receptors in human breast cancer. Cancer Res 38:4289–4291
Kirkpatrick AF, Kaiser N, Milholland RJ, Rosen F (1972) Glucocorticoid-binding macromolecules in normal tissue and tumors: stabilization of the specific binding component. J Biol Chem 247:70–74

Kirkpatrick AF, Milholland RJ, Rosen F (1971) Stereospecific glucocorticoid binding to subcellular fractions of the sensitive and resistant lymphosarcoma P1798. Nature (New Biol) 232:216–218

Kisling S, Adler VV, Dmitrieva LV, Shapot VS (1979) The existence of specific receptors for glucocorticoid on the plasma membranes of the rat liver. Biochemistry (Biokhimiia) 44:1600–1604

Knight WA, Livingston RB, Gregory EJ, McGuire WL (1977) Estrogen receptor as an independent prognostic factor for early recurrence in breast cancer. Cancer Res 37:4669–4671

Konior GS, Lippman ME, Johnson GE, Leventhal BG (1977a) Correlation of glucocorticoid receptor levels and complete remission duration in "poor prognosis" acute lymphatic leukemia. Proc Am Soc Clin Oncol 18:353

Konior GS, Lippman ME, Johnson GE, Owens AH, Leventhal BG (1977b) Glucocorticoid receptors in acute non-lymphocytic leukemia. Proc Am Assoc Cancer Res 18:235

Konior-Yarbro GS, Lippman ME, Johnson GE, Leventhal BG (1977) Glucocorticoid receptors in subpopulations of childhood acute lymphocytic leukemia. Cancer Res 37:2688–2695

Laing L, Calman KC, Smith MG, Smith DC, Reake RE (1977) Nuclear oestrogen receptors and treatment of breast cancer. Lancet 2:168–169

Lampkin JM, Potter M (1958) Response to cortisone and development of cortisone resistance in a cortisone-sensitive lymphosarcoma of the mouse. J Natl Cancer Inst 20:1091–1111

Lampkin-Hibbard JM (1966) Lymphomas: Regression, carcinogenesis and prevention. LS Haines, Miami

Leclercq G, Heuson JC (1977) Therapeutic significance of sex-steroid hormone receptors in the treatment of breast cancer. Eur J Cancer 13:1205–1215

Leclercq G, Heuson JC (1980) Estrogen-linked cytotoxic agents of potential value for the treatment of breast cancer: binding affinity for estrogen receptors. In: Genazzani E, DiCarlo F and Mainwaring WIP (eds) Pharmacological modulation of steroid action, Raven, New York, pp 217–226

Lee SH (1979) Cancer cell estrogen receptor of human mammary carcinoma. Cancer 44:1–12

Levy-Wilson B, Baxter JD (1976) Distribution of thyroid and glucocorticoid hormone receptors in transcriptionally active and inactive chromatin. Biochem Biophys Res Comm 68:1045–1051

Lippman ME, Halterman RH, Leventhal BG, Perry S, Thompson EB (1973) Glucocorticoid-binding proteins in human acute lymphoblastic leukemic blast cells. J Clin Invest 52:1715–1725

Lippman ME, Perry S, Thompson EB (1975) Glucocorticoid binding proteins in myeloblasts of acute myelogenous leukemia. Am J Med 59:224–227

Lippman ME, Allegra JC, Thompson EB, Simon R, Barlock A, Green L, Huff KK, Do HMT, Aitken S, Warren R (1978) The relation between estrogen receptors and response rate to cytotoxic chemotherapy in metastatic breast cancer. N Engl J Med 298:1223–1228

Maass H, Engel B, Trams G, Nowakowski H, Stolzenbach G (1975) Steroid hormone receptors in human breast cancer and the clinical significance. J Steroid Biochem 6:743–749

Mainwaring WIP, Symes EK, Higgins SJ (1976) Nuclear components responsible for the retention of steroid-receptor complexes, especially from the standpoint of the specificity of hormonal responses. Biochem J 156:129–141

Marsland TA, Rosenbaum C, Stolbach LL, Cohen JL (1979) Estrogen receptors and chemotherapy in breast cancer. Proc Am Soc Clin Oncol 20:367

Martin PM, Rolland PH, Jacquemier J, Rolland AM, Toga M (1979) Multiple steroid receptors in human breast cancer. III. Relationships between steroid receptors and the state of differentiation and the activity of carcinomas throughout the pathologic features. Cancer Chemotherap Pharmacol 2:115–120

Massol N, Lebeau M-C, Baulieu E-E (1978) Estrogen receptor in hen oviduct chromatin digested by micrococcal nuclease. Nucleic Acids Res 5:723–738

Mayer M, Nir S, Milholland RJ, Rosen F (1976) Effect of temperature on glucocorticoid uptake and glucocorticoid-receptor translocation in rat thymocytes. Arch Biochem Biophys 176:28–36

Maynard PV, Davies CJ, Blamey RW, Elston CW, Johnson J, Griffiths K (1978) Relationship between oestrogen-receptor content and histological grade in human primary breast tumors. Br J Cancer 38:745–748

McGuire WL (1978) Steroid receptors in human breast cancer. Cancer Res 38:4289–4291

McGuire WL (1980) Steroid hormone receptors in breast cancer treatment strategy. Recent Prog Horm Res 36:135–146

McGuire WL, Carbone PP, Sears ME, Escher GC (1975) Estrogen receptors in human breast cancer: an overview. In: McGuire WL, Carbone PP, Vollmer EP (eds) Estrogen receptors in human breast cancer. Raven, New York, pp 1–7

McGuire WL, Horwitz KB, Zava DT, Garola RE, Chamness GC (1978) Hormones in breast cancer: update 1978. Metabolism 27:487–501

McPartland RP, Milholland RJ, Rosen F (1977) Nuclear binding of steroid-receptor complex to lymphosarcoma P1798 resistant and sensitive cells and effect of concanavalin A on receptor levels. Cancer Res 37:4256–4260

Meyer JS, Lee JY (1980) Relationships of S-phase fraction of breast carcinoma in relapse to duration of remission, estrogen receptor content, therapeutic responsiveness and duration of survival. Cancer Res 40:1890–1896

Meyer JS, Bauer WC, Rao BR (1978) Subpopulations of breast carcinoma defined by S-phase fraction, morphology and estrogen receptor content. Lab Invest 39:225–235

Milgrom E, Atger M, Bailly A (1976) Interaction of rat liver glucocorticoid receptor with DNA. Eur J Biochem 70:1–6

Milholland RJ, Ip MM, Rosen F (1979) The effect of hydrocortisone treatment on the in vivo phosphorylation of a subgroup of non-histone nuclear proteins in the mouse lymphosarcoma P1798. Biochem Biophys Res Comm 88:993–997

Morgan L, Laggatt PR, DeSouza I, Salih H, Hobbs JR (1977) Prolactin receptors in human breast tumors. J Endocrinol 73:17P

Muller RE, Sheard BE, Traish A, Wotiz HH (1980) Effect of chemotherapeutic agents on the formation of estrogen receptor complex in human breast tumor cytosol. Cancer Res 40:2941–2942

Nicholson ML, Young DA (1978) Effect of glucocorticoid hormones in vitro on the structural integrity of nuclei in corticosteroid-sensitive and -resistant lines of lymphosarcoma P1798. Cancer Res 38:3673–3680

Nicholson ML, Young DA (1979) Independence of the lethal actions of glucocorticoids on lymphoid cells from possible hormone effects on calcium uptake. J Supramol Struct 10:165–174

Nicholson ML, Voris BP, Young DA (1979) Lethal actions of glucocorticoids in lymphoid cells: a protein associated with emergence of the resistant state. Cancer Treat Rep 63:1196

Nomura Y, Yamagata J, Kondo H (1979) Significance of estrogen receptor assay in cytotoxic chemotherapy in relation to previous endocrine therapy of advanced breast cancer patients. Gann 70:473–482

Nomura Y, Takatani O, Sugano H, Matsumoto K (1980) Oestrogen and progesterone receptors and response to endocrine therapy in Japanese breast cancer. J Steroid Biochem 13:565–566

Panko WB, MacLeod RM (1978) Uncharged nuclear receptors for estrogen in breast cancers. Cancer Res 38:1948–1951

Parl FF, Wagner RK (1980) The histological evaluation of human breast cancers in correlation with estrogen receptor values. Cancer 46:362–367

Partridge RK, Hahnel R (1979) Prolactin receptors in human breast carcinoma. Cancer 43:643–646

Pearson OH, Eliel LP (1950) Use of pituitary adrenocorticotropic hormone (ACTH) and cortisone in lymphomas and leukemias. JAMA 144:1349–1353

Persijn JP, Korsten CB, Engelsman E (1975) Oestrogen and androgen receptors in breast cancer and response to endocrine therapy. Br Med J 4:503

Pfahl M, Kelleher RJ, Bourgeois S (1978) General features of steroid resistance in lymphoid cell lines. Mol Cell Endocrinol 10:193–207

Plagemann PGW, Erbe J (1976) Glucocorticoids – uptake by simple diffusion by cultured Reuber and Novikoff rat hepatoma cells. Biochem Pharmacol 25:1489–1494

Puca GA, Nola E, Hibner U, Cicala G, Sica V (1975) Interaction of the estradiol receptor from calf uterus with its nuclear acceptor sites. J Biol Chem 250:6452–6459

Raina PN, Rosen F (1969) Selective effect of cortisol on deoxyribonuclease II activity of lymphosarcoma P1798. Arch Int Pharmacodyn 182:14–23

Ranney HM, Gellhorn A (1957) The effect of massive prednisone and prednisolone therapy on acute leukemia and malignant lymphomas. Am J Med 22:405–413

Rao BR, Wiest WG (1971) Estradiol-17β stimulation of progesterone binding in rabbit uterus (abstract). Fed Proc 30:1213

Rao ML, Rao GS, Holler M, Breuer H, Schattenberg PJ, Stein WD (1976) Uptake of cortisol by isolated rat liver cells. A phenomenon indicative of carrier-mediation and simple diffusion. Hoppe Seylers Z Physiol Chem 357:573–584

Rao ML, Rao GS, Eckel J, Breuer H (1977) Factors involved in uptake of corticosterone by rat liver cells. Biochim Biophys Acta 500:322–332

Rich MA, Furmanski P, Brooks SC (1978) Prognostic value of estrogen receptor determinations in patients with breast cancer. Cancer Res 38:4296–4298

Roath S, Israels MCG, Wilkinson JF (1964) The acute leukemias: a study of 580 patients. Q J Med 33:257–283

Rochefort H, Garcia M (1976) Androgen on the estrogen receptor: I. Binding and in vivo nuclear translocation. Steroids 28:549–560

Romic-Stojkovic R, Gamulin S (1980) Relationship of cytoplasmic and nuclear estrogen receptors and progesterone receptors in human breast cancer. Cancer Res 40:4821–4825

Rosen JM, Fina JJ, Milholland RJ, Rosen F (1970a) Inhibition of glucose uptake in lymphosarcoma P1798 by cortisol and its relationship to the biosynthesis of deoxyribonucleic acid. J Biol Chem 245:2074–2080

Rosen JM, Rosen F, Milholland RJ, Nichol CA (1970b) Effects of cortisol on DNA metabolism in the sensitive and resistant lines of mouse lymphoma P1798. Cancer Res 30:1129–1136

Rosen JM, Fina JJ, Milholland RJ, Rosen F (1972) Inhibitory effect of cortisol in vitro on 2-deoxyglucose uptake and RNA and protein metabolism in lymphosarcoma P1798. Cancer Res 32:350–355

Rosner D, Nemoto T (1979) A randomized study of 2 and 3 drug regimen in relation with estrogen receptors in metastatic breast cancer. Proc Am Assoc Cancer Res 20:46

Rubens RD, King RJB, Sexton S, Minton MJ, Hayward JL (1980) Oestrogen receptors and response to cytotoxic chemotherapy in advanced breast cancer. Cancer Chemother Pharmacol 4:43–45

Ruh TS, Wassilak SG, Ruh MF (1975) Androgen-induced nuclear accumulation of the estrogen receptor. Steroids 25:257–273

Samal B, Singhakowinta H, Brooks SC, Vaitkevicius VK (1978) Estrogen receptors and response of breast cancer to chemotherapy. N Engl J Med 299:604

Samuels HH, Tomkins GM (1970) Relation of steroid structure to enzyme induction in hepatoma tissue culture cells. J Mol Biol 52:57–74

Schmidt TJ, Thompson EB (1978) Glucocorticoid receptor function in leukemic cells. In: Sharma RK, Criss WE (eds) Endocrine control in neoplasia. Raven, New York, pp 263–290

Schmidt TJ, Harmon JM, Thompson EB (1980) "Activation-labile" glucocorticoid-receptor complexes of a steroid-resistant variant of CEM-C7 human lymphoid cells. Nature 286:507–510

Schmidt WN, Sadler MA, Katzenellenbogen BS (1976) Androgen-uterine interaction: nuclear translocation of the estrogen receptor and induction of the synthesis of the uterine-induced protein (IP) by high concentrations of androgens in vitro but not in vivo. Endocrinology 98:702–716

Scott RW, Frankel FR (1980) Enrichment of estradiol-receptor complexes in a transcriptionally active fraction of chromatin from MCF-7 cells. Proc Natl Acad Sci 77:1291–1295

Shanbrom E, Miller S (1962) Critical evaluation of massive steroid therapy of acute leukemia. N Engl J Med 266:1354–1358

Sherman MR, Corval PL, O'Malley BW (1970) Progesterone-binding components of chick oviduct. I. Preliminary characterization of cytoplasmic components. J Biol Chem 245:6085–6096

Sibley CH, Yamamoto KR (1979) Mouse lymphoma cells: mechanisms of resistance to glucocorticoids. In: Baxter JD, Rousseau GG (eds) Glucocorticoid hormone action. Springer, Berlin Heidelberg New York, pp 357–376

Silfversward C, Gustafsson JA, Gustafsson SA, Humla S, Nordenskjold B, Wallgren A, Wrange O (1980) Estrogen receptor concentrations in 269 cases of histologically classified human breast cancer. Cancer 45:2001–2005

Silvestrini R, Daidone MG, DiFronzo G (1979) Relationship between proliferative activity and estrogen receptors in breast cancer. Cancer 44:665–670

Simons Jr SS (1979) Factors influencing association of glucocorticoid receptor-steroid complexes with nuclei, chromatin and DNA: interpretation of binding data. In: Baxter JD, Rousseau GG (eds) Glucocorticoid hormone action, Springer, Berlin Heidelberg New York, pp 161–187

Skinner LG, Barnes DM, Ribeiro GG (1978) Cited by WL McGuire in Steroid receptors in human breast cancer. Cancer Res 38:4289–4291

Socher SH, Krall JF, Jaffee RC, O'Malley BW (1976) Distribution of binding sites for the progesterone receptor within chick oviduct chromatin. Endocrinology 99:891–900

Spelsberg TC, Thrall C, Webster R, Pikler G (1977) Isolation and characterization of the nuclear acceptor that binds the progesterone-receptor complex in hen oviduct. J Toxicol Environ Health 3:309–337

Stevens J, Stevens YW (1979) Physicochemical differences between glucocorticoid-binding components from the corticoid-sensitive and -resistant strains of mouse lymphoma P1798. Cancer Res 39:4011–4021

Stevens J, Stevens YW, Hollander VP (1974) Substrate requirements and kinetic analysis of the cortisol effects on uridine uptake and incorporation by mouse lymphoma P1798 cells in vitro. Cancer Res 34:2330–2337

Stevens J, Stevens YW, Rhodes J, Steiner G (1978) Differences in nuclear glucocorticoid binding between corticoid-sensitive and corticoid-resistant lymphocytes of mouse lymphoma P1798 and stabilization of nuclear hormone receptor complexes with carbobenzyoxy-L-phenylalanine. J Nat Cancer Inst 61:1477–1485

Stevens J, Stevens YW, Rosenthal RL (1979) Characterization of cytosolic and nuclear glucocorticoid binding components in human leukemic lymphocytes. Cancer Res 39:4939–4948

Terenius L, Simonsson B, Nilsson K (1976) Glucocorticoid receptors, DNA synthesis, membrane antigens and their relation to disease activity in chronic lymphatic leukemia. J Steroid Biochem 7:905–909

Teulings FAG, van Gilse HA, Henkelman MS, Portengen H, Alexieva-Figusch J (1980) Estrogen, androgen, glucocorticoid and progesterone receptors in progestin-induced regression of human breast cancer. Cancer Res 40:2557–2561

Thompson EA, Moore WM, Sawyer RH (1980) Glucocorticoid effects of lymphosarcoma P1798 on DNA replication and growth of subcutaneous tumors in mice. J Natl Cancer Inst 65:477–483

Thompson EB (1979) Report on the International Union against Cancer Workshop on steroid receptors in leukemia. Cancer Treat Rep 63:189–195

Thorsen T (1979) Occupied and unoccupied nuclear oestradiol receptor in human breast tumours: relation to oestradiol and progesterone cytosol receptors. J Steroid Biochem 10:661–668

Thrall CL, Spelsberg TC (1980) Factors affecting the binding of chick oviduct progesterone receptor to deoxyribonucleic acid: evidence that deoxyribonucleic acid alone is not the nuclear acceptor site. Biochemistry 19:4130–4138

Toft DO, O'Malley BW (1972) Target tissue receptors for progesterone: the influence of estrogen treatment. Endocrinology 90:1041–1045

Tsai T-LS, Katzenellenbogen BS (1977) Antagonism of development and growth of 7,12-dimethylbenz(a)anthracene-induced rat mammary tumors by the antiestrogen U23, 469, and effects on estrogen and progesterone receptors. Cancer Res 37:1537–1543

Turnell RW, Burton AF (1974) Studies on the mechanism of resistance to lymphocytolysis induced by corticosteroids. Cancer Res 34:39–42

Turnell RW, Burton AF (1975) Glucocorticoid receptors and lymphocytolysis in normal and neoplastic lymphocytes. Mol Cell Biochem 9:175–189

Turnell RW, Clarke LH, Burton AF (1973) Studies on the mechanism of corticosteroid-induced lymphocytolysis. Cancer Res 33:203–212

Voris BP, Nicholson ML, Young DA (1979) Resistance to lethal effects of glucocorticoids: increased synthesis of the same proteins may be responsible for the emergence of resistance in P1798 mouse lymphosarcoma and normal rat thymus cells. Fed Proc 38:512

Wagner RK, Gorlich L, Jungblut PW (1973) Dihydrotestosterone receptor in human mammary cancer. Acta Endocrinol [Suppl] 173:65

Walt AJ, Singhakowinta A, Brooks SC, Cortez A (1976) The surgical implications of estrophile protein estimations in carcinoma of the breast. Surgery 80:506–512

Webster DJT, Bronn DG, Minton JP (1978) Estrogen receptors and response of breast cancer to chemotherapy. N Engl J Med 299:604

Westley B, Rochefort H (1979) Estradiol induced proteins in the MCF-7 human breast cancer cell line. Biochem Biophys Res Comm 90:410–416

Wittliff JL, Lewko WM, Park DC, Kute TE, Baker DT, Kane LN (1978) Steroid binding proteins of mammary tissues and their clinical significance in breast cancer. In: McGuire WL (ed) Hormones, receptors and breast cancer. Raven, New York, pp 325–359

Yamamoto KR, Stampfer MR, Tomkins GM (1974) Receptors from glucocorticoid-sensitive lymphoma cells and two classes of insensitive clones: physical and DNA-binding properties. Proc Natl Acad Sci 71:3901–3905

Yamamoto KR, Gehring U, Stampfer MR, Sibley CH (1976) Genetic approaches to steroid hormone action. Recent Prog Horm Res 32:3–32

Young PCM, Einhorn LH, Ehrlich CE, Cleary RE, Rohn RJ (1978) Progesterone receptor as a marker of hormone responsive human breast tumor. Proc Am Assoc Cancer Res 19:204

Zava DT, McGuire WL (1977) Estrogen receptor. Unoccupied sites in nuclei of a breast tumor cell line. J Biol Chem 252:3703–3708

Section VII: Modification of Resistance

CHAPTER 24

Collateral Sensitivity and Cross-Resistance

B. T. HILL

A. Introduction

During the past 10 years cancer chemotherapy has established a valuable role in the management of many human malignancies. Its introduction has significantly improved the prognosis of patients with breast, ovarian and oat-cell lung cancers, and has resulted in long-term survivors or "cures" in cases of testicular teratomas, leukaemias, lymphomas and certain paediatric solid tumours (CARTER 1978; ZUBROD 1979). However, the overall success rate for many solid tumours remains low. Further progress depends on identifying factors which influence our failures and finding ways of overcoming or circumventing them. Drug resistance, once considered a rather academic enigma, now poses a major practical clinical problem. The high response rates of many tumours to chemotherapy reported in the literature are too often accompanied by very short durations of remission and failure to respond to subsequent therapy. Similarly overgrowth of drug-resistant tumour cells from initially predominantly sensitive populations is commonly seen with a variety of murine solid tumours used as predictive models for drug therapy (SCHABEL et al. 1980).

A knowledge of the establishment and regrowth patterns of drug-resistant populations is vital. Whilst the search for potential new agents continues we need to use the drugs already available more effectively. For example: (a) a knowledge of how readily resistance to particular drugs emerges, which conditions favour its development and whether this can be influenced adversely by the presence of other drugs could provide information for optimal drug scheduling; (b) details of cross-resistance between various agents could allow exclusions when selecting drugs for combinations or sequential schedules; (c) positive attempts to eradicate drug-resistant populations might involve using drugs to which these cells are collaterally sensitive.

This chapter aims to review our knowledge of patterns of collateral sensitivity and cross-resistance amongst experimental animal tumours, in vivo and in vitro, to a range of antitumour drugs. Only those drugs which are used clinically are considered in detail. An attempt is then made to link data from animal laboratory studies to those obtained with human tumour biopsy material in the laboratory or in phase II clinical trials. Finally the implications this knowledge has for altering the strategy of subsequent clinical studies are discussed.

Table 1. Agents tested in vivo

Mammalian tumour lines resistant in vivo to:		Actinomycin D	Adriamycin	Daunomycin	mAMSA	Mithramycin	5-Azacytidine	araC	Methotrexate
Actinomycin D	P388	R	S[a]						S[a]
	Ridgeway osteogenic sarcoma	R	CR[b]						
Adriamycin	P388	CR[c]	R	CR[c]	CR[c]	CR[c]	S[c]	S[c]	S[c]
	Ehrlich ascites		R	CR[d]				CS[d]	S[d]
	Sarcoma 180		R	CR[e]					S[e]
Daunomycin	P388	CR[c]	CR[c]	R					
	Ehrlich ascites		CR[d]	R					S[d]
	Yoshida sarcoma	CR[f]	CR[f]	R					
	L1210		CR[f]	R					
Vinblastine	P815			CR[g]				S[g]	
	Ehrlich ascites		CR[d]	CR[d]				CS[d]	S[d]
Vincristine	P388	CR[i]	S[g]	CR[i]				S[a]	S[g]
	Ehrlich ascites		CR[d]	CR[d]				S[d]	S[d]
Asparaginase	L5178Y							S[g]	S[j], CS[g] S[j] CS[g]

[a] SCHABEL et al. (1980)
[b] KAYE and BODEN (1980)
[c] JOHNSON et al. (1978)
[d] DANO (1976)
[e] VOLM and LINDNER (1978)
[f] HOSHINO et al. (1972)
[g] HUTCHINSON and SCHMID (1973)
[h] HUTCHISON (1965)
[i] BOSMANN and KESSEL (1970)
[j] SCHMID and HUTCHISON (1971)
[k] SCHABEL (1979)
[l] JAYARAM et al. (1979)

B. Definition of Terms

Resistant cells are selected or derived from a population originally responsive to drug treatment. These resistant cells are characterised by their lack of susceptibility to the cytotoxic effects of this specific drug. Cross-resistance is identified when the resistant population, unlike the parent from which it was selected, also exhibits resistance to other related or unrelated drugs (HUTCHISON and SCHMID 1973). Collateral sensitivity describes a cell population that is resistant to one or more drugs but is more sensitive to the cytotoxic effects of another drug or drugs than the drug-sensitive parent population (SZYBALSKI and BRYSON 1952).

These definitions rely heavily on accurate evaluation of susceptibility to the drugs tested. Just as the degree of resistance can vary for any particular agent and within any cell population so the terms "collateral sensitivity" and "cross-resistance" should not be taken as "all or none" phenomena.

Table 1 (continued)

5-Fluorouracil	6-Mercaptopurine	BCNU	*cis*-Platinum	Cyclophosphamide	HN2	Mitomycin C	Melphalan	Vinblastine	Vincristine	Vindesine	Maytansine	VM26	VP-16-213	Asparaginase
		S[a]	S[a]	S[a]			S[a]		CR[a]				S[a]	
									CR[b]					
S[c]		S[c]	S[c]	S[c]	S[c]	S[c]	S[c]	CR[c]	CR[c]	CR[c]		CR[c]	CR[c]	
	S[d]							CR[d]	CR[d]					
				S[e]										
S[c]									CR[c]	CR[c]				
								CR[d]	CR[d]					
									CR[f]					
								R	CR[h]					
	S[d]	CS[d]						R	CR[d]					
		S[a]		S[a]			S[a]	CR[h]	R	CR[a]	CR[a]		S[g]	
	S[d]	S[d]						CR[d]	R				S[d]	
				S[g]										R

[m] LASTER and SCHABEL (1979)
[n] BROCKMAN (1974)
[o] WODINSKY and KENSLER (1964)
[p] HUTCHISON (1963)
[q] SCHABEL (1980, unpublished data)
[r] SCHMID and STOCK (1976)
[s] KLINE et al. (1971)
[t] GOLDENBERG (1975)
[u] TSUKAGOSHI and HASHIMOTO (1973)
[v] RIECH and BRADNER (1979)
[w] SCHABEL et al. (1978)

C. Incidence of Collateral Sensitivity and Cross-Resistance in Experimental Animal Tumours

I. In Vivo Studies

Data obtained from transplantable animal tumours rendered resistant to a particular drug, generally by serial passage of the tumour through animals treated with increasing doses of drug, are summarised in Tables 1–3. A comparison is made of the effects of subsequent drug treatment on both the parent tumour line and the resistant line and their responses have been classified: *S* indicates that the drug was equally effective against both tumour lines, *CR* indicates cross-resistance and *CS* collateral sensitivity. In most of the studies the effects of drug therapy were monitored by standard procedures involving a recording of survival times or gross tumour measurements. However, for example, in the studies of

Table 2. Agents tested in vivo

Mammalian tumour lines resistant in vivo to:		Actinomycin D	Adriamycin	Daunomycin	Neocarcinostatin	5-Azacytidine	Deazauridine	Azaserine	araC	Methotrexate
Azaserine	L1210							R		
	Plasma cell							R		CS[g]
Cytosine arabinoside	P388					S[a]	CS[k]		R	
	P815								R	
	L1210					S[a]	CS[n]	S[o]	R	S[g]
	L5178Y								R	S[g]
Methotrexate	L1210	CS[f]	CS[f]	S[g]	CR[g]			CR[g]	S[g]	R
	Ehrlich ascites									R
	P388							S[g]	S[g]	R
	L5178Y									R
Hydroxyurea	L1210								S[k]	
5-Fluorouracil	P388									CR[h]
	P815							S[g]	S[g]	S[g]
	L1210	CS[p]	S[f]	S[f]						S[p]
	Yoshida sarcoma		S[f]							
6-Mercaptopurine	L1210	S[p]			CS[g]			CS[p]	S[g]	CS[p]
	Ehrlich ascites							CS[p]		CS[n]
	Yoshida sarcoma		S[f]							
	Sarcoma 180				CS[g]				S[g]	
Thioguanine	L1210							S[g]		S[g] CS[p]
	Ehrlich ascites							S[p] CS[p]		S[p]

[a] SCHABEL et al. (1980)
[b] KAYE and BODEN (1980)
[c] JOHNSON et al. (1978)
[d] DANO (1976)
[e] VOLM and LINDNER (1978)
[f] HOSHINO et al. (1972)
[g] HUTCHINSON and SCHMID (1973)
[h] HUTCHISON (1965)
[i] BOSMANN and KESSEL (1970)
[j] SCHMID and HUTCHISON (1971)
[k] SCHABEL (1979)
[l] JAYARAM et al. (1979)

SCHABEL, SKIPPER and their colleagues (SCHABEL et al. 1980; SKIPPER et al. 1978, 1979) the net log change in viable tumour-cell population after drug treatment was recorded, allowing a more critical evaluation of the range and extent of sensitivity, collateral sensitivity, resistance or cross-resistance. For example, Table 4 shows that all four cell lines exhibit similar sensitivities to cyclophosphamide, 1,3-bis(2-chloroethyl)-1-nitrosourea (BCNU), melphalan and methotrexate. Com-

Table 2 (continued)

Hydroxyurea	5-Fluorouracil	6-Mercaptopurine	6-Thioguanine	PALA	Pyrazofurin	BCNU	Cyclophosphamide	DTIC	HN2	Myleran	Melphalan	Thiotepa	Vincristine	Asparaginase
	S[g]	CR[g]							S[g]			S[g]		
	S[g]		S[g]				CR[g]		S[g]		CS[g]			
	S[a]			CS[m]	CS[k]		S[a]							
	CS[l]													
S[g]														
S[g]	S[o]	S[o]	S[o]			S[g]	S[g]		S[o]	S[o]			S[o]	
		CS[a]												
							S[j]							CS[j]
S[a]	S[g]	S[g]	CR[g]				S[g]		CS[g]		CS[g]	S[g]		S[g]
		CS[p]					CS[p]							
	CS[p]													
	S[g]		CR[g]				CR[g]		S[g]		CS[g]	S[g]		
							S[g]							S[g]
														CS[g]
R														
	R			CS[m]										
	R		S[g]				S[g]		S[g]		CS[g]	CR[g]		
	R	CS[p]					CR		S[p]					
	R													
	S[p]	R	CR[p]				CS[g]	S[p]	CS[p]					
							S[p]		S[p]					
		R	CR[p]											
		R							S[p]					
		R	CR[p]											
	CR[g]	CR[p]	R				S[g]		CS[g]		CS[g]	CS[g]		
		CR[g]	R											

[m] Laster and Schabel (1979)
[n] Brockman (1974)
[o] Wodinsky and Kensler (1964)
[p] Hutchison (1963)
[q] Schabel (1980, unpublished data)
[r] Schmid and Stock (1976)
[s] Kline et al. (1971)
[t] Goldenberg (1975)
[u] Tsukagoshi and Hashimoto (1973)
[v] Riech and Bradner (1979)
[w] Schabel et al. (1978)

plete cross-resistance is shown to daunomycin by the vincristine- and adriamycin-resistant lines and to vincristine by the adriamycin- and actinomycin-D-resistant cell lines. However, the lines differ in their responses to *cis*-platinum, with the adriamycin- and actinomycin-D-resistant lines being as sensitive as the parent line, whilst the vincristine-resistant line shows limited cross-resistance. Similarly the adriamycin-resistant line differs from the other lines, showing marked

Table 3. Agents tested in vivo

Mammalian tumour lines resistant in vivo to:		Actinomycin D	Adriamycin	Daunomycin	mAMSA	5-Azacytidine	araC	Methotrexate	5-Fluorouracil	6-Mercaptopurine
BCNU	L1210									
	P388									
Methyl CCNU	Lewis lung							S[g]		S[g]
cis-Platinum	L1210									
Cyclophosphamide	L1210							CR[g]	CR[a]	
	P388	S[a]	S[a]		S[a]				CR[a]	
	Yoshida sarcoma		S[f]							
	Fortner plasmacytoma							S[f]		
DTIC	L1210			S[s]			S[s]	S[s]		S[s]
HN2	L5178Y									
	Yoshida sarcoma									
Mitomycin	L1210		S[v]							
	Yoshida sarcoma	S[f]	S[f]	S[f]						CS[p]
Myleran	Yoshida sarcoma		S[f]							
Melphalan	L1210	S[a]	S[a]			S[a]				
	P388		S[a]							
	Dunning leukaemia	S[p]						S[g]		S[g]
	Walker 256									
Peptichemio	L1210						CS[r]			
Thiotepa	Yoshida sarcoma		S[f]							

[a] SCHABEL et al. (1980)
[b] KAYE and BODEN (1980)
[c] JOHNSON et al. (1978)
[d] DANO (1976)
[e] VOLM and LINDNER (1978)
[f] HOSHINO et al. (1972)
[g] HUTCHINSON and SCHMID (1973)
[h] HUTCHISON (1965)
[i] BOSMANN and KESSEL (1970)
[j] SCHMID and HUTCHISON (1971)
[k] SCHABEL (1979)
[l] JAYARAM et al. (1979)

cross-resistance to 4'demethyl-epipodophyllotoxin-9-(4,6-*O*-ethylidene-*β*-D-glycopyranoside (VP-16-213). These data illustrate the range of drug sensitivities being considered.

The data in Tables 1–3 allow certain general conclusions: (a) cross-resistance is most frequently noted amongst the following drugs: actinomycin D, adriamycin, daunomycin and the *Vinca* alkaloids; (b) collateral sensitivity was only noted when treating "alkylating agent"- or "antimetabolite"-resistant tumours with other "alkylating agents" or "antimetabolites;" (c) no general patterns of cross-resistance are apparent with the "alkylating agents" or "antimetabolites", with the exception of most of the nitrosoureas, which appear cross-resistant to each

Table 3 (continued)

PALA	BCNU	CCNU	Methyl CCNU	Chlorozotocin	Streptozotocin	*cis*-Platinum	Cyclophosphamide	Dianhydrogalacticol	DTIC	HN2	Mitomycin C	Myleran	Melphalan	Peptichemio	Thiotepa	Vincristine	VP-16-213
	R	CR[a]	CR[a]		S[a]	S[a]	S[a]	S[a]	S[a]				S[a]		CR[a]		
	R					S[a]	S[a]	S[a]					S[a]				
			R				S[g]										
	S[q]	S[q]	S[q]	S[q]		R	S[q]	S[q]					S[q]				
	S[a]	S[a]	S[a]	S[a]	CR[a]	S[a]	R	S[a]			S[a]		C[a]	S[a]	CR[a]		
													CS[r]	CS[r]			
CR[a]	S[a]					S[a]	R	S[a]			S[a]		S[a]	S[a]		S[a]	S[a]
							R										
	CR[h]						R			CR[h]	CR[h]	CR[h]					
	CS[s]	S[s]					S[s]		R				S[s]				
	CR[t]						CR[t]			R							
CS[u]										R							
											R						
										CR[p]	R				CR[p]		
												R					
	S[a]	S[a]	S[a]			CR[a]	S[a]	S[a]		S[a]	S[a]		R	CR[a]	CR[n]		
	S[a]					CR[a]	S[a]				S[a]		R	CR[a]		CR[a]	S[a]
							CR[g]			CR[g]		CR[g]	R		CR[g]		
						CR[g]	CR[a]			CR[h]			R	CR[h]			
							S[r]			S[r]			CR[r]	R			
															R		

[m] LASTER and SCHABEL (1979)
[n] BROCKMAN (1974)
[o] WODINSKY and KENSLER (1964)
[p] HUTCHISON (1963)
[q] SCHABEL (1980, unpublished data)
[r] SCHMID and STOCK (1976)
[s] KLINE et al. (1971)
[t] GOLDENBERG (1975)
[u] TSUKAGOSHI and HASHIMOTO (1973)
[v] RIECH and BRADNER (1979)
[w] SCHABEL et al. (1978)

other. This latter point, arising mainly from the work of SCHABEL et al. (1978), emphasises how mistaken is the widely held belief that all "alkylating agents" have similar biochemical mechanisms whereby they kill cells and that tumour cells resistant to one "alkylating agent" probably are cross-resistant to other "alkylating agents." The individuality of action of chlorambucil, melphalan and myeleran was pointed out in earlier studies using drug-sensitive and drug-resistant strains of the Yoshida ascites sarcoma (HARRAP and HILL 1969a, 1969b).

SKIPPER (1972), however, emphasised earlier that "it is not intended to imply that the patterns of cross-resistance or lack of cross-resistance obtained to date and reviewed... will hold for all tumours." Although it can be seen that where

Table 4. Net $\log_{10}$ change in viable P388 leukemia cells following optimal treatment of mice implanted i.p. with 10^6 tumour cells. (After SCHABEL et al. 1980)

Agent	Treatment schedule	Parent cell line	Vincristine-resistant line	Adriamycin-resistant line	Actinomycin-D-resistant line
Cyclophosphamide	A	−7	−7	−7	−7
BCNU	A	−7	−7	−7	−7
Melphalan	A	−7	−7	−7	−7
cis-Platinum	C	−6	−4	−6	−6
Adriamycin	A	−6	−4	−2	−5
Daunomycin	A	−6	0	−1	ns
Actinomycin D	A	−5	−3	−1	−2
Vincristine	B	−6	+2	+3	+3
VP-16-213	B	−7	−6	+1	−5
Methotrexate	D	−3	−4	−2	−3

A, single dose; B, every 4 days × 3; C, daily for 5 days; D, every 3 h × 8, every 4 days × 3; ns, not stated

different tumour types were selected, as shown in these tables, remarkably similar patterns of sensitivity or resistance were observed. This is in spite of the fact that not only may the extent of resistance vary, but it may have been derived using different treatment schedules and the tumour may have been maintained in the continued presence or absence of the specific agents. There were of course a few exceptions. For example: (a) the actinomycin-D- (SCHABEL et al. 1980) and vincristine-resistant lines of the P388 leukaemia (BOSMANN and KESSEL 1970) were sensitive to adriamycin, unlike the actinomycin-D-resistant Ridgeway osteogenic sarcoma (KAYE and BODEN 1980) and the vincristine-resistant Ehrlich ascites tumour (DANO 1976), which were both cross-resistant to adriamycin. (b) The methotrexate-resistant L1210 leukaemia was cross-resistant to azaserine, unlike the methotrexate-resistant P388 leukaemia, which was sensitive (HUTCHISON and SCHMID 1973). However, caution is essential when attempting to interpret these animal tumour data relating to drug resistance and collateral sensitivity, since for most of these experiments it has not been possible to establish and employ optimal drug schedules. Drug scheduling and the size of the body burden of tumour cells are of course critical factors in planning curative chemotherapy with effective drugs (SCHABEL et al. 1980).

II In Vitro Studies

Table 5 summarises data obtained from in vitro studies, which are far less extensive than reports using tumour-bearing animals. The following points may be noted: (a) examples of collateral sensitivity were quoted only for methotrexate-resistant, adriamycin-resistant or 5-fluorouracil-resistant tumour cell lines. The collateral sensitivity of methotrexate-resistant tumours to adriamycin was also observed in vivo (Table 1). (b) Cross-resistance has most frequently been observed amongst the following drugs: actinomycin D, adriamycin, daunomycin, vincristine and vinblastine. This corresponds with in vivo data (see Tables 1–3). (c) Whilst HN2-resistant L5178Y cells exhibit cross-resistance to a number of other "alkylating agents" (GOLDENBERG 1975), similar cross-resistance patterns were not seen with cyclophosphamide- and BCNU-resistant L1210 cells (ALEXANDER et al. 1980). (d) The vincristine-resistant CHO (BIEDLER et al. 1980) and P388 leukaemia lines (WILKOFF and DULMADGE 1978 b) showed cross-resistance to VP-16-213. This differs from in vivo data using the P388 and Ehrlich ascites tumour cells (HUTCHISON and SCHMID 1973).

D. Mechanisms Implicated in Determining Collateral Sensitivity or Cross-Resistance

Mechanisms invoked to attempt to explain collateral sensitivity are often simple reversions of the postulated mechanisms of resistance (HUTCHISON and SCHMID 1973). For example: elevated "target" enzyme levels may confer drug resistance whilst decreased enzyme activity could be associated with increased sensitivity. The validity of this statement remains uncertain mainly because of lack of data. Cross-resistance is generally ascribed to a shared pattern of resistance often involving a transport defect. For example, the mechanism of resistance of adriamycin-resistant and daunomycin-resistant P388 leukaemia appears to be identical and this is reflected in a qualitatively similar pattern of cross-resistance (JOHNSON et al. 1978). In contrast, differences in the mechanism of resistance between adriamycin-resistant and vincristine-resistant tumours are associated with differences in the pattern of cross-resistance. However, these authors point out that mechanisms of resistance may differ in vivo and in vitro. A decreased drug uptake has often been implicated in in vitro studies but recent data suggest that this may not be particularly relevant to in vivo resistance. For example: (a) enhanced drug efflux rather than impaired influx may underlie resistance in vivo (INABA and JOHNSON 1979), and (b) whilst uptake of PALA in vitro was reduced in a refractory L1210 leukaemia, 24 h after drug administration in vivo nearly identical intratumoural drug concentrations were observed in representative, sensitive and refractory tumours (JAYARAM et al. 1979).

Various mechanisms of collateral sensitivity were listed originally by HUTCHISON and SCHMID (1973) (see Table 6) and most of these will have been discussed in earlier chapters. Collateral sensitivity may be conferred as a result of a biochemical alteration accompanying the development of resistance. For example, BROCKMAN (1974) suggested that the increased sensitivity to deazauridine of a cytosine arabinoside (araC)-resistant L1210 line could be accounted for by the resistant cells' incapacity to utilise exogenous deoxycytidine as a consequence of their loss of deoxycytidine kinase or their relatively smaller pool of deoxycytidine-5-triphosphate (dCTP). It is, however, conceivable that alternative or distinctive mechanisms may be involved in determining the expression of collateral sensitivity or cross-resistance, without being centrally implicated in the original resistance mechanism. HILL et al. (1975) showed the value of a combination of 2,4-diamino-5-(3′,4′-dichlorophenyl)-6-methylpyrimidine (DDMP) and leucovorin in selectively reducing the survival of methotrexate-resistant L5178Y cells. This

Table 5. Agents tested in vitro

Mammalian cell lines resistant in vitro to:		Actinomycin D	Adriamycin	Daunomycin	mAMSA	Bleomycin	Mithramycin	araC	Azaserine	Methotrexate	DDMP
Actinomycin D	CHO	R	CR[a]	CR[b]			CR[b]			S[b]	
Adriamycin	CHO		R							CS[c]	
	S180		R	CR[d]							
Daunomycin	CHO	CR[b]	CR[a]	R							
Bleomycin	CHO					R					
Vincristine	CHO	CR[f]		CR[f]							
	P388	CR[g]	CR[g]	CR[g]							
	L5178Y	CR[i]	CR[i]								
Methotrexate	ALL-MOLT 3			S[j]				S[j]		R	CS[j]
	L5178Y		CS[k]					S[l]		R	CS[m]
	L1210		S[k]							R	
	CHO		CS[c]							R	
DDMP	L1210									S[p]	R
5-Fluorouracil	L5178Y		CS[n]		CS[n]					S[n]	
BCNU	L1210										
Cyclophosphamide	L1210										
HN2	L5189Y										
ICRF 159	BHK	S[s]	S[s]	S[s]	S[s]	S[s]	S[s]	S[s]		S[s]	S[s]

[a] RIEHM and BIEDLER (1971)
[b] BIEDLER und RIEHM (1970)
[c] HERMAN et al. (1979)
[d] SIEGFRIED et al. (1980)
[e] BRABBS and WARR (1979)
[f] BIEDLER et al. (1980)
[g] WILKOFF and DULMADGE (1978a)
[h] WILKOFF and DULMADGE (1978b)
[i] HILL and WHELAN (1982)
[j] OHNOSHI et al. (1980)

selectivity takes advantage of a membrane change in the methotrexate-resistant cells which appears to render leucovorin ineffective as a competitor for DDMP influx, compared with a marked competition of leucovorin for DDMP uptake in sensitive cells. This finding suggests that properties of the resistant cell might be exploited to increase its killing while protecting the normal sensitive cell. To establish whether this is a more general phenomenon, fundamentals of drug action must be studied specifically in these drug treated populations rather than just working with the parent cell lines as has been done mainly in the past.

Another possible approach to establishing molecular mechanisms of resistance is to work with the range of stable drug-resistant phenotypes involving many drugs used in clinical practice, which have been established in culture. Although these mutants may not have an exact counterpart in the human body they

Table 5 (continued)

Hydroxyurea	5-Fluorouracil	6-Mercaptopurine	BCNU	Chlorozotocin	Dibromodulcitol	*cis*-Platinum	Cyclophosphamide	Chlorambucil	HN2	Mitomycin C	Melphalan	ICRF 159	Vinblastine	Vincristine	Vondesine	VM26	VF-16-213
										CR[b]			CR[b]	CR[b]			
										S[d]				CR[d]			
														CR[b]			
													CR[e]				
														R			CR[f]
														R			CR[h]
													CR[i]	R	CR[i]		
	S[j]					S[j]											
CR[n]	S[n]				S[n]							CS[o]				CR[n]	
												S[n]					
	R	CS[n]			S[n]	S[n]				CS[n]	CS[n]	S[n]		CR[n]	CR[n]	S[n]	S[n]
			R	S[q]													
			S[q]	S[q]			R										
			CR[r]					CR[r]	R	CR[r]	CR[r]						
		S[s]				S[s]		S[s]				R	S[s]				

[k] Hill et al. (1976)
[l] Fischer (1962)
[m] Hill et al. (1973)
[n] Hill B.T. (unpublished data)
[o] Hill and Hellmann (1977)
[p] Brownman and Lazarus (1980)
[q] Alexander et al. (1980)
[r] Goldenberg (1975)
[s] White (1979)

have proved valuable in providing evidence for a genetic basis for drug resistance (Siminovitch 1976), but also have demonstrated the involvement of non-genetic factors (DeMars 1974). Studies with methotrexate-resistant Chinese hamster ovary (CHO) cells have shown also that different phenotypes, which may be distinguished genetically and biochemically as representing different mechanisms of resistance, can be obtained from the same cell line (Flintoff 1976). The alteration that confers colchicine resistance also results in a display of cross-resistance to adriamycin, vinblastine and melphalan but collateral sensitivity to cyclophosphamide, steroids and acronycine (Ling 1975).

The last two proposals listed in Table 6 are those most generally invoked as relating specifically to the development of collateral sensitivity and have been reviewed in detail by Hutchison and Schmid (1973) and Mihich (1973). It has been

Table 6. Possible mechanisms for collateral sensitivity. (After HUTCHISON and SCHMID 1973)

1. Mechanisms which may be associated with the mode of action of the drug:
   a) Decreased activity of the "target" enzyme
   b) Increased affinity of the "target" enzyme for the inhibitor
   c) Increased dependence upon a "drug-sensitive" pathway
   d) Increased activity of an enzyme that carries out "lethal" synthesis
2. Mechanisms which may be associated with specific drugs:
   a) Modification of DNA so that drugs bind more firmly or at more sites
   b) Increased requirement for a specific metabolite
3. Mechanisms which need not be associated with the mode of action of the drug:
   a) Increased cellular permeability
   b) Loss of a drug-detoxifying enzyme
   c) Antigenic alteration of the malignant cell
   d) Loss of oncogenic potential of the malignant cell

proposed that cells undergo changes in oncogenic potential or immunogenicity, resulting in an expression of collateral sensitivity or cross-resistance when challenged with another drug. It has been noted that the mice bearing drug-resistant leukaemias have increased survival times (HUTCHISON and SCHMID 1973). Heterotransplantation studies where L5178Y or L1210 cells were injected into X-irradiated hamsters also revealed that the animals receiving drug-resistant cells had a longer mean survival time than those receiving cells of the parent line (HUTCHISON and SCHMID 1973). In vitro studies have also shown the loss of transplantability back into animals of induced drug-resistant cells (SUGIMURA 1970). These results have been interpreted as a demonstration of a decreased oncogenic potential in the drug-resistant cells (HUTCHISON and SCHMID 1973). However, published data of the growth rates of a number of murine leukaemias selected for drug resistance have indicated that drug-resistant tumour cells have approximately the same growth kinetics as the parent drug-sensitive line from which they were derived (SCHABEL et al. 1980). Indeed other workers have provided examples of a lack of detectable differences in intrinsic oncogenic potential between the parent and a subline of L1210 resistant to methylglyoxal bis(guanylhydrazone), with both lines having comparable growth patterns in X-irradiated mice (MIHICH and KITANO 1971). In this case resistance is accompanied by enhanced and different antigenic specificities. It is possible that resistance to chemotherapy may be associated with increased tumour immunogenicity. This effect may arise as a result of decreased immunoselection occurring during treatments with the resistance-selecting agent which also may exert immunosuppressive action (MIHICH 1973). Alternative mechanisms which cannot be excluded invoke mutation induction by the selecting drugs. Increased cell susceptibility to immune responses may also play a role in determining the different responses seen as suggested by TSUKAGOSHI and HASHMOTO (1973) using a HN2-resistant Yoshida sarcoma which exhibited collateral sensitivity to 6-mercaptopurine.

These studies have led to the hope that with the right combination of events during the development of drug resistance a population might emerge which would either no longer be tumourigenic because of a decrease in oncogenic potential or would allow such manipulation of the "antigenic stimulus" as to lead to immunological rejection. Such approaches depend on a deeper understanding of the biological controlling mechanisms of tumour growth and more specifically on how they are influenced or modified in resistant tumour populations. It is therefore disappointing that with little new data published recently work in this area has not been pursued.

E. Establishment, Stability and Reversion of Collateral Sensitivity and Cross-Resistance

Drug-resistant mutants to all known anticancer drugs may occur spontaneously in vivo and/or in vitro. The rates of mutation to resistance vary markedly, ranging from 10^{-5} to 10^{-8} (BROCKMAN 1974), being highest for vincristine, less frequent for araC and lowest for cyclophosphamide (SCHABEL et al. 1980). This frequency can often be increased by (a) treatment with known chemical mutagens, for example, ethyl methane sulphonate has been used to increase the frequency of resistance to bleomycin in CHO cells (BRABBS and WARR 1979), or (b) exposure to particular antitumour agents, a number of which are considered to be mutagenic under certain conditions (THOMPSON and BAKER 1973). However, these studies have produced evidence for multiple genetic loci underlying drug-resistant phenotypes. Clones of baby hamster kidney (BHK) cells isolated for resistance to aminopterin after treatment with chemical mutagens display a different mechanism of resistance from lines occurring spontaneously (ORKIN and LITTLEFIELD 1971).

The rate and extent of development of resistance by exposure to antitumour drugs and its stability vary widely and the reasons remain unclear. In a number of lines developed in vivo by drug treating tumour-bearing mice over successive transplant generations resistance was established by the 12th passage, e.g., resistance to melphalan in L1210 leukaemia (SCHABEL et al. 1978) and resistance to vincristine or adriamycin in the P388 leukaemia (JOHNSON et al. 1978). However, FOX (1969) has reported that resistance to methylene di-methanesulphonate in the Yoshida tumour developed as a single-step process in vivo and resistance to mitomycin C was established after only one transfer generation (HOSHINO et al. 1972). DANO (1976) also noted variability, reporting that whilst resistance to daunomycin occurred readily in the Ehrlich ascites tumour it was a more gradual process with adriamycin. Clearly the influence of dosage and scheduling on the rate of selection of drug-resistant tumour cells must be established and this may well provide information of value in designing future clinical studies. For example, it is known that with the L1210 leukaemia repetitive doses of various "antimetabolites" and "alkylating agents" fail to cure (under certain circumstances) because they specifically select out resistant tumour cells (SKIPPER et al. 1978).

Maintenance of lines in vivo involves either continued drug treatment at each passage, for example in the L1210 leukaemia resistant to melphalan (SCHABEL et al. 1978) and the Ehrlich ascites tumour resistant to vincristine (DANO 1976), or in other cases drug treatment is discontinued since resistance is considered stable, for example in the vincristine- and adriamycin-resistant P388 leukaemias (JOHN-

SON et al. 1978). Resistant cells have also been transferred successfully from tumour-bearing animals into culture, reflecting their stable character. However, the stability of resistance in vitro appears more variable. In five clones of CHO cells resistant to bleomycin, resistance was stable in three but unstable in the other two (BRABBS and WARR 1979). Many resistant lines are maintained in vitro in the continuous presence of the drug. This is the policy of my laboratory with L5178Y lines resistant to methotrexate, 5-fluorouracil or vincristine. However, this may be unnecessary since these lines grown in the absence of the selecting agents showed no sign of reversion within 6 months. This contrasts with the report of COURTENAY and ROBINS (1972) concerning a line of methotrexate-resistant L5178Y cells, but perhaps serves to emphasise that cells with different mechanisms of resistance may also have different stabilities. For example, both lines of methotrexate-resistant L5178Y cells have elevated dihydrofolate reductase levels but in addition our line has a drug transport defect. This point is further illustrated by recent findings of SCHIMKE and his colleagues (KAUFMAN et al. 1979). They concluded that in stably amplified methotrexate-resistant lines the dihydrofolate reductase genes are chromosomal and segregate equally at mitosis, whereas in unstably amplified cell variants the genes are largely extrachromosomal and as a result of unequal distribution at mitosis can be lost from the population in subsequent generations.

In the few cases reported where resistance has been lost, details concerning patterns of cross-resistance or collateral sensitivity in the revertants have often not been provided. However, BECH-HANSEN et al. (1976), working with colchicine-resistant CHO cells, reported that spontaneous revertants which had lost resistance to colchicine also lost their cross-resistance and collateral sensitivity to other drugs.

F. Clinical Studies Concerned with the Evaluation of Drug Sensitivity or Cross-Resistance

One aim of clinical studies is to identify drugs of value in treating recurrent disease, hence avoiding sequential use of drugs exhibiting cross-resistance. Any potentially new antitumour agent undergoes evaluation predominantly in patients heavily pretreated with drugs as single agents or in combinations and/or radiotherapy who have failed or ceased to respond. Table 7 summarises some recently published results (predominantly from the Proceedings of the American Association for Cancer Research and the American Society of Clinical Oncology, 1979 and 1980) in a range of human malignancies which provide some basis for identifying promising new drugs, for indicating which second line drugs may be valuable in treating recurrent disease and which might be best avoided. These results make the point previously shown in animal studies of the danger of grouping together drugs with apparently similar chemical structures and assuming a common mechanism of action. For example: (a) patients pretreated with adriamycin frequently subsequently responded to m-9-acridinylamino-ethanosulfon-m-anisidide (mAMSA) (AHMANN et al. 1980); (b) peptichemio was effective in patients with breast cancer who had failed on cyclophosphamide, another so-

Table 7. Results from some recent clinical studies indicating "valuable" or "ineffective" secondary drugs in releasing patients

Tumour type	Pretreatment with single drugs or combinations including:	Valuable second line drugs	References	Non-effective drugs	References
Breast	CYC	Peptichemio	HUG et al. (1980)		
	CYC+ADR			CYC+MTX +5FU	WENDT et al. (1980)
	CYC+ADR+5FU +MTX	VLB (as infusion)	YAP et al. (1980b)	Rubidazone	INGLE et al. (1979)
		VDS	SKELLEY et al. (1980)		
	CYC+ADR+5FU +MTX	AMSA+Peptichemio	BUZDAR et al. (1980)		
		AMSA	SAMAL et al. (1980)		
	CYC+MTX+5FU +VCR+PRED	ADR+VP-16-213	VAN ECHO et al. (1979)		
		cis-Pt	HAKES et al. (1979)		
Colorectal	5-FU	DBD	BIERMANN et al. (1979)	VDS	ROSSOF et al. (1979)
		Ftorofur	ANSFIELD et al. (1980)	ICRF 159	DOUGLASS et al. (1979)
	5-FU			AMSA	LEICHMAN et al. (1980)
Cervix	Not stated			VP-16-213	SLAYTON et al. (1979a)
Germinal	VLB	VP-16-213	WILLIAMS et al. (1979)	VDS	REYNOLDS et al. (1979)
Melanoma	AMSA+DTIC	PALA	CREAGAN et al. (1980)		
	ADR	AMSA	AHMANN et al. (1980)		
	DTIC	AMSA	HALL et al. (1979)		
Osteogenic sarcoma	ADR+MTX	*cis*-Pt	ROSEN et al. (1979)		
Ovarian	"Alkylating agents"	*cis*-Pt	THIGPEN et al. (1979)	VP-16-213	SLAYTON et al. (1979b)
				ADR	OZOLS et al. (1980)
				AMSA	DOMBROWSKY and HAUSEN (1980)
Lung "non-oat" cell	PROC:VCR:CYC:CCNU	VDS	STAMBAUGH (1980)	AMSA	FUKS et al. (1980)
	VP-16-213:ADR:MTX	*cis*-Pt	ROSENFELT et al. (1980)		
Sarcoma	ADR	VDS	MAGILL et al. (1980)		
		AMSA	AHMANN et al. (1980)		
Testicular	VLB+ActD+BLEO +MTX	*cis*-Pt	ROZENCWEIG et al. (1978)		
Acute leukemia	VCR:PRED:ADR:-AraC:Asp	AMSA	LAWRENCE et al. (1980)	Rubidazone	DASGUPTA et al. (1979)
		VDS	BAYSSAS et al. (1979)		
Non-Hodgkin's lymphoma	CYC+VCR+PRED +BLEO	VLB (as infusion)	TIBER et al. (1980)		

CYC, cyclophosphamide; ADR, Adriamycin; 5FU, 5-fluorouracil; MTX, methotrexate; VCR, vincristine; PRED, prednisolone; VLB, vinblastine; AMSA, 9-acridinylamino-methanesulfon-m-anisidide; DTIC, 5-(3,3-dimethyl-1-triazeno)-imidazole-4-carboxamide; PROC, procarbazine; ActD, actinomycin D; BLEO, bleomycin; Asp, L-asparaginase; VDS, vindesine; DBD, dibromodulcitol; *cis*-Pt, *cis*-Platinum

Table 8. In vitro detection of cross-resistance and sensitivity in relapsing ovarian cancer with the human tumour stem-cell assay. (After Alberts et al. 1980a)

Drug treatment on which patient relapsed (drug I)	Second line drug tested (drug II)	Number of samples showing:		% of S tests
		CR between drugs I and II	S to drug II	
Melphalan	Adriamycin	30	4	12
Melphalan	Bleomycin	20	3	13
Melphalan	*cis*-Platinum	28	7	20
Melphalan	Methotrexate	15	4	21
Melphalan	Vinblastine	18	9	33
Adriamycin	Methotrexate	13	3	19
Adriamycin	*cis*-Platinum	27	6	18
Adriamycin	Vinblastine	19	9	32
Methotrexate	Adriamycin	ns	ns	12
Methotrexate	*cis*-Platinum	ns	ns	22
Methotrexate	Vinblastine	ns	ns	20
Bleomycin	*cis*-Platinum	ns	ns	32
Vindesine	Vinblastine	ns	ns	0
mAMSA	Adriamycin	ns	ns	29

ns, not stated

called alkylating agent (Hug et al. 1980); (c) vinblastine as 5-day infusions produced responses in patients who had received a prior combination including vincristine (Yap et al. 1980b; Tiber et al. 1980) and (d) some responses to Ftorofur were noted in patients not responding to 5-fluorouracil (Ansfield et al. 1980). However, results from these clinical studies are rarely precise and responses are often difficult to assess and interpret. Responses are influenced not only by the stage of the tumour being treated but also by the drug scheduling. For example, responses were seen to 5-fluorouracil or vindesine given by prolonged infusion in patients who had failed to respond to these drugs given as bolus injections (Gorton et al. 1980; Yap et al. 1980a). This raises the old problem of how to equate therapies in mice and man. However, with this type of data attempts can be made to see whether results from the laboratory are relevant to clinical experience.

One encouraging recent development concerns the evaluation of drug sensitivities and cross-resistance in human tumours in vitro using the stem-cell assay devised by Hamburger and Salmon (1977). This system has already proved useful for quantitating and predicting drug sensitivity and resistance to standard anticancer drugs with a high degree of accuracy in certain tumour types, predominantly ovarian ascites, myeloma and melanoma (Salmon et al. 1978; Alberts et al. 1980b; von Hoff et al. 1980). Recently Alberts et al. (1980a) evaluated survival of ovarian tumour colony-forming units from 69 relapsing patients. The patterns of cross-resistance and sensitivity observed are listed in Table 8. These results show that (a) vinblastine was the most active of the second line drugs in vitro against tumour colony-forming units from melphalan- or adriamycin-resistant patients, (b) *cis*-platinum and methotrexate show some in vitro activity in these drug-resistant patients in percentages similar to those observed clinically, (c) there was no evidence of collateral sensitivity between adriamycin and methotrexate, unlike that observed in some in vivo and in vitro animal models, (d) cross-resistance between vindesine and vinblastine was complete and (e) adriamycin was not cross-resistant with mAMSA. These results were used to select agents for treatment of relapsed patients on an individual basis. The authors point out that a clinical study to identify active agents with a similar degree of accuracy would have required 215 evaluable patients.

In a similar study by OZOLS et al. (1980) using 26 patients, three different patterns of sensitivity to adriamycin were observed: (a) in 75% of previously untreated patients there was >70% reduction in survival of colony-forming cells after exposure to adriamycin (1 μg/ml), a level approximating the peak plasma level after i.v. therapy; (b) in all patients with progressive disease while on a regimen without adriamycin a >70% reduction in colony-forming cells was observed only at a concentration of 10 μg/ml, a level not achievable by i.v. administration; and (c) in 80% of patients with progressive disease after treatment with adriamycin, as part of the primary regimen, a 70% reduction in tumour colony-forming cells could not be achieved even at 10 μg/ml. These in vitro results agree with clinical observations regarding the effectiveness of adriamycin in previously untreated patients (42% response rate) with ovarian cancer as well as its ineffectiveness (0%–6% response rate) as a second line therapy in relapsed patients (OZOLS et al. 1980). This work is sufficiently encouraging to hope that further studies with other tumour types will be initiated.

G. Implications of Collateral Sensitivity and Cross-Resistance

A knowledge of patterns of collateral sensitivity and cross-resistance is potentially valuable in the following areas: (a) scheduling antitumour agents to perhaps prevent the emergence of resistance, (b) designing optimal drug combinations to overcome cross-resistance or exploit collateral sensitivity, (c) devising specific second line therapies in relapsing patients to avoid drugs unlikely to be useful, (d) developing new antitumour drugs which can overcome resistance and lack cross-resistance, and (e) screening for new agents to which resistant tumours exhibit collateral sensitivity.

The success of chemotherapy both experimentally and clinically is greatly influenced not only by the stage of the disease being treated but also by the schedule employed. In animals bearing tumours the selecting out of specifically drug-resistant tumour cells is a major cause of treatment failure (SKIPPER et al. 1978). For example, repetitive doses of certain "alkylating agents" and several "antimetabolites" favour the emergence of drug-resistant cells. Thus treatment with a low dose of these agents on a prolonged daily basis is avoided in animal experiments, but unfortunately is still used in some clinical studies. SCHABEL et al. (1980) have also pointed out that the development of drug resistance is influenced by the drug doses used. A full dose combination of cyclophosphamide and 6-mercaptopurine, which resulted in complete regression and cure after four courses in the Ridgeway osteogenic sarcoma, when given in lower doses to animals carrying similarly staged advanced tumours, still produced regression but allowed tumour regrowth during continued treatment and all the animals died. Similarly, the growth of the drug-resistant population in a tumour is favoured by the practice of continuing with initially effective single drugs or combinations until it is overtly obvious that treatment is becoming less effective or failing before instituting alternative therapy (SCHABEL et al. 1980). One way of helping here is to use two different non-cross-resistant sequential schedules. This procedure has been tested experimentally and more recently in the clinic. For example, for squamous-cell carcinoma of the lung adriamycin, procarbazine and VP-16-213 have been shown to be non-cross-resistant with a combination of methotrexate, vincristine, cyclophosphamide and 1-(2-chloroethyl)-3-cyclohexyl-1-nitrosourea (CCNU) (LIVINGSTON 1980).

In general the emphasis of experimental studies has been to prevent the emergence of drug-resistant tumour-cell populations. Resistance has been found to develop to certain drugs more easily than others either spontaneously (discussed above) or following specific drug exposure. This fact is also almost certainly reflected in the examples cited in Tables 1–5 since failures to establish drug-resistant populations are generally not reported, although HUTCHISON and SCHMID (1973) stated that 15–20 generations of the Ridgeway osteogenic sarcoma were treated with cyclophosphamide, mitomycin C or nitrogen mustard (HN2) with absolutely no increase in resistance noted. Certain drug-resistant derived populations are not generally cross-resistant to other agents, for example: in vivo the araC-resistant (WODINSKY and KENSLER 1964) and the mitomycin-C-resistant L1210 leukaemias (REICH and BRADNER 1979) and the asparaginase-resistant L5178Y lymphomas (HUTCHISON and SCHMID 1977) and in vitro the 1-2-bis(3,5-dioxpiperazine-1-yl)propane (ICRF 159)-resistant BHK cells (WHITE 1979). Furthermore cross-resistance between drugs with similar chemical structures is by no means always observed either experimentally or clinically. This of course, as pointed out by BROCKMAN (1974), argues against the "lumping" together of certain drugs and dismissing their usefulness as has been frequently done with the "alkylating agents" (CONNORS et al. 1974; SCHABEL et al. 1978). These observations point to other factors which should be considered when selecting drugs for clinical studies.

Another factor is that whilst reciprocal cross-resistance may be expressed between two particular drugs, for example between actinomycin D and adriamycin or vincristine and daunomycin, this is not always the case. For example, in tumour-bearing animals, cells resistant to cyclophosphamide have been shown to be cross-resistant to methotrexate and 5-fluorouracil (see Table 3); however, cells resistant to methotrexate or 5-fluorouracil retain sensitivity to cyclophosphamide (see Table 2). Clinically it has also been observed that whilst some drugs are valuable as second line therapies in some tumours they are ineffective in others. Of course many factors including tumour site and histology, variable drug access and metabolism may well be involved. However, it has been shown that adriamycin with or without additional vincristine is valuable in recurrent breast tumours previously treated with combinations of cyclophosphamide, methotrexate and 5-fluorouracil (HENDERSON and CANELLOS 1980) but is ineffective in treating ovarian tumours relapsing after therapy with certain "alkylating agents," for example melphalan, chlorambucil and low-dose cyclophosphamide (HUBBARD et al. 1978), whilst *cis*-platinum appears a valuable drug in both previously untreated patients and relapsing patients with ovarian carcinomas (THIGPEN et al. 1979) or head and neck cancer (WITTES et al. 1979). Further data of this type may help in deciding which agent should be used as initial therapy and which could be used for second line treatment.

In this respect the concept of collateral sensitivity is extremely appealing. By allowing resistance to one agent to develop and so producing a tumour with known collateral sensitivity to another available agent this phenomenon could be exploited and so diminish a major obstacle to successful chemotherapy. However, this approach suggested by various workers (FOX 1977; KAYE and BODEN 1980) must be considered carefully since, whilst evidence for collateral sensitivity in certain animal system is available, it is not an "all or none" phenomenon (RUTMAN 1964) and its clinical relevance remains speculative. It has even been suggested that collateral sensitivity might be a chance occurrence or purely a laboratory phenomenon (HAKIMI and BOSMANN 1977). However, demonstration of collateral sensitivity in clinical studies, as defined, is hardly to be expected since it is unlikely that a patient developing resistance would be retreated with a drug to which they had originally shown a poor or no response. It is possible though that examples of therapeutic synergy might involve an expression of collateral sensitivity. For example: (a) whilst prednisolone was ineffective in Hodgkin's disease, its addition to MOP (nitrogen mustard, vincristine and procarbazine) resulted in a significantly enhanced response rate (DEVITA et al. 1970) and (b) a 33% response rate was recorded in patients with advanced pancreatic cancer receiving a combination of 5-fluorouracil and BCNU when 5-fluorouracil alone produced a response of only 16% and BCNU was completely inactive (KOVACH et al. 1974).

In the search for valuable second line agents it has been shown experimentally that whilst a drug may be inactive as initial therapy this should not necessarily preclude its testing in resistant tumours. For example, with *N*-phosphonacetyl-L-aspartate (PALA) collateral sensitivity has been shown in a P388 leukaemia line resistant to araC, although this drug was considered ineffective in initial screening of the parent line (LASTER and SCHABEL 1979). This of course raises the major question as to whether our experimental and clinical screening procedures are adequate. If there are indeed such agents these procedures would need to be modified. Experimentally drug-resistant populations would have to be screened. Clinically, although the current design of phase-II clinical studies would pick up effective second line agents, these would then be used in phase-III trials predominantly in previously untreated patients and would be rejected if they lacked activity.

Account must also be taken of the fact that multiple drug combinations are commonly employed. The influence of such combinations on the development of resistance or collateral sensitivity, the mechanisms involved and the response of such populations to subsequent therapy are questions that now need to be addressed. Experimentally a few tumour lines resistant to more than one particular agent have been developed (HUTCHISON and SCHMID 1973, 1974; BIEDLER and RIEHM 1970) but this is an area needing further attention.

The search for agents which will overcome specific drug-resistance, fail to show cross-resistance to other drugs and/or exhibit collateral sensitivity to currently available agents will probably centre on new compounds. It is, however, also important not to reject the agents we already have, since many have not been adequately evaluated in several tumour types. Undoubtedly better use can be made of these drugs which have a major advantage over newer compounds since it is known that they can be administered safely to people. The gradually increasing experimental work with human tumours as established lines in vitro, or in short-term cloning tests using biopsy material or in nude mice as xenografts, will provide a more rapid screening process for these drugs than can be achieved in clinical studies, although the direct relevance of this type of experimental model to trials in patients remains uncertain due to lack of data. This is a fruitful area for cooperative studies between the laboratory and the clinic.

H. Concluding Remarks

This review has emphasised that our attempts to establish patterns of collateral sensitivity and cross-resistance have only just begun. We should be encouraged that some of the in vitro and in vivo animal data appear to be corroborated by early clinical experience. Further work is needed particularly with human tumour material; and laboratory-clinical correlations using the in vitro assay systems, which can provide quantitative data most readily, will be of great importance. One exciting idea suggested by preliminary experimental work is the possibility that certain drugs will be more valuable as initial treatment whilst others will be more or equally effective as second line therapies. If confirmed, such information would be of value to the clinician in tailoring distinct cancer chemotherapy protocols not only against particular tumour types as at present, but also for use either as adjuvant therapy or for the treatment of advanced recurrent or untreated disease.

Acknowledgments. I am extremely grateful to the late Dr. F.M. Schabel and to Drs. L.A. Price, M. Fox, H.T. Rupniak and A.M. Creighton for their helpful advice and criticism in the preparation of this manuscript. I am indebted to Drs. F.M. Schabel and D. Alberts for allowing me to include some of their current unpublished data. The valuable assistance and patience of Mrs. E. Simmons and Miss G. Yiangou in typing the manuscript is greatly appreciated.

References

Ahmann F, Meyskens F, Jones S, Durie B, Alberts D, Salmon S (1980) A broad phase-II trial of AMSA with in vitro stem-cell culture drug sensitivity correlations. Proc Am Soc Clin Oncol 21:369

Alberts DS, Salmon SE, Chen HSG, Surwit EA, Soehnlein B, Young L (1980a) In vitro detection of cross-resistance and sensitivity in relapsing ovarian cancer with the human stem-cell assay. Proc Am Assoc Cancer Res 21:181

Alberts DS, Salmon SE, Chen HSG, Surwit EA, Soehnlein B, Young L, Moon TE (1980b) In vitro clonogenic assay for predicting response of ovarian cancer to chemotherapy. Lancet II:340–342

Alexander J, Adamson DJ, Wheeler GP (1980) Effects of two nitrosoureas upon cultured sensitive and resistant L1210 cells. Proc Am Assoc Cancer Res 21:13

Ansfield FJ, Callas G, Singson J, Uy B (1980) Further phase I–II studies with oral tegafur (Ftorafur). Proc Am Soc Clin Oncol 21:347

Bayssas M, Gouveia J, De Vassal F, Misset JL, Machover D, Schwarzenberg L, Schnieder M, Mathe G (1979) Phase-II clinical trials with vindesine for remission induction in leukemias and lymphomas. Apparent absence of cross resistance with vincristine. Proc Am Assoc Cancer Res 20:48

Bech-Hansen NT, Till JE, Ling V (1976) Pleiotropic phenotype of colchicine-resistant CHO cells: Cross-resistance and collateral sensitivity. J Cell Physiol 88:23–32

Biedler JL, Riehm H (1970) Cellular resistance to actinomycin-D in Chinese hamster cells in vitro: cross-resistance, radioautographic and cytogenetic studies. Cancer Res 30:1174–1184

Biedler JL, Meyers MB, Peterson RHF, Spengler BA (1980) Marker chromosome with a homogenously staining region in vincristine-resistant cells. Proc Am Assoc Cancer Res 21:292

Biermann WA, Catalano RB, Engstrom PF (1979) A positive phase-II study of dibromodulcitol in previously treated patients with advanced colorectal carcinoma. Proc Am Soc Clin Oncol 20:373

Bosmann HB, Kessel D (1970) Altered glycosidase levels in drug-resistant mouse leukemias. Mol Pharmacol 6:345–349

Brabbs S, Warr JR (1979) Isolation and characterisation of bleomycin-resistant clones of CHO cells. Genet Res 34:269–279

Brockman RW (1974) Circumvention of resistance. In: Pharmacological basis of cancer chemotherapy. 27th Annual symposium on fundamental cancer research. Williams and Wilkins, Baltimore, pp 695–711

Brockman RW, Yajisawa Y, Ling V, Schabel FM, DiMarco A, Harrap KR, Holland JF (1978) Modes of acquiring resistance to chemotherapeutic agents. In: Siegenthaler W, Luthy (eds) Current chemotherapy. American Society for Microbiology, pp 97–102

Browman GP, Lazarus H (1980) Combination antifol therapy: observations on the development of resistant L1210 leukemic cells in vivo. Cancer Treat Rep 64:231–236

Buzdar AU, Legha SS, Hortobagyi GN, Blumenschein GR, Bodey GP (1980) Phase-II evaluation of AMSA in combination with peptichemio in metastatic breast cancer resistant to conventional chemotherapy. Proc Am Assoc Cancer Res 21:181

Carter SK (1978) Cancer chemotherapy as it approaches middle age. Cancer Chemother Pharmacol 1:1–4

Connors TA (1974) Mechanisms of clinical drug resistance to alkylating agents. Biochem Pharmacol 23 [Suppl 2]:89–100

Courtenay VD, Robins AB (1972) Loss of resistance to methotrexate in L5178Y mouse leukemia grown in vitro. J Natl Cancer Inst 49:45–53

Creagan ET, Ahmann DL, Ingle JN, Purvis III JD (1980) Phase II study of *N*-(phosphonoacetyl)-L-asparate (PALA) in disseminated malignant melanoma. Proc Am Soc Clin Oncol 21:344

Dano K (1976) Experimentally developed cellular resistance to daunomycin. Acta Pathol Microbiol Scand [A] [Suppl 256]:1–78

Dasgupta I, Steinherz L, Steinherz P, Tan C (1979) Trial of rubidazone in children with cancer. Proc Am Assoc Cancer Res 20:156

DeMars R (1974) Resistance of cultured human fibroblasts and other cells to purine and pyrimidine analogs in relation to mutagenesis detection. Mutation Res 24:335–364

Devita VT, Serpick AA, Carbone PP (1970) Combination chemotherapy in the treatment of advanced Hodgkin's disease. Ann Intern Med 73:881–895

Dombernowsky P, Hansen HH (1980) m-AMSA in advanced ovarian carcinoma – a phase-II study. Proc Am Soc Clin Oncol 21:426

Douglass HO, Kaufmann J, Engstrom PF, Klaassen DJ, Carbone PP (1979) Single agent chemotherapy of advanced colorectal cancer with ICRF-159, Yoshi-864, piperazinedione, CCNU, actinomycin D, L-PAM or methotrexate. Proc Am Soc Clin Oncol 20:434

Fischer GA (1962) Defective transport of amethopterin(methotrexate) as a mechanism of resistance to the antimetabolite in L5178Y leukemic cells. Biochem Pharmacol 11:1233–1234

Flintoff WF, Davidson SV, Siminovitch L (1976) Isolation and partial characterization of three methotrexate-resistant phenotypes from Chinese hamster ovary cells. Somatic Cell Genet 2:245–261
Fox BW (1969) The sensitivity of the Yoshida sarcoma to methylene dimethane sulphonate. Int J Cancer 4:54–60
Fox BW (1977) Collateral sensitivity between methylene dimethane sulfonate and halogenated methotrexate derivatives in the Yoshida sarcoma in vivo and in vitro. J Natl Cancer Inst 58:955–958
Fuks JZ, Van Echo DA, Aisner J, Kravitz S, Wiernik PN (1980) A phase II trial of AMSA in patients with renal cell carcinoma and refractory small cell carcinoma of the lung. Proc Am Soc Clin Oncol 21:477
Goldenberg GJ (1975) The role of drug transport in resistance to nitrogen mustard and other alkylating agents in L5178Y lymphoblasts. Cancer Res 35:1687–1692
Gorton SJ, Zelkowitz L, Agrawal BL, Stott PB (1980) Treatment of breast cancer patients who have failed cytoxan, methotrexate and 5-fluorouracil with cytoxan and 5-fluorouracil. Proc Am Soc Clin Oncol 21:347
Hakes TB, Wittes JT, Wittes RE, Knapper WH (1979) *cis*-Platinum diamminedichloroplatinum II in breast cancer: high versus low dose. Proc Am Assoc Clin Oncol 20:304
Hakimi J, Bosmann HB (1977) Collateral sensitivity: problems of demonstration in murine leukaemia cells. Biochem Pharmacol 26:1094–1096
Hall SW, Benjamin RS, Legha SS, Gutterman JU, Burgess MA, Bodey GP (1979) AMSA: A new acridine derivative with activity against metastatic melanoma. Proc Am Soc Clin Oncol 20:372
Hamburger AW, Salmon SE (1977) Primary bioassay of human tumor stem cells. Science 197:461–463
Harrap KR, Hill BT (1969a) The selectivity of action of alkylating agents and drug resistance. I. Biochemical changes occurring in sensitive and resistant strains of Yoshida ascites sarcoma following chemotherapy. Br J Cancer 23:210–226
Harrap KR, Hill BT (1969b) The selectivity of action of alkylating agents and drug resistance. II. A comparison of the effects of alkylating drugs on growth inhibition and cell size in sensitive and resistant strains of the Yoshida ascites sarcoma. Br J Cancer 23:227–234
Henderson IC, Canellos GP (1980) Cancer of the breast – the past decade. N Engl J Med 302:78–90
Herman TS, Cress AE, Gerner EW (1979) Collateral sensitivity to methotrexate in cells resistant to adriamycin. Cancer Res 39:1937–1942
Hill BT, Hellmann K (1977) Razoxane and methotrexate resistance. Lancet I:47
Hill BT, Whelan RDH (1982) Establishment of vincristine-resistant and vindesine-resistant lines of murine lymphoblasts in vitro and characterisation of their patterns of cross-resistance and drug sensitivities. Cancer Chemother Pharmacol 8:163–169
Hill BT, Goldie JH, Price LA (1973) Studies concerned with overcoming resistance to methotrexate: A comparison of the effects of methotrexate and 2,4-diamino-5-(3′,4′-dichlorophenyl)-6-methylpyrimidine on the colony-forming ability of L5178Y cells. Br J Cancer 28:262–268
Hill BT, Price LA, Goldie JH (1975) Methotrexate resistance and uptake of DDMP by L5178Y cells – selective protection with folinic acid. Eur J Cancer 11:545–553
Hill BT, Price LA, Goldie JH (1976) The value of adriamycin in overcoming resistance to methotrexate in tissue culture. Eur J Cancer 12:541–549
Hoshino A, Kato T, Amo H, Ota K (1972) Antitumour effects of adriamycin on Yoshida rat sarcoma and L1210 mouse leukaemia – cross-resistance and combination chemotherapy. In: Carter SK, DiMarco A, Ghione M, Krakoff IH, Mathe E (eds) International symposium on adriamycin. Springer, Berlin Heidelberg New York, pp 75–89
Hubbard SM, Barkes P, Young RC (1978) Adriamycin therapy for advanced ovarian carcinoma recurrent after chemotherapy. Cancer Treat Rep 62:1375–1377
Hug V, Hortobagyi GN, Buzdar AU, Blumenschein GR, Grose W, Burgess MA, Bodey GP (1980) A phase-II study of peptichemio in advanced breast cancer. Cancer 45:2524–2528

Hutchison DJ (1963) Cross resistance and collateral sensitivity studies in cancer chemotherapy. Adv Cancer Res 7:235–350
Hutchison DJ (1965) Studies on cross-resistance and collateral sensitivity. Cancer Res 25:1581–1595
Hutchison DJ, Schmid FA (1973) Cross resistance and collateral sensitivity. In: Mihich E (ed) Drug resistance and selectivity – biochemical and cellular basis. Academic, New York, pp 73–126
Hutchison DJ, Schmid FA (1974) Collateral sensitivity of drug treated and drug-resistant lines of L1210 leukaemia. Prog Chemother III:849–853
Inaba M, Johnson RK (1977) Decreased retention of actinomycin D as the basis for cross-resistance in anthracycline-resistant sublines of P388 leukaemia. Cancer Res 37:4629–4634
Ingle JN, Ahmann DL, Bisel HF, Rubin J, Kvols LK (1979) Randomized phase-II trial of rubidazone and adriamycin in women with advanced breast cancer. Proc Am Assoc Clin Oncol 20:427
Jayaram HN, Cooney DA, Vistica DT, Kariya S, Johnson RK (1979) Mechanisms of sensitivity or resistance of murine tumors to *N*-(phosphonacetyl)-L-aspartate (PALA). Cancer Treat Rep 63:1291–1302
Johnson RK, Chitnis MP, Embrey WM, Gregory EB (1978) In vivo characteristics of resistance and cross-resistance of an adriamycin-resistant subline of P388 leukemia. Cancer Treat Rep 62:1535–1547
Kaufman RJ, Brown PC, Schimke RT (1979) Amplified dihydrofolate reductase genes in unstably methotrexate-resistant cells are associated with double minute chromosomes. Proc Natl Acad Sci USA 76:5669–5673
Kaye SB, Boden JA (1980) Cross-resistance between actinomycin D, adriamycin and vincristine in a murine solid tumour in vivo. Biochem Pharmacol 29:1081–1084
Kline I, Woodman RJ, Gang M, Venditti JM (1971) Effectiveness of anti-leukaemic agents in mice inoculated with leukaemia L1210 variants resistant to 5-(3,3-dimethyl-1-triazeno) imidazole-4-carboxamide or 5-[3,3-bis(2-chloroethyl)-1-triazeno]imidazole-4-carboxamide. Cancer Chemother Rep 55:9–28
Kovach JS, Moertel CG, Schutt AJ, Hahn RG, Reitemeier RJ (1974) A controlled study of combined 1,3-bis-(2-chloroethyl)-1-nitrosourea and 5-fluorouracil therapy for advanced gastric and pancreatic cancer. Cancer 33:563–567
Laster WR, Schabel FM (1979) Collateral sensitivity of P388/Ara-C and P388/5-FU to *N*-(phosphonacetyl)-L-aspartate (PALA). Proc Am Assoc Cancer Res 20:95
Lawrence HJ, Ries CA, Reynolds RD, Lewis JP, Koretz MM (1980) m-AMSA: a promising new agent in refractory acute leukemia. Proc Am Soc Clin Oncol 21:438
Leichman L, Buroker TR, O'Bryan RM, Baker LH (1980) A phase-II trial of AMSA in disseminated adenocarcinoma of the colon and rectum. Proc Am Soc Clin Oncol 21:355
Ling V (1975) Drug resistance and membrane alteration in mutants of mammalian cells. Can J Genet Cytol 17:503–515
Livingston RB (1980) Small-cell carcinoma of the lung. Blood 56:575–584
Magill GB, Sordillo P, Gralla R, Golbey RB (1980) Phase-II trials of DVA, AMSA and DCNU as single agents in adult sarcomas. Proc Am Soc Clin Oncol 21:362
Mihich E (1973) Tumor immunogenicity in therapeutics. In: Mihich E (ed) Drug resistance and selectivity, biochemical and cellular basis. Academic, New York, pp 391–412
Mihich E, Kitano M (1971) Differences in the immunogenicity of leukemia L1210 sublines in DBA/2 mice. Cancer Res 31:1999–2003
Ohnoshi T, Ohnuma T, Holland JF (1980) Establishment of methotrexate-resistant human acute lymphocytic leukemia cells in culture and effects of various antifols. Proc Am Assoc Cancer Res 21:298
Orkin SH, Littlefield JW (1971) Mutagenesis to aminopterin resistance in cultured hamster cells. Exp Cell Res 69:174–180
Ozols RF, Willson JKV, Weltz MD, Grotzinger KR, Myers CE, Young RC (1980) Inhibition of human ovarian cancer colony formation by adriamycin and its major metabolites. Cancer Res 40:4109–4112

Reich SD, Bradner WT (1979) Responses of mitomycin-C-resistant lines of L1210 leukemia to treatment with chemotherapeutic drugs. Proc Am Assoc Cancer Res 20:214
Reynolds TF, Cvitkovic E, Golbey RB, Young CW (1979) Phase-II trial of vindesine in patients with germ cell tumors. Proc Am Soc Clin Oncol 20:338
Riehm H, Biedler JL (1971) Cellular resistance to daunomycin in Chinese hamster cells in vitro. Cancer Res 31:409–412
Rosen G, Nirenberg A, Juergens H, Tan C (1970) Phase-II trial of *cis*-platinum in oesteogenic sarcoma. Proc Am Soc Clin Oncol 20:363
Rosenfelt FP, Sikic BI, Daniels JR, Rosenbloom BE (1980) Phase II evaluation of *cis*-diamminedichloroplatinum in small cell carcinoma of lung. Proc Am Soc Clin Oncol 21:449
Rossof AH, Chandra G, Wolter J, Showel J (1979) Phase II trial of vindesine in advanced metastatic cancer. Proc Am Assoc Cancer Res 20:146
Rozencweig M, Von Hoff DD, Muggia FM (1978) New agents – selected problems in drug development and clinical testing. In Brodsky I, Kahn S, Conroy JF (eds) Cancer chemotherapy III. The 46th Hahneman Symposium. Grune and Stratton, New York, pp 75–85
Rutman RJ (1964) Experimental chemotherapy studies. V. The collateral sensitivity to alkylating agents of several antimetabolite-resistant ascites tumors in mice. Cancer Res 24:634–638
Salmon SE, Hamburger AW, Soehnlein B, Durie BGM, Alberts DS, Moon TE (1978) Quantitation of differential sensitivity of human-tumor stem cells to anticancer drugs. N Engl J Med 298:1321–1327
Samal BA, McDonald B, Kim PM, McKenzie M, Baker L (1980) m-AMSA for treatment of disseminated breast cancer. Proc Am Soc Clin Oncol 21:363
Schabel FM (1979) Test systems for evaluating the antitumor activity of nucleoside analogs. In: Walker RT, De Clercq E, Eckstein F (eds) Nucleoside analogues. Plenum, New York, pp 363–394
Schabel FM, Trader MW, Laster WR, Wheeler GP, Witt MH (1978) Patterns of resistance and therapeutic synergism among alkylating agents. In: Schabel FM (ed) Fundamentals in cancer chemotherapy, antibiotics and chemotherapy, vol 23. Karger, Basel, pp 200–215
Schabel FM, Trader MW, Laster WR, Corbett TH, Griswold DP (1979) *cis*-Dichlorodiammineplatinum II. Combination chemotherapy and cross-resistance studies with tumors of mice. Cancer Treat Rep 63:1459–1473
Schabel FM, Skipper HE, Trader MW, Laster WR, Corbett TH, Griswold DP (1980) Concepts for controlling drug-resistant tumour cells. In: Mouridsen HT, Palshof T (eds) Breast cancer: Experimental and clinical aspects. Pergamon, Oxford, pp 199–212
Schmid FA, Hutchison DJ (1971) Induction and characteristics of resistance to L-asparaginase (NSC-109229) in mouse leukemia L5178Y. Cancer Chemother Rep 55:115–121
Schmid FA, Stock CC (1976) Antitumor activity of peptichemio. Proc Am Assoc Cancer Res 17:49
Siegfried JM, Kennedy KA, Tritton TR (1980) Investigation of adriamycin-resistant cell lines with respect to proposed mechanisms of drug action. Proc Am Assoc Cancer Res 21:12
Siminovitch L (1976) On the nature of hereditable variation in cultured somatic cells. Cell 7:1–11
Skelley M, Tormey D, Robins HI, Falkson G, Crowley J, Falkson H, Ansfield F (1980) Phase-II trial of vindesine in advanced breast cancer patients. Proc Am Assoc Cancer Res 21:172
Skipper HE, Hutchison DJ, Schabel FM, Schmidt LH, Goldin A, Brockman RW, Venditti JM, Wodinsky I (1972) A quick reference chart on cross-resistance between anticancer agents. Cancer Chemother Rep 56:493–498
Skipper HE, Schabel FM, Lloyd HH (1978) Experimental therapeutics and kinetics: selection and overgrowth of specifically and permanently drug-resistant tumour cells. Semin Haematol 15:207–219

Skipper HE, Schabel FM, Lloyd HH (1979) Dose-response and tumor-cell repopulation rate in chemotherapeutic trials. In: Rosowsky A (ed) Advances in cancer chemotherapy, vol 1. Marcel Dekker, New York, pp 205–253
Slayton R, Creasman W, Bundy B (1979a) Phase-II trial of VP-16 in treatment of advanced squamous cell carcinoma of the cervix. Proc Am Soc Clin Oncol 20:365
Slayton R, Petty W, Blessing J (1979b) Phase-II trial of VP-16 in treatment of advanced ovarian adenocarcinoma. Proc Am Assoc Cancer Res 20:190
Stambaugh JE (1980) Vindcsinc in thc trcatmcnt of paticnts with advanccd ncoplastic disease. Proc Am Soc Clin Oncol 21:344
Sugimura T (1970) In: Nakahara W (ed) Chemical tumour problems. Jap Soc for the Promotion of Sci, Tokyo, pp 269–284
Szybalski W, Bryson V (1952) Genetic studies on microbial cross-resistance to toxic agents I. Cross-resistance of *Escherichia coli* to fifteen antibiotics. J Bacteriol 64:489–499
Thigpen T, Lagasse L, Bundy B (1979) Phase-II trial of *cis*-platinum in treatment of advanced ovarian adenocarcinoma. Proc Am Assoc Cancer Res 20:84
Thompson LH, Baker RM (1973) Isolation of mutants of cultured mammalian cells. In: Prescott DM (ed) Methods in cell biology, vol 6 Academic, London, pp 209–281
Tiber C, Conrad F, Hagemeister R (1980) Continuous vinblastine for previously treated non-Hodgkin's lymphoma. Proc Am Assoc Cancer Res 21:162
Tsukagoshi S, Hashimoto Y (1973) Increased immunosensitivity in nitrogen mustard-resistant Yoshida sarcoma. Cancer Res 33:1038–1042
Van Echo DA, Aisner J, Wirnik PH (1979) Combination chemotherapy of advanced breast cancer with adriamycin and VP16-213. Proc. Am Assoc Cancer Res 20:228
Volm M, Lindner C (1978) Detection of induced resistance in short term tests. Adriamycin-resistant sarcoma 180. Z Krebsforsch 91:1–10
Von Hoff DD, Casper J, Bradley E, Trent JM, Hodach A, Reichert C, Makuch R, Altman A (1980) Direct cloning of human neuroblastoma cells in soft agar culture. Cancer Res 40:3591–3597
Wendt AJ, Jones SE, Salmon SE (1980) Salvage treatment of patients relapsing after breast cancer adjuvant chemotherapy. Cancer Treat Rep 64:269–273
White K (1979) Studies on the mechanism of cellular resistance to the antitumour agent ICRF-159. PhD Thesis, London University
Wilkoff LJ, Dulmadge EA (1978a) Resistance and cross-resistance of cultured leukemia P388 cells to vincristine, adriamycin, adriamycin analogs and actinomycin-D. J Natl Cancer Inst 61:1521–1524
Wilkoff LJ, Dulmadge EA (1978b) Sensitivity and resistance of cultured leukemia P388 cells to vincristine and 4′-demethyl podophyllotoxin. Proc Am Assoc Cancer Res 19:37
Williams SD, Einhorn LH, Greco A, Oldham R, Fletcher R, Bond WH (1979) VP-16-213: an active drug in germinal neoplasms. Proc Am Assoc Cancer Res 20:72
Wittes RE, Cvitkovic E, Shah J, Gerold FP, Strong EW (1979) *cis*-Dichlorodiammine-platinum (II) in the treatment of epidermoid carcinoma of the head and neck. Cancer Treat Rep 61:359–366
Wodinsky I, Kensler CJ (1964) Activity of selected compounds in subline of leukaemia L1210 resistant to cytosine arabinoside. Cancer Chemother Rep 43:1–3
Yap HY, Blumenschein GR, Bodey GP, Hortobagyi GN, Buzdar AU, Distefano A (1980a) Continuous 5-day infusion vindesine – improvement in therapeutic index in the treatment of refractory breast cancer. Proc Am Soc Clin Oncol 21:408
Yap HY, Blumenschein GR, Keating MJ, Horotbagyi GN, Tashima CK, Loo TL (1980b) Vinblastine given as a continuous 5-day infusion in the treatment of refractory advanced breast cancer. Cancer Treat Rep 64:279–283
Zubrod CG (1979) Historic milestones in curative chemotherapy. Semin Oncol 6:490–505

Subject Index

Handbook of Experimental Pharmacology

Continuation of "Handbuch der experimentellen Pharmakologie"

Volume 28: Part 1
Concepts in Biochemical Pharmacology I

Part 3
Concepts in Biochemical Pharmacology III

Volume 29
Oral wirksame Antidiabetika

Volume 30
Modern Inhalation Anesthetics

Volume 32: Part 2
Insulin II

Volume 34
Secretin, Cholecystokinin Pancreozymin and Gastrin

Volume 35: Part 1
Androgene I

Part 2
Androgens II and Antiandrogens/Androgene II und Antiandrogene

Volume 36
Uranium - Plutonium - Transplutonic Elements

Volume 37
Angiotensin

Volume 38: Part 1
Antineoplastic and Immunosuppressive Agents I

Part 2
Antineoplastic and Immunosuppressive Agents II

Volume 39
Antihypertensive Agents

Volume 40
Organic Nitrates

Volume 41
Hypolipidemic Agents

Volume 42
Neuromuscular Junction

Volume 43
Anabolic-Androgenic Steroids

Volume 44
Heme and Hemoproteins

Volume 45: Part 1
Drug Addiction I

Part 2
Drug Addiction II

Volume 46
Fibrinolytics and Antifibronolytics

Volume 47
Kinetics of Drug Action

Volume 48
Arthropod Venoms

Volume 49
Ergot Alkaloids and Related Compounds

Volume 50: Part 1
Inflammation

Part 2
Anti-Inflammatory Drugs

Volume 51
Uric Acid

Volume 52
Snake Venoms

Springer-Verlag
Berlin
Heidelberg
New York
Tokyo

Handbook of Experimental Pharmacology

Continuation of "Handbuch der experimentellen Pharmakologie"

Springer-Verlag
Berlin
Heidelberg
New York
Tokyo

MIX
Papier aus verantwortungsvollen Quellen
Paper from responsible sources
FSC® C105338
FSC
www.fsc.org

If you have any concerns about our products,
you can contact us on
ProductSafety@springernature.com

In case Publisher is established outside the EU,
the EU authorized representative is:
Springer Nature Customer Service Center GmbH
Europaplatz 3, 69115 Heidelberg, Germany

Printed by Libri Plureos GmbH
in Hamburg, Germany